CARDIOVASCULAR PHARMACOLOGY

Second Edition

Cardiovascular Pharmacology

Second Edition

Editor

Michael J. Antonaccio, Ph.D.

Vice President
Cardiovascular Research
Bristol Myers Company
Evansville, Indiana

Raven Press ▪ New York

Raven Press, 1140 Avenue of the Americas, New York, New York 10036

Made in the United States of America

Library of Congress Cataloging in Publication Data
Main entry under title:

Cardiovascular pharmacology

   Includes bibliographical references and index.
   1. Cardiovascular agents. 2. Cardiovascular system--
Diseases--Chemotherapy. I. Antonaccio, Michael J.
[DNLM: 1. Cardiovascular diseases--Drug therapy.
2. Cardiovascular system--Drug effects. 3. Cardiovascular
agents--Therapeutic use. QV 150 C275]
RM345.C376 1984 615'.71 83-23087
ISBN 0-89004-872-X

To my parents, Frances and Mario Antonaccio,
My wife, Patty, and my son, Nicky,
For their love and support through the years

Preface

The first edition of *Cardiovascular Pharmacology* sought to fill a need for a single text containing the basic elements of cardiovascular pharmacology useful to both graduate students and experienced investigators. The success of the first edition clearly demonstrated the existence of such a need, and the second edition is intended to build and expand upon the original publication.

Most of the original chapters have been retained and brought up to date. Others have been divided where appropriate so that topics that have grown in importance could be adequately covered. For instance, there are now entire chapters devoted to the topics of hypertensive vascular pathophysiology, antihypertensives, calcium antagonists, and the control of renin release. Recent findings in presynaptic modulation of neurotransmitter release are considered important enough to be treated independently. In 1977, this area of research was in its infancy.

This volume, like the first edition, will be of interest to both new and established investigators in cardiovascular pharmacology who wish to broaden their general knowledge, as well as to practicing and teaching clinicians.

Michael J. Antonaccio

Preface to the First Edition

In a relatively few years, the study of the cardiovascular system and the drugs that affect it has undergone some rather remarkable and exciting changes. Entirely new classes of compounds, such as those that selectively inhibit various steps in the process that allows the enzyme renin to eventually form the peptide angiotensin II, have only recently been discovered and put to use as analytical and clinical tools. Agents such as these have created a renaissance of interest in the physiology and pharmacology of the renin-angiotensin system—especially in relation to hypertension—and have even led to the discovery of probable new hormones such as angiotensin III.

The recent national emphasis on hypertension as an insidious, dangerous disease of epidemic proportions and the importance of early, effective treatment with antihypertensive agents in decreasing morbidity and mortality have given a new impetus to the search for causes and treatment of hypertension. This, in turn, has resulted in the discovery of newer and better antihypertensives and increased emphasis on the importance of the extraordinary number of physiological systems involved in the homeostasis of normotension. The central nervous system has only recently been implicated in the genesis of peripheral cardiovascular disorders, with new and provocative findings being published daily. The incredibly burgeoning field of prostaglandins, their newly discovered endoperoxide intermediates, and their potential role in circulatory function has provided a good deal of valuable information as well as raised many questions concerning the final role of these agents under normal as well as pathological conditions. The kidney has once again become an obviously important organ for study, and its paramount role in maintaining the proper ionic and hormonal milieu necessary for normal cardiovascular control is once again being emphasized. The study of cardiac muscle and those parameters of the circulation that affect it, directly or indirectly, has grown enormously in the last few years and the knowledge that has accumulated and resulted in new drugs for the treatment of arrhythmias, myocardial infarction, angina pectoris, and shock is indeed overwhelming.

The need, then, for a convenient source of this material becomes obvious. Even more obvious is the lack of a single text that contains the basic elements of cardiovascular pharmacology. Thus, the main thrust of this book, which seeks to provide a summary of the important areas of cardiovascular pharmacology. Furthermore, it seeks to do this in an integrated logical manner by demonstrating the interrelationship of various aspects of cardiovascular pharmacology and, it is hoped, conveying the means by which these seemingly different aspects are all part of a natural and integrated whole. Hence, the book is suited for use as a textbook for graduate students in the biological sciences who have heretofore had no comprehensive reference source or logically presented material on which to rely. Each chapter provides background information necessary for the understanding of newer and more complex developments in a particular field. The contents may range from basic physiology to theoretical pharmacology and from basic diagnostic procedures to guarded speculation, thereby providing both a broad range of coverage and a historical perspective as to where we have been, where we are now, and where we are headed in the future. The extensive use of summary tables and figures should be particularly useful for teaching purposes.

It is hoped, however, that the usefulness of this book will not be limited to students. Although not designed to provide an exhaustive coverage of any particular area, the book's range and depth of material should be valuable to both new and established investigators in the field of cardiovascular pharmacology who wish to broaden their general knowledge, as well as to practicing and teaching clinicians.

I would like to express my gratitude to the late Dr. Ronald Hill whose enthusiasm and assistance made this book possible.

My thanks to Mrs. Betty Dooley and Mrs. Jean Phillips for their perseverance in the typing of manuscripts and correspondence, to Mrs. Jeanne Halley for her editorial assistance, and to many friends for their encouragement and assistance in evaluating manuscripts.

Special acknowledgment is given to the contributing authors who have made the book a reality.

Michael J. Antonaccio

Contents

Contributors

Michael J. Antonaccio
Cardiovascular Research
Bristol Myers Company
Evansville, Indiana 47721

Michael Armstrong
Synthelabo L.E.R.S.
Paris, France 75013

Thomas Baum
Schering Corporation
Pharmaceutical Research Division
Bloomfield, New Jersey 07003

Edward H. Blaine
Merck Institute for Therapeutic Research
West Point, Pennsylvania 19486

William B. Campbell
Department of Pharmacology
University of Texas Health Science Center at Dallas
Dallas, Texas 75235

Jay N. Cohn
University of Minnesota Hospital
Minneapolis, Minnesota 55455

Gary S. Francis
University of Minnesota Hospital
Minneapolis, Minnesota 55455

Robert Z. Gussin
McNeil Pharmaceutical
Spring House, Pennsylvania 19477

Jerry B. Hook
Center for Environmental Toxicology
Michigan State University
East Lansing, Michigan 48824

Albert L. Hyman
Department of Surgery
Tulane University School of Medicine
New Orleans, Louisiana 70112

Philip J. Kadowitz
Department of Pharmacology
Tulane University School of Medicine
New Orleans, Louisiana 70112

T. Kent Keeton
Department of Pharmacology
University of Texas Health Science Center at San Antonio
San Antonio, Texas 78284

Salomon Z. Langer
Synthelabo L.E.R.S.
Paris, France 75013

Allan M. Lefer
Department of Physiology
Jefferson Medical College
Thomas Jefferson University
Philadelphia, Pennsylvania 19107

Howard L. Lippton
Department of Pharmacology
Tulane University School of Medicine
New Orleans, Louisiana 70112

Benedict R. Lucchesi
Department of Pharmacology
University of Michigan Medical School
Ann Arbor, Michigan 48109

Dennis B. McNamara
Department of Pharmacology
Tulane University School of Medicine
New Orleans, Louisiana 70112

S. Moncada
Department of Prostaglandin Research
Wellcome Research Laboratories
Langley Court, Beckenham
Kent BR33BS, U.K.

Eugene S. Patterson
Department of Pharmacology and the
Upjohn Center for Clinical Pharmacology
University of Michigan Medical School
Ann Arbor, Michigan 48109

Ravinder K. Saini
Squibb Institute for Medical Research
Princeton, New Jersey 08540

Alexander Scriabine
Miles Institute for Preclinical Pharmacology
P.O. Box 1956
New Haven, Connecticut 06509

Friedel Seuter
Bayer AG
Institute of Pharmacology
5600 Wyppertol 1, F.R.G.

James A. Spath, Jr.
Department of Physiology
Jefferson Medical College
Thomas Jefferson University
Philadelphia, Pennsylvania 19107

Charles S. Sweet
Merck Institute for Therapeutic Research
West Point, Pennsylvania 19486

D. G. Taylor
Miles Institute for Preclinical Pharmacology
P.O. Box 1956
New Haven, Connecticut 06509

R. Clinton Webb
Department of Physiology
University of Michigan
Ann Arbor, Michigan 48109

B. J. R. Whittle
Department of Prostaglandin Research
Wellcome Research Laboratories
Langley Court, Beckenham
Kent BR33BS, U.K.

Michael S. Wolin
Department of Pharmacology
Tulane University School of Medicine
New Orleans, Louisiana 70112

Cardiovascular Pharmacology, Second Edition,
edited by Michael Antonaccio.
Raven Press, New York © 1984.

Fundamental Principles Governing Regulation of Circulatory Function

Thomas Baum

Pharmaceutical Research Division, Schering Corporation, Bloomfield, New Jersey 07003

AUTONOMIC NERVOUS SYSTEM

The autonomic nervous system plays a central role in the regulation of cardiovascular function. Although the system is not essential to life, it does enable organs to respond rapidly and efficiently to changing requirements. In its absence, overall adaptation to stressful situations may be severely compromised, although function at rest may remain within normal limits.

The system consists of two major divisions: the parasympathetic and the sympathetic (1,2). Autonomic outflow originates from "centers" (i.e., nuclei or more diffusely arranged groups of cells) in the midbrain and hypothalamus. These regions are closely interrelated and are further subject to excitatory and inhibitory input from afferents and from higher brain structures and the cerebellum. Preganglionic fibers emerge from the brainstem or cord and synapse or relay in ganglia (Fig. 1). These structures contain cell bodies of postganglionic fibers that innervate target organs. Activation of autonomic fibers results in the release of chemical substances (transmitters, mediators) from their terminals. The transmitter binds to a sensitive region (receptor) on the membrane of the target cell and initiates a complex series of events resulting in a response. Many organs (e.g., the viscera) are innervated by both divisions of the autonomic nervous system, which may exert opposing actions either directly or by modifying mediator release from opposing fibers. Other structures, such as most blood vessels, are predominantly supplied by fibers from only the sympathetic system. Some cells receive both sympathetic and parasympathetic innervation (e.g., in the sinoatrial node). Other organs, such as the iris, are also innervated by both systems, but sympathetic fibers supply the radial muscle and parasympathetic fibers the circular muscle. During the resting state, individual autonomic nerves may be quiescent or may fire at a relatively low rate. Activity of an organ may be initiated or enhanced by increasing the "tone" (i.e., firing rate) of the excitatory system and/or by reducing the activity of the inhibitory system. Cell bodies of afferent fibers lie in dorsal root ganglia or in the sensory ganglia of cranial nerves.

Parasympathetic Nervous System

Preganglionic fibers arise from the midbrain, medulla oblongata, and the sacral portion of the spinal cord (Fig. 1) (1). The third, seventh, ninth, and tenth cranial nerves contain fibers emanating from the brainstem. The sacral outflow forms the pelvic nerve and innervates the bladder, sexual organs, and terminal portions of the intestinal tract. Preganglionic parasympathetic fibers synapse in ganglia located in proximity to the target innervated. Consequently, postganglionic nerves are relatively short. On activation, both pre-

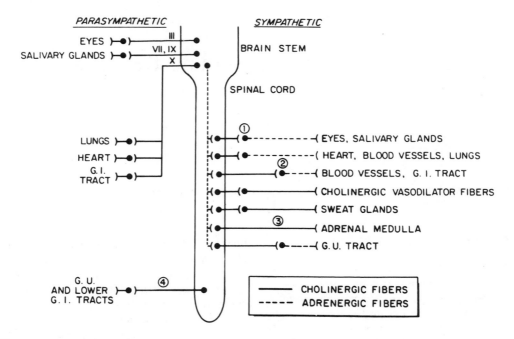

FIG. 1. Schematic representation of autonomic outflow. Various outflow patterns are illustrated in a highly schematic form. Roman numerals refer to cranial nerves. (1) Synapses in ganglia of the paravertebral sympathetic chain. (2) Synapses in more distal ganglia (e.g., celiac, superior and inferior mesenteric). (3) Preganglionic fibers in the splanchnic nerve. (4) Sacral parasympathetic outflow.

ganglionic and postganglionic fibers release acetylcholine (ACh) from their terminals.

Choline is transported into nerve terminals by an active process (2). Choline acetyltransferase catalyzes its synthesis into ACh, which is then stored in discrete vesicles within nerve endings. The enzyme is synthesized in the perikaryon and transported along the axon to the terminal by the microtubules. Small quantities of ACh are continuously released. Nerve activation results in dramatic changes in the permeability characteristics of the neuronal membrane, with consequent influx of ions (predominantly sodium and calcium) and depolarization (3). These events cause the migration of ACh-containing vesicles toward and fusion with the neurolemma, and extrusion of their contents (exocytosis). The released ACh combines with its receptors on target cells (*vide infra*). Acetylcholine esterase rapidly degrades free ACh. The enzyme is located on the postsynaptic membrane and, in some structures, also on the presynaptic side.

The cholinergic transmission process has a high degree of efficiency. Prolonged stimulation does not reduce tissue ACh content. The ACh release process is subject to modulation by numerous factors. It is highly dependent on calcium influx and can be inhibited by agents that depress nerve transmission (tetrodotoxin) or calcium entry. Several substances, including morphine, enkephalins, prostaglandins, botulism toxin, and adenosine triphosphate (ATP), diminish exocytotic release of ACh. Hemicholinium inhibits ACh synthesis by blocking its membrane transport system.

Sympathetic Nervous System

Anatomy

Descending tracts originating primarily from the medulla oblongata but also from the hypothalamus innervate, directly or via interneurons, cell bodies of preganglionic neurons located in the intermediolateral column of the thoracolumbar spinal cord (C-8 to L2–3). Preganglionic myelinated fibers emerge via the anterior roots and white rami and synapse in the paravertebral sympathetic chain or traverse the chain and relay in more peripheral ganglia (1,2). The former consists of 22 pairs of ganglia lying parallel to the vertebral column and extending from the superior cervical ganglion to the lumbar region. Individual segments carry descending and ascending efferent and afferent fibers. Gray rami convey postganglionic fibers from the chain to spinal nerves. Preganglionic fibers not synapsing in the paravertebral chain usually do so in more peripheral ganglia in the abdomen (i.e., celiac, superior and inferior mesenteric, and aorticorenal). Some fibers may synapse in even more distal ganglia lying in proximity to the organs innervated (e.g., genitourinary tract, rectum). Fibers to the adrenal medulla do not synapse on route. Most sympathetic postganglionic fibers release norepinephrine (NE, noradrenaline) at their endings and consequently are considered "adrenergic" or "noradrenergic" (4–7). These fibers form an extensive terminal plexus in the organ innervated. Varicosities appear periodically along the terminal network. Some sympathetic fibers liberate ACh (e.g., fibers to sweat glands and vasodilator fibers to skeletal muscle). Sympathetic cholinergic vasodilator pathways originate in the cortex and hypothalamus.

Adrenergic Synthesis, Storage, and Release Mechanisms

NE synthesis, storage, and release occur in the varicosities of the terminal fibers (2,5). These structures contain mitochondria as well as catecholamine-containing vesicles (Fig. 2). The vesicles are formed within the cell body and are transported peripherally.

Hydroxylation of tyrosine to form 3,4-dihydroxyphenylalanine (DOPA) initiates the enzymatic synthesis of NE and occurs in the axoplasm of the varicosity (2,5–9). The reaction is catalyzed by tyrosine hydroxylase utilizing a pteridine cofactor and constitutes the rate-limiting step. DOPA is decarboxylated to form dopamine, which is then transported into the vesicle, where β-hydroxylation to form NE occurs. Dopamine β-hydroxylase (DBH), a copper-containing enzyme, catalyzes the latter step. NE is stored within vesicles partially as a complex with ATP and the protein chromogranin, as well as in a more loosely bound form in both the vesicle and cytoplasm. Turnover studies have demonstrated that newly synthesized NE is incorporated into a more mobile pool and is preferentially released by nerve stimulation.

Uptake of catecholamines into vesicles is an active transport process requiring ATP and magnesium (10). NE can be highly concentrated within these structures and thereby protected from degradative enzymes. Several substances, including reserpine, tetrabenazine, and prenylamine, inhibit the uptake mechanism into vesicles and consequently prevent storage of NE.

Conducted action potentials induce influx of sodium and calcium into adrenergic nerve endings. As in cholinergic terminals, calcium promotes the migration of vesicles toward the neurolemma, fusion of the vesicular membrane with the neurolemma, and extrusion of the vesicular contents (NE, ATP, DBH, and chromogranin) into the extracellular space (2,7). Autonomic fibers can release more than one type of transmitter (e.g., an amine and a peptide) (11).

Released NE can exert a negative feedback on its own liberation (7,12,13). Receptors (α_2) (*vide infra*) on the presynaptic membrane mediate this inhibition (Fig. 2). The process is probably physiologically relevant at low rates of sympathetic firing. However, contradictory views have been offered (14). A β-receptor-mediated facilitory mechanism also exists on the presynaptic membrane (7,12). Its physiologic role remains uncertain, but it may be activated by circulating epinephrine. Angiotensin II (AII) can also facilitate NE release (7,15). Several other substances, including ACh, dopamine, prostaglandins of the E series, 5-hydroxytryptamine (serotonin, 5HT),

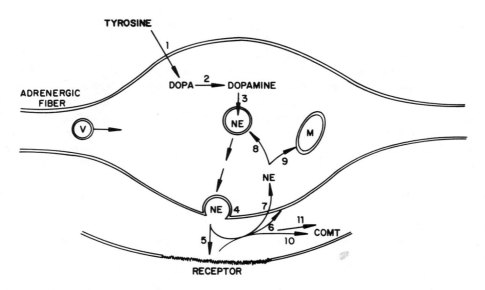

FIG. 2. Schematic representation of the adrenergic transmission process. The diagram illustrates a varicosity in a terminal sympathetic fiber and the effector cell. Tyrosine is transported across the axoplasmic membrane into the cytoplasm and hydroxylated to form DOPA by tyrosine hydroxylase (1). DOPA is then decarboxylated by DOPA decarboxylase to form dopamine (2). The latter is transported into the vesicles (V), where it is hydroxylated to form NE by dopamine β-hydroxylase (3). Vesicles are synthesized within the cell body and transported peripherally. NE is stored in vesicles partly in association with ATP and the protein chromogranin. An action potential results in the extrusion of the contents of the varicosity into the synaptic cleft (4). The released NE may then activate α- or β-adrenergic receptors on the effector cell (5). It also participates in a negative-feedback loop by activating α receptors on the presynaptic membrane, resulting in inhibition of the release process (6). NE is also returned to the fiber by the uptake-1 process (7). Free intracellular NE may then be transported into vesicles (8) or metabolized by mitochondria (M, 9). NE in the synaptic cleft is susceptible to metabolism by catecholamine-o-methyltransferase (COMT, 10), or it may diffuse away from the synaptic region (11).

adenosine, and opiate peptides, attenuate NE release. Their contribution to the regulation of adrenergic transmission is even more speculative. In the heart, however, vagally released ACh can inhibit responses to sympathetic stimulation, probably by a presynaptic mechanism (6,7), as well as by physiologic postsynaptic antagonism.

In contrast to the situation with action-potential-induced NE liberation, tyramine and similar substances release NE most probably by displacement from the cytoplasmic pool rather than by exocytosis (2,5). These agents do not simultaneously liberate DBH, ATP, and chromogranin along with NE. Further, the process does not depend on availability of extracellular calcium.

The adrenergic transmission mechanism is remarkably efficient. Prolonged physiologic or electrical activation of sympathetic nerves does not reduce tissue NE levels (9). Enhanced turnover, in conjunction with a highly effective reuptake process of released transmitter and accelerated synthesis, maintains tissue concentrations. Tyrosine hydroxylase is subject to feedback inhibition by free NE in the cytoplasm (9). Nerve activation accelerates synthesis partially by attenuating this feedback. More prolonged periods of enhanced sympathetic activity result in the synthesis of additional quantities of enzymes (9,17,18).

A major factor contributing to the overall efficiency of sympathetic transmission is a mechanism for the reuptake of released mediator. An active process in the axoplasmic membrane termed "uptake-1" transports NE from the extracellular space back into the nerve terminal (10). The carrier requires energy, is linked to Na-K ATPase, and exhibits stereospecificity. However, other phenolic phenethylamines in addition to NE (e.g., metaraminol, α-methyl NE, α-methylepinephrine, tyramine, and octopamine) are also transported across the nerve membrane, although at slower rates. Several classes of compounds inhibit uptake-1. These include phenethylamines lacking a phenolic hydroxyl group (e.g., amphetamine), as well as structurally diverse substances such as ouabain, cocaine, imipramine, and guanethidine. Inhibitors of the axoplasmic transport system also attenuate the actions of agents capable of gaining access to the interior of the nerve ending and subsequently causing the release of NE (i.e., indirectly acting sympathomimetic amines such as tyramine). 6-Hydroxydopamine is also a substrate for the membrane pump. After uptake, it causes the destruction of the adrenergic fiber.

In contrast to the normal state, continuous sympathetic activation rapidly leads to depletion of tissue stores of NE after blockade of the membrane pump. On the other hand, pump inactivation can lead to potentiation and prolongation of effects of sympathetic nerve stimulation and injected NE.

NE can also be taken up into extraneuronal sites in smooth muscle, heart, glandular tissue, and other organs ("uptake-2") (10). The capacity of this mechanism to store NE exceeds that of uptake-1; however, its affinity for NE and epinephrine is more limited. Consequently, uptake-1 predominates at relatively lower concentrations. Amines taken up by the second process are rapidly metabolized. Uptake-2 can be blocked by drugs such as phenoxybenzamine and metanephrine.

Several drugs inhibit action-potential-evoked release of NE. Both guanethidine and bretylium rapidly attenuate NE release, but probably by different mechanisms (19). In addition, guanethidine produces a long-lasting depletion of tissue stores of NE, probably by blocking both the axoplasmic and vesicular uptake mechanisms. The initial short-latency inhibitory action of guanethidine can be rapidly reversed by administration of substances that have an affinity for uptake-1, such as amphetamine (20). Displacement of guanethidine from its inhibitory site probably accounts for restoration of the transmission process. The efficacy of these release inhibitors varies with the frequency of nerve activation.

Certain substances can affect the transmission process by acting as "false transmitters." For example, α-methyldopa is incorporated into storage vesicles after transformation into α-methylnorepinephrine, which in turn is released by physiologic impulses (19). Octopamine, formed by β-hydroxylation of tyramine, and, indeed, guanethidine, can be released in a similar fashion. The end-organ response to the false transmitter may be subnormal and may lead to reduced responsiveness, as in the case of octopamine.

Reduction or depletion of tissue stores of NE can alter organ responses to sympathetic nerve activation. Reserpine diminishes the NE content of nerve endings by inhibiting the vesicular membrane pump (10). NE not sequestered into vesicles is exposed to the action of degradative enzymes. However, total tissue NE content must be greatly reduced in order to depress transmission. For example, organ responses to nerve stimulation recover much more rapidly after reserpine than do tissue stores of NE.

As discussed earlier, reuptake of released NE is the major process for terminating the response to sympathetic nerve activation. NE is metabolized by two major pathways (7). Extracellular NE is subject to *o*-methylation by catechol-*o*-methyltransferase. Monoamine oxidase also deactivates NE rapidly; the enzyme resides primarily within mitochondria in nerve terminals and participates in the control of levels of free NE within nerve endings. NE may also diffuse from the synaptic site into the circulation.

Autonomic Ganglia

Activation of preganglionic fibers initiates a complex series of events in postganglionic neurons. An initial fast negative potential (excitatory postsynaptic potential, EPSP), a positive potential (inhibitory postsynaptic potential, IPSP), a late negative potential, and a late-late negative potential can be recorded from autonomic ganglia (21–23). ACh, the primary excitatory transmitter in ganglia, induces the initial fast EPSP and the late EPSP by activating nicotinic and muscarinic receptors, respectively (*vide infra*). The nature of the IPSP remains uncertain; it may be generated either monosynaptically by ACh or by ACh-induced release of dopamine or NE from interneurons (22,23). Exogenous dopamine and NE can hyperpolarize postganglionic membranes under appropriate circumstances. Preganglionic stimulation can elevate cyclic adenosine 3',5'-monophosphate (cAMP) levels in ganglia. The late-late EPSP may be mediated by a peptide (22).

Adrenal Medulla

Synthetic processes in the adrenal medulla follow the scheme outlined earlier for catecholamines. Final methylation of NE to epinephrine by phenylethanolamine-N-methyltransferase occurs in the cytoplasm. Activation of preganglionic nerves results in the liberation of ACh, depolarization of the chromaffin cells, calcium influx, and release of the contents of the storage granules: catecholamines (primarily epinephrine), ATP, chromogranin, and enkephalins (24). Although epinephrine can markedly influence many organ systems, the precise physiologic role of the adrenal medulla remains obscure.

Receptors

Biologically active substances (transmitters, hormones, some drugs) interact with specific proteins called "receptors," resulting in various biophysical, biochemical, and ultimately physiologic consequences (25–27). Three general classes of receptors have been identified: (a) receptors located on the external surface of the plasma membrane in nerves, muscle,

and glands activated by amines and peptides; chemically, these are glycoproteins associated with lipids; (b) receptors for steroids that are located intracellularly in the soluble compartment; (c) receptors located within the cell nucleus (e.g., for thyroid hormone). In some instances, the agonist-receptor complex (e.g., peptides, insulin, growth hormone, prolactin, as well as low-density lipoproteins) can be internalized by endocytosis to form a vesicle within the cell (25–28).

Ligands interact with receptors by highly specific binding processes resulting in changes in the conformation or charge distribution of the receptor or neighboring region. These, in turn, result in changes in membrane permeability, alteration of the conformation of enzymes, or alteration of their associated regulatory subunits. Quantitatively, binding of agonists to membrane receptors depends on the number of receptors present and their affinity state. Binding of several classes of agonists (β-adrenergic, opiate) is markedly attenuated by guanosine triphosphate (GTP) and by sodium. GTP converts these receptors from high-affinity states to low-affinity states. In contrast, GTP does not alter binding of antagonists.

Physiologic responses vary with the number of receptors occupied. However, activation of a relatively small proportion of membrane receptors usually results in maximal physiologic responses.

The number and affinity of receptors are subject to negative feedback, leading to desensitization (down-regulation) or supersensitivity (up-regulation). Down-regulation may involve reduced synthesis of receptors. Not all agonist-receptor interactions are subject to down-regulation (e.g., aldosterone release by AII). Binding can alter the conformation of receptors in such a manner that the affinity of remaining receptors decreases (negative cooperativity). Large numbers of receptor systems utilizing amines, peptides, and steroids as agonists have been identified. These include receptors for NE, epinephrine, dopamine, ACh, 5HT, histamine, adenosine, AII, vasopressin, oxytocin, γ-aminobutyric acid, enkephalins, substance P, glycine, glutamate, etc. (25–30).

Antagonists can inhibit the actions of agonists by combining with agonist binding sites on the receptor or by binding to adjacent (allosteric) sites. Competitive blockade is surmountable, and the usual organ responses are obtained if the concentration of the agonist is increased; i.e., the dose–response curve is shifted to the right, but the maximum obtainable response remains unaltered. Noncompetitive blockade involves covalent binding to receptors. Maximum responses are depressed, and restoration of activity requires synthesis of new receptors.

Cholinergic Receptors

Acetylcholine is an agonist for two major types of receptors. These were originally classified as "muscarinic" or "nicotinic" on the basis of their similarities to responses to the alkaloid muscarine and nicotine. Cholinergic receptors in skeletal muscle and most of those on the cell bodies of postganglionic neurons and on nonmyelinated C fibers respond to nicotine and are considered "nicotinic." In contrast, receptors innervated by postganglionic cholinergic fibers, such as in smooth muscle and glands, are termed "muscarinic" (Table 1). Nicotinic receptors in ganglia and skeletal muscle are inhibited by competitive blockers such as hexamethonium and d-tubocurarine, respectively. Atropine exemplifies a blocker of muscarinic receptors (Table 2).

Activation of cholinergic receptors results in changes in cell membranes ultimately leading to various responses such as hyperpolarization of cells in the sinoatrial node or depolarization of ganglia (as indicated earlier) and intestinal smooth muscle. Biochemically, muscarinic receptors (e.g., in the heart) may be negatively coupled to adenylate cyclase and indirectly linked to guanylate cyclase, resulting in elevated concentrations of cyclic guanosine monophosphate (cGMP).

Adrenergic Receptors

On the basis of qualitative and quantitative organ responses to various sympathomimetic amines, Ahlquist concluded that two distinct adrenergic receptors, α and β, exist (33). Subsets of these (α_1, α_2, β_1, β_2) have been identified by binding studies and the use of appropriate antagonists.

Both α_1- and α_2-adrenoceptors subserve arterial vasoconstriction. The finding that constrictor responses to sympathetic nerve stimulation are selectively attenuated by α_1 blockers, whereas parenterally administered NE is most susceptible to α_2 blockers, has led to the hypothesis that neuronally released NE gains access primarily to α_1 receptors at postjunctional sites but that circulating NE activates both (12,34). Activation of α_2 receptors on adrenergic, cholinergic, and tryptaminergic nerve terminals can inhibit the release of these transmitters (7,12). Adrenergic inhibition of intestinal motility is partially mediated by reduction of ACh release from cholinergic fibers.

NE and phenylephrine are potent agonists for α_1 receptors, which can in turn be blocked relatively selectively by prazosin and corynanthine (Table 2); α_2 receptors are activated by norepinephrine and guanabenz and blocked by rauwolscine.

Numerous biophysical and biochemical consequences of α-adrenoceptor activation have been observed, including inhibition of adenylate cyclase in some organs (e.g., platelets), elevation of cAMP in the brain, and indirect linkage to guanylate cyclase (12,31). α_1 receptor activation has been shown to augment the breakdown of phosphatidyl inositol (35). α_2 stimulation may specifically enhance calcium influx in vascular smooth muscle.

Activation of β_1-adrenoceptors causes augmentation of cardiac rate and contractility and relaxation of intestinal tone (37). Stimulation of β_2 receptors results in vasodilatation and bronchial and uterine relaxation (Table 1). Propranolol blocks both receptors, whereas metoprolol and atenolol block β_1 receptors relatively selectively (Table 2).

TABLE 1. *Organ responses to autonomic mediators[a]*

Organ	Adrenergic	Cholinergic
Heart		
Sinoatrial node	Rate + (β)	Rate −
Atrioventricular node	Automaticity + (β)	Automaticity −
	Conduction + (β)	Conduction −
His-Purkinje system	Automaticity + (β)	
Atria	Contractile force + (β)	Contractile force −
Ventricles	Contractile force + (β)	Contractile force −
Blood vessels		
Skeletal muscle	Constriction (α)	Dilatation
	Dilatation (β)	
Skin	Constriction (α)	Slight dilatation
Kidney, intestine	Constriction (α)	Dilatation
	Slight dilatation (β)	
Intestine	Motility and tone −	Motility and tone
Urinary bladder		
Detrussor	Relaxation (β)	Contraction
Trigone and sphincter	Contraction (α)	Relaxation
Uterus	Relaxation (β)	
	Contraction (α)	
Eye		
Radial muscle	Contraction (α)	
Sphincter		Contraction
Lacrimal glands		Secretion
Salivary glands	Viscous secretion (α)	Watery secretion
Sweat glands		Secretion
Metabolic	Glycogenolysis, lipolysis +	

[a] A plus sign indicates an increase or enhancement; a minus sign indicates a decrease or slowing; α and β refer to the type of adrenergic receptor that mediates the response. Constrictor responses in blood vessels are mediated by α receptors and dilator responses by β receptors. Epinephrine usually reduces vascular resistance of skeletal muscle, because the β-response predominates. Norepinephrine exerts relatively weak effects on vascular β receptors. As a result, sympathetic stimulation usually results in constriction. Responses of the uterus vary greatly and depend on the stage of the menstrual cycle, etc. Activation of both α and β receptors in the intestine results in inhibition of motility and tone. Species variation exists in the type of receptor involved in metabolic responses.

Adrenergic receptors are subject to feedback phenomena characteristic of receptors in general, such as up- and down-regulation and interaction with other systems (e.g., stimulation of α receptors can lower the affinity of β receptors) (25–28). Receptor density can vary widely among and within organs. Within the heart, the left atrium contains the highest concentration, followed by the right atrium and right and left ventricles (38).

Biochemical consequences of β receptor activation have been extensively studied (25–27). The β receptor, a guanine nucleotide regulatory protein, and the enzyme adenylate cyclase exist as a complex in the cell membrane. Binding by agonists to β receptors results in conformational changes that promote the exchange of guanosine diphosphate (GDP) bound to the regulatory protein for GTP. The regulatory-protein–GTP complex combines with the inactive catalytic subunit of the enzyme, forming an active complex capable of catalyzing the conversion of ATP to cAMP. The latter promotes the dissociation of regulatory subunits of protein kinases from their catalytic subunits, thereby activating them. Protein kinases, in turn, phosphorylate various proteins, leading to activation or inactivation

TABLE 2. *Receptor agonists and antagonists*

Receptor	Agonist	Antagonist
Adrenergic		
α_1	NE, phenylephrine, tramazoline	Prazosin, corynanthine
α_2	NE, guanabenz, clonidine	Rauwolscine
β_1	NE, isoproterenol	Metoprolol, atenolol
β_2	NE, isoproterenol, terbutaline	Propranolol (nonselective)
Dopamine$_1$	Dopamine, aminotetralins	Bulbocapnine, bromocriptine
Dopamine$_2$	Dopamine, apomorphine	Haloperidol, *S*-sulpiride
5HT$_1$	5HT	Methysergide
5HT$_2$	5HT	Ketanserin
Cholinergic-muscarinic	ACh	Atropine
Cholinergic-nicotinic	ACh	Tetraethylammonium, hexamethonium, curare
Histamine$_1$	Histamine, 2-methylhistamine	Mepyramine
Histamine$_2$	Histamine, 4-methylhistamine, dimaprit	Cimetidine
Angiotensin II	Angiotensin II	Saralasin

of particular enzymes. The enzyme phosphodiesterase degrades cAMP and thereby participates in the regulation of its tissue levels.

GTP decreases the affinity of β receptors as well as other adenyl-cylase-linked receptors for their agonist.

Dopamine

Ascending dopaminergic tracts originating in the brainstem have been identified (6). Peripherally injected dopamine stimulates the heart and constricts blood vessels by β- and α-adrenoceptor activation, respectively. In addition, it can activate distinct receptors in the renal and mesenteric beds, leading to vasodilation (39). Dopamine receptor activation can inhibit NE release and ganglionic transmission, as indicated earlier.

Dopamine receptors have been classified according to their linkage to adenyl cyclase. DA$_1$ receptors are linked, whereas DA$_2$ receptors are not. Agonists and antagonists are listed in Table 2 (39–42). Renal and mesenteric receptors resemble the DA$_1$ subgroup, but their linkage to adenyl cyclase remains uncertain.

Interactions of Other Endogenous Substances with the Cardiovascular and Autonomic Nervous Systems

AII, which will be discussed again later, can release epinephrine from the adrenal medulla, stimulate autonomic ganglia and intramural nerves in various organs, and enhance release of NE during sympathetic nervous stimulation (7,16,43,44).

Members of the prostaglandin family, particularly of the E series, inhibit NE release from sympathetic nerves by a presynaptic action in some organs (7,45–47). However, under certain circumstances they may potentiate the response of smooth muscle to various agonists, including NE, ACh, and 5HT, and at other times may diminish responses (34–36). Prostaglandins may play a physiologic regulatory role at sympathetic nerve endings, because inhibitors of their synthesis enhance organ responses to sympathetic nerve stimulation under appropriate conditions. Prostaglandins have also been reported to inhibit cardiac responses to vagal nerve stimulation (45).

5HT-containing neurons and tracts exist in

the brain and spinal cord and in the intestinal tract. 5HT both constricts and dilates blood vessels by direct actions, and it can enhance the pressor effects of other agonists. Dilatation resulting from inhibition of sympathetic tone can also occur. 5HT receptors have also been subclassified: $5HT_1$ and $5HT_2$ (Table 2) (48,49). The former is adenylate-cyclase-linked.

Histamine stored in mast cells and platelets can be released by several agents, including compound 48/80, morphine, and curare. Histamine exerts numerous actions, including release of adrenal epinephrine, ganglionic stimulation, and contraction or relaxation of various smooth-muscle cells. Activation of H_2 receptors leads to gastric secretion and cardiac stimulation. Blood vessels contain H_1 as well as H_2 receptors. Both must be blocked in order to completely obtund the vasodilator action of histamine.

Purinergic Nerves

A nonadrenergic inhibitory system has been demonstrated in the intestine (50). Activation of the system results in hyperpolarization and relaxation of smooth-muscle cells. Cell bodies of these neurons originate in Auerbach's plexus and, in at least some portions of the intestine, are subject to control by preganglionic vagal nerves. Evidence suggests that ATP serves as the inhibitory mediator.

PERIPHERAL CIRCULATION

Tissue perfusion is the primary role of the circulation. The heart generates the force required to propel blood throughout peripheral vessels and must also provide an output adequate for the widely varying and rapidly changing demands of the organism.

Characteristics of Vascular Smooth Muscle

Vascular smooth-muscle cells possess characteristics generally typical of excitable cells.

Their plasma membrane contains several specific ion channels and a number of active transport systems. These result in differences in ionic concentration and a potential difference across the membrane (50–70 mV, inside negative). Changes in the conformation or charge distribution within channels form "gating" mechanisms that regulate ion fluxes. The number of open channels and their kinetics are influenced by membrane voltage, mediators, hormones, cyclic nucleotides, and drugs (50–56).

The association of electrical membrane phenomena and mechanical activity has been demonstrated in several types of smooth muscle (51,52). Spontaneous rhythmic electrical activity and associated contractions occur in several isolated vessels, including mesenteric arteries and veins and portal veins. Slow fluctuations appear in the membrane potential, and spikes resembling action potentials arise from the peaks of the slow waves. Action potentials of long duration (up to 30 sec) have been observed in the turtle aorta and vena cava. Electrical activity arises in pacemaker areas in numerous isolated preparations, such as the rabbit portal vein, and then spreads over the entire tissue. Constrictor substances usually produce depolarization and initiate or increase the frequency of action potentials in spike-generating tissue.

Some tissues appear to respond to excitatory stimuli by graded depolarization rather than by spike generation. NE has been shown to produce depolarization and contraction in rat caudal, cat basilar, and rabbit pulmonary arteries (57–59). Papaverine and isoproterenol exert opposite effects (hyperpolarization and relaxation) (60). Inhibition of the sarcolemmal sodium pump by inhibition of Na-K ATPase results in depolarization.

Contractile mechanisms in vascular smooth muscle bear numerous similarities to those in skeletal and cardiac muscle (55,56,62–66). All contain the major proteins myosin and actin, but the arrangement of these two filaments is not as regular in smooth muscle, resulting in the absence of clear cross-striations. Myosin is composed of two "heavy" chains and two pairs of "light" chains. Extensions of the myosin molecule containing the light chains form cross-bridges toward the actin filament. The cross-bridges also possess a magnesium-dependent ATPase and an actin binding site.

Calcium binds to the protein calmodulin during initiation of the contractile process in vascular smooth muscle. The calcium-calmodulin complex then binds to the inactive catalytic subunit of myosin light-chain kinases, resulting in its activation. This enzyme phosphorylates the myosin light chain, permitting the activation of the magnesium-dependent ATPase on the myosin cross-bridges by actin. Hydrolysis of ATP ensues and results in tension development due to conformational changes in the cross-bridges and the relative movement of the myosin and actin filaments. Tension varies with the number of active cross-bridges and their cycling rate. Myosin light-chain phosphatase removes phosphate from the light chain and restores the two filaments to their "dormant" state. An alternative mode of activating myosin ATPase by the protein leiotonin has been proposed.

In cardiac and skeletal muscle the proteins tropomyosin and the troponins are associated with actin and exert an inhibitory role on its activity. Binding of calcium to troponin C removes this inhibition and permits activation of myosin ATPase.

Thus, calcium assumes a central role in the contractile process of all forms of muscle. During the resting state its concentration approximates 10^{-7} M or less. Concentration related activation occurs at 10^{-7} to 10^{-5} M. This calcium derives primarily from the sarcoplasmic reticulum (SR) in skeletal muscle. In cardiac muscle, influx of calcium occurs during the plateau of the action potential and is also released from the SR. In smooth muscle, calcium enters the cells through "voltage"-activated channels that become operative on membrane depolarization or through receptor-activated channels. Calcium can also be released from the SR and other intracellular binding sites. The contributions of these sources of calcium vary in different blood vessels and also depend on the mode of activation (53,55).

Biologically active substances such as NE, AII, and 5HT contract vascular smooth muscle by enhancing calcium influx through receptor-operated channels as well as release from intracellular stores. Agonist-induced depolarization provides another mechanism for calcium entry through the voltage-sensitive channels.

Relaxation occurs on sequestration of calcium into the SR or other stores or by efflux. Relaxant substances can act by influencing one or more of these processes. cAMP promotes the uptake of calcium by the SR and has also been shown to inhibit myosin light-chain kinase. Vasodilation produced by nitroglycerin and nitroprusside correlates with increases in cGMP (67,68).

Characteristics of Blood Vessels and Vascular Beds

Vascular smooth-muscle cells are arranged in series and in parallel with elastic components (69–71). Their contraction generates tension within the vessel wall. Tension generation and velocity of shortening vary with muscle length up to an optimal value (e.g., 150% of resting length in some vascular tissue) and then declines. Stretch affects the number of myosin cross-bridges capable of interacting with actin. Compared with skeletal and cardiac muscle, smooth muscle contracts very slowly but can generate great force at a relatively low energy cost.

Vascular smooth muscle is subject to influences by numerous local and extrinsic factors and at any one time may be in a relaxed state (i.e., possess little "tone"), whereas in other circumstances it may be contracted and possess a high degree of tone. Basal tone (i.e., the degree of intrinsic contraction in the absence of known external factors) varies considerably among different vessels.

Blood vessel caliber is determined by the interplay of two opposing forces: transmural distending pressure and tangential wall tension (71). Laplace described the relationship between the radius and wall tension in hollow circular structures as follows: tension = pressure × radius. Neither his formulation nor equations incorporating an additional factor relating to wall thickness are totally applicable to the circulation. However, they provide an extremely useful concept in describing vessel behavior as well as cardiac behavior.

Poiseuille studied the flow of liquids through rigid tubes and concluded that flow (F) varies directly with effective driving pressure (P) and the fourth power of the vessel radius (R) and inversely with the viscosity (V) of the fluid and the length (L) of the tube: $F = \pi PR^4/8VL$. Again, this formulation serves only as an approximation for the circulation, because blood vessels are distensible rather than rigid, flow is pulsatile, and blood consists of liquid as well as corpuscular components. Nevertheless, the equation highlights the critical factors influencing flow in a vascular bed, such that (other factors remaining constant) flow varies directly with driving pressure and inversely with resistance.

The content of contractile and elastic elements in arterial and venous vessels varies. Relative smooth-muscle content increases progressively from the aorta to precapillary sphincters. Veins contain a higher proportion of elastic elements than arteries and have a smaller wall/lumen ratio. Arterial and arteriolar segments control the resistance of vascular beds. However, under certain circumstances, postcapillary vessels can assume a relatively large proportion of the total resistance in some beds.

Compliance or distensibility represents a passive property of blood vessels that depends primarily on the elastic constituents of the vessel wall and accounts for the change in radius in response to altered distending pressure (74). Smooth-muscle tone, as well as disease processes, can influence overall elasticity and compliance. Venous capacitance greatly exceeds that of precapillary vessels. Thus, small changes in intravascular pressure can produce large changes in vein radius. Veins contain

approximately 65% of total blood volume. Consequently, small changes in venous tone can translocate relatively large quantities of blood. Events on the arterial side are also capable of influencing venous mechanics. At constant systemic pressure, arterial constriction results in a fall in transmural pressure in postcapillary vessels. The latter, in turn, causes a reduction of venous volume as a result of passive recoil of the venous wall.

Small precapillary vessels and sphincters relax and contract spontaneously (74). This vasomotion persists after denervation but is under the influence of local metabolic factors. The opening and closing of sphincters results in intermittent flow in individual capillaries, and only a fraction are patent at any instant. During increased metabolic activity of an organ, the proportion of open capillaries increases markedly.

Bidirectional fluid movement occurs across capillaries and consists of filtration into the interstitial space and reabsorption into the capillary. Several factors influence these fluxes (74). The pressure gradient across the vessels walls tends to drive fluid out, whereas the colloid osmotic pressure difference favors reabsorption. At a given aortic pressure, the ratio of precapillary resistance to postcapillary resistance determines capillary pressure in individual beds. Thus, arteriolar dilation unaccompanied by venous relaxation tends to increase capillary pressure and enhance filtration. Venous constriction produces a similar change. Filtration predominates at the arterial end of a capillary, and reabsorption predominates at the venous end. However, because of periodic opening and closing of precapillary sphincters, filtration may occur across the entire length of an individual capillary at any one time, whereas reabsorption may predominate in others. The lymphatic system returns excess filtrate to the main circulation.

Arteriovenous anastomoses or shunts connecting small arteries to small veins and bypassing capillaries occur in some tissues, particularly in skin (74). Blood flowing through these channels serves no metabolic function.

Closure of cutaneous shunts by sympathetic stimuli diverts flow into capillaries and facilitates heat loss during exercise.

Control of Flow in Vascular Beds

The peripheral circulation consists of numerous vascular beds connected in parallel. The relative resistance of each bed determines the proportion of cardiac output it will receive. As in a parallel electrical circuit, the reciprocal of total resistance $(1/R)$ equals the sum of the reciprocals of individual resistances $(1/r_1 + \ldots + 1/r_n)$. At rest, the kidneys and intestinal organs each receive approximately 20% of cardiac output, the brain and skeletal muscle 15%, and heart and skin 5%. During exercise, flow to muscle increases greatly. On the other hand, proportional (although not necessarily absolute) flow to some other organs (e.g., intestinal tract and kidneys) declines. Other activities that augment individual organ requirements for blood can also result in flow redistribution.

The state of vascular smooth-muscle contraction or tone is the major determinant of resistance. In vessels with minimal ability to constrict or relax, flow will tend to depend on the arterial–venous pressure gradient. The magnitude of intrinsic precapillary vessel tone varies considerably in different organs. Therefore, a given stimulus will not produce the same degree of dilatation or constriction in all beds.

Numerous local, neurogenic, and humoral factors influence vascular resistance. Trophic factors (e.g., NE) produce more long-term effects (75). Vascular smooth-muscle cells readily respond to alterations in tissue P_{O_2}, P_{CO_2}, and pH (73–75). Hypoxia, hypercarbia, and reduced pH result in vasodilatation, whereas changes in the opposite direction cause constriction. Overall, a correlation exists between metabolic activity and blood flow or vascular resistance under normal conditions. Venous blood emerging from normally perfused organs usually is vasodilator relative to arterial blood. However, the perfusion of various vascular beds with hypoxic blood results in dilatation only when P_{O_2} is greatly reduced; i.e., to approximately 40 mm Hg (73). Thus, tissue oxygen, carbon dioxide, or hydrogen ion concentrations cannot individually be responsible for resistance regulation. However, carbon dioxide tension is of critical importance in the cerebral circulation (77–79). Other factors contributing to local regulation include metabolites, nucleotides such as adenosine, potassium ion, and changes in osmolarity (73, 75,80,81). Metabolic vasodilation in skeletal muscle also results in the opening of additional capillary channels. In contrast, postcapillary vessels appear to remain unaffected by local regulatory mechanisms. The pulmonary circulation displays a somewhat atypical response to hypoxia in that pulmonary arterial pressure increases. Augmented blood flow may contribute to the pressure elevation. Numerous other locally generated factors (prostaglandins, bradykinin, 5HT, histamine, etc.) also influence vascular tone.

The power of local regulatory mechanisms is illustrated by the phenomenon of autoregulation of blood flow. Changes in arterial transmural pressure or inflow result in changes in smooth-muscle tone and vessel resistance in the same direction, and these, in turn, tend to maintain blood flow constant (82). Autoregulation usually prevails in the pressure range of 60 to 140 mm Hg in most organs. Regulatory mechanisms become inadequate at the extremes, and flow will vary in proportion to driving pressure. The degree of autoregulation varies in different organs, being particularly powerful in the kidney and brain, somewhat less so in skeletal muscle, and almost negligible in skin. Passive mechanisms tend to counteract autoregulation to some extent, because changes in distending pressure modify vessel radius and, thereby, resistance.

At least three major mechanisms have been proposed to account for the process. The tissue-pressure hypothesis suggests that increasing perfusion pressure leads to increased capillary filtration and an elevation of extravascular pressure, and thus an increase in resistance. However, most evidence supports the metabolic and myogenic theories. The former is based on the supposition that a decrease in perfusion pressure will initially lower blood flow and reduce tissue PO_2 and cause an accumulation of metabolites. These factors, in turn, dilate smaller arterial vessels, reduce resistance, and tend to raise blood flow toward original levels. Myogenic theories of autoregulation extend the original observations of Bayliss and are based on the hypothesis that vascular smooth muscle responds to changes in distending pressure by contraction or relaxation. Isolated strips of small mesenteric and cerebral arteries have been shown to contract when quickly stretched. Distension also increases rhythmicity of isolated strips that normally display periodic contractions. Further, elevation of distending pressure increases vasomotion in small arterial vessels.

The relative roles of metabolic and myogenic factors in autoregulation remain controversial, and neither can account for the phenomenon alone. Their respective contributions probably vary from organ to organ as well as from time to time as circumstances change. Normal vascular tone is a prerequisite for autoregulation, because reactive hyperemia or the administration of vasodilators or metabolic inhibitors obtunds the process.

The cerebral circulation is principally under the control of intrinsic factors, with only minor contributions by extrinsic, including nervous, factors (77–79,83). A unique feature of the cerebral circulation is the highly selective permeability of the capillary endothelium, establishing a "blood-brain barrier." The barrier apparently depends on glial cells. Large arteries contribute significantly to the total resistance of this bed. Renal blood flow, unlike that to other organs, greatly exceeds metabolic requirements; yet the organ displays vigorous autoregulation.

Autonomic Control of the Peripheral Circulation

Adrenergic Influence

Most blood vessels are richly innervated by sympathetic nerves. Nerve terminals form a network of anastomosing filaments that run along the periphery of vessels. Adrenergic innervation is usually limited to the junction of the adventitia and the media. However, neurons have been demonstrated to penetrate for a short distance into the media in some vessels (e.g., the proximal saphenous artery of the rabbit) (4,84–86). In general, arteries are more densely innervated than veins. However, the density of innervation of individual arteries and veins varies considerably. Terminal axons have also been shown to innervate precapillary sphincters.

The preponderant limitation of adrenergic fibers to the adventitial-medial junction raises the question of the mode of activation of the more medial smooth-muscle cells. This could be accomplished by (a) diffusion of the mediator, (b) inward electrotonic spread of the excitatory potential from innervated cells, and (c) conduction by smooth-muscle cells along low-resistance pathways (84). The relative importance of these mechanisms remains unsettled. It has been demonstrated that impulse propagation can occur in isolated vascular tissue but that vessels differ greatly in their ability to conduct (86).

Stimulation of sympathetic nerves to most organs, or intraarterial administration of NE, results in vasoconstriction and an increase in vascular resistance, as indicated by a reduction in blood flow or by an increase in perfusion pressure when flow is maintained by a pump. Sympathetic stimulation also causes venous constriction, resulting in a reduction in venous capacitance and an increase in resistance (74). Maximal responses usually appear at frequencies of 10 to 20 Hz or less (74). Even lower frequencies result in peak effects in venous preparations. It has been estimated that stimulation at 0.5 to 2 Hz approximates the level of spontaneous tonic activity usually encountered in anesthetized animals.

Sympathetic stimulation may affect vessels in different organs or even vessels within an organ differentially. For example, blood is distributed away from the renal cortex during stimulation. Along similar lines, stimulation at equivalent frequencies produces larger increases in resistance in the kidney than in the forelimb (87).

The preponderant role of local factors in the regulation of the cerebral circulation was indicated earlier. In general, cerebrovascular responses to sympathetic nerve stimulation are weak (77,78,83). Coronary arteries are innervated by sympathetic fibers, stimulation of which can produce vasoconstriction. However, local metabolic factors predominate (88). Stimulation of sympathetic fibers to the intestine can result in intense vasoconstriction, which then "escapes" because of accumulation of locally produced dilator factors.

The ability to record pressures from small vessels has permitted more detailed studies of vascular responses to sympathetic nerve stimulation. These methods have revealed that the initial increment in total vascular resistance of the gastrocnemius muscle during sympathetic nerve activation results from constriction of the more distal arterial vessels. During continued stimulation, however, the distal vessels tend to relax while the larger proximal segment constricts progressively (89).

Responses to sympathetic stimulation in the perfused dog forelimb have also been studied in detail and have demonstrated even greater complexity (87,90). It was found that stimulation increased the overall vascular resistance, but changes in the constituent muscle and cutaneous beds differed considerably. Vascular resistance of the large arterial segments increased in muscle and particularly in skin. Small-vessel resistance, comprising effects in small arteries, arterioles, and smaller veins, did not change greatly in muscle but fell markedly in skin. Resistance of the venous segment composed of the larger veins increased very greatly in skin, but the increase was considerably smaller in muscle. These responses resulted in a net redistribution of blood flow from skin to muscle.

Sympathetic stimulation has also been shown to cause a net constriction of precapillary sphincters, resulting in reduced capillary surface area. During prolonged stimulation, accumulation of metabolites overcomes the decline in capillary filtration. In contrast, tonic sympathetic activity may not influence precapillary sphincters greatly or play a role in the regulation of capillary filtration surface area (91).

Arterial and venous constrictor responses to sympathetic stimulation and NE are mediated predominantly by α_1-adrenoceptor activation, as indicated earlier, but α_2 receptors may assume a greater role in large veins (92). Arterial smooth-muscle cells also possess β receptors (β_2). These probably are not innervated or do not respond greatly to neuronally released NE but may be activated by circulating epinephrine (93).

Intravenous infusion of NE elevates total peripheral resistance. On the other hand, total resistance usually falls during epinephrine infusion, mainly because of β-mediated dilation of vessels in skeletal muscle. NE has been reported to exert a trophic effect on vascular smooth muscle (76). Dopaminergic vasodilator receptors exist in the mesenteric and renal beds, as indicated earlier (39).

Sympathetic Vasodilator Fibers

Sympathetic nerves to skin and skeletal muscle also contain vasodilator fibers. The latter compose a system that originates in the cerebral cortex, relays in the hypothalamus and midbrain collicular region, but not in the medulla, and emerges from the thoracolumbar cord. Activation of the system by hypothalamic stimulation results in dilatation in muscle, but constriction in most other beds, as well as cardiac augmentation (94,95). Stimulation of these sites in conscious animals produces sham rage. Cholinergically mediated vasodilatation can be readily demonstrated in muscle on sympathetic nerve stimulation after pretreatment with adrenergic neuron blocking agents (96–98).

Parasympathetic Vasoactive Fibers

Cholinergic vasodilator fibers emerge from the sacral cord and innervate the genitals, bladder, and large intestine. Control of penile erection is one of the primary functions of this system. Activation of cholinergic fibers dilates resistance vessels in the penis, leading to greatly augmented blood flow and filling of the cavernous tissue under high pressure (99). Parasympathetic stimulation results in local vasodilatation in salivary glands through the mediation of bradykinin (*vide infra*).

Other Vasodilator Systems

Complex vasodilator systems exist in cutaneous beds such as the canine paw. After administration of adrenergic neuron blockers, sympathetic nerve stimulation results in a "sustained" noncholinergic vasodilator response that exceeds the duration of nerve activation (96–98). Transmural stimulation of isolated cerebral arteries causes relaxation that cannot be attributed to known mediators (100).

Histamine is widely distributed in the body in mast cells, leukocytes, and platelets and can be released from these depots by drugs and other stimuli. The substance dilates precapillary vessels and may also increase capillary filtration rate. It has been postulated that a histaminergic vasodilator system may participate in the reflex regulation of resistance of muscle beds (96,101).

Other Regulatory Systems

Renin-Angiotensin System

Renin is a proteolytic enzyme found principally in the kidney; it forms the decapeptide angiotensin I (from a circulating α_2-globulin) Angiotensin converting enzyme (ACE), an exopeptidase, splits two amino acids from the decapeptide and forms the octapeptide AII. Juxtaglomerular cells located at the vascular pole on renal glomeruli form and release renin into the circulation (44,102). Renin is also present in numerous other organs, including blood vessels, the brain, uterus, etc. (103,104). Several mechanisms control renin release from juxtaglomerular cells. Release is inversely related to the distension of "baroreceptors" or

stretch receptors in the afferent arteriole. Mechanisms in the macula densa sense the amount of sodium in the distal tubule and regulate renin release. Activation of β-adrenoceptors on juxtaglomerular cells causes elaboration of renin. Prostaglandins also release renin and may constitute a critical link in several of the foregoing mechanisms. AII exerts negative feedback on release. Dopamine and vasopressin also inhibit.

AII is a powerful constrictor of vascular smooth muscle, probably mediated by influx and intracellular release of calcium. Infusion of subpressor quantities of AII can increase blood pressure in experimental animals after a latency of a few days (105). The peptide is one of the principal regulatory mechanisms for aldosterone release. In the kidney, AII affects the distribution of blood flow and the glomerular filtration rate and enhances tubular sodium reabsorption (44,106,107). AII also facilitates release of NE at adrenergic neuroeffector junctions (7,15,44). The various components of the renin-angiotensin system are present in the brain. Central mechanisms will be discussed later.

In intact humans and animals, stress (e.g., sodium depletion, upright posture, hemorrhage, etc.) elevates plasma renin activity (PRA). The AII generated participates in cardiovascular adjustments to these interventions.

Several peptide competitive blockers of AII receptors have been synthesized, e.g., the 1-sarosine-8-alanine analogue (saralasin). Inhibitors of ACE have also been developed (108). The renin-angiotensin system is discussed in greater detail elsewhere in this volume.

Prostaglandins

Two families of highly active substances are derived from arachidonic acid: prostaglandins and leukotrienes (109–111). Prostaglandins (PGs) are a group of unsaturated acidic lipids containing a 20-carbon skeleton. Arachidonic acid is released from membrane phospholipids by phospholipases. In the PG pathway, cyclooxygenase forms the intermediate endoperoxides PGG_2 and PGH_2 from arachidonic acid. These, in turn, and depending on the tissue, are transformed into thromboxane A_2 (TxA_2) (e.g., in platelets), into prostacyclin (PGI_2) (in the walls of blood vessels), or into PGE_2 or $PGF_{2\alpha}$.

In the lipoxygenase pathways, arachidonic acid is converted into hydroxyperoxy eicosatetraenoic acid (HPETE) and then into several leukotrienes. Leukotrienes have been found in leukocytes, in mast cells, and in lung tissue. These substances compose the "slow-reacting substance of anaphylaxis" (SRS-A). Their cardiovascular role remains to be elucidated. However, they have been shown to constrict coronary arteries (112).

TxA_2 is the major metabolite of arachidonic acid in platelets and may also be formed in the lungs and spleen. It is an extremely potent aggregator of platelets, an effect probably mediated by reduction of cAMP levels (109, 110,113). Prostacyclin, the principal metabolite of arachidonic acid in blood vessels, inhibits platelet aggregation and produces vasodilatation (109,110,114). Locally formed PGs may participate in regulation of blood flow. Their role in modulation of sympathetic transmission and renin release was discussed earlier.

Kinins

Kinins are potent vasodilator peptides formed from globulins (kininogens) by kininases (e.g., kallikrein). Salivary glands, pancreas, kidney, and plasma contain high concentrations of kallikrein (115,116). Glandular kallikrein forms kallidin (lysyl-bradykinin), which in turn is converted to the nonapeptide bradykinin by an aminopeptidase. Bradykinin is inactivated by kininase II, an enzyme identical with ACE. Kinins affect blood clotting mechanisms, fibrinolysis, and capillary permeability, in addition to participating in local control of blood flow. In the kidney, kinins influence water and electrolyte excretion. AII and PGs can release bradykinin in organs such as the kidney. Bradykinin, in turn, is capable of releasing PGs.

Vasopressin

The nonapeptide vasopressin (antidiuretic hormone, ADH) is formed in the hypothalamus and stored and released from the posterior pituitary (117). Its primary physiologic role involves renal water reabsorption by controlling the permeability of collecting ducts to water. Although vasopressin exerts potent vasoconstrictor activity, its role in circulatory control remains unsettled, because much higher doses are required to raise blood pressure than to produce antidiuresis (118). However, this difference may be attributable to buffering by the baroreceptors. Nevertheless, vasopressin probably contributes to circulatory regulation in stressful states such as hemorrhage and may provide a backup mechanism to the renin-angiotensin system (118–120). Development of hypertension in models using sodium overload involves vasopressin (121).

5-Hydroxytryptamine

5HT is released from aggregating platelets. It is concentrated in the lungs, in the gastrointestinal tract, and in various brain pathways. 5HT has complex vascular actions (49,122). Vasoconstriction predominates, but dilatation can occur through direct means or secondary to inhibition of sympathetic-mediator release. 5HT can also enhance the constrictor actions of other agonists.

Other Vasoactive Substances

A substance released from the endothelium of isolated blood vessels has been shown to mediate the relaxant responses to ACh and bradykinin (123). Expansion of blood volume causes the release of a circulating natriuretic factor that increases renal sodium excretion subsequent to inhibition of Na-K ATPase. Inhibition of this enzyme also affects intracellular ion concentrations in cardiac and vascular smooth muscle. The hormone has been implicated in the development of hypertension (124,125). Evidence indicates that it may be released from the anterior hypothalamus. It may also be related to the postulated endogenous digitalislike substance "endoxin."

THE HEART

The primary function of cardiac muscle is generation of the force required to propel blood into peripheral organs. The actual volume of blood pumped by the heart results from the interplay of numerous complex factors.

Mechanical Properties of Cardiac Muscle Fibers

Depolarization of cardiac tissue results from rapid but brief influx of sodium. Calcium influx occurs during the plateau phase of the action potential, and repolarization is caused by potassium efflux (126). Contractile mechanisms in cardiac muscle resemble those outlined earlier for smooth muscle in regard to the general interaction of myosin and actin. However, activation results from the binding of calcium to troponin C and negation of its inhibitory influence on actin. The transverse tubular system and the SR are highly developed in cardiac muscle, and intracellular calcium stores play a greater role in the contractile process than in smooth muscle. Depolarization releases calcium from the SR (62,65,127).

Cardiac muscle consists of contractile and elastic elements arranged in series and in parallel. The contractile elements shorten on activation and stretch the series elastic elements. The external length of the muscle will diminish when the tension generated exceeds the imposed load.

Increasing the length of cardiac muscle up to its optimum maximizes the possibility for cross-bridge interaction and augments the extent and rate of force generation. This length–tension relationship forms the basis for the Frank-Starling "law of the heart," which states that the energy of contraction, however measured, is a function of the length of the muscle fiber prior to contraction (Fig. 3).

As just indicated, increasing the resting length (up to a point) augments the rate of tension development of isometric contraction and the velocity of shortening of isotonic contraction (128–131). On the other hand, an increase in the afterload (i.e., the load against which the muscle contracts) reduces the shortening velocity (Fig. 3). Isometric contraction results when the afterload is so great that the velocity of external shortening equals zero. Shortening velocity becomes maximal rapidly after initiation of contraction but then declines

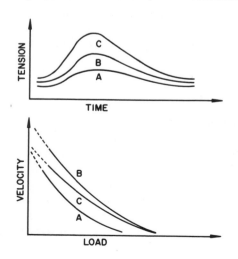

FIG. 3. Tension generation during isometric contraction and characteristics of the force–velocity relationship of isolated ventricular muscle. **Top panel:** Schematic representation of tension development during isometric contraction. Resting muscle length was increased progressively from *A* to *C,* causing rises in resting tension, rate of tension development, and peak tension during contraction. The time to peak tension did not change. **Bottom panel:** Schematic representation of the force–velocity relationship during shortening. Increasing the afterload reduces the peak velocity of shortening (curve *A*). Increasing the resting length shifts the curve upward (*C*) so that the velocity of shortening at a given afterload rises. However, extrapolation of the curve back to zero load provides the same value for V_{max}. A positive inotropic intervention shifts the curve upward, as from *A* to *B*. Under these circumstances, peak observed velocity, as well as V_{max}, increases. (Adapted from Sonnenblick et al., ref. 128, with permission.)

as the muscle decreases in length. The velocity of shortening at any time during contraction varies with muscle length at that instant and is no longer dependent on the initial length of the muscle. Theoretically, the maximal velocity of shortening (V_{max}) occurs when muscle contracts against no external load. V_{max} can be approximated by extrapolation of the velocity–load curve to zero. V_{max} varies with the contractile state of the muscle but, according to several investigators, is independent of preload and afterload (Fig. 3).

Force generation depends on its rate of development and the duration of the active state. The rate of tension development or the intensity of the active state depends critically on the concentration of calcium in the vicinity of the contractile proteins. Changes in resting length do not alter the basic "contractility" of cardiac muscle, which can be defined as the force developed at a given fiber length or, alternatively, as the rate of tension development or the velocity of contraction at a given length, or as V_{max}.

Increasing the number of contractions per unit time up to an optimum rate will augment contractility, as exemplified by the extent and velocity of shortening and the V_{max} of muscle. Relaxation also accelerates. The rate of tension development of an isometric contraction also rises, but the total tension generated may not increase, because the time to peak tension declines. Appropriately timed extrasystoles tend to potentiate the ensuing regular beats. The interpolation of a second stimulus soon after the termination of the refractory period of every regular beat (i.e., "paired pacing") usually results in only a small distinct increase in tension in its own right, but it greatly enhances the force generated by the subsequent primary beat (114,115).

Chemical substances that exert a positive inotropic effect increase the extent and velocity of shortening, V_{max}, and, in isometrically contracting muscle, the rate of force development. The total tension generated depends on both the rate of its development and the time to peak tension.

Mechanical Properties of the Intact Heart

The properties of myocardial fibers just outlined apply in principle to the whole heart. However, the geometry of the organ and the complex arrangement of muscle fibers introduce complicating factors. Nevertheless, the intact ventricle can be considered to function as a preloaded and afterloaded muscle. End-diastolic pressure (EDP), in conjunction with diastolic compliance, determines the resting length of muscle fibers (preload). Activation results in the development of force or tension within the myocardial wall and elevation of intracavity pressure. When intraventricular pressure exceeds aortic pressure (afterload), ejection ensues, and the ventricular volume declines. Prior to opening of the outflow valves, the ventricular volume remains unaltered, but the ventricle changes shape; i.e., the base-to-apex length shortens, and circumferential dimensions increase. Thus, some muscle fibers shorten even at this time. Wall tension follows the Laplace relationship during contraction: tension = pressure × radius. However, it must be emphasized that the Laplace formulation was developed for thin-wall vessels. During ejection, the ventricular radius shortens, and the myocardial tension required to maintain internal pressure declines according to the Laplace relationship (Fig. 4) (110,132,134).

Length–Tension Relationship and Starling's Law of the Heart

The mechanical properties of the intact heart can be viewed in terms of the rate of tension development and the force–velocity relationship of contractile elements. However, because the function of the heart is to contract and propel blood into the periphery, the more obvious parameters of pressure, flow, work, and force of contraction can also be used to evaluate mechanical activity. Just as in isolated muscle, the resting or diastolic length of the ventricle determines the force generated during contraction. The latter can be ex-

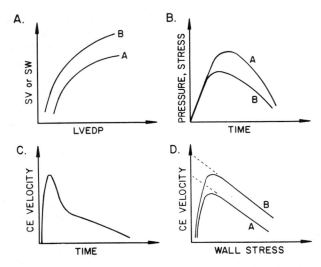

FIG. 4. Schematic representation of determinants of stroke volume, wall stress, intraventricular pressure, and contractile-element velocity in the intact heart. **A:** The Frank-Starling relationship between LVEDP or fiber length and stroke volume (SV) at constant outflow resistance or stroke work (SW). A positive inotropic intervention shifts the control curve (*A*) upward and to the left (*B*), so that greater SV or SW results from a given or even lower LVEDP. **B:** The time courses of left ventricular pressure development (*A*) and wall stress (*B*) during contraction. Wall stress declines as ventricular diameter shortens during ejection. **C:** The time course of the velocity of shortening of contractile elements (CE). Velocity rises rapidly after activation and reaches its peak early during the isovolumic phase. Velocity then declines as wall tension or stress rises. **D:** Relationships between CE velocity and wall stress or tension. After reaching an initial peak, an inverse relationship exists between CE velocity and wall stress. V_{max}, the theoretical maximal value for CE velocity, can be derived by extrapolating the descending portion of the curve back to the zero-stress axis. A positive inotropic intervention shifts the curve, as well as V_{max}, upward (*B*). (Adapted from Sonnenblick et al., ref. 128, with permission.)

pressed as stroke output at constant outflow pressure or as stroke work: stroke volume × (systolic pressure − EDP). Segment length is difficult to determine precisely in many circumstances; therefore, EDP has been used instead. EDP and segment length vary in the same direction, but discrepancies occur at higher pressures (e.g., above 12–15 mm Hg) or after changes in compliance.

A hyperbolic relationship exists between EDP or fiber length and stroke volume at constant afterload, as a consequence of the Frank-Starling relationship (Fig. 4) (132). Up to a point, the healthy heart will eject whatever quantity of blood flows into it by altering its EDP and fiber length. Increasing inflow elevates EDP, which, within limits, increases fiber length, resulting in a more forceful ventricular contraction and increases in stroke

volume and ejection velocity. An elevation of outflow resistance results in incomplete emptying of the ventricle, leading to an increase in EDP, which in turn will tend to return stroke volume to its original level. In addition, it has been suggested that an increased afterload may produce a small augmentation of contractile force in its own right (homeometric autoregulation) (135,136). At very high EDP, particularly in diseased hearts, stroke volume or work may diminish. The heart may then function on the "descending limb" of the Starling curve (not illustrated in Fig. 4).

Many factors, such as heart rate, temperature, autonomic impulses, drugs, and disease states, influence the basic Frank-Starling mechanism and indeed may obscure it in conscious animals and humans. In the normal conscious reclining dog, left ventricular end-diastolic diameter is near maximum, so that further lengthening will not necessarily augment force. Loading with intravenous infusions in conscious dogs with low prevailing heart rate does not increase stroke volume (137).

Factors controlling ventricular filling also contribute to performance. These include atrial pressure, ventricular compliance, and duration of diastole. Changes in compliance occur in disease states (e.g., hypertension) (138,139).

Rates of Pressure Development and the Force–Velocity Relationship in the Intact Heart

As intraventricular pressure rises during isovolumic contraction, the rate of pressure development (dP/dt) mounts steadily. Maximum dP/dt occurs before or at valve opening, provided that aortic pressure is not excessive. A rise in aortic pressure will delay valve opening and lead to an increase in dP/dt (132, 140–142). Maximum dP/dt depends on left ventricular EDP (LVEDP) as well as peak ventricular pressure.

The velocity of shortening of contractile elements (V_{ce}) can be calculated from the stresses and velocities of change in ventricular geometry during contraction (128,132,134). Wall stress can be derived from intraventricular pressures and contours using the Laplace relationship: tension = (pressure × radius)/(2 × wall thickness). Stress increases quickly during isovolumic contraction, but then starts to decline, whereas pressure may continue to rise (Fig. 4). Calculated V_{ce} increases very rapidly after the onset of activation, but after reaching an early peak it diminishes as wall tension rises. During this period, an inverse relationship exists between V_{ce} and tension or stress. Extrapolation of this force–velocity relationship to the velocity axis (zero force) provides a maximum value for V_{ce}: i.e., V_{max}. Increases in LVEDP or in aortic pressure elevate the force–velocity curve but alter its shape, so that extrapolated V_{max} remains constant.

Several indices of contractility employing

aspects of the force–velocity relationship have been developed for use in humans and intact animals: the maximum of the continuously computed dP/dt/instantaneous P, comparison of dP/dt at a given pressure (e.g., at 40 mm Hg), or V_{ce}. These indices attempt to minimize the influences of changes in preload and afterload (128,132).

Inotropic Interventions

Numerous factors, including pH and other ions, tissue oxygen and metabolite concentrations, temperature, pacing rate and sequence, drugs, etc., influence the cardiac contractile state. Positive inotropic interventions alter the force–velocity relationship. They increase the rate of force development at equivalent muscle length or augment pressure development at a given LVEDP (or end-diastolic diameter) and speed the rate of relaxation. Indices of contractility, such as $V_{ce\ max}$, $dP/dt/P$, etc., are increased, and the Frank-Starling curve is shifted upward and to the left by positive inotropic interventions (128,132,134,140,142). Total force may not change if the increase in force development is matched by an equivalent reduction in the duration of the active state. In general, inotropic stimuli produce more profound responses in anesthetized animals than in conscious animals and in depressed hearts than in normal or healthy hearts.

Function of the Atrium

Atrial muscle has properties similar to those of ventricular muscle. The atrium has been likened to a "booster pump" in that it augments the transfer of fluid from the feeder line or venous bed into the main pump, permitting adequate ventricular filling at relatively low venous pressure. An increase in atrial pressure enhances contractile force according to the Frank-Starling relationship and results in the transfer of greater amounts of blood into the ventricle (135,143,144). Atrial contraction produces a small elevation in ventricular EDP and usually a larger change in fiber length. At low ventricular rates, the atrial contribution to ventricular stroke volume may be relatively minor in normal hearts. At elevated rates and in diseased hearts, appropriately timed atrial systole assumes greater importance (144,145). In addition, atrial contraction promotes the closure of A-V valves.

Factors Regulating Cardiac Output

Cardiac minute volume represents the product of heart rate and stroke volume. Isolated changes in rate produce variable changes in cardiac output. In the midrange (i.e., 80–140 beats/minute), output usually remains independent of rate in humans as well as in animals (142,146,147). Output diminishes at much slower or faster rates. However, an increase in rate contributes greatly to the elevation of output during exercise or, as shown in conscious dogs, during infusion of a volume load (137). Stroke volume declines progressively above optimal rates of about 60 to 90 beats per minute, all other factors remaining constant.

Numerous factors, including preload (EDP, end-diastolic volume, fiber length), afterload (outflow impedance), cardiac contractility, activation sequence, etc., influence stroke volume.

As stated earlier, the healthy heart can readily accommodate an increased inflow. Increased "venous return" resulting from an elevated pressure gradient from the venous capacity vessels to the right atrium tends to enhance stroke volume by the Starling mechanism. A fall in atrial pressure also augments the gradient for venous return. However, changes in preload (e.g., during blood infusion) do not always elevate cardiac output, because of countervailing reflex mechanisms.

Changes in outflow impedance can influence steady-state stroke volume. This effect is probably minimal in healthy hearts, but it assumes much greater importance in disease states such as congestive failure (132). On the other hand,

outflow impedance influences end-systolic and end-diastolic dimensions and ejection fraction.

The force of contraction in a healthy heart usually accommodates adequately to changing preload and afterload and is not the limiting factor in determining stroke volume. Slight or even relatively moderate changes in contractility usually do not modify cardiac output. Thus, cardiac glycosides or paired ventricular pacing most often fail to augment output in healthy humans or animals (148).

The sequence of activation of cardiac muscle assures its optimum function as a pump. The importance of appropriately timed atrial contraction, particularly at rapid heart rates, was stressed earlier. Major disturbances in ventricular conduction, such as bundle branch block or ventricular extrasystoles, can reduce output.

Postural changes can influence cardiac output and dimensions partly as a result of reflex mechanisms. Output usually declines as the subject moves from the supine to the sitting and standing positions. Heart size diminishes during anesthesia and even more so after thoracotomy.

Numerous compensatory mechanisms exist that enable a weakened heart to meet metabolic demand (132). Initial or short-term adjustments include the Frank-Starling mechanism and reflexly induced changes in autonomic outflow. Cardiac output may be restored to acceptable levels, but indices of contractility remain depressed. Excessive volume loads or increases in outflow resistance can rapidly lead to ventricular dilatation and failure. Long-term compensatory adjustments result in hypertrophy due to the synthesis of additional myofibrils and contractile units. Hypertrophy reduces ventricular compliance and thus can modify the Frank-Starling mechanism. Dilatation augments myocardial oxygen consumption according to the Laplace relationship because the internal ventricular diameter increases. Hypertrophy also tends to encroach on oxygen supply. Autonomic adjustments to cardiac weakness or failure result in tachycardia and arterial and venous constriction, leading to redistribution of available cardiac output to the most vital organs.

Autonomic Influence

Atria and junctional tissues are richly innervated by parasympathetic and sympathetic fibers, whereas the latter predominate in ventricles (149,150). Vagal stimulation reduces sinus rate and depresses atrial contractility and conduction through the atrioventricular node (135,143). Cholinergic fibers also exert negative inotropic effects on the ventricles, but the magnitude of the response tends to be rather small. These fibers also have the capability of depressing ventricular automaticity.

Sympathetic activation augments contractility of atria and ventricles by β-adrenoceptor- and cAMP-mediated elevation of intracellular calcium concentration that is due, in part, to an increase in the number of calcium channels, as indicated earlier. Sympathetic stimuli increase the sinus rate, as well as that of other automatic tissues, and enhance transmission through the atrioventricular node and can constrict veins, leading to increased "venous return." Cholinergic and adrenergic stimuli react in a complex manner as outlined earlier. In addition, simultaneous excitation of both systems can produce cardiac dysrhythmias.

The relative contributions of parasympathetic and sympathetic systems to reflex changes in heart rate in conscious and anesthetized subjects vary considerably (149). Neurally mediated increases in rate may occur as a result of augmented sympathetic tone and/ or reduced vagal tone, whereas opposite changes in firing of these fibers reduce the heart rate. Although considerable evidence exists for simultaneous and reciprocal changes in the two systems, increases in rate occur predominantly as a result of augmented sympathetic activity, whereas enhanced vagal firing is mainly responsible for reducing the rate. However, different levels of sympathetic tone and vagal tone exist under varying circumstances. Pentobarbital-anesthetized dogs have high sympathetic tone but relatively low vagal tone. Consequently, reduction of vagal activity plays a lesser role in raising heart rate in these animals than in conscious animals.

Elevated sympathetic tone contributes to the increases in heart rate and output during exercise. However, cardiac denervation does not seem to greatly diminish the running performances of dogs. Heart rate and output still increase in these animals, although changes may occur more slowly and may not reach the same peak levels as before denervation. However, propranolol has been shown to reduce the capacity for strenuous exertion in humans and to attenuate the accompanying increases in heart rate and output (151). Further, it was found that cardiac denervation combined with β blockade reduced the running performances of greyhounds considerably, whereas β blockade alone exerted only a slight effect (152). Thus, the autonomic nervous system plays an important but by no means indispensable role in the cardiovascular response to exercise.

Cardiac Energetics

Myocardial cells consume oxygen in their resting state to maintain their integrity, as do all other cells. Contraction necessitates far greater oxygen utilization. Major determinants of oxygen consumption in cardiac fibers are the rate and extent of shortening and, in the intact heart, systolic tension and its rate of development. The latter will vary with preload, afterload, end-diastolic dimensions, and inotropic state (132,153). Cardiac dimensions influence oxygen consumption, because more wall tension is required to generate a given intraventricular pressure in a large heart than in a small heart (Laplace relationship). Thus, inotropic drugs may reduce the oxygen consumption of dilated hearts because they diminish heart size. Heart rate is also one of the major determinants of oxygen consumption.

Overall, increases in stroke volume require relatively less oxygen than increases in pressure. Thus, "volume work" is more efficient than "pressure work."

Coronary Circulation

Coronary blood flow is subject to the same regulatory factors prevalent in other beds, i.e., driving pressure and vascular resistance. However, myocardial systole produces a high extravascular pressure gradient from the epicardium toward the endocardium (154). Consequently, flow occurs mainly during diastole in the deeper regions. Perfusion of subendocardial areas of the left ventricle may be particularly compromised during stress in patients with coronary atherosclerosis. Partial occlusion of a coronary vessel by mechanical measures or disease causes progressive dilatation of the resistance vessels in the subservient area. Under these conditions, flow becomes more and more dependent on the pressure gradient across the bed (arterial minus atrial or ventricular end-diastolic), as well as on the degree of extravascular compression. Dilatation of resistance vessels in normally perfused areas can divert blood away from the ischemic regions (coronary "steal").

Coronary vessels respond to autonomic stimuli directly, as do other beds, but cardiac oxygen consumption is the major determinant of coronary resistance. Adenosine may serve as a link in the metabolic regulation of resistance (81).

Spasm of coronary arteries, due to either local or exogenous factors, has been demonstrated angiographically and can precipitate episodes of angina pectoris (155).

BLOOD VOLUME

The volume and composition of blood greatly influence the circulation. Hematocrit, viscosity, and vascular resistance are intimately related, as outlined earlier. Plasma volume, in relation to the tone of resistance and capacitance vessels, determines the pressures within these compartments and thus, sec-ondarily, modifies most aspects of circulatory function. For example, blood pressure of anephric patients is markedly sensitive to changes in plasma volume.

The balance between ingestion and excretion determines body water content. In turn, blood volume is determined by (a) fluid exchange between plasma and the interstitial space, (b) exchange between plasma and the external environment, and (c) erythrocyte volume. Factors responsible for capillary fluid fluxes were outlined earlier.

Numerous regulatory mechanisms exist for the maintenance of optimal plasma volume. These operate primarily by modifying renal excretion of sodium and water. "Osmoreceptors" in the hypothalamus detect variations in plasma osmolality and respond by initiating appropriate changes in the rate of ADH (vasopressin) secretion (117). Increases in left atrial pressure activate stretch receptors in the atrial wall that result in a vagally mediated reduction in ADH secretion, leading to enhanced renal elimination of water and sodium (*vide infra*). Baroreceptor reflexes also affect ADH release. Aldosterone plays a major role in plasma volume control by regulating renal handling of sodium. Aldosterone secretion, in turn, is controlled by numerous factors, including plasma potassium concentration, angiotensin, ACTH, etc. The "natriuretic factor" discussed earlier also influences blood volume. Disease states can alter blood volume by many mechanisms, such as modifying secretion and degradation rates of aldosterone and ADH.

NEURAL CONTROL OF THE CIRCULATION

The nervous system has the ability to rapidly and profoundly modify cardiovascular function. Emotional stress tends to elevate blood pressure and heart rate, whereas the opposite changes occur during sleep. The central nervous system regulates the circulation primarily by varying sympathetic and parasympathetic outflow and by modifying the release of numerous hormones.

Central Pathways and Mechanisms

Neurons in the hypothalamus and medulla oblongata predominate in central cardiovascular regulation, but higher brain areas, the midbrain, pons, cerebellum, and spinal cord participate. Groups of nuclei subserving excitatory and inhibitory functions exist in the anterior and posterior hypothalamus. Nuclei and more diffusely grouped cells in the dorsal and ventrolateral regions of the medulla predominate in cardiovascular control. The dorsal vagal nuclei and the nuclei ambiguus contain cell bodies of cardiac vagal efferents (156–159).

Descending excitatory and inhibitory fibers form discrete tracts within the spinal cord (159,160). These impinge, either monosynaptically or polysynaptically, on preganglionic neurons located primarily in the intermediolateral column of the cord. Some descending hypothalamic tracts project directly to the cord without synapsing in the medulla.

It has been proposed that oscillatory circuits in the medulla generate firing with a periodicity of 2 to 6 Hz and that spinal neurons generate oscillatory activity with a periodicity of 10 Hz (161). It has been further suggested that input from other areas entrains these basic rhythms.

Baroreceptor afferents (*vide infra*) terminate in the nuclei of the solitary tracts (NTS), which in turn project to other cardiovascular "regions" in the medulla, as well as the hypothalamus, pons, and spinal cord (159–162). Baroreceptor reflexes are integrated at both supraspinal levels and spinal levels (159).

A large and diverse group of putative neurotransmitters modulate central cardiovascular mechanisms. Noradrenergic fibers originating in various cell groups in the brainstem innervate "cardiovascular" neurons in the hypothalamus, medulla, and spinal cord (158,159, 163–165). Depletion of brain NE does not disrupt normal central regulatory mechanisms but does prevent the development of several forms of experimental hypertension (166).

Excitatory as well as inhibitory functions for noradrenergic fibers have been postulated (156,159,163,167). NE applied iontophoretically inhibits firing of spinal preganglionic neurons (168). Injection of NE into the NTS or anterior hypothalamus lowers blood pressure (156,163). Epinephrine-containing fibers originating in the brainstem also contribute to central control (164).

Ascending and descending serotonergic fibers originate in the raphe nuclei. Evidence indicates that spinal 5HT pathways are excitatory to preganglionic neurons, although contradictory views have been offered (156, 165,168–170).

The various components of the renin-angiotensin system, including renin, its substrate, ACE, and AII receptors, exist in the central nervous system and are intimately involved with thirst mechanisms (133). Infusion of AII into the vertebral artery or its administration into the brain ventricular system elevates blood pressure by augmenting sympathetic outflow and by vasopressin release (44,171). Neural structures in the midbrain and medulla mediate the response in dogs and cats. Cells in the anterior hypothalamus (i.e., periventricular tissue in the anterior and ventral regions of the third ventricle, AV3V) participate in thirst mechanisms as well as centrally mediated responses to AII and several forms of experimental hypertension in rats (166). This region may directly or indirectly regulate elaboration of the natriuretic factor.

Other systems and mediators participate in central cardiovascular mechanisms: cholinergic, opiate peptide, γ-aminobutyric acid, substance P, glycine, glutamate, etc. (172–178). The great complexity of these is illustrated by evidence indicating that opiate peptides may mediate the hypotensive response to central α_2-adrenoceptor stimulation by clonidine (179).

Sensors exist within the circulation that detect changes in pressure, wall stretch, pH, P_{CO_2}, P_{O_2}, etc., and initiate compensatory reflex adjustments.

High-Pressure (Baroreceptor) Reflexes

The carotid sinuses and aortic arch contain specialized sensory fibers that are activated by distension of the vessel wall. Changes in luminal pressure alter the strain on these fibers and influence their firing rate in direct proportion to the distension. An increase in intraluminal pressure augments the firing rate of individual fibers and also recruits additional elements. The rate of change of pressure also determines the level of nerve firing. Thus, pulsatile pressure results in greater nerve activity than steady pressure at comparable mean levels. Changes in the ionic environment (sodium, potassium, calcium) of the nerve endings can alter their sensitivity (181). In dogs and cats the carotid sinus mechanism has a lower threshold and operates at a lower range of pressures than aortic receptors. Myelinated afferents have a lower threshold than nonmyelinated fibers (181,183).

Carotid sinus and aortic depressor afferents project to the NTS and result in inhibition of sympathetic outflow and frequently enhancement of vagal outflow. These lead to vasodilatation, reduction in blood pressure, and usually a decrease in heart rate. Thus, an increase in sinus and aortic arch pressure reflexly inhibits sympathetic outflow, whereas a fall in pressure produces opposite effects.

Baroreceptor reflexes modify cardiac contractility in anesthetized animals (132, 135,157,180). However, experiments in conscious animals and humans suggest that these reflexes do not have a great influence on the mechanical activity of the heart (184,185). Venous tone and venous capacity are subject to baroreceptor control (186). However, studies in conscious animals and in humans suggest only minimal participation of the venous system in baroreceptor reflexes (184).

Baroreceptors adapt relatively slowly (i.e., in a matter of hours or days) to sustained changes in pressure. Prolonged changes, however, result in a shift in the sensitive range. Upward resetting of baroreceptors in chronic hypertension probably results from reduced distensibility of the vascular wall (187). Reduction of pressure by long-term drug administration has been shown to return sensitivity to normal levels (188).

Sectioning of carotid sinus and aortic arch fibers results in an acute rise in blood pressure, which then tends to decline slowly. Blood pressure in conscious dogs after sinoaortic baroreceptor denervation is exquisitely sensitive to external stimuli, and continuously monitored pressure varies to a much greater extent over a 24-hr period in these animals than in controls. However, pressures are not greatly elevated in a quiet environment (189). These results have led to the conclusion that the primary function of the baroreceptors is not to set the long-term level of blood pressure but to minimize short-term fluctuations.

Pressure-sensitive areas along the common carotid and subclavian arteries and in the descending aorta have also been described, but their physiologic roles remain uncertain.

Cardiopulmonary Receptors

Reflexes originate from numerous cardiopulmonary regions (182,190). Receptors in tracheobronchial passages detect irritant substances and trigger the cough reflex. Pulmonary stretch receptors sensitive to inflation and deflation participate in the Hering-Breuer reflex. Deflation or "J" receptors can be activated by forced deflation or pulmonary congestion. Activation of these receptors can lower blood pressure and heart rate, but they are primarily concerned with respiration.

Three major groups of afferent fibers (two vagal, one sympathetic) emanate from the heart. Myelinated vagal fibers (A and B fibers) arising from the junctions of venae cavae and the right atrium and the pulmonary arteries and the left atrium compose one of these (182,190,191). The A fibers are activated by tension in the atrial wall, and they fire during atrial systole. The B fibers are more sensitive to changes in volume, and they discharge during rapid inflow. Mechanical distension of these junctional areas, particularly on the left side, reflexly increases heart rate (Bainbridge reflex) (191). Volume loading raises the heart rate when it is low in conscious baboons, but it exerts the opposite effect when the prevailing rate is high (192). Left atrial distension also inhibits ADH release.

Nonmyelinated vagal afferents originate from throughout the atrial and ventricular walls. They are activated by distension and cause sympathoinhibition and vagal firing. Although they exhibit a low rate of spontaneous discharge, they contribute to cardiovascular regulation and assume considerable importance in adjustments to hemorrhage and venous pooling (190,193,194). Myelinated fibers also originate from the ventricular myocardium. Vagal fibers with similar function originate from the pulmonary artery.

Coronary artery occlusion can stimulate nonmyelinated fibers and initiate reflex bradycardia and hypotension. A similar reflex response can occur during myocardial infarction.

Afferent impulses from the heart are also carried over sympathetic nerves (181,190). Activation of these fibers by mechanical or chemical means enhances efferent sympathetic outflow to the heart.

Chemoreceptors and Chemoreflexes

Medullary hypoxia profoundly ehances sympathetic outflow to blood vessels and the heart, resulting in vasoconstriction and cardiac augmentation (157). Discrete chemosensitive organs exist in the carotid sinus and aortic arch regions (195,196). Afferent fibers run with the carotid sinus and aortic depressor nerves. Reduced pH and P_{O_2} and elevated P_{CO_2}, as well as chemical substances such as cyanide, nicotine, and phenyldiguanide, activate the carotid and aortic bodies, resulting in stimulation of respiration and complex car-

diovascular effects. The respiratory response is probably the most important.

Perfusion of the carotid and aortic bodies with hypoxic blood usually elevates peripheral resistance but reduces heart rate and atrial and ventricular contractility. Variable changes in systemic blood pressure occur. Injection of nicotine and cyanide into carotid arterial blood activates chemoreceptors and generally produces similar cardiovascular responses. These agents have also been shown to constrict muscular beds and dilate cutaneous and coronary beds (197).

Intravenous or intra-coronary-artery injection of veratrum alkaloids initiates the coronary chemoreflex or Bezold-Jarisch reflex, leading to decreases in blood pressure and heart rate. These substances have the ability to activate or sensitize numerous myelinated and nonmyelinated mechanoreceptor fibers. Other compounds, such as 5HT, bradykinin, lobeline, nicotine, phenyldiguanide, and aconitine, can also activate these fibers (198,199).

Spinal Reflexes

Somatic afferents can also modify cardiovascular function by facilitating or inhibiting preganglionic neurons at spinal levels (200). In addition, ascending projections from segmental levels influence bulbar control of sympathetic outflow and thus modulate input from other areas. Purely spinal cardiovascular reflexes can be demonstrated in experimental preparations and in paraplegic humans.

OVERALL REGULATION OF THE CIRCULATION

Guyton and associates have analyzed overall circulatory control critically and evaluated the roles of the baroreceptors, the chemoreceptors, the central and autonomic nervous systems, the renin-angiotensin-aldosterone system, capillary fluid shifts, and renal excretory function (201). Nervous control mechanisms are ideally suited to short-term circulatory control because they respond very quickly and can profoundly affect function. They are directed predominantly toward maintenance of systemic blood pressure rather than cardiac output. For example, blood pressure will tend to remain relatively constant in the face of induced changes in cardiac output or during infusion of fluids as a consequence of reflexly mediated changes in vascular resistance. After baroreceptor denervation or destruction of the central nervous system, these interventions result in wide variations in pressure. Local regulatory factors then control vascular resistance, and the circulation is transformed from a pressure-regulated system to a flow-regulated system. Thus, the primary function of nervous mechanisms probably is to mediate the rapid circulatory adjustments to changing situations rather than long-term setting of blood pressure levels.

The renin-angiotensin-aldosterone system participates in short- as well as longer-term blood pressure control by influencing renal sodium reabsorption and by direct and possibly centrally mediated effects on blood vessels, as discussed earlier. According to Guyton and associates, the kidney is the primary regulator of blood pressure in the long term. A direct relationship exists between systemic blood pressure and sodium and urine outputs. Thus, any variation in pressure initiates a compensatory change in urinary volume and, in turn, plasma volume, which will tend to return pressure to normal levels. These adaptations, of course, imply adequate renal function. Disease states that compromise renal function may severely strain this homeostatic process.

There are numerous other examples of cardiac and vascular adaptation to changing internal environment and to disease. Cardiac dilatation and hypertrophy in response to chronically increased volume and pressure loads were mentioned earlier. Blood vessels also hypertrophy in the presence of persistently elevated pressure (202).

Numerous cardiovascular control mechanisms are outlined in the foregoing, and it is evident that considerable redundancy exists. The autonomic nervous system contributes to the rapid adjustment to exercise. Yet animals or humans subjected to cardiac denervation or pharmacologic blockade increase their output markedly during exercise, although the response may not be as great or occur as rapidly as in the normal situation. Although extensively studied, the importance of the adrenal medulla in normal circulatory control remains uncertain. However, its role may be crucial after inhibition of sympathetic vasoconstrictor responsiveness (203). The renin-angiotensin system assumes a critical regulatory role during sodium depletion and hemorrhage. Vasopressin probably provides an additional backup system.

Responses to Drugs

Many of the mechanisms outlined earlier can be modified by drugs. However, responses to equivalent doses may vary widely under differing physiologic conditions and in disease states. Effects of autonomic blocking agents will naturally depend greatly on prevailing levels of sympathetic and parasympathetic outflow. Sympathetic tone is very low in a quietly resting dog; therefore, sympatholytic drugs will exert negligible effects on blood pressure and cardiac function. On the other hand, animals anesthetized with barbiturates exhibit a high degree of sympathetic tone but low vagal tone. Under these conditions, sympatholytics affect function markedly. Drugs that depress cardiac contractility slightly probably do not influence cardiac output in healthy conscious animals or humans, because of considerable reserve capacity. However, in hearts depressed by disease or anesthesia, these substances can produce pronounced effects. It is clear that the state of the circulation at any instant will profoundly influence the qualitative and quantitative nature of drug responses. Regulatory mechanisms will attempt to nullify drug-induced changes.

REFERENCES

1. Kuntz, A. (1953): *The Autonomic Nervous System.* Lea & Febiger, Philadelphia.

2. Mayer, S. E. (1980): Drugs acting at synaptic and neuroeffector junctional sites. Neurohumoral transmission and the autonomic nervous system. In: *The Pharmacological Basis of Therapeutics,* edited by A. G. Gilman, L. S. Goodman, and A. Gilman, pp. 56–90. Macmillan, New York.

3. Ceccarelli, B., and Hurlbut, W. P. (1980): Vesicle hypothesis of the release of quanta of acetylcholine. *Physiol. Rev.,* 60:396–434.

4. Fuxe, K., and Sedvall, G. (1965): The distribution of adrenergic nerve fibers to blood vessels in skeletal muscle. *Acta Physiol. Scand.,* 64:75–86.

5. Smith, A. D. (1973): Mechanisms involved in the release of noradrenaline from sympathetic nerves. *Br. Med. Bull.,* 29:123–129.

6. Livett, B. G. (1973): Histochemical visualization of peripheral and central adrenergic neurons. *Br. Med. Bull.,* 29:93–99.

7. Vanhoutte, P. M., Verbeuren, T. J., and Webb, R. C. (1981): Local modulation of adrenergic neuroeffector interaction in the blood vessel wall. *Physiol. Rev.,* 61:151–247.

8. Cotten, M. deV. (editor) (1972): Regulation of catecholamine metabolism in the sympathetic nervous system. *Pharmacol. Rev.,* 24:161–434.

9. Weiner, N., Cloutier, G., Bjur, R., and Pfeffer, R. I. (1972): Modification of norepinephrine synthesis in intact tissue by drugs during short-term adrenergic nerve stimulation. *Pharmacol. Rev.,* 24:203–221.

10. Iversen, L. (1973): Catecholamine uptake processes. *Br. Med. Bull.,* 29:130–135.

11. Pelletier, G., Steinbusch, H. W. M., and Verhofstad, A. A. J. (1981): Immunoreactive substance P and serotonin present in the same dense-core vesicles. *Nature,* 293:71–72.

12. Langer, S. Z. (1981): Presynaptic regulation of the release of catecholamines. *Pharmacol. Rev.,* 32:337–362.

13. Weiner, N. (1979): Multiple factors regulating the release of norepinephrine consequent to nerve stimulation. *Fed. Proc.,* 38:2193–2202.

14. Kalsner, S., Suleiman, M., and Dobson, R. E, (1980): Adrenergic presynaptic receptors: An overextended hypothesis? *J. Pharm. Pharmacol.,* 32:2990–2992.

15. Zimmerman, B. G. (1981): Adrenergic facilitation by angiotensin: Does it serve a physiological function? *Clin. Sci.,* 60:343–348.

16. Muscholl, E. (1980): Peripheral muscarinic control of norepinephrine release in the cardiovascular system. *Am. J. Physiol.,* 239:H713–H720.

17. Pletscher, A. (1972): Regulation of catecholamine turnover by variation of enzyme levels. *Pharmacol. Rev.,* 24:225–232.

18. Zigmond, R. E. (1980): The long-term regulation of ganglionic tyrosine hydroxylase by preganglionic nerve activity. *Fed. Proc.,* 39:3003–3008.

19. Laverty, R. (1973): The mechanism of action of some antihypertensive drugs. *Br. Med. Bull.,* 29:152–157.

20. Day, M. D., and Rand, M. J. (1963): Evidence for a competitive antagonism of guanethidine by dexamphetamine. *Br. J. Pharmacol.,* 20:17–28.

21. Volle, R. L., and Hancock, J. C. (1970): Transmission in sympathetic ganglia. *Fed. Proc.,* 29:1913–1918.

22. Dunn, N. J. (1980): Ganglionic transmission: Electrophysiology and pharmacology. *Fed. Proc.,* 39:2982–2989.

23. McAfee, D. A., Hennon, B. K., Whiting, G. J., Horn, J. P., Jarowsky, P. J., and Turner, D. K. (1980): The action of cAMP and catecholamines in mammalian sympathetic ganglia. *Fed. Proc.,* 39:2997–3002.

24. Wilson, S. P., Klein, R. L., Chang, K.-J., Gasparis, M. S., Viveros, O. H., and Yang, W. S. (1980): Are opioid peptides co-transmitters in noradrenergic vesicles of sympathetic nerves? *Nature,* 228:707–709.

25. Baxter, J. D., and Funder, J. W. (1979): Hormone receptors. *N. Engl. J. Med.,* 304:1149–1161.

26. Lefkowitz, R. J., Caron, M. G., Michel, T., and Stadel, J. M. (1982): Mechanisms of hormone receptor-effector coupling: The α-adrenergic receptor and adenylate cyclase. *Fed. Proc.,* 41:2664–2670.

27. Pollet, R. J., and Levey, G. S. (1980): Principles of membrane receptor physiology and their application to clinical medicine. *Ann. Intern. Med.,* 92:663–680.

28. Snyder, S. H., and Goodman, R. R. (1980): Multiple neurotransmitter receptors. *J. Neurochem.,* 35:5–15.

29. Demeyts, P., and Rousseau, G. G. (1980): Receptor concepts. A century of evolution. *Circ. Res. [Suppl. I],* 46:I-3–I-9.

30. Snyder, S. H., Bruns, R. F., Daly, J. W., and Innis, R. B. (1981): Multiple neurotransmitter receptors in the brain: Amines, adenosine and cholecystokinin. *Fed. Proc.,* 40:142–146.

31. Sabol, S. L., and Nirenberg, M. (1979): Regulation of adenylate cyclase of neuroblastoma $\times$ glioma hybrid cells by α-adrenergic receptors. *J. Biol. Chem.,* 254:1913–1920.

32. Rosenberger, L. B., Yamamura, H. I., and Roeske, W. R. (1980): The regulation of cardiac muscarinic cholinergic receptors by isoproterenol. *Eur. J. Pharmacol.,* 65:129–130.

33. Ahlquist, R. P. (1948): A study of the adrenotropic receptors. *Am. J. Physiol.,* 153:586–600.

34. Drew, G. M., and Whiting, S. B. (1979): Evidence for two distinct types of postsynaptic α-adrenoceptor in vascular smooth muscle in vivo. *Br. J. Pharmacol.,* 67:207–215.

35. Jacobs, K. H., and Schultz, G. (1982): Signal transformation involving adrenoceptors. *J. Cardiovasc. Pharmacol.,* 4:S63–S67.

36. VanMeel, J. C. A., DeJonge, A., Kalkman, H. O., Wilffert, B., Timmermans, P. B. M. W. M., and Van Zwieten, P. A. (1981): Vascular smooth muscle contraction initiated by postsynaptic α-adrenoceptor activation is induced by an influx of extracellular calcium. *Eur. J. Pharmacol.,* 69:205–208.

37. Lands, A. M., Arnold, A., McAuliff, J. P., Luduena, F. P., and Brown, T. G., Jr. (1967): Differentiation of receptor systems activated by sympathomimetic amines. *Nature,* 214:597–598.

38. Baker, S. P., Boyd, H. M., and Potter, L. T. (1980): Distribution and function of α-adrenoceptors in dif-

ferent chambers of the canine heart. *Br. J. Pharmacol.,* 68:57–63.

39. Goldberg, L. I., Kohli, J. D., Kotake, A. N., and Volkman, P. H. (1978): Characteristics of the vascular dopamine receptor: Comparison with other receptors. *Fed. Proc.,* 37:2396–2402.

40. Creese, I., Sibley, D. R., Leff, S., and Hamblin, M. (1981): Dopamine receptors: Subtypes, localization and regulation. *Fed. Proc.,* 40:147–152.

41. Brodde, O.-E. (1982): Vascular dopamine receptors: Demonstration and characterization by in vitro studies. *Life Sci.,* 31:289–306.

42. Cavero, I., Massinghamn, R., and Lefèvre-Borg, F. (1982): Peripheral dopamine receptors, potential targets for a new class of antihypertensive agents. *Life Sci.,* 31:939–948.

43. Regoli, D., Park, W. K., and Rioux, F. (1974): Pharmacology of angiotensin. *Pharmacol. Rev.,* 26:69–123.

44. Peach, M. J. (1977): Renin-angiotensin system: Biochemistry and mechanisms of action. *Physiol. Rev.,* 57:313–370.

45. Hedqvist, P. (1973): Autonomic neurotransmission. In: *The Prostaglandins,* edited by P. W. Ramwell, pp. 101–131. Plenum Press, New York.

46. Moncada, S., and Vane, J. R. (1979): Pharmacology and endogenous roles of prostaglandin endoperoxides, thromboxane A_2, and prostacyclin. *Pharmacol. Rev.,* 30:293–331.

47. Brody, M. J., and Kadowitz, P. J. (1974): Prostaglandins as modulators of the autonomic nervous system. *Fed. Proc.,* 33:48–60.

48. Leysen, J. E., Awouters, F., Kennis, L., Laduron, P. M., Vandenberk, J., and Janssen, P. A. J. (1981): Receptor binding profile of R 41 468, a novel antagonist at 5-HT receptors. *Life Sci.,* 28:1015–1022.

49. VanNeuten, J. M., Janssen, P. A. J., VanBeek, J., Xhonneux, R., Verbeusen, T. J., and Vanhoutte, P. M. (1981): Vascular effects of ketanserin (R41 468), a novel antagonist of 5-HT$_2$ serotonin receptors. *J. Pharmacol. Exp. Ther.,* 218:217–230.

50. Burnstock, G. (1972): Purinergic nerves. *Pharmacol. Rev.,* 24:509–581.

51. Somlyo, A. P., and Somlyo, A. V. (1968): Vascular smooth muscle. I. Normal structure, pathology, biochemistry, and biophysics. *Pharmacol. Rev.,* 20:197–272.

52. Holman, M. E. (1969): Electrophysiology of vascular smooth muscle. *Ergeb. Physiol.,* 61:137–177.

53. Casteels, R. (1980): Electro- and pharmacomechanical coupling in vascular smooth muscle. *Chest [Suppl.],* 78:150–156.

54. Katz, A. M., Messineo, F. C., and Herbette, L. (1982): Ion channels in membranes. *Circulation [Suppl. I],* 65:I-2–I-10.

55. VanBreemen, C., Aaronson, P., Loutzenhiser, R., and Meisheri, K. (1980): Ca^{+2} movement in smooth muscle. *Chest [Suppl.],* 78:157–165.

56. Webb, R. C., and Bohr, D. F. (1981): Regulation of vascular tone, molecular mechanisms. *Prog. Cardiovasc. Dis.,* 24:213–242.

57. Hermsmeyer, K., Abel, P. W., and Trapani, A. J. (1982): Membrane sensitivity and membrane potentials of caudal arterial muscle in DOCA-salt, Dahl, and SHR hypertension in the rat. *Hypertension [Suppl. II],* 4:II-49–II-51.

58. Harder, D. R., Abel, P. W., and Hermsmeyer, K. (1981): Membrane electrical mechanism of basilar artery constriction and pial artery dilatation by norepinephrine. *Circ. Res.,* 49:1237–1242.

59. Häusler, G. (1982): α-Adrenoceptor mediated contractile and electrical responses of vascular smooth muscle. *J. Cardiovasc. Pharmacol.,* 4:S97–S100.

60. Itoh, T., Kajiwara, M., Kitamura, K., and Kurijama, H. (1981): Effects of vasodilator agents on smooth muscle cells of the coronary artery of the pig. *Br. J. Pharmacol.,* 74:455–468.

61. Brock, T. A., Smith, J. B., and Overbeck, H. W. (1982): Relationship of vascular sodium-potassium pump activity to intracellular sodium in hypertensive rats. *Hypertension [Suppl. II],* 4:II-43–II-48.

62. Adams, R. J., and Schwartz, A. (1980): Comparative mechanisms for contraction of cardiac and skeletal muscle. *Chest [Suppl.],* 78:123–139.

63. Hartshorne, D. J. (1980): Biochemical basis for contraction of vascular smooth muscle. *Chest [Suppl.],* 78:140–149.

64. Stull, J. T., and Sanford, C. F. (1981): Differences in skeletal, cardiac and smooth muscle contractile element regulation by calcium. In: *New Perspectives on Calcium Antagonist,* edited by G. B. Weiss, pp. 35–46. American Physiological Society, Bethesda.

65. Bárány, M., and Bárány, K. (1981): Protein phosphorylation in cardiac and vascular smooth muscle. *Am. J. Physiol.,* 241:H117–H128.

66. Murphy, R. A. (1982): Myosin phosphorylation and crossbridge regulation in arterial smooth muscle. *Hypertension [Suppl. II],* 4:II-3–II-7.

67. Axelsson, K. L., Wikberg, J. E. S., and Andersson, R. G. G. (1979): Relationship between nitroglycerin, cyclic GMP and relaxation of vascular smooth muscle. *Life Sci.,* 24:1779–1786.

68. Keith, R. A., Burkman, A. M., Sokoloski, T. D., and Fertel, R. H. (1982): Vascular tolerance to nitroglycerin and cyclic GMP generation in rabbit aortic smooth muscle. *J. Pharmacol. Exp. Ther.,* 221:525–531.

69. Rhodin, H. P. (1980): Architecture of the vessel wall. In: *Handbook of Physiology, Section 2, The Cardiovascular System, Vol. 2, Vascular Smooth Muscle,* edited by D. F. Bohr, A. P. Somlyo, and H. V. Sparks, Jr., pp. 1–31. American Physiological Society, Bethesda.

70. Somlyo, A. V. (1980): Ultrastructure of vascular smooth muscle. In: *Handbook of Physiology, Section 2, The Cardiovascular System, Vol. 2, Vascular Smooth Muscle,* edited by D. F. Bohr, A. P. Somlyo, and H. V. Sparks, Jr., pp. 33–67. American Physiological Society, Bethesda.

71. Dobrin, P. B. (1978): Mechanical properties of arteries. *Physiol. Rev.,* 58:397–460.

72. Rüegg, J. A. (1971): Smooth muscle tone. *Physiol. Rev.,* 51:201–248.

73. Haddy, F. J., and Scott, J. B. (1968): Metabolically linked vasoactive chemicals in local regulation of blood flow. *Physiol. Rev.,* 48:688–707.

74. Mellander, S., and Johansson, B. (1968): Control of resistance, exchange, and capacitance functions

in the peripheral circulation. *Pharmacol. Rev.,* 20:117–196.

75. Sparks, H. R., Jr. (1980): Effect of local metabolic factors. In: *Handbook of Physiology, Section 2, The Cardiovascular System, Vol. 2, Vascular Smooth Muscle,* edited by D. H. Bohr, A. P. Somlyo, and H. V. Sparks, Jr., pp. 475–513. American Physiological Society, Bethesda.

76. Abel, P. W., Trapani, A., Aprigliano, O., and Hermsmeyer, K. (1980): Trophic effect of norepinephrine on the rat portal vein in organ culture. *Circ. Res.,* 47:770–775.

77. Kuschinsky, W., and Wahl, M. (1978): Local chemical and neurogenic regulation of cerebral vascular resistance. *Physiol. Rev.,* 58:646–689.

78. Abboud, F. M. (1981): Special characteristics of the cerebral circulation. *Fed. Proc.,* 40:2296–2300.

79. Sokoloff, L. (1981): Relationships among local functional activity, energy metabolism, and blood flow in the central nervous system. *Fed. Proc.,* 40:2311–2316.

80. Dobson, J. G., Jr., Rubio, R., and Berne, R. M. (1971): Role of adenine nucleotides, adenosine, and inorganic phosphate in the regulation of skeletal muscle blood flow. *Circ. Res.,* 29:375–384.

81. Berne, R. (1980): The role of adenosine in the regulation of coronary blood flow. *Circ. Res.,* 47:807–813.

82. Johnson, P. C. (1980): The myogenic response. In: *Handbook of Physiology, Section 2, The Cardiovascular System, Vol. 2, Vascular Smooth Muscle,* edited by D. F. Bohr, A. P. Somlyo, and H. R. Sparks, Jr., pp. 409–442. American Physiological Society, Bethesda.

83. Heistad, D. D., Busija, D. W., and Marcus, M. L. (1981): Neural effects on cerebral vessels: Alteration of pressure-flow relationship. *Fed. Proc.,* 40:2317–2321.

84. Burnstock, G., Gannon, B., and Iwayama, T. (1970): Sympathetic innervation of vascular smooth muscle in normal and hypertensive animals. *Circ. Res.,* [*Suppl. II*], 27:5–23.

85. Bevan, J. A., and Purdy, R. E. (1973): Variations in adrenergic innervation and contractile responses to the rabbit saphenous artery. *Circ. Res.,* 32:746–751.

86. Bevan, J. A., and Ljung, B. (1974): Longitudinal propagation of myogenic activity in rabbit arteries and in the rat portal vein. *Acta Physiol. Scand.,* 90:703–715.

87. Abboud, F. M. (1972): Control of the various components of the peripheral vasculature. *Fed. Proc.,* 31:1226–1239.

88. Mohrman, D. E., and Feigl, E. O. (1978): Competition between sympathetic vasoconstriction and metabolic vasodilatation in the canine coronary circulation. *Circ. Res.,* 42:79–86.

89. Folkow, B., Sonnenschein, R. R., and Wright, D. L. (1971): Loci of neurogenic and metabolic effects on precapillary vessels of skeletal muscle. *Acta Physiol. Scand.,* 81:4459–4471.

90. Abboud, F. M., and Eckstein, J. W. (1966): Comparative changes in segmental vascular resistance in response to nerve stimulation and to norepinephrine. *Circ. Res.,* 18:263–277.

91. Honig, C. R., Frierson, J. L., and Patterson, J. L. (1970): Comparison of neural controls of resistance and capillary density in resting muscle. *Am. J. Physiol.,* 218:937–942.

92. Vanhoutte, P. M. (1982): Heterogeneity of postjunctional vascular α-adrenoceptors and handling of calcium. *J. Cardiovasc. Pharmacol.,* 4:S91–S96.

93. Russell, M. P., and Moran, N. C. (1980): Evidence for lack of innervation of β_2-adrenoceptors in the blood vessels of the gracilis muscle of the dog. *Circ. Res.,* 46:344–352.

94. Uvnas, B. (1966): Cholinergic vasodilator nerves. *Fed. Proc.,* 25:1618–1622.

95. Folkow, B., Lisander, B., Tuttle, R. S., and Wang, S. C. (1968): Changes in cardiac output upon stimulation of the hypothalamic defense area and the medullary depressor areas in the cat. *Acta Physiol. Scand.,* 72:220–233.

96. Beck, L., Pollard, A. A., Kayaalp, S. O., and Weiner, L. M. (1966): Sustained dilatation elicited by sympathetic nerve stimulation. *Fed. Proc.,* 25:1596–1606.

97. Ballard, D. R., Abboud, F. M., and Mayer, H. E. (1970): Release of a humoral vasodilator substance during neurogenic vasodilatation. *Am. J. Physiol.,* 219:1451–1457.

98. Rolewicz, T. F., and Zimmerman, B. G. (1972): Peripheral distribution of cutaneous sympathetic vasodilator system. *Am. J. Physiol.,* 223:939–944.

99. Weiss, H. D. (1972): The physiology of human penile erection. *Ann. Intern. Med.,* 76:763–799.

100. Lee, T. J.-F., Hume, W. R., Su, C., and Bevan, J. A. (1978): Neurogenic vasodilatation of cat cerebral arteries. *Circ. Res.,* 42:535–542.

101. Ryan, M. J., and Brody, M. J. (1972): Neurogenic and vascular stores of histamine in the dog. *J. Pharmacol. Exp. Ther.,* 181:83–91.

102. Keeton, T. K., and Campbell, W. B. (1980): The pharmacologic alteration of renin release. *Pharmacol. Rev.,* 31:81–227.

103. Ganten, D., Schelling, P., and Ganten, V. (1977): Tissue isorenins. In: *Hypertension: Pathology and Treatment,* edited by J. Genest, E. Koiw, and O. Kuchel, pp. 240–256. McGraw-Hill, New York.

104. Asaad, M. M., and Antonaccio, M. J. (1982): Vascular wall renin in spontaneous hypertensive rats. Potential relevance to hypertension maintenance and antihypertensive effect of captopril. *Hypertension,* 4:487–493.

105. McCubbin, J. W., Soares deMoura, R., Page, I. H., and Olmsted, F. (1965): Arterial hypertension elicited by subpressor amounts of angiotensin. *Science,* 149:1395–1396.

106. Freeman, R. H., and Davis, J. O. (1979): Physiological actions of angiotensin II on the kidney. *Fed. Proc.,* 38:2276–2279.

107. Ploth, D. W., and Navar, G. (1979): Intrarenal effects of the renin-angiotensin system. *Fed. Proc.,* 38:2280–2285.

108. Antonaccio, M. J., and Cushman, D. W. (1981): Drugs inhibiting the renin-angiotensin system. *Fed. Proc.,* 40:2275–2284.

109. Moncada, S., and Vane, J. R. (1979): Pharmacology and endogenous roles of prostaglandin endoperox-

ides, thromboxane A_2, and prostacyclin. *Pharmacol. Rev.,* 30:293–331.

110. Moncada, S. (1982): Biological importance of prostacyclin. *Br. J. Pharmacol.,* 76:3–31.

111. Sirois, P., and Borgeat, P. (1980): From slow reacting substance of anaphylaxis (SRS-A) to leukotriene D_4 (LTD$_4$). *Int. J. Immunopharmacol.,* 2:281–293.

112. Michelassi, F., Landa, L., Hill, R. D., Lowenstein, E., Watkins, W. D., Petkau, A. J., and Zapol, W. M. (1982): Leukotriene D_4: A potent coronary artery vasoconstrictor associated with impaired ventricular contraction. *Science,* 217:841–843.

113. Gorman, R. R. (1979): Modulation of human platelet function by prostacyclin and thromboxane A_2. *Fed. Proc.,* 328:83–88.

114. Feigen, L. P. (1981): Actions of prostaglandins in peripheral vascular beds. *Fed. Proc.,* 40:1987–1990.

115. Regoli, D., and Barabé, J. (1980): Pharmacology of bradykinin and related kinins. *Pharmacol. Rev.,* 32:1–46.

116. Carretero, O. A., and Scicli, A. G. (1981): Possible roles of kinins in circulatory homeostatis. *Hypertension [Suppl. II],* 3:I-4–I-12.

117. Bie, P. (1980): Osmoreceptors, vasopressin, and control of renal water excretion. *Physiol. Rev.,* 60:962–1048.

118. Johnston, C. I., Newman, M., and Woods, R. (1981): Role of vasopressin in cardiovascular homeostasis and hypertension. *Clin. Sci.,* 61:129s–139s.

119. Cowley, A. W., Switzer, S. J., and Guinn, M. M. (1980): Evidence and quantification of the vasopressin arterial pressure control system in the dog. *Circ. Res.,* 46:58–67.

120. Gavras, H., Hatzinikolaou, P., North, W. G., Bresnahan, M., and Gavras, I. (1982): Interaction of the sympathetic nervous system and renin in the maintenance of blood pressure. *Hypertension,* 4:400–405.

121. DiPette, D. J., Gavras, I., North, W. G., Brunner, H. R., and Gavras, H. (1982): Vasopressin in salt induced hypertension of experimental renal insufficiency. *Hypertension [Suppl. II],* 4:II-125–II-130.

122. VanNeuten, J. M., Janssen, P. A. J., deRidder, W., and Vanhoutte, P. M. (1982): Interactions between 5-hydroxytryptamine and other vasoconstrictor substances in the isolated femoral artery of the rabbit; effect of ketanserin (R41 468). *Eur. J. Pharmacol.,* 77:281–287.

123. Chand, N., and Altura, B. M. (1981): Acetylcholine and bradykinin relax intrapulmonary arteries by acting on endothelial cells: Role in lung vascular disease. *Science,* 213:1376–1379.

124. Panmani, M., Huot, S., Buggy, J., Clough, D., and Haddy, F. (1981): Demonstration of a humoral inhibitor of the Na^+-K^+ pump in some models of experimental hypertension. *Hypertension [Suppl. II],* 3: II-96–II-101.

125. Gruber, K. A., Rudel, L. L., and Bullock, B. C. (1982): Increased circulating levels of an endogenous digoxin-like factor in hypertensive monkeys. *Hypertension,* 4:348–354.

126. Carmeliet, E., and Vereeck, J. (1979): Electrogenesis of the action potential and automaticity. In: *Handbook of Physiology, Section 2, The Cardiovascular*

System, Vol. 1, The Heart, edited by R. M. Berne, pp. 269–334. American Physiological Society, Bethesda.

127. Winegrad, S. (1979): Electromechanical coupling in heart muscle. In: *Handbook of Physiology, Section 2, The Cardiovascular System, Vol. 1, The Heart,* edited by R. M. Berne, pp. 393–428. American Physiological Society, Bethesda.

128. Sonnenblick, E. H., Parmley, W. W., and Urschel, C. W. (1969): The contractile state of the heart as expressed by force-velocity relations. *Am. J. Cardiol.,* 23:488–503.

129. Jewell, B. R. (1977): A reexamination of the importance of muscle length on myocardial performance. *Circ. Res.,* 40:221–230.

130. Brady, A. J. (1979): Mechanical properties of cardiac fibers. In: *Handbook of Physiology, Section 2, The Cardiovascular System, Vol. 1, The Heart,* edited by R. M. Berne, pp. 461–474. American Physiological Society, Bethesda.

131. Strobeck, J. E., Kreuger, J., and Sonnenblick, E. H. (1980): Load and time considerations in the force-length relation of cardiac muscle. *Fed. Proc.,* 39:175–182.

132. Braunwald, E., and Ross, J., Jr. (1979): Control of cardiac performance. In: *Handbook of Physiology, Section 2, The Cardiovascular System, Vol. 1, The Heart,* edited by R. M. Berne, pp. 533–580. American Physiological Society, Bethesda.

133. Weber, K. T., and Hawthorne, E. W. (1981): Descriptors and determinants of cardiac shape: An overview. *Fed. Proc.,* 40:2005–2010.

134. Weber, K. T., and Janicki, J. S. (1980): The dynamics of ventricular contraction: Force, length, and shortening. *Fed. Proc.,* 39:188–195.

135. Sarnoff, S. J., and Mitchell, J. H. (1961): The regulation of the performance of the heart. *Am. J. Med.,* 30:747–771.

136. Vatner, S. F., Monroe, R. G., and McRitchie, R. J. (1974): Effects of anesthesia, tachycardia, and autonomic blockade on the Anrep effect in intact dogs. *Am. J. Physiol.,* 226:1450–1456.

137. Vatner, S. F., and Boettcher, D. H. (1978): Regulation of cardiac output by stroke volume and heart rate in conscious dogs. *Circ. Res.,* 42:557–561.

138. Janicki, J. S., and Weber, K. T. (1980): Factors influencing the diastolic pressure-volume relation of the cardiac ventricles. *Fed. Proc.,* 39:133–140.

139. Rankin, J. S., Arentzen, C. E., Ring, W. S., Edwards, C. H., II, McHale, P. A., and Anderson, R. W. (1980): The diastolic mechanical properties of the intact left ventricle. *Fed. Proc.,* 39:141–147.

140. Mason, D. T., Braunwald, E., Covell, J. W., Sonnenblick, E., and Ross, J., Jr. (1971): Assessment of cardiac contractility. The relation between the rate of pressure rise and ventricular pressure during isovolumic systole. *Circulation,* 44:47–58.

141. Peterson, K. L., Uther, J. B., Shabetai, R., and Braunwald, E. (1973): Assessment of left ventricular performance in man. Instantaneous tension-velocity-length relations obtained with the aid of an electromagnetic velocity catheter in the ascending aorta. *Circulation,* 47:924–935.

142. Mason, D. T., Spann, J. F., Jr., and Zelis, R. (1970):

Quantification of the contractile state of the intact human heart. Maximal velocity of contractile element shortening determined by the instantaneous relation between the rate of pressure rise and pressure in the left ventricle during isovolumic systole. *Am. J. Cardiol.,* 26:248–257.

143. Mitchell, J. H., Gilmore, J. P., and Sarnoff, S. J. (1962): The transport function of the atrium. Factors influencing the relation between mean left atrial pressure and left ventricular end diastolic pressure. *Am. J. Cardiol.,* 9:237–247.

144. Skinner, N. S., Jr., Mitchell, J. H., Wallace, A. G., and Sarnoff, S. J. (1963): Hemodynamic effects of altering the timing of atrial systole. *Am. J. Physiol.,* 205:499–503.

145. Lister, J. W., Klotz, D. H., Jomain, S. L., Stuckey, J. H., and Hoffman, B. F. (1964): Effect of pacemaker site on cardiac output and ventricular activation in dogs with complete heart block. *Am. J. Cardiol.,* 14:494–503.

146. Ross, J., Jr., Linhart, J. W., and Braunwald, E. (1965): Effects of changing heart rate in man by electrical stimulation of the right atrium. Studies at rest, during exercise, and with isoproterenol. *Circulation,* 32:549–558.

147. Bishop, V. S., Stone, H. L., and Horwitz, L. D. (1971): Effects of tachycardia and ventricular filling pressure on stroke volume in the conscious dog. *Am. J. Physiol.,* 220:436–439.

148. Vatner, S. F., Higgins, C. B., Patrick, T., Franklin, D., and Braunwald, E. (1971): Effects of cardiac depression and of anesthesia on the myocardial action of a cardiac glycoside. *J. Clin. Invest.,* 50:2585–2595.

149. Higgins, C. B., Vatner, S. F., and Braunwald, E. (1973): Parasympathetic control of the heart. *Pharmacol. Rev.,* 25:119–155.

150. Levy, M. N., and Martin, P. J. (1979). Neural control of the heart. In: *Handbook of Physiology, Section 2, The Cardiovascular System, Vol. 1, The Heart,* edited by R. M. Berne, pp. 581–620. American Physiological Society, Bethesda.

151. Epstein, S. E., Robinson, B. F., Kahler, R. L., and Braunwald, E. (1965): Effects of beta-adrenergic blockade on the cardiac response to maximal and submaximal exercise in man. *J. Clin. Invest.,* 44:1745–1753.

152. Donald, D. E., Ferguson, D. A., and Milburn, S. E. (1968): Effect of beta-adrenergic receptor blockade on racing performance of greyhounds with normal and with denervated hearts. *Circ. Res.,* 22:127–134.

153. Gibbs, C. L. (1978): Cardiac energetics. *Physiol. Rev.,* 58:174–254.

154. Moir, T. W. (1972): Subendocardial distribution of coronary blood flow and the effect of antianginal drugs. *Circ. Res.,* 30:621–627.

155. Braunwald, E. (1981): Coronary artery spasm as a cause of myocardial ischemia. *J. Lab. Clin. Med.,* 97:299–312.

156. Calaresu, F. R., Faiers, A. A., and Mogenson, G. J. (1975): Central neural regulation of heart and blood vessels in mammals. *Prog. Neurobiol.,* 5:1–35.

157. Korner, P. I. (1979): Central nervous control of autonomic cardiovascular function. In: *Handbook of Physiology, Section 2, The Cardiovascular System, Vol. 1, The Heart,* edited by R. M. Berne, pp. 691–739. American Physiological Society, Bethesda.

158. Smith, O. A., Astley, C. A. S., DeVito, J. L., Stein, J. M., and Walsh, K. E. (1980): Functional analysis of hypothalamic control of the cardiovascular responses accompanying emotional behavior. *Fed. Proc.,* 39:2487–2494.

159. Dampney, R. A. L. (1981): Functional organization of central cardiovascular pathways. *Clin. Exp. Pharmacol. Physiol.,* 8:241–259.

160. Foreman, R. D., and Wurster, R. D. (1973): Localization and functional characteristics of descending sympathetic spinal pathways. *Am. J. Physiol.,* 225:212–217.

161. Gebber, G. L. (1980): Central oscillators responsible for sympathetic nerve discharge. *Am. J. Physiol.,* 239:H143–H155.

162. Ross, C. A., Ruggiero, D. A., and Reis, D. J. (1981): Afferent projections to cardiovascular portions of the nucleus of the tractus solitarius in the rat. *Brain Res.,* 223:402–408.

163. Elliott, J. M. (1979): The central noradrenergic control of blood pressure and heart rate. *Clin. Exp. Physiol. Pharmacol.,* 6:569–579.

164. Chalmers, J. P., Blessing, W. W., West, M. J., Howe, P. R. C., Costa, M., and Furness, J. B. (1981): Importance of new catecholamine pathways in control of blood pressure. *Clin. Exp. Hypertens.,* 3:396–416.

165. Loewy, A. D., and Neil, J. J. (1981): The role of descending monoaminergic systems in central control of blood pressure. *Fed. Proc.,* 40:2778–2785.

166. Brody, M. J., Haywood, J. R., and Touw, K. B. (1980): Neural mechanisms in hypertension. *Annu. Rev. Physiol.,* 42:441–453.

167. Szabadi, E. (1979): Adrenoceptors on central neurones: Microelectrophoretic studies. *Neuropharmacology,* 18:831–843.

168. Coote, J. H., Macleod, V. H., Fleetwood-Walker, S., and Gilbey, M. P. (1981): The response of individual sympathetic preganglionic neurones to microelectrophoretically applied endogenous amines. *Brain Res.,* 215:135–145.

169. Kuhn, D. M., Wolf, W. A., and Lovenberg, W. (1980): Review of the role of the central serotonergic neuronal system in blood pressure regulation. *Hypertension,* 2:243–255.

170. Franz, D. N., Madsen, P. W., Peterson, R. G., and Sangdee, C. (1982): Functional roles of monoaminergic pathways to sympathetic preganglionic neurons. *Clin. Exp. Hypertens.,* A4:543–562.

171. Phillips, M. I., Weyhenmeyer, J., Felix, D., Ganter, D., and Hoffman, W. E. (1979): Evidence for an endogenous brain renin-angiotensin system. *Fed. Proc.,* 38:2260–2266.

172. Buccafusco, J. J., and Brezenoff, H. E. (1979): Pharmacological study of a cholinergic mechanism within the rat posterior hypothalamic nucleus which mediates a hypertensive response. *Brain Res.,* 165:295–310.

173. Schaz, K., Stock, G., Simon, W., Schlör, K.-H., Unger, T., Rockhold, R., and Gant, D. (1980):

Enkephalin effects on blood pressure, heart rate, and baroreceptor reflex. *Hypertension,* 2:395–407.

174. Persson, B. (1980): GABAergic mechanisms in blood pressure control. A pharmacologic analysis in the rat. *Acta Physiol. Scand.* [*Suppl.*], 491:1–54.

175. Williford, D. J., DiMicco, J. A., and Gillis, R. A. (1980): Evidence for the presence of a tonically active forebrain GABA system influencing central sympathetic outflow in the cat. *Neuropharmacology,* 19:245–250.

176. Häusler, G., and Osterwalder, R. (1980): Evidence suggesting a transmitter or neuromodulatory role for substance P at the first synapse of the baroreceptor reflex. *Naunyn Schmiedebergs Arch. Pharmacol.,* 314:111–121.

177. Gillis, R. A., Helke, C. J., Hamilton, B. L., Norman, W. P., and Jacobowitz, D. M. (1980): Evidence that substance P is a transmitter of baro- and chemoreceptor afferents in the nucleus tractus solitarius. *Brain Res.,* 181:476–481.

178. Reis, D. J., Granata, A. R., Perrone, M. H., and Talman, W. T. (1981): Evidence that glutamic acid is the neurotransmitter of baroreceptor afferents terminating in the nucleus of the tractus solitarius (NTS). *J. Autonom. Nervous Syst.,* 3:321–334.

179. Farsang, C., Ramirez-Gonzales, M. D., Mucci, L., and Kunos, G. (1980): Possible role of an endogenous opiate in the cardiovascular effects of central alpha adrenoceptor stimulation in spontaneously hypertensive rats. *J. Pharmacol. Exp. Ther.,* 214:203–208.

180. Downing, S. E. (1979): Baroreceptor regulation of the heart. In: *Handbook of Physiology, Section 2, The Cardiovascular System, Vol. 1, The Heart,* edited by R. M. Berne, pp. 621–652. American Physiological Society, Bethesda.

181. Brown, A. M. (1980): Receptors under pressure. An update on baroreceptors. *Circ. Res.,* 46:1–10.

182. Paintal, A. S. (1973): Vagal sensory receptors and their reflex effects. *Physiol. Rev.,* 53:159–227.

183. Jones, J. V., and Thorén, P. N. (1977): Characteristics of aortic baroreptors with non-medullated afferents arising from the aortic arch of rabbits with chronic renovascular hypertension. *Acta Physiol. Scand.,* 101:286–293.

184. Epstein, S. E., Beiser, G. D., Goldstein, R. E., Stampfer, M., Wechsler, A. S., Glick, G., and Braunwald, E. (1969): Circulatory effects of electrical stimulation of the carotid sinus nerves in man. *Circulation,* 40:269–276.

185. Vatner, S. F., Higgins, C. B., Franklin, D., and Braunwald, E. (1972): Extent of carotid sinus regulation of the myocardial contractile state in conscious dogs. *J. Clin. Invest.,* 51:995–1008.

186. Shoukas, A. A., and Sagawa, K. (1973): Control of total systemic vascular capacity by the carotid sinus baroreceptor reflex. *Circ. Res.,* 33:22–33.

187. Kezdi, P. (1967): Resetting of the carotid sinus in experimental renal hypertension. In: *Baroreceptors and Hypertension,* edited by P. Kezdi, pp. 301–308. Pregamon Press, Oxford.

188. Sapru, H. N. (1974): Prevention and reversal of baroreceptor resetting in the spontaneously hypertensive rat. *Fed. Proc.,* 33:359.

189. Cowley, A. W., Jr., Liard, J. F., and Guyton, A. C. (1973): Role of the baroreceptor reflex in daily control of arterial blood pressure and other variables in dogs. *Circ. Res.,* 32:564–576.

190. Brown, A. M. (1979): Cardiac reflexes. In: *Handbook of Physiology, Section 2, The Cardiovascular System, Vol. 1, The Heart,* edited by R. M. Berne, pp. 677–689. American Physiological Society, Bethesda.

191. Linden, R. J. (1973): Function of cardiac receptors. *Circulation,* 48:463–480.

192. Vatner, S. F., and Zimpfer, M. (1981): Bainbridge reflex in conscious, unrestrained, and tranquilized baboons. *Am. J. Physiol.,* 240:H164–H167.

193. Thorén, P. N. (1977): Characteristics of left ventricular receptors with nonmedullated vagal afferents in cats. *Circ. Res.,* 40:415–421.

194. Abboud, F. M., Eckberg, D. L., Johannsen, U. J., and Mark, A. L. (1979): Carotid and cardiopulmonary baroreceptor control of splanchnic and forearm vascular resistance during venous pooling in man. *J. Physiol.,* 286:173–184.

195. Biscoe, T. J. (1971): Carotid body: Structure and function. *Physiol. Rev.,* 51:437–495.

196. Coleridge, J. C. G., and Coleridge, H. M. (1979): Chemoreflex regulation of the heart. In: *Handbook of Physiology, Section 2, The Cardiovascular System, Vol. 1, The Heart,* edited by R. M. Berne, pp. 621–652. American Physiological Society, Bethesda.

197. Hackett, J. G., Abboud, F. M., Mark, A. L., Schmid, P. G., and Heistad, D. D. (1972): Coronary vascular responses to stimulation of chemoreceptors and baroreceptors. Evidence for reflex activation of vagal cholinergic innervation. *Circ. Res.,* 31:17–18.

198. Kaufman, M. P., Baker, D. G., Coleridge, H. M., and Coleridge, J. C. G. (1980): Stimulation by bradykinin of afferent vagal C-fibers with chemosensitive endings in the heart and aorta of the dog. *Circ. Res.,* 46:476–484.

199. Felder, R. B., and Thames, R. D. (1982): Responses to activation of cardiac sympathetic afferents with epicardial bradykinin. *Am. J. Physiol.,* 242:H148–H153.

200. Sato, A., and Schmidt, R. F. (1973): Somatosympathetic reflexes: Afferent fibers, central pathways, discharge characteristics. *Physiol. Rev.,* 53:916–947.

201. Guyton, A. C. (1980): *Arterial Pressure and Hypertension.* W. B. Saunders, Philadelphia.

202. Folkow, B. (1982): Physiological aspects of primary hypertension. *Physiol. Rev.,* 62:347–504.

203. deChamplain, J., and Van Amerigen, M. R. (1972): Regulation of blood pressure by sympathetic nerve fibers and adrenal medulla in normotensive and hypertensive rats. *Circ. Res.,* 31:617–628.

Cardiovascular Pharmacology, Second Edition,
edited by Michael Antonaccio.
Raven Press, New York © 1984.

Renal Physiology and Pharmacology

*Jerry B. Hook and **Robert Z. Gussin

*Center for Environmental Toxicology, Michigan State University, East Lansing, Michigan 48824; and
**McNeil Pharmaceutical, Spring House, Pennsylvania 19477

The kidney is a highly dynamic organ that functions to maintain salt and water balance within rather narrow limits even though dietary intake may fluctuate markedly. There are conditions, however, when because of a primary renal disorder or a nonrenal pathologic condition (e.g., congestive heart failure, cirrhosis, etc.) the capacity of the kidney to maintain salt and water balance is overwhelmed; salt and water are retained, and edema and/or ascites develop. The clinically prudent course for the physician is to treat the underlying cause of the disorder and allow the kidneys to reestablish homeostasis. However, in many cases the imbalance may be immediately threatening to the well-being of the patient, and pharmacological intervention is required. Diuretics are used because they act directly on the kidney to enhance the excretion of salt and water.

With few exceptions, little is known about the biochemical mechanisms whereby diuretics enhance salt and water excretion. It is clear, however, that the clinical effects arise from drug-induced inhibition of normal salt and water reabsorption and that the location where a drug acts along the nephron determines the magnitude and major side effects of its action. Consequently, an understanding of normal physiology of the nephron is the critical component in understanding renal pharmacology. Thus, this chapter is designed to first describe normal renal function and then discuss groups of diuretics.

It is hoped that this chapter will serve as a starting point for those interested in renal pharmacology. The references cited may aid in guiding the reader to sources of more extensive explanations of each topic covered.

PHYSIOLOGIC CONSIDERATIONS IN RENAL FUNCTION

Homeostasis and Electrolyte Metabolism

A study of renal physiology and pharmacology requires some understanding of body fluid and electrolyte distribution and balance, because the kidneys are primarily responsible for maintenance of the consistency of body fluid composition in both healthy and disease states.

The total volume of body water varies between 45 and 70% of body weight, being higher in children and lean adults and lower in obese persons. The total volume is divided into two major compartments (the extracellular and intracellular) and a much smaller third component (the transcellular). This last component represents only about 2.5% of the total body water and includes the fluids in the tracheobronchial tree, the kidneys and glands, the cerebrospinal fluid, the aqueous humor of the eye, and the fluid within the gastrointestinal tract. The intracellular compartment accounts for the largest volume and represents more than half the total body water. It is a heterogeneous compartment made up of the sum of the fluid of all cells of the body. Because different types of cells (e.g., liver cells, fat cells, muscle cells) vary greatly in water content as well as chemical composition, it is impossible to provide a simplified representation of this compartment. The extracellular compartment accounts for about one-third of the total body water and represents all fluid that exists outside of cells, with the exception of the transcellular fluid. The extracellular compartment is further subdivided into two components: the vascular or plasma compartment and the interstitial fluid. The interstitial fluid accounts for about 75% of the extracellular compartment; plasma makes up the remaining 25%.

There are marked differences in the compositions of extracellular and intracellular fluids. Naturally, the composition of extracellular fluid has been more completely defined, because this compartment is more readily accessible for study. Plasma samples can be obtained with great ease, and the interstitial fluid is essentially an ultrafiltrate of plasma, lacking only the protein component. A tabular summary of the fluid compartments and some average values to describe ionic composition, where reasonable, are shown in Table 1.

The kidneys regulate the volume, osmolality, and ionic composition of the extracellular fluid. This is accomplished by retaining and excreting the appropriate amounts of the appropriate species to maintain normal composition. The plasma is in ionic equilibrium with the interstitial fluid compartment, which in turn influences the composition of the intracellular compartment. This oversimplified view of the kidneys' role actually reflects a complex and multifaceted process that begins with the ultrafiltration of plasma at the glomerulus.

Before entering into a more detailed description of renal function, it is necessary to review briefly the anatomy of the kidneys (Fig. 1). The kidneys are somewhat flattened, bean-shaped organs located retroperitoneally on either side of the vertebral column against the posterior abdominal wall. Together, the two kidneys weigh about 300 g. Although the kidneys represent only about 0.4% of the weight of the body, their blood requirement accounts for 20 to 25% of cardiac output at rest. This is the greatest blood flow, in proportion to weight, supplied to any organ of the body. This high flow is a requisite for the kidneys' function of regulating the composition of body fluids.

Blood enters and leaves the kidney almost solely through two major vessels: the renal artery and vein. After entering the renal pelvis, the renal artery subdivides several times and

TABLE 1. *Distribution of body water and electrolytes*

Compartment	Percentage of total body water	Major cations (mEq/liter)	Major anions (mEq/liter)
Intracellular	55	Na (10), K (160), Mg (40)[a]	Cl (2), HCO$_3$ (10), PO$_4$ and SO$_4$ (150),[a] protein (50)
Extracellular	35		
Plasma	7	Na (140), K (4), Ca (5), Mg (2.0)	Cl (100), PO$_4$ and SO$_4$ (3.5), HCO$_3$ (28), organic anions (5), protein (17)
Interstitial fluid	28	Na (144), K (4), Ca (2.5), Mg[b] (1.5)	Cl (115), PO$_4$ and SO$_4$ (3.0),[b] HCO$_3$ (30), organic anions (5), protein (0)
Transcellular water	2.5		
Inaccessible bone water	7.5		

[a] Roughly estimated for muscle tissue in mEq/liter H_2O.
[b] Rough approximations by calculation.

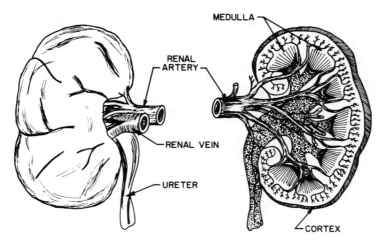

FIG. 1. Diagram of human kidneys showing the outer portion (cortex) and the inner portion (medulla) and the major vascular supply.

eventually forms the afferent arterioles, which lead to the glomerular capillary tuft, and the efferent arteriole, leading from the glomerular capillary tuft and proceeding to branch into the richly anastomosing peritubular capillary network.

Each kidney is made up of an exceedingly large number of similar units called nephrons, operating in parallel (Fig. 2). Each human kidney contains approximately 1 million nephrons. The nephron is the functional unit of the kidney and consists of a renal corpuscle, a proximal convoluted tubule, a loop of Henle, a distal convoluted tubule, and a multibranched collecting duct that is common to and drains a number of units. The renal corpuscle consists of the glomerular capillary tuft surrounded by a blind epithelial pouch, Bowman's capsule, into which the ultrafiltrate of plasma flows and begins its journey into the proximal tubule and throughout the remainder of the nephron. The postglomerular capillaries surrounding tubules of the cortical nephrons form a peritubular network.

The loops of Henle of the juxtamedullary nephrons are supplied by recurrent vascular loops, the vasa recta, which parallel the tubule. Blood is supplied to the glomerular capillary tufts by short, direct, wide-bore vessels, the

afferent arterioles, which ensure a high filtration pressure. The peritubular capillary system is a portal system, operating at low pressure. This low pressure, along with an elevated colloid osmotic pressure due to concentration of plasma proteins by expression of fluid at the glomerulus, favors the entry of reabsorbed fluids and solutes into the vascular system from the peritubular interstitial fluid.

Three discrete processes are involved in the formation of urine: glomerular filtration, tubular reabsorption, and tubular secretion.

Glomerular Filtration

Simple filtration removes particulate matter, whereas ultrafiltration carries the process even further and effects the removal of proteins and lipids. Urine formation begins with the ultrafiltration of large volumes of plasma through the glomerular capillary tufts. The glomerulus is similar to other capillary beds, and filtration at this site is subject to the same physical laws that govern the transport of fluid and permeant ions and molecules across any capillary membrane. The driving force for the filtration process is the hydrostatic pressure of the blood derived from the work of the heart. The pressure in the glomerular capillar-

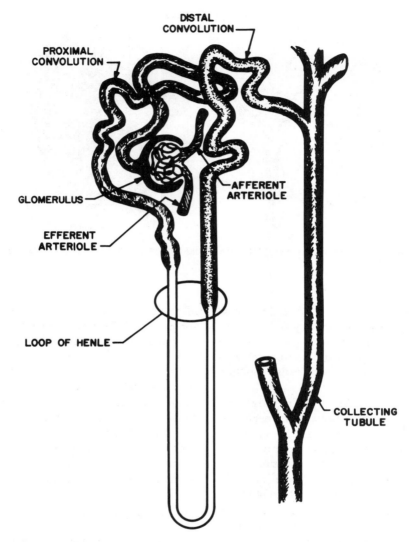

FIG. 2. The nephron. Cortical nephrons have short loops of Henle, whereas juxtamedullary nephrons have much longer loops.

ies is about 60% of the arterial pressure. Plasma proteins and lipids, as stated earlier, do not penetrate the glomerular membrane to an appreciable extent, but all other plasma constituents do penetrate.

The rate of glomerular filtration averages about 125 ml/min per 1.73 m² surface area in the adult male and about 110 ml/min per 1.73 m² in the adult female. The glomerular filtration rate is quite stable even during rela-

tively wide fluctuations in systemic blood pressure. Because the average pressure in the glomerular capillaries is about 60% of the systemic arterial pressure, it is estimated that the mean systemic blood pressure would have to drop to about 40 mm Hg before glomerular filtration would cease.

The rate of glomerular filtration can be determined by measuring excretion and plasma concentration of a substance that is freely filtered through the glomeruli and is neither secreted nor reabsorbed by the tubules. The amount of such a substance that appears in the urine per unit of time must be derived by filtering exactly the number of milliliters of plasma that contain this amount of substance. This is called renal clearance. Thus, if one uses the polysaccharide inulin, for example, a measure of the urinary concentration (U_{in}) and the urinary volume (V) for a given period of time will provide the amount of inulin excreted ($U_{in} \times V$). If this is then divided by the plasma concentration of inulin, one obtains the volume of plasma cleared of inulin:[1]

$$C_{in} = \frac{U_{in}V}{P_{in}}$$

Because inulin is not reabsorbed, secreted, or metabolized, the inulin clearance is a measure of the glomerular filtration rate. Inulin is accepted as the best substance for measuring glomerular filtration rate.

It is evident from the glomerular filtration rate that if the entire filtrate were excreted, the urinary volume in a 24-hr period would be approximately 180 liters. This, of course, would be incompatible with life, because the total extracellular fluid volume is only about 12.5 liters, an amount filtered in about 100 min. In actuality, the average 24-hr urinary volume is about 1.5 liters, or less than 1% of the volume of fluid filtered. Over 99% of the filtered fluid is reabsorbed.

Tubular Reabsorption

The importance of renal tubular reabsorption was emphasized by the preceding example. The composition of the reabsorbate must be very close to that of the glomerular filtrate to prevent extensive changes in the composition of the extracellular fluid. It is obvious from the magnitude of the reabsorptive process that drugs that slightly modify tubular

reabsorption can greatly affect urinary volume and composition.

The 160 to 180 liters of fluid that are filtered at the glomerulus in 24 hr contain more than 1,000 g of sodium chloride, 500 g of sodium bicarbonate, 180 g of glucose, 100 g of free amino acids, 4 g of vitamin C, and significant quantities of a variety of other constituents. Many relatively discrete mechanisms are involved in reabsorption of the various components of the glomerular filtrate. For example, one mechanism is responsible for the reabsorption of glucose, fructose, galactose, and xylose; another for sulfate and thiosulfate; a third for arginine, lysine, ornithine, and cystine; and others for various ions, certain other amino acids, etc. Some substances compete for a common step or steps in transport processes.

It is impossible to describe the characteristics of all of the various transport systems in this chapter. The reader is directed to any one of a number of textbooks on renal physiology, such as that by Valtin (1). However, it is necessary to discuss briefly the reabsorption of some of the major electrolytes in order to set the stage for a discussion of diuretic agents.

The reabsorption of ions and water in the proximal segment of the renal tubule is isosmotic. This simply means that both the fluid reabsorbed and that remaining in the tubular lumen have the same osmotic pressure as plasma. Because sodium, bicarbonate, and chloride account for 90 to 95% of the osmotic activity of the plasma and glomerular filtrate, it is evident that ions and water must be reabsorbed at osmotically equivalent rates. The proximal reabsorption of sodium is thought to be active, requiring the expenditure of metabolic energy. Reabsorption of chloride in the proximal tubule is believed to be a passive process, occurring down an electrochemical gradient. Water is reabsorbed passively as a result of the osmotic force created by the reabsorption of sodium and chloride ions. Water diffuses readily in both directions across the proximal tubular epithelium, and hence the osmotic pressures of the tubular contents and the blood plasma remain equal. The proximal

---

[1] C_{in} = clearance of inulin (ml/min); U_{in} = urinary inulin concentration (mg/ml); V = urine flow (ml/min); P_{in} = plasma concentration of inulin (mg/ml).

tubule performs no osmotic work (it neither dilutes nor concentrates the tubular urine), but four-fifths to seven-eighths of the glomerular filtrate is normally reabsorbed in this area.

The thick ascending limb of Henle's loop is one portion of the nephron where the luminal fluid is diluted by the reabsorption of more sodium chloride than water. This transport property is important for both urinary dilution and concentration, and it accounts for a substantial fraction of the total sodium chloride reabsorption from the nephron. Burg and Green (2) and Rocha and Kokko (3) demonstrated that, contrary to earlier beliefs, the electrical-potential difference in the thick ascending limb of Henle's loop is oriented lumen-positive, so that sodium chloride transport in this segment consists of active chloride transport plus passive sodium movement along the resulting electrical-potential gradient. Although their studies did not exclude the possibility of some active sodium transport, they could find no convincing evidence for its existence.

The thick ascending limb of the loop of Henle is relatively impermeable to water. This has two consequences: First, the sodium chloride concentration in the tubular fluid falls, reaching a minimum value usually in the first portion of the distal convolution. Second, the sodium chloride concentration becomes elevated in the interstitial fluid. Thus, a concentration gradient is established across the tubular epithelium by electrolyte transport at a site of low water permeability. The small horizontal gradient then becomes multiplied in a vertical direction as a result of the architecture of the loop of Henle and the vasa recta and the presence of a countercurrent mechanism. Movements of water from the descending limb of the loop of Henle in response to the hyperosmolality of the interstitial fluid, as well as diffusions of Na and Cl from the medullary interstitium back into the tubular fluid of the descending limb, contribute to a progressive rise in osmotic pressure of the fluid as it flows toward the tip of the loop (Fig. 3). After the fluid moves around the bend at the tip of the loop, it enters the area of the ascending limb, where salt is actively moved out of the tubule without an osmotic equivalent of water, and hence, as seen in Fig. 3, the osmotic pressure of the fluid begins to fall. The hairpin construction of the blood vessels in the renal medulla (the vasa recta) and the relatively low rate of blood flow in these vessels allow them to act as countercurrent exchangers. They parallel the loops of Henle and allow maintenance of the osmotic gradient. If the architecture of these vessels were similar to that in the cortex and the blood flow were faster, the osmotic gradient would be washed out, and the multiplier system of the nephron would not function. A detailed description of the countercurrent system is presented in the text by Valtin (1) and in a review of medical physiology by Ganong (4).

Fluid in the ascending limb becomes isosmotic with plasma at approximately the cortico-medullary junction. From this point until it passes the glomerulus (cells of the tubule referred to as the macula densa actually make contact with the glomerulus of the same tubule), NaCl continues to be reabsorbed subsequent to active chloride transport. It appears that after the macula densa, NaCl reabsorption is again due to Na transport, although the point of transition from active Cl transport to active Na transport is not clearly defined. Regardless, from approximately the corticomedullary junction to the point of joining a collecting duct, NaCl is reabsorbed much more avidly than water, and the urine is rendered dilute. This area is termed the cortical diluting segment; whatever the state of hydration of the individual, urine entering the collecting ducts will be dilute.

Fine control of salt and water excretion is effected in the latter part of the distal tubule and collecting duct and is regulated by the actions of at least two hormones. A peptide hormone from the posterior pituitary, vasopressin (or antidiuretic hormone, ADH), is released in response to systemic dehydration or increased plasma osmolality. In the absence of ADH, the cells of the collecting duct are

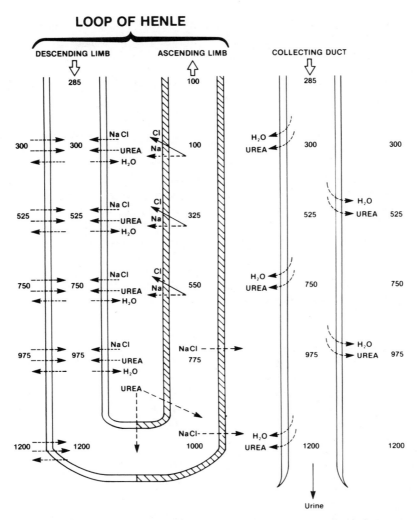

FIG. 3. Countercurrent multiplier system. Areas of the nephron shown cross-hatched are impermeable to water. Solid arrows indicate sites of active electrolyte transport; broken arrows indicate passive movement. Numbers represent osmolality. Peritubular capillaries (vasa recta) parallel the tubular loop.

relatively impermeable to water. As fluid flows down the duct, more electrolytes are reabsorbed, but the water is retained in the lumen, and a dilute urine is excreted. In the presence of ADH, the permeability of the collecting duct to water is enhanced, and water is reabsorbed in response to the osmotic gradient established by the loop of Henle, with a small volume of concentrated urine being formed.

Sodium reabsorption in the latter part of the distal tubule is enhanced by the mineralo-corticoid aldosterone. Fluid entering the latter parts of the nephron is quite low in chloride concentration, and anions like sulfate and phosphate in the urine are not readily reabsorbed with sodium. Thus, as sodium is reabsorbed, a steep electrical gradient (lumen-negative) is established that favors movement of potassium and hydrogen ions into the urine. It follows that any procedure that enhances reabsorption of sodium in this part of the nephron will enhance excretion of potassium.

Tubular Secretion

Tubular secretion resembles tubular reabsorption, but its processes are oriented in the opposite direction, moving substances from the peritubular blood through the tubular cells and into the luminal fluid. Active tubular secretion occurs against an electrochemical gradient and requires a constant supply of energy. There are three types of secretory processes that occur and are analogous to reabsorptive counterparts: (a) active secretion, with an absolute limitation of transport capacity, i.e., transport-maximum-limited (T_m-limited) systems; (b) active secretory processes that exhibit gradient/time limitation of transport capacity; (c) passive secretory processes that involve diffusion of materials down gradients of concentration. A detailed description of these processes is provided in the textbook by Valtin (1).

Organic acids and organic bases are transported by separate systems in the proximal tubule that are T_m-limited; raising the blood or intracellular concentration above a certain level does not result in further increases in secretory rate. Within each of these two transport systems (organic acid and organic base), substances compete with each other for transport sites. However, there is no cross-competition, that is, an acid competing with a base. Para-aminohippurate (PAH) and uric acid are examples of organic acids transported by one system, and choline and catecholamines are examples of organic bases transported by the other system. Some substances do exist as *Zwitterions* and are transported by the appropriate system for each form simultaneously, rather than by a complex dual carrier (5).

Hydrogen ions are secreted by a gradient/time-limited system in the distal portion of the nephron. That the secretion of hydrogen ions is gradient-limited is supported by the observation that large quantities of hydrogen ions are secreted if the intracellular levels are high and if the transtubular gradient is maintained by the presence in the urine of large amounts of buffer of favorable pK. If large amounts of potassium are present in the cell and the amount of hydrogen is low, potassium will be excreted to the exclusion of hydrogen.

A series of weak bases and some weak acids are passively secreted in their nonionic form and are trapped in the lumen if the urinary pH is such that the ionic form of the acid or base is formed. The tubules are not permeable to the ionic form, which cannot diffuse back to the blood. Accordingly, the clearance of weak bases, such as ammonia, quinine, and quinacrine, is greater in acid urine than in alkaline urine, whereas the clearance of weak acids, such as salicylic acid and phenobarbital, is greater in alkaline urine than in acid urine. Passive secretion occurs primarily in the distal portion of the nephron, where the highest hydrogen ion gradients are established.

The transport systems in the renal tubule participate in the excretion of drugs as well as naturally occurring substances. They can be modified by inhibitors in order to influence the rate of elimination of substances, such as maintenance of high circulating levels of penicillin by administration of probenecid, a competitive inhibitor of the renal tubular secretion of organic acids.

Renal Regulation of Acid–Base Balance

The processes of renal tubular acid secretion, NH_4^+ production, and bicarbonate excretion can produce urine that varies from pH 4.5 to about pH 8.0 in humans. The excretion of urine whose pH differs from the pH of body fluids is an important factor in the body's maintenance of electrolyte and acid–base balance.

Acids are buffered in both plasma and cells by sodium bicarbonate through the following reaction: $HA(acid) + NaHCO_3 \leftrightharpoons NaA(salt) + H_2CO_3$. The H_2CO_3, in turn, forms CO_2 and H_2O. The CO_2 is expired; the NaA reaches the renal tubular fluid in the glomerular filtrate. Some of the Na^+ is replaced by H^+ as titratable acid or NH_4^+, and the Na^+ is reabsorbed for conservation in the body. The availability of H^+ in this procedure is due in large part to the reaction $H_2O + CO_2$ $\leftrightarrows H_2CO_3 \leftrightarrows H^+ + HCO_3^-$, a reaction that is catalyzed by the enzyme carbonic anhydrase. When this enzyme is inhibited, the H^+ is less readily available to replace Na^+ in the tubular fluid, and more Na^+ is excreted in the urine. This is the mechanism of action of a class of diuretics to be discussed later.

For each H^+ that is excreted as titratable acid or NH_4^+ there is a net gain of one HCO_3^- in the blood, replenishing the supply of this important buffer anion. When base is added to the body, the OH^- ions are buffered, and plasma HCO_3^- increases. When plasma HCO_3^- levels rise above 28 mEq/liter, the extra HCO_3^- is excreted in the urine.

The renin-angiotensin-aldosterone system is discussed in detail in another chapter. This discussion will deal only with aldosterone and its effect on the renal tubules. Suffice it to state here that renin release from the kidney due to a variety of stimuli leads to the conversion of angiotensinogen to angiotensin I, a decapeptide that is then converted to angiotensin II, an octapeptide. Angiotensin II, in turn, acts on the zona glomerulosa of the adrenal cortex to stimulate the release of aldosterone, whose structure is shown.

Aldosterone plays an important role in the regulation of sodium and potassium balance. A review of aldosterone and angiotensin by Gross and Mohring (6) provides an extensive description of the release and activity of aldosterone.

Adrenocorticotropic hormone (ACTH) from the anterior pituitary also plays a role in the secretion of aldosterone, but the fine control is believed to be under the influence of the renin-angiotensin system. Plasma potassium concentration, as well as some humoral factors not yet identified, may also participate in the control of aldosterone secretion.

The theory that angiotensin II is the primary regulator of aldosterone secretion was initially met with great enthusiasm, but additional findings have cast some doubt on the importance of this role of angiotensin. For example, in intact and hypophysectomized rats, angiotensin has no effect on aldosterone production (7,8) except in very high doses (9) or during sodium deficiency (10). In humans, sodium deficiency induces much greater increases in plasma aldosterone levels than are produced by infusions of angiotensin that provide levels as high as those obtained during sodium deficiency (11). Bilateral nephrectomy does not affect aldosterone excretion in either sheep (12) or humans (13). In anephric patients, plasma aldosterone has been found to correlate with plasma potassium concentration (14).

Aldosterone is the mineralocorticoid hormone of the adrenal cortex. It regulates Na^+ and K^+ excretion by the kidney and influences Na^+ transport in other secretory glands and epithelial systems. In the kidney, aldosterone acts on the renal tubule to enhance Na^+ reabsorption directly and potassium excretion indirectly. Aldosterone also affects urinary acid excretion. In humans, aldosterone has been shown to enhance net acid secretion (15,16).

When mineralocorticoids are administered repeatedly, or when the endogenous plasma concentration of aldosterone is high, the kidney escapes from the sodium-retaining effects, but not the potassium-wasting effects. A comprehensive review of this escape phenomenon and also the mechanism by which aldosterone regulates electrolyte transport through the stimulation of RNA and protein synthesis has been presented by Gross and Mohring (6).

Erythrogenin

Erythrogenin is also referred to as the renal erythropoietic factor (REF). REF is released into the bloodstream by the kidney and stimulates bone marrow to increase its rate of production of red blood cells. REF also produces an increase in reticulocytes in peripheral blood and accelerates the rate of iron incorporation into heme of newly formed red blood cells. Gordon et al. (17) have extensively reviewed the status of erythrogenin. Both clinical and experimental studies have indicated a relationship between the kidney and erythropoiesis, although the role of the kidney in the day-to-day control of erythropoiesis is still not clear. In rats, nephrectomy markedly reduces the production of the erythropoiesis stimulating factor (ESF, erythropoietin) in response to stimuli (18,19). In humans, anemia often accompanies renal deficiency states (20,21), and erythrocytosis may occur in humans with hypernephroma (22) or hydronephrosis (23).

Experiments in animals have ruled out the possibility that the lowered erythropoietic response to oxygen deficiency in nephrectomized or renal-deficient animals is due to unexcreted wastes that are present in the renoprival state. Bilateral ureteral ligation or implantation of the ureter into the iliac vein does not result in depression of the erythropoietic response to hypoxia in these animals.

sues. The levels of the circulating substrate for erythrogenin are believed to be controlled through its own negative-feedback system. The scheme proposed by Gordon et al. (17) to describe the system has been shown.

Prostaglandins

The origins and roles of the prostaglandins in circulatory control are covered in detail in another chapter. It does appear that prostaglandins produced in the kidney may influence renal function in several ways. Although much has been made of the natriuretic effect of infusions of prostaglandins, the direct tubular effects are probably slight. Vasodilator prostaglandins are released by adrenergic stimuli and probably serve to maintain renal circulation in conditions of low blood flow, shock, etc. A major role of renal prostaglandins (probably prostacyclin) appears to be as an important step in renin release. Early work with renal medullary prostaglandins suggested an important antihypertensive role for these compounds. This has not been unequivocally doc-

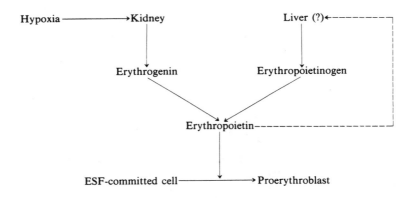

Erythrogenin can be extracted in concentrated form from light-mitochondrial and microsomal fractions of kidneys. It is released from the kidney in response to a variety of hypoxic stimuli. Erythrogenin then activates a substrate in the serum to produce ESF, which in turn stimulates erythropoietic tis-

umented, however. It does appear that in some way renal medullary PGE_2 may be an endogenous inhibitor of ADH, possibly via an intrinsic negative-feedback mechanism. The various aspects of the renal actions of prostaglandins provided the subject for a recent symposium (24).

Endogenous Substances Affecting Renal Function

Aldosterone

Aldosterone has been discussed previously. It is a steroid released from the zona glomerulosa of the adrenal cortex in response to various stimuli. Aldosterone acts on the renal tubules to promote the reabsorption of sodium. Reabsorption of sodium produces an electrical gradient that favors diffusion of potassium into the tubular urine. The activity of aldosterone, once released, is slow, requiring 30 to 90 min for onset. This delay is believed to be due to a requirement for protein synthesis as part of the action of the hormone. Hyperaldosteronism may occur because of an adrenal cortical tumor (primary) or in response to excessive sodium loss, as may occur during diuretic therapy (secondary). It can lead to sodium retention and edema formation, excess potassium loss leading to muscle weakness and cardiac arrhythmias, and refractoriness to ongoing classic diuretic therapy. Hypoaldosteronism, as may occur in adrenal insufficiency, can lead to a salt-wasting syndrome.

Vasopressin (Antidiuretic Hormone)

Vasopressin is a nonapeptide (considering each half-cystine as a single amino acid) from the posterior lobe of the pituitary gland.

$$\text{Cys—Try—Phe—Gln—Asn—Cys—Pro—Arg—Gly—NH}_2$$
$$\phantom{\text{Cys}}123456789$$

with an S——S bridge connecting positions 1 and 6.

This hormone is identical in all mammals studied, with the exception of the pig and the hippopotamus, in which lysine replaces arginine in position 8 of the molecule. In the posterior pituitary, vasopressin is stored bound to a polypeptide known as a neurophysin. Storage granules in the posterior pituitary contain vasopressin, neurophysin, and ATP, and all three substances are released on stimulation. Once released, vasopressin acts on the distal portion of the nephron (distal convoluted tubule and collecting duct) to increase its permeability to water. Vasopressin may also play a minor role in electrolyte transport in the mammalian renal tubule, but this role is poorly understood. Various stimuli increase vasopressin secretion. Some of these are increased effective osmotic pressure of plasma, decreased extracellular fluid volume, certain drugs (such as morphine, nicotine, and barbiturates), and some additional factors such as pain, emotion, stress, and exercise. Factors that may decrease vasopressin secretion are decreased effective osmotic pressure of plasma, increased extracellular fluid volume, and alcohol.

The osmoreceptors responsible for vasopressin release are located in the hypothalamus (primarily in the supraoptic nucleus) and are sensitive to changes in plasma osmolality. Vasopressin secretion is thus controlled by a delicate feedback mechanism that continuously operates to maintain normal plasma osmolality. There is a steady level of vasopressin secretion even when plasma osmolality is normal. This results in a continuous plasma vasopressin concentration of about 3 microunits (equivalent to about 10^{-10} M). Significant changes in vasopressin secretion can occur in response to osmolality changes as small as 2%. Thus, plasma osmolality in normal individuals is maintained very close to 290 mOsm/liter.

There are instances of inappropriate vasopressin hypersecretion leading to hyponatremia. These are seen in some pulmonary diseases, such as lung cancer, and in certain cerebral diseases, such as pseudotumor cerebri.

Diabetes insipidus is the syndrome that results when vasopressin deficiency occurs as a result of injury or diseases involving the supraoptic nuclei, the hypothalamo-hypophyseal tract, or the posterior pituitary gland, or when the kidney is unresponsive to vasopressin. The symptoms of this syndrome are extreme polyuria and polydipsia, provided that the thirst mechanism is intact. If the sense of thirst is depressed, severe dehydration and death may ensue.

Natriuretic Hormone

During extracellular fluid expansion for any one of a number of reasons, sodium reabsorption in the proximal tubule has been shown to decrease. Some controversy exists as to whether this decrease in reabsorption results purely from physical factors such as hemodynamic changes or hydrostatic or oncotic pressure or whether there is truly a natriuretic hormone, or third factor, as it has been called (factors one and two are glomerular filtration rate and aldosterone, both of which can affect the rate of sodium excretion). Because the third factor has not yet been isolated or identified, consideration of its role must await further research. Those interested in additional information on this subject are referred to the work of Cort and Lichardus (25).

DIURETICS

The important homeostatic role of the kidney in maintaining the volume and composition of the body fluids has been discussed. When, for any reason, the kidneys can no longer provide sufficient fluid and salt excretion, excessive fluid will build up within the tissues. In order to remove this edema, diuretic drugs can be used. Ideally, of course, the treatment of edema or ascites should be directed toward control of the primary disease and reversal of the pathophysiologic processes that lead to expansion of the extracellular fluid.

Diuretics are loosely defined as agents that increase the rate of urine formation. Common usage of the term "diuresis" has resulted in two connotations: One refers to the increase in urine volume; the other, certainly the more important usage, refers to an increase in the excretion of sodium and either chloride or bicarbonate along with water, which is eliminated secondarily.

Although all diuretics in common use may alter the glomerular filtration rate, their actions generally are independent of this effect, and their major influence is on the tubular reabsorption of electrolytes.

Diuretic agents vary widely in terms of chemical structure, efficacy, and the patterns of electrolyte excretion that they induce. They have been categorized in numerous ways, including classification based on structure, efficacy, site of action, or mechanism of action. No single classification system has been entirely satisfactory. In order to cover the major diuretics presently in use, the agents discussed in this chapter will be classified as follows: (a) osmotic agents, (b) xanthines, (c) acid-forming salts, (d) organomercurials, (e) carbonic anhydrase inhibitors, (f) thiazides, (g) high-ceiling diuretics (ethacrynic acid and furosemide), (h) aldosterone antagonists/antikaliuretics (spironolactone and triamterene), (i) miscellaneous (quinethazone, metolazone, chlorthalidone, and bumetanide).

Methods for Studying Diuretics

Before entering into a discussion of the diuretic agents, it is helpful to describe some of the methods used to determine the site or sites within the nephron where these agents act. These methods include (a) clearance techniques, (b) micropuncture, (c) stop-flow, and (d) miscellaneous *in vitro* techniques.

Clearance Techniques

The concept of renal clearance was first described by Moller et al. (26) in 1929. Clearance is an empiric measure of the ability of the kidney to remove a substance from the blood, although it tells us nothing about the mechanism of removal. However, when the clearance of a substance is compared to the clearance of a standard substance that is known to be handled by the kidney in a specific way, clearance can tell us a great deal. For example, let us suppose that there exists a substance with the following properties: (a) It is freely filterable through glomerular capillary membranes; i.e., it is not bound to plasma proteins or sieved in the process of ultrafiltration. (b) It is biologically inert and is neither reabsorbed nor secreted by the renal tubules; an indication of this is given by a linear relationship between plasma concentration and urinary excretion rate. (c) It is nontoxic and does not alter renal function when infused in quantities that allow adequate quantification in plasma and urine. (d) It can be quantified in plasma and urine with a high degree of accuracy.

The clearance of such a substance measures the glomerular filtration rate; that is, it can be used as an indicator of the volume of plasma filtered through the glomerular capillaries per minute. Substances with the properties previously described do exist. A fructose polysaccharide, inulin, is the most popular of these substances. The renal clearance of inulin provides a measure of glomerular filtration rate.

This information can be used in several ways. If a substance exists freely in the plasma (not bound to proteins) and has a renal clearance higher than that for inulin, it is assumed to be secreted by the renal tubules, as well as filtered at the glomerulus. If its clearance is lower than the inulin clearance, it is assumed that the substance is filtered and reabsorbed. It must be remembered that because tubular secretion and reabsorption can occur simultaneously, the clearance provides the net result.

In addition to using clearance to determine how substances are handled by the kidney, one can also use it to examine electrolyte and water excretion and the magnitude of the effect of a diuretic. For example, if plasma sodium concentration and glomerular filtration rate are known, the amount of sodium filtered at the glomerulus per minute can be calculated. Then, by determining the amount of sodium excreted in the urine per minute, it becomes possible to calculate the amount of sodium being reabsorbed by the renal tubules. Generally, this amount is greater than 99% of the sodium filtered. Using this type of information, one can examine quantitatively the effects of diuretic agents on sodium excretion. This type of determination can be performed for any measurable substance.

The total osmolar clearance (C_{osm}) and the magnitude of the excretion of nonosmotically obligated water (free water) are important in determining the sites of action of diuretic drugs. In addition to the free-water clearance (C_{H_2O}), negative free-water clearance, more commonly referred to as solute-free water reabsorption (Tc_{H_2O}), is used to determine tubular sites of diuretic action. Basically, C_{H_2O} and Tc_{H_2O} represent deviations of urine osmolality from the osmolality of plasma in terms of plasma water. Thus, when urine and plasma are isosmotic with one another, the C_{H_2O} and Tc_{H_2O} are zero. In the well-hydrated state, a dilute urine is excreted. Water is excreted in excess of solute. The volume of this excess is free-water clearance. It is calculated by subtracting the osmolar clearance from the total volume of urine excreted. The calculation can be represented as follows:

$$C_{osm} = \frac{U_{osm}V}{P_{osm}}$$

$C = V - C_{osm}$, where C_{osm} is osmolar clearance, U_{osm} is urinary osmolality (mOsm/liter), P is plasma osmolality (mOsm/liter), V is urine volume (ml/min), and C_{H_2O} is free-water clearance.

The osmolar clearance is a measure of solute excretion. Free-water clearance provides a quantitative measurement of the diluting ability of the kidney. Urinary dilution is a consequence of removal of solute from tubular fluid at two water-impermeable sites: the thick ascending limb of Henle's loop and the distal convoluted tubule. The solute removed at the thick ascending limb of Henle's loop contributes to the hypertonic medullary interstitium, which would normally provide the driving force for fluid to move from the collecting duct back into the interstitium and hence be reabsorbed. However, in the highly hydrated state, the collecting duct is impermeable to water because of the absence of antidiuretic hormone, and the fluid cannot move in response to the hypertonic stimulus. Thus, the sodium-deficient fluid continues on through the tubular system and emerges as dilute urine with a measurable amount of free water.

On the other hand, solute-free water reabsorption provides a measure of the concentrating ability of the kidney in the dehydrated subject. During dehydration, the collecting ducts are maximally permeable, and water does move passively out of the collecting ducts in response to the hypertonic medullary interstitium. The amount of water passing from the collecting ducts into the medullary interstitium and then into the blood is directly related to the degree of hypertonicity of the medullary interstitium. The urine excreted by the dehydrated subject has a higher osmolar clearance than volume, indicating that solute-free water was reabsorbed. The degree of solute-free water reabsorption can be calculated by subtracting urinary volume from osmolar clearance: $Tc_{H_2O} - C_{osm} - V$.

Measuring the effects of diuretics on free-water clearance and solute-free water reabsorption can provide much useful information about the tubular sites of action. A drug that inhibits sodium reabsorption in the proximal tubule only causes an increase in the amount of isosmotic fluid leaving the proximal tubule. The increased amount of sodium reaching the loop of Henle results in the removal of greater amounts of sodium and, in the hydrated individual, an increase in free-water clearance. In the dehydrated subject, this type of drug will provide additional sodium chloride to the loop of Henle, which will lead to an increase in the medullary hypertonicity and will cause more water to move out of the collecting ducts, resulting in increased solute-free water reabsorption.

In contrast, drugs that depress solute reabsorption at either of the two diluting sites (thick ascending limb of Henle's loop and distal convoluted tubule) will decrease the free-water clearance in the hydrated subject. However, only an action at the first diluting site will also reduce solute-free water reabsorption in the dehydrated subject, because only solute removed at this site contributes to the medullary tonicity. Both the thick ascending limb of Henle's loop and the distal convoluted tubule participate in urinary dilution, but only

the former contributes to urinary concentration. The effects of diuretics acting at different tubular sites on C_{H_2O} and Tc_{H_2O} are shown schematically in Fig. 4.

The use of C_{H_2O} and Tc_{H_2O} to determine the sites of action of diuretics becomes less clear when the drugs act at multiple sites. For example, if a drug decreases C_{H_2O} and Tc_{H_2O}, it does act on the loop of Henle, but there could also be a masked proximal tubular effect, or it could be acting at both diluting sites. Under these circumstances, additional studies are required to clarify the sites of activity.

Additional information about sites of action can sometimes be obtained using C_{H_2O} by superimposing the effect of the drug under study on a maximal diuresis produced by a drug with a known site of action. For instance, a drug acting in the distal convoluted tubule could further lower C_{H_2O} after it was lowered by a drug acting only on the ascending limb of the loop of Henle. If the agent under study affected only the loop site, it would not cause an additional decrease in C_{H_2O} unless it acted at a different point in a biochemical chain of events, even though its effect was at the same anatomical site as that of the standard.

Micropuncture

Micropuncture provides another way of examining the renal tubular sites and the mechanisms of action of diuretics. The method involves the removal of fluid samples from single renal tubules by use of micropipettes inserted during transillumination of the kidney. The method is difficult, and it examines surface nephrons, but not deeper nephrons.

The most important measurement for evaluation of the sites of action of diuretics when micropuncture techniques are used is the ratio of inulin concentration in the tubular fluid to that in the plasma (*TF/P*), which is used to measure fractional fluid reabsorption. The determination, however, has limitations, for the combined analytical and sampling error alone may lead to errors in the estimation of fractional reabsorption in the proximal tubule

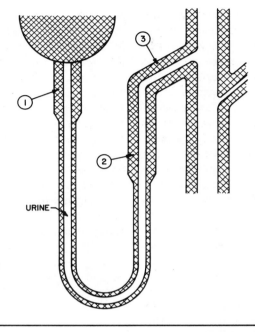

	Hydrated subject	Dehydrated subject
1. Proximal tubule	$\uparrow C_{H_2O}$	$\uparrow Tc_{H_2O}$
2. Thick ascending limb of Henle's loop	$\downarrow C_{H_2O}$	$\downarrow Tc_{H_2O}$
3. Distal tubule	$\downarrow C_{H_2O}$	$- Tc_{H_2O}$

FIG. 4. The influences of diuretics acting at various renal tubular sites on free-water clearance (C_{H_2O}) and solute-free water reabsorption (Tc_{H_2O}).

as large as 10%. Artifacts associated with the technique of collection pose a serious potential hazard. The dangers of altered flow proximal to the puncture site as a result of tubular obstruction or excessive suction, as well as of retrograde fluid collection from distal points, must be avoided. Another limitation has been the difficulty of obtaining valid control data for comparison with a set of experimental data. A more recent approach to micropuncture provides a solution to this latter problem by using recollection of proximal tubular fluid samples from the same puncture site even several hours apart (27). Therefore, each tubule serves as its own control.

Whereas free-flow inulin concentration ratios are important for examination of the net effects of diuretics at various sites within the nephron, more detailed information is made available through use of the split-oil-droplet technique originally described by Gertz (28). In this method, a drop of oil is injected into a tubule, and then the droplet is split by the introduction of a measured volume of an aqueous electrolyte solution into it. After a known length of time, the aqueous solution trapped by the two oil droplets is removed, and the volume is determined. Comparison of the times required for the droplet to be reduced to 50% of its original volume (half-time) before and after a diuretic, combined with the influence of the diuretic on flow rate as determined by the transit time for a bolus of a dye, usually lissamine green, provides useful information on the effect of the drug on the reabsorptive capacity of the tubule.

Studies designed to demonstrate inhibition of sodium reabsorption in the proximal tubule using micropuncture suffer from several major difficulties. When urinary fluid and electrolyte losses are not replaced, extracellular fluid (ECF) volume decreases, and fractional reabsorption increases, thus masking any effect of a drug. In addition, the decrease in ECF volume, as well as increased intratubular pressure produced by the experimental technique, can lead to a decrease in glomerular filtration rate that also increases fractional reabsorption. Third, the increased intratubular pressure can cause inadvertent retrograde collection of tubular fluid with a high concentration of inulin, providing a falsely high fractional reabsorption.

Isolated tubule preparation. The most direct method of examining the renal tubular sites and mechanisms of action of diuretics is with the isolated perfused tubule procedure. This technique was first developed by Burg (2). Individual tubules are gently teased out of the renal tissue and immersed in ice-cold rabbit serum. An individual tubule segment is mounted on specialized glass micropipettes and held in place by gentle suction. Fluid is perfused through the tubule with a microsyringe pump or simple hydrostatic pressure and collected into a micropipette mounted at the other end of the tubule. The reabsorption of tubular fluid can then be determined by measuring the concentration of inulin in the collected fluid and comparing it to the initial perfusate inulin concentration. Transtubule electrical-potential difference and transtubule resistance can also be measured by inserting a microelectrode into the tubule lumen.

The rabbit nephron has been most extensively studied with this technique. In the isolated proximal tubule, ouabain will inhibit net fluid reabsorption, which is consistent with the notion that proximal fluid reabsorption is linked to the active transport of solute. Several diuretics are sulfonamides and possess some degree of carbonic anhydrase inhibitory activity (29). In the isolated perfused convoluted proximal tubule these agents will all inhibit fluid reabsorption to some degree. In 1973, using this technique with the isolated ascending limb, two research groups (2,3) independently observed that as sodium chloride was reabsorbed the lumen remained electrically positive in relation to the bath and that removal of chloride from the perfusate and bath (substituted with sulfate) decreased the transtubular potential difference to zero; removal of sodium and substitution with choline increased the transtubular potential difference. This was accepted as unequivocal evidence for active transport of chloride in this portion of the nephron. The isolated cortical collecting tubule demonstrated a transtubular potential of -38.5 mV that represents the profound driving force for potassium secretion in this area of the nephron.

Stop-Flow

Stop-flow provides a technically simpler alternative to micropuncture studies of isolated tubules for the determination of sites of action of diuretics. The theory behind the stop-flow technique is that if one arrests the flow of urine in the tubule, the persistence of passive and active processes will eventually permit the attainment of limiting concentration gradients for all components in the static column of urine. Analysis of serially collected samples of urine after release of the obstruction will provide a profile related to the various areas of the renal tubule and will allow localization of transport processes within the nephron.

The experiments, as originally reported by Malvin et al. (30), were conducted as follows: The ureter in the appropriate animal was cannulated; an osmotic diuresis was induced by intravenous infusion of mannitol, and after sufficient equilibration time, some free-flow urine was collected for analysis and the ureter was occluded. The occlusion was maintained for a variable length of time, usually 3 to 6 min, during which it is believed that the composition of the stationary column of fluid was altered by continuing active and passive processes until a steady state was reached. The obstruction was then released, and serial urine samples were collected in rapid succession. The concentrations of the various constituents as functions of sample number or time were plotted, and the concentration profiles served to localize the transport processes as shown in Fig. 5. The first few samples collected represented urine that was trapped in dead-space areas such as the renal pelvis and contained a sodium concentration equal to that of free-flow samples. The sodium concentration then fell precipitously to a minimum level before returning once again to free-flow levels. The area at which the minimum sodium concentration occurred was believed to represent the samples from the distal tubule and collecting duct. The sodium concentration plateau in later samples represented urine derived from

the proximal tubule, as evidenced by the PAH profile. Because PAH is secreted only in the proximal tubule, and glucose is reabsorbed at this site, the samples containing the highest PAH concentrations and lowest glucose concentrations must have been in contact with the proximal tubular epithelium for the greatest length of time. The appearance of new filtrate in stop-flow experiments can be marked by the injection of inulin or another marker during the period of stop-flow.

Stop-flow provides the possibility of examining concentration patterns for various urinary constituents from occlusions before and after administration of a diuretic in the same animal. A drug that impairs the distal tubule's ability to reabsorb sodium will elevate the distal minimum for sodium in the stop-flow pattern. However, because all urine from the

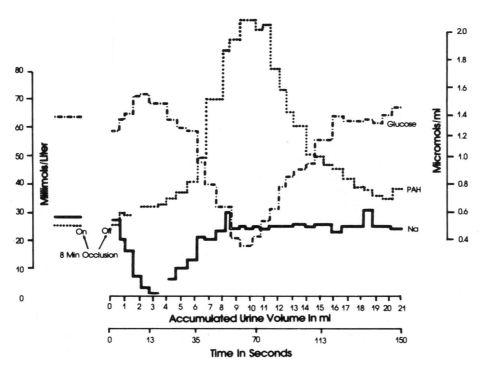

FIG. 5. Concentration patterns developed for PAH, sodium, and glucose during stop-flow in the dog. Vertical scale on the right for PAH only. The minimum concentration of sodium that occurred at 3 ml of accumulated urine represents the purest sample from distal tubular areas, whereas the maximum PAH concentration and minimum glucose concentration occurred at about 10 ml of accumulated urine and depict samples from the proximal tubule area (30).

proximal portion of the nephron must pass the distal tubule during collection, impairment of the ability of the distal tubule to reabsorb sodium could alter the concentrations of electrolytes in samples derived from the proximal tubule. A modification of the stop-flow procedure applicable to drugs that are secreted by the proximal tubular cells and are rapidly acting has been developed to avoid the problem of distal modification of proximal samples (31). The modification involves administration of the diuretic after ureteral occlusion and cessation of filtration. Therefore, the drug can gain access to the tubular fluid only by secretion and thus enters the proximal tubule, but not the distal tubule. This technique provides the opportunity to observe the influence of a proximal effect at a time when no drug has reached distal tubular cells; hence, the distal minimum for sodium remains unchanged.

Although stop-flow does provide a relatively simple method of examining tubular sites of action, it is a method that involves average values for many nephrons of various lengths. Thus, when urine from distal areas of longer nephrons reaches the renal pelvis, it mixes with urine from more proximal areas of shorter nephrons. The stop-flow pattern represents average values and hence involves some smearing. It is useful only in defining distal and proximal portions of the nephron; it cannot distinguish more finely, such as between the ascending limb of the loop of Henle and the early distal convoluted tubule, or between the proximal convoluted tubule and the descending limb of the loop of Henle.

Provided that the shortcomings of stop-flow are recognized, the technique provides a tool for easily gaining insight into the sites of action of diuretics.

Miscellaneous Techniques for Studying Diuretics

The sites and mechanisms of action of diuretics have also been examined using a variety of other techniques. Slices of renal cortex from a variety of species are used to examine how the drug itself is handled by the kidney (active transport, passive movement, transport by an acid or base transport mechanism, etc.) and also to learn something about the receptor and about how the agent influences electrolyte transport.

The ability of diuretics to influence electrolyte transport has been examined in isolated frog skin, toad bladders, red blood cells, barnacle muscle fibers, and a variety of other "transporting" tissues. Of recent interest is the cornea of the toad, which can be used as an *in vitro* model of active chloride transport.

In addition, certain species are useful for examining different aspects of renal pharmacology. For example, the presence in the chicken of a renal portal system makes it possible to administer substances to the renal tubules of one kidney and to determine tubular secretion without concern for systemic cardiovascular effects.

Pharmacology of Diuretics

The mechanism of fluid and electrolyte retention that accompanies congestive heart failure differs from that of hepatic or renal failure. These, in turn, differ from the localized edemas such as cerebral or pulmonary edema. Although diuretics may be effective in all types of edema because they function at the kidney to alter the tubular reabsorption of electrolytes, either directly or indirectly, or by influencing those hormones that regulate active tubular transport mechanisms, an understanding of their mechanisms of action can allow one to choose the best agent for a particular pathologic entity.

The drugs to be considered include osmotic diuretics, xanthines, acid-forming salts, mercurials, carbonic anhydrase inhibitors, thiazides, loop-acting diuretics, aldosterone antagonists, and some miscellaneous agents.

Osmotic Diuretics

Osmotic diuretics are primarily nonelectrolytes, such as mannitol, that are (a) freely filterable at the glomerulus, (b) not reabsorbed along the nephron to any great extent, and (c) pharmacologically inert.

Mechanism and site of action. Solutes that are not reabsorbed in the proximal tubule exert significant osmotic effects as the volume of tubular fluid decreases and their concentrations within the lumen increase. Because reabsorption in the proximal tubule is isotonic, reabsorption of proximal tubular fluid is reduced because of the presence of this added solute. In addition to increasing urine volume by retaining fluid in the tubular lumen, these agents may also increase the rates of electrolyte excretion, particularly for sodium, chloride, and potassium. Enhanced electrolyte excretion occurs only after large doses and is related to reduced reabsorption in the proximal tubule. Under normal conditions, sodium is actively reabsorbed from the proximal tubule, and water follows passively, maintaining the isosmotic composition of the proximal tubular fluid. However, in the presence of nonreabsorbable solute, the diffusion of water is impaired relative to sodium movement. Consequently, the concentration of sodium in the tubule decreases, the gradient of tubular sodium concentration to plasma sodium concentration is increased, and sodium reabsorption is depressed.

Therapeutic indications. Osmotic diuretics are not effective in the mobilization of edema fluid. They usually are given intravenously as concentrated, hyperosmotic solutions. Their main clinical applications include reduction of vitreous volume prior to iridectomy, reduction of intraocular pressure, and reduction of intracranial pressure. Mannitol can be administered, usually in combination with furosemide, to prevent renal failure following trauma to the kidney. Mannitol is extensively used prophylactically to prevent acute renal failure during a wide variety of surgical procedures in which urine flow may fall precipitously because of a decrease in filtration rate.

Toxic reactions. Although headache, nausea, vomiting, chills, lethargy, dizziness, polydipsia, confusion, and chest pains have all been observed following mannitol administration, the major toxic reaction is related to its effects on the extracellular volume compartment. Because mannitol will equilibrate with the total body extracellular space, administration to patients with cardiac decompensation or edematous conditions associated with diminished cardiac reserve can cause an acute expansion of the extracellular space, resulting in congestive heart failure or pulmonary edema, a risk that may outweigh any potential benefit in certain patients.

Xanthines and Aminouracil Diuretics

The diuretic properties of xanthines, such as caffeine and theophylline, have been recognized for many years. Early observations of the cardiac-stimulating properties of these substances led to the belief that the diuretic activity resulted from increased renal blood flow and glomerular filtration rate. In addition, direct renal tubular effects of the xanthines have been demonstrated.

Mechanism and site of action. Administration of a xanthine diuretic results in small increases in urine flow and sodium and chloride excretion, with no appreciable effect on urinary acidification or potassium excretion. The actions of the xanthines are potentiated by carbonic anhydrase inhibitors but are only slightly affected by acid–base disturbances.

Therapeutic indications. Clinically, the xanthines and related compounds may be given orally or parenterally, but they are used very sparingly because of their limited efficacy and the development of tolerance. These agents are, however, used as bronchodilators in asthma patients.

Toxic reactions. Mild gastrointestinal irritation is the most common side effect of the xanthines and related compounds. Excessive doses may result in nausea, vomiting, and epigastric pain.

Acid-forming Salts

Acidifying salts such as ammonium chloride are combinations of a labile cation and a fixed anion. Their use was first described in the early 1900s. These salts produce a diuresis that cannot be accounted for by an osmotic action, and this led to the conclusion that their acid-forming properties are responsible for the diuretic action.

Mechanism and site of action. The ammonium salts owe their acid-forming properties to the ability of the body to convert the ammonium ion to urea. Calcium chloride functions as an acidifying agent because the calcium ion is poorly absorbed and is mostly excreted in the feces as insoluble carbonate and phosphate after an oral dose. The chloride ion is readily absorbed in exchange for bicarbonate. The net effect is equivalent to the ingestion of hydrochloric acid. When ammonium chloride is absorbed, transported to the liver, and converted to urea, the by-product is again hydrochloric acid. The hydrogen that results from administration of either ammonium or calcium chloride reacts with the body buffers. Interaction with bicarbonate leads to the formation of CO_2, which can be excreted through the lungs, thus resulting in the replacement of bicarbonate, a labile ion, by chloride, a fixed ion, and the production of metabolic acidosis.

The increased chloride concentration in the extracellular fluid leads to an increased load to the renal tubules, with subsequent escape from reabsorption of some of the excess chloride. This chloride carries with it an equivalent amount of cation and an isosmotic quantity of water and hence produces a net loss of extracellular fluid.

The acidosis produced by the acidifying agents triggers renal mechanisms to compensate and normalize the acid–base balance. This is accomplished by the excretion of chloride unaccompanied by a fixed cation. The kidney increases its elaboration of ammonia, secretes more hydrogen ion, and excretes chloride in combination with ammonium. When the compensation is complete and as much ammonium chloride is excreted in the urine as is ingested orally, the drug no longer mobilizes edema fluid. This tolerance is a major problem with the use of acid-forming salts. Complete renal compensation can occur in as little as 2 days.

Therapeutic indications. The usefulness of acidifying salts as primary diuretics is limited, mostly because of the quickly developing tolerance to their diuretic action. They can be administered orally to counteract the metabolic alkalosis produced by mercurials, loop diuretics, and sometimes thiazides (although metabolic alkalosis is not common in the latter). There is no justification for chronic administration of acidifying salts as primary diuretic agents.

Toxic reactions. Oral administration of acid-forming salts can cause gastric irritation, nausea, and vomiting. Use of ammonium nitrate can result in methemoglobinemia. Acidifying salts should not be used during a marked reduction in renal function, for uncompensated acidosis can result. The use of acidifying salts is contraindicated during severe hepatic failure.

Carbonic Anhydrase Inhibitors

The carbonic anhydrase inhibitors are rarely used as primary diuretics, but they are of historical interest, for they played a major role in our understanding of fundamental renal physiology and pharmacology. Acetazolamide is the prototype of this class of agents.

$$CH_3CONH - \underset{N-N}{\overset{S}{\diamondsuit}} - SO_2NH_2$$

Acetazolamide

Carbonic anhydrase was first described by Roughton (32) in the early 1930s as an enzyme present in red blood cells that catalyzes the reversible reaction of carbon dioxide with water to form carbonic acid: $CO_2 + H_2O \rightleftharpoons H_2CO_3$. The dissociation of carbonic acid to hydrogen and bicarbonate ions and the association of these ions are instantaneous ionic reactions ($H_2CO_3 \rightleftharpoons H^+ + HCO_3^-$) that are uninfluenced by the enzyme. In the absence of carbonic anhydrase, the hydration of carbon dioxide in an aqueous medium at body temperature is relatively slow, requiring about

200 sec to come within 10% of equilibrium. The amount of carbonic anhydrase in erythrocytes is theoretically sufficient to accelerate the rate of reaction in whole blood 7,500-fold. Carbonic anhydrase has since been found in many sites, including the renal cortex, gastric mucosa, pancreas, eye, and central nervous system. An excellent review of the role of carbonic anhydrase has been provided by Maren (33).

When sulfanilamide was introduced as a chemotherapeutic agent, Strauss and Southworth (34) observed that patients receiving this drug showed transient alkaline diuresis and metabolic acidosis. A year later, Mann and Keilin (35) demonstrated that sulfanilamide and other N'-unsubstituted sulfonamides inhibit carbonic anhydrase activity *in vitro*. This, coupled with the observation of Davenport and Wilhelmi (36) that the enzyme is highly concentrated in the renal cortex, paved the way for an explanation of the way in which sulfanilamide produces an alkaline urine and metabolic acidosis. Subsequent work led to the synthesis of acetazolamide by Roblin and Clapp (37) in 1950.

Mechanism and site of action. Oral or parenteral administration of acetazolamide will result in a rapid increase in urine volume, accompanied by increases in urinary bicarbonate, sodium, and potassium excretion and a decrease in urinary chloride excretion. However, the diuretic effect of carbonic anhydrase is both weak and short-lived. The maximal amount of sodium that can be excreted after administration of acetazolamide is only approximately 2 to 4% of the filtered load. The urinary pH, which is normally acidic, becomes alkaline, accompanied by a decrease in the excretion of ammonia and titratable acid. As a result, acetazolamide will cause a decrease in the extracellular bicarbonate concentration and thus induce metabolic acidosis. Loss of bicarbonate in the urine can result in a state of equilibrium in which the small amount of hydrogen ion that is being secreted is sufficient to reabsorb the reduced amount of filtered bicarbonate. There is, therefore, no longer a sufficient loss of bicarbonate with its associated cation and water. This phenomenon may partially explain why tolerance develops. However, there must be additional factors other than decreased filtration of bicarbonate to account for tolerance, because potassium depletion, which results in extracellular alkalosis, also decreases the diuretic response (33).

In the kidney, carbonic anhydrase is located predominantly in the brush border of the proximal tubule. Although early experiments localized the site of action of acetazolamide exclusively to the distal tubule, subsequent micropuncture and free-water-clearance data indicate a pronounced effect in the proximal tubule, a minor effect in the distal tubule, and no effect in the ascending limb. The enzyme is present in vast excess; in fact, 99% of the enzyme activity must be inhibited in the kidney before any physiologic manifestations will occur. Acetazolamide is also actively secreted by the anionic transport mechanism of the proximal tubule and will therefore inhibit the secretion of other organic acids as well.

Therapeutic indications. The use of carbonic anhydrase inhibitors as diuretic agents is of more experimental value than therapeutic value. Recent discoveries of more effective and less toxic diuretics have largely replaced the once widely prescribed carbonic anhydrase inhibitors. These agents have recently been found useful for decreasing intraocular pressure in glaucoma. They have also been used as anticonvulsants for both grand mal and petit mal epilepsy.

Other applications for carbonic anhydrase inhibitors include alkalinization of the urine to enhance renal excretion of lipid-soluble weak organic acids.

Toxic reactions. Although serious side effects are rare with the carbonic anhydrase inhibitors, anorexia, weight loss, gastrointestinal distress, weakness, loss of libido, impotence, and general malaise can result (38). The malaise may be the result of systemic acidosis and can be relieved by bicarbonate administration. With large doses, drowsiness and paresthesias can occur.

Mercurial Diuretics

The use of mercury compounds as diuretics dates back to the sixteenth century, when Paracelsus observed that calomel (mercurous chloride) would increase the rate of urination. Calomel was also one of the components of the famous nineteenth-century "Guy's Hospital pill" (digitalis, squill, calomel), and it is believed to be responsible for the diuretic action of this preparation. It was not until 1920, when Saxl and Heilig noticed that merbaphen, an antisyphilitic agent containing mercury in organic linkage, caused a marked diuresis, that the diuretic effects of organic mercurials became evident (39). Subsequently, in 1924, mersalyl was introduced into therapeutics; it was followed by the production of many other organomercurials. These agents remained the drugs of choice for selective removal of edema fluid for over 30 years. However, the more recent development of less toxic diuretics has resulted in discontinuation of clinical use of the mercurials. The basic structural formula of the mercurials is pictured.

$$\begin{array}{c} \overset{\displaystyle OY}{\underset{\displaystyle |}{}} \\ R{-}CH{-}CH_2{-}Hg^+ \end{array}$$

When the beta carbon is substituted with an alkyl group, the $Hg^{2+}{-}CH_2$ bond is acid-labile, and the compound displays diuretic activity. However, when the beta carbon is unsubstituted, the $Hg^+{-}CH_2$ bond is acid-stable, and no diuretic activity is present. Mercurials usually contain a methyl or some other alkyl group at site Y and a complex organic moiety at site R. Increasing the length of the alkyl group generally will decrease the potency, and the R substitution usually will determine the distribution and excretion of the mercurial.

Mechanism and site of action. Mercurial diuretics cause an increase in the excretion of chloride, with an almost equivalent amount of sodium. However, the effects of potassium excretion are more complex. Generally, organomercurials depress potassium excretion. However, when the initial excretion rate is low, mercurials will cause a paradoxical increase in potassium excretion. The chloride loss, not accompanied by an equal loss of bicarbonate, leads to hypochloremic alkalosis. Because the disruption of the carbon-to-mercury bond is dependent on an acid environment, resistance to drug therapy can develop during long-term therapy with organomercurials. This resistance is also termed refractoriness. Administration of sodium bicarbonate, with resultant metabolic alkalosis, will render the mercurials ineffective, whereas metabolic acidosis induced by ammonium chloride will potentiate the diuretic action.

Organomercurials may act in the proximal tubule; an action there could result in a 50% reduction in the reabsorption of proximal tubular fluid. Mersalyl can cause impairment in the ability of the kidney to reabsorb solute-free water, indicating an action in the ascending limb of the loop of Henle. Stop-flow studies have also indicated that organomercurials are capable of acting in the distal tubule. Thus, the exact site of action of organomercurials remains controversial; in fact, the action may be the result of inhibition of solute and water reabsorption at multiple sites along the nephron.

As mentioned earlier, the presence of an acid-labile carbon-mercury bond appears to be essential for the diuretic activity of the mercurials. This phenomenon has been attributed to *in vivo* intrarenal release of inorganic mercury from the parent compound and involves only a small fraction of the administered dose. Rupture of the carbon-mercury bond may be catalyzed by thiols, and the postulated diuretic receptor for mercury may be a two-subunit site in which one unit is a thiol and the second is a different group. Thus, the diuretic activity would involve the release of mercuric ions ($R{-}C{-}Hg^+ \rightarrow Hg^{2+}$), which in turn would bind to the two subsites at the receptor in the renal tubule. Compounds such as dithiol and dimercaprol (BAL) have sites with greater affinity for mercury than does the renal tubular receptor. In fact, administration of these compounds will terminate the diuretic action of organomercurials.

Therapeutic indications. Because of the development of less toxic oral diuretics that are effective, organomercurials are rarely used in clinical practice, although they retain some experimental interest.

Toxic reactions. Organomercurials can produce toxic signs in the kidney, heart, skin, liver, and mucous membranes of the mouth. Intravenous injections can cause sudden death due to ventricular arrhythmias. After a rapid injection of organomercurials, intraventricular conduction can be depressed (increased QRS interval). Atrioventricular dissociation, extrasystoles, and ventricular tachycardia may precede ventricular fibrillation. In the kidney, early signs of toxicity can include albuminuria, hematuria, and cast formation. There may also be decreased glomerular filtration rate and renal plasma flow. After multiple doses of mercurials, tubular necrosis and degeneration may be evident. In the late stages of nephrotoxicity, anuria, azotemia, and edema may be present. Death can occur from renal failure. Nonfatal toxic reactions can include cloudy swelling of the hepatic parenchyma, flushing, urticaria, dermatitis, fever, nausea and vomiting, neutrophilia, and thrombocytopenia.

Thiazides

The thiazides, or benzothiadiazines, are a large group of compounds, most of which are analogues of 1,2,4-benzothiadiazine-1,1-dioxide. The structure of chlorothiazide, the first member of this class to be extensively studied, is shown.

Chlorothiazide

The discovery of the thiazides illustrates how unanticipated activity can occur in new but structurally similar chemical entities. The synthesis was an outgrowth of a search for a more potent carbonic anhydrase inhibitor.

The resulting structure was found to have increased diuretic activity and to produce a diuresis with different characteristics than that produced by carbonic anhydrase inhibitors.

Mechanism and site of action. Thiazides cause increased excretion of sodium, chloride, potassium, magnesium, water, and, to a small extent, bicarbonate ions (the latter effect probably is due to inhibition of carbonic anhydrase). In addition, chronic thiazide therapy can reduce calcium excretion. Thiazides are well absorbed from the gastrointestinal tract, and their diuretic activity is unaffected by acid–base disturbances. Thiazides, like many organic anions, are actively secreted into the proximal tubule, an event that can be blocked by probenecid. When administered during hydropenia, thiazides have no effect on free-water reabsorption (Tc_{H_2O}), suggesting that they do not act in the medullary ascending limb. When administered during water diuresis, the magnitude of the increase in urine osmolality is greater than the increase in urine volume, thus decreasing free-water excretion (C_{H_2O}). A decrease in C_{H_2O} with no corresponding effect on Tc_{H_2O} indicates a primary site of action in the cortical diluting segment. This hypothesis is supported by stop-flow and micropuncture experiments.

The thiazides have an important effect on potassium excretion. In most patients, a satisfactory diuresis is accompanied by a significant kaliuresis that, if extended, could lead to hypokalemia. Separation of the effects of thiazides on sodium and potassium has been difficult to achieve. However, at all but minimally diuretic doses, thiazides will increase potassium excretion, presumably by enhancing distal tubular secretion.

The basic pharmacologic action of all the thiazide diuretics is the same as for chlorothiazide. Individual thiazide agents will differ in their potency (milligrams necessary for effect), onset and duration of action, and effects on carbonic anhydrase. For example, bendroflumethiazide is 100 times more potent than chlorothiazide and has very little effect on carbonic anhydrase. In maximally effective doses, all thiazides are capable of inhibiting about 10% of sodium reabsorption.

Therapeutic indications. The widespread success of the thiazides is due mainly to their low toxicity and their effectiveness as outpatient medications. In patients with normal renal function, combination therapy with thiazides and potassium-sparing diuretics is effective in treating nephrotic or cirrhotic edema with ascites. They are the drugs of choice for maintenance therapy in ambulatory patients with cardiac edema. Thiazides are occasionally used to control the edema associated with premenstrual tension and corticosteroid or estrogen therapy. However, thiazides are not effective in patients with markedly impaired renal function (glomerular filtration rate less than 30 ml/min); in fact, they can exacerbate the renal insufficiency. Metolazone has been purported to be more effective than thiazides in patients with chronic renal failure. Thiazides are used extensively in the treatment of essential hypertension. This use of thiazides is discussed in Chapter 8.

Thiazides are paradoxically useful in the management of diabetes insipidus (DI). They are less effective than vasopressin in treating pituitary DI, but they are important in controlling nephrogenic DI and can result in a 50% reduction in urine output in these patients. The mechanism of action is believed to involve enhanced proximal tubular reabsorption of NaCl and water due to a diuretic-induced contraction of the extracellular space.

Toxic reactions. In experimental animals, the toxic dose of the thiazides is much larger than the pharmacologic dose. Clinical toxicity is rarely seen but can be expressed as a hypersensitivity reaction, dizziness, weakness, fatigue, and leg cramps. During chronic thiazide therapy, serum sodium, potassium, chloride, and bicarbonate concentrations should be checked periodically. Serum potassium usually falls slightly (to 3–3.5 mEq/liter) and may be associated with hypochloremic alkalosis. Although the thiazide-induced hypokalemia is not progressive and may demonstrate no

overt symptoms, episodes of diarrhea, vomiting, and anorexia can further reduce serum potassium concentrations and pose a serious threat to the patient. This is a particular problem in patients receiving digitalis who are extremely sensitive to alterations in serum potassium. In the digitalized patient, diuretic-induced alterations in serum potassium can result in serious arrhythmias. However, in the healthy ambulatory patient with mild hypertension, the observed hypokalemia due to thiazide therapy may be asymptomatic, and a potassium supplement may not be indicated (40).

Thiazides can induce hyperglycemia. This reaction usually is not clinically important, except in patients with preexisting or subclinical diabetes. Thiazides will also produce an asymptomatic hyperuricemia. The mechanism is unknown, but it may involve direct competitive inhibition of the uric acid secretory mechanism by thiazides.

Loop Diuretics

Loop diuretics, also called "high-ceiling" diuretics, are a group of chemically distinct compounds that share similar pharmacologic actions. These drugs also have the characteristic of producing a peak diuresis greater than that produced by any of the other diuretic agents. Ethacrynic acid and furosemide are the prototype compounds. Ethacrynic acid was first described by Schultz et al. (41) in 1962 in an attempt to find a compound that reacts with sulfhydryl groups in a manner similar to the mercurials. Subsequently, Beyer and associates described its unique biologic activity. Furosemide was later developed as a sulfonamide-type diuretic. Two newer agents presently available in Europe, bumetanide (now available in the United States) and muzolimine, have actions very similar to those of ethacrynic acid (*left*) and furosemide acid (*right*).

Mechanism and site of action. Administration of loop diuretics results in a prompt, profound diuresis that is greater than that produced by other diuretic agents. Following maximal doses, as much as 40 to 50% of the filtered load of sodium can be excreted at the peak of diuresis, with chloride as the accompanying anion. Potassium, magnesium, and calcium excretions are also increased. The increased potassium excretion is a result of increased distal secretion and correlates with the increase in flow rate to this segment (42).

Administration of furosemide or ethacrynic acid will result in marked decreases in both Tc_{H_2O} and C_{H_2O}, along with dissipation of the renal medullary osmotic gradient. The presence of an effect with these characteristics indicated a site of action in the ascending limb of the loop of Henle. This was further substantiated by micropuncture studies. Unequivocal proof of this site of action was provided by Burg and Green, who demonstrated that furosemide (10^{-5} M) caused a 75% decrease in the electrical-potential difference across the isolated perfused ascending limb (2) and that this was due to inhibition of chloride transport. Ethacrynic acid, like furosemide, decreased the potential difference in the isolated ascending limb. In fact, the cysteine adduct of ethacrynic acid was more effective than the parent compound in inhibiting ascending-limb chloride transport, suggesting that it may be the active form.

Both furosemide and ethacrynic acid have alternate sites of action in the proximal tubule. This proximal site for furosemide has been substantiated with micropuncture techniques (43) and can be attributed to inhibition of carbonic anhydrase. This phenomenon occurs at high doses and probably is not clinically relevant in most cases. Gussin and Cafruny (31), using a modified stop-flow technique, demonstrated that ethacrynic acid has activity in the proximal tubule also. However, early attempts to substantiate this observation with micropuncture failed to demonstrate any proximal effect of ethacrynic acid (44). In this latter experiment, urinary losses were not replaced, which resulted in a decrease in ECF volume and glomerular filtration rate. When the glomerular filtration rate was stabilized in later experiments (45), a proximal tubular site of action was demonstrated for ethacrynic acid.

Ethacrynic acid is an inhibitor of Na-K ATPase. However, it would appear that this phenomenon is not related to its diuretic activity, because, as pointed out by Hook and Williamson (46), this inhibition is seen in rats, a species that is highly resistant to the diuretic activity of ethacrynic acid. Additional evidence that inhibition of Na-K ATPase is not related to the diuretic action of ethacrynic acid was supplied by Inagaki et al. (47). They examined the binding of ethacrynic acid to a membrane preparation containing Na-K ATPase *in vitro,* as well as the influence of intrarenal infusion of ethacrynic acid on Na-K ATPase in dogs, and they concluded that their results did not support the concept that Na-K ATPase is a pharmacologic receptor for ethacrynic acid.

Loop diuretics have variable effects on renal blood flow, depending on the dosage and the rate of drug administration. After furosemide, the resulting increase in total renal blood flow is associated with a shift in flow from the medulla to the cortex. This action may involve prostaglandins and renin, because loop diuretics cause increased excretion of these agents, and indomethacin, at doses that inhibit prostaglandin synthesis, will block the prostaglandin secretion and the increase in renal blood flow caused by furosemide.

Therapeutic indications. Furosemide has received wider therapeutic acceptance than ethacrynic acid because of its lower incidence of gastrointestinal disturbances and wider dose–response curve. The loop diuretics are effective in treating the edema associated with hepatic cirrhosis and ascites, renal failure, and cardiac failure. They are particularly useful for rapid dissipation of pulmonary congestion in congestive heart failure. Furosemide, given with mannitol, is a useful tool in oliguric patients for diagnosing acute renal failure. During nephrosis or chronic renal failure, the dose of furosemide required may be higher than the usual therapeutic dose (48). The reason for this is not clear, but it may involve decreased tubular secretion or increased binding to plasma proteins.

Toxic reactions. Because of their extreme potency, the loop diuretics will quickly cause dehydration and serious losses of electrolytes that can result in hypokalemia, hypotension, and hypochloremic alkalosis. Side effects unrelated to their primary renal action, although rare, include gastrointestinal distress, skin rashes, hepatic dysfunction, paresthesias, and depression of the formed elements of blood. Hyperuricemia is quite common but is usually asymptomatic. Ototoxicity is also a side effect of these diuretics. Deafness, both transient and permanent, is a rare but serious side effect of ethacrynic acid. Furosemide has also been reported to cause transient deafness. The use of other potentially ototoxic drugs, such as aminoglycosides, in conjunction with the loop diuretics is not advisable.

Furosemide can be metabolized to a reactive intermediate that may produce hepatic or renal toxicity. This has been shown in experimental animals after massive doses. However, therapeutic treatment of renal failure may involve larger doses that may result in potentially toxic intermediates (49).

Potassium-sparing Diuretics

The diuretic therapy discussed thus far can result in increased potassium loss and hypokalemia. Potassium-sparing diuretics and supplemental potassium salts are commonly used to correct this side effect. Recently, the therapeutic value of potassium replacement in nonedematous patients has been questioned (40). In these patients, the observed hypokalemia is usually asymptomatic, and replacement therapy can (in rare instances) lead to life-threatening hyperkalemia if not properly administered. There is little justification in prescribing measures to replace potassium losses if serum potassium remains above 3 mEq/liter

unless clear symptoms develop. In edematous patients, as well as digitalized patients, potassium replacement may be necessary.

Mechanism and site of action. Spironolactone (*below left*) is a competitive inhibitor of aldosterone. Triamterene (*below right*) also acts in the distal nephron, but independent of aldosterone, to depress tubular secretion of potassium. These latter compounds will interfere with distal sodium reabsorption, re-

sulting in increased excretion of sodium and conservation of potassium. The potassium-sparing drugs are therefore not very effective diuretics, because only a small fraction of the filtered load of sodium is absorbed in the distal nephron. Spironolactone, because of its mechanism of action, is most effective when elevated circulating aldosterone levels are involved in the sodium and fluid retention. This is frequently the case following chronic therapy with one of the more potent diuretic agents. A compensatory increase in aldosterone secretion occurs in response to the diuretic-induced sodium loss, and refractoriness to the diuretic may result. Spironolactone, used either intermittently or in combination with other diuretics, is effective in preventing or overcoming the refractoriness. The evidence for this competitive nature of spironolactone for the aldosterone receptor is indirect. Spironolactone is effective only in the presence of endogenous or exogenous aldosterone. Also, the antagonistic properties of spironolactone can be overcome by increasing the concentration of aldosterone (50,51).

Triamterene produces increased excretion of sodium and chloride but has no other significant pharmacologic actions. Triamterene is not an antagonist of aldosterone and acts independent of the hormone. When administered alone to a normal patient, triamterene has minimal effect on potassium excretion. However, when given simultaneously with other diuretic agents that promote potassium loss, triamterene will cause a sharp decrease in potassium excretion. The transtubular electrical-potential difference in the distal nephron is the normal driving force for potassium secretion (52). Triamterene, by decreasing sodium reabsorption, reduces this potential difference, leading to decreased potassium excretion.

Therapeutic indications. The major therapeutic use of these agents involves their ability to reduce excessive potassium losses induced by other diuretic agents. As mentioned earlier, their value in nonedematous patients is questionable. However, their use in edematous or digitalized patients may be highly beneficial in preventing symptomatic hypokalemia and digitalis toxicity. Spironolactone is also used in the management of edema refractory to other diuretic agents.

Toxic reactions. The most serious side effect of these drugs is hyperkalemia. This may occur particularly in patients with high potassium intake, in patients with severe renal insufficiency, and in the elderly. Triamterene can produce nausea, vomiting, dizziness, and leg cramps. Spironolactone can cause minor gastrointestinal distress and gynecomastia.

Miscellaneous Diuretics

Thiazidelike Diuretics

Metolazone, quinethazone, and chlorthalidone are sulfonamide diuretics that differ slightly in structure from the thiazides. However, their pharmacologic action is essentially identical with that of the thiazides. These agents act primarily to inhibit sodium chloride reabsorption in the cortical diluting segment and in the proximal convoluted tubule. Metolazone may have a therapeutic advantage over the thiazides in that it has been reported to produce marked diuresis in patients with severely reduced glomerular filtration rate (less than 20 liters/min). Chlorthalidone is noted for its prolonged duration of action and is widely used in treatment of hypertension.

Uricosuric Agents

Many diuretics currently in use lead to urate retention and hyperuricemia due to a diuretic-induced decrease in urate excretion. This can result in acute attacks of gout in those disposed to this condition, and hyperuricemia may itself be a risk factor in the development of cardiovascular disease, urate-induced nephropathy, and carbohydrate intolerance. Ticrynofen was approved for use in the United States in 1979 as an antihypertensive agent. However, because of several reports of renal failure and death due to hepatic toxicity, this drug was voluntarily removed from the market in January 1980. Indacrynic acid is not yet available in the United States.

Mechanism and site of action. Ticrynofen, also called tienilic acid, causes prompt diuresis characterized by increases in sodium and chloride excretion and a small increase in potassium excretion. Ticrynofen is structurally similar to ethacrynic acid, but it does not appear to act at the same site. Ticrynofen causes impairment in the renal diluting mechanism, but not the concentrating mechanism, suggesting an action in the cortical diluting segment of the distal tubule. However, ticrynofen will enhance the diuresis produced by maximal doses of hydrochlorothiazide and may therefore be acting by a different biochemical mechanism than thiazides. This agent is transported into the tubule by the anionic transport system, an event that can be blocked with probenecid. In fact, in experiments with a variety of species that have either net urate excretion or reabsorption, ticrynofen has an action on urate handling similar to that of probenecid. Ticrynofen is capable of producing a fivefold increase in the clearance of uric acid.

Indacrynic acid, like ticrynofen, can inhibit proximal tubular urate reabsorption; however, unlike ticrynofen, it can also block the reabsorption of NaCl in the ascending limb.

Therapeutic indications. Ticrynofen is used mainly as an antihypertensive agent and is equal in efficacy to the thiazides (see Chapter 8). It can be used as a diuretic agent, as well as to reduce serum urate in nonedematous normotensive patients. However, because there are many other nondiuretic uricosuric agents available, a diuretic uricosuric may not be indicated. Ticrynofen is useful in relieving the symptoms of chronic congestive heart failure, particularly for those patients with a history of gout who require a diuretic similar to the thiazides in potency.

Toxic reactions. Ticrynofen can cause gastrointestinal distress, dizziness, leg cramps, and fatigue. Increases in serum creatinine and BUN may also occur. Ticrynofen also causes hypokalemia similar in magnitude to that caused by the thiazides, and, when indicated, potassium supplement may be necessary. Potassium-sparing diuretics should be avoided in this case because of the exaggerated elevation in BUN that can occur when ticrynofen is given with triamterene. Glucose intolerance and hyperglycemia can also occur. Salicylates can also inhibit the uricosuric effects of ticrynofen. As noted earlier, this drug is no longer available because of its apparent renal and hepatic toxicity.

REFERENCES

1. Valtin, H. (1973): *Renal Function: Mechanisms Preserving Fluid and Solute Balance in Health.* Little, Brown, Boston.
2. Burg, M. B., and Green, N. (1973): Function of the thick ascending limb of Henle's loop. *Am. J. Physiol.*, 224:659–668.
3. Rocha, A. S., and Kokko, J. P. (1973): Sodium chloride and water transport in the medullary thick ascending limb of Henle. Evidence for active chloride transport. *J. Clin. Invest.*, 52:612–623.
4. Ganong, W. F. (1973): *Review of Medical Physiology.* Lange Medical, Los Altos, California.
5. Rennick, B., and Quebbemann, A. J. (1971): Renal tubular excretion of drugs: Proximal tubule secretion and metabolism. In: *Renal Pharmacology,* edited by J. W. Fisher and E. J. Cafruny, pp. 68–84. Appleton-Century-Crofts, New York.
6. Gross, F., and Mohring, J. (1973): Renal pharmacology, with special emphasis on aldosterone and angiotensin. In: *Annual Reviews of Pharmacology,* edited

by H. W. Elliot, R. Okun, and R. George, pp. 57–90. Annual Reviews, Palo Alto, California.
7. Eilers, E. A., and Peterson, R. E. (1964): In: *Aldosterone. A Symposium,* edited by E. E. Baulieu and P. Robel, pp. 251–264. Blackwell Scientific, Oxford.
8. Marieb, N. J., and Mulrow, P. J. (1965): Role of the renin-angiotensin system in the regulation of aldosterone secretion in the rat. *Endocrinology,* 76:657–664.
9. Dufau, M. L., and Kliman, B. (1968): Pharmacologic effects of angiotensin-II-amide on aldosterone and corticosterone secretion by the intact anesthetized rat. *Endocrinology,* 82:29–36.
10. Kinson, G. A., and Singer, B. (1968): Sensitivity to angiotensin and adrenocorticotrophic hormone in the sodium deficient rat. *Endocrinology,* 83:1108–1116.
11. Boyd, G. W., Adamson, A. R., Arnold, M., James, V. H. T., and Peart, W. D. (1972): The role of angiotensin II in the control of aldosterone in man. *Clin. Sci.,* 42:91–104.
12. Blair-West, J. R., Coghlan, J. P., Denton, D. A., Goding, J. R., Wintour, M., and Wright, R. D. (1968): The effect of nephrectomy on aldosterone secretion in the conscious sodium-depleted hypophysectomized sheep. *Aust. J. Exp. Biol. Med. Sci.,* 46:295–318.
13. Balikian, H. M., Brodie, A. H., Dale, S. L., Melby, J. C., and Tait, J. F. (1968): Effect of posture on the metabolic clearance rate, plasma concentration and blood production rate of aldosterone in man. *J. Clin. Endocrinol. Metab.,* 28:1630–1640.
14. Bayard, R., Cooke, C. R., Tiller, D. J., Beitins, I. Z., Kowarski, A., Walker, W. G., and Migeon, C. J. (1971): The regulation of aldosterone secretion in anephric man. *J. Clin. Invest.,* 50:1585–1595.
15. Fourman, P., Reifenstein, E. C., Kepler, E. J., Dempsey, E., Bartter, R., and Albright, F. (1952): Effect of desoxycorticosterone acetate on electrolyte metabolism in a normal man. *Metabolism,* 1:242–253.
16. Lemann, J., Jr., Piering, W. F., and Lennon, E. J. (1970): Studies of the acute effects of aldosterone and cortisol on the interrelationship between renal sodium, calcium and magnesium excretion in normal man. *Nephron,* 7:117–130.
17. Gordon, A., Zanjani, E., and McLaurin, W. (1971): The renal erythropoietic factor. In: *Renal Pharmacology,* edited by J. W. Fisher and E. J. Cafruny, pp. 141–165. Appleton-Century-Crofts, New York.
18. Jacobson, L. O., Goldwasser, E., Fried, W., and Plzak, L. (1957): Role of the kidney in erythropoiesis. *Nature,* 179:633–634.
19. Jacobson, L. O., Goldwasser, E., Gurney, C. W., Fried, W., and Plzak, L. (1959): Studies on erythropoietin: The hormone regulating red cell production. *Ann. N.Y. Acad. Sci.,* 77:551–573.
20. Brown, G. E., and Roth, G. M. (1922): The anemia of chronic nephritis. *Arch. Intern. Med.,* 30:817.
21. Loge, J. P., Lange, R. D., and Moore, C. V. (1950): Characterization of the anemia associated with chronic renal insufficiency. *J. Clin. Invest.,* 29:830.
22. Forssel, J. (1954): Polycythemia and hypernephroma. *Acta Med. Scand.,* 150:155.
23. Cooper, W. M., and Tuttle, W. B. (1957): Polycythemia associated with a benign kidney lesion. Report

of a case of erythrocytosis with hydronephrosis with remission of polycythemia following nephrectomy. *Ann. Intern. Med.,* 42:1008.

24. Scriabine, A., Lefer, A. M., and Kuehl, F. A., Jr. (editors) (1980): *Prostaglandins in Cardiovasular and Renal Function.* SP Medical and Scientific, New York.

25. Cort, J. H., and Lichardus, B. (editors) (1970): *Regulation of Body Fluid Volumes by the Kidney: A Symposium on Natriuretic Hormone.* I. Karger, Basel.

26. Moller, E., MacIntosh, J. R., and Van Slyke, D. D. (1929): Studies of urea excretion: II. Relationship between urine volume and rate of urea excretion by normal adults. *J. Clin. Invest.,* 6:427.

27. Berliner, R. S., Dirks, J. H., and Cirksena, W. J. (1965): Mechanism of drug action upon kidney. XXIII International Congress. *Proc. Int. Union Physiol. Sci.,* 4:122.

28. Gertz, K. H. (1963): Transtubular sodium chloride transport and permeability for nonelectrolytes in the proximal and distal convolution of the rat kidney. *Pfluegers Arch.,* 276:336–356.

29. Baer, F. E., and Beyer, K. H. (1966): Renal pharmacology. *Ann. Neu-Pharmacol.,* 6:261–292.

30. Malvin, R. L., Wilde, W. S., and Sullivan, L. P. (1958): Localization of nephron transport by stopflow analysis. *Am. J. Physiol.,* 194:135–142.

31. Gussin, R. Z., and Cafruny, E. J. (1966): Renal sites of action of ethacrynic acid. *J. Pharmacol. Exp. Ther.,* 158:148–158.

32. Roughton, F. J. W. (1934): Recent work on carbon dioxide transport by the blood. *Physiol. Rev.,* 15:241–296.

33. Maren, T. H. (1967): Carbonic anhydrase: Chemistry, physiology and inhibition. *Physiol. Rev.,* 47:595–781.

34. Strauss, M. B., and Southworth, H. (1938): Urinary changes due to sulfanilamide administration. *Bull. Johns Hopkins Hosp.,* 63:41–51.

35. Mann, T., and Keilin, D. (1940): Sulfanilamide as a specific inhibitor of carbonic anhydrase. *Nature,* 146:164–165.

36. Davenport, H. W., and Wilhelmi, A. E. (1941): Renal carbonic anhydrase. *Proc. Soc. Exp. Biol. Med.,* 48:53–56.

37. Roblin, R. O., Jr., and Clapp, J. W. (1950): The preparation of heterocyclic sulfonamides. *J. Am. Chem. Soc.,* 72:4890–4892.

38. Grant, W. (1973): Antiglaucoma drugs: Problems with carbonic anhydrase inhibitors. In: *Symposium on Ocular Therapy, Vol. 6,* edited by I. H. Leopold, pp. 19–38. C. V. Mosby, St. Louis.

39. Vogl, A. (1950): The discovery of the organic mercurial diuretics. *Am. Heart J.,* 39:881–883.

40. Kassirer, J. P., and Harrington, J. T. (1977): Diuretics and potassium metabolism: A reassessment of the need, effectiveness and safety of potassium therapy. *Kidney Int.,* 11:505–515.

41. Schultz, E. M., Cragoe, E. J., Bicking, J. B., Balhofer, W. A., and Sprague, J. A. (1962): Alpha,beta-unsaturated ketone derivatives of aryloxyacetic acids, a new class of diuretics. *J. Med. Pharm. Chem.,* 5:660–662.

42. Giebisch, G. (1976): Effects of diuretics on renal transport of potassium. In: *Methods in Pharmacology, Vol. 4A, Renal Pharmacology,* edited by M. Martinez-Maldonado, pp. 121–164. Plenum Press, New York.

43. Morgan, T., Tadokoro, M., Martin, D., and Berliner, R. W. (1970): Effect of furosemide on Na^+ and K^+ transport studied by microperfusion of the rat nephron. *Am. J. Physiol.,* 218:292–297.

44. Berliner, R. W., Dirks, J. H., and Cirksena, W. J. (1966): Action of diuretics in dogs studied by micropuncture. *Ann. N.Y. Acad. Sci.,* 139:424–432.

45. Clapp, J. R., Nottebohm, G. A., and Robinson, R. R. (1971): Proximal site of action of ethacrynic acid: Importance of filtration rate. *Am. J. Physiol.,* 220:1355–1360.

46. Hook, J. B., and Williamson, H. E. (1965): Lack of correlation between natriuretic activity and inhibition of renal Na-K-activated ATPase. *Proc. Soc. Exp. Biol. Med.,* 120:358–360.

47. Inagaki, C., Martinez-Maldonado, M., and Schwartz, A. (1973): Some *in vivo* and *in vitro* effects of ethacrynic acid on renal Na-K-ATPase. *Arch. Biochem. Biophys.,* 158:421–434.

48. Muth, R. G. (1973): Diuretics in chronic renal insufficiency. In: *Modern Diuretic Therapy in the Treatment of Cardiovascular and Renal Disease,* edited by A. F. Lant and G. M. Wilson, pp. 294–305. Excerpta Medica, Amsterdam.

49. Mitchell, J. R., Potter, W. F., Hinson, J. A., and Follow, D. J. (1974): Hepatic necrosis caused by furosemide. *Nature,* 251:508–511.

50. Kagawa, C. M., Sturtevant, F. M., and Van Arman, C. G. (1959): Pharmacology of a new steroid that blocks salt activity of aldosterone and desoxycorticosterone. *J. Pharmacol. Exp. Ther.,* 126:123–130.

51. Liddle, G. W. (1961): Specific and non-specific inhibition of mineralocorticoid activity. *Metabolism,* 10:1021–1030.

52. Gatzy, J. T. (1971): The effect of K^+-sparing diuretics on ion transport across the excised toad bladder. *J. Pharmacol. Exp. Ther.,* pp. 580–594.

Cardiovascular Pharmacology, Second Edition, edited by Michael Antonaccio. Raven Press, New York © 1984.

Control of Renin Release and Its Alteration by Drugs

*T. Kent Keeton and **William B. Campbell

* Department of Pharmacology, University of Texas–Health Science Center at San Antonio, San Antonio, Texas 78284; and ** Department of Pharmacology, University of Texas–Health Science Center at Dallas, Dallas, Texas 75235

In 1898, Tigerstedt and Bergman (1) discovered that injection of crude extracts of rabbit kidney could raise blood pressure in anesthetized rabbits, and they suggested that this renal pressor substance, which they called "renin," might be of importance in the control of the circulation. Almost four decades passed before interest in renin was rekindled. In 1934, Goldblatt et al. (2) reported that persistent arterial hypertension could be produced by constriction of the renal artery, and they suggested that a circulating pressor substance of renal origin served as a mediator of the hypertension. It was soon determined that the substance "renin" was actually an enzyme that catalyzed the formation of a peptide with potent vasoconstrictor properties (3). Braun-Menendez et al. (4) confirmed that the pressor substance found in the venous blood in ischemic kidneys was the same as that formed when renin was incubated with blood proteins. This peptide was called either "angiotonin" or "hypertensin" until 1958, when the compromise term "angiotensin" was suggested. After synthetic angiotensin became available in 1957, it was discovered that the compound possessed numerous pharmacologic activities, each of which could contribute to the elevation and maintenance of blood pressure.

With the development of sensitive radioimmunoassay techniques for the measurement of angiotensin I (AI) and angiotensin II (AII), a great volume of literature appeared concerning the physiologic control of renin release and its relationship to human hypertension. In the course of these studies it became apparent that the amount of renin circulating in the blood was the major rate-limiting step in the formation of AII. Finally, interest in the relationship between the renin-angiotensin system and hypertension was spurred by the advent of selective competitive antagonists of AII in the early 1970s. These receptor blocking agents soon became major tools in defining the role of angiotensin in experimental hypertension [see Davis et al. (5) for a review] and clinical hypertension (6). As clinical and experimental studies on the role of the renin-angiotensin system in the causation of hypertension have progressed, it has become apparent that antihypertensive drugs and other therapeutic agents alter the rate at which renin is released from the kidney. More important, these drug-induced changes in circulating renin activity can limit or alter pharmacologic responses to antihypertensive agents.

The scientific literature concerning the role of the renin-angiotensin system in health and disease, the pharmacology of angiotensin II, and the control of renin release and its alteration by drugs is voluminous, and all facets of this subject cannot be covered in this chapter. Therefore, we shall direct the reader to pertinent review articles, with the aim of providing more detailed information for those interested in specific aspects of the renin-angiotensin system. This chapter will emphasize the physiologic control of renin release and its alteration by drugs, especially those agents used in the treatment of cardiovascular disease.

DEFINITIONS

We shall use the term "renin release" to indicate the movement of renin molecules from the granular juxtaglomerular cells of the kidney, where renin is synthesized and stored, into the blood flowing through the afferent glomerular arteriole. We have assumed that changes in plasma or serum renin activity, as measured in samples of peripheral blood, are a faithful reflection of changes in the amount of renin released into the renal afferent arterioles. Furthermore, we have used the word "renin" to refer to the proteolytic enzyme released from the kidney, not the renin

isozymes found in other tissues such as the uterus, brain, and salivary gland. Renin also has been identified in the arterial wall, and a portion of this renin is of renal origin.

ANATOMY OF THE JUXTAGLOMERULAR APPARATUS

A brief description of the anatomic relationships of the structures composing the juxtaglomerular (JG) apparatus or complex is prerequisite for any discussion of the mechanisms controlling renin release. Each nephron has a region known as the JG apparatus that is composed of (a) granular cells, (b) the macula densa, (c) agranular cells, and (d) mesangial cells (Fig. 1).

The granular JG cells, which synthesize, store, and secrete renin, are differentiated smooth-muscle cells that are usually found in the media of the renal afferent arteriole just

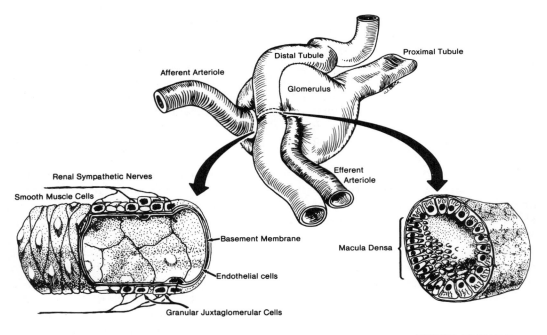

AFFERENT ARTERIOLE   **DISTAL TUBULE**

FIG. 1. Anatomic relationships of the granular JG cells, which synthesize and release renin, and the afferent arteriole, renal sympathetic nerves, and macula densa cells of the distal tubule. (Adapted from Barajas, ref. 24 and Netter, ref. 258).

adjacent to the glomerulus. Granular JG cells are sometimes found in the wall of the efferent arteriole and among the mesangial cells, but their presence in the afferent arteriole is more prominent. Myofibrils, which are characteristic of vascular smooth-muscle cells, are observed in the granular JG cells. The granules found in these cells are relatively homogeneous and dense and are membrane-bound. The granular JG cells have a well-developed endoplasmic reticulum and Golgi membranes, cytologic characteristics that are consistent with an endocrine function. The renal sympathetic nerves innervate the granular JG cells (Fig. 1).

The macula densa segment of the distal tubule, a specialized group of heavily nucleated cells located on the glomerular side of the tubule, always lies in close contact with the vascular pole of the glomerulus, from which the tubule originates (Fig. 1). The cells of the macula densa, which may be columnar or cuboidal, depending on the species studied, mark the transition from the ascending limb of the loop of Henle to the distal tubule. As the ascending limb of the loop of Henle approaches the glomerulus, it runs parallel with the efferent arteriole for some distance and then comes into brief contact with the afferent arteriole before becoming the convoluted portion of the distal tubule. The cells of the macula densa are in close contact with the granular JG cells of the afferent arteriole.

It also should be pointed out that at the hilus of the glomerulus, both the afferent and efferent arterioles have a lumen that is about two to five times the thickness of the vascular wall, but the wall of the efferent arteriole quickly thins to the point that the vessel resembles a thin-walled venule. The efferent arteriole then courses for some distance before branching into the peritubular capillaries.

RENIN

A brief description of the enzymic steps involved in the renin-angiotensin system is another important prerequisite for readers not familiar with the subject of renin release. Renin is a proteolytic enzyme of approximately 40,000 MW that is released into the bloodstream in response to certain physiologic stimuli. Once in the blood, renin cleaves the leucylleucine bond that joins the amino-terminal decapeptide AI to the remainder of the renin substrate (also called angiotensinogen) (Fig. 2). Renin is synthesized and stored in the JG cells that line the afferent glomerular arteriole (Fig. 1), whereas renin substrate (approximately 60,000 MW) is produced in the liver and is widely distributed in the blood and other extracellular fluids. After AI is released from renin substrate, converting enzyme (also known as kininase II) removes two amino acid residues from its carboxy terminus to yield AII. The conversion of AI to AII once was thought to occur predominantly in lung tissue, but it is now known that this reaction occurs in vascular endothelium throughout the body. The heptapeptide des-Asp-AII, which is formed from AII *in vivo,* also possesses many of the pharmacologic actions of AII and has been called angiotensin III (AIII).

Angiotensin II has a very short half-life

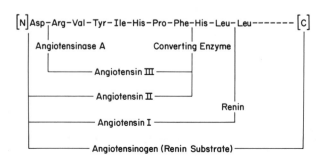

FIG. 2. Amino acid sequences of AI, AII, and AIII.

(~30 sec) in the blood, and its continued production is dependent on the presence of renin substrate and renin. However, the concentration of renin substrate in the blood is usually constant, and, in point of fact, it is the amount of renin circulating in the blood that is the major rate-limiting step in the production of AII *in vivo*. On the other hand, despite the fact that renin has a much longer half-life in the circulation (~4–15 min), a constant stimulus still is required to chronically increase the rate of renin release from the kidney.

Those readers interested in a more comprehensive review of the biochemistry of the renin-angiotensin system should consult Erdos (7) and Peach (8).

ROLE OF THE RENIN-ANGIOTENSIN SYSTEM IN REGULATION OF ARTERIAL BLOOD PRESSURE AND PLASMA VOLUME

The octapeptide AII is a potent compound that has numerous pharmacologic effects, all of which are directed at increasing blood pressure (Fig. 3). Its principal effect is that of vaso-

constriction due to a direct action on vascular smooth muscle. In addition, AII increases cardiac contractility *in vitro* both by a direct action on the myocardium (9) and by potentiating the release of norepinephrine from the cardioaccelerator nerves (10). It should be noted that the direct positive inotropic and chronotropic effects of AII usually are masked *in vivo* because of the fact that the systemic pressor effects of AII elicit a baroreflex-mediated increase in cholinergic tone to the heart. By an action in the central nervous system, AII elicits an increase in efferent nerve activity to the peripheral sympathetic nervous system that results in increases in cardiac output and total peripheral resistance (11), the two major determinants of blood pressure. Because the area postrema, which has been identified as one site of action of the central cardiovascular effects of AII, lies outside the blood-brain barrier, circulating AII has the potential to elicit these central-nervous-system-mediated events. In addition, AII has a dipsogenic effect when injected into the ventricular system of the brain (12), but it is not known at this time whether or not circulating AII has free access

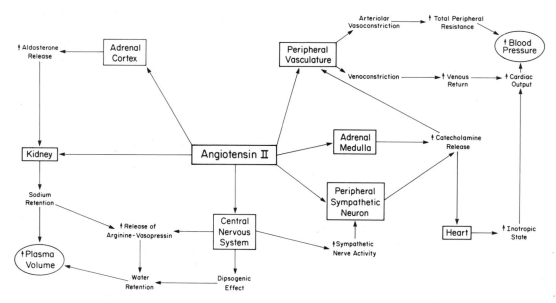

FIG. 3. Role of the renin-angiotensin-aldosterone system in regulation of arterial blood pressure and plasma volume.

to the receptors involved. In addition to increasing efferent sympathetic nerve activity through an action in the central nervous system, AII causes the release of epinephrine and norepinephrine from the adrenal medulla (13), facilitates the release of norepinephrine from the peripheral sympathetic neurons (14), and blocks the uptake of norepinephrine by peripheral sympathetic neurons (15).

Aside from its direct and indirect vasoconstrictor effects, AII increases steroidogenesis in the zona glomerulosa of the adrenal cortex (16). This action results in increased synthesis and release of the mineralocorticoid aldosterone. Although AII is a major determinant of the rate of synthesis and release of aldosterone, it should be appreciated that adrenocorticotropic hormone and an increase in plasma potassium concentration also increase the adrenal production of aldosterone. Aldosterone acts at specific receptors in the distal tubule and collecting duct of the kidney to increase the reabsorption of sodium and the secretion of potassium. Because aldosterone causes an increase in the urinary excretion of potassium, aldosterone is one of the major factors that protects the body from hyperkalemia. Thus, it is not surprising that an increase in plasma potassium concentration stimulates the synthesis and release of aldosterone. As total body sodium content increases under the influence of aldosterone, water reabsorption in the collecting duct is increased because of an increase in circulating arginine vasopressin (AVP). In this particular situation, two events lead to an increase in the release of AVP from the pituitary gland. First, the continued increase in sodium reabsorption caused by aldosterone would result in hypernatremia if plasma volume remained constant. However, as plasma sodium concentration begins to increase, osmoreceptors located in the hypothalamus are stimulated, resulting in increased release of AVP from the pituitary gland. Second, circulating AII directly causes the release of AVP from the neurohypophysis (17). The increased reabsorption of water prevents hypernatremia and at the same time causes expansion of the extracellular fluid (ECF) volume. Finally, AII itself exerts a direct antinatriuretic effect in the kidney when administered in small doses (18).

All of these effects of AII help to restore and maintain blood pressure when the body is threatened by hypovolemia and/or hypotension. Each of these effects of AII has a different response time and produces a different amount of gain in the maintenance of blood pressure. Thus, the direct and indirect "pressor" effects of AII represent a major homeostatic mechanism involved in long-term maintenance and control of blood pressure. Against this background, it is apparent that drug-induced alterations of renin release are of great importance in experimental and clinical medicine.

MEASUREMENT OF PLASMA (SERUM) RENIN ACTIVITY AND PLASMA (SERUM) RENIN CONCENTRATION

Plasma renin activity (PRA) is a measure of the ability of plasma to generate AI *in vitro* given the amounts of renin and renin substrate present in the sample. The same considerations apply to serum renin activity (SRA), and determinations of PRA and SRA yield comparable values. PRA usually is expressed in units of nanograms of AI generated per milliliter of plasma per hour of incubation at 37°C (ng AI/ml/hr) and generally is accepted as being a reflection of the level of activity of the renin-angiotensin system *in vivo*. Plasma renin concentration (PRC) is a measure of the ability of plasma to generate AI *in vitro* given the amount of renin present in plasma, but with an excess of exogenous renin substrate (usually homologous) added to the sample. PRC usually is expressed in units of nanograms of AI generated per milliliter of undiluted plasma sample per hour of incubation at 37°C (ng AI/ml/hr) and generally is accepted as being a reflection of the amount of renin circulating *in vivo*. With few exceptions, an increase in PRA is accompanied by an increase in PRC. Despite this high degree of correlation between PRA and PRC, the values for PRC always are higher than the corresponding values for PRA. This difference stems from the fact that the reaction of renin and renin substrate in plasma samples, as during the determination of PRA, does not obey zero-order (substrate-independent) kinetics. This adherence to first-order kinetics by renin results from the fact that the concentration of renin substrate in plasma is not high enough to result in substrate saturation (19). Thus, an increase in the circulating levels of renin substrate can lead to an increase in PRA, even though the amount of renin in the plasma remains constant.

During short-term experiments with animals and humans, changes in PRA are almost always due to a change in the rate of renin release from the kidney, because the concentration of plasma renin substrate is not subject to rapid changes. However, during long-term therapy with certain drugs (e.g., oral contraceptives), an increase in PRA potentially may be due to an increase in the production of renin substrate by the liver.

PATHOPHYSIOLOGIC STATES ASSOCIATED WITH INCREASE OR DECREASE IN RENIN RELEASE

Many pathophysiologic states are associated with an increase or decrease in renin release (Table 1). As a result, many of the abnormalities of blood pressure, renal function, plasma electrolyte balance, and intravascular and extravascular volumes observed in these pathophysiologic states can be attributed to an increase or a decrease in the level of activity of the renin-angiotensin-aldosterone system.

TABLE 1. *Pathophysiologic states associated with an increase or decrease in renin release*

Increased renin release	Decreased renin release
Hemorrhage	Water immersion
Acute and chronic sodium depletion	Primary aldosteronism (Conn's syndrome)
Thoracic caval constriction	Congenital adrenal hyperplasia
Congestive heart failure	Cushing's syndrome
Renal artery stenosis	Liddle's syndrome
Coarctation of the aorta	Excessive ingestion of licorice
Hypertension after renal transplantation	Hypothyroidism
Acute pyelonephritis	Salt loading
Cirrhosis with ascites	Iodiopathic autonomic insufficiency
Hepatorenal syndrome	Diabetic neuropathy
Hemodialysis	Potassium loading
Acute metabolic acidosis	Low-renin hypertension
Acute respiratory acidosis	
Dehydration	
Ethanol intoxication and hangover	
Adrenalectomy	
Addison's disease	
Increased ureteral pressure	
Malignant hypertension with renal failure	
Tumors of the JG cells	
Wilms' tumor	
Hyperthyroidism	
Acute renal failure	
Salt-wasting nephritis	
Nephrotic syndrome	
Insulin-induced hypoglycemia	
Toxemia of pregnancy	
Chronic potassium depletion	
High-renin hypertension	
Bartter's syndrome	

PHYSIOLOGIC CONTROL OF RENIN RELEASE

Because all drugs ultimately affect renin release by altering one or more of the physiologic mechanisms controlling renin release, a brief discussion of these mechanisms is important. During the past 20 years, five basic mechanisms controlling renin release have been described. They are (a) an intrarenal baroreceptor, (b) the sympathetic nervous system and humorally released catecholamines, (c) the amount of sodium (or possibly chloride) ion sensed by the macula densa segment of the distal tubule, (d) other hormonal factors (e.g., AII, prostaglandins, steroids), and (e) plasma electrolytes (e.g., potassium, calcium).

Intrarenal Vascular Receptor or Baroreceptor

In 1959, Tobian et al. (20) proposed the existence of a renal baroreceptor that either increased or decreased renin release in response to a decrease or an increase in mean renal perfusion pressure, respectively. According to Tobian's "stretch-receptor" hypothesis, an increase in renal perfusion pressure or renal (afferent arteriolar) vasodilation will stretch the wall of the afferent arteriole. The granular JG cells also will be stretched, because they are located in the media of the afferent arterioles, and this increased stretch will result in a decrease in renin release. Conversely, a decrease in renal perfusion pressure or renal vasoconstriction will lead to a decrease in renin release. In the ensuing years, many experiments have been conducted to test this hypothesis, and although changes in renal perfusion pressure per se have been shown to alter renin release, considerable controversy has existed concerning the nature of the physical factors sensed by this renal baroreceptor (21). However, when all of the results are taken collectively, renal baroreceptor-mediated renin release appears to involve physical changes in the afferent arteriole and possibly changes in the synthesis of renal prostaglandins (22). The release of renin is inversely related to the "stretch" of the afferent arteriole, and the amount of stretch can be described by wall tension (circumferential stress) or volume strain (21,23), which are affected by changes in intraluminal and interstitial pressures and the internal and external radii of the afferent arteriole. The most important determinants of wall tension, however, appear to be changes in intraluminal pressure (renal perfusion pressure) or the transmural pressure gradient (the difference between intraluminal pressure and renal interstitial pressure). In short, an increase in renal perfusion pressure inhibits renin release, whereas a decrease in renal perfusion pressure elevates renin release. Prostaglandins seem to mediate a large portion of renal baroreceptor-mediated renin release when renal perfusion pressure is decreased, as long as the capacity of the kidney to autoregulate blood flow is not exceeded (22). Because physical distortion of tissues has been found to stimulate prostaglandin synthesis, it is tempting to speculate that renal prostaglandins are a chemical link between changes in wall tension (or volume strain) and the increased renin release seen during renal arteriolar hypotension.

Sympathetic Nervous System

One of the most important factors controlling renin release is the level of activity of the renal sympathetic nerves, which have been shown to innervate the granular JG cells (24). Either direct or indirect stimulation of the renal nerves leads to an increase in renin release (21). Moreover, this sympathetically mediated renin release has been shown to be the result of stimulation by norepinephrine of β-adrenergic receptors located on the granular JG cells. For example, Taher et al. (25) stimulated the renal nerves of anesthetized dogs at a frequency that consistently increased renin secretion 5- to 10-fold without altering renal blood flow (RBF), glomerular filtration rate (GFR), or sodium excretion. The increase in renin secretion seen during nerve stimulation was blocked by *l*-propranolol or *d,l*-propranolol, but not by *d*-propranolol, which possesses only 1/100th of the β-adrenergic receptor blocking potency of *l*-propranolol. Because no significant change in mean arterial pressure (MAP), RBF, GFR, or urinary electrolyte excretion occurred in any of these experiments, the increase in renin secretion could not have occurred via activation of the renal baroreceptor or macula densa. Again, the stereospecific blockade of nerve-stimulated renin release by propranolol emphasized the fact that the norepinephrine released by the renal sympathetic nerves impinged on β-adrenergic receptors located on the granular JG cells of the kidney.

The physiologic stimulation of the renal nerves *in vivo* originates within the central nervous system, and several neural reflexes involved in cardiovascular homeostasis affect renin release. A decrease in arterial pressure in the carotid sinus leads to a reflex activation of the renal sympathetic nerves, and, accordingly, bilateral occlusion of the carotid arteries has been shown to elicit renin release in anesthetized dogs (26). As would be expected, a decrease in systemic blood pressure, as seen after the administration of vasodepressor drugs, also reflexly activates the renal sympathetic nerves, leading to a neurally mediated increase in renin release (27). In addition to the carotid baroreflex, other neural pathways that affect the level of activity of the peripheral sympathetic nervous system originate in one or more receptors located in the cardiopulmonary region. In years past, the role of the arterial (carotid and aortic) baroreceptors in controlling peripheral sympathetic outflow has been stressed, but more recently cardiopulmonary receptors in the atria, ventricles, and lungs have been found to affect the firing rate of the noradrenergic nerves that innervate the peripheral vascular beds, including the kidney. Consistent with these observations, Mancia et al. (28) discovered the existence of vagally innervated receptors in the cardiopulmonary region that tonically restrain renin release by suppressing efferent renal nerve activity. That is, interruption of afferent vagal nerve impulses, by bilateral cooling of the cervical vagi (28) or bilateral cervical vagotomy (29), increased PRA in anesthetized dogs.

Suppression of renin release by cardiopulmonary receptors occurs rapidly. Zehr et al. (30) found that mechanical distension of the left atrial-pulmonary region of sodium-depleted anesthetized dogs suppressed renin secretion by 50% within 5 min after distension had begun. Central venous pressure, MAP, and RBF were unchanged. This rapid suppression of renin secretion was prevented by either renal denervation or bilateral cervical vagotomy, which indicated that left atrial distension reduced renin secretion via vagal afferent and renal sympathetic efferent nerve pathways.

Because both the arterial baroreceptors and cardiopulmonary receptors can alter renin release by affecting sympathetic neurotransmission, Thames et al. (31) studied the relationship between these two neural pathways in the control of renin release. On the basis of studies with anesthetized dogs, it was concluded that (a) cardiopulmonary receptors with vagal afferent pathways tonically inhibit renin release even in the presence of a normally functioning carotid baroreceptor system, (b) these cardiopulmonary receptors can respond to a decrease in central blood volume that does not activate the arterial baroreceptors, and (c) the normal buffering effects of the arterial baroreceptors can inhibit the increase in renin secretion that normally results from complete interruption of vagal afferent nerve traffic originating in the cardiopulmonary receptors.

The exact nature of the stimulus for these cardiopulmonary receptors cannot be stated with certainty, but inhibitory signals from heart and lungs appear to be associated with the increase in stretch or volume associated with the filling of the chambers of the heart or the pulmonary artery. Because venous return is an important determinant of cardiac output, many investigators believe that these cardiopulmonary receptors help to maintain blood pressure at a constant value during changes in blood volume. That is, when venous return to the heart is reduced as a result of a decrease in blood volume, fewer inhibitory vagal afferent signals travel to the brain to suppress sympathetic nerve activity and renin release. As a result, the disinhibition of efferent sympathetic nerve activity increases vasomotor tone by releasing norepinephrine and stimulating renin release. Thus, blood pressure is maintained by increasing venous return (venoconstriction) and total peripheral resistance (arteriolar constriction).

With these facts in mind, the reader can discern that the arterial and cardiopulmonary baroreceptors share one common feature, viz., the phasic stimulation of these receptors during the cardiac cycle sends neural signals to the brain that restrain the activity of the peripheral sympathetic nervous system. These two sets of baroreceptors work in concert to monitor the functional status of the cardiovascular system, and interruption of afferent neural signals from one set of baroreceptors results in an increase in afferent inhibitory signals from the other set of baroreceptors.

It is important to note that the majority of the studies aimed at discovering the functional significance of cardiopulmonary receptors have been conducted with dogs. The existence of cardiopulmonary-volume receptors that control renin release in humans has been questioned. Hesse et al. (32) reported that an acute 10% reduction in blood volume in humans did not increase PRA even though right atrial pressure was decreased. Previous investigators (33) also had reported that the removal of 400 to 600 ml of blood from humans, which would be expected to decrease venous return to the heart, did not increase PRA. When two groups of clinical investigators (34,35) attempted to assess the control of renin release by low-pressure cardiopulmonary receptors in humans, conflicting conclusions were reported. However, as pointed out by Mark et al. (35), it may be difficult to demonstrate the neural control of renin release by cardiopulmonary receptors in the presence of the tonic inhibition from the arterial barore-

ceptors. Despite the controversy surrounding this issue, the reader should keep in mind the possibility that drugs that elevate renin release by reflexly mediated activation of the renal sympathetic nerves may do so by affecting the afferent input from the arterial and/or cardiopulmonary receptors.

In addition to neurally released norepinephrine in kidney, circulating catecholamines have been shown to increase renin release (21). One problem in demonstrating an increase in renin release by infusing norepinephrine and epinephrine is the fact that sufficiently large quantities of these catecholamines will increase systemic blood pressure, an effect that will tend to suppress renin release by increasing renal perfusion pressure. However, Vander (36) found that both norepinephrine and epinephrine stimulated renin release in anesthetized dogs in which renal perfusion pressure was held at the control level. At first it was believed that the renal vasoconstriction (37) and decrease in sodium excretion (36) caused by the catecholamines were responsible for the rise in renin release, but Ueda et al. (38) proved otherwise. When norepinephrine was infused intravenously into anesthetized dogs, PRA increased threefold as blood pressure rose. RBF, GFR, and sodium excretion dropped. However, dibenamine, an α-adrenergic antagonist, completely reversed the effects of norepinephrine on RBF, GFR, and sodium excretion but did not alter the ability of norepinephrine to elicit renin release. Propranolol did impair norepinephrine-induced renin release. Therefore, Ueda et al. (38) concluded that circulating catecholamines elevated PRA by direct stimulation of β-adrenergic receptors located on the granular JG cells.

Consistent with the latter conclusion, Weinberger et al. (39) found that both norepinephrine and epinephrine caused a concentration-related increase in renin secretion from rat renal cortical slices *in vitro* when added at concentrations ranging from 10^{-9} to 10^{-7} M. Thus, Weinberger et al. (39) demonstrated that norepinephrine and epinephrine were capable of stimulating renin release *in vitro* in concentrations that were comparable to those observed in the plasma in conscious rats. Norepinephrine- and epinephrine-stimulated renin secretion was inhibited by *d,l*-propranolol and *l*-propranolol but was not affected by *d*-propranolol or phentolamine, an α-adrenergic antagonist (39). As with the studies in animals, intravenous infusion of both norepinephrine and epinephrine into normal and hypertensive humans has been shown to increase PRA (40). Isoproterenol, a nonselective β-adrenergic agonist, has been shown in many studies to stimulate renin release in rabbits, cats, rats, dogs, and humans (21).

Although dopamine is a naturally occurring catecholamine, its ability to alter renin release is unclear. Dopamine has been shown to increase renin secretion from rat renal cortical slices *in vitro* (41). Because dopamine-induced renin release was blocked by *d,l*-propranolol, but not by the dopamine antagonist haloperidol, Henry et al. (41) concluded that dopamine stimulated renin release by interacting with renal β-adrenergic receptors rather than dopaminergic receptors. On the other hand, Imbs et al. (42) found that the increase in renin secretion seen during intrarenal arterial infusion of dopamine into the denervated kidneys of anesthetized dogs was blocked by haloperidol, a dopamine antagonist, but not by *d,l*-propranolol. Intravenous infusion of dopamine has not been demonstrated to have a consistent effect on renin release in humans (21).

In summary, the renal sympathetic nerves exert a marked effect on renin release, and renal nerve activity is, in turn, controlled by several neural reflex arcs. Circulating catecholamines also stimulate renin release. It should be mentioned that accelerated renal sympathetic nerve activity has been implicated as a cause for the increased renin release that accompanies or follows a number of stimuli: psychosocial stimuli, auditory stimuli, intermittent electrical shock, and exercise in rats; immobilization stress in rabbits; heat stress and avoidance operant conditioning in ba-

boons; heat stress, running exercise, the hypnotic suggestion of running, mental arithmetic, psychosocial stimuli, operant conditioning for cardioacceleration, ethanol intoxication and hangover, passive tilt, the assumption of upright posture, and high-renin hypertension in humans.

Renal Sodium Metabolism and the Macula Densa Segments of the Distal Tubule

As pointed out earlier, the macula densa segment of the distal tubule is composed of a specialized group of columnar or cuboidal cells that are in close contact with the granular JG cells of the glomerulus from which the tubule originates. The macula densa usually is found at the boundary of the ascending limb of the loop of Henle and the distal tubule. Both light and electron microscopy have revealed that the macula densa and the granular JG cells of a single nephron are so intimately related that at times only an incomplete basement membrane separates them. Vander (43) has presented an excellent review of the anatomic and biochemical evidence that suggests a functional relationship between the macula densa cells and the granular cells of the JG apparatus. Although some researchers believe that the single-nephron GFR is in some way controlled by the ionic composition of the tubular urine at the macula densa via the release of renin by the granular JG cells, the role of the macula densa as a sensor for renin secretion into the blood will be considered here.

In 1963, Brown et al. (44) discovered that sodium depletion in humans elevated PRA and that sodium loading suppressed PRA. In subsequent years, this observation has been corroborated in humans, dogs, rats, rabbits, and sheep. Total daily sodium excretion falls to very low levels during sodium depletion because of a decrease in the fractional excretion of filtered sodium. Because much of the increase in the efficiency of sodium reabsorption occurs in the proximal tubule, the tubular sodium concentration and sodium load (the product of sodium concentration and the flow rate of the tubular fluid) passing the macula densa segment of the distal tubule will be decreased. Conversely, sodium loading results in an increase in total daily sodium excretion. Fractional reabsorption of sodium decreases in the proximal tubule, and, as a result, the tubular sodium concentration and sodium load passing the macula densa are increased. Because sodium depletion results in a decrease in intravascular volume, it would be reasonable to believe that the stimulation of renin release by sodium depletion occurs in order to increase and/or maintain sodium reabsorption and intravascular volume via aldosterone. Based on these observations, it also would be reasonable to conclude that a decrease in sodium transport into the macula densa cells would constitute a stimulus to renin release, whereas an increase in sodium transport at the macula densa cells would suppress renin release.

Original studies of Vander and Miller (45) indicated that renin release was indeed inversely related to the tubular sodium concentration or load in the region of the macula densa. Most subsequent investigations of this mechanism involved the use of physiologic or pharmacologic perturbations to alter renal sodium excretion in an attempt to relate the rate of renin release to changes in sodium metabolism. Unfortunately, the pharmacologic approach proved to be of limited value, because it initially led to the establishment of two schools of thought. One group (46–48) proposed that an increase in renin release resulted from an increase in sodium transport at the macula densa, whereas the other (49–55) believed that renin release was inversely related to sodium transport at the macula densa.

Because the "loop" diuretics were known to inhibit sodium reabsorption in the thick ascending limb of the loop of Henle and to cause a large increment in the sodium content of the tubular urine passing the macula densa, the former group of researchers (46–48) examined the effects of furosemide and ethacrynic acid on renin release in anesthetized animals.

Based on the data from these studies, it was concluded that the rate of renin release was directly related to amount of sodium passing the macula densa. Although later we shall discuss in greater detail the mechanisms by which furosemide and ethacrynic acid increase renin secretion, the reader should be apprised at this time that both drugs increase renin release by mechanisms that are not directly related to their diuretic activity but probably are mediated via the renal baroreceptor, the renal sympathetic nerves, renal prostaglandins, and/or a direct effect on the granular JG cells of the afferent arteriole. In addition, both furosemide and ethacrynic acid appear to inhibit ion transport at the macula densa cells and thus prevent the macula densa from sensing the increases in tubular sodium concentration and load caused by these drugs. These facts being considered, the observations of these investigators (46–48) are easily reconciled with the original hypothesis (45) that renin release is inversely related to the sodium concentration or load passing the macula densa.

Fortunately, a great deal of research in this area has involved physiologic manipulation of sodium excretion that did not involve the administration of diuretics. The studies of Nash et al. (52), Humphreys et al. (54), and Churchill et al. (55) have indicated that renin secretion, as controlled by the macula densa, is inversely related to tubular sodium concentration or load. More recently, Churchill et al. (49,50) conducted elegant micropuncture experiments that strongly supported the idea that sodium load, rather than tubular sodium concentration, is the factor controlling renin release by the macula densa. In addition, Shade et al. (56) reported that glomerular filtration was necessary for sodium loading to inhibit renin release. Therefore, this inhibition is mediated by a renal tubular mechanism rather than a direct effect on sodium on the granular JG cells. The latter conclusion is supported by observations made with renal cortical slices and renal cortical cell suspensions *in vitro* (57,58). If one considers only the range of sodium concentrations that are observed *in vivo* (i.e., 100–160 mEq/liter), changes in sodium concentration had only slight effects on renin release *in vitro*. Studies conducted with sheep, dogs, and humans have indicated that the expansion of ECF volume per se that occurs during saline infusion is not a factor in the suppression of renin release caused by this intervention. Lastly, Kotchen et al. (59) have presented convincing evidence that chloride, rather than sodium, is the ion sensed by the macula densa in the control of renin release. In this respect, it is interesting to note that the cells of the macula densa are morphologically similar to the epithelial cells of the thick ascending limb of Henle's loop, and chloride, rather than sodium, is the ion actively transported in the ascending limb of Henle's loop (60).

When all of these observations are considered collectively, it is apparent that renin secretion is inversely related to the tubular sodium and/or chloride load sensed by the macula densa cells of the distal tubule. This relationship, as established in animal experiments, is consistent with the observations made during sodium depletion and loading in humans.

Other Plasma Electrolytes

Potassium

Potassium loading suppresses renin release (61), and potassium depletion increases renin release (62). Small changes in serum potassium concentration have been shown to exert profound effects on the release of renin, and this control mechanism may be of physiologic significance. This inverse relationship has been noted between potassium balance and renin release in rats, dogs, and humans. The mechanism by which potassium suppresses renin release appears to involve an increase in the delivery of sodium to the macula densa, because potassium had no inhibitory effects in dogs with a single nonfiltering kidney or in rat renal cortical slices *in vitro*. Although it is unclear whether or not potassium inhibits proximal tubular reabsorption of sodium, intrarenal arterial administration of potassium consistently induces a natriuresis. Because it is this increase in sodium excretion that appears to suppress renin release, potassium must inhibit sodium reabsorption at some point proximal to the macula densa, possibly in the ascending limb of the loop of Henle. On the other hand, the suppression of PRA in humans by chronic potassium loading appears to be independent of whether or not this dietary alteration induces a natriuresis. Although studies in adrenalectomized animals and Addisonian patients suggest that an increase in the circulating level of aldosterone is required for potassium loading to inhibit renin release, further studies are necessary to clarify this point. Because inhibitors of prostaglandin synthesis have been found to inhibit the renin release caused by potassium depletion in dogs and the hypokalemia and hyperreninemia in patients with Bartter's syndrome, a role for renal prostaglandins must be considered in the control of renin release by potassium.

Calcium

The presence of calcium ion in secretory and smooth-muscle cells is an important requirement for stimulus-secretion coupling and excitation-contraction coupling. Because the granular JG cells are both secretory cells and smooth-muscle cells, it is not surprising that calcium ion affects renin release. When considering the role of calcium in renin release, it appears that intracellular, rather than extracellular, calcium is the most important determinant. If intracellular calcium levels are decreased by β-adrenergic stimuli (63), calcium chelators such as EDTA or EGTA (64), or the absence of extracellular calcium (64), renin release is stimulated. In contrast, if the intracellular levels of calcium are elevated by decreasing the efflux of calcium with lanthanum (65) or by increasing calcium influx with high potassium concentration (64), ouabain (66), AII (67), or calcium ionophores (68), renin release is inhibited. It is puzzling why the secretory activity of the granular JG cells evolved so differently from that of other secretory cells, in which an increase in intracellular calcium concentration stimulates secretion. Churchill et al. (69) have suggested that renin secretion is a function of the transmembrane sodium gradient of the granular JG cells, which in turn governs the influx and efflux of calcium from the cells.

Magnesium

From the available data, it appears that an increase in plasma magnesium concentration stimulates the release of renin, whereas a decrease in plasma magnesium concentration lowers renin release. Although the mechanism by which magnesium effects these changes is unknown, much of the evidence points to a direct effect of magnesium on the granular JG cells. In this respect, magnesium may elevate renin release by inhibiting the movement of calcium across the membrane of the granular JG cells. The physiologic, pharmacologic, and pathophysiologic importance of magnesium in the control of renin release remains to be determined.

Circulating Hormones

AII

In 1965, Vander and Geelhoed (70) proposed a pressure-independent mechanism by which circulating levels of AII would inhibit renin release by a direct intrarenal action. Subsequent studies conducted in animals (71) and humans (72,73) have supported the idea that AII inhibits renin release by a direct action on the granular JG cells. Subpressor doses of AII, given intravenously, have been shown to inhibit renin release in humans (72,73) by a mechanism independent of aldosterone. Carey et al. (72) found AII and AIII to be equipotent in suppressing renin release in normotensive humans on a normal or low-sodium diet. Several research groups have described the ability of AII to inhibit renin release from renal cortical slices *in vitro* (74) and from isolated perfused rat kidney (67). In the latter studies, it was concluded that AII inhibited basal and stimulated renin release by a mechanism dependent on the presence of extracellular calcium (67). Because AII elicits vasoconstriction by increasing the intracellular concentration of calcium in vascular smooth-muscle cells, direct inhibition of renin release by AII also may result from the ability of this peptide to increase the intracellular concentration of calcium in the granular JG cells.

This direct negative-feedback inhibition of AII on renin release is referred to as the "short-loop" mechanism (75) to distinguish it from the indirect inhibitory effect of increased levels of aldosterone. In the latter case, called the "long-loop" mechanism, AII stimulates the secretion of aldosterone, and the resultant retention of sodium and ECF volume expansion eventually suppress renin release. Thus, the short-loop effects of AII provide immediate modulation of renin release, whereas the long-loop mechanism provides feedback control over longer periods of time.

AVP

Because AVP causes renal vasoconstriction, increases blood pressure, inhibits water secretion, and increases sodium excretion, it is not surprising that this hormone alters renin release. In fact, AVP has been found to suppress renin release in rats, dogs, and humans. Although AVP has been noted to have variable effects on basal renin release, it has been shown to inhibit stimulated renin release consistently, whether the stimulus was sodium depletion (76), a decrease in renal perfusion pressure (77), isoproterenol (78), diuretic agents, (79) or ureteral occlusion (80). Endogenously synthesized AVP appears to have a similar effect on PRA, because PRA is elevated in rats with hereditary diabetes insipidus and suppressed in patients with the syndrome of inappropriate secretion of AVP. In the dog, this peptide appears to inhibit renin secretion by a direct action on the granular JG cells, but in humans it is unclear whether this inhibition of renin release is due to a direct action on the granular JG cells or to the expansion of plasma volume. Despite this uncertainty concerning the mechanism of action of AVP, variations in the plasma concentrations of AVP in the pathologic range, and most likely in the physiologic range, are involved in the control of renin release.

Prostaglandins

Like almost every other physiologic process, renin release is affected by prostaglandins (PG). Both PGE_1 and PGE_2 were found to increase renin release, urinary volume, urinary sodium excretion, and RBF when infused intrarenally into anesthetized dogs (81). Later observations indicated that the stimulation of renin release by an intrarenal infusion of PGE_2 was not dependent on the sympathetic nervous system or macula densa (82). Because PGE_1 and PGE_2 had no stimulatory effect on renin release from rat and rabbit renal cortical slices in vitro (83), the release of renin by PGE appears to be due to an indirect action, most likely related to the renal baroreceptor (21), but the exact mechanism cannot be stated with certainty. Although the effects of $PGF_{2\alpha}$ on renin release have not been studied extensively, this prostaglandin has been shown to cause a dose-related inhibition of renin secretion from rabbit renal cortical slices in vitro (83). This inhibition by $PGF_{2\alpha}$, which appears to occur via a direct action on the granular JG cells, has been observed in vivo (84).

The prostaglandin precursor arachidonic acid and the cyclic endoperoxides PGG_2 and PGH_2 have been demonstrated to elicit renin release in rats, rabbits, and dogs (21). Arachidonic acid also stimulated the release of renin from rabbit renal cortical slices in vitro, and this stimulatory effect was blocked by indomethacin, an inhibitor of the enzyme prostaglandin synthetase. Because PGE_2 did not enhance renin release in vitro, and because $PGF_{2\alpha}$ inhibited renin release, investigators reasoned that some product of prostaglandin synthesis other than PGE_2 or $PGF_{2\alpha}$ must mediate the renin release caused by arachidonic acid.

Two other prostaglandins discovered in subsequent years proved likely candidates as the mediators of arachidonic-acid-induced renin release. When PGD_2 was infused intrarenally in dogs, both renin release and RBF were elevated, but urinary volume and urinary sodium excretion were not altered (21). However, PGD_2 had no effect on renin release from renal cortical slices in vitro (85) and seemed to elevate renin release via the renal baroreceptor (21). An intrarenal arterial infusion of prostacyclin (PGI_2) caused increases in renin release, RBF, urinary volume, and urinary sodium excretion in dogs (86), and the stimulation of renin release by PGI_2 was not dependent on the presence of a functional macula densa (82). Furthermore, PGI_2 increased the release of renin from rabbit renal cortical slices in vitro (87), and arachidonic-acid-induced renin release from renal cortical slices in vitro was antagonized by the prostacyclin synthetase inhibitor 9,11-azoprosta-5,13-dienoic acid (85).

In summary, PGE_1, PGE_2, PGA_2, PGD_2, PGI_2, PGG_2, PGH_2, and arachidonic acid stimulate the release of renin, whereas $PGF_{2\alpha}$ inhibits renin release. It appears that the renin release elicited by PGE_2, PGD_2, PGI_2, and arachidonic acid in vivo occurs via activation of the renal baroreceptor, possibly because of an increase in renal interstitial pressure and a resultant fall in the transmural pressure gradient at the afferent arteriole (21). Because arachidonic acid and PGI_2 stimulate the release of renin from renal cortical slices in vitro, these compounds seem to possess an additional direct effect on the granular JG cells. On the basis of these findings, and the ability of the prostacyclin synthetase inhibitor 9,11-azoprosta-5,13-dienoic acid to inhibit arachidonic-acid-induced renin release in vitro, PGI_2 is the most likely candidate for the renin-releasing metabolite of arachidonic acid.

Cyclic Adenosine 3',5'-Monophosphate

Numerous investigations have delineated the role of the sympathetic nervous system and renal β-adrenergic receptors in the control of renin release (21). Because stimulation of β-adrenergic receptors activates adenyl cyclase in many tissues, and because this activation leads to an increase in the intracellular concentration of cyclic adenosine 3',5'-monophosphate (cyclic AMP), it is not surprising that the role of cyclic AMP in renin release has been studied. Cyclic AMP and dibutyryl cyclic AMP (a more lipid-soluble form) appear to elicit renin release *in vivo* (88,89) and *in vitro* (90) by a direct action on the granular JG cells. No effect of cyclic guanosine 3',5'-monophosphate on renin release has been noted. Even though the stimulation of renin release by cyclic AMP is believed to mimic β-adrenergically mediated renin release, the effects of cyclic AMP and dibutyryl cyclic AMP, even in the presence of inhibitors of phosphodiesterase, are quite weak as compared with those of renal nerve stimulation and catecholamines.

Adenosine

In recent years, a potential role for endogenous adenosine in the control of renin release, renal hemodynamics, and renal electrolyte metabolism has been recognized (91). The rate of production of adenosine in the isolated kidney appears to be quite high, and numerous stimuli have been shown to cause further increments in renal adenosine release. In addition to renal nerve stimulation, other factors (norepinephrine and AII, a decrease in renal perfusion pressure, and renal hypoxia) have been demonstrated to cause rapid increases in the release of adenosine from the kidneys of rabbits *in vitro* and the kidneys of rats, cats, and dogs *in vivo* (21). Experiments have revealed that adenosine suppresses renin release, and this action is directly related to the level of activity of the renin-angiotensin system (92). The only renal actions of adenosine that would account for its ability to inhibit renin release are an attenuation of the release of norepinephrine from the renal sympathetic nerves and a direct effect on the granular JG cells. Although many different stimuli elicit the production of adenosine in the kidney, the role of endogenous adenosine in the control of renal hemodynamics and hydrodynamics and renin release remains to be defined.

PHARMACOLOGIC ALTERATION OF RENIN RELEASE

Anesthetics

Because anesthetic agents are used widely in animal experimentation, it is not surprising that a number of studies have focused on the effects of anesthetics on the release of renin. Anesthetic drugs, when used in doses that produce a surgical plane of anesthesia, stimulate the release of renin in humans and experimental animals. In this respect, pentobarbital, phenobarbital, ketamine, urethane, chloralose, urethane plus chloralose, morphine, droperidol plus fentanyl, ether, halothane, nitrous oxide, methoxyflurane, cyclopropane, enflurane, and fluroxene have been found to elevate PRA in humans or experimental animals (21). Each anesthetic agent appears to alter renin release by a different mechanism, and the chronology of this renin release is different in each case. Additionally, under certain circumstances, the presence of anesthesia will affect the secretory response of the granular JG cells to physiologic or pathologic stimuli that increase or decrease the release of renin (21).

Drugs Affecting the Autonomic Nervous System

α-Adrenergic Receptor Agonists

Several factors have engendered interest in the effects of α-adrenergic receptor agonists on renin release. The popularity of the α-adrenergic agonist clonidine and α-methyldopa as antihypertensive agents and as research tools in cardiovascular studies led researchers to determine the mechanism by which these agents inhibited renin release and the importance of this inhibition in the lowering of blood pressure. In addition, evidence from studies performed *in vivo* and *in vitro* led to the idea that α-adrenergic receptor stimulation in the kidney suppressed renin release by an action on the granular JG cells.

Clonidine

The imidazoline compound clonidine exhibits activity at both peripheral and central α-adrenergic receptors. For example, intravenous administration of clonidine to anesthetized dogs has been shown to result in an initial transient increase in blood pressure, associated with decreases in heart rate and cardiac output and a rise in total peripheral resistance, which is followed by a prolonged period of vasodepression. During this prolonged period of vasodepression, heart rate and cardiac output remained suppressed, whereas total peripheral resistance returned to the control level. The initial pressor effect of clonidine was shown to be due to a direct effect of clonidine on vascular α-adrenergic receptors, but the subsequent fall in blood pressure was demonstrated to result from an action of the drug on the vasomotor and cardiac centers of the brain. Clonidine, in concentrations that have no direct effect on vascular tone, reversibly reduces nerve-stimulated norepinephrine release from sympathetic neurons. This action is known to be due to the activation of prejunctional α-adrenergic receptors that are inhibitory to the release of norepinephrine, and it has been shown to diminish as the frequency of stimulation is increased.

Clonidine has been reported to decrease renin release in normotensive (93) and hypertensive (94) humans, conscious (95) and anesthetized (96) dogs, and conscious (97) and anesthetized (98) rats. Data from clinical studies have indicated that the vasodepressor effect of clonidine does not appear to be related to the suppression of renin release by this drug,

and long-term therapy with clonidine does not necessarily result in the continued attenuation of renin release. Single-dose or short-term administration of clonidine has been shown to produce a more consistent inhibition of renin release (93). The centrally acting clonidinelike drug ST-600 produced a hemodynamic profile similar to that of clonidine and decreased PRA in hypertensive patients (99). Because clonidine appeared to lower PRA, blood pressure, and heart rate by the centrally mediated withdrawal of sympathetic tone, it was only natural for researchers to try to relate changes in these values to changes in the metabolism of catecholamines. The inhibition of renin release by clonidine in hypertensive patients was associated with large decrements in the urinary excretion of norepinephrine, epinephrine, and vanillylmandelic acid (100). The plasma levels of catecholamines also were decreased. Therefore, clonidine was believed to lower PRA by a centrally mediated decrease in the peripheral release of norepinephrine, but a direct action of the drug at the renal level could not be excluded.

The mechanism by which clonidine suppresses renin release has been studied extensively in animals, but researchers have come to different conclusions. Basically, two schools of thought exist. Reid et al. (96) have presented evidence indicating that clonidine suppresses renin release by centrally mediated withdrawal of renal sympathetic tone. On the other hand, Pettinger et al. (97) and other investigators (101) believe that clonidine inhibits renin release by stimulating intrarenal α-adrenergic receptors, possibly located on the granular JG cells. Evidence has been presented to support both the central and intrarenal theories regarding the mode of action of clonidine (21), but the use of anesthetized animals and possibly species differences have confounded the efforts of researchers to come to an agreement.

Methyldopa

Methyldopa lowers arterial blood pressure by an action in the central nervous system.

Peripherally administered methyldopa is taken up by noradrenergic nerves in the central nervous system and converted enzymatically to methylnorepinephrine, which then lowers blood pressure by stimulating central α-adrenergic receptors.

Methyldopa has been observed to decrease PRA in hypertensive patients (102), but this is not a universal observation (103). Methyldopa did not attenuate the rise in PRA seen in response to orthostasis or furosemide (104). Moreover, the efficacy of methyldopa as an antihypertensive agent was not related to its ability to suppress renin release (102). In studies conducted with anesthetized dogs, the suppression of renin release by methyldopa appeared to occur by a peripheral action related to the presence of the renal sympathetic nerves (105). Carbidopa, a compound that inhibits L-aromatic amino acid decarboxylase but does not enter the central nervous system, blocked the decrease in PRA caused by intravenous injection of methyldopa (105).

Levodopa

Although levodopa itself is not an α-adrenergic agonist, it is converted into norepinephrine in sympathetic neurons. This compound is used most frequently in the treatment of Parkinson's disease. During long-term therapy of these patients with levodopa, PRA is decreased (106). Levodopa did not affect the rise in PRA caused by orthostasis or salt depletion. Results from experiments conducted with anesthetized dogs indicated that the suppression of renin release by levodopa results from the central conversion of levodopa to norepinephrine, which causes a decrease in the level of activity of the renal sympathetic nerves (107).

Other α-adrenergic agonists

Phenylephrine and methoxamine also inhibit renin release *in vivo* under most circumstances, but it is not known whether this inhibition results from systemic or renal hemodynamic changes or a direct effect on the granular JG cells (21). The effect of the indirectly acting agonist tyramine on renin release *in vivo* is dose-dependent. The small amount of norepinephrine released by small doses of tyramine stimulates renin release, but larger doses of tyramine cause the release of quantities of norepinephrine sufficient to stimulate α-adrenergic receptors in the kidney that inhibit renin release (21).

α-Adrenergic Receptor Antagonists

Phenoxybenzamine

The noncompetitive α-adrenergic blocking agent phenoxybenzamine, when administered systemically, has been reported to increase PRA in anesthetized (108) and conscious rats (109), anesthetized dogs (110), and hypertensive patients (111). Loeffler et al. (110) noted that phenoxybenzamine caused PRA to triple as it lowered blood pressure by 30% in anesthetized dogs. Pretreatment with the β-adrenergic antagonist propranolol did not alter the fall in blood pressure but did block the rise in PRA. As a result, it was concluded that the decrement in blood pressure caused by peripheral α-adrenergic receptor blockade triggered a reflexly mediated increase in the activity of the renal sympathetic nerves. This conclusion is consistent with the known ability of phenoxybenzamine to increase plasma norepinephrine concentration and urinary norepinephrine excretion in animals and humans. In addition, intrarenal injection of phenoxybenzamine *in vivo* does not elicit renin release, and this drug has no effect on renin release in the isolated perfused rat kidney and rat renal cortical slices *in vitro*. In the ensuing years, administration of phenoxybenzamine to experimental animals has been found to potentiate the increase in renin release caused by physostigmine, insulin-induced hypoglycemia, stimulation of the renal nerves, and infusion of epinephrine, norepinephrine, and isoproterenol (21). The fact that the renin release brought about by each of these stimuli was blocked by propranolol strengthened the idea that phenoxybenzamine-induced renin release involved indirect stimulation of intrarenal β-adrenergic receptors.

Phentolamine

Phentolamine is a short-acting competitive α-adrenergic antagonist that possesses some direct vasodilating effects. Phentolamine has been shown to stimulate renin release in anesthetized (112) and conscious (109) rats, anesthetized cats (113), and normotensive (114) and hypertensive (115) humans. In conscious rats, phentolamine caused a dose-related elevation of PRA that developed rapidly and was associated with a marked rise in heart rate. Phentolamine-induced renin release in humans occurs in association with a decrease in blood pressure and an increase in heart rate.

As with phenoxybenzamine, a wealth of evidence indicates that phentolamine elicits renin release by reflex activation, via the carotid baroreflex, of the renal sympathetic nerves. Meyer et al. (112) noted that phentolamine-induced renin release in the anesthetized rat was blocked by *l*-propranolol but not *d*-propranolol. Desipramine and amitriptyline, two compounds that inhibit the neuronal uptake of norepinephrine but have no effect on renin release themselves, potentiated phentolamine-induced but not isoproterenol-induced renin release. The rise in PRA seen after the administration of phentolamine also was prevented or greatly attenuated by pretreatment with reserpine, with the noradrenergic neurotoxin 6-hydroxydopamine, or with the ganglionic blockers pempidine or camphidonium. Later, Keeton and Pettinger (109) studied the roles of the sympathetic neuronal, the renal baroreceptor, and the macula densa mechanisms in phentolamine-induced renin release in the conscious rat. Pretreatment with propranolol impaired 90% of the renin release and all of the tachycardia caused by phentolamine without altering the decrement in blood pressure caused by phentolamine. Therefore, it was concluded that the decrement in renal perfusion pressure sensed by the afferent arteriolar baroreceptor did not contribute to the rise in PRA seen when blood pressure was decreased with phentolamine. Because the vasodepression caused by phentolamine was known to decrease GFR, renal plasma flow (RPF), urinary volume, and urinary sodium excretion in conscious rats, the effect of phentolamine on renin release was examined in salt-loaded rats. Salt loading by pretreatment with deoxycorticosterone (a mineralocorticoid) and saline drinking water greatly suppressed basal PRA and blunted the vasodepressor effect of phentolamine but did not impair the ability of phentolamine to increase renin release or heart rate. Based on these data, it was concluded that the decrease in sodium reaching the macula densa during phentolamine-induced vasodepression had little to do with the renin release caused by this agent. Clinical studies with hypertensive patients support this conclusion.

Prazosin

Although prazosin was originally believed to lower blood pressure by active vasodilation, it is now known to elicit vasodepression by α-adrenergic blockade. Accordingly, prazosin is classified as an α-adrenergic antagonist rather than as a peripheral vasodilator. When given to hypertensive humans, prazosin has been found to lower blood pressure and total peripheral resistance, to cause little or no change in heart rate, and to increase cardiac index, GFR, and RPF. Thus, unlike phentolamine and phenoxybenzamine, prazosin-induced hypotension does not result in a reflexly mediated tachycardia.

As a general rule, either short- or long-term treatment of hypertensive patients with prazosin leads to no change or a decrease in PRA. When patients with hypertension were divided into high-, normal-, and low-renin subgroups and treated with prazosin, PRA decreased in all of the high-renin patients and in 4 of the 12 normal-renin patients. The remainder of the normal-renin patients and the 2 low-renin patients exhibited no change in PRA. Prazosin did not elevate heart rate in any of these studies (21). The reason for a lack of increase in renin release and heart rate during the administration of prazosin to hypertensive humans is unknown.

Prazosin does elicit a tachycardia in conscious rats, and consistent with the mechanism by which α-adrenergic antagonists increase PRA, prazosin stimulates renin release in this species (116). Graham and Pettinger (116) observed that both phentolamine and prazosin brought about dose-related decreases in MAP and increases in SRA and heart rate. For a given reduction in MAP, phentolamine caused greater increases in SRA and heart rate than did prazosin. These authors believed that the difference in the magnitudes of the rises in SRA caused by equihypotensive doses of phentolamine and prazosin resulted from the fact that prazosin had little or no activity in blocking the prejunctional α-adrenergic receptors that have been shown to attenuate nerve-stimulated norepinephrine release.

In summary, α-adrenergic antagonists stimulate the release of renin by reflex activation of the renal sympathetic nerves secondary to a decrease in MAP. This increase in renin release is blocked by β-adrenergic antagonists. Prazosin is the exception to this generalization, because it may lower blood pressure in some cases without eliciting an increase in renin release or heart rate.

Other drugs with α-adrenergic receptor blocking activity

The neuroleptic agents chlorpromazine and clozapine have been shown to be antagonists at α-adrenergic receptors. Chlorpromazine did increase PRA in humans, and clozapine decreased blood pressure and increased SRA in conscious rats.

The renin-releasing properties of other α-adrenergic antagonists such as tolazoline, azapetine, and piperoxane are unknown. Similarly, the ability of other neuroleptic agents with marked activity at α-adrenergic receptors to alter renin release has not been tested.

Importance of Prejunctional and Postjunctional α-Adrenergic Blockade in the Renin Response to α-Adrenergic Antagonists

During the past decade, evidence has accumulated to support the existence of prejunc-
tional α-adrenergic receptors that modulate the neuronal release of norepinephrine. Stimulation of these receptors by α-adrenergic agonists inhibits the exocytotic liberation of norepinephrine, and the blockade of these prejunctional α-adrenergic receptors results in a greater release of norepinephrine at low frequencies of nerve stimulation. α-Adrenergic antagonists differ in their ability to cause receptor blockade at prejunctional and postjunctional α-adrenergic receptors. For example, yohimbine preferentially antagonizes norepinephrine at prejunctional sites, with postjunctional blockade occurring only at higher concentrations of the drug. In contrast, prazosin appears to be a preferential postjunctional α-adrenergic antagonist, and phentolamine appears to possess equal activity at both sites. These conclusions are based mostly on data obtained from experiments conducted *in vitro,* but recently the results of studies conducted *in vivo* have given strong support to the functional significance of prejunctional α-adrenergic modulation of sympathetic function (117).

Graham et al. (117) measured the reflexly mediated increase in plasma norepinephrine concentration that resulted from giving equihypotensive doses of hydralazine, prazosin, phenoxybenzamine, and phentolamine to conscious rats. Hydralazine, a peripheral vasodilator that does not block α-adrenergic receptors, elicited a 4.2-fold increase in the amount of norepinephrine found in the plasma. Prazosin, phenoxybenzamine, and phentolamine elevated plasma norepinephrine concentrations by 5.5-, 7.5-, and 8.9-fold, respectively. Thus, the relative abilities of these three α-adrenergic antagonists to increase the plasma level of norepinephrine were in the same rank order as their abilities to block prejunctional α-adrenergic receptors *in vitro*. These data also help to explain the observation that for a given reduction in MAP, phentolamine caused a greater increase in SRA than did prazosin (116). The exceptional prejunctional selectivity of yohimbine was evidenced by the fact that a small dose of this drug did not lower blood pressure but did elicit a tachycardia and a 3.6-fold elevation in the circulating levels of norepinephrine (117). More recently, yohimbine has been found to cause dose-related increases in SRA and heart rate in conscious rats, even though blood pressure was not decreased. The increases in SRA and heart rate caused by yohimbine were blocked by propranolol (21). Thus, α-adrenergic antagonists, by acting at prejunctional sites, increase the release of norepinephrine onto postjunctional renal and cardiac β-adrenergic receptors, rather than stimulating them directly.

β-Adrenergic Antagonists and Agonists

As seen previously, the renal sympathetic nerves play an important role in the stimulation of renin release, and this response is mediated via β-adrenergic receptors located on the granular JG cells. In fact, much of the evidence for the latter conclusion is based on the fact that β-adrenergic receptor blocking drugs prevent sympathetically mediated renin release, irrespective of whether the renal nerves are activated directly or indirectly (*vide supra*). In addition, the renin response to β-adrenergic antagonists has been a subject of great interest ever since Buhler et al. (118) suggested that the magnitude of the vasodepressor effect of these drugs was dependent on the initial PRA value and the magnitude of suppression of renin release. Thus, the renin responses to the various β-adrenergic antagonists are of interest in basic and clinical research as well as in clinical therapeutics.

In 1969, some 5 years after propranolol was first synthesized, it was discovered that propranolol blocked orthostasis-induced renin release in normal humans without lowering supine PRA values (119). A year later, Stokes et al. (120) reported that propranolol lowered peripheral and renal venous PRA in hypertensive patients. In 1972, Michelakis and McAllister (121) found that therapy with multiple small doses of propranolol suppressed PRA in hypertensive and normotensive humans

without affecting blood pressure. The suppression of renin release by propranolol was dose-related, and propranolol lowered both supine PRA and upright PRA by 50% in the normal and salt-depleted states. At the same time, propranolol was found to lower PRA by 60 to 70% in salt-deprived and normal anesthetized dogs (122). Buhler et al. (118) then hypothesized a relationship between the ability of propranolol to lower renin release and its ability to lower blood pressure. In the same year, Salvetti et al. (123) reported that oxprenolol decreased renin release in the supine and upright positions in patients with normal-renin hypertension but was without effect in low-renin hypertension. Since 1972, hundreds of papers have been published concerning the effects of β-adrenergic antagonists on renin release, and the major findings of these studies will be presented here.

All β-adrenergic antagonists tested to date inhibit renin release in animals and humans, but these drugs differ in terms of efficacy and potency. Propranolol usually is used as the standard of comparison for all other β-adrenergic antagonists. Some general points can be made concerning the effects of β-adrenergic antagonists on renin release. First, renal β-adrenergic receptor blockade does not suppress basal (supine) renin release to zero in humans; therefore, factors other than renal nerve activity maintain renin release in the supine position. Second, many of these drugs block the increase in PRA that results from the attainment of upright posture in humans. This blockade of orthostasis-induced renin release has been demonstrated with propranolol, acebutolol, atenolol, metoprolol, oxprenolol, penbutolol, pindolol, practolol, and labetalol (21). In a similar fashion, exercise-induced renin release in humans has been prevented by pretreatment with propranolol, atenolol, bufuralol, metoprolol, oxprenolol, penbutolol, pindolol, practolol, timolol, tolamolol, and labetalol (21). Next, and in accord with the original suggestion of Buhler et al. (118), other clinicians observed that β-adrenergic receptor blockade with propranolol, bunolol, oxprenolol, pindolol, and sotalol lowered PRA by a greater percentage in high-renin hypertensive patients than in low-renin hypertensive patients. It is important to note, however, that these differing responses of renin release to β-adrenergic blockade were detected when the patients were in the upright position. Usually, no difference in renin suppression was observed in recumbent high- and low-renin hypertensive patients after β-adrenergic blockade.

β-Adrenergic antagonists have the ability to lower the elevated PRA values found in sodium-depleted animals and humans. For example, propranolol lowered PRA by 50 to 70% in salt-depleted humans, dogs, and rats (21). In like fashion, pindolol and oxprenolol lowered PRA in sodium-depleted humans. However, even with this degree of inhibition of renin release in the salt-depleted state, the absolute PRA values encountered are usually greater than, or at least equal to, the PRA values found in the states of normal sodium balance in the absence of β-adrenergic blockade. In each of these experiments, sodium depletion was achieved primarily by the ingestion of a low-salt diet, with only minimal use of diuretic drugs. In each case, diuretic therapy had been withdrawn several days before administration of the β-adrenergic antagonist. This inhibition of renin release by β-adrenergic blockers during sodium depletion is comparable to the effects of these drugs on thiazide-induced renin release (*vide infra*), and this suppression has been taken as evidence that the stimulatory effect of the renal sympathetic nerves on renin release is increased during sodium depletion and the subsequent contraction of plasma volume.

Although it was originally reported that propranolol blocked renal baroreceptor-stimulated renin release in anesthetized dogs (124), other investigators (125) have been unable to confirm this finding. In a well-designed study in conscious dogs, Hanson et al. (125) elicited a twofold increase in PRA by decreasing renal perfusion pressure with an inflatable cuff implanted around the renal artery. Pretreatment with propranolol had no effect on this renal baroreceptor-mediated renin release.

Analogous studies have been conducted in humans in that the effects of oxprenolol on orthostasis-induced renin release were examined in patients with functioning renal allografts, i.e., denervated kidneys (126). In these patients, the increase in PRA after attainment of the upright position is not as rapid as it is in humans with intact renal innervation, but the magnitude of the increase is the same. This increase in PRA might result from the release of catecholamines by the adrenal gland or activation of the renal baroreceptor. Salvetti et al. (126) observed that 5 of 6 patients with functioning renal transplants exhibited increases in PRA with orthostasis some 3 to 5 months after surgery. After the administration of oxprenolol, the postural rise in renin release was reduced in only 2 of 6 patients. Therefore, it is not known whether or not β-adrenergic antagonists can block renal baroreceptor-mediated renin release in humans.

The advent of the cardioselective β-adrenergic antagonists generated a great deal of interest in the pharmacologic characterization of the renal β-adrenergic receptor controlling renin release. In 1967, Lands et al. (127) presented evidence that β-adrenergic receptors can be subdivided into β_1 and β_2 subtypes, with the β_1 receptors mediating positive chronotropic and inotropic responses in the heart and β_2 receptors subserving bronchodilation and vasodilation. During the last few years, researchers have used β_1- and β_2-adrenergic antagonists and agonists, either singly or in combination, in an attempt to determine whether renin release is mediated via β_1- or β_2-adrenergic receptors.

With this aim in mind, Weber et al. (128) studied the effects of *d,l*-propranolol, *d*-propranolol, pindolol, oxprenolol, metoprolol, practolol, and H35/25 on both basal and isoproterenol-stimulated renin release in conscious rabbits. With the exception of *d*-propranolol and pindolol, all of these anta------ lowered basal PRA during the cour: 6-hr intravenous infusion. The decrem

PRA with the cardioselective blockers metoprolol (−31%) and practolol (−22%) were significantly less than with the nonselective drugs d,l-propranolol (−64%) and oxprenolol (−57%). In addition, practolol and metoprolol inhibited the chronotropic effects of isoproterenol, but not the increase in PRA caused by isoproterenol. In an opposite fashion, the β_2-adrenergic receptor blocker H35/25 prevented the rise in PRA, but not the increase in heart rate, elicited by isoproterenol. Oxprenolol, pindolol, and d,l-propranolol blocked the renin release and tachycardia caused by isoproterenol. The d isomer of propranolol did not alter basal or stimulated renin release, and pindolol caused a 3.4-fold increase in PRA in association with a marked tachycardia. If PRA, MAP, and heart rate had previously been lowered by an intravenous infusion of d,l-propranolol, the addition of pindolol to the infusate raised PRA and heart rate back to the prepropranolol control values without affecting blood pressure. Because pindolol stimulated renin release and reversed the ability of propranolol to suppress PRA, but prevented isoproterenol-induced renin release, it was concluded that the stimulatory effects of pindolol on PRA and heart rate resulted from the marked intrinsic sympathomimetic activity of pindolol. Therefore, those drugs that possess prominent β_2-adrenergic blocking activity (d,l-propranolol, oxprenolol, pindolol, and H35/25) had greater inhibitory effects on basal and isoproterenol-stimulated renin release than did those agents with β_1-adrenergic receptor activity (practolol and metoprolol). Weber et al. (128) concluded that the effects of β-adrenergic blockers on renin release in rabbits depended on the sum of their direct effects, either agonistic or antagonistic, on β_2-adrenergic receptors in the kidney.

More recently, Weber et al. (129) found that pindolol infused directly into the renal artery in conscious rabbits brought about a 2.5-fold increase in renin secretion without altering RBF and MAP. The same dose given intravenously did not affect renin secretion. The ability of small doses of pindolol to elevate renin

secretion was thought to be due to the marked sympathomimetic effect of pindolol. A single bolus injection of pindolol or oxprenolol also has been shown to elevate renin release and heart rate in conscious rabbits. The intrinsic activities of pindolol and oxprenolol are 56 and 29%, respectively, of that of isoproterenol at cardiac chronotropic receptors, and the agonistic properties of these drugs are fully expressed in the rabbit kidney (128) and partially expressed in the human kidney (21). Although it was originally thought that renin release was mediated by β_2-adrenergic receptors in the cat (130), more recent studies (131) have indicated that β_1-adrenergic receptors mediate sympathetically induced renin release in the cat.

Atenolol, a β_1-adrenergic antagonist, was found to block the renin release and tachycardia caused by intravenous infusion of isoproterenol in conscious dogs (132). The vasodepression caused by isoproterenol was not affected. Conversely, the selective β_2-adrenergic antagonist IPS-339 prevented the decrease in blood pressure caused by isoproterenol but did not impair isoproterenol-induced renin release or tachycardia. In these studies, d,l-propranolol blocked the renin release, tachycardia, and vasodepression seen with isoproterenol, but d-propranolol did not. Based on these data, it was concluded that β_1-adrenergic receptors mediated renin release in the dog.

More recent observations have supported the belief that β_1-adrenergic receptors mediate renin secretion in the dog. Osborn et al. (133) found that direct low-level (0.5-Hz) stimulation of the renal nerves in anesthetized dogs increased renin secretion without altering MAP, RBF, GFR, and urinary sodium excretion. This increase in renin secretion was blocked by the β_1-adrenergic antagonist atenolol but was not affected by the β_2-adrenergic antagonist butoxamine. The β_1-adrenergic agonist prenalterol increased renin secretion in anesthetized dogs by 2.5-fold without changing MAP, RBF, GFR, urinary volume, and urinary sodium excretion (134). Pretreatment with the β_1-adrenergic antagonist metoprolol abolished the ability of prenalterol to increase renin secretion.

Oates et al. (135) studied the effects of several β-adrenergic antagonists on renin release in anesthetized rats. Atenolol, metoprolol, and propranolol, at doses that produced equal β_1-adrenergic receptor blockade, suppressed basal PRA by 35, 41, and 40%, respectively, despite the fact that these doses of atenolol and metoprolol exhibited no β_2-adrenergic receptor blocking activity. If the doses of atenolol and metoprolol were increased by eightfold to achieve β_2-adrenergic receptor blockade, little additional suppression of renin release was noted. Conversely, when equipotent β_2-adrenergic receptor blocking doses of atenolol, metoprolol, propranolol, and butoxamine were tested, PRA was lowered by atenolol and metoprolol but not by propranolol and butoxamine. Neither β_1- nor β_2-adrenergic receptor blocking doses of practolol affected PRA, and this lack of effect was attributed to the high intrinsic activity of practolol. It was concluded that sympathetically mediated renin release in the rat occurred via β_1-adrenergic receptors (135). The work of Desaulles et al. (136) and Campbell et al. (88) supports this contention. In the former case, a positive correlation was found between the degree of inhibition of isoproterenol-induced renin release in rat renal cortical slices *in vitro* and the pA_2 values for propranolol, atenolol, practolol, and IPS 339 at cardiac β_1 receptors (136). More recently, the cardioselective β_1-adrenergic receptor agonist prenalterol, at doses that increased heart rate but did not affect blood pressure, was found to increase PRA eightfold in conscious rats. Taken collectively, these results (88,135,136) indicate that β_1-adrenergic receptors are involved in the control of renin release in rats.

Similar attempts have been made to assess the type of β-adrenergic receptor controlling renin release in humans. Based on the observation that practolol blocked orthostasis-induced renin release in normal subjects, Salvetti et al. (123) first suggested that renin

release was a β_1-adrenergic receptor event in humans. Later, Buhler et al. (137) determined the activities of a group of β-adrenergic receptor blockers on supine and exercise-induced renin release in normotensive humans. The cardioselective agents atenolol, bufuralol, practolol, and metoprolol, the nonselective antagonists LL/21945, oxprenolol, pindolol, propranolol, and timolol, and the combined α- and β-adrenergic receptor blocker labetalol were administered in doses that caused equal blockade of exercise-induced tachycardia. All of these drugs lowered stimulated PRA by 30 to 55%. With the exceptions of oxprenolol, pindolol, and labetalol, all of these β-adrenergic receptor blockers also caused significant suppression of supine PRA. After comparing the data, it was concluded that cardioselective β receptor antagonists with no intrinsic activity, such as atenolol, suppressed basal PRA best. The least inhibition of PRA under basal conditions occurred with nonselective β blockers that possessed a significant amount of intrinsic activity, such as pindolol.

The β_2-adrenergic receptor agonist salbutamol also has been used to identify the type of β-adrenergic receptors controlling renin release in humans. Johnson et al. (138) chose doses of isoproterenol and salbutamol that elicited equal increments in systolic blood pressure, heart rate, and PRA and equal decrements in diastolic blood pressure in supine normal subjects. The infusions of these β-adrenergic receptor agonists were repeated after 3 days of treatment with practolol. The elevations in heart rate and PRA elicited by either agonist were blocked by practolol in a competitive fashion, as was the fall in diastolic blood pressure caused by isoproterenol. However, practolol did not prevent the decrement in diastolic blood pressure elicited by salbutamol. In another study in normal recumbent humans, isoproterenol and salbutamol lowered MAP by 14% and elevated heart rate by 47 and 27 beats per minute, respectively. PRA was increased 80% by isoproterenol, but salbutamol failed to alter PRA, despite its equal hypotensive effect. Salbutamol is a partial agonist at renal β-adrenergic receptors, because this drug markedly attenuated isoproterenol-induced renin release in humans (139). Metaproterenol, another β-adrenergic receptor agonist with moderate selectivity for β_2-adrenergic receptors, was found to stimulate renin release in normal humans, and this stimulatory effect was prevented by pretreatment with propranolol (140). However, the doses of metaproterenol used in these studies (140) were sufficient to increase heart rate, indicating a considerable amount of β_1-adrenergic receptor activation. Thus, studies (138,140) with β_2-adrenergic receptor agonists have given support to the belief that β_1-adrenergic receptors mediate renin release in humans.

In conclusion, β-adrenergic receptor antagonists suppress basal renin release in animals and humans, and this inhibition appears to be due to the blockade of β-adrenergic receptors located on the granular JG cells of the kidney. β_2-Adrenergic receptors appear to mediate renin release in rabbits, whereas renin release in rats, cats, dogs, and humans is subserved by β_1-adrenergic receptors.

Phosphodiesterase Inhibitors

Several investigators have attempted to determine the role of endogenous cyclic AMP in the control of renin release by using inhibitors of phosphodiesterase such as papaverine and theophylline. The idea was that by inhibiting the degradation of cyclic AMP to 5'-adenosine monophosphate, these drugs should elevate the concentration of cyclic AMP in the granular JG cells. The results obtained with papaverine are not consistent. Papaverine has variously been reported to cause an increase, a decrease, and no change in PRA. In one study, papaverine elicited renin release from canine renal cortical slices *in vitro,* and this stimulation was associated with a rise in the cellular content of cyclic AMP (141). On the other hand, Churchill et al. (142) found that papaverine inhibited both basal and isoproterenol-stimulated renin release from rat renal cortical slices *in vitro.* Another inhibitor of phosphodiesterase, 3-isobutyl-1-methylxan-

thine, increased basal renin secretion but had no effect on isoproterenol-induced renin release (142). Theophylline was found to elevate renin release in humans (143) and animals and in the isolated perfused kidneys of animals (144), but it had no effect on renin release from renal cortical slices *in vitro* (145). Although some investigators believe that intact renal innervation is necessary for theophylline to increase renin release, propranolol does not inhibit theophylline-induced renin release (144). In addition, indomethacin did not affect the rise in PRA caused by theophylline (146). Theophylline also appears to be a specific antagonist of the effects of adenosine in the kidney, but it is not known whether the ability of theophylline to stimulate renin release is related to the antagonism of the inhibitory action of adenosine, a direct effect on cyclic AMP levels in the granular JG cells, or the renal hemodynamic effects of the compound. Caffeine has been shown to elicit a modest increase in PRA in supine humans (147).

Other Drugs That Effect the Sympathetic Nervous System and Endogenous Catecholamines

Reserpine

Reserpine is an alkaloid of natural origin that depletes both central and peripheral catecholamines and indoleamines by "poisoning" the storage granules in the nerves. The effects of reserpine on renin release have not been well characterized. Although reserpine decreases the concentration of norepinephrine in the kidney and lowers blood pressure in experimental animals, no consistent pattern of change in renin release has been observed (21).

Guanethidine and bretylium

Guanethidine and bretylium prevent the release of norepinephrine from peripheral sympathetic neurons but do not inhibit the release of catecholamines from the adrenal medulla. In addition, guanethidine also depletes catecholamine stores in peripheral sympathetic neurons. Both drugs block the neuronal uptake of catecholamines and thus produce supersensitivity toward circulating catecholamines.

Guanethidine has been reported both to increase (148) and to decrease (149) renin release in experimental animals. Meyer et al. (148) found that guanethidine increased PRC in conscious normal and adrenalectomized rats. Blood pressure was not altered by guanethidine in either group of animals, but a significant decrease in heart rate occurred. Guanethidine also potentiated the elevation of PRC caused by isoproterenol.

When blood for the determination of PRA was obtained from rats after anesthesia with ether, guanethidine and bretylium decreased PRA by 25 to 45% (149). Guanethidine depleted the renal stores of norepinephrine by 35% but did not cause a change in renal renin concentration. Guanethidine potentiated the renin release elicited by phentolamine, and bretylium accentuated the renin release caused by hydralazine. As a result, Meyer et al. (149) suggested that guanethidine and bretylium decreased PRA by preventing the release of norepinephrine from peripheral sympathetic neurons and potentiated the renin-releasing effects of phentolamine and hydralazine by enhancing the action of catecholamines released from the adrenal medulla.

In hypertensive patients treated chronically with guanethidine, renin release was stimulated in association with a decrease in the urinary excretion of norepinephrine (21). Guanethidine elevated PRA into the normal range in patients with low-renin hypertension, and this stimulation appeared to be related to the vasodepressor action of the drug (21).

Inhibitors of neuronal catecholamine uptake

The effects of these agents on renin release have been studied very little. Meyer and Hertting (150) measured PRC in ether-anesthetized rats pretreated with cocaine, desipramine, and amitriptyline. These inhibitors of uptake-1 had no effect on basal PRC or the renin release caused by isoproterenol. However, as might be expected, these drugs did enhance the renin release elicited by phentolamine. The latter observation is consistent with the fact that phentolamine stimulates renin release by reflexly increasing the release of norepinephrine from the renal sympathetic nerves. Cocaine caused a 45% elevation of renin release from rat renal cortical slices *in vitro,* presumably by preventing neuronal uptake of norepinephrine being released spontaneously by the tissue.

6-Hydroxydopamine

The neurotoxin 6-hydroxydopamine is taken up by the peripheral sympathetic neurons, which are then destroyed by an intracellular action of the compound. Because 6-hydroxydopamine is frequently used to produce functional adrenergic denervation in cardiovascular studies, it is important to know how this agent affects renin release.

Meyer et al. (112) gave multiple intravenous doses of 6-hydroxydopamine to rats and found that cardiac norepinephrine stores were decreased by 84%, whereas the concentration of epinephrine in the adrenal gland rose by 33%. Basal PRC, after ether anesthesia, was unchanged. The renin release elicited by isoproterenol was enhanced, but the rise in PRC caused by phentolamine was greatly reduced. When blood for the measurement of SRA was obtained from 6-hydroxydopamine-treated animals after decapitation, basal SRA was unchanged, even though the norepinephrine concentration of the kidneys was decreased by 35% (T. K. Keeton, *unpublished observations*). Porlier et al. (151) administered 6-hydroxydopamine to conscious normotensive dogs and noted that blood pressure decreased rapidly. This hypotension was accompanied by a sixfold elevation of PRA and a threefold increase in plasma catecholamine levels. PRA remained elevated for 1 week, but had returned to the control levels, as had MAP, by the end of 2 weeks. The stimulation of renin release after 6-hydroxydopamine was thought to be the result of (a) a decrease in blood pressure, (b) an increase in the circulating levels of catecholamines, and/or (c) a decrease in the sodium load at the macula densa (151).

Ganglionic stimulants

Dimethylphenylpiperazinium, given either intravenously or intrarenally, has been reported to increase renin release in anesthetized dogs (152). In urethane-anesthetized rats, Alexandre et al. (108) found that the pressor effects of physostigmine were accompanied by a rise in PRA. The β-adrenergic antagonists propranolol, oxprenolol, and pindolol inhibited the increase in PRA but enhanced the hypertension caused by physostigmine. Conversely, phenoxybenzamine blocked the pressor effects of physostigmine but did not alter the ability of this drug to elevate PRA. Thus, the generalized increase in peripheral sympathetic nerve activity caused by physostigmine appeared to result in an increase in the stimulation of β-adrenergic receptors located on the granular JG cells. In this particular case, it must be assumed that the stimulatory effect of nerve activity on renin release overrode the inhibitory effect on renin release of an increase in renal perfusion pressure.

Cholinergic antagonists

Ganglionic blocking drugs inhibit neurotransmission in the paravertebral ganglia by occupying nicotinic receptors. The changes in heart rate and blood pressure seen after these drugs have been administered are dependent on the preexisting state of sympathetic and cholinergic tone. In humans, where vagal tone usually predominates, a mild tachycardia often accompanies ganglionic blockade, but in the rat, where sympathetic tone predominates, a bradycardia is observed after ganglionic blockade. Similarly, the high incidence of orthostatic hypotension in humans treated with ganglionic blockers emphasizes the importance of existing sympathetic tone in determining the magnitude of the vasodepressor response. Ganglionic blockade had been demonstrated to decrease the concentration of norepinephrine in the plasma of humans and rats.

Pettinger et al. (153) found that chlorisondamine brought about a dose-related elevation of SRA in conscious rats that was not affected by pretreatment with propranolol. Chlorisondamine also increased SRA by twofold in sodium-depleted rats (97). Although pempidine did not alter PRC in anesthetized rats, Meyer et al. (112,148) observed that trimethidinium elevated PRC by threefold in conscious rats, and phenylephrine prevented this effect of trimethidinium. The same investigators found that camphidonium elevated PRC by twofold in one group of anesthetized rats (154) but had no effect in another series of experiments (112).

In more recent studies designed to determine the mechanism by which ganglionic blockade stimulates renin release, Keeton and Pettinger (109) found, in conscious rats, that chlorisondamine increased SRA by twofold and decreased MAP and heart rate by 40 and 14%, respectively. Because propranolol did not alter the renin-releasing effects of chlorisondamine, it was reasoned that the reduction in MAP caused by this drug activated renin release via the renal baroreceptor and/or the macula densa. To test the latter possibility, animals were treated with deoxycorticosterone acetate and saline drinking water for 2 days. Even though salt loading lowered basal SRA by 90%, the ability of chlorisondamine to stimulate renin release was not blunted. In fact, the elevation of SRA by chlorisondamine after salt loading was actually much greater than the percentage increase seen after chlorisondamine in states of normal sodium balance. In salt-loaded rats, chlorisondamine decreased MAP and heart rate by 30 and 11%, respectively. Based on these data, these authors concluded that chlorisondamine elevated renin release by the hypotensive activation of the renal baroreceptor. Chlorisondamine also was found to inhibit by 72% the rise in SRA induced by phentolamine.

Prostaglandins appear to play an important role in chlorisondamine-induced renin release. Campbell et al. (88) discovered that the 2.7-fold increase in SRA seen after administration of chlorisondamine to conscious rats was completely blocked by a dose of indomethacin that prevented arachidonate-induced hypotension and markedly suppressed the urinary excretion of PGE_2 and $PGF_{2\alpha}$. The hypotension and bradycardia caused by chlorisondamine were not affected by indomethacin.

When MAP was lowered from 140 to 65 mm Hg with trimethaphan in conscious renal-hypertensive dogs, PRA increased threefold (155). Lifschitz and Horwitz (156) noted that PRA increased by 60% when blood pressure of conscious dogs was lowered by 17 to 37 mm Hg with pentolinium.

In hypertensive patients, pentolinium (111) and trimethaphan (157) decreased blood pressure by 20 to 25 mm Hg but did not change PRA. In one of these studies (111), plasma norepinephrine content decreased by 32% after pentolinium. It is conceivable that in humans the decrement in renin release that occurred after decreasing sympathetic nerve activity was counterbalanced by the stimulation of renin release by the renal baroreceptor. Kaneko et al. (158) found that the increase in PRA and decrease in RBF caused by the administration of a vasodepressor dose of sodium nitroprusside to normotensive and hypertensive humans were prevented by either pentolinium or trimethaphan.

Diuretics

The scientific literature concerning the effects of diuretic agents on renin release, like that concerning renin release in general, is almost overwhelming. We have already noted that changes in sodium (and possibly chloride) transport within the renal tubule have a profound effect on renin release, and, as would be expected from this observation, diuretic drugs have the ability to alter renin release. In general, diuretic drugs increase renin release because they decrease plasma volume and thus cause activation of the renal baroreceptor and sympathetic nervous system mechanisms controlling renin release. After prolonged treatment with diuretics, the depletion of total body sodium leads to activation of the macula densa. It is also possible for diuretic agents to cause an immediate increase in renin release by inhibiting sodium and/or chloride transport at the macula densa, by direct activation of the renal baroreceptor, by altering renal sympathetic nerve traffic, or by a direct effect on the granular JG cells. Therefore, we must try to distinguish between the direct effects of the drugs on renin release and their indirect effects on renin release that are mediated via changes in salt and water balance.

Furosemide, Ethacrynic Acid, and Bumetanide

Furosemide and ethacrynic acid, which were introduced for clinical use in the mid-1960s, and the more recently developed drug bumetanide, are powerful natriuretic and diuretic drugs that are commonly referred to as "loop" or "high-ceiling" diuretics. Furosemide has been demonstrated to increase renin release in rabbits, cats, dogs, rats, and sheep. Ethacrynic acid was shown to increase renin release in dogs, and bumetanide increased renin release in dogs and rats. Both ethacrynic acid and bumetanide have low diuretic potency in the rat, and, as a result, the ability of these two drugs to alter renin release in this species has not been studied extensively. All three agents significantly increase PRA in humans.

The elevation of PRA elicited by these loop diuretics, furosemide in particular, is of great interest for three reasons. First, furosemide enjoys widespread use in clinical medicine, and this drug can cause iatrogenic changes in renin and aldosterone secretion. Second, furosemide is used diagnostically to determine renin responsiveness for the classification of patients with low-renin hypertension. Lastly, furosemide alters renin release by several different mechanisms that appear to be preferentially activated as a function of the dose and time after administration.

The renal effects of furosemide (159), ethacrynic acid (159), and bumetanide (160) have been reviewed recently, but their actions on ion transport and RBF are of more immediate importance in our discussion, because these actions can affect renin release. In 1973, Burg and Green (161) and Rocha and Kokko (60) presented firm evidence for the active transport of chloride, rather than sodium, in the medullary and cortical segments of the thick ascending limb of the loop of Henle. Sodium reabsorption in this segment of the renal tubule appears to occur passively. Subsequently it was demonstrated that both furosemide and ethacrynic acid inhibit active chloride transport, and thus sodium reabsorption, in the ascending limb of Henle's loop. Because the cellular effects of bumetanide in this region of the renal tubule are very similar to those of furosemide, it is probable that bumetanide also inhibits active chloride transport in the ascending limb of Henle's loop. In addition, tubuloglomerular feedback of urine flow rate in the early proximal tubule in the rat is critically dependent on chloride transport across the macula densa cells, and this feedback is blocked by furosemide. Wright and Schnermann (162) found that ethacrynic acid failed to alter tubuloglomerular feedback in rat nephrons, but this drug is also relatively ineffective in inhibiting chloride transport in the loop of Henle in this species. Therefore, it is tempting to speculate that all loop diuretics will inhibit chloride transport at the macula densa if they have the ability to inhibit chloride transport in the loop of Henle. In this respect, it is of interest to note that the cells of the macula densa are morphologically similar to the epithelial cells of the thick ascending limb of Henle's loop.

It is also important to realize that furosemide, ethacrynic acid, and bumetanide have direct effects on RBF that are not related to their diuretic activity. Soon after furosemide and ethacrynic acid were introduced, it was learned that these drugs increased renal cortical blood flow and decreased flow in the juxtamedullary cortex and outer renal medulla. Many investigators have noted that furosemide, ethacrynic acid, and bumetanide increase total RBF in several species of animals by lowering renal vascular resistance. In fact, Dluhy et al. (163) have suggested that renal

vasodilation might be a characteristic effect of diuretic agents that act at the loop of Henle. The exact mechanism by which furosemide, ethacrynic acid, and bumetanide elevate RBF cannot be stated with certainty, but it appears that this hemodynamic effect is mediated via prostaglandins, the kallikrein-kinin system, an increase in proximal tubular pressure, or some combination of these factors. It is generally agreed that inhibitors of prostaglandin synthetase will prevent the increment in RBF elicited by these drugs.

Results from many studies with experimental animals have indicated that the loop diuretics appear to increase renin release by both a direct effect and indirect effect on the macula densa (21). The direct effect appears to involve the blockade of sodium or chloride transport into these chemoreceptor cells, whereas the indirect effect develops slowly as a result of salt and water losses. These conclusions are supported by the fact that furosemide-induced renin release was prevented by volume repletion when small doses were used, whereas it was not affected by fluid replacement when larger doses were used. Larger doses of loop diuretics also increase renin release via the renal baroreceptor, possibly by elevating renal interstitial pressure. In addition, ongoing renal nerve activity appears to amplify the ability of these drugs to increase renin release. It is possible that the renin release caused by loop diuretics is mediated by renal prostaglandins, because blockade of prostaglandin synthesis prevents the stimulation of renin release. Finally, loop diuretics can directly stimulate the release of renin from the granular JG cells by an unknown mechanism. Activation of each of these control mechanisms may depend on the dose of these drugs, the time after injection, and the species involved. It is easy to see why investigators in this field have presented so many different, and often conflicting, theories to explain the effects of loop diuretics on renin release.

In 1965, Fraser et al. (164) reported that furosemide caused an immediate twofold elevation of PRA in normotensive humans. In the ensuing years, many groups of investigators have reported similar results in normotensive and hypertensive humans. Unfortunately, most of these studies are purely descriptive and fail to give any insight into the mechanism by which loop diuretics increase renin release in humans. Furosemide, in single and multiple doses of 0.29 to 1.14 mg/kg (assuming an average patient weight of 70 kg), caused 1.3- to 5-fold increases in PRA in both normotensive and hypertensive humans. In similar fashion, bumetanide (0.03 mg/kg) and ethacrynic acid (1.4–4.3 mg/kg) elevated PRA by twofold to fivefold in normotensive humans. Unfortunately, in many of these studies the administration of furosemide was followed by variable periods of ambulation before collecting blood for PRA measurements. Because attainment of upright posture in humans increases renin release through activation of the renal sympathetic nerves and the renal afferent arteriolar baroreceptor, mainly those studies conducted with patients in the supine position should be considered in the analysis of the mechanism of furosemide-induced renin release in humans. The route and duration of treatment with furosemide are other factors that may determine the mechanism by which furosemide alters renin release. With regard to the direct renin-releasing effects of furosemide in humans, we consider those studies involving the measurement of PRA soon after intravenous injection of furosemide to recumbent subjects to be the most meaningful for purposes of pharmacologic analysis. It should be pointed out that the doses of furosemide (0.29–1.14 mg/kg) used in these studies correspond to the small doses of the drug used in the animal studies.

A single intravenous dose of furosemide (0.29–1.14 mg/kg) was observed to cause a twofold to fivefold peak elevation of PRA within 10 to 20 min in supine normotensive and hypertensive humans, and renin release remained elevated during the next 1 to 2 hr. Several investigators have noted a biphasic increase in PRA after either intravenous or oral administration of furosemide (21). After an

average threefold elevation of PRA at 10 to 20 min after furosemide, PRA declined to about twice the control values. Approximately 90 to 120 min after furosemide, PRA began to rise again.

In general, the loop diuretics stimulate renin release in humans by the same mechanisms that have been identified in animal studies, i.e., by activation of (a) the macula densa, (b) the renal sympathetic nerves, and (c) the renal prostaglandin system (21). The strongest evidence, although indirect, supports an action of these saluretic agents on the renal sympathetic nerves and the renal prostaglandin system. Keeton and Campbell (21) should be consulted for an extensive analysis of the mechanism(s) by which the loop diuretics stimulate renin release in humans.

Thiazides

Prolonged administration of thiazide diuretics to normal and hypertensive humans results in an elevation of PRA. At first it was thought that hydrochlorothiazide elevated PRA only during the initial stages of therapy, with PRA later returning to control levels, but the advent of more accurate techniques for measurement of PRA revealed that this drug raised PRA by twofold to sixfold when given daily for 6 to 24 weeks. Similar changes in PRA were seen after continued treatment with the other thiazide diuretics. It is of interest to note that treatment of hypertensive patients with either chlorothiazide or furosemide elevated PRA to the same extent after long-term therapy.

The effects of β-adrenergic antagonists on thiazide-induced renin release give some support to the idea that these diuretics stimulate renin release by indirectly activating the sympathetic nervous system. For instance, propranolol was shown to block the renin release brought about by intravenous injection of chlorothiazide into anesthetized dogs. Later, Sweet and Gaul (165) found that timolol completely blocked the fourfold rise in PRA that usually accompanied hydrochlorothiazide treatment in conscious dogs. Timolol also attenuated the hypokalemia that usually developed during long-term treatment with this thiazide, but it was not known if this increase in plasma potassium concentration was involved in the suppression of renin release (165). Similarly, in renal-hypertensive and normotensive dogs and spontaneously hypertensive (SH) and normotensive rats, bendroflumethiazide increased PRA by fourfold to sixfold, and timolol prevented 40 to 90% of this elevation of PRA (166). The ability of timolol to lessen the rise in PRA caused by bendroflumethiazide in rats was especially interesting in light of the fact that timolol potentiated the natriuresis elicited by bendroflumethiazide. Again, timolol attenuated the hypokalemia caused by this thiazide (166).

Timolol, pindolol, oxprenolol, propranolol, and atenolol have been reported to lessen or prevent the increase in PRA that results from prolonged treatment of humans with thiazide diuretics. Chalmers et al. (167) found that hydrochlorothiazide raised PRA from 1.7 to 3.2 ng AI/ml/hr in seated hypertensive patients, whereas timolol suppressed PRA by 65% relative to the control values. Combined treatment with timolol and hydrochlorothiazide resulted in no change in PRA, as compared with the pretreatment values. Similar changes were found by Nielsen et al. (168), who reported PRA to be 3.5, 6.4, 1.7, and 3.5 ng AI/ml/hr during the control, bendroflumethiazide, propranolol, and bendroflumethiazide plus propranolol periods, respectively. Such clearcut findings, however, are not always obtained, because in many cases thiazide-induced renin release was only partially attenuated by β-adrenergic blockade. It also should be pointed out that other investigators have indicated that timolol and oxprenolol are incapable of suppressing the renin release caused by hydrochlorothiazide. Methyclothiazide had no effect on renin secretion from rat renal cortical slices *in vitro*.

Chlorthalidone is a sulfonamide diuretic with properties very similar to those of the thiazides. Chlorthalidone has been shown to increase PRA when given to hypertensive patients for 4 to 14 weeks. Chlorthalidone-induced renin release in hypertensive patients has been shown to be blocked or attenuated by propranolol and sotalol, especially in the standing position. Zanchetti et al. (169) found that continued therapy with chlorthalidone potentiated orthostasis-induced renin release, and, moreover, propranolol was more efficacious in suppressing the renin release caused by chlorthalidone when the patients were in the upright position. Unfortunately, differences in posture cannot account for the differing effects of β-adrenergic blockade on thiazide-induced renin release. For example, some investigators have reported that timolol and oxprenolol lower PRA in thiazide-treated patients in the standing position, but other researchers have found timolol and oxprenolol to have little effect under apparently identical conditions.

Other Diuretic Agents

The mercurial diuretics mercaptomerin and chlormerodrin appear to elevate renin release by promoting the loss of sodium and by depleting plasma volume. Meralluride may raise PRA by another mechanism, possibly the renal baroreceptor.

No information is available concerning the effects of acetazolamide on basal PRA values in animals or humans.

Clopamide inhibits sodium reabsorption in the proximal tubule and does not alter RPF or GFR. Imbs et al. (170) found that clopamide suppressed renin secretion by 50% in anesthetized dogs and attributed this inhibition of renin secretion to an increase in salt load at the macula densa. The effects of long-term treatment with clopamide on basal PRA in animals and humans have not been described.

Metolazone inhibits sodium reabsorption in the proximal tubule and cortical diluting segment, and thus it is similar in its actions to chlorthalidone and the thiazide diuretics. Metolazone-induced renin release in hypertensive humans was lessened by propranolol, and metolazone appeared to increase PRA by a mechanism similar to that of the thiazide diuretics.

Amiloride and triamterene act mainly on the distal tubule and are termed "potassium-sparing" diuretics. Both amiloride and triamterene have been shown to elevate PRA in hypertensive patients.

Spironolactone, a competitive receptor antagonist of the mineralocorticoid aldosterone, blocks the reabsorption of sodium in exchange for potassium and hydrogen in the distal tubule. Spironolactone has been reported to stimulate renin release in hypertensive patients after 3 to 8 weeks of therapy (171). Weinberger and Grim (171) found that spironolactone elicited a dose-related elevation of PRA. Propranolol, but not aspirin, greatly attenuated spironolactone-induced renin release in hypertensive humans. Canrenone, a major active metabolite of spironolactone, elevated PRA and caused sodium loss and potassium retention (like spironolactone) in hypertensive patients.

In conclusion, the non-loop diuretics appear to increase renin release by depleting intravascular volume and thus activating the renal sympathetic nerves.

Vasodilators

The peripheral vasodilating drugs are used widely in the treatment of hypertension, and the increase in renin release by these agents has proved to be of great clinical significance, because the resulting increases in blood levels of AII have been shown to antagonize the antihypertensive effects of these drugs. Hydralazine, minoxidil, diazoxide, sodium nitroprusside, and bupicomide increase renin release in animals and humans by reflex activation of the sympathetic nervous system.

Hydralazine

Hydralazine increases renin release in rats, rabbits, dogs, and normotensive and hypertensive humans. The evidence indicates that hydralazine elicits renin release in animals and humans by reflex activation of the renal sympathetic nerves. Ueda et al. (172) found that intravenous administration of hydralazine to 20 hypertensive patients lowered MAP by 16%, increased heart rate by 16%, and elevated renin secretion by 6.5-fold. RBF rose by 34% as renal vascular resistance dropped by 37%, but GFR was unchanged. Sodium excretion fell by 20%, and medullary RBF increased. The increase in renin secretion did not correlate with changes in MAP, RBF, renal medullary blood flow, renal vascular resistance, filtration fraction, or sodium excretion, but a strong correlation with the increase in heart rate was noted. In order to test the hypothesis that hydralazine elicited renin release via the sympathetic nervous system, hydralazine was injected directly into the kidneys of 3 patients, followed by intravenous hydralazine some 10 min later. Intrarenally administered hydralazine did not alter the renal venous PRA of the injected kidneys, but the subsequent intravenous dose of hydralazine resulted in significant increases in renal venous PRA from both kidneys. In addition, hydralazine failed to stimulate renin release in a patient with a functioning renal allograft. Therefore, Ueda et al. (172) proposed that the reflexly induced increase in renal sympathetic tone precipitated by the vasodilatory properties of hydralazine was the stimulus to renin release.

The importance of the renal sympathetic nerves in hydralazine-induced renin release became more apparent when it was determined that β-adrenergic antagonists inhibited this renin release. In the first experiments of this type, Meyer et al. (149) discovered that pretreatment with propranolol blocked 85% of the ninefold increase in renin release seen when a large dose of hydralazine was given to anesthetized rats. Blood pressure and heart rate were not measured in these studies, and the inhibition by propranolol was thought to be due to blockade of renal β-adrenergic receptors.

In a more comprehensive series of studies conducted with conscious and normotensive and SH rats, Pettinger et al. (27,173,174) found that hydralazine elicited a dose-related elevation of SRA. The peak increase (fivefold) after 1 mg/kg hydralazine occurred at 20 min, and SRA remained elevated (twofold to three-fold) for the next 5 hr. Pretreatment of normal rats with 0.3 and 1.5 mg/kg propranolol, which resulted in serum propranolol levels of 40 and 220 ng/ml, respectively, inhibited this rise in SRA by 85 and 91%, respectively. In concert with earlier investigators (149,172), Pettinger et al. (27) concluded that hydral-azine-induced vasodepression reflexly activated the noradrenergic nerves innervating the gran-ular JG cells. These same researchers also demonstrated that hydralazine caused a 4.5-fold rise in SRA in conscious SH rats that was blocked by 95% when the animals were pretreated with propranolol (173,174). When the ability of propranolol to prevent the rise in SRA caused by hydralazine was examined in greater detail, it was discovered that pre-treatment with a higher dose of propranolol (15 mg/kg), which gave plasma propranolol concentrations of 750 ng/ml, resulted in less impairment of renin release than did lower doses of propranolol (173). Furthermore, higher doses of hydralazine were capable of overriding the inhibition of renin release by propranolol. In both normotensive and SH rats, propranolol potentiated the vasodepres-sor effects of hydralazine and blocked the re-flex tachycardia. For instance, in normoten-sive rats hydralazine and propranolol lowered blood pressure by 21 and 5%, respectively, but the combination of these two drugs low-ered blood pressure by 39%. Thus, proprano-lol inhibited hydralazine-induced renin release even though systemic blood pressure was low-ered to a greater extent than with hydralazine alone. These observations in conscious ani-mals again emphasize the importance of the renal sympathetic nerves, rather than the af-ferent arteriolar baroreceptor, in the stimula-tion of renin release by hydralazine.

More recently, Campbell et al. (88,175,176) discovered that inhibitors of prostaglandin synthesis prevented the 10-fold increase in re-nin release elicited by hydralazine in rats (88,175) and rabbits (176). Pretreatment of conscious rats with indomethacin or meclofe-namate, in doses that reduced the urinary ex-cretion of PGE_2 and $PGF_{2\alpha}$ by 89 and 74%, respectively, inhibited hydralazine-induced re-nin release by 100 and 77%, respectively. Be-cause pretreatment with a combination of in-domethacin and propranolol did not inhibit hydralazine-induced renin release to a greater extent than did either blocker alone, these au-thors concluded that indomethacin and pro-pranolol inhibited hydralazine-induced renin release by a common mechanism that involved the sympathetic nervous system. These same investigators also found that hydralazine caused a twofold increase in PRA, which was accompanied by a threefold elevation of plasma norepinephrine concentration, in con-scious rabbits (176). Indomethacin, in a dose that lowered renal venous PGE_2 levels by 56%, blocked hydralazine-elicited renin re-lease but not the increment in plasma norepi-nephrine concentration. Indomethacin did not affect the fall in blood pressure brought about by hydralazine, but the reflex increase in heart rate was attenuated. Thus, in the rat and the rabbit, renal prostaglandins appear to be in-volved in the renin release that accompanies reflex activation of the renal sympathetic nerves by hydralazine.

Because both renal nerve stimulation (177) and an intrarenal arterial infusion of isoproter-enol (178) have been demonstrated to elicit a greater renin response at a low renal perfu-sion pressure than at a normal renal perfusion pressure, the fall in renal perfusion pressure that results from the decrease in systemic blood pressure after hydralazine may serve to potentiate the renin-releasing effects of the reflex increase in noradrenergic nerve activity at the granular JG cells. Such an interaction between these mechanisms controlling renin release also might explain the greater stimula-tion of renin release from the affected kidney in patients with unilateral renal artery stenosis after therapy with hydralazine. However, be-cause β-adrenergic blockade inhibited hydralazine-induced renin release while potentiating hydralazine-induced vasodepression (173), the amplifying effects of the renal baroreceptor on vasodilatory drug-induced renin release appear to be of little importance.

Minoxidil

The newly released peripheral vasodilator minoxidil has been reported to elevate PRA in conscious rats and hypertensive humans, and, as with hydralazine, this stimulation of renin release by minoxidil has been found to be blocked by propranolol.

After the initial reports of minoxidil-induced renin release in patients, Pettinger et al. (27,173) demonstrated that minoxidil elicited a dose-related elevation of SRA in normotensive rats. At higher doses, minoxidil was much more potent than hydralazine in increasing renin release. The peak increase in SRA occurred at 45 min, and renin release remained stimulated over the next 5 hr. Pretreatment with 0.3 and 1.5 mg/kg propranolol inhibited minoxidil-induced renin release by 78 and 89%, respectively. As with hydralazine, the ability of propranolol to mitigate the elevation of SRA caused by minoxidil waned as the dose of propranolol was increased, but, unlike hydralazine, higher doses of minoxidil did not override the inhibition of renin release produced by propranolol. Concerning hemodynamic changes in normal rats, propranolol and minoxidil reduced blood pressure by 3 and 15%, respectively, whereas propranolol decreased heart rate, and minoxidil, when given alone, markedly increased heart rate. Propranolol potentiated the vasodepressor effect of minoxidil (a 24% decrement in blood pressure) and prevented the associated tachycardia.

Minoxidil-induced renin release also has been studied extensively in hypertensive patients. Pettinger and Mitchell (179) found PRA to be elevated in severely hypertensive patients during long-term therapy with minoxidil. When propranolol was withdrawn from patients receiving propranolol and minoxidil, both supine PRA and upright PRA increased.

In another study of patients with malignant hypertension, it was noted that propranolol lowered supine PRA and upright PRA by 80%, and the addition of minoxidil resulted in a twofold rise in PRA (180). However, even though minoxidil stimulated renin release in the presence of propranolol, the supine and upright PRA values were still 60 to 70% lower than the prepropranolol levels.

When O'Malley et al. (181) used minoxidil to lower blood pressure in patients with essential hypertension, PRA rose to six to seven times the control values, and the addition of propranolol to the drug regimen blocked 60 to 75% of the stimulatory effect of minoxidil. Minoxidil lowered MAP (-27%) and total peripheral resistance (-45%) and raised heart rate ($+31\%$) and cardiac index ($+47\%$). The addition of propranolol further lowered blood pressure, and heart rate and cardiac index returned to the control levels. Total peripheral resistance rose after propranolol but remained significantly lower (-25%) than the value observed during the predrug period. Sodium excretion fell by 16% after minoxidil alone, and propranolol caused no further change in renal function.

Diazoxide

Diazoxide is effective in causing a rapid fall in blood pressure and is used in the treatment of hypertensive crisis. Treatment with diazoxide has been demonstrated to elevate PRA in rats (182), dogs (183), and normotensive (119) and hypertensive (184) humans.

In a group of supine hypertensive patients, diazoxide elicited a fivefold increase in PRA (184). Blood pressure fell and heart rate increased. Whereas the attainment of upright posture brought about a twofold rise in PRA, orthostasis after diazoxide resulted in little additional increment in renin release. Salt depletion raised supine PRA values by fivefold, and PRA increased another 56% when the patients stood up. Injection of diazoxide at this point caused an additional threefold increase in PRA; therefore, sodium depletion potentiated the renin-releasing effects of diazoxide.

It was concluded that diazoxide elicited renin release via activation of the sympathetic nervous system, and this conclusion was supported by the previous observation that diazoxide increased the circulating level of catecholamines in rats. Consistent with the belief that diazoxide stimulated renin release via the sympathetic nervous system (184), propranolol prevented diazoxide-induced renin release in normal humans (119).

A large dose of diazoxide brought about an 11-fold increase in PRA in anesthetized rats, and this stimulatory effect was reduced by one-half by prior adrenal demedullation or treatment with oxprenolol (182). Although a single dose of guanethidine and multiple doses of reserpine and 6-hydroxydopamine had essentially no effect on basal renin release, each of these treatments blocked the renin response to diazoxide by approximately 50%. These data further support the belief that diazoxide-stimulated renin release results from activation of the sympathetic nervous system in response to a decrease in blood pressure.

On the other hand, Vandongen and Greenwood (185) detected an increase in renin release when diazoxide was injected into the isolated perfused rat kidney, but this drug was a comparatively weak stimulus when compared with isoproterenol. Because the decrease in renal perfusion pressure, which occurred with time, was similar in control and diazoxide-treated kidneys, it was believed that diazoxide had a direct action on the granular JG cells that might involve a competition for calcium binding sites.

Sodium Nitroprusside

Like diazoxide, sodium nitroprusside rapidly lowers blood pressure and has been used in hypertensive emergency. Because the vasodepressor effect of sodium nitroprusside is short-lived, this drug must be given by continuous intravenous infusion in order to lower blood pressure to an acceptable level. In a recent collaborative study, no significant increase in heart rate was observed during sodium-nitroprusside-induced vasodepression,

but some clinicians found that the drug produced a tachycardia. Because a standardized preparation of sodium nitroprusside has become available only recently, the number of studies concerning the effects of sodium nitroprusside on renin release is small. However, sodium nitroprusside has been shown to increase PRA in rats (186) and in normotensive (187) and hypertensive (188) humans.

The renin release induced by sodium nitroprusside, like that induced by hydralazine, minoxidil, and diazoxide, appears to result from the fact that the vasodepressor effects of sodium nitroprusside elicit a reflex activation of the renal sympathetic nerves.

Other Vasodilators

Bupicomide, a compound with systemic hemodynamic effects similar to those of hydralazine, was shown to elevate PRA in hypertensive patients (189). This stimulation of renin release was thought to occur as a result of an increase in sympathetic nerve activity and a decrease in renal perfusion pressure (189).

The inhalation of amyl nitrite by recumbent normal humans lowered blood pressure and raised heart rate, but no perceptible change in PRA was observed. However, after PRA had been elevated by treatment with phentolamine, amyl nitrite caused a further increase in PRA.

Calcium Antagonists

In recent years, the slow-channel calcium antagonists have been found to be useful in the treatment of angina and certain types of cardiac arrhythmias. Limited clinical observations have been made concerning the effects of these drugs on renin release, but the calcium antagonists have been employed more extensively in studies of the role of calcium in renin secretion in vitro.

Aoki et al. (190) found that nifedipine lowered diastolic blood pressure by 26% when given sublingually to hypertensive patients. Heart rate increased and PRA doubled. The renin responses of 2 patients with malignant hypertension and 1 patient with renovascular hypertension did not differ from those of patients with essential hypertension, but 2 patients with primary aldosteronism failed to exhibit a rise in PRA. In the latter case, a marked fall in blood pressure was not accompanied by an increase in heart rate. Later, propranolol was shown to prevent the increases in PRA and heart rate caused by nifedipine (191). The effects of a single sublingual dose of nifedipine on blood pressure, heart rate, PRA, and plasma norepinephrine and epinephrine concentrations were studied in normotensive and hypertensive patients (192). In normal subjects, nifedipine increased PRA, heart rate, and plasma norepinephrine and epinephrine concentrations but had no effect on blood pressure. Although blood pressure decreased and plasma norepinephrine concentration increased in hypertensive patients, PRA and heart rate were not changed. After 3 weeks of oral treatment with nifedipine, hypertensive patients exhibited a decrease in blood pressure and an increase in plasma norepinephrine concentration in both the supine and upright position, but neither PRA nor heart rate was increased. The renin release caused by nifedipine *in vivo* appears to result from reflex activation of the renal sympathetic nerves.

The effects of the calcium antagonists on renin secretion *in vitro* do not necessarily reflect their effects on renin secretion *in vivo*. As stated previously, an increase in intracellular calcium concentration is associated with a decrease in renin release, whereas a decrease in intracellular calcium concentration is associated with an increase in renin release. Accordingly, depolarization of the granular JG cells in rat renal cortical slices *in vitro* suppresses renin secretion by causing an increase in calcium influx. Churchill (193) found that the compound D-600, the methoxy derivative of verapamil, reversed the inhibition of renin release caused by 60-mM potassium. AII also inhibited renin secretion *in vitro,* and this inhibition required the presence of extracellular

calcium. However, D-600 did not reverse the inhibition of renin secretion caused by AII. In later studies with diltiazem, Churchill et al. (194) noted that this calcium antagonist also reversed the inhibition of renin secretion caused by the depolarization of rat renal cortical slices *in vitro*. Lowering the extracellular calcium concentration enhanced the efficacy of diltiazem. In the presence of concentrations of diltiazem that blocked the inhibitory effects of potassium-induced depolarization, AII and AVP still suppressed renin secretion *in vitro*. From these studies, Churchill et al. (193,194) concluded that calcium influx through voltage-sensitive calcium channels mediates the inhibitory effects of depolarization and that AII and AVP inhibit renin secretion by mechanisms that are independent of the voltage-sensitive calcium channels. On the other hand, Park et al. (195) reported that verapamil prevented the suppression of renin secretion caused by potassium-induced depolarization, AII, and AVP. The reasons for these disparate results (194,195) are not known.

Cardiac Glycosides

Despite the widespread use of cardiac glycosides in the treatment of congestive heart failure and cardiac arrhythmias in humans, little is known of the effects of this class of drugs on renin release. In a brief report published in 1976, Antonello et al. (196) reported that PRA decreased by 50% within 30 min after intravenous injection of digoxin into supine hypertensive patients. Plasma renin activity remained suppressed by 40% for up to 3 hr and then slowly increased during the next 2-hr period. The inhibition of renin release was related to the plasma concentration of digoxin. In a more recent brief report (197) from the same laboratory, the rise in PRA brought about by administration of a single oral dose of furosemide to hypertensive patients was greatly attenuated by subsequent administration of digoxin. The inhibitory effect of digoxin developed rapidly, when the concentration of digoxin in the plasma was still quite low, and was thought to be related to the concentration of digoxin in the tubular urine. Pretreatment of the patients with the β-adrenergic antagonist oxprenolol partially blocked furosemide-induced renin release, but digoxin was not able to prevent the residual response to furosemide (197). As pointed out by Ferrari (197), the digitalis glycosides could affect renin release by inhibiting ion transport (presumably at the granular JG cells or the macula densa), causing hemodynamic changes, or exerting an antiadrenergic effect. The last mechanism was favored because of the data obtained with oxprenolol and furosemide. An intrarenal infusion of ouabain has also been demonstrated to prevent furosemide-stimulated renin secretion in conscious sheep (198).

The idea that cardiac glycosides inhibit renin release by altering sympathetic neurotransmission is supported by data obtained in experimental animals (199). For example, both digitoxin and acetyldigitoxin reduced the cardiac chronotropic response to sympathetic nerve stimulation and epinephrine in anesthetized dogs with denervated hearts. Thames (199) demonstrated that intracoronary injection or epicardial application of acetylstrophanthidin caused a reflex reduction in renal sympathetic nerve activity via cardiac receptors with vagal afferent fibers. Decrements in renal nerve activity were evoked by small doses of acetylstrophanthidin that did not reflexly lower MAP or heart rate. It was also mentioned that intracoronary injection of ouabain caused bradycardia, hypotension, and a decrease in renin release, but this effect of ouabain on renin release was not studied systematically. In addition, the reflex hemodynamic responses to acetylstrophanthidin were similar to those observed after intracoronary injection of the veratrum alkaloid cryptenamine. Cryptenamine also lowered heart rate, blood pressure, and renin secretion in anesthetized dogs by the activation of ventricular receptors with vagal afferents. These similar effects of digitalis and veratrum alkaloids, as pointed out by Thames (199), may result from the marked structural similarities between the two

classes of compounds. Evidence supports the belief that the renal nerves are responsible for the renal vasoconstriction and augmented renin release seen in congestive heart failure, and cardiac receptors with vagal afferent fibers may have a reduced sensitivity in heart failure. This being the case, Thames (199) suggested that the effect of digitalis on renin release would be greatest in congestive heart failure, because basal renal nerve activity would be high and basal cardiac receptor stimulation would be low. In this respect, the relative ability of cardiac glycosides to inhibit renin release in normal humans and patients with congestive heart failure needs to be determined.

Ouabain did not affect basal renin release in anesthetized dogs (200) or conscious sheep (198), but intrarenal infusion of ouabain did block the rise in renin secretion caused by ureteral occlusion or a decrease in renal perfusion pressure (200). Because ouabain was known to increase the intracellular concentration of sodium ion, it was concluded that ouabain inhibited the stimulation of renin release caused by these two interventions by increasing the intracellular concentration of sodium in the cells of the macula densa. This conclusion gained support from the observation that renin release from rat renal cortical slices *in vitro* did appear to be inversely related to the intracellular concentration of sodium (201). Renin release from the slices was directly related to the sodium concentration of the medium; however, when the normal extrusion of sodium from the cells was impaired by inhibiting sodium-potassium ATPase with ouabain, renin release was inversely related to the sodium content of the medium (201).

A slightly different ionic mechanism of action was suggested to account for the blockade by ouabain of furosemide-induced renin release in conscious sheep (198). Presumably, furosemide decreased the transport of chloride into the macula densa cells, thus enhancing renin release, and ouabain blocked this action by depolarizing the macula densa cells and allowing the passive redistribution of chloride into these cells (202). However, it should be pointed out that ouabain did not change the magnitude or the duration of the renin release that followed the addition of ethacrynic acid to isolated, superfused rat glomeruli (203). Ouabain did not affect the basal release of renin from isolated, superfused rat glomeruli (203) or renal cortical cell suspensions *in vitro* (57), but it did suppress renin release from renal cortical slices *in vitro* (64,66). The suppression of renin release in the latter case was shown to be dependent on the presence of extracellular calcium.

More recently, Park et al. (195) found that ouabain inhibited epinephrine-induced renin secretion from rat renal cortical slices *in vitro*. The following explanation, mainly derived from knowledge of the mechanism by which β-adrenergic receptor stimulation causes relaxation of vascular smooth muscle, was put forward to explain this observation. Epinephrine activates the sodium-potassium pump by phosphorylating membrane proteins, an action mediated by cyclic AMP and its dependent protein kinase. The increased electrochemical gradient of sodium resulting from the increased activity of the sodium-potassium pump enhances the efflux of calcium in exchange for the influx of sodium. As intracellular calcium concentration decreases, renin release is increased. Ouabain prevents the activation of the sodium-potassium pump by epinephrine and thus blocks epinephrine-induced renin release.

Inhibitors of the Renin-Angiotensin System

The successful synthesis of specific competitive antagonists of AII and specific inhibitors of AI converting enzyme during the past decade has enabled researchers to define more accurately the physiologic role of the renin-angiotensin system, as well as its role in experimental and clinical hypertension. In 1970, Marshall et al. (204) demonstrated that 4-Phe-8-Tyr-AII was a competitive receptor antagonist of AII. In the ensuing years, other analogues of AII, with aliphatic amino acids (alanine, isoleucine, and glycine) substituted for the phenylalanine residue in the 8-position of AII, were produced in other laboratories. In addition, in most of these compounds the 1-position was occupied by the nonmammalian amino acid sarcosine, because this substitution was found to prolong the half-life of the peptides and thereby increase their potency. The most extensively characterized receptor antagonist of AII is 1-Sar-8-Ala-AII, also known as saralasin. A nonapeptide (Pyr-Trp-Pro-Arg-Pro-Gln-Ile-Pro-Pro) that has been shown to inhibit AI converting enzyme was isolated from the venom of the fer-de-lance snake (*Bothrops jararaca*) by Ondetti et al. (205) in 1971. The synthetic form of this compound (Glu-Trp-Pro-Arg-Pro-Gln-Ile-Pro-Pro) was designated SQ 20,881 (teprotide). Because teprotide was liable to enzymic degradation, and thus had to be given intravenously in order to have an effect, a program to develop an orally active inhibitor of AI converting enzyme was initiated by Ondetti et al. (206). In 1977 these researchers (206) indicated that some mercaptoalkanoyl and carboxyalkanoyl derivatives of amino acids were effective and selective inhibitors of AI converting enzyme, with SQ 14,225 (D-3-mercapto-2-methylpropranoyl-L-proline; captopril) being the most potent compound. Other authors have reviewed in detail the pharmacology of the AII receptor antagonists (5,207), teprotide (208) and captopril (209), and in the discussion that follows we shall consider the effects of these agents on renin release in animals and humans.

Antagonists of AII

Antagonists of AII, primarily saralasin, have been shown to increase renin release in anesthetized (210) and conscious (211) dogs, conscious rabbits (212), and anesthetized (213) and conscious (75,214) rats. In the majority of these studies the renin release caused by saralasin was attributed to the ability of saralasin to block the AII-mediated negative-feedback loop controlling renin release. In those situations in which saralasin lowered blood pressure, such as sodium depletion (211), no relationship was noted between the decrease in MAP and the rise in PRA. Keeton et al. (75) made a thorough study of the effects of salt balance and adrenergic blockade on the renin release elicited by saralasin in conscious rats and concluded that (a) the major portion of saralasin-induced renin release in conscious normal and sodium-depleted rats results from this disinhibition of AII-mediated suppression of renin release, (b) the importance of the "short-loop" suppression of renin release by intrarenally generated AII is amplified by sodium deprivation, (c) the short-loop negative-feedback mechanism controlling renin release is closely associated with intrarenal β-adrenergic receptors, presumably located on the granular JG cells, and (d) saralasin, under certain circumstances, acts temporarily as an agonist at the intrarenal AII receptors inhibitory to renin release and thereby decreases renin release. It should be pointed out that the agonistic properties of saralasin are modulated by dietary sodium and that sodium depletion minimizes the ability of saralasin to act as a partial agonist. Lastly, because AII had been shown to inhibit adenylate cyclase in rat tail artery, and because β-adrenergically mediated renin release appeared to involve the production of cyclic AMP, it was suggested that saralasin increased renin release by releasing granular JG cell adenylate cyclase from the inhibitory effect of AII. Because inhibitors of prostaglandin synthesis prevented other forms of sympathetically mediated renin release (88), Campbell et al. (214) probed the role of prostaglandins in saralasin-induced renin release in normal rats. Both indomethacin and meclofenemate blocked saralasin-induced renin release in conscious normal and sodium-depleted rats. When doses of indomethacin and propranolol that did not completely inhibit saralasin-induced renin release were given together, the rise in SRA caused by saralasin was inhibited by 100%. Campbell et al. (214) concluded that the renin release caused by saralasin in conscious rats appeared to be intimately associated with renal

β-adrenergic receptors and possibly was mediated by renal prostaglandins.

Concerning the effects of AII antagonists on renin release in vitro, Vandongen et al. (215) found that nonpressor derivatives of AII, including saralasin, increased perfusate renin activity by fourfold in the isolated perfused rat kidney. A slight decrement in renal perfusion pressure occurred. Hofbauer et al. (216) noted that small doses of saralasin caused a slight amount of vasodilation and renin release in the isolated perfused rat kidney, but larger doses, which completely blocked AII-induced vasoconstriction, elicited vasoconstriction and inhibition of renin release. Plasma saralasin levels of similar magnitude were associated with increased renin release in vivo (75). If a high concentration of AII was used to depress renal perfusate flow and renin release in the isolated perfused rat kidney, saralasin reversed the vasoconstriction but not the inhibition of renin release. It was concluded that saralasin possessed a high degree of intrinsic activity at the AII receptors of granular JG cells. Even though saralasin reversed AII-mediated inhibition of renin release from rat renal cortical slices in vitro, saralasin by itself did not cause a significant elevation of renin release (217).

In normotensive and hypertensive humans, saralasin and other receptor antagonists of AII were observed to elevate PRA, and the ability of these agents to stimulate renin release appeared to be a function of both the pretreatment level of PRA and sodium intake (21). As a general rule, those patients with higher than normal PRA values exhibited a rise in PRA during the administration of saralasin. In like fashion, when basal PRA was elevated by salt depletion in humans who had not previously shown a renin response to saralasin, this AII antagonist elicited renin release. Saralasin, and other AII antagonists such as 1-Sar-8-Ile-AII, are partial agonists at AII receptors located in the vasculature, adrenal gland, and granular JG cells, and the expression of the agonistic and antagonistic properties of saralasin is dependent on the basal value of PRA and sodium intake. Thus, saralasin decreased PRA and increased blood pressure in normal humans on a high-salt diet, in normal-renin hypertensive patients on a high-salt diet, and in low-renin hypertensive patients on either a normal or low-salt diet. Conversely, AII receptor blockade increased renin release and decreased blood pressure in patients with high-renin hypertension on a normal or low-salt diet, in normal-renin hypertensive and normotensive humans on a salt-restricted diet, in hypertensive patients with coarctation of the thoracic aorta, in patients with renovascular hypertension, in hypertensive patients being treated with vasodilators, in some hypertensive patients on maintenance hemodialysis, in cases of pheochromocytoma, and in other hyperreninemic conditions not associated with an elevation of blood pressure. In the last category, normotensive patients with Bartter's syndrome, renal tubular acidosis, and cirrhosis with ascites experienced a fall in blood pressure and a rise in PRA during the antagonism of AII receptors.

Although many investigators have reported saralasin-induced renin release in humans, a major disagreement exists concerning the mechanism by which this stimulation occurs. On the one hand, saralasin was thought to elicit renin release only in those situations in which it caused vasodepression. On the other hand, many researchers have voiced the opinion that the renin-releasing effects of saralasin are not dependent on the ability of this compound to lower blood pressure. In the former case, saralasin-induced vasodepression was thought to stimulate renin release via activation of the renal baroreceptor and/or the renal sympathetic nerves, whereas in the latter case saralasin was thought to increase renin release by blocking the negative feedback of AII on the secretory function of the granular JG cells. However, studies of the effects of saralasin on renin release and renal hemodynamics during alterations in sodium intake have indicated that the renal baroreceptor does not appear to play a crucial role in saralasin-induced renin release in humans.

The sympathetic ner[...] play a role in saralasin-i[...] in humans. It is not unusual [...] agents to stimulate renin releas[...] fall in blood pressure results in re[...] tion of the renal sympathetic nerves. H[...] this generalized increase in sympathetic [...] charge usually results in an increase in hea[...] rate, and saralasin-induced vasodepression is notable for its inconsistent effects on heart rate. Despite this fact, Pettinger and Mitchell (218,219) found that infusion of saralasin into hypertensive patients receiving minoxidil caused a threefold rise in PRA that was clearly related to the fall in blood pressure. A single dose of propranolol that yielded an average plasma propranolol level of 150 ng/ml did not alter basal PRA or the vasodepressor action of saralasin but did prevent the previously observed rise in PRA. Chronic therapy with propranolol decreased basal PRA and blood pressure; however, under these conditions, saralasin had little effect on blood pressure or renin release. It was suggested that PRA was elevated by saralasin as a result of blockade of the AII-mediated short-loop inhibition of renin release and that the intrarenal AII receptors responsible for the suppression of renin release were closely related to the β-adrenergic receptors located on the granular JG cells (218). These conclusions are in accord with the results obtained in animal studies (75,214).

Inhibitors of AI Converting Enzyme

Both teprotide and captopril have been shown to prevent the conversion of AI to AII and the degradation of bradykinin. Therefore, just as the partial agonist activity of the AII receptor antagonists was found to limit their use as pharmacologic tools in the study of physiologic and pathophysiologic phenomena, the dual effects of the converting enzyme inhibitors on angiotensin and kinin metabolism also have presented problems of interpretation. For example, a portion of the vasodepressor effect of teprotide in anesthetized, two-kid-

teprotide increased ..., odium
excretion in sodium-deprived dogs but had no
effect on these parameters after a high-salt
diet. The presence of elevated renin release
in the face of an increase in sodium excretion
makes it unlikely that teprotide stimulated renin release via the macula densa. Pretreatment
with propranolol did not block the increase
in PRA caused by teprotide in conscious sodium-depleted dogs (222). In each of these
studies it was concluded that the nonapeptide
inhibitor of AI converting enzyme stimulated
renin release by blockade of the short-loop
feedback system mediated by AII.

The AI converting enzyme inhibitor captopril, which is more potent than teprotide and
has no direct effect on vascular smooth muscle, elicited renin release in normotensive
(223,224) and SH rats (223,225). In normotensive rats, captopril did not affect blood pressure (225), and yet chronic administration of
this drug resulted in a continual elevation of
PRA over a 6-month period. Chronic treatment of SH rats with captopril for 6 months
caused a large decrement in blood pressure
and a 15-fold increment in PRA. In contrast,
a dose of hydralazine that produced a lesser
degree of vasodepression over a 6-month period caused only a threefold increase in PRC.
These observations are similar to those obtained when saralasin and hydralazine were
compared in sodium-depleted normotensive
rats (75).

Antonaccio et al. (223) studied the effects
of treatment with either propranolol or in-

domethacin on the renin release seen in SH
and Wistar-Kyoto (normotensive) rats after
3 days of oral therapy with captopril. Captopril elevated PRA to a greater extent in SH
rats (eightfold increase) as compared with normotensive animals (threefold increase). Indomethacin alone suppressed PRA by 60 and
70% in both SH and normal rats, respectively,
but did not block the stimulation of renin release caused by captopril. Propranolol alone
lowered basal PRA by 70 and 40% in SH
and normal rats, respectively. During combined administration of propranolol and captopril to SH rats, PRA rose sevenfold relative
to the values seen with propranolol alone, but
the absolute PRA values were significantly less
than those observed after captopril alone. In
like fashion, propranolol did not impair the
ability of captopril to elicit renin release in
normal rats. Neither propranolol nor indomethacin altered the 20% decrease in MAP
caused by captopril in the two strains of rats.
Conversely, Schiffrin et al. (224) found captopril-induced renin release to be attenuated
greatly by propranolol in normotensive
Sprague-Dawley rats. AII also blocked the rise
in PRA caused by captopril, but indomethacin
was without effect. Thus, Antonaccio et al.
(223) and Schiffrin et al. (224) agreed that
prostaglandins were not involved in the renin
release elicited by captopril. Captopril appeared to elevate PRA by interruption of the
short-loop feedback control of renin release
and activation of the renal sympathetic nerves.

Captopril also has been shown to elicit renin
release in anesthetized dogs (226) and conscious dogs on a normal (227) and sodium-
restricted (228) diet. In conscious normotensive dogs, captopril caused a moderate dose-
related decrease in MAP without affecting
heart rate (227). In parallel fashion, this drug
elicited a dose-related elevation of PRA (up
to 15-fold increase), and both the level of PRA
achieved and the duration of the effect were
dose-dependent. Plasma renin activity was
thought to increase in response to the interruption of the short-loop feedback mechanism
and the fall in arterial pressure.

The nonapeptide teprotide increased PRA in both normotensive (229) and hypertensive (230,231) humans. In like fashion, treatment with captopril stimulated renin release in normotensive (232) and hypertensive (233) humans. Gavras et al. (230,231) suggested that the stimulation of renin release by teprotide resulted from a combination of blockade of the short-loop feedback controlling renin release and the fall in blood pressure. In these studies, PRA increased in supine hypertensive patients on a low- or normal-salt diet, and orthostasis-induced renin release also was potentiated by teprotide. Sancho et al. (229) observed a twofold to threefold elevation of PRA after teprotide was given to supine normotensive patients on a low- or normal-salt diet. Blood pressure fell slightly in the former case, but did not change in the latter case. Thus, the stimulation of renin release was believed to be due to a decrease in the concentration of AII at the granular JG cells (229).

In 1977, Ferguson et al. (232) reported that a single dose of captopril elicited a twofold increase in PRA in normotensive humans without lowering blood pressure. Because blood pressure did not fall, the rise in PRA was conjectured to be the result of blockade of the short-loop feedback of renin release. It should be pointed out that a recent study by Kono et al. (234) supports the idea that captopril-induced renin release in humans results from the removal of the inhibitory effects of AII on renin release. These investigators found that subpressor doses of AII, given intravenously, prevented the rise in PRA caused by the administration of a single oral dose of captopril to normotensive and hypertensive humans. However, Case et al. (233) found that the increase in PRA seen after the administration of a single oral dose of captopril to seated hypertensive patients was closely correlated with the decrement in arterial pressure and the pretreatment PRA value. During chronic oral therapy with captopril, PRA was elevated in both the supine and upright positions. In other clinical studies (235), chronic treatment of hypertensive patients with captopril lowered MAP by 21% and increased PRA by fivefold. A greater stimulation of renin release was observed in patients with renovascular hypertension as compared with those with essential hypertension, and a slight elevation of pulse rate was seen in all patients. As a result, it was concluded that captopril stimulated renin release by blockade of the short-loop control system and by activation of the renal sympathetic nerves.

Abe et al. (236) reported that indomethacin blocked the increase in PRA seen after chronic treatment of normotensive and hypertensive humans with captopril. Captopril lowered MAP by 18% in hypertensive patients but had no effect on blood pressure in the normotensive subjects. The hemodynamic responses to captopril were not affected by the addition of indomethacin. Urinary excretion of PGE increased by 48% during therapy with captopril, and addition of indomethacin resulted in a 50% decrease in the urinary concentration of PGE. Abe et al. (236) concluded that captopril elevated PRA by interrupting the inhibition of renin release by AII and that endogenous prostaglandins were involved in the short-loop feedback inhibition of renin release. The latter conclusion is consistent with the observation that indomethacin blocked saralasin-induced renin release in conscious rats (214), but it does not agree with the observations made with captopril in rats (223,224).

To summarize, AII receptor antagonists and inhibitors of AI converting enzyme increase renin release in normotensive and hypertensive animals and humans. In general, the ability of these drugs to stimulate renin release is dependent on the pretreatment level of PRA, which is in turn affected by changes in salt intake. In situations in which PRA is increased by these agents, and yet blood pressure is unaltered, the stimulation of renin release is probably the result of blockade of the negative-feedback effect of AII on the secretory function of the granular JG cells. The importance of this short-loop inhibition of renin release is amplified by sodium deprivation, but, in addition, the stimulation of renin release in sodium-depleted states is partly attributable to the vasodepressor effects of these drugs. In certain situations, the partial agonist effect of saralasin actually causes a decrease in renin secretion. β-Adrenergic receptor blockade prevents saralasin-induced renin release in rats and humans, and inhibition of prostaglandin synthesis prevents this drug action in rats. Teprotide-induced renin release was not affected by β-adrenergic blockade in dogs. Propranolol inhibited the rise in PRA caused by captopril in some studies (rats, dogs) but not in other studies (rats, rabbits). Indomethacin inhibited captopril-induced renin release in humans but not in rats.

Nonsteroidal Antiinflammatory Drugs (Prostaglandin Synthesis Inhibitors)

Since the discovery by Vane (237) in 1971 that nonsteroidal antiinflammatory drugs such as aspirin and indomethacin inhibited the synthesis of prostaglandins, a monumental number of studies have been performed with these drugs in an attempt to delineate the contribution of endogenous prostaglandins to various physiologic phenomena. Along these lines, a number of investigators have used these prostaglandin synthesis inhibitors to probe the involvement of renal prostaglandins in the control of renin release (238). In reviewing these studies, however, the reader must bear in mind that these drugs have a number of actions, in addition to inhibiting prostaglandin synthesis, that may alter the release of renin. For instance, various inhibitors of prostaglandin synthesis have been shown to antagonize the actions of calcium, elicit salt and water retention, and inhibit the enzymes phosphodiesterase and 1-aromatic amino acid decarboxylase. Thus, even in studies in which suppression of prostaglandin synthesis has been clearly demonstrated, the evidence for a prostaglandin-mediated mechanism of action is indirect, and the conclusions should be viewed with appropriate caution.

The prostaglandin synthetase inhibitors have been shown to inhibit basal renin release.

For example, indomethacin has been reported to suppress basal PRA by about 50% in conscious (88,239) and anesthetized (240) rats, conscious rabbits (241), anesthetized dogs (242), and normotensive (243) and hypertensive (244) humans. Meclofenamate suppressed basal PRA in conscious rats (88,239), and both aspirin and diclofenac sodium lowered basal renin release in normotensive humans. These studies indicate that renal prostaglandins exert a tonic stimulatory influence on renin release.

In addition to altering basal renin release, these drugs inhibit renin release that has been elevated by a number of physiologic, pharmacologic, and pathologic stimuli. Inhibitors of prostaglandin synthetase blocked the increase in PRA associated with the attainment of upright posture in humans (243). Reflex-induced activation of the renal sympathetic nerves is thought to be the major factor in orthostasis-induced renin release in humans, with the renal baroreceptor playing a minor role (245). Other types of β-adrenergically mediated renin release have been found to be inhibited by prostaglandin synthetase inhibitors. Pretreatment with indomethacin blocked the increase in PRA caused by isoproterenol in conscious rats (88), conscious dogs (246), anesthetized cats (247), and normal humans (248). However, in other studies with anesthetized dogs (249) and sodium-depleted humans (248), indomethacin did not alter isoproterenol-induced renin release. Campbell et al. (88) found that the renin release elicited by administration of hydralazine, prenalterol (a β_1-adrenergic agonist), and dibutyryl cyclic AMP was prevented by indomethacin and meclofenamate in doses that reduced the urinary excretion of PGE_2 and $PGF_{2\alpha}$ by 65 and 89%, respectively. Based on the results of this study, Campbell et al. (88) concluded that renal prostaglandins, by acting at a site distal to the β-adrenergic receptors of the granular JG cells, serve as mediators of sympathetically induced renin release in the conscious rat.

In later studies, these same investigators (176) noted that indomethacin, in a dose that lowered renal venous PGE_2 levels by 56%, blocked the rise in PRA, but not the increases in plasma norepinephrine and epinephrine concentrations, seen when hydralazine was given to conscious rabbits. Subsequently, indomethacin was shown to inhibit insulin-induced renin release in conscious rats (250). The increase in plasma epinephrine levels and the decrease in plasma glucose concentration caused by insulin were not affected by indomethacin.

Inhibitors of prostaglandin synthesis also have been shown to reduce hemorrhage-induced renin release, which probably is mediated by the renal sympathetic nerves and the renal baroreceptor. However, these drugs only reduced the rise in PRA caused by nonhypotensive hemorrhage. The increase in PRA seen during hypotensive hemorrhage in anesthetized dogs was not altered by indomethacin. The disparate results reported in these two studies can be reconciled by assuming that renal prostaglandins mediate the release of renin that occurs following nonhypotensive hemorrhage in which RBF and GFR are maintained. However, following hypotensive hemorrhage, in which RBF and GRF are significantly reduced, the release of renin is controlled by factors other than the prostaglandins. This situation would be analogous to that observed with baroreceptor-mediated renin release, in which renal prostaglandins mediate the renin release only within the autoregulatory range of RBF (vide supra).

As discussed previously, prostaglandins appear to be involved in the mediation of renal baroreceptor-stimulated renin release. Because ureteral occlusion in anesthetized dogs was thought to elevate renin release by activation of the renal baroreceptor mechanism, and because this maneuver increased RBF and the urinary excretion of PGE_2 in anesthetized dogs, Blackshear and Wathen (22) tested the effects of indomethacin on PRA and RBF during ureteral occlusion in anesthetized hydropenic dogs. Blockade of renal prostaglandin synthesis prevented the increase in RBF and markedly blunted the increase in renin se-

cretion normally observed during ureteral clamping. After ureteral occlusion had increased renin secretion and RBF in untreated animals, an intrarenal arterial infusion of PGE_2 did not further elevate RBF or renin secretion. However, infusion of PGE_2 in indomethacin-treated dogs after ureteral occlusion resulted in renal vasodilation and increased renin secretion. It was concluded that renal prostaglandins caused the increase in RBF seen during ureteral occlusion. Furthermore, these prostaglandins, either directly or indirectly through vasodilation, appeared to stimulate renin secretion during an increase in ureteral pressure (22). The elevation of SRA caused by administration of the ganglionic blocker chlorisondamine to conscious rats, which has been shown to be the result of activation of the renal baroreceptor (109), was completely blocked by pretreatment with indomethacin (88). Although indomethacin may inhibit renal vasodilation and renin secretion by actions that do not involve the inhibition of prostaglandin synthesis, it does appear that these inhibitors have the potential to alter baroreceptor-mediated renin secretion.

Indomethacin was found to decrease the renin release elicited by endotoxic shock, glycerol-induced renal failure, and severe potassium depletion. Indomethacin also has been found to inhibit furosemide-induced renin release in humans and animals. Furosemide-induced renin release is biphasic, with the first increase in PRA occurring within 10 min, followed by another larger increase in PRA occurring 60 to 120 min later (251). In the most comprehensive study, Frolich et al. (251) found in normal humans that intravenous furosemide produced a 2.6-fold increase in PRA that reached its peak level at 10 min. Indomethacin, in doses that caused 55% suppression of the urinary excretion of PGE, completely inhibited the initial increase in PRA caused by furosemide. Indomethacin also reduced the natriuretic effect of furosemide by 28% but did not alter urinary excretion or plasma levels of furosemide. Abe et al. (252) observed a 2.5-fold increase in the urinary excretion of PGE in normal and hypertensive humans within the first 2 hr after intravenous furosemide. These changes in PGE excretion were accompanied by a 4.5-fold increase in PRA and a sixfold increase in sodium excretion. Therefore, the initial elevation of PRA caused by furosemide appeared to result from increased production of prostaglandins, possibly PGE, and indomethacin prevented this initial increase in PRA. In addition, pretreatment with indomethacin inhibited by 50 to 80% the later rise in PRA caused by furosemide in humans and animals. As a result, indomethacin can modify the results obtained with the furosemide stimulation test used to identify low-renin hypertensive patients (251,253). For instance, Tan and Mulrow (253) administered furosemide orally to 12 normotensive humans the night before and the morning of the test, followed by 4 hr of ambulation to elevate PRA further. Indomethacin, in doses that suppressed urinary excretion of PGE_2 by 97%, prevented 78% of the stimulated renin release. Thus, it is clear that indomethacin inhibited the late rise in PRA elicited by furosemide; however, in the absence of studies in which the urinary losses of salt and water caused by furosemide were replaced, it is not known if indomethacin reduced the late rise in PRA by inhibiting furosemide-induced natriuresis and/or renal prostaglandin synthesis.

The role of renal prostaglandins in macula-densa-mediated renin release has received little attention to date. Williams et al. (254), using a stop-flow technique in anesthetized dogs, found the peak concentrations of urinary PGE to be located in the portion of the tubular fluid that would correspond to a nephron segment located between the proximal and distal tubule. Therefore, PGE, and possibly other renal prostaglandins, enters the renal tubular fluid at a site proximal to the macula densa. If the PGE reaching the macula densa inhibits the active reabsorption of sodium and chloride, as it does in the ascending limb of the loop of Henle and the collecting duct, then the rate of renin release will be enhanced.

Perhaps the disease in which the effects of prostaglandin synthesis inhibitors have been studied most extensively is Bartter's syndrome, a condition characterized by hyperreninemia, hyperaldosteronism, normotension, hypokalemia, juxtaglomerular hyperplasia, insensitivity to the pressor effects of AII, and increased production of renal prostaglandins (255). In 1976, Verberckmoes et al. (256) reported that indomethacin reversed the hypokalemia, hyperreninemia, hyperaldosteronism, and angiotensin insensitivity in Bartter's syndrome. Since that time, a number of reports, involving 12 patients of various ages, have revealed that administration of the prostaglandin synthesis inhibitors indomethacin, aspirin, or ibuprofen resulted in reversal of the abnormalities observed in Bartter's syndrome.

In summary, these studies indicate that nonsteroidal antiinflammatory drugs inhibit the release of renin by a mechanism most likely related to inhibition of synthesis of renal prostaglandins. Furthermore, it would appear that endogenous renal prostaglandins are involved in baroreceptor-mediated and sympathetically mediated renin release. Their involvement in the renin release mediated by the macula densa is not known at present. Overproduction of renal prostaglandins seems to mediate the hyperreninemia of Bartter's syndrome, and inhibitors of prostaglandin synthesis have been shown to lessen the biochemical changes that characterize this disease. Although renal prostaglandins appear to mediate the elevated PRA values observed in other pathologic conditions, there is no evidence to date that this mediation is related to an underlying abnormality of the renal prostaglandin system.

Steroids

Based on both clinical and experimental observations, researchers realized many years ago that steroids, particularly those from the adrenal gland, have the ability to alter the release of renin. In fact, it is now appreciated that aldosterone is one of the principal long-term physiologic regulators of renin release.

Both naturally occurring and synthetic steroids have effects on the renin-angiotensin system, but the different classes of steroids elicit these changes in PRA by different mechanisms (21). For instance, mineralocorticoids, by virtue of their action on renal sodium metabolism, appear to suppress renin release by expansion of the ECF and plasma volumes. Aldosterone is one of the major factors controlling renin release on a long-term basis. In contrast, glucocorticoids have been found to cause an increase, decrease, or no change in PRA (21). The increase in PRA occasionally observed after glucocorticoids has been attributed to sodium depletion or an increase in the plasma concentration of renin substrate, whereas the decrease in PRA was supposedly due to an increase in ECF volume. Like mineralocorticoids, glucocorticoids do not seem to have any direct effects on renin release, but the effects of glucocorticoids on renin release are in need of systematic investigation. Androgens have little effect on PRA or PRC, but, again, the effects of this class of steroids on renin release have not been studied widely. Estrogens increase PRA by elevating the concentration of renin substrate in the plasma (21). However, PRC often does not change or even decreases, because the rise in PRA increases the production of AII, which in turn directly inhibits renin release via the short-loop negative-feedback system. This is one of the few cases in which PRA and PRC do not change in concert after a pharmacologic intervention. Progesterone appears to stimulate renin release by causing sodium depletion, but other progestins may elevate PRA by a direct effect on the granular JG cells (megestrol) or by increasing the hepatic synthesis of renin substrate (norethisterone). Many of the other synthetic progestins do not change PRA. The increase in PRA elicited by oral contraceptives reflects the effect of the estrogenic component of this steroid mixture on plasma renin substrate levels (21).

Inactive Renin and Its Alteration by Drugs

One of the original techniques developed for measurement of PRC involved the prior destruction of plasma angiotensinases and endogenous renin substrate by lowering the pH of plasma to less than 4 (257). Exogenous renin substrate was then added, and PRC was calculated from the amount of AI generated at pH 7.4. However, recent studies have indicated that human plasma contains both an active form and an inactive form of renin, and the latter can be converted into an enzymatically active form by acid activation or cryoactivation. Thus, prior acidification followed by neutralization may artifactually increase the activity of renin in plasma from humans, dogs, and pigs. Inactive renin also has been reported to be present in renal tissue from humans. In fact, it has been suggested that the inactive form of renin may be the intrarenal storage form of this enzyme.

At this time, many questions concerning the physicochemical characteristics and pathophysiologic significance of the inactive renin in the blood are unanswered. Nevertheless, the following facts have been established: (a) The increase in the enzymatic activity of plasma renin after acid treatment does indeed appear to be due to the activation of a proenzyme rather than the removal of an inhibitor. (b) The values determined for inactive renin in human and porcine plasma are considerably greater than those of active renin. (c) The values of active and inactive renin in human plasma are well correlated under steady-state conditions. (d) Bilateral nephrectomy causes marked decreases in both active and inactive renin in the blood. (e) The half-life of inactive renin in the circulation is much longer than the half-life of active renin. (f) The reaction of acid-activated human plasma renin and renal renin with either homologous or heterologous renin substrate revealed identical K_m values. (g) Plasma AII levels are well correlated with active renin (PRA) but not with inactive renin. (h) The kidney may play a role in the activation of inactive renin in the blood.

(i) Under basal conditions, renin is secreted from the human kidney mainly in the active form. (j) The renal release of active and inactive renin in response to various stimuli can be dissociated. (k) Changes in the release of active renin in response to stimuli occur rapidly, whereas changes in inactive renin release occur more slowly.

With these observations in mind, we shall briefly consider the physiologic and pharmacologic alterations of the release of inactive renin from the kidney. The β-adrenergic antagonists propranolol and metoprolol lowered PRA without affecting PRC [measured as "total plasma renin" by the method of Skinner et al. (257)] in hypertensive patients. In like fashion, atenolol did not lower "total plasma renin activity" (TPRA) in hypertensive humans. In more recent studies, researchers have measured active renin (PRA), total renin (TPRA), and inactive renin (TPRA − PRA) after physiologic perturbations or administration of various drugs to healthy and hypertensive humans and experimental animals. In many cases, stimulation of the release of active renin (PRA) is accompanied by a decrease in the circulating level of inactive renin. On the other hand, certain interventions, sodium depletion in particular, tend to elicit increases in PRA, TPRA, and inactive renin. Some species differences also may occur. For example, isoproterenol increases PRA and decreases inactive renin in humans, whereas this drug elevates both active and inactive renin in pigs. Until the exact importance of inactive renin in health and disease is determined, the significance of these drug-induced changes in the release of inactive renin cannot be stated with any certainty.

REFERENCES

1. Tigerstedt, R., and Bergman, P. G. (1898): Niere und Kreislauf. *Skand. Arch. Physiol.*, 8:223–271.
2. Goldblatt, H., Lynch, J., Hanzal, R. F., and Summerville, W. (1934): Studies on experimental hypertension. 1. The production of persistent elevation of systolic pressure by means of renal ischemia. *J. Exp. Med.*, 59:347–379.
3. Page, I. H., and Helmer, O. M. (1940): A crystalline pressor substance, angiotensin, resulting from the reaction between renin and renin activator. *J. Exp. Med.*, 71:29–42.
4. Braun-Menendez, E., Fasciolo, J. C., Leloir, C. F., and Munoz, J. M. (1940): The substance causing renal hypertension. *J. Physiol. (Lond.)*, 98:283–298.
5. Davis, J. O., Freeman, R. H., Johnson, J. A., and Speilman, W. S. (1974): Agents which block the action of the renin-angiotensin system. *Circ. Res.*, 34:279–285.
6. Brunner, H. R., Gavras, H., Laragh, J. H., and Keenan, R. (1973): Angiotensin II-blockade in man by sar¹-ala⁸angiotensin II for understanding and treatment of high blood pressure. *Lancet*, 2:1045–1048.
7. Erdos, E. G. (1975): Angiotensin I converting enzyme. *Circ. Res.*, 36:247–255.
8. Peach, M. J. (1977): Renin-angiotensin system: Biochemistry and mechanisms of action. *Physiol. Rev.*, 57:313–370.
9. Blumberg, A. L., Ackerly, J. A., and Peach, M. J. (1975): Differentiation of neurogenic and myocardial angiotensin II receptors in isolated rabbit atria. *Circ. Res.*, 36:719–726.
10. Starke, K., Werner, U., and Schumann, H. J. (1969): Effect of angiotensin on the function of isolated rabbit hearts and/or nonadrenaline release at rest and during sympathetic nerve stimulation. *Arch. Exp. Pathol. Pharmacol.*, 264:170–186.
11. Scroop, G. C., Katic, F., Joy, M. D., and Lowe, R. D. (1971): Importance of central vasomotor effects in angiotensin-induced hypertension. *Br. Med. J.*, 1:324–326.
12. Severs, W. B., and Daniels-Severs, A. E. (1973): Effects of angiotensin on the central nervous system. *Pharmacol. Rev.*, 25:415–449.
13. Peach, M. J., Cline, W. H., and Watts, D. T. (1966): Release of adrenal catecholamines by angiotensin II. *Circ. Res.*, 19:571–575.
14. Zimmerman, B. G., and Gisslen, J. (1968): Pattern of renal vasoconstriction and transmitter release during sympathetic stimulation in the presence of angiotensin and cocaine. *J. Pharmacol. Exp. Ther.*, 163:320–329.
15. Khairallah, P. A. (1972): Action of angiotensin on adrenergic nerve endings: Inhibition of norepinephrine uptake. *Fed. Proc.*, 31:1351–1357.
16. Biron, P., Koiw, E., Nowaczynski, W., Broulet, J., and Genest, J. (1961): The effects of intravenous infusion of valine-5-angiotensin II and other pressor agents on urinary electrolytes and corticosteroids including aldosterone. *J. Clin. Invest.*, 40:338–347.
17. Ramsy, D. J., Keil, L. C., Sharpe, M. C., and Shinsako, J. (1978): Angiotensin II infusion increases vasopressin, ACTH, and 11-hydroxycorticosteroid secretion. *Am. J. Physiol.*, 234:R66–R71.
18. Navar, L. G., and Langford, H. D. (1974): Effects of angiotensin on the renal circulation. In: *Angiotensin, Handbook of Experimental Pharmacology, Vol. 37*, edited by I. H. Page and F. M. Bumpus, pp. 455–474. Springer-Verlag, New York.
19. Poulsen, K. (1973): Kinetics of the renin system. *Scand. J. Clin. Lab. Invest. [Suppl. 132]*, 31:1–83.

20. Tobian, L., Tomboulian, A., and Janecek, J. (1959): Effect of high perfusion pressure on the granulation of juxtaglomerular cells in an isolated kidney. *J. Clin. Invest.*, 38:605–610.

21. Keeton, T. K., and Campbell, W. B. (1980): The pharmacologic alteration of renin release. *Pharmacol. Rev.*, 32:81–227.

22. Blackshear, J. L., and Wathen, R. L. (1978): Effects of indomethacin on renal blood flow and renin secretory responses to ureteral occlusion in the dog. *Mineral Electrolyte Metab.*, 1:271–278.

23. Fray, J. C. S. (1976): Stretch receptor model for renin release with evidence from perfused rat kidney. *Am. J. Physiol.*, 231:936–944.

24. Barajas, L. (1979): Anatomy of the juxtaglomerular apparatus. *Am. J. Physiol.*, 237:F333–F343.

25. Taher, M. S., McLain, L. G., McDonald, K. M., and Schrier, R. W. (1976): Effect of beta-adrenergic blockage on renin response to renal nerve stimulation. *J. Clin. Invest.*, 57:459–465.

26. McPhee, M. S., and Lakey, W. H. (1971): Neurologic release of renin in mongrel dogs. *Can. J. Surg.*, 14:142–147.

27. Pettinger, W. A., Campbell, W. B., and Keeton, K. (1973): Adrenergic component of renin release induced by vasodilating antihypertensive drugs in the rat. *Circ. Res.*, 33:82–86.

28. Mancia, G., Romero, J. C., and Shepherd, J. T. (1975): Continuous inhibition of renin release in dogs by vagally innervated receptors in the cardiopulmonary region. *Circ. Res.*, 36:529–535.

29. Yun, J. C. H., Delea, C. S., Bartter, F. C., and Kelly, G. D. (1977): Increase in renin release after sinoaortic denervation and cervical vagotomy in anesthetized dogs. *Proc. Soc. Exp. Biol. Med.*, 156:186–191.

30. Zehr, J. E., Hasbargen, J. A., and Kurz, K. D. (1976): Reflex suppression of renin secretion during distention of cardiopulmonary receptors in dogs. *Circ. Res.*, 38:232–239.

31. Thames, M. D., Jarecki, M., and Donald, D. E. (1978): Neural control of renin secretion in anesthetized dogs: Interaction of cardiopulmonary and carotid baroreceptors. *Circ. Res.*, 42:237–245.

32. Hesse, B., Nielsen, I., Ring-Larsen, H., and Hansen, J. F. (1978): The influence of acute blood volume changes on plasma renin activity in man. *Scand. J. Clin. Lab. Invest.*, 38:155–161.

33. Bull, M. B., Hillman, R. S., Cannon, P. J., and Laragh, J. H. (1970): Renin and aldosterone secretion in man as influenced by changes in electrolyte balance and blood volume. *Circ. Res.*, 27:953–960.

34. Kiowski, W., and Julius, S. (1978): Renin response to stimulation of cardiopulmonary mechanoreceptors in man. *J. Clin. Invest.*, 62:656–663.

35. Mark, A. L., Abboud, F. M., and Fitz, A. E. (1978): Influence of low- and high-pressure baroreceptors on plasma renin activity in humans. *Am. J. Physiol.*, 235:H29–H33.

36. Vander, A. J. (1965): Effect of catecholamines and the renal nerves on renin secretion in anesthetized dogs. *Am. J. Physiol.*, 209:659–662.

37. Wathen, R. L., Kingsbury, W. S., Stouder, D. A.,

Schneider, E. G., and Rostorfer, H. H. (1965): Effects of infusions of catecholamines and angiotensin II on renin release in anesthetized dogs. *Am. J. Physiol.*, 209:1012–1024.

38. Ueda, H., Yasuda, H., Takabatake, Y., Iizuka M., Iizuka, T., Ihori, M., and Sakamoto, Y. (1970): Observations on the mechanism of renin release by catecholamines. *Circ. Res.* [Suppl. I.], 26/27:195–200.

39. Weinberger, M. H., Aoi, W., and Henry, D. P. (1975): Direct effect of beta-adrenergic stimulation on renin release by the rat kidney slice *in vitro*. *Circ. Res.*, 37:318–324.

40. Gordon, R. D., Kuchel, O., Liddle, G. W., and Island, D. P. (1967): Role of the sympathetic nervous system in regulating renin and aldosterone production in man. *J. Clin. Invest.*, 46:599–605.

41. Henry, D. P., Aoi, W., and Weinberger, M. H. (1977): The effects of dopamine on renin release *in vitro*. *Endocrinology*, 101:279–283.

42. Imbs, J. L., Schmidt, M., and Schwartz, J. (1975): Effect of dopamine on renin secretion in the anesthetized dog. *Eur. J. Pharmacol.*, 33:151–157.

43. Vander, A. J. (1967): Control of renin release. *Physiol. Rev.*, 47:359–382.

44. Brown, J. J., Davies, D. L., Lever, A. F., and Robertson, J. I. S. (1963): Influence of sodium loading and sodium depletion on plasma renin in man. *Lancet*, 1:278–279.

45. Vander, A. J., and Miller, R. (1964): Control of renin secretion in the anesthetized dog. *Am. J. Physiol.*, 207:537–546.

46. Birbari, A. (1972): Intrarenal factors in the control of renin secretion. *Pfluegers Arch.*, 337:29–37.

47. Cooke, C. R., Brown, T. C., Zacherle, B. J., and Walker, W. G. (1970): Effect of altered sodium concentration in the distal nephron segments on renin release. *J. Clin. Invest.*, 49:1630–1638.

48. Meyer, P., Menard, J., Papanicolaou, N., Alexander, J. M., Devaux, C., and Millez, P. (1968): Mechanism of renin release following furosemide diuresis in rabbits. *Am. J. Physiol.*, 215:908–915.

49. Churchill, P. C., Churchill, M. C., and McDonald, F. D. (1979): Effects of saline and mannitol on renin and distal tubule Na in rats. *Circ. Res.*, 45:786–792.

50. Churchill, P. C., Churchill, M. C., and McDonald, F. D. (1978): Renin secretion and distal tubule Na⁺ in rats. *Am. J. Physiol.*, 235:F611–F616.

51. Freeman, R. H., Davis, J. O., Gotshall, R. W., Johnson, J. A., and Spielman, W. S. (1974): The signal perceived by the macula densa during changes in renin release. *Circ. Res.*, 35:307–315.

52. Nash, F. D., Rosterfa, H. H., Bailin, M. D., Wathern, W. L., and Schneider, E. G. (1968): Renin release: Relation to renal sodium load and dissociation from hemodynamic changes. *Circ. Res.*, 22:473–487.

53. Vander, A. J., and Carlson, J. (1964): Mechanism of the effects of furosemide on renin release in anesthetized dogs. *Circ. Res.*, 25:145–152.

54. Humphreys, M. H., Reid, I. A., Ufferman, R. C., Lieberman, R. A., and Earley, L. E. (1975): The relationship between sodium excretion and renin secretion by the perfused kidney. *Proc. Soc. Exp. Biol. Med.*, 150:728–734.

55. Churchill, P. C., Churchill, M. C., Hoskins, H. A., and McDonald, F. D. (1975): Renin and distal tubule Na⁺ during stop flow in dogs. *Proc. Soc. Exp. Biol. Med.*, 148:734–738.

56. Shade, R. E., Davis, J. O., Johnson, J. A., and Witty, R. T. (1972): Effects of arterial infusion of sodium and potassium on renin secretion in the dog. *Circ. Res.*, 31:719–727.

57. Lyons, H. J., and Churchill, P. C. (1975): Renin secretion from rat renal cortical cell suspension. *Am. J. Physiol.*, 228:1835–1839.

58. Lyons, H. J., and Churchill, P. C. (1975): The influence of ouabain on *in vitro* secretion and intracellular sodium. *Nephron*, 14:442–450.

59. Kotchen, T. A., Gallas, J. H., and Luke, R. G. (1978): Contribution of chloride to the inhibition of plasma renin by sodium chloride in the rat. *Kidney Int.*, 13:201–207.

60. Rocha, A. S., and Kokko, J. P. (1973): Sodium chloride and water transport in the medullary thick ascending limb of Henle: Evidence for active chloride transport. *J. Clin. Invest.*, 52:612–623.

61. Abbrecht, P. H., and Vander, A. J. (1970): Effects of chronic potassium deficiency on plasma renin activity. *J. Clin. Invest.*, 49:1510–1516.

62. Brunner, H. R., Baer, L., Sealey, J. E., Ledingham, J. G. G., and Laragh, J. H. (1970): The influence of potassium administration and of potassium deprivation on plasma renin in normal and hypertensive subjects. *J. Clin. Invest.*, 49:2128–2138.

63. Harada, E., and Rubin, R. P. (1978): Stimulation of renin secretion and calcium efflux from the isolated perfused cat kidney by noradrenaline after prolonged calcium deprivation. *J. Physiol. (Lond.)*, 274:367–379.

64. Park, C. S., and Malvin, R. L. (1978): Calcium in the control of renin release. *Am. J. Physiol.*, 235:F22–F25.

65. Logan, A. G., Tenyi, I., Quesada, T., Peart, W. S., Breathnach, A. S., and Martin, B. G. H. (1975): Blockade of renin release by lanthanum. *Clin. Sci. Mol. Med.*, 48:31s–32s.

66. Churchill, P. C. (1979): Possible mechanism of the inhibitory effect of ouabain on renin secretion from rat renal cortical slices. *J. Physiol. (Lond.)*, 294:123–134.

67. Vandongen, R., and Peart, W. S. (1974): Calcium dependence of the inhibitory effect of angiotensin on renin secretion in the isolated perfused kidney of the rat. *Br. J. Pharmacol.*, 50:125–129.

68. Baumbach, L., and Leyssac, P. P. (1977): Studies on the mechanism of renin release from isolated superfused rat glomeruli: Effects of calcium, calcium ionophore and lanthanum. *J. Physiol. (Lond.)*, 273:745–764.

69. Churchill, P. C., McDonald, F. D., and Churchill, M. C. (1979): Phenytoin stimulates renin secretion from rat kidney slices. *J. Pharmacol. Exp. Ther.*, 211:615–619.

70. Vander, A. J., and Geelhoed, G. W. (1965): Inhibition of renin secretion by angiotensin II. *Proc. Soc. Exp. Biol. Med.*, 120:339–403.

71. McDonald, K. M., Taher, S., Aisenbrey, G., deTorrente, A., and Schrier, R. W. (1975): Effect of angiotensin II and an angiotensin II inhibitor on renin secretion in the dog. *Am. J. Physiol.*, 228:1562–1567.

72. Carey, R. M., Vaughan, E. D., Jr., Peach, M. J., and Ayers, C. R. (1978): Activity of [Des-Aspartyl]-angiotensin II and angiotensin II in man. *J. Clin. Invest.*, 61:20–31.

73. Williams, G. H., Hollenberg, N. K., Moore, T. J., Dluhy, R. G., Bauli, S. Z., Solomon, H. S., and Mersey, J. H. (1978): Failure of renin suppression by angiotensin II in hypertension. *Circ. Res.*, 42:46–52.

74. Capponi, A. M., Gourjon, M., and Vallotton, M. B. (1977): Effect of beta-blocking agents and angiotensin II on isoproterenol-stimulated renin release from rat kidney slices. *Circ. Res. [Suppl. I]*, 40:89–93.

75. Keeton, T. K., Pettinger, W. A., and Campbell, W. B. (1976): The effects of altered sodium balance and adrenergic blockade on renin release induced in rats by angiotensin antagonism. *Circ. Res.*, 38:531–539.

76. Johnson, M. D., Kinter, L. B., and Beeuwkes, R., III (1979): Effects of AVP and DDAVP on plasma renin activity and electrolyte excretion in conscious dogs. *Am. J. Physiol.*, 236:F66–F70.

77. Bunag, R. D., Page, I. H., and McCubbin, J. W. (1967): Inhibition of renin release by vasodepressin and angiotensin. *Cardiovasc. Res.*, 1:67–73.

78. Meyer, D. K., Boll, H., Lauterwein, B., and Hertting, G. (1975): Inhibition of isoprenaline-induced increase in plasma renin concentration by vasoconstrictors. *Experientia*, 31:1071–1072.

79. Lauterwein, B., Boll, H., Meyer, D. K., and Hertting, G. (1975): Inhibition of furosemide-induced renin release by vasoconstrictors. *Naunyn Schmiedebergs Arch. Pharmacol.*, 290:307–314.

80. Vander, A. J. (1968): Inhibition of renin release in the dog by vasopressin and vasotocin. *Circ. Res.*, 23:605–609.

81. Vander, J. J. (1968): Direct effect of prostaglandin on renal function and renin release in anesthetized dogs. *Am. J. Physiol.*, 214:218–221.

82. Gerber, J. G., Branch, R. A., Nies, A. S., Gerkens, J. F., Shand, D. G., Hollifield, J., and Oates, J. A. (1978): Prostaglandins and renin release: II. Assessment of renin secretion following infusions of PGI₂, E₂, and D₂ into the renal artery of anesthetized dogs. *Prostaglandins*, 15:81–88.

83. Weber, P. C., Larsson, C., Anggard, E., Hamberg, M., Corey, E. J., Nicolaou, K. C., and Samuelsson, B. (1976): Stimulation of renin release from rabbit renal cortex by arachidonic acid and prostaglandin endoperoxides. *Circ. Res.*, 39:868–874.

84. Soveri, P., Fyhrquist, F., and Widholm, O. (1976): Plasma renin activity in abortion. *Acta Obstet. Gynecol. Scand.*, 55:175–177.

85. Whorton, A. R., Lazar, J. D., Smigel, M. D., and Oates, J. A. (1980): Prostaglandin-mediated renin release from renal cortical slices. In: *Advances in Prostaglandin and Thromboxane Research, Vol. 7*, edited by B. Samuelsson, P. W. Ramwell, and R. Paoletti, pp. 1123–1129. Raven Press, New York.

86. Bolger, P. M., Eisner, G. M., Ramwell, P. W., Slotkoff, L. M., and Corey, E. J. (1978): Renal actions of prostacyclin. *Nature*, 271:467–469.

87. Whorton, A. R., Misono, K., Hollifield, J., Frolich, J. C., Inagami, T., and Oates, J. A. (1977): Prostaglandins and renin release: I. Stimulation of renin release from rabbit renal cortical slices by PGI_2. *Prostaglandins,* 14:1095–1104.

88. Campbell, W. B., Graham, R. M., and Jackson, E. K. (1979): Role of renal prostaglandins in sympathetically mediated renin release in the rat. *J. Clin. Invest.,* 64:448–456.

89. Okahara, T., Abe, Y., and Yamamoto, K. (1977): Effects of dibutyryl cyclic AMP and propranolol on renin secretion in dogs. *Proc. Soc. Exp. Biol. Med.,* 156:213–218.

90. Michelakis, A. M., Caudle, J., and Liddle, G. W. (1969): In vitro stimulation of renin production by epinephrine, norepinephrine and cyclic AMP. *Proc. Soc. Exp. Biol. Med.,* 130:748–753.

91. Spielman, W. S., and Thompson, C. I. (1982): A proposed role for adenosine in the regulation of renal hemodynamics and renin release. *Am. J. Physiol.,* 242:F423–435.

92. Osswald, H., Schmitz, H. -J., and Kemper, R. (1978): Renal action of adenosine: Effect on renin secretion in the rat. *Naunyn Schmiedebergs Arch. Pharmacol.,* 303:95–99.

93. Brod, J., Horbach, L., Just, H., Rosenthal, J., and Nicolescu, R. (1972): Acute effects of clonidine on central and peripheral hemodynamics and plasma renin activity. *Eur. J. Clin. Pharmacol.,* 4:107–114.

94. Karlberg, B. E., Nilsson, O., and Tolagen, K. (1977): Clonidine in primary hypertension: Effects on blood pressure, plasma renin activity, plasma and urinary aldosterone. *Curr. Ther. Res.,* 21:10–20.

95. Crayton, S., Keeton, T. K., and Pettinger, W. A. (1976): Clonidine suppression of renin release in the conscious dog. *Pharmacologist,* 18:138 (abstract).

96. Reid, I. A., Morris, B. J., and Ganong, W. F. (1978): The renin-angiotensin system. *Annu. Rev. Physiol.,* 40:377–410.

97. Pettinger, W. A., Keeton, T. K., Campbell, W. B., and Harper, D. C. (1976): Evidence for a renal α-adrenergic receptor inhibiting renin release. *Circ. Res.,* 38:338–346.

98. Oates, H. F., Stoker, L. M., MacCarthy, E. P., Monaghan, J. C., and Stokes, G. S. (1978): Comparative haemodynamic effects of clonidine and guanfacine. *Arch. Int. Pharmacodyn. Ther.,* 231:148–156.

99. Kho, T. L., Schalekamp, M. A. D. H., Zaal, G. A., Wester, A., and Birkenhager, W. H. (1975): Comparison between the effects of ST-600 and Catapres. *Arch. Int. Pharmacodyn. Ther.,* 214:347–350.

100. Hokfelt, B., Hedeland, H., and Hansson, B. -G. (1975): The effect of clonidine, respectively on catecholamines in blood and urine, plasma renin activity and urinary aldosterone in hypertensive patients. *Arch. Int. Pharmacodyn. Ther.,* 213:307–321.

101. Chevillard, C., Pasquier, R., Duchene, N., and Alexandre, J. -M. (1978): Mechanism of inhibition of renin release by clonidine in rats. *Eur. J. Pharmacol.,* 48:451–454.

102. Gavras, H., Gavras, I., Brunner, H. R., and Laragh, J. H. (1977): The antihypertensive action of methyldopa in relation to its effect on the renin-aldosterone system. *J. Clin. Pharmacol.,* 17:372–378.

103. Weidmann, P., Hirsch, D., Maxwell, M. H., Okun, R., and Schroth, P. (1974): Plasma renin and blood pressure during treatment with methyldopa. *Am. J. Cardiol.,* 34:671–676.

104. Lowder, S. C., and Liddle, G. W. (1975): Effects of guanethidine and methyldopa on standardized test for renin responsiveness. *Ann. Intern. Med.,* 82:757–760.

105. Frankel, R. J., Reid, I. A., and Ganong, W. F. (1977): Role of central and peripheral mechanisms in the action of alpha-methyldopa on blood pressure and renin secretion. *J. Pharmacol. Exp. Ther.,* 201:400–405.

106. Barbeau, A., Gillo-Joffroy, L., Boucher, R., Nowaczynski, W., and Genest, J. (1969): Renin-aldosterone system in Parkinson's disease. *Science,* 165:291–292.

107. Blair, M. L., Reid, I. A., and Ganong, W. F. (1977): Effect of L-dopa on plasma renin activity with and without inhibitor of extracerebral dopa decarboxylase in dogs. *J. Pharmacol. Exp. Ther.,* 202:209–215.

108. Alexandre, J. M., Menard, J., Chevillard, C., and Schmitt, H. (1970): Increased plasma renin activity induced in rats by physostigmine and effects of alpha and beta-receptor blocking drugs thereon. *Eur. J. Pharmacol.,* 12:127–131.

109. Keeton, T. K., and Pettinger, W. A. (1979): The dominance of adrenergic mechanisms in mediating hypotensive drug-induced renin release in the conscious rat. *J. Pharmacol. Exp. Ther.,* 208:303–309.

110. Loeffler, J. R., Stockigt, J. R., and Ganong, W. F. (1972): Effect of alpha- and beta-adrenergic blocking agents on the increase in renin secretion produced by stimulation of the renal nerves. *Neuroendocrinology,* 10:129–138.

111. Johnston, C. I., Anavekar, N., Chua, K. G., and Louis, W. J. (1973): Plasma renin and angiotensin levels in human hypertension following treatment. *Clin. Sci. Mol. Med.,* 45:287s–290s.

112. Meyer, D. K., Rauscher, W., Peskar, B., and Hertting, G. (1973): The mechanism of the drinking response to some hypotensive drugs. Activation of the renin-angiotensin system by direct or reflex-mediated stimulation of β-receptor. *Naunyn Schmiedebergs Arch. Pharmacol.,* 276:13–24.

113. Coote, J. H., Johns, E. J., MacLeod, V. H., and Singer, B. (1972): Effect of renal nerve stimulation, renal blood flow, and adrenergic blockade on plasma renin activity in the cat. *J. Physiol. (Lond.),* 226:15–36.

114. Levy, S. B., Holle, R., Hsu, L., Lilley, J. J., and Stone, R. A. (1977): Physiologic and pharmacologic influence on adrenergic regulation of renin release. *Clin. Pharmacol. Ther.,* 22:511–518.

115. Drayer, J. I. M., Weber, M. A., Atlas, S. A., and Laragh, J. H. (1977): Phentolamine testing for alpha-adrenergic participation in hypertensive patients: Independence from renin profiles. *Clin. Pharmacol. Ther.,* 22:286–292.

116. Graham, R. M., and Pettinger, W. A. (1979): Effects of prazosin and phentolamine on arterial pressure, heart rate, and renin activity: Evidence in the conscious rat for the functional significance of the pre-

synaptic alpha-receptor. *J. Cardiovasc. Pharmacol.,* 1:497–502.

117. Graham, R. M., Stephenson, W. H., and Pettinger, W. A. (1980): Pharmacological evidence for a functional role of the pre-synaptic alpha-adrenoceptor in noradrenergic neurotransmission in the conscious rat. *Naunyn Schmiedebergs Arch. Pharmacol.,* 311:497–502.

118. Buhler, F. R., Laragh, J. H., Baer, L., Vaughn, E. D., Jr., and Brunner, H. R. (1972): Propranolol inhibition of renin secretion. A specific approach to diagnosis and treatment of renin-dependent hypertensive disease. *N. Engl. J. Med.,* 287:1209–1214.

119. Winer, N., Chokshi, D. S., Yoon, M. S., and Freedman, A. D. (1969): Adrenergic receptor mediation of renin secretion. *J. Clin. Endocrinol. Metab.,* 29:1168–1175.

120. Stokes, G. S., Gentle, J. L., Stoker, L. M., Goldsmith, R. F., and Hayes, J. M. (1970): Effects of alpha- and beta-adrenergic blockade on peripheral and renal vein renin activity in hypertensive patients. *Proc. Aust. Soc. Med. Res.,* 2:354 (abstract).

121. Michelakis, A. M., and McAllister, R. G. (1972): The effect of chronic adrenergic receptor blockade on plasma renin activity in man. *J. Clin. Endocrinol.,* 34:386–394.

122. Zehr, J. E., and Feigl, E. O. (1972): Attenuation of renin activity by beta receptor blockade. *Fed. Proc.,* 31:825 (abstract).

123. Salvetti, A., Arzilli, F., and Baccini, C. (1973): The effect of a beta-blocker on plasma renin activity of hypertensive patients. *J. Nucl. Biol. Med.,* 17:142–150.

124. Winer, N. (1972): Mechanism of increased renin secretion associated with adrenalectomy, hemorrhage, renal artery constriction, and sodium depletion. In: *Hypertension '72,* edited by J. Genest and E. Koiw, pp. 25–36. Springer-Verlag, New York.

125. Hanson, R. C., Davis, J. O., and Freeman, R. H. (1976): Effects of propranolol on renin release during chronic thoracic caval constriction or acute renal artery stenosis in dogs. *Proc. Soc. Exp. Biol. Med.,* 152:224–228.

126. Salvetti, A., Arzilli, F., Sassano, P., Gazzetti, P., and Rindi, P. (1975): Postural changes in plasma renin activity after renal transplantation. *Clin. Sci. Mol. Med.,* 48:283s–286s.

127. Lands, A. M., Arnold, A., McAuliff, J. P., Ludena, F. P., and Brown, T. G., Jr. (1967): Differentiation of receptor systems activated by sympathomimetic amines. *Nature,* 214:597–598.

128. Weber, M. A., Stokes, G. S., and Gain, J. M. (1974): Comparison of the effects on renin release of beta adrenergic antagonists with differing properties. *J. Clin. Invest.,* 54:1413–1419.

129. Weber, M. A., Graham, R. M., Gain, J. M., and Stokes, G. S. (1977): Pharmacological stimulation of renin secretion within the kidney. *Arch. Int. Pharmacodyn. Ther.,* 227:343–350.

130. Johns, E. J., and Singer, B. (1974): Comparison of the effects of propranolol and ICI 66082 in blocking the renin releasing effect of renal nerve stimulation in the cat. *Br. J. Pharmacol.,* 52:315–318.

131. Johns, E. J. (1981): An investigation into the type of β-adrenoceptor mediating sympathetically activated renin release in the cat. *Br. J. Pharmacol.,* 73:749–754.

132. Himori, N., Hayakawa, S., and Ishimori, T. (1979): Role of β-1 and β-2 adrenoceptors in isoproterenol-induced renin release in conscious dogs. *Life Sci.,* 24:1953–1958.

133. Osborn, J. L., DiBona, G. F., and Thames, M. D. (1981): Beta-1 receptor mediation of renin secretion elicited by low-frequency renal nerve stimulation. *J. Pharmacol. Exp. Ther.,* 216:265–269.

134. Kopp, U., Aurell, M., Svensson, L., and Ablad, B. (1981): Effect of prenalterol, a β-1-adrenoceptor agonist, on renin secretion rate in the anesthetized dog. *Acta Pharmacol. Toxicol.,* 49:230–235.

135. Oates, H. F., Stoker, L. M., Monaghan, J. C., and Stokes, G. S. (1978): The beta-adrenoceptor controlling renin release. *Arch. Int. Pharmacodyn. Ther.,* 234:205–213.

136. Desaulles, E., Miesch, F., and Schwartz, J. (1978): Evidence for the participation of beta₁-adrenoceptors in isoprenaline-induced renin release from rat kidney slices *in vitro. Br. J. Pharmacol.,* 63:421–425.

137. Buhler, F. R., Burkhart, F., Lutold, B. E., Kung, M., Marbet, G., and Pfisterer, M. (1975): Antihypertensive beta blocking action as related to renin and age: A pharmacologic tool to identify pathogenetic mechanisms in essential hypertension. *Am. J. Cardiol.,* 36:653–669.

138. Johnson, B. F., Smith, I. K., LaBrooy, J., and Bye, C. (1976): The nature of the beta-adrenoreceptor controlling plasma renin activity in man. *Clin. Sci. Mol. Med.,* 51:113s–115s.

139. Wiggins, R., Davies, R., Basar, I., and Slater, J. D. H. (1978): The inhibition of adrenergically provoked renin release by salbutamol in man. *Br. J. Clin. Pharmacol.,* 5:213–215.

140. Borner, V. H., Falkenhagen, D., Rohmann, H., and Kruger, M. (1976): Das Verhalten der Plasma-Renin-Aktivitat, hamodynamischer Parameter und der Clearancewerte unter dem Einfluss von Orciprenalin und Propranolol bei Patienten mit eingeschrankter Nierenfunktion. *Z. Urol.* 69:877–884.

141. Gaal, K., Siklos, J., Mozes, T., and Toth, G. F. (1978): Effect of papaverine on renin release in dogs *in vivo* and *in vitro. Acta Physiol. Acad. Sci. Hung.,* 51:305–314.

142. Churchill, P. C., McDonald, F. D., and Churchill, M. C. (1980): Effects of papaverine on basal and on isoproterenol-stimulated renin secretion from rat kidney slices. *Life Sci.,* 27:1299–1305.

143. Zehner, J., Klaus, D., Klumpp, F., Lemke, R., Schneider, J., and Kapert, A. (1974): Einfluss von β-Synpathikolytika auf die Stimulierbarkeit der Reninsekretion durch Theophyllin. *Verh. Dtsch. Ges. Inn. Med.,* 80:266–268.

144. Peart, W. S., Quesada, T., and Tenyi, I. (1975): The effects of cyclic adenosine 3′,5′-monophosphate and guanosine 3′,5′-monophosphate and theophylline on renin secretion in the isolated perfused kidney of the rat. *Br. J. Pharmacol.,* 54:55–60.

145. Nolly, H. L., Reid, I. A., and Ganong, W. F. (1974):

Effect of theophylline and adrenergic blocking drugs on the renin response to norepinephrine *in vitro. Circ. Res.,* 35:575–579.

146. Oliw, E., Anggard, E., and Fredholm, B. B. (1977): Effect of indomethacin on the renal actions of theophylline. *Eur. J. Pharmacol.,* 43:9–16.

147. Robertson, D., Frolich, J. C., Carr, R. K., Throck-Watson, J., Hollifield, J. H., Shand, D. G., and Oates, J. A. (1978): Effects of caffeine on plasma renin activity, catecholamines, and blood pressure. *N. Engl. J. Med.,* 298:181–186.

148. Meyer, D. K., Kempter, A., Boll, H., Eisenreich, M., and Hertting, G. (1977): α-Adrenoceptor-mediated inhibitory effect of the sympathetic nervous system on the isoprenaline-induced increase in plasma renin concentration. *Naunyn Schmiedebergs Arch. Pharmacol.,* 299:77–82.

149. Meyer, D. K., Peskar, B., Tauchmann, U., and Hertting, G. (1971): Potentiation and abolition of the increase in plasma renin activity seen after hypotensive drugs in rats. *Eur. J. Pharmacol.,* 16:278–282.

150. Meyer, D. K., and Hertting, G. (1973): Influence of neuronal uptake-blocking agents on the increase in water intake and in plasma concentrations of renin and angiotensin I induced by phentolamine and isoprenaline. *Naunyn Schmiedebergs Arch. Pharmacol.,* 280:191–200.

151. Porlier, G. A., Nadeau, R. A., deChamplain, J., and Bichet, D. G. (1977): Increased circulating plasma catecholamines and plasma renin activity in dogs after chemical sympathectomy with 6-hydroxydopamine. *Can. J. Physiol. Pharmacol.,* 55:724–733.

152. Bunag, R. D., Page, I. H., and McCubbin, J. W. (1966): Neural stimulation of release of renin. *Circ. Res.,* 19:851–858.

153. Pettinger, W. A., Augusto, L., and Leon, A. S. (1972): Alteration of renin release by stress and adrenergic receptor and related drugs in unanesthetized rats. In: *Comparative Pathophysiology of Circulatory Disturbances,* edited by C. M. Bloor, pp. 105–117. Plenum Press, New York.

154. Meyer, D. K., Abele, M., and Hertting, G. (1974): Influence of serotonin on water intake and the renin-angiotensin system in the rat. *Arch. Int. Pharmacodyn. Ther.,* 212:130–140.

155. Ayers, C. R., Harris, R. H., Jr., and Lefer, L. G. (1969): Control of renin release in experimental hypertension. *Circ. Res. [Suppl. I],* 24/25:103–113.

156. Lifschitz, M. D., and Horwitz, L. D. (1976): Plasma renin activity during exercise in the dog. *Circ. Res.,* 38:483–487.

157. Morganti, A., Leonetti, G., Terzolo, L., Bernasconi, M., and Zanchetti, A. (1975): Dosaggio dell'attivita reninica plasmatica nelle vene renali nell' ipertensione arteriosa essenziale e nefrovascolare: effetto dell'infusione di trimetafano. *Boll. Dell. Soc. Ital. Cardiol.,* 20:1159–1167.

158. Kaneko, Y., Takeda, T., Ikeda, T., Tagawa, H., Ishii, M., Takabatake, Y., and Ueda, H. (1970): Effect of ganglion-blocking agents on renin release in hypertensive patients. *Circ. Res.,* 27:97–103.

159. Williamson, H. E. (1977): Furosemide and ethacrynic acid. *J. Clin. Pharmacol.,* 17:663–672.

160. Olsen, U. B. (1977): The pharmacology of bumetanide. *Acta Pharmacol. Toxicol. [Suppl. III],* 41:1–31.

161. Burg, M. B., and Green, N. (1973): Function of the thick ascending limb of Henle's loop. *Am. J. Physiol.,* 224:659–667.

162. Wright, F. A., and Schnermann, J. (1974): Interference with feedback control of glomerular filtration rate by furosemide, triflocin, and cyanide. *J. Clin. Invest.,* 53:1695–1708.

163. Dluhy, R. G., Wolf, G. L., and Lauler, D. P. (1970): Vasodilator properties of ethacrynic acid in the perfused dog kidney. *Clin. Sci.,* 38:347–357.

164. Fraser, R., James, V. H. T., Brown, J. J., Isaac, P., Lever, A. F., and Robertson, J. I. S. (1965): Effect of angiotensin and of furosemide on plasma aldosterone, corticosterone, cortisol and renin in man. *Lancet,* 2:989–991.

165. Sweet, C. S., and Gaul, S. L. (1975): Attenuation of hydrochlorothiazide-induced hypokalemia in dogs by a beta-adrenergic blocking drug, timolol. *Eur. J. Pharmacol.,* 32:370–374.

166. Nielsen, C. K., Olsen, U. B., Anhfelt-Ronne, I., and Arrigoni-Martelli, E. (1976): Investigation on the antihypertensive activity of timolol and bendroflumethiazide and the combination in dogs and rats. *Acta Pharmacol. Toxicol.,* 39:500–512.

167. Chalmers, J., Tiller, D., Horvath, J., and Bune, A., (1976): Effects of timolol and hydrochlorothiazide on blood-pressure and plasma renin activity. *Lancet,* 2:328–331.

168. Nielsen, I., Steiness, E., and Hesse, B. (1977): Plasma renin activity and blood pressure during long-term treatment with propranolol and diuretic. *Acta Med. Scand. [Suppl.],* 602:97–101.

169. Zanchetti, A., Leonetti, G., Morganti, A., Terzoli, L., Schwarz, E., Manfrin, M., and Bernasconi, M. (1976): Longitudinal study of plasma renin activity in hypertensive patients under anti-hypertensive treatment including diuretics. In: *Systemic Effects of Antihypertensive Agents,* edited by M. P. Sambhi, pp. 251–264. Stratton, New York.

170. Imbs, J. L., Desaulles, E., Velly, J., Bloch, R., and Schwartz, J. (1972): Action du clopamide et de l'acide ethacrynique sur la secretion de renine chez la chien. *Pfluegers Arch.,* 331:294–306.

171. Weinberger, M. H., and Grim, C. E. (1976): Effects of spironolactone and hydrochlorothiazide on blood pressure and plasma renin activity in hypertension. In: *Systemic Effects of Antihypertensive Agents,* edited by M. P. Sambhi, pp. 481–493. Stratton, New York.

172. Ueda, H., Kaneko, Y., Takeda, T., Ikeda, T., and Yagi, S. (1970): Observations on the mechanisms of renin release by hydralazine in hypertensive patients. *Circ. Res. [Suppl. II],* 26/27:201–206.

173. Pettinger, W. A., and Keeton, K. (1975): Altered renin release and propranolol potentiation of vasodilatory drug hypotension. *J. Clin. Invest.,* 55:236–243.

174. Pettinger, W. A., Keeton, T. K., Campbell, W. B., Berthelsen, S., and Morris, M. (1976): Further studies on abnormalities of renin release in spontaneously hypertensive rats (SHR). *Clin. Exp. Pharmacol. Physiol. [Suppl.],* 3:135–139.

175. Campbell, W. B., Graham, R. M., and Jackson, E. K. (1980): Indomethacin inhibition of hydralazine-induced renin release in the rat. *Arch. Int. Pharmacodyn. Ther.*, 246:315–323.

176. Campbell, W. B., Jackson, E. K., Graham, R. M., Pettinger, W. A., and Loisel, D. P. (1980): Effect of indomethacin on hydralazine-induced renin and adrenal catecholamine release in conscious rabbits. *Br. J. Pharmacol.*, 71:529–531.

177. Thames, M. D., and DiBona, G. F. (1979): Renal nerves modulate the secretion of renin mediated by non-neural mechanisms. *Circ. Res.*, 44:645–652.

178. Eide, E., Loyning, E., and Kiil, F. (1974): Potentiation of renin release by combined renal arterial constriction and beta-adrenergic stimulation. *Scand. J. Clin. Lab. Invest.*, 34:301–310.

179. Pettinger, W. A., and Mitchell, H. C. (1976): Additive effect of beta-adrenergic blockers in combination with vasodilators in lowering blood pressure. *Aust. N.Z. J. Med. [Suppl. 3]*, 6:76–82.

180. Mutterperl, R. E., Diamond, F. B., and Lowenthal, D. T. (1976): Long-term effects of minoxidil in the treatment of malignant hypertension in chronic renal failure. *Clin. Pharmacol.*, 16:498–509.

181. O'Malley, K., Velasco, M., Wells, J., and McNay, J. L. (1976): Mechanism of the interaction of propranolol and a potent vasodilator antihypertensive agent-minoxidil. *Eur. J. Clin. Pharmacol.*, 9:355–360.

182. Kaul, C. L., and Grewal, R. S. (1976): Effect of some antihypertensive drugs and catecholamine depletors on the plasma renin activity in the rat. *Arch. Int. Pharmacodyn. Ther.*, 224:91–101.

183. Graham, R. M., Muir, M. R., and Hayes, J. M. (1976): Differing effects of the vasodilator drugs, prazosin and diazoxide on plasma renin activity in the dog. *Clin. Exp. Pharmacol. Physiol.*, 3:173–177.

184. Kuchel, O., Fishman, L. M., Liddle, G. W., and Michelakis, A. (1967): Effect of diazoxide on plasma renin activity in hypertensive patients. *Ann. Intern. Med.*, 67:791–799.

185. Vandongen, R., and Greenwood, D. M. (1975): The stimulation of renin secretion by diazoxide in the isolated rat kidney. *Eur. J. Pharmacol.*, 33:197–200.

186. Miller, E. D., Jr., Ackerly, J. A., Vaughan, E. D., Jr., Peach, M. D., and Epstein, R. M. (1977): The renin-angiotensin system during controlled hypotension with sodium nitroprusside. *Anesthesiology*, 47:257–262.

187. Kaneko, Y., Ikeda, T., Takeda, T., and Ueda, H. (1967): Renin release during acute reduction of arterial pressure in normotensive subjects and patients with renovascular hypertension. *J. Clin. Invest.*, 46:705–716.

188. Kaneko, Y., Ikeda, T., Takeda, T., Inoue, G., Tagawa, H., and Ueda, H. (1968): Renin release in patients with benign essential hypertension. *Circulation*, 38:353–362.

189. Velasco, M., and McNay, J. L. (1977): Physiologic mechanisms of bupicomide and hydralazine-induced increase in plasma renin activity in hypertensive patients. *Mayo Clin. Proc.*, 52:430–432.

190. Aoki, K., Yoshida, T., Kato, S., Tazumi, K., Sato, I., Takikawa, K., and Hotta, K. (1976): Hypotensive action and increased plasma renin activity of Ca^{2+} antagonist (nifedipine) in hypertensive patients. *Jpn. Heart J.*, 17:479–484.

191. Aoki, K., Kondo, S., Mochizuki, A., Yoshida, T., Kato, S., Kato, K., and Takikawa, K. (1978): Antihypertensive effect of cardiovascular Ca^{2+}-antagonist in hypertensive patients in the absence and presence of beta-adrenergic blockade. *Am. Heart J.*, 96:218–226.

192. Corea, L., Miele, N., Bentivoglio, M., Boschetti, E., Agabiti-Rosei, E., and Muiesan, G. (1979): Acute and chronic effects of nifedipine on plasma renin activity and plasma adrenaline and noradrenaline in controls and hypertensive patients. *Clin. Sci.*, 57:115s–117s.

193. Churchill, P. C. (1980): Effect of D-600 on inhibition of *in vitro* renin release in the rat by high extracellular potassium and angiotensin II. *J. Physiol. (Lond.)*, 304:449–458.

194. Churchill, P. C., McDonald, F. D., and Churchill, M. C. (1981): Effect of diltiazem, a calcium antagonist, on renin secretion from rat kidney slices. *Life Sci.*, 29:383–389.

195. Park, C. S., Han, D. S., and Fray, J. C. S. (1981): Calcium in the control of renin secretion: Ca^{2+} influx as an inhibitory signal. *Am. J. Physiol.*, 240:F70–F74.

196. Antonello, A., Cargnielli, G., Ferrari, M., Melacini, P., and Montanaro, D. (1976): Effect of digoxin and plasma-renin-activity in man. *Lancet*, 2:850.

197. Ferrari, M. (1979): Effects of digoxin and digoxin plus furosemide on plasma renin activity of hypertensive patients. *Circ. Res.*, 44:295.

198. Blaine, E. H., and Zimmerman, M. B. (1978): Renal function and renin secretion after administration of ouabain and ouabain plus furosemide in conscious sheep. *Circ. Res.*, 43:36–43.

199. Thames, M. D. (1979): Acetylstrophanthidin-induced reflex inhibition of canine renal sympathetic nerve activity mediated by cardiac receptors with vagal afferents. *Circ. Res.*, 44:8–15.

200. Churchill, P. C., and McDonald, F. D. (1974): Effect of ouabain on renin secretion in anesthetized dogs. *J. Physiol.*, 242:635–646.

201. Lyons, H. J., and Churchill, P. C. (1974): The influence of ouabain on *in vitro* renin secretion. *Proc. Soc. Exp. Biol. Med.*, 145:1148–1150.

202. Blaine, E. H. (1977): Renin secretion after papaverine and furosemide in conscious sheep. *Proc. Soc. Exp. Biol. Med.*, 154:232–237.

203. Baumbach, L., Leyssac, P. P., and Skinner, S. L. (1976): Studies on renin release from isolated superfused glomeruli: Effects of temperature, urea, ouabain, and ethacrynic acid. *J. Physiol. (Lond.)*, 258:243–256.

204. Marshall, G. R., Vine, W., and Needleman, P. (1970): Specific competitive inhibitor of angiotensin II. *Proc. Natl. Acad. Sci. U.S.A.*, 67:1624–1630.

205. Ondetti, M. A., Williams, N. J., Sabo, E. F., Pluscec, J., Weaver, E. R., and Kocy, O. (1971): Angiotensin-converting enzyme inhibitors from the venom of *Bothrops jararaca*. Isolation, elucidation of structure, and synthesis. *Biochemistry*, 10:4033–4039.

206. Ondetti, M. A., Rubin, B., and Cushman, D. W.

(1977): Design of specific inhibitors of angiotensin-converting enzyme: A new class of orally active antihypertensive agents. *Science,* 196:441–444.

207. Regoli, D., Park, W. K., and Rioux, F. (1973): Pharmacology of angiotensin antagonist. *Can. J. Physiol. Pharmacol.,* 51:114–121.

208. Bianchi, A., Evans, D. B., Cobb, M., Peschka, M. T., Schaeffer, T. R., and Laffan, R. J. (1973): Inhibition by SQ 20881 of vasopressor response to angiotensin I in conscious animals. *Eur. J. Pharmacol.,* 23:90–96.

209. Rubin, B., Antonaccio, M. J., and Horovitz, Z. P. (1978): Captopril (SQ 14,225) (D-3-mercapto-2-methylpropranoyl-L-proline); a novel orally active inhibitor of angiotensin-converting enzyme and antihypertensive agent. *Prog. Cardiovasc. Dis.,* 21:183–194.

210. Beatty, O., III, Sloop, C. H., Schmid, H. E., Jr., and Buckalew, V. M., Jr. (1976): Renin response and angiotensinogen control during graded hemorrhage and shock in the dog. *Am. J. Physiol.,* 231:1300–1307.

211. Bravo, E. L., Khosla, M. C., and Bumpus, F. M. (1976): Comparative studies of the humoral and arterial pressure responses to Sar^1-ala^8-, Sar^1-Ile^8- and Sar^1-Thr^8-angiotensin II in the trained, unanesthetized dog. *Prog. Biochem. Pharmacol.,* 12:33–40.

212. Steele, J. M., Jr., and Lowenstein, J. (1974): Differential effects of an angiotensin II analogue on pressor and adrenal receptors in the rabbit. *Circ. Res.,* 35:592–600.

213. Bing, J., and Poulsen, K. (1975): Time course of changes in plasma renin after blockade of the renin-system. *Acta Pathol. Microbiol. Scand. [Suppl.],* A83:454–466.

214. Campbell, W. B., Jackson, E. K., and Graham, R. M. (1979): Saralasin-induced renin release: Its blockade by prostaglandin synthesis inhibitors in the conscious rat. *Hypertension,* 1:637–642.

215. Vandongen, R., Peart, W. S., and Boyd, G. W. (1974): Effect of angiotensin II and its non-pressor derivatives on renin secretion. *Am. J. Physiol.,* 226:277–282.

216. Hofbauer, K. G., Bauereiss, K., Zschiedrich, H., and Gross, F. (1976): Effects of saralasin on renal function in the rat. *Prog. Biochem. Pharmacol.,* 12:63–83.

217. Naftilan, A. J., and Oparil, S. (1978): Inhibition of renin release from rat kidney slices by the angiotensins. *Am. J. Physiol.,* 235:F62–F68.

218. Pettinger, W. A., and Mitchell, H. C. (1975): Renin release, saralasin and the vasodilator-beta-blocker drug interaction in man. *N. Engl. J. Med.,* 292:1214–1217.

219. Pettinger, W. A., and Mitchell, H. C. (1976): Clinical pharmacology of angiotensin antagonists. *Fed. Proc.,* 35:2521–2525.

220. Thurston, H., and Swales, J. D. (1978): Converting enzyme inhibitor and saralasin infusion in rats. Evidence for an additional vasodepressor property of converting enzyme inhibitor. *Circ. Res.,* 42:588–592.

221. Kimbrough, J. M., Vaughn, E. D., Jr., Carey, R. M., and Ayers, C. R. (1977): Effect of intrarenal

angiotensin II blockade on renal function in conscious dogs. *Circ. Res.,* 40:174–178.

222. Samuels, A. I., Miller, E. D., Jr., Fray, J. C. S., Haber, E., and Barger, A. C. (1976): Renin-angiotensin antagonists and the regulation of blood pressure. *Fed. Proc.,* 35:2512–2520.

223. Antonaccio, M. J., Harris, D., Goldenberg, H., High, J. P., and Rubin, B. (1979): The effects of captopril, propranolol and indomethacin on blood pressure and plasma renin activity in spontaneously hypertensive and normotensive rats. *Proc. Soc. Exp. Biol. Med.,* 162:429–433.

224. Schiffrin, E. L., Gutkowska, J., and Genest, J. (1981): Mechanism of captopril-induced renin release in conscious rats. *Proc. Soc. Exp. Biol. Med.,* 167:327–332.

225. Horovitz, Z. P., Rubin, B., Antonaccio, M. J., High, J., Schaffer, T., and Harris, D. (1978): Antihypertensive effects of SQ 14,225 (D-3-mercapto-2-methyl-propanoyl-L-proline), and orally active angiotensin I-converting enzyme inhibitor, in spontaneously hypertensive rats (SHR) during chronic therapy. *Fed. Proc.,* 37:718 (abstract).

226. Waldron, T. L., and Murthy, V. S. (1978): Hemodynamic effects of SQ 14,225, an orally effective angiotensin converting enzyme (ACE) inhibitor, in dogs. *Fed. Proc.,* 37:718 (abstract).

227. Harris, D. N., Heran, C. L., Goldenberg, H. J., High, J. P., Laffan, R. J., Rubin, B., Antonaccio, M. J., and Goldberg, M. E. (1978): Effects of SQ 14,225 on orally active inhibitor of angiotensin converting enzyme on blood pressure, heart rate and plasma renin activity of conscious normotensive dogs. *Eur. J. Pharmacol.,* 51:345–349.

228. McCaa, R. E. (1977): Aldosterone and blood pressure response to an orally active inhibitor of angiotensin I converting enzyme (SQ-14,225) in sodium deficient dogs. *I.R.C.S. Med. Sci.,* 5:207.

229. Sancho, J., Re, R., Buront, J., Barger, A. C., and Haber, E. (1976): The role of the renin-angiotensin aldosterone system in cardiovascular homeostasis in normal human subjects. *Circulation,* 53:400–405.

230. Gavras, H., Brunner, H. R., Laragh, J. H., Sealey, J. E., Gavras, I., and Vukovich, R. A. (1974): An angiotensin converting-enzyme inhibitor to identify and treat vasoconstrictor and volume factors in hypertensive patients. *N. Engl. J. Med.,* 291:817–821.

231. Gavras, H., Gavras, I., Textor, S., Volicer, L., Brunner, H. R., and Rucinska, E. J. (1978): Effect of angiotensin converting enzyme inhibition on blood pressure, plasma renin activity and plasma aldosterone in essential hypertension. *J. Clin. Endocrinol. Metab.,* 46:220–226.

232. Ferguson, R. K., Turini, G. A., Brunner, H. R., Gavras, H., and McKinstry, D. N. (1977): A specific orally active inhibitor of angiotensin-converting enzyme in man. *Lancet,* 1:775–778.

233. Case, D. B., Atlas, A. S., Laragh, J. H., Sealey, J. E., Sullivan, P. A., and McKinstry, D. N. (1978): Clinical experience with blockade of the renin-angiotensin-aldosterone system by an oral converting-enzyme inhibitor (SQ 14,225, captopril) in hypertensive patients. *Prog. Cardiovasc. Res.,* 21:195–206.

234. Kono, T., Ikeda, F., Oseko, F., Imura, H., and Endo,

J. (1981): Suppression of captopril-induced increase in plasma renin activity by des-Asp[1]-Ileu[8]-angiotensin II in man. *J. Clin. Endocrinol. Metab.*, 52:354–358.

235. Gavras, H., Brunner, H. R., Turini, G. A., Kershaw, G. R., Tifft, C. P., Cuttelod, S., Gavras, I., Vukovich, R. A., and McKinstry, D. N. (1978): Antihypertensive effect of the oral angiotensin converting-enzyme inhibitor SQ 14,225 in man. *N. Engl. J. Med.*, 198:991–995.

236. Abe, K., Itoh, T., Satoh, M., Haruyama, T., Imai, Y., Goto, T., Satoh, K., Otsuka, Y., and Yoshinaga, K. (1980): Indomethacin (IND) inhibits an enhanced renin release following the captopril, SQ 14,225, administration. *Life Sci.*, 26:561–565.

237. Vane, J. R. (1971): Inhibition of prostaglandin synthesis as a mechanism of action for aspirin-like drugs. *Nature [New Biol.]*, 231:232–235.

238. Henrich, W. L. (1981): Role of prostaglandins in renin secretion. *Kidney Int.*, 19:822–830.

239. Campbell, W. B., Gomez-Sanchez, C. E., Schmitz, J. M., Adams, B. V., and Itskovitz, H. D. (1979): Attenuation of angiotensin II and III induced aldosterone release by prostaglandin synthesis inhibitors. *J. Clin. Invest.*, 64:1552–1557.

240. Leyssac, P. O., Christensen, P., Hill, R., and Skinner, S. L. (1975): Indomethacin blockade or renal PGE synthesis. Effect on total renal and tubular function and plasma renin concentration in hydropenic rats and on their response to isotonic saline. *Acta Physiol. Scand.*, 94:484–496.

241. Romero, J. C., and Strong, C. G. (1977): The effect of indomethacin blockade of prostaglandin synthesis on blood pressure of normal rabbits and rabbits with renovascular hypertension. *Circ. Res.*, 40:35–41.

242. Yun, J. C., Kelly, G., Bartter, F. C., and Smith, H., Jr. (1977): Role of prostaglandins in the control of renin secretion in the dog. *Circ. Res.*, 40:459–464.

243. Rumpf, K. W., Frenzel, S., Lowitz, H. D., and Scheler, F. (1975): The effect of indomethacin on plasma renin activity in man under normal conditions and after stimulation of the renin angiotensin system. *Prostaglandins*, 10:641–648.

244. Patak, R. V., Mookerjee, B. K., Bentzel, C. J., Hysert, P. E., Babej, M., and Lee, J. B. (1975): Antagonism of the effects of furosemide by indomethacin in normal and hypertensive man. *Prostaglandins*, 10:649–659.

245. Beckerhoff, R., Uhlschmid, G., Vetter, W., Armbruster, H., and Siegenthaler, W. (1974): Plasma renin and aldosterone after renal transplantation. *Kidney Int.*, 5:39–46.

246. Seymour, A. A., and Zehr, J. E. (1979): Influence of renal prostaglandin synthesis on renin control mechanisms in the dog. *Circ. Res.*, 45:13–25.

247. Feuerstein, G., and Feuerstein, N. (1980): The effect of indomethacin on isoprenaline-induced renin secretion in the cat. *Eur. J. Pharmacol.*, 61:85–88.

248. Frolich, J. C., Hollifield, J. W., Michelakis, A. M., Vesper, B. S., Wilson, J. P., Shand, D. G., Seyberth, H. G., Frolich, W. H., and Oates, J. A. (1979): Reduction of plasma renin activity by inhibition of the fatty acid cyclooxygenase in human subjects: Independence of sodium retention. *Circ. Res.*, 44:781–787.

249. Berl, T., Henrich, W. L., Erickson, A. L., and Schrier, R. W. (1979): Prostaglandins in the beta-adrenergic and baroreceptor-mediated secretion of renin. *Am. J. Physiol.*, 236:F472–477.

250. Campbell, W. B., and Zimmer, J. (1980): Insulin-induced renin release: Blockade by indomethacin in the rat. *Clin. Sci.*, 58:415–418.

251. Frolich, J. C., Hollifield, J. W., Dormois, J. C., Frolich, B. L., Seyberth, H., Michelakis, A. M., and Oates, J. A. (1976): Suppression of plasma renin activity by indomethacin in man. *Circ. Res.*, 39:447–452.

252. Abe, K., Yasujima, M., Chiba, S., Irokawa, N., Ito, T., and Yoshinaga, K. (1977): Effect of furosemide on urinary excretion of prostaglandin E in normal volunteers and patients with essential hypertension. *Prostaglandins*, 14:512–521.

253. Tan, S. Y., and Mulrow, P. J. (1977): Inhibition of renin-aldosterone response to furosemide by indomethacin. *J. Clin. Endocrinol. Metab.*, 45:174–176.

254. Williams, W. M., Frolich, J. C., Nies, A. S., and Oates, J. A. (1977): Urinary prostaglandins: Site of entry into renal tubular fluid. *Kidney Int.*, 11:256–260.

255. McGiff, J. C. (1977): Bartter's syndrome results from an imbalance of vasoactive hormones. *Ann. Intern. Med.*, 87:369–372.

256. Verberckmoes, R., van Damme, B., Clement, J., Amery, A., and Michielsen, P. (1976): Bartter's syndrome with hyperplasia of renomedullary cells. Successful treatment with indomethacin. *Kidney Int.*, 9:302–307.

257. Skinner, S. L. (1967): Improved assay methods for renin "concentration" and "activity" in human plasma. Methods using selective denaturation of renin substrate. *Circ. Res.*, 20:392–402.

258. Netter, F. H. (1973): In: *Kidneys, Ureters, and Urinary Bladder*. The Ciba Collection of Medical Illustrations, Vol. 6, edited by R. K. Shapter and F. F. Yonkman, p. 7, Ciba Pharmaceutical Co., Summit, N.J.

Cardiovascular Pharmacology, Second Edition,
edited by Michael Antonaccio.
Raven Press, New York © 1984.

Angiotensin-Converting Enzyme and Renin Inhibitors

Charles S. Sweet and Edward H. Blaine

Merck Institute for Therapeutic Research, West Point, Pennsylvania 19486

Interest in the renin-angiotensin system has intensified in recent years because new drugs have been introduced that have considerably aided in clarifying the role of angiotensin in experimental and human hypertension. Figure 1 illustrates the various components of the renin-angiotensin system and sites of inhibition. Renin antibodies were first used to inhibit the system, but because of lack of pure renin preparations, this approach has been slow to develop. However, other approaches to develop renin inhibitors appear promising. With the elucidation of the structure of angiotensin II, potent and specific inhibitors of angiotensin II were developed (1,2). Unfortunately, the therapeutic utility of such compounds is limited by the lack of oral absorption. A major advance in the development of effective inhibitors of the renin-angiotensin system was discovery of angiotensin-converting enzyme inhibitors. These compounds have been widely used to investigate the role of the renin-angio-tensin system in the pathogenesis of hypertension and have proved remarkably effective. This chapter will highlight converting enzyme and renin inhibitors—two therapeutic categories that appear to be particularly promising for the treatment of hypertension.

ANGIOTENSIN-CONVERTING ENZYME INHIBITORS

Enzyme Properties

Angiotensin-converting enzyme (ACE), or kininase II, is the component of the renin-angiotensin system that is responsible for hydrolyzing the carboxyl-terminal dipeptide from angiotensin I. Skeggs et al. (3) were the first to identify ACE, and they later purified this enzyme that is responsible for the conversion of angiotensin I to angiotensin II. Helmer (4) and Skeggs et al. (5) demonstrated that

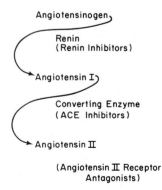

FIG. 1. Renin-angiotensin system showing sites of inhibition.

angiotensin I lacked inherent biological activity and that the pressor product of the enzyme reaction was angiotensin II. Several years later, Ng and Vane (6), using bioassay techniques, showed that the conversion of angiotensin I to angiotensin II took place in the lungs and other vascular beds, but not much in plasma. The bioassay technique was followed by more specific methods, and these have led to more precise quantitation of the levels of converting enzyme activity in tissue and in plasma. Cushman and Ondetti (7), Erdos (8), Soffer (9), and Skeggs et al. (10) have reviewed many of these methods, as well as some of the historical developments in the elucidation of the role of converting enzyme in the activity of the renin-angiotensin system.

The most important substrates for converting enzyme are angiotensin I and bradykinin. Further characterization of converting enzyme has revealed that it hydrolyzes angiotensin I to angiotensin II and inactivates bradykinin by cleaving the C-terminal dipeptides (11). The enzyme isolated from hog or guinea pig plasma, kininase II, differs from another enzyme, kininase I, which removes only the C-terminal arginine of bradykinin. The importance of this dual function has significant implications for understanding the antihypertensive actions of inhibitors of this enzyme. Inhibition of the catabolism of bradykinin (a potent vasodilator) and/or inhibition of the formation of angiotensin II (a potent vasoconstrictor) have been proposed to explain the blood-pressure-lowering effects subsequent to inhibition of this enzyme.

Throughout this chapter, the name angiotensin-converting enzyme inhibitors (as opposed to inhibitors of kininase II) will be used when referring to those pharmacologic agents that inhibit this enzyme, because the majority of evidence suggests that these compounds act by inhibition of the formation of angiotensin II.

Cheung and Cushman (12) and Das and Soffer (13) have described in detail the structural and catalytic properties of ACE. Recognition of mechanistic similarities between ACE and carboxypeptidase A was a key factor in the development of a hypothetical model for ACE that led to the design of the first nonpeptidic inhibitors of converting enzyme (14).

In 1965, Ferreira (15) described a factor obtained from the venom of *Bothrops jararaca* that inhibited plasma kininase II and potentiated the hypotensive or contractile effects of bradykinin. This bradykinin-potentiating factor (BPF) was later shown to be a mixture of nine peptides that enhanced the effect of bradykinin and inhibited the hypertensive action of angiotensin I. Several inhibitors of ACE have been isolated from BPF, and a number of these peptides have been synthesized by the research team at the Squibb Institute (16). The two most impressive compounds in terms of *in vivo* inhibition of angiotensin I and duration of action are a nonapeptide and an octapeptide with the following structures: Pyr-Trp-Pro-Arg-Pro-Gln-Ile-Pro-Pro (SQ 20,881) and Pyr-Asn-Trp-Pro-His-Pro-Gln-Ile-Pro-Pro (SQ 20,858). The venom of *Agkistrodon halys blomhoffi* also contains peptides that inhibit converting enzyme.

The nonapeptide SQ 20,881 (Teprotide®) synthesized and characterized by Ondetti et al. (16) was the first ACE inhibitor to be tested clinically. Green et al. (17) designated this peptide as bradykinin-potentiating peptide 9a (BPP$_{9a}$), because studies showed that it enhanced the contractile response to bradykinin. This agent, however, did not possess activity when given orally. SQ 20,881 inhibited the rabbit lung enzyme with an IC$_{50}$ of 1 μg/ml. It attenuated the contractile response of the excised guinea pig ileum to angiotensin I and potentiated the contractile response of this tissue to bradykinin at 0.07 and 0.0017 μg/ml, respectively. The compound's specificity of action in selectively blocking the pressor action of angiotensin I was confirmed, and other studies showed that it did not inhibit a variety of enzymes, nor did it interfere with the contractile properties of acetylcholine or angiotensin II.

BPP$_{5a}$
(SQ 20,475)

<Glu-Lys-Trp-Ala-Pro

BPP$_{9a}$ Teprotide
(SQ 20,881)

<Glu-Trp-Pro-Arg-Pro-Gln-Ile-Pro-Pro

Captopril

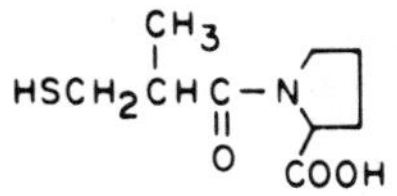

SA-446
(Santen)

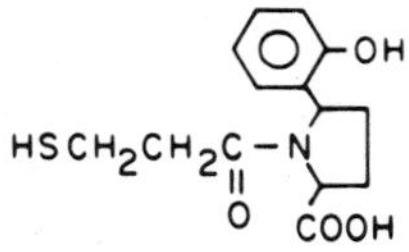

RHC 3659
(Revlon Health Care)

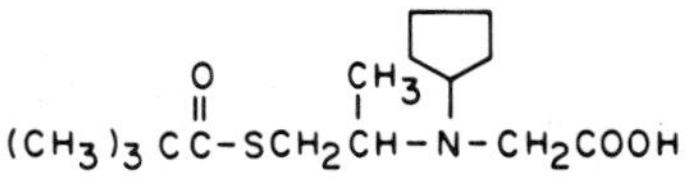

Keto-ACE
(Almquist)

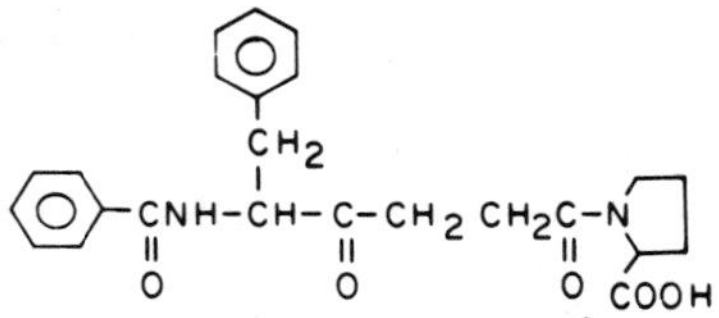

YS-980
(Yoshitomi)

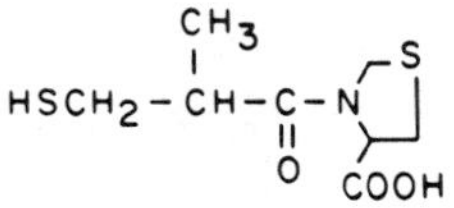

ENALAPRIL
(Merck)

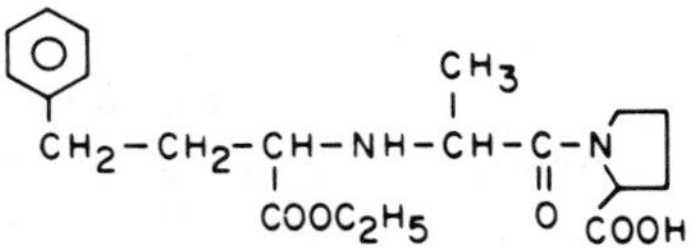

MK-521
(Merck)

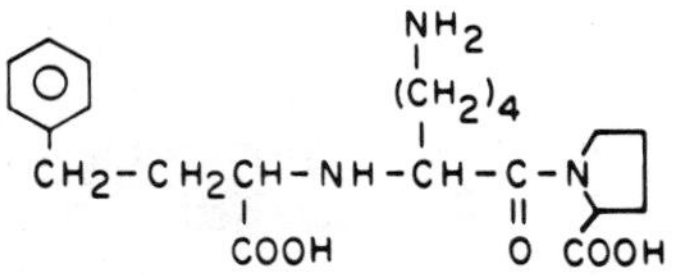

A Phosphoramide
(Galardy)

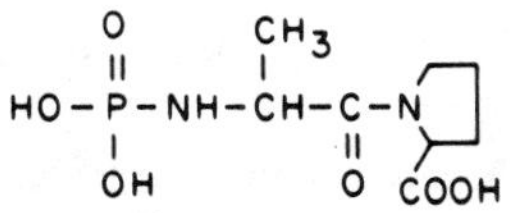

FIG. 2. Structures of converting enzyme inhibitors.

Converting Enzyme Assay Methods

Before proceeding to consideration of other specific peptide inhibitors, a discussion of the methods for assessing converting enzyme activity is warranted. The basis for some of the *in vitro* assays is the ability of isolated tissues to convert angiotensin I to angiotensin II and to induce an increase in smooth-muscle tone. Application of ACE inhibitors in such systems will prevent the smooth-muscle response to subsequent administration of angiotensin I. The blood-bathed-organ technique has been used by Ng and Vane (6) to estimate the conversion of angiotensin I to angiotensin II in the lungs. This system can also be used to identify circulating humoral substances. In this system, several different isolated smooth-muscle strips (rat colon, rat stomach, chick rectum), selected because of their differential sensitivities to biologically active substances, are superfused in series with blood. The rat colon, for example, will contract in response to angiotensin II as well as in response to prostaglandins, whereas the chick rectum is sensitive to the latter but not the former. The conversion of angiotensin I to angiotensin II can be quantified *in vitro* using the rat colon superfused in series with an isolated lung. The colon contracts to angiotensin II but not angiotensin I. The conversion of angiotensin I to angiotensin II is estimated by comparing the contractile response to angiotensin I injected into the pulmonary artery versus the response to angiotensin I added directly to the tissues. One common technique involves measurement of angiotensin-I-induced contraction of the guinea pig ileum. The isolated tissue contracts because of conversion of angiotensin I to angiotensin II. Potential ACE inhibitors can be introduced into the bath at single or cumulative concentrations, with ED_{50} values being computed based on percentage inhibition of the contractile response. Bradykinin also produces a contraction in this system that is enhanced by ACE inhibitors. The basis for this augmentation, as mentioned previously, is the blockade of bradykinin breakdown.

In vivo test systems often involve blockade of the pressor or vasoconstrictor response to angiotensin I or measurement of the enhanced vasodepressor response to bradykinin. By comparing the amounts of angiotensin I and angiotensin II required to produce equivalent decreases in blood flow in a selected vascular bed, the activity of ACE can be estimated. Some workers have measured the formation of radiolabeled histidyl-leucine from angiotensin I. A spectrophotometric assay has been used that measures hippuric acid from the substrate hippuryl-L-histidyl-L-leucine (HHL).

Design of New ACE Inhibitors

In 1974 the utility of converting enzyme inhibitors as antihypertensive drugs became apparent, and the search for an effective oral agent began. Cushman and Ondetti (7) have described the development and rationale for the design of nonapeptide inhibitors of converting enzyme. Their approach in designing these newer orally effective agents was to develop a hypothetical model of the active site on the enzyme (14). The substrate specificity of ACE suggested that it was a zinc metallopeptidase with a mechanism similar to that of the digestive enzyme pancreatic carboxypeptidase A. Using an analogue of the byproduct inhibitors previously described for carboxypeptidase A (succinyl-L-proline), the Squibb researchers began to formulate a hypothetical active site for converting enzyme using succinyl-L-proline as a prototype inhibitor. Extensive structure-activity experiments with hundreds of analogues were performed, and finally a compound with 20,000 times the inhibitory potency of succinyl-L-proline on ACE was found. This agent was captopril (Fig. 2).

A somewhat modified hypothetical model of the active site for ACE is shown in Fig. 3. The top portion of the figure shows a schematic representation of the binding of sub-

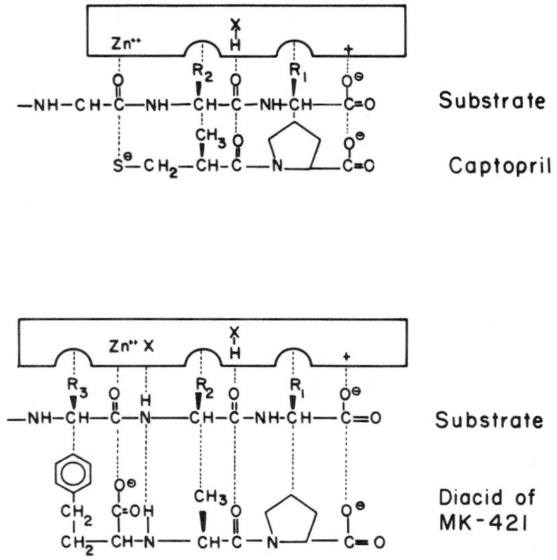

FIG. 3. Modified hypothetical Squibb model for the active site of ACE as proposed by Ondetti et al. (14). **Top:** Schematic representation of the binding of substrate (angiotensin I) and the inhibitor captopril to converting enzyme. The circular clefts represent subsites that can potentially interact with specific amino acids of substrates or inhibitors (captopril). **Bottom:** MSDRL model of Schematic representation of binding of MK-421 diacid to active site of enzyme as proposed by Patchett et al. (18).

strate (angiotensin I) and the inhibitor captopril to converting enzyme (14). The circular clefts represent subsites that can potentially interact with specific amino acids of substrates or inhibitors. Substrates apparently bind to the enzyme at their carboxyl-terminal tripeptide. Enalapril (MK-421), a new ACE inhibitor (18), with its theoretical binding sites, is also shown in Fig. 3.

Converting Enzyme Inhibitory Characteristics of Captopril

In Vitro

Captopril at 0.10 to 0.04 μM inhibits ACE from a variety of species. The inhibitor is 200 times more potent than SQ 20,881 on a weight basis. Captopril does not inhibit other enzymes such as chymotrypsin, trypsin, carboxypeptidase A and B, and leucine aminopeptidase; for a review, see Cushman and Ondetti (7).

Reference has been made to the use of the guinea pig ileum for evaluation of converting enzyme inhibitors. Rubin et al. (19) were the first to demonstrate that captopril ($IC_{50} = 5$ ng/ml) was more potent than SQ 20,881

against angiotensin-I-induced contraction in the guinea pig ileum. They reported that captopril at a concentration of 0.7 ng/ml augmented the contractile response to bradykinin by 50%. Importantly, the contractile responses to 11 other agonists, including acetylcholine and angiotensin II, were not altered by captopril.

In Vivo

Captopril is active in blunting the pressor effect of angiotensin I in rats and dogs. The doses of captopril that inhibited the pressor response to angiotensin I by 50% were 20μg/kg i.v. for rats and 37 μg/kg i.v. for dogs (19). Gross et al. (20) reported a somewhat higher value, which may reflect differences in experimental procedures.

The short duration of action of single intravenous doses of captopril in dogs is illustrated in Fig. 4. These data show that maximum inhibitory activity was immediate, and recovery of the angiotensin I pressor response occurred by 15 min. As shown in Fig. 5, the minimally effective dose of captopril in rats was 0.1 mg/kg; the onset was rapid, and the duration of action was dependent on the dose.

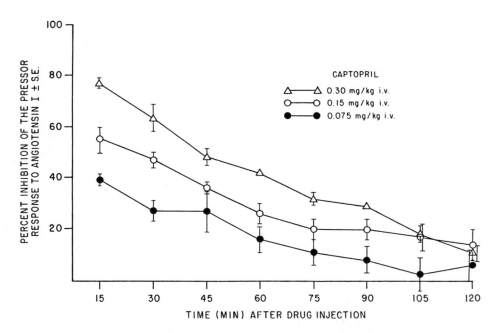

FIG. 4. Durations of action of single intravenous doses of captopril in anesthetized dogs. Captopril was administered at time zero, and angiotensin was injected at the various time intervals shown. The percentage inhibition of the pressor response was computed from the initial pretreatment pressor responses.

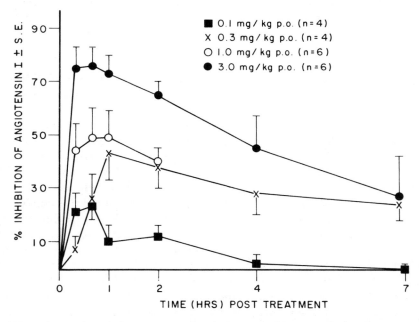

FIG. 5. Oral ACE inhibitory activity of captopril in unanesthetized rats: Percentage inhibition of angiotensin I pressor responses in rats at 1, 2, and 7 hr after treatment at 0.1 to 3 mg/kg orally.

Antihypertensive Activity in Spontaneously Hypertensive Rats

Captopril was developed and designed to bind specifically to the active site of converting enzyme. From the initial pharmacologic studies (14,19) it was clear that the principal mechanism of action of this compound was enzyme inhibition. The compound did not interact directly with the autonomic nervous system, did not block or potentiate adrenergic receptors, and did not interact with central nervous system mechanisms (e.g., clonidine).

There is currently no strong evidence to indicate that there is an excessive level of a circulating pressor substance or a decreased level of a depressor substance in spontaneously hypertensive rats (SHR). The level of plasma renin activity (PRA), despite extensive study, has been reported to be normal or below normal (21). Thus, it is still uncertain whether or not the renin-angiotensin system plays an important role in genetic hypertension. Furthermore, SHR of the Okamoto-Wistar strain were found to have reduced angiotensin-I-converting enzyme in serum, kidney, and anterior pituitary (22). Thus, it seems surprising that captopril would reduce blood pressure in SHR simply by inhibiting the renin system. Yet, there have been several studies that have demonstrated that acute and chronic administration of captopril results in a significant reduction in blood pressure (23–25).

Acute and Chronic Studies in Established Hypertension

The first demonstration of the antihypertensive effects of captopril in Okamoto SHR was made by Laffan et al. (23). The doses of captopril that reduced blood pressure were larger than required to block the pressor response to angiotensin I. They also showed that the antihypertensive dose–response regression line was flat.

Captopril also has been shown to reduce blood pressure by about 12% in the New Zealand genetic hypertensive rat, a strain that seems to be most similar to the Okamoto SHR (26). In the stroke-prone substrain of SHR, Watanabe and Sokabe (27) reported that captopril decreased blood pressure by 21%. The somewhat larger decrement in blood pressure in this study may have been due to the higher initial plasma renin levels.

Chronic administration of captopril for 6 months causes a progressive fall in arterial pressure to essentially normotensive levels (28). The maintenance of the antihypertensive effect of captopril with prolonged treatment indicates that the tolerance that can be demonstrated with many antihypertensive drugs does not occur with these agents that inhibit the renin-angiotensin system. Interestingly, the antihypertensive effect of captopril was not attended by tachycardia (28).

Development of Hypertension in SHR

Several studies (29–31) have demonstrated that captopril can slow and essentially prevent the development of hypertension in SHR by a mechanism that involves a decrease in peripheral resistance rather than a reduction in cardiac output. The hemodynamic mechanisms associated with the reversal of the development of genetic hypertension by captopril have been partially elucidated. Studies using tracer microspheres (29) demonstrated that captopril-induced attenuation of the rise in blood pressure was associated with an increase in cardiac output, a reduction in mean arterial pressure, and therefore a fall in total peripheral resistance. An expansion of blood volume that would have been predicted because of the prolonged hypotension did not occur, because of the increase in renal function associated with ACE inhibitor treatment (*vide infra*).

One interesting characteristic of the blood pressure profile when captopril was discontinued during 6 months of treatment in SHR was that blood pressure slowly returned toward hypertensive levels at about the same rate regardless of whether treatment ended at 4, 8, 12, or 16 weeks (Fig. 6). These findings

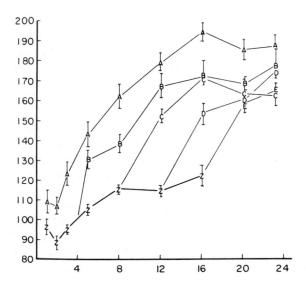

FIG. 6. Effects of captopril (100 mg/kg/day) on systolic blood pressure in SHR. Curve Z represents all of the animals on captopril therapy (initially 60 rats). In curve A, rats (*N* = 10) were maintained on water for duration of study. From the group, rats were randomly removed from drug 4 (B), 8 (C), 12 (D), and 16 (E) weeks after dosing. Ordinate: systolic blood pressure (mm Hg). Abscissa: weeks of dosing. (From Ferrone and Antonaccio, ref. 30, with permission.)

indicate that captopril suppressed but did not eliminate the underlying mechanism responsible for this form of hypertension. Although it is clear that the antihypertensive mechanism is not understood completely, it was suggested that inhibition of the arterial-wall renin-angiotensin system might account for the blood-pressure-lowering effect (30). This system has some of the same characteristics as the renal renin-angiotensin system, but the half-life of renin in blood vessels is considerably longer than that of renin in plasma. Other mechanisms, such as reduction in plasma of the angiotensin II concentration and a central nervous system effect of captopril, were discounted.

In addition to the antihypertensive effect of captopril in SHR, reversal of cardiac hypertrophy has been observed (31,32). Thus, captopril behaves much like methyldopa in this ability to decrease cardiac hypertrophy. The mechanisms responsible for reversal of cardiac hypertrophy are not understood but probably are due to a reduction in afterload secondary to a decrease in peripheral vascular resistance, although an effect on cardiac adrenergic drive or a direct biochemical effect cannot be excluded (32).

Discrepancies between Inhibition in Plasma Converting Enzyme and Blood Pressure Reduction

Reference has been made to the fact that PRA values in adult SHR are either similar to or slightly lower than those in normotensive adult rats. It is not yet understood why captopril is able to lower blood pressure in genetically hypertensive rats by inhibiting the renin-angiotensin system, in view of the observation that angiotensin antibodies or saralasin, an angiotensin II receptor antagonist administered acutely (33,34), did not reduce blood pressure in this model. It is conceivable that PRA activity is not the best determinant of the extent to which the renin system is supporting or maintaining blood pressure in SHR. The assumption that inhibition of circulating ACE is an index of the efficacy of these compounds may not be correct. It is known, for instance, that plasma conversion of angiotensin I to angiotensin II plays only a minor role in the total rate of conversion and that tissue-bound ACE (e.g., in the lungs) is the principal site of conversion (6). Only limited information is available correlating the reductions in ACE activity in plasma and tissue after enzyme inhibition, and although these data do suggest a positive correlation, they must be considered preliminary.

In some patients, blood pressure has remained low for up to 14 hr after the last dose of captopril, despite resumption of normal plasma converting enzyme activity (35). Other clinical (36) and nonclinical (37,38) studies have confirmed that the effects of captopril on blood pressure and angiotensin-I-converting enzyme do not run in parallel. It has been pointed out that measurements of converting enzyme from stored ($-20°C$) plasma samples under-estimate the inhibition of this enzyme in plasma, which may, in part, explain the discrepancies noted earlier (36).

We have observed that there is a discrepancy between the extent of blockade of the pressor response to angiotensin I and the decrement in mean arterial pressure induced by captopril (39). Figure 7 shows data indicating that the time courses for blockade of angiotensin I and the blood pressure reduction did not correspond. In addition, the finding that enalapril (MK-421), a new ACE inhibitor, is more potent than captopril in lowering blood pressure, but equally active in its ability to block angiotensin I pressor responses, suggests that a mechanism other than inhibition of the conversion of angiotensin I to angiotensin II is involved in the decrease in blood pressure in SHR.

In one clinical study (104), chronic captopril treatment produced a sustained decrease in blood pressure, but plasma angiotensin II levels did not remain suppressed, suggesting a discrepancy between the blood pressure effects and a component of the renin-angiotensin system. However, ACE inhibition by captopril increased renin secretion and angiotensin I levels (40). One of the problems, therefore, in the measurement of angiotensin II after inhibition of ACE is an increased concentration of angiotensin I that potentially could cross-react with the angiotensin II antibody. This interaction could result in falsely high values for angiotensin II (37).

Acute administration of captopril causes similar inhibitions of the pressor response to i.v. angiotensin I and fluorometrically measured ACE (38). However, with prolonged (4 months) oral treatment, plasma ACE activity can be dissociated from the i.v. pressor response to angiotensin I (38). Some studies have shown that chronic oral captopril treatment increases converting enzyme in plasma, brain, and lung (41–43). In most of these studies, ACE activity was increased only after captopril had been removed from the assay by N-ethylmaleimide (NEM), dialysis, or storage. Thus, caution must be exercised when interpreting data in which plasma converting enzyme activity is used as an indication of the state of the renin-angiotensin system.

Central Antihypertensive Effects in SHR

In contrast to the results with peripheral administration, central nervous system administration of angiotensin II receptor antagonists reduces blood pressure (45). Furthermore, Stamler et al. (46) and Hutchinson et al. (47) demonstrated that captopril administered into the lateral brain ventricle (intracerebroventricular injection, i.c.v.) lowered blood pressure. In stroke-prone SHR (a model with somewhat higher PRA values), captopril caused a biphasic response in blood pressure at high doses and only a depressor response at low doses. Thus, at 500 μg i.c.v., captopril caused a sharp rise (50 mm Hg) in blood pressure, followed by a fall in blood pressure lasting 4 hr.

Suzuki et al. (51) compared the central antihypertensive properties of saralasin and captopril in normotensive rats and SHR and found that both inhibitors of the renin-angiotensin system caused small but significant lowering of blood pressure. Similar findings were obtained in renal-hypertensive rats but not DOCA/salt-hypertensive or normotensive rats.

It should be pointed out that several studies (48–50) have shown that orally administered captopril or enalapril does not pass the blood-brain barrier in sufficient quantities to interfere with the effects of centrally administered angiotensin I.

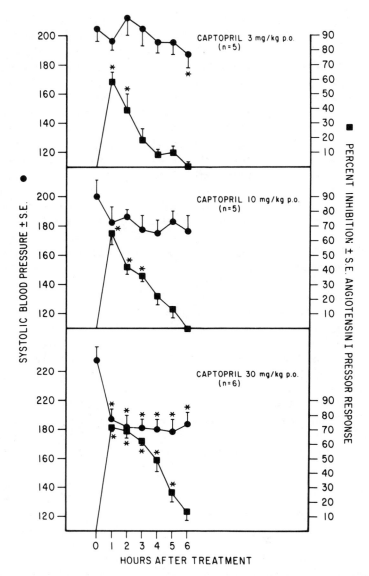

FIG. 7. Relationship between angiotensin I blockade and fall in blood pressure in SHR with high (single) doses of captopril. The figure shows changes in systolic pressure ± SEM (circles), measured directly from indwelling arterial catheters, and percentage inhibition ± SEM (squares) of the pressor response to angiotensin I, 300 ng/kg i.v., following captopril, 3, 10, and 30 mg/kg p.o. An asterisk represents a statistically significant change in systolic pressure from the pretreatment control values or a statistically significant increase in the percentage inhibition of the angiotensin I pressor response. The initial pressor responses to angiotensin I before captopril were 61 ± 3, 67 ± 3, and 63 ± 4 mm Hg, respectively.

Effect of Nephrectomy in SHR

The kidneys play a central role in the pathogenesis of hypertension in several animal models. Because this organ is the principal source of renin, it would be expected that removal of the kidney would render ACE inhibitors ineffective if their mechanism of action is to block one of the blood-borne components of this system. There is some controversy whether or not the kidneys in SHR are essential for demonstrating the acute antihypertensive response to ACE inhibitors. Bilateral nephrectomy performed shortly before administration of captopril (23) or enalapril (52) prevented the acute hypotensive response. Hutchinson et al. (47), in contrast, showed that bilateral nephrectomy did not significantly alter the mean arterial pressure response to intravenous captopril. The slow progressive hypotensive response in these animals was identical with that observed in the intact SHR.

In anephric subjects, Schalekamp et al. (53) found that blood pressure fell after captopril treatment, provided the patients were not overloaded with fluid. Because the primary source of renin was removed in these patients, and angiotensin II levels were low, it was concluded that the effects of the drug did not depend on circulating levels of this peptide. The concept that captopril acts in the blood vessel wall or in close contact with it, rather than in circulating blood, was proposed as a mechanism to explain the hypotensive effect of captopril in these patients. Additional evidence to support this hypothesis has been presented by Thurston and Swales (54), who demonstrated that an infusion of the nonapeptide inhibitor SQ 20,881 decreased blood pressure by 25% in nephrectomized renal-hypertensive rats.

Vasopressin and Prostaglandins in SHR

There is some evidence that young SHR have slightly higher urinary excretion of vasopressin. Crofton et al. (55) showed that administration of captopril decreased urinary excretion of vasopressin over a 4-week period. The decreases in plasma angiotensin II levels may have been responsible for the reduction in vasopressin levels. Alternatively, the increase in water intake that occurred with treatment could have inhibited vasopressin release through a change in plasma osmolality. Ap-

parently an elevation in kinin levels subsequent to ACE inhibition would not be involved, because an elevation in kinin would be expected to increase the level of vasopressin. At this time, it is difficult to assess the role of the elevated plasma vasopressin levels in maintenance of the hypertension in SHR. The magnitude of this elevation is small, but SHR have an increased sensitivity to the pressor effects of vasopressin. In the malignant phase of two-kidney Goldblatt hypertension in DOCA/salt-hypertensive rats and stroke-prone SHR, considerably more evidence has been accumulated to indicate that vasopressin may participate in a more substantial manner in the control of blood pressure. Prostaglandins appear to play no role in the ability of captopril to lower blood pressure in SHR. According to Antonaccio et al. (56), indomethacin (2.5 mg/kg/day for 3 days) did not affect the reduction in blood pressure induced by captopril.

Antihypertensive Effects in Renal-Hypertensive Rats

Since the development of the renal-hypertensive model by Goldblatt, extensive studies have been conducted on the role of the renin-angiotensin system in the development of hypertension in this model. In one form of renal hypertension, one kidney is removed, and the renal artery of the remaining kidney is constricted (1K-1C). In this model there is an initial increase in PRA (acute phase) that correlates well with the degree of blood pressure elevation. After several days, PRA returns to normal or lower levels, and the blood pressure elevation appears not to be directly related to the circulating renin levels. If ACE inhibitors work by inhibiting the blood-borne renin-angiotensin system, this model would be expected to be refractory to ACE inhibitor treatment in the chronic phase of hypertension. In another form of renal hypertension, one renal artery is constricted, and the contralateral kidney remains intact (2K-1C). In this model, PRA is elevated in the acute and chronic phases of the hypertension, and it would be anticipated that ACE inhibitors would be more efficacious in this model than in 1K-1C hypertension.

Two-Kidney-One-Clipped (2K-1C) Hypertension

A variety of studies using angiotensin II antagonists or continuous converting enzyme blockade have demonstrated a role for the renin-angiotensin system in the initiation (Fig. 8) and to some extent in the maintenance of elevated blood pressure in the 2K-1C model (57–60).

The 2K-1C model is characterized by elevated plasma renin activity, high kidney renin activity in the clipped kidney, and low intrarenal renin activity in the nonclipped kidney (61–64). Despite some observations (57, 69,70,74) that short-term infusions of angiotensin II antagonists failed to lower blood pressure in chronic 2K-1C rats, it is important to consider that most angiotensin II antagonists have inherent agonist activity. Another explanation for the lack of acute effect of these inhibitors could be that there is a slower angiotensinogenic mechanism that is not mediated by circulating angiotensin II. As an illustration, Riegger et al. (75) infused saralasin, an angiotensin II receptor antagonist, and the nonapeptide converting enzyme inhibitor continuously for 11 hr in chronic 2K-1C rats made hypertensive about 6 weeks previously.

Saralasin and the ACE inhibitor produced a small reduction in blood pressure within the first hour, but when infused for 11 hr they produced a dramatic fall in blood pressure, which approached normotensive levels. Other studies with prolonged administration of captopril (76,77) have indicated that this agent is effective in reducing blood pressure in chronic 2K-1C hypertension.

In addition to the participation of the renin system in the pathogensis of 2K-1C hypertension, the sympathoadrenal system also contributes to the blood pressure elevation (78) in this model. However, the antihypertensive response to captopril was not modified by 6-OH-dopamine treatment (79).

The site of action of ACE inhibitors in reducing blood pressure in 2K-1C rats is not known. Interruption of the renin-angiotensin system not only blocks the vasoconstrictor actions of angiotensin II on blood vessels but also may blunt the action of angiotensin II on the nonclipped contralateral kidney. A number of researchers have shown that this kidney has altered tubular function and hemodynamics (63–68). As will be discussed later, administration of converting enzyme inhibitors often dramatically improves renal function, resulting in an increase in sodium excretion. Another site of action of ACE inhibitors might be the vascular-wall renin system, which might take on greater significance in the chronic stages of 2K-1C renal hypertension. A reduction in angiotensin II concentra-

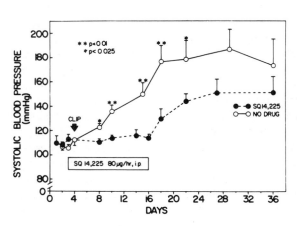

FIG. 8. Development of hypertension in two groups of rats with left renal artery clipped and contralateral kidney untouched. One group (open circles, $N = 7$) was untreated, and the other group (filled circles, $N = 7$) was infused continuously from day 3 to 16 with SQ 14,225 (80 μg/hr i.p.). Rats were clipped on day 4. Asterisks denote differences between the two groups. (From Freeman et al., ref. 60, with permission.)

tion at this site might reduce blood vessel reactivity.

One-Kidney-One-Clipped (1K-1C) Hypertension

In rats with one kidney removed, renal artery constriction causes an acute increase in PRA that is followed by the release of aldosterone from the adrenals. Aldosterone then acts on the kidney to cause sodium and water retention. As the hypertension becomes established, plasma renin and angiotensin II levels return toward normal (80–83), and hypervolemia becomes a predominant mechanism in maintaining the elevated blood pressure (57). An increase in cardiac output has been implicated in some studies (84–86). Gavras et al. (59) placed 1K-1C renal-hypertensive rats on a low-sodium diet and showed that an infusion of an angiotensin inhibitor caused a marked reduction in blood pressure. With sodium repletion (food containing salt, and 0.9% saline to drink), the renin dependency of the hypertension was eliminated, and the fall in blood pressure caused by the angiotensin antagonist was completely prevented.

In the clinical treatment of hypertension, diuretics modify the volume component of hypertension and induce renin release. In a sense, diuretics convert a volume-dependent hypertension to a vasoconstrictor hypertension. To a large extent this explains the greater efficacy of ACE inhibitors in diuretic-treated patients.

In rats with 1K-1C renal hypertension it is possible to delay the rise of blood pressure following a renal artery clip provided that both vasoconstrictor and volume mechanisms are blocked (Fig. 9). Seymour et al. (87) used simultaneous ACE blockade with captopril (infused via Alza minipumps) and sodium depletion to minimize both the vasoconstrictor and volume components. These interventions prevented blood pressure from increasing above normal levels on the 12th day after nephrectomy and clipping. If volume depletion is not employed, as illustrated in Fig. 10, elevated blood pressure in 1K-1C rats develops even in the presence of converting enzyme blockade with captopril (60).

Mineralocorticoid Hypertension

This model of experimental hypertension is produced by administration of DOCA (desoxycorticosterone) and 1% saline in uninephrectomized rats. The reduced renal mass and mineralocorticoid administrations produce retention of sodium and water and consequently expansion of intracellular spaces. The model is associated with an increase in the activity of the peripheral sympathetic nervous system and adrenal medulla. The characteristics of DOCA/salt hypertension include increased water intake, increased intravascular volume, and reduced hematocrit. The renin-

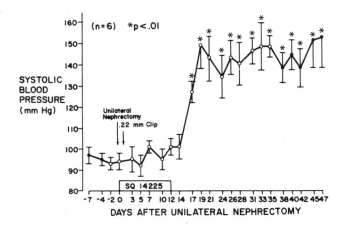

FIG. 9. Systolic blood pressure (SBP) changes after contralateral nephrectomy and renal artery clipping in sodium-restricted rats. Filled circles represent measurements obtained while rats were sodium-replete; unfilled circles represent those measurements obtained while rats were sodium-restricted. A horizontal bar indicates the period in which converting enzyme inhibitor SQ 14,225 was delivered at 80 μg/hr via constant intraperitoneal infusion. Asterisks mark days on which SBP was significantly different from sodium-replete control values. (From Seymour et al, ref. 87, with permission.)

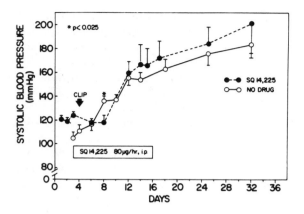

FIG. 10. Development of hypertension in two groups of rats with left renal artery clipped and right nephrectomy. One group was untreated (open circles, $N = 6$), and the other group (filled circles, $N = 6$) was infused continuously from day 3 to 16 with SQ 14,225 (80 μg/hr i.p.). Rats were clipped on day 4. Asterisk denotes difference between the two groups. (From Freeman et al., ref. 60, with permission.)

angiotensin system is suppressed in the plasma and kidney, and the kallikrein-kinin axis is enhanced (88–90).

Because of the low plasma renin levels in DOCA/salt hypertension, it might be expected that the antihypertensive effects of captopril would be modest or absent. Indeed, it was reported that captopril did not lower blood pressure in established DOCA/salt hypertension (91,93), nor did it prevent the development of DOCA/salt hypertension (91). However, Miyamori et al. (92) found that captopril slightly reduced blood pressure by a mechanism that may involve the release of prostaglandins, because indomethacin pretreatment significantly blunted the antihypertensive effect of captopril.

In another hypertensive model with a suppressed renin-angiotensin system (Heymann nephritis-DOCA/salt rat), captopril prevented the expected rise in systolic pressure, but it did not do so in DOCA/salt rats (93). The contrasting effects of captopril in these two low-renin models could not be explained by changes in electrolyte and fluid balance or urinary kallikrein excretion.

Antihypertensive Actions in Dogs

Vollmer et al. (96) used the two-kidney perinephritis model of hypertension (94,95) and showed that captopril caused a sustained reduction in blood pressure when plasma renin activity was normal. A direct cause–effect re-

lationship between the captopril-induced fall in plasma angiotensin II level and the blood pressure decrement was not found, but there was a relationship between the rise in PRA (which comes about because of the interruption of the short loop feedback system on renin release) and the peak hypotensive response to captopril.

Several workers have demonstrated that ACE inhibitors will reduce blood pressure in normotensive dogs (97–101). Captopril administered intravenously consistently reduced mean arterial pressure 14 to 25 mm Hg and usually increased heart rate. In dogs nephrectomized 12 to 18 hr previously, captopril produced a fall in mean arterial pressure that was slightly less than that observed in intact dogs (97,100). In dogs pretreated with the angiotensin receptor antagonist saralasin, captopril decreased the blood pressure (100). This observation is consistent with the interpretation that captopril's hypotensive response in dogs cannot be attributed entirely to blockade of the vasoconstrictor effects of circulating angiotensin II. In anesthetized dogs, the mechanisms involved in captopril-induced hypotensive effects have not been fully elucidated, but some workers have reported that it decreases renal vascular resistance and hindlimb vascular resistance (99). Some of these hemodynamic effects have been observed in nephrectomized dogs without an intact sympathetic nerve supply. An interesting observation is that hindlimb responses to activation of the baroreceptor reflex (reflex vasodilation and carotid occlusion responses) were blunted by large doses of captopril. It is not yet clear if captopril, when administered in such large doses, exerts an effect independent of its ability to inhibit converting enzyme. In summary, the antihypertensive responses to captopril in nephrectomized and normotensive dogs suggest that there are additional mechanisms that may contribute to the blood-pressure-lowering effects of ACE inhibitors in dogs. It is conceivable that bradykinin may be involved as a hypotensive mechanism in these experiments.

Sodium deprivation results in activation of the renin-angiotensin system and increases in aldosterone biosynthesis. Studies involving long-term infusions of converting enzyme inhibitors [captopril or enalapril (MK-421)] or angiotensin II antagonists have demonstrated that changes in urinary sodium excretion during dietary sodium restriction are independent of changes in the salt-retaining hormone aldosterone but are highly dependent on the activity of the renin-angiotensin system (102,103). These studies also have shown that the renin-angiotensin system contributes to the level of blood pressure in animals fed a diet deficient in sodium. As illustrated in Fig. 11, blockade of angiotensin II formation with enalapril at 80 mg/day in conscious dogs resulted in a rapid decline in arterial pressure, an increase in urinary sodium excretion, and decreases in plasma angiotensin II and aldosterone concentrations. These experiments and others like them have revealed several important mechanisms by which the renin-angiotensin system supports blood pressure and renal function during chronic changes in sodium intake. The decrease in aldosterone concentration after captopril treatment apparently does

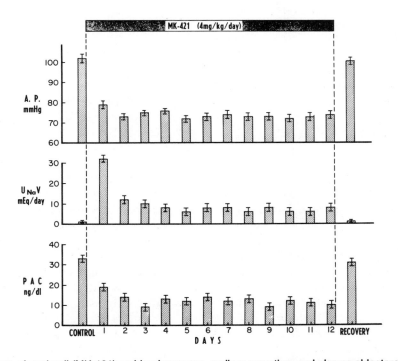

FIG. 11. Effects of enalapril (MK-421) on blood pressure, sodium excretion, and plasma aldosterone concentration in sodium-restricted dogs. Enalapril at 4 mg/kg p.o. reduced arterial pressure, produced a transient elevation in urinary sodium excretion, and reduced aldosterone plasma levels. Blood pressure was restored to pretreatment values during simultaneous infusion of angiotensin II at a dosage that sufficiently restored plasma aldosterone levels. (Data from McCaa).

not contribute to its antihypertensive effect, because chronic replacement of this steroid does not alter blood pressure in captopril-treated dogs (102). On the other hand, restoration of circulating angiotensin II (by continuous intravenous administration) completely restores blood pressure to normal, in addition to normalizing renal function.

Inhibition of angiotensin II formation with ACE inhibitors or increased circulating and renal tissue concentrations of kinins can elicit hypotensive and natriuretic responses. Despite evidence from short-term experiments that circulating kinins increased after ACE inhibition (103), Hall et al. (102) ruled out kinin potentiation as a factor in the antihypertensive mechanism in these experiments. With the aldosterone level as an index for restoration of the renin-angiotensin system, Hall et al. (102) infused angiotensin II in captopril-treated dogs and showed that blood pressure returned to a normal level at a dose of angiotensin II that was sufficient to return the aldosterone level to normal. If bradykinin was responsible for the fall in blood pressure, they reasoned that more angiotensin II would be needed to restore blood pressure than to restore the aldosterone level.

Role for Bradykinin in the Action of ACE Inhibitors

Bradykinin is believed to be essentially a tissue hormone. In blood, kinins are rapidly destroyed, and their plasma concentrations may not reflect important local changes at vascular sites. Therefore, an understanding of the physiologic role of tissue bradykinin in the regulation of blood flow or blood pressure or in the mechanism of action of ACE inhibitors must await progress in understanding the site of action of bradykinin. Progress in this area has also been slow, in part because of a lack of specific antagonists of bradykinin. Despite these limitations, the "kinin hypothesis" as an explanation for the antihypertensive properties of ACE inhibitors is still attractive, because bradykinin, in addition to its direct vaso-

dilator properties, acts indirectly through stimulation of prostaglandin synthesis. As pointed out previously, bradykinin and angiotensin I share a common point of metabolism, because converting enzyme is functionally identical with kininase II. Bradykinin (a vasodilator) and angiotensin II (a potent vasoconstrictor) have opposing actions on vascular tone—thus the speculation that the antihypertensive effect of converting enzyme inhibitors might be caused by inhibition of the conversion of angiotensin I to angiotensin II and/or by inhibition of the destruction of kinins. Because ACE inhibitors influence both the renin-angiotensin system and kallikrein-kinin system, blood pressure and vascular responses must be interpreted cautiously.

At present, there are three approaches that have been used to determine the contribution of kinins in mediating the antihypertensive action of ACE inhibitors.

Plasma Bradykinin Levels

An unresolved problem is whether or not an increase in plasma bradykinin within the physiologic range can exert a significant vasodepressor effect. Furthermore, bradykinin has a short half-life and is very difficult to measure. It is not surprising that measurements of plasma bradykinin by radioimmunoassay after acute or subacute administration of converting enzyme inhibitors have yielded conflicting results in humans (104–107). Interestingly, chronic administration of captopril has not resulted in any long-term increase in circulating venous bradykinin levels in humans (107).

Increases in urinary kinins in patients treated with SQ 20,881 suggest that renovascular tissue kinins may have increased, even though plasma levels of bradykinin are normal (106). Tissue levels of kinins may increase after ACE inhibitors and could represent an important site of action for this class of agents. Unfortunately, there is little published information about changes in tissue concentrations of bradykinin after ACE inhibitors.

There are reasons why bradykinin levels may not actually change with ACE inhibitors. First, the affinity of bradykinin for ACE is higher than that for angiotensin II, such that bradykinin would be degraded at a faster rate than would angiotensin I. Also, metabolic changes induced by ACE inhibitors, such as an increase in blood or tissue extraction, could alter the production and/or clearance of bradykinin. Another possibility is that kininase I, an enzyme also responsible for the destruction of bradykinin, might become active during ACE inhibition.

Inhibition of Kallikrein-Kinin System with Aprotinin

Glandular kallikrein activity is modulated by endogenous inhibitors present in many organs, including the kidneys. Aprotinin (Trasylol®) is an example of such an inhibitor prepared from bovine lungs; see Levinsky (108) for a review. It is important to point out that aprotinin is not a specific inhibitor of the kinin system, but inhibits trypsin, chymotrypsin, and plasmin as well.

Therefore, studies using this inhibitor must be cautiously interpreted. Because aprotinin blocks kinin formation, inhibition of ACE with captopril should not cause an accumulation of kinins. In some limited clinical studies in renovascular hypertension patients (109), aprotinin infusion significantly increased arterial pressure that had been lowered by converting enzyme inhibitor treatment. Other studies demonstrated that reduction of kinin formation by aprotinin completely blocked the acute blood pressure response to captopril in low- and normal-renin hypertension (110). Long-term clinical studies with a kallikrein inhibitor in combination with a converting enzyme inhibitor are needed to confirm the findings of the acute experiments reported earlier.

Antikinin Antibodies

A third approach to defining the role of kinins in the antihypertensive response to ACE inhibitors has been the use of antibodies directed against lysbradykinin. In sodium-depleted rats, the acute vasodepressor effects of captopril were similar in rats treated with rabbit globulins and those treated with antikinin globulins (111). In contrast, in 2K-1C rats, the acute depressor response to captopril was attenuated, suggesting that the acute fall in blood pressure in 2K-1C rats is due, in part, to an increase in kinin concentration. There are limitations in using kinin antibodies as pharmacologic tools. These antibodies probably block only circulating kinins, not tissue kinins. Furthermore, they have a short half-life, being cleared from the circulation by the reticuloendothelial system within 4 hr (111). It is important that data from kinin antibody experiments be interpreted with caution, because antigen-antibody complexes may cause anaphylactoid reactions, with release of histamine and decrease in blood pressure.

Converting Enzyme Inhibition and the Kidney

Several observations have indicated that angiotensin II may have important regulatory functions within the kidney. Indeed, a tissue-bound intrarenal renin-angiotensin system located within the juxtaglomerular apparatus (112) has recently been demonstrated by immunohistofluorescence techniques, and such an enzyme system could exert local regulation of renal function (113–115), in addition to the several physiologic functions of angiotensin II that can be ascribed to the peptide generated systemically.

Kimbrough et al. (116) infused SQ 20,881 into the renal artery in unanesthetized dogs fed a low-sodium diet and observed increased renal blood flow and glomerular filtration. Meggs and Hollenberg (117) similarly observed increases in renal function after direct intrarenal artery administration of SQ 20,881 into patients.

Kimbrough et al. (116) showed that similar changes in renal blood flow and glomerular filtration rate were observed with SQ 20,881 or with a specific angiotensin II antagonist, saralasin. Thus, in sodium deficiency, it appears likely that the renal vascular response after an ACE inhibitor is due to an angiotensin II mechanism. Hall et al. (102) came to a similar conclusion based on more elaborate studies in which ACE was inhibited for several days by continuous intravenous infusion of captopril into sodium-deficient dogs. In these studies, renal plasma flow increased significantly and remained elevated for the duration of the captopril infusion. Glomerular filtration rate, on the other hand, decreased significantly for the duration of the infusion. Presumably, the principal renal vasoconstrictor effect of angiotensin II is exerted on the efferent arteriole, the relaxation of which reduces glomerular filtration pressure. Superimposing a low-dose angiotensin II infusion during the captopril infusion restored renal plasma flow and glomerular filtration to pretreatment levels. The ability of angiotensin II to reverse the captopril-induced changes in renal function suggests that the mechanism of action of captopril is through inhibition of the formation of angiotensin II.

In contrast to the pronounced renal effects of ACE inhibitors in animals and humans on a sodium-restricted diet, there is little response to converting enzyme inhibitors when the renin-angiotensin system is suppressed by an increased sodium intake (117).

In addition to the renovasodilator effect of converting enzyme inhibition in low-salt states, similar changes in renal blood flow have been observed in conditions in which the prevailing PRA is high, e.g., after nonhypotensive hemorrhage, in renovascular-hypertensive dogs, and in pentobarbital-anesthetized dogs (118–122).

Also, studies with a thiazolidine analogue of captopril (YS-980) have shown that there is a redistribution of renal cortical blood flow favoring the inner cortex (123).

Whereas the studies of Kimbrough et al. (116), Hall et al. (102) and McCaa et al. (103) strongly suggest that inhibition of angiotensin II is the mediator of the renal vascular effects of ACE inhibitors, other investigators have suggested that the renal vasodilating actions of the kinins and prostaglandins may play a role in these effects (123). In acute studies, bradykinin levels have been observed to increase in renal venous blood (104) following converting enzyme inhibition. It is known that renal production of the vasodilator prostacyclin occurs in response to an elevated kinin level (124). Inhibition of prostaglandin production by indomethacin markedly attenuates the potentiation of the bradykinin-induced hypotension or renal vasodilator action of ACE inhibitors, suggesting the possibility of a prostaglandin mediation of this response (120, 124). Importantly, the observation of Abe et al. (123) that indomethacin abolishes the renovasodilator effect of YS-980 needs confirmation with other ACE inhibitors.

Sodium Excretion

The second major renal effect of ACE inhibitors is their ability to increase sodium excretion. Elsewhere the hypothesis is advanced that the renin-angiotensin system contributes to sodium homeostasis by regulating aldosterone biosynthesis and modulating renal blood flow and glomerular filtration. It has been speculated that angiotensin II may directly influence sodium transport within the kidney, and therefore inhibition of the formation of angiotensin II could result in an increase in sodium excretion, in addition to inhibition of aldosterone biosynthesis. In addition to this direct effect of inhibition of angiotensin II formation, ACE inhibitors increase renal blood flow, which could contribute to the natriuretic action of these drugs. Hall's study showed that urinary sodium excretion was increased during chronic blockade of angiotensin II formation, even in the face of large decreases in arterial pressure that would be expected to depress sodium excretion (102). In short-term dog experiments, the glomerular filtration rate increased with SQ 20,881, and the increase in sodium excretion in this circumstance could have been due to an increase in the filtered load of sodium that followed the rise in glomerular filtration rate (116). However, during chronic blockade of converting enzyme, Hall et al. (102) observed a reduction in glomerular filtration rate; so the natriuresis could not have been due to an increase in the filtered load of sodium.

Renin Release

Renin secretion is regulated by a variety of stimuli that affect renal perfusion pressure, sodium reabsorption, or β-adrenergic receptors. Volume expansion, such as occurs secondary to aldosterone-stimulated sodium reabsorption, can decrease renin release. Also, renin release can be suppressed directly by a short-loop feedback of angiotensin II on juxtaglomerular cells (125–129). In sodium-replete animals in which renin levels are normal, administration of ACE inhibitors results in only a small rise in renin. In sodium-depleted dogs, large increases in PRA have been demonstrated. The mechanism for the enhanced renin release is principally inhibition of the short-loop feedback inhibition of angiotensin II on renin release, as well as a decrease in renal perfusion pressure and stimulation of β-adrenergic receptors (116).

In conscious rats treated with captopril, PRA rises after several days and reaches a peak on day 5. Schiffrin et al. (130) found evidence that the sympathetic nervous system and the short-loop feedback of angiotensin II are involved in the effects of captopril on renin release, because both an infusion of angiotensin II (administered via osmotic minipumps) and propranolol administration suppressed PRA. There was no evidence for a role of endogenous prostaglandins in captopril-induced renin secretion in this study. These findings conflict with the results of the study of Abe et al. (131), who demonstrated that indomethacin abolished the increase in PRA induced by YS-980 in dog (123) and captopril in humans (131).

Interaction with Noradrenergic Mechanisms

There is some information suggesting that the antihypertensive mechanism of action of captopril might be related to an inhibition of sympathetic function. In pithed normotensive rats, for example, high doses of captopril suppressed the vasopressor effect of intravenous norepinephrine (132,133) and blocked the vasoconstrictor response to nerve stimulation in isolated arteries (134). In pithed SHR, a prejunctional site of action on blood vessel was proposed to explain the finding that captopril blunted the pressor responses to sympathetic nerve stimulation (135,136). There apparently are two types of α-adrenergic receptors (α_1 and α_2) that subserve vasoconstriction in this model. Accordingly, DeJonge et al. (137) found that captopril blocked norepinephrine only after preferential blockade of vascular α_1 receptors with prazosin. Their study suggested that the renin system modulates that part of the vascular tone that is maintained by postsynaptic α_2-adrenoceptors (137).

New ACE Inhibitors

Enalapril was the first new ACE inhibitor to be widely studied after the introduction of captopril (18,20,39,41,50,52). The most common side effects accompanying the clinical use of captopril were rashes and loss of taste, both of which usually cleared on withdrawal or reduction of the dosage. Because similar side effects were observed with penicillamine, a mercapto-containing drug with side effects similar to those of captopril, the Merck group (18) searched for potent specific inhibitors of ACE lacking a mercapto function and characterized by weak chelating properties (Fig. 1). These new inhibitors were substituted *N*-carboxymethyl dipeptides that were active in inhibiting ACE in the nanomolar levels. A number of thioesters or sulfhydryl compounds that have a modified proline, such as SA-446 (142), RHC-3659 (140), YS-980 (123,131) and CL-242,817 (143), have been described. Keto

ACE, a tripeptide in which the central nitrogen atom has been replaced by a methylene group (138), and a phosphoramide inhibitor (141) are representative of still other structural modifications.

SUMMARY

There is no direct evidence to indicate that the currently available ACE inhibitors, when administered at reasonable doses, have a mechanism of action other than specific inhibition of converting enzyme kininase II. Less understood are the events following inhibition of this enzyme.

A consistent observation has been that ACE inhibitors reduce blood pressure most effectively in models of hypertension in which the prevailing PRA is high (2K-1C, sodium-restricted, acute 1K-1C models) and less effectively in models in which PRA is low (DOCA/salt, chronic 1K-1C, and sodium-replete). This favors a primary role for the reduction of angiotensin II as the mechanism of action. In addition, if low-renin models are subjected to salt depletion with diuretics or dietary manipulation, they become highly responsive to ACE inhibitors. The possibility of complementary actions of angiotensin II antagonists and converting enzymes can be questioned on the basis of duration of treatment. Only in acute studies was this complementary action observed, and it could be due to non-steady-state conditions or partial agonist activity.

The one study (75) in which an angiotensin II antagonist was infused for an extended period indicated similar blood-pressure-lowering effects of angiotensin II antagonist and converting enzyme inhibitor.

Additional compelling evidence for a role for an angiotensin-II-mediated mechanism has been the finding of angiotensin II replacement with converting enzyme inhibitor. These studies have shown that angiotensin II replacement restores blood pressure aldosterone and renal function to normal (102,144).

Evidence to support a kinin-mediated

mechanism based on kinin antibodies or aprotinin are of interest. However, only limited studies have been conducted using these compounds. More extensive studies will be required before these initial observations can be considered convincing evidence for a role for kinins in the antihypertensive action of ACE inhibitors.

Most studies have used changes in plasma levels of angiotensin II or bradykinin as indices of ACE inhibition. However, it is well established that these substances can function as local hormones. This aspect has not been adequately investigated, and further studies are needed to define a possible action of ACE inhibitors at a local level.

In summary, there have been some acute studies supporting the view that there is an additional mechanism of action of ACE inhibitors other than reduction of circulating angiotensin II levels. As of this time, the mechanisms that contribute to the *chronic* hypotensive response to ACE inhibitors seem to be explained by a reduction in plasma angiotensin II levels.

RENIN INHIBITORS

The previous sections of this chapter discussed the antihypertensive actions of ACE inhibitors, and the evidence favors an angiotensinogenic mechanism as their mode of action, but other factors, such as potentiation of bradykinin, could be involved. Resolution of this question, and indeed the more fundamental question of the role of the renin-angiotensin system in the pathogenesis of hypertension, can be achieved only with the use of more specific inhibitors of the renin-angiotensin system.

Even before the discovery of ACE inhibitors, considerable effort had been expended to develop specific inhibitors of renin. Several classes of compounds have been studied, including renin antibodies, endogenous phospholipids, pepstatin, and renin substrate analogues.

The following sections review some of these

findings and suggest a fundamental role for the renin-angiotensin system in the cause of hypertension.

Renin Antibodies

The first efforts to define the role of the renin-angiotensin system in hypertension used passive immunization procedures in which antibodies to renin were produced in rabbits by injection of crude extract of dog renal cortex (145). The antiserum thus obtained was effective in blocking the pressor response to partially purified dog renin in dogs. The antiserum did not block the pressor response to posterior pituitary extracts, suggesting specificity for the renin-angiotensin system.

One of the most serious problems associated with antibody production and use involves the side effects, especially anaphylaxis, that can occur secondary to injection of crude tissue extract. Lamfrom et al. (146) partially overcame this problem by purifying renin and by using small quantities of antiserum for the passive immunization. These investigators injected partially purified hog renin into humans and successfully produced anti-hog-renin antibodies. Unfortunately, anti-hog-renin antibodies did not cross-react with human renin and therefore did not lower arterial pressure in hypertensive patients. It was clear from these studies that antibodies directed against renin from a given species did not cross-react equally well with renin in all species. In humans, they did not cross-react at all.

One of the most striking demonstrations of the efficacy of renin antibodies to reduce arterial blood pressure was presented by Helmer (147). In this study, chronic treatment of renal-hypertensive dogs with a renal cortical extract normalized blood pressure for 5 years. The decrease in arterial blood pressure was correlated with the appearance of a high titer of renin antibodies, but in those dogs that did not develop an antirenin titer, blood pressure was not affected. These animals presumably had chronic low-renin hypertension, because both kidneys were wrapped in silk (Page hypertension)—a model that is the equivalent of the 1K-1C model more extensively used in later studies. Other investigators have also demonstrated the antihypertensive properties of antirenin antibodies (148,149), but in some instances dogs have demonstrated high titers of renin antibodies yet remained hypertensive (148).

Thus, the failure of some animals to respond to renin antibodies with a decrease in arterial pressure and the potential for anaphylaxis have prevented general acceptance of these data as evidence for a fundamental role for the renin-angiotensin system in the pathogenesis of arterial hypertension. Additionally, Romero et al. (150) found that anti-hog-renin antibodies lowered arterial blood pressure in the acute phase of 1K-1C hypertension in rabbits but were ineffective in the chronic phase. Thus, the question remains unanswered whether or not renin antibodies are an effective antihypertensive treatment in chronic low-renin hypertension. A major advance in this area has been made recently with the purification to homogeneity of renin from several animal species and humans. It is now possible to produce specific antirenin antibodies and determine their antihypertensive properties. Dzau et al. (151) purified dog renin 600,000-fold and produced antibodies in goats to this homogeneous material. The antiserum reduced mean arterial pressure and inhibited renin activity in sodium-depleted dogs and was an effective antihypertensive in acute 1K-1C hypertension. Studies in chronic low-renin hypertension have not been reported, but it seems likely that the long-sought answer to the question of the role of renin in chronic hypertension is imminent.

Endogenous Phospholipid Renin Inhibitor

The concept of naturally occurring inhibitors or activators of the renin-angiotensin system originated with the earliest work on the identification of renin from the kidney. Tigerstedt and Bergman (152) observed that saline extracts of kidneys produced a greater pressor response when injected into nephrectomized animals than when injected into normal animals. Later experiments revealed that if normal plasma was transfused into a nephrectomized animal before renin was injected, the subsequent pressor response was diminished (153), and constant quantities of renin added to plasma samples from different individuals generated varying amounts of angiotensin (154,155). Although these observations were consistent with the loss of a renin inhibitor after nephrectomy, alternative explanations also were possible, the most likely being that the increased renin substrate produced after nephrectomy was responsible for increased angiotensin generation. Smeby et al. (156) showed that the plasma angiotensinogen concentration reached maximum levels within 24 hr after nephrectomy, but the potentiation of the reaction of renin with its substrate continued for up to 48 hr. These studies argued strongly for loss of an inhibitor in plasma after nephrectomy, rather than increased angiotensinogen, as the cause of the augmented angiotensin generation.

Such observations led several workers to investigate the possibility that the kidney elaborates an inhibitory substance that limits the reaction of renin with its substrate and subsequent generation of angiotensin. An inhibitor of this type would potentially be important in modulating all of the actions of the renin-angiotensin system.

Sen et al. (157) first isolated a phospholipid from dog kidneys that appeared to possess the requisite renin inhibitory activity. *In vitro,* this phospholipid reduced angiotensin generation when added to a standard mixture of dog renin and dog renin substrate. Although not identified, the compound(s) had properties very similar to those of phosphatidylserine.

Although this renal phospholipid was not very active *in vitro* (1–2 mg added to a reaction mixture of renin and angiotensinogen inhibited angiotensin production by 50%), when it was administered to hypertensive rats their arterial blood pressure fell substantially (157). The decrease in blood pressure required 2 to 4 days of treatment for its full expression and was sustained for the duration of the treatment (5 days). It is important to note that blood pressure slowly returned to normal after cessation of the injections. The antihypertensive activity of renal phospholipid extracts was confirmed after intravenous (159,160) and oral (159) administration. No blood-pressure-lowering activity was observed in normal rats receiving the extract. Specificity of the inhibitor for renin was indicated by its ability to reduce plasma renin activity *in vivo* (160) and its ability to block the pressor response to renin, but not to angiotensin II (158).

The original material extracted from dog kidneys by Sen et al. (157) was found to be an inactive precursor called renin preinhibitor (156) that had to be converted to the active lysophospholipid for expression of its renin inhibitory activity.

Of interest was the finding that the level of renin preinhibitor did not decrease after nephrectomy (161), indicating that the kidney was not the source of the inhibitor. Also, there were high levels of renin preinhibitor in red blood cells that may even have increased after nephrectomy (162). Osmond et al. (163) confirmed the presence of the renin preinhibitor in human plasma and erythrocytes. By thin-layer chromatography, the preinhibitor from dog plasma and erythrocytes and that from human plasma migrated similarly. Likewise, the dog plasma inhibitor appeared similar to the material that had earlier been extracted from dog kidneys (157). Large amounts of preinhibitor were found in plasma and red cells (1 and 9% of total lipid phosphorus, respectively). This could be interpreted to indicate that even a relatively poor inhibitor, if present in large concentrations, could be effective in inhibiting renin activity. On the other hand, such relatively large quantities of so specific a substance as a renin inhibitor would seem unlikely to occur naturally.

The fact that the kidney was not the source of the renin inhibitor was surprising, because its presence had been postulated on the basis of greater renin activity in nephrectomized plasma that was independent of renin substrate concentration. According to observations by Osmond et al. (162), not only the kidney but also the heart, liver, and red blood cells contain large amounts of renin preinhibitor. Whether or not any or all of these organs are sources of the preinhibitor remains unknown.

With the kidney ruled out as a sole source for renin preinhibitor, it must follow that the kidney plays a paramount role in converting the preinhibitor to its active lysophospholipid form. The initial suggestion that renal phospholipase was the activating enzyme was made by Smeby et al. (156) and subsequently confirmed by Osmond et al. (163). Baggio et al. (164) found significant conversion of the inactive renin preinhibitor to the active lysophospholipid by rat kidney phospholipase A_2. Similar findings of conversion of inactive inhibitor to active inhibitor after addition of crude extracts of human kidney further supported a primary role for the kidney in activating the renin preinhibitor (165). Renin preinhibitor added to plasma did not form the active lysophospholipid (166). Osmond et al. (166), on the other hand, studied the ability of nephrectomized rat plasma to convert phosphatidylethanolamine to lysophosphatidylethanolamine and found no reduction in the capacity to form the active inhibitor. Osmond et al. (166) questioned the concept of a phospholipid renin preinhibitor on the basis of this study, because they could deduce no central role for the kidney either in elaborating the preinhibitor (nephrectomy did not reduce it) or in activating the preinhibitor (nephrectomy did not reduce the ability of plasma to activate the preinhibitor). It should be pointed out, however, that the source of preinhibitor used in this study was liver phosphatidylethanolamine, and because the true identity of the renin preinhibitor has not been established, it is possible that the material used in this study differed from that originally studied by Sen et al. (157,159,160) and by Baggio et al. (165).

Additional evidence has been presented questioning the existence of a naturally occurring renin inhibitor. Poulson (167) studied the kinetics of the renin-angiotensinogen reaction in plasma and serum from normal, salt-depleted, 24- and 48-hr nephrectomized rats and hypertensive rats and found no evidence to support the idea of a naturally occurring inhibitor of the renin reaction. Tinker et al. (168) also questioned the existence of phospholipid renin inhibitors after observing that phosphatidylethanolamine from dog kidney did not inhibit renin *in vivo* and was no more active *in vitro* than ox brain phosphatidylserine.

Lack of specificity of phosphatides is an important consideration, especially in view of the observation by Turcotte et al. (169) that a phosphoglyceride from shark kidney is active as a renin inhibitor *in vitro,* despite the fact that sharks do not have a renin-angiotensin system. Bŭnag and Walaszek (170) found that acid/ether extracts of rabbit kidney reduced the pressor response to renin but not to angiotensin II, suggesting a specific renin inhibitor. However, synthetic oleyl and palmityl phospholipids had the same effect. These observations led to the suggestion that phospholipids might form micelles around the renin molecule, thus denying access to angiotensinogen, and inhibit the reaction in this nonspecific manner.

Interestingly, sodium deoxycholate, a vehicle frequently used to administer phospholipid renin inhibitors, was found to inhibit the renin-angiotensin reaction with a K_i of 7×10^{-4} M (171).

Despite questions raised concerning the existence of phosphatide renin inhibitors, several laboratories undertook to synthesize analogues that would have renin inhibitory activity. Rakhit (172) characterized the phospholipid from renal tissue and found the substance to be phosphatidylethanolamine containing a large percentage of polyunsaturated fatty acids. The general structure is shown in Fig. 12. The material isolated and characterized by Rahkit appeared to be identical with the original material studied by Sen et al. (157) and was equipotent with the original inhibitory substance. Subsequent synthesis efforts

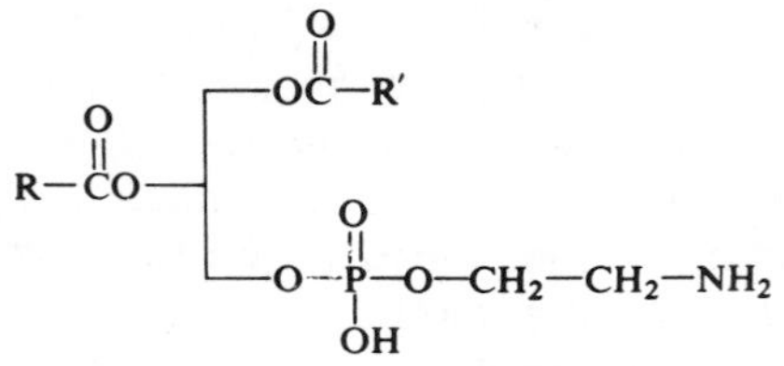

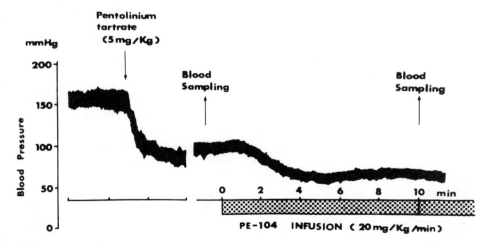

FIG. 12. General structure of phospholipid inhibitor. (From Rakhit, ref. 172, with permission.)

by this group produced dilinolenyl phosphatidylethanolamine, which was equipotent with the natural inhibitor in preventing the formation of angiotensin I *in vitro* (173). From a large series of ethanolamine derivatives, compounds containing a 1-adamantyl moiety and ethanolamine side chain were found to have renin inhibitory activity only slightly less than that of the natural hog kidney lysophosphatidylethanolamine (174,175). Miyazaki et al. (176,177) and Hosoki et al. (178) developed a series of phosphatidylethanolamine derivatives that were active both *in vitro* and *in vivo* to block the pressor action of renin and also were effective antihypertensive agents. The compound that has the greatest *in vivo* activity is 2-[4-(4'-chlorophenoxy)phenoxyacetyl-amino]-ethylphosphorylethanolamine (PE-104). *In vitro,* PE-104 was found to be a competitive inhibitor of renin, with a K_i of 2 mM. The intact compound was the active entity, because structural fragments were not inhibitors of renin. This compound is relatively specific for renin and does not inhibit the proteolytic activities of papain or trypsin, and it inhibits pepsin only modestly at a concentration of 10 mM (178). Further *in vivo* studies with PE-104 documented its ability to inhibit the pressor response to renin injected into anesthetized, ganglion-blocked rats and its ability to lower arterial blood pressure of anesthetized, two-kidney renal-hypertensive rats (20 mg/kg/min) by approximately 25 mm Hg (Fig. 13). PE-104 also

FIG. 13. Effect of PE-104 on blood pressure in a male Wistar strain, two-kidney model, renal-hypertensive rat weighing about 250 g. After treatment with pentobarbital (50 mg/kg i.p.), atropine (1 mg/kg s.c.), and pentolinium tartrate (5 mg/kg i.v.), infusion of PE-104 was started at a rate of 20 mg/kg/min. (From Hosoki et al., ref. 178, with permission.)

decreased endogenous plasma renin activity during the period of infusion.

Turcotte et al. (179) synthesized a series of lysophosphatidylethanolamine analogues, the most active of which was eicosatetraenyl-(3-aminopropyl) phosphonate. Comparison of this compound (URI-73A) with other inhibitors of the renin-angiotensin system, namely, [Sar[1],Thr[8]]-angiotensin II (a competitive antagonist of angiotensin II) and SQ 14,225 (captopril) (a converting enzyme inhibitor), indicated that the compound had good antihypertensive activity in both acute (Fig. 14) and chronic (Fig. 15) two-kidney hypertensive rats (58). URI-73A was only slightly less active than captopril in both the acute and chronic models, whereas [Sar[1],Thr[8]]-angiotensin II was active only in the acute phase of hypertension. Likewise, in one-kidney chronic hypertensive rats, URI-73A and captopril had similar antihypertensive efficacies. URI-73A appeared to inhibit renin, rather than converting enzyme, or to directly antagonize angiotensin II, because during treatment the PRA was suppressed in the presence of URI-73A, whereas it was increased during treatment with either the converting enzyme in-

hibitor or the angiotensin II antagonist. This later effect presumably was due to loss of the short-loop negative feedback of angiotensin II on renin release.

Pepstatin

During a search for inhibitors of pepsin as antiulcer drugs, culture broths of *Streptomyces* species were found to contain a peptide with the requisite pepsin inhibitory property. The compound, pepstatin, was unique in that it contained an unusual amino acid, 4-amino-3-hydroxy-6-methylheptanoic acid (180), presently known as statine. Mass-spectrographic analysis showed that the structure of pepstatin was isovaleryl-L-valyl-L-valyl-statyl-L-alanyl-statine (181). In addition to its activity as an inhibitor of pepsin, pepstatin also inhibits cathepsins and renin. Despite the fact that pepstatin is less active as a renin inhibitor than as an inhibitor of pepsin (IC_{50} 6.6×10^{-6} M versus 1.4×10^{-8} M, respectively), it was, until recently, the most potent inhibitor of renin discovered. This relatively high degree of activity against renin led to its use as a tool to investigate the physiologic actions of the re-

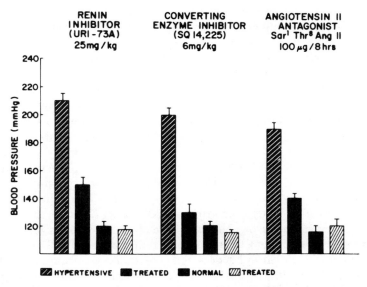

FIG. 14. Effects of inhibitors of renin-angiotensin system on two-kidney (high-renin) hypertensive rats 6 weeks following clipping. (From Sen et al., ref. 58, with permission.)

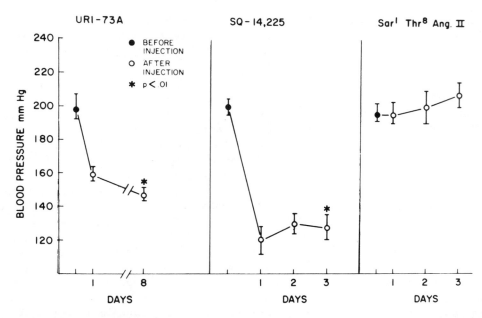

FIG. 15. Effects of inhibitors of renin-angiotensin system on blood pressure of two-kidney Goldblatt chronic hypertensive rats 36 weeks after clipping. **Left:** Effects of renin inhibitor URI-73A at 25 mg/kg/24 hr. **Center:** Effects of converting enzyme inhibitor SQ 14,225 at 20 mg/kg/24 hr. **Right:** Effects of angiotensin II antagonist [Sar¹,Thr⁸]-angiotensin II at 100 mg/kg/8 hr. (From Sen et al., ref. 58, with permission.)

nin-angiotensin system and as a lead compound in the development of pharmacologic inhibitors of renin.

Gross et al. (182) first reported the renin inhibitory effects of pepstatin *in vitro* and *in vivo*. Pepstatin is a specific inhibitor of the blood-pressure-elevating effect of intravenously administered renin, and it does not significantly inhibit the pressor effects of angiotensin II or norepinephrine in anesthetized intact or nephrectomized rats (183).

In vitro studies by most investigators have found the IC_{50} for pepstatin to be in the range of 10^{-6} to 10^{-7} M (184), and the evidence favors noncompetitive inhibition (184–186); but see Guyene et al. (187). McKown et al. (185) reported a K_i for pepstatin against human renin of 1×10^{-10} M, but that study used synthetic substrate. Other studies using human plasma with endogenous renin and substrate found 50% inhibition of angiotensin I generation in the range of 10^{-6} to 10^{-7} M (187).

Pepstatin significantly reduced blood pressure when injected into intact or nephrecto-mized rats whose blood pressure had been elevated by infusion or injection of renin (182,183,188). Pepstatin is relatively short-lived in the circulation, and blood pressure returns to control levels within minutes. Norepinephrine and angiotensin II pressor responses are not inhibited by pepstatin, suggesting specificity of its action to inhibit the formation of angiotensin I (183). In addition to its ability to inhibit renin, pepstatin may have slight nonspecific hypotensive actions, as shown by its ability to lower blood pressure slightly in nephrectomized rats (183).

In acute 1K-1C hypertensive rats whose blood pressure appears to be sustained by elevated renin levels, pepstatin is an effective antihypertensive agent. In one study, pepstatin at 200 μg/kg i.v. lowered arterial blood pressure of an anesthetized renal-hypertensive rat from approximately 127 mm Hg to 105 mm Hg, with blood pressure recovering to control levels within 10 min. No hypotensive effect was observed in similarly treated normotensive rats (188) (Fig. 16). Scholkens and Jung

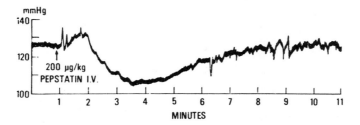

FIG. 16. Blood pressure record of a Goldblatt rat. Blood pressure before anesthesia was 206 mm Hg. Pepstatin sample was 124 μg/ml. Time of recovery to elevated blood pressure level was dose-related. (From Miller et al., ref. 188, with permission.)

(189) studied conscious, unrestrained rats with spontaneous or chronic renal hypertension and found pepstatin to be a modest hypotensive agent (10–15 mm Hg pressure decrease) with a short duration of action. In a model of acute renal hypertension secondary to occlusion of the renal pedicle, pepstatin had a more profound blood-pressure-lowering effect (189). Recently, a more soluble form of pepstatin, *N*-acetyl pepstatin, was infused into the cerebral ventricles by small implantable osmotic minipumps, and it delayed the onset of hypertension in SHR and lessened the blood pressure elevation (200).

One of the most serious problems with the use of pepstatin to study the renin-angiotensin system has been its relative insolubility, preventing maximally effective doses from being administered *in vivo*. Several investigators have sought to render pepstatin more soluble by formation of the arginine salt of pepstatin (201) or synthesis of pepstatinyl-arginine-*o*-methyl ester (191,192). The arginine salt of pepstatin is approximately 50 times more soluble in water than pepstatin, and the arginine-*o*-methyl ester derivative is 30 times more soluble (191). Both compounds are effective inhibitors of renin *in vitro*, with K_i of 1×10^{-7} M for pepstatin and 3.15×10^{-7} M for pepstatinyl-Arg-*o*-Me (192). Both synthetic compounds are active *in vivo* to lower arterial blood pressure secondary to renin injection or in renin-dependent models of hypertension (191,192). Miyazaki et al. (193) isolated a natural product, *N*-acetyl pepstatin, from *Streptomyces* culture broth that proved to be more

soluble than pepstatin and to be an effective inhibitor of renin both *in vitro* and *in vivo*.

Further work with more soluble derivatives of pepstatin may well yield useful tools to study the role of the renin-angiotensin system in hypertension, but it is doubtful if pepstatin will be a useful antihypertensive drug, because of its low potency and short duration of action.

Pepstatin has proved to be an extremely useful compound for purifying renin and has found extensive use in affinity chromatography for isolating renin from kidney and salivary gland (194–196).

Substrate Analogues

Enzyme inhibitors that are modeled after natural substrates have been developed for a number of enzyme systems, and this same course has been followed in the development of specific renin inhibitors. Angiotensinogen, the endogenous substrate for renin, is a large α_2-globulin produced by the liver and, as such, does not provide a good model for developing synthetic analogues. Fortunately, the terminal 14-amino-acid sequence of angiotensinogen is a full substrate for renin (197,198), and this tetradecapeptide (Fig. 17) has proved most useful for modeling of peptide renin inhibitors.

The object of developing useful substrate analogues that inhibit renin is to develop compounds that bind to the enzyme but do not cleave the peptide bond between the amino acids at positions 10 and 11. Early studies focused on the leucyl-leucine bond at the cleavage position, and numerous Leu-Leu-

```
     1    2    3    4    5    6    7    8    9   10   11   12  13   14
   Asp-Arg-Val-Tyr-Ileu-His-Pro-Phe-His-Leu-Leu-Val-Tyr-Ser
```

$$\downarrow \text{Renin}$$

Asp-Arg-Val-Tyr-Ileu-His-Pro-Phe-His-Leu + Leu-Val-Tyr-Ser

Angiotensin I

$$\downarrow \text{Converting Enzyme}$$

Asp-Arg-Val-Tyr-Ileu-His-Pro-Phe + His-Leu

Angiotensin II

FIG. 17. The cascade leading to the formation of angiotensin II beginning with tetradecapeptide substrate. The amino acid sequence illustrated for tetradecapeptide is of equine origin (195). The sequence for human tetradecapeptide is Asp-Arg-Val-Tyr-Ileu-His-Pro-Phe-His-Leu-Val-Ileu-His-Thr (197).

containing di-, tri-, and tetrapeptide analogues were synthesized (200,201). Of these, only the methyl or ethyl esters of the tetrapeptides Leu-Leu-Val-Tyr and Leu-Leu-Val-Phe were active as renin inhibitors. The compounds exhibited competitive-type inhibition but were active only in the millimolar range *in vitro* against rabbit renin. Further development of the compounds was undertaken by Parry et al. (202), who synthesized "bio-isosteres" of the tetrapeptide inhibitors of the following type:

$$\begin{array}{c} \text{CH}_2\text{CHMe}_2 \\ | \\ \text{H}_2\text{N---CH---CH}_2\text{---Leu-Val-Phe-}o\text{-Me} \end{array}$$

This compound was found to be superior to the tetrapeptides synthesized by Kokubu's group described earlier, and it decreased blood pressure by 33% in acute 1K-1C hypertensive rats.

Another approach taken to develop useful inhibitors was to replace the naturally occurring L-amino acids at the 10–11 positions in the tetradecapeptide substrate with their D-enantiomorphs. Such compounds were synthesized by Parikh and Cuatrecasas (203) and also were effective competitive inhibitors of renin *in vitro*, with a K_i of about 10^{-6} M.

At about the same time, Poulsen et al. (204) reported studies in which a previously synthesized octapeptide (197) was used to model other substrate analogue inhibitors of renin. This peptide, His-Pro-Phe-His-Leu-Leu-Val-Tyr,

corresponding to amino acid residues 6–13 of the tetradecapeptide renin substrate, was a competitive inhibitor of renin, with a K_i of 39 μM. Several analogues of this model octapeptide were synthesized, including D-Leu substitutions at positions 6 and 7. The [D-Leu[6]] octapeptide had a K_i of 3 μM, and unlike many of the other analogues it was not a partial substrate. This compound also inhibited the reaction between human renin and its endogenous plasma substrate.

One serious problem encountered in developing peptide inhibitors of renin was their poor solubility, probably due to the presence of hydrophobic amino acid residues such as leucine, valine, and phenylalanine (205). This problem was partially overcome by synthesizing compounds with additional proline residues on the *N* terminus to increase solubility (206). Interestingly, there is a strong pH dependence on inhibitory activity demonstrated by many of these substrate analogues, such that compounds that are active at acid pH lose all activity at physiologic pH of 7.5. One of the best compounds of this series, considering both inhibitory activity and solubility at pH 7.5, is Pro-His-Phe-His-Leu-Phe-Val-Tyr.

In addition to difficulties related to the solubility and activity of these peptides at physiologic pH, significant specificity exists among renins and renin substrates of different species. Whereas human renin cleaves substrate from most other species, the reverse is not true. Likewise, peptide renin inhibitors modeled af-

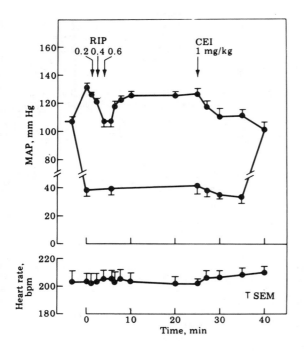

FIG. 18. After 1 hr of aortic cuff inflation, mean arterial pressure (MAP) above the aortic cuff (*upper curve*) rose from 107 to 131 mm Hg in six studies of renin-dependent hypertension. Aortic pressure below the cuff was maintained at approximately 40 mm Hg (*lower curve*). Renin-inhibitory peptide (RIP) was given as a graded infusion in 0.2-mg/kg/min increments. At 0.6 mg/kg/min, MAP was restored to prehypertensive levels ($p < 0.004$). After a brief period, infusion was discontinued, and MAP increased to 127 mm Hg. Converting enzyme inhibitor (CEI) at 1 mg/kg reduced MAP to 111 mm Hg ($p < 0.002$). The MAP responses to RIP and to CEI were similar (difference not statistically significant). Heart rate was consistent throughout. (From Burton et al., ref. 209, with permission.)

ter the amino acid sequence of human renin substrate do not inhibit renin from species other than primates (207).

Further synthesis efforts yielded a peptide renin substrate analogue, Pro-His-Pro-Phe-His-Phe-Phe-Val-Tyr-Lys, in which both valine residues at the cleavage site of renin were replaced by phenylalanine. This compound virtually completely inhibited the pressor response to human renin when injected into primates, but it had no effect on angiotensin I or II pressor responses. In addition, this compound, at 2 mg/kg i.v., reduced arterial blood pressure in sodium-deficient primates to the same degree as the ACE inhibitor SQ 20,881 at 1 mg/kg (208), while having no effect on blood pressure in sodium-replete monkeys (209). In acute one-kidney renovascular hypertension this peptide renin inhibitor restored mean arterial blood pressure to normal levels (Fig. 18), similarly to SQ 20,881.

Peptide renin inhibitors appear to be promising candidates as antihypertensive drugs and should display greater specificity than converting enzyme inhibitors (they do not potentiate kinin). Whether or not this greater specificity will be an advantage remains to be determined. However, before these compounds can be considered for therapeutic use, their durations of action must be increased, and they must be active when taken orally. That these are not insurmountable obstacles is attested to by the development of ACE inhibitors that also were initially small peptides suffering from these same deficiencies.

REFERENCES

1. Khosla, M. C., Smeby, R. R., and Bumpus, F. M. (1974): Structure activity relationship in angiotensin II analogs. In: *Angiotensin*, edited by I. H. Page and F. M. Bumpus, pp. 126–161. Springer-Verlag, New York.
2. Khosla, M. C., Page, I. H., and Bumpus, F. M. (1979): Interrelations between various blood pressure regulatory systems and mosaic theory of hypertension. *Biochem. Pharmacol.*, 28:2867–2882.
3. Skeggs, L. T., Marsh, W. H., Kahn, J. R., and Shumway, N. P. (1954): The purification of hypertensin I. *J. Exp. Med.*, 100:363–370.
4. Helmer, O. M. (1957): Differentiation between two forms of angiotonin by means of spirally cut strips of rabbit aorta. *Am. J. Physiol.*, 188:571–577.
5. Skeggs, L. T., Kahn, J. R., and Shumway, N. P.

(1956): The purification of hypertension II. *J. Exp. Med.*, 103:301–307.

6. Ng, K. K. F., and Vane, J. R. (1967): Conversion of angiotensin I to angiotensin II. *Nature,* 216:762–766.

7. Cushman, D. W., and Ondetti, M. A. (1980): Inhibitors of angiotensin-converting enzyme. *Prog. Med. Chem.,* 17:43–104.

8. Erdos, E. G. (1976): Conversion of angiotensin I to angiotensin II. *Am. J. Med.,* 60:749–759.

9. Soffer, R. L. (1976): Angiotensin converting enzyme and the regulation of vasoactive peptides. *Annu. Rev. Biochem.,* 45:45–94.

10. Skeggs, L. T., Dorer, F. E., Kahn, J. R., Lentz, K. E., and Levine, M. (1976): The biochemistry of the renin-angiotensin system and its role in hypertension. *Am. J. Med.,* 60:737–748.

11. Yang, H. Y. T., Erdos, E. G., and Levin, Y. (1971): Characterization of a dipeptide hydrolase (kininase II: angiotensin I converting enzyme). *J. Pharmacol. Exp. Ther.,* 177:291–300.

12. Cheung, H. S., and Cushman, D. W. (1973): Inhibition of homogeneous angiotensin-converting enzyme of rabbit lung by synthetic venom peptides of *Bothrops jararaca. Biochim. Biophys. Acta,* 293:451–463.

13. Das, M., and Soffer, R. L. (1975): Pulmonary angiotensin-converting enzyme (structural and catalytic properties). *J. Biol. Chem.,* 250:6762–6768.

14. Ondetti, M. A., Rubin, B., and Cushman, D. W. (1977): Design of specific inhibitors of angiotensin-converting enzyme: New class of orally active antihypertensive agents. *Science,* 196:441–444.

15. Ferreira, S. H. (1965): Bradykinin-potentiating factor (BFP) present in the venom of *Bothrops jararaca. Br. J. Pharmacol. Chemother.,* 24:163–169.

16. Ondetti, M. A., Williams, N. J., Sabo, E. F., Pluscec, J., Weaver, E. R., and Kocy, O. (1971): Angiotensin-converting enzyme inhibitors from the venom of *Bothrops jararaca.* Isolation, elucidation of structure and synthesis. *Biochemistry,* 19:4033–4039.

17. Green, L. J., Camargo, A. C. M., Kreiger, E. M., Stewart, J. M., and Ferreira, S. H. (1972): Inhibition of the conversion of angiotensin I to angiotensin II and potentiation of the conversion of angiotensin I to II and potentiation of bradykinin by small peptides present in *Bothrops jararaca* venom. *Circ. Res.* [*Suppl. II*], 31:II-62–II-71.

18. Patchett, A., Harris, E., Tristram, E., Wyvratt, M., Wu, M. T., Taub, D., Peterson, E., Ikeler, T., ten Broeke, J., Payne, L., Ondeyka, D., Thorsett, E., Greenlee, W., Lohr, N., Maycock, A., Hoffsommer, R., Joshua, H., Ruyle, W., Rothrock, J., Aster, S., Robinson, F. M., Sweet, C. S., Ulm, E. H., Gross, D. M., Vassil, T. C., and Stone, C. A. (1980): A new class of angiotensin converting enzyme inhibitors. *Nature,* 288:280–283.

19. Rubin, B., Laffan, R. J., Kotler, D. G., O'Keefe, E. H., DeMaio, D. A., and Goldberg, M. E. (1978): SQ 14,225 (D-3-mercapto-2-methylpropanoyl-L-proline), a novel orally active inhibitor of angiotensin I-converting enzyme. *J. Pharmacol. Exp. Ther.,* 204:271–280.

20. Gross, D. M., Sweet, C. S., Ulm, E. H., Backlund, E. P., Morris, A. A., Weitz, D., Bohn, D. L., Wen-

ger, H. C., Vassil, T. C., and Stone, C. A. (1980): Effect of N-[(S)-1-carboxy-3-phenylpropyl]-L-Ala-L-Pro and its ethyl ester (MK-421) on angiotensin converting enzyme *in vitro* and angiotensin I pressor responses *in vivo. J. Pharmacol. Exp. Ther.,* 216:552–557.

21. Trippodo, N. C., and Frohlich, E. D. (1981): Similarities of genetic (spontaneous) hypertension man and rat. *Circ. Res.,* 48:309–319.

22. Polsky-Cynkin, R., Reichlin, S., and Fanburg, B. L. (1980): Angiotensin I-converting enzyme activity in the spontaneously hypertensive rat. *Proc. Soc. Exp. Biol. Med.,* 164:242–247.

23. Laffan, R. J., Goldberg, M. E., High, J. P., Schaffer, T. R., Waugh, M. H., and Rubin, B. (1978): Antihypertensive activity in rats of SQ 14,225, an orally active inhibitor of angiotensin I-converting enzyme. *J. Pharmacol. Exp. Ther.,* 204:281–288.

24. Muirhead, E. E., Prewitt, R. L., Jr., Brooks, B., and Brosius, W. L., Jr. (1978): Antihypertensive action of the orally active converting enzyme inhibitor (SQ 14,225) in spontaneously hypertensive rats. *Circ. Res.,* 43:53–59.

25. Antonaccio, M. J., Rubin, B., Horovitz, L. P., Laffan, R. J., Goldberg, M. E., High, J. P., Harris, D. N., and Laidi, S. (1979): Effects of chronic treatment with captopril (SQ 14,225), an orally active inhibitor of angiotensin I-converting enzyme, in spontaneously hypertensive rats. *Jpn. J. Pharmacol.,* 29:285–294.

26. Andrews, D. I. (1979): Effects of saralasin and captopril on the blood pressure of conscious genetically hypertensive and normotensive rats. *Med. J. Aust.* [*Specl. Suppl.*], 2:vii–ix.

27. Watanabe, T. X., and Sokabe, H. (1979): Acute vasodepressor effect of D-3-mercapto-2-methylpropanoyl-L-proline (SQ 14,225) in the stroke-prone substrain of spontaneously hypertensive rats. *Jpn. J. Pharmacol.,* 29:133–135.

28. Antonaccio, M. J., Rubin, B., and Horovitz, Z. P. (1980): Effects of captopril in animal model of hypertension. *Clin. Exp. Hypertension,* 2:613–637.

29. Koike, H., Sto, K., Mujamoto, M., and Nishino, H. (1980): Effect of long-term blockade of angiotensin-converting enzyme with captopril (SQ 14,225) on hemodynamics and circulating blood volume in SHR. *Hypertension,* 2:299–303.

30. Ferrone, R. A., and Antonaccio, M. J. (1979): Prevention of the development of spontaneous hypertension in rats by captopril (SQ 14,225). *Eur. J. Pharmacol.,* 60:131–137.

31. Giudicelli, J. F., Freslon, J. L., Glasson, S., and Richer, C. (1980): Captopril and hypertension development in the SHR. *Clin. Exp. Hypertension,* 2:1083–1096.

32. Sen, S., Tarazi, R. C., and Bumpus, F. M. (1980): Effect of converting enzyme inhibitor (SQ 14,225) on myocardial hypertrophy in spontaneously hypertensive rats. *Hypertension,* 2:169–176.

33. Christlieb, A. R., and Hickler, R. B. (1972): Blood pressure response and antibody formation in spontaneously hypertensive rats and in normal albino rats after immunization against angiotensin II. *Endocrinology,* 91:1064–1070.

34. Pals, D. T., Masucci, F. D., Denning, G. S., Jr., Sipos, F., and Fessler, D. C. (1971): Role of the pressor action of angiotensin II in experimental hypertension. *Circ. Res.*, 29:673–681.

35. Waeber, B., Brunner, H. R., Brunner, D. B., Curtet, A.-L., Turini, G. A., and Gavras, H. (1980); Discrepancy between antihypertensive effect and angiotensin converting enzyme inhibition by captopril. *Hypertension*, 2:236–242.

36. Boomsma, F., DeBruyn, J. H. B., Derkx, F. H. M., and Schalekamp, M. A. D. H. (1981): Opposite effects of captopril on angiotensin I-converting enzyme "activity" and "concentration"; relation between enzyme inhibition and long-term blood pressure response. *Clin. Sci.*, 60:491–498.

37. Morton, J. J., Tree, M., and Casals-Stenzel, J. (1980): The effect of captopril on blood pressure and angiotensin I, II and III in sodium-depleted dogs: Problems associated with the measurement of angiotensin II after inhibition of converting enzyme. *Clin. Sci.*, 58:445–450.

38. Unger, T., Scholl, B., Hubner, D., Yukimura, T., Lang, R. E., Rascher, W., and Ganten, D. (1981): Plasma-converting enzyme activity does not reflect effectiveness of oral treatment with captopril. *Eur. J. Pharmacol.*, 72:255–259.

39. Sweet, C. S., Arbegast, P. T., Gaul, S. L., Blaine, E. H., and Gross, D. M. (1981): Relationship between angiotensin I blockade and antihypertensive properties of single doses of MK-421 and captopril in spontaneous and renal hypertensive rats. *Eur. J. Pharmacol.*, 76:167–176.

40. Schiffrin, E. L., Gutkowska, J., and Genest, J. (1981): Mechanism of captopril-induced renin release in conscious rats. *Proc. Soc. Exp. Biol. Med.*, 167:327–332.

41. Ulm, E. H., and Vassil, T. C. (1982): Total serum angiotensin converting enzyme activity in rats and dogs after enalapril maleate (MK-421). *Life Sci.*, 30:7225–7230.

42. Fyhrquist, F., Forslund, T., Tikkanen, S., and Gronhagen-Riska, C. (1980): Induction of angiotensin I-converting enzyme in rat lung by captopril (SQ 14,225). *Eur. J. Pharmacol.*, 67:473–475.

43. Kokubu, T., Veda, E., Ono, M., Kawabe, T., Hayashi, Y., and Kan, T. (1980): Effect of captopril (SQ 14,225) on the renin-angiotensin-aldosterone system in normal rats. *Eur. J. Pharmacol.*, 62:269–275.

44. Lai, F. M., Tanikella, T., Herzlinger, H., and Cervoni, P. (1980): Effect of the time interval between blood sampling and assay on serum angiotensin I-converting enzyme activity from captopril-treated rats. *Eur. J. Pharmacol.*, 67:97–99.

45. Ganten, D., Hutchinson, J. S., and Schelling, P. (1975): The intrinsic brain iso-renin-angiotensin system in the rat: Its possible role in central mechanisms of blood pressure regulation. *Clin. Sci. Mol. Med.*, 48:265s–268s.

46. Stamler, J. F., Brody, M. J., and Phillips, M. I. (1980): The central and peripheral effects of captopril (SQ 14,225) on the arterial pressure of spontaneously hypertensive rats. *Brain Res.*, 186:499–504.

47. Hutchinson, J. S., Mandelsohn, F. A. O., and Doyle, A. E. (1980): Blood pressure responses of conscious normotensive and spontaneously hypertensive rats to intracerebroventricular and peripheral administration of captopril. *Hypertension*, 2:546–550.

48. Vollmer, R. R., and Boccagno, J. A. (1977): Central cardiovascular effects of SQ 14,225, an angiotensin I converting enzyme inhibitor in chloralose-anesthetized cats. *Eur. J. Pharmacol.*, 45:117–125.

49. Mann, J. F. E., Rascher, W., Dietz, R., Schomig, A., and Ganten, D. (1979): Effects of an orally active converting enzyme inhibitor, SQ 14,225 on the pressor response to angiotensin administered into the brain ventricles of spontaneously hypertensive rats. *Clin. Sci.*, 56:585–589.

50. Gaul, S. L., Martin, G. E., and Sweet, C. S. (1982): Comparative central actions of enalapril and captopril in spontaneously hypertensive rats. *Fed. Proc.*, 41:1663.

51. Suzuki, H., Kondo, H., Handa, M., and Saruta, T. (1981): Role of brain isorenin-angiotensin system in experimental hypertension in rats. *Clin. Sci.*, 61:175–180.

52. Sweet, C. S., Gross, D. M., Arbegast, P. T., Gaul, S. L., Britt, P. M., Ludden, C. T., Weitz, D., and Stone, C. A. (1981): Antihypertensive activity of *N*-[(*S*)-1-(ethoxycarbonyl)-3-phenylpropyl]-L-Ala-L-Pro (MK-421), an orally active converting enzyme inhibitor. *J. Pharmacol. Exp. Ther.*, 216:558–566.

53. Man in't Veld, A. J., Schicht, I. M., Derky, H. M. F., DeBruyn, J. H. B., and Schalekamp, M. A. D. H. (1980): Effects of an angiotensin-converting enzyme inhibitor (captopril) on blood pressure in anephric subjects. *Br. Med. J.*, 280:288–290.

54. Thurston, H., and Swales, J. D. (1977): Blood pressure response of nephrectomized hypertensive rats to converting enzyme inhibitor: Evidence for persisting vascular renin activity. *Clin. Sci. Mol. Med.*, 53:299–304.

55. Crofton, J. T., Share, L., and Horovitz, L. P. (1979): The effect of SQ 14,225 on systolic blood pressure and urinary excretion of vasopressin in developing spontaneously hypertensive rats. *Hypertension*, 1:462–467.

56. Antonaccio, M. J., Harris, D., Goldenberg, H., High, J. P., and Rubin, B. (1979): The effects of captopril, propranolol and indomethacin on blood pressure and plasma renin activity in spontaneously hypertensive and normotensive rats. *Proc. Soc. Exp. Biol. Med.*, 162:429–433.

57. Brunner, H. R., Kirshman, J. D., Sealey, J. E., and Laragh, J. H. (1973): Hypertension of renal origin: Evidence for two different mechanisms. *Science*, 174:1344–1346.

58. Sen, S., Smeley, R. R., Bumpus, M., and Turcotte, J. G. (1979): Role of renin-angiotensin system in chronic renal hypertensive rats. *Hypertension*, 1:427–434.

59. Gavras, H., Brunner, H. R., Vaughan, E. D., Jr., and Laragh, J. H. (1973): Angiotensin-sodium interaction in blood pressure maintenance of renal hypertensive and normotensive rats. *Science*, 180:1369–1371.

60. Freeman, R. H., Davis, J. O., Watkins, B. C., Stephens, G. A., and DeForrest, J. M. (1979): Effects of continuous converting enzyme blockade on reno-

vascular hypertension in the rat. *Am. J. Physiol.*, 236:F21–F24.

61. Huang, W.-C., Ploth, D. W., Bell, P. D., Work, J., and Navar, L. G. (1981): Bilateral renal function responses to converting enzyme inhibitor (SQ 20,881) in two-kidney, one-clip Goldblatt hypertensive rats. *Hypertension*, 3:285–293.

62. Ploth, D. W., Schnermann, J., Dahlheim, H., Hermle, M., and Schmidmeier, E. (1977): Autoregulation and tubulo-glomerular feedback in normotensive and hypertensive rats. *Kidney Int.*, 12:253–267.

63. Brunner, H., DeSaulles, P. A., Regoli, D., and Gross, F. (1962): Renin content and excretory function of kidney in rats with experimental hypertension. *Am. J. Physiol.*, 202:795–799.

64. Fourcade, J. C., Navar, L. J., and Guyton, A. C. (1971): Possibility that angiotensin resulting from unilateral kidney disease affects contralateral renal function. *Nephron*, 8:1–16.

65. Schweitzer, G., and Gertz, K. H. (1979): Changes of hemodynamics and glomerular ultrafiltration in renal hypertension of rats. *Kidney Int.*, 15:134–143.

66. Kramer, P., and Ochwadt, B. (1972): Sodium excretion in Goldblatt hypertension: Long term separate kidney function studies in rats by means of a new technique. *Pfluegers Arch.*, 332:332–345.

67. Lowitz, H. D., Stumpe, K. O., and Ochwadt, B. (1968): Natrium- und Wasser-Resorption in den verschiedenen Abschnitten des Nephrons beim experimenteller renalen Hochdruck der Ratte. *Pfluegers Arch.*, 304:322–335.

68. Peters, G., Brunner, H., and Gross, F. (1964): Isotonic saline diuresis and urinary concentrating ability in renal hypertensive rats. *Nephron*, 1:295–309.

69. Fernandes, M., Fiorentine, R., Onesti, G., Bellini, G., Gould, A. B., Hessan, H., Kim, K. E., and Swartz, C. (1978): Effect of administration of Sar^1-Ala^8-angiotensin II during the development and maintenance of renal hypertension in the rat. *Clin. Sci. Mol. Med.*, 54:633–637.

70. Mann, S. E., Phillips, M. I., Dietz, R., Harbara, H., and Ganten, D. (1978): Effects of central and peripheral angiotensin blockade in hypertensive rats. *Am. J. Physiol.*, 234:H629–H637.

71. Bumpus, F. M., Sen, S., Smelz, R. R., Sweet, C., Ferrario, C. M., and Khosla, M. C. (1973): Use of angiotensin II antagonists in experimental hypertension. *Circ. Res. [Suppl. I]*, 32–33:I-150–I-158.

72. Coleman, T. G., and Guyton, A. C. (1975): The pressor role of angiotensin in salt deprivation and renal hypertension in rats. *Clin. Sci. Mol. Med.*, 48:45s–48s.

73. Thurston, H., and Swales, J. D. (1974): Comparison of angiotensin II antagonist and antiserum infusion with nephrectomy in the two-kidney Goldblatt hypertensive rat. *Circ. Res.*, 35:325–329.

74. Brown, J. J., Fraser, R., Lever, A. F., Morton, J. J., Robertson, J. S. S., and Schalekamp, M. A. D. H. (1977): Mechanisms in hypertension: A personal view. In: *Hypertension*, edited by J. Genest, E. Kow, and O. Kuchel, p. 529. McGraw-Hill, New York.

75. Riegger, A. J. G., Millar, J. A., Lever, A. F., Morton, J. J., and Slack, B. (1977): Correction of renal hypertension in the rat by prolonged infusion of angiotensin inhibitors. *Lancet*, 2:1317–1319.

76. Antonaccio, M. J., Rubin, B., Horovitz, Z. P., Mackaness, G., and Panasevich, R. (1979): Long-term efficacy of captopril (SQ 14,225) in 2-kidney renal hypertensive rats. *Clin. Exp. Hypertension*, 1:505–517.

77. Rubin, B., Antonaccio, M. J., Goldberg, M. E., Harris, D. N., Atkin, A. G., Horovitz, Z. P., Panasevich, R. E., and Laffan, R. J. (1978): Chronic antihypertensive effects of captopril (SQ 14,225) on orally active angiotensin I-converting enzyme inhibitor in conscious 2-kidney renal hypertensive rats. *Eur. J. Pharmacol.*, 51:377–388.

78. Bellini, G., Fiorentini, R., Fernandez, M., Onesti, G., Hessan, H., Gould, A. B., Bianchi, M., Kim, K. E., and Swartz, C. (1979): Neurogenic activity angiotensin II interaction during development and maintenance of renal hypertension in the rat. *Clin. Sci.*, 57:25–29.

79. Antonaccio, M. J., Ferrone, R. A., Waugh, M., Harris, D., and Rubin, B. (1980): Sympathoadrenal and renin-angiotensin systems in the development of two-kidney, one-clip renal hypertension in rats. *Hypertension*, 2:723–731.

80. Bianchi, G., Tilde Tenconi, L., and Lucca, R. (1970): Effect in the conscious dog of constriction of the renal artery to a sole remaining kidney on haemodynamics, sodium balance, body fluid volumes, plasma renin concentration and pressor responsiveness to angiotensin. *Clin. Sci.*, 38:741–766.

81. Brown, T. C., Davis, J. O., Olichney, M. J., and Johnston, C. S. (1966): Relation of plasma renin to sodium balance and balance arterial pressure in experimental renal hypertension. *Circ. Res.*, 18:475–483.

82. Midsche, L. W., Miksche, U., and Gross, F. (1970): Effect of sodium restriction on renal hypertension and on renin activity in the rat. *Circ. Res.*, 27:973–984.

83. Sen, S., Smelz, R. R., Bumpus, F. M., and Turcotte, J. P. (1979): Role of renin-angiotensin system in chronic renal hypertensive rats. *Hypertension*, 1:427–431.

84. Ledingham, J. M., and Cohen, R. D. (1964): Changes in the extracellular fluid volume and cardiac output during the development of experimental renal hypertension. *Can. Med. Assoc. J.*, 90:292–294.

85. Lucas, J., and Floyer, M. A. (1974): Changes in body fluid distribution and interstitial fluid compliance during the development and reversal of experimental renal hypertension in the rat. *Clin. Sci. Mol. Med.*, 47:1–11.

86. Ferrario, C. M., and Page, I. H. (1978): Current views concerning cardiac output in the genesis of experimental hypertension. *Circ. Res.*, 43:821–831.

87. Seymour, A. A., Davis, J. O., Freeman, R. H., DeForrest, J. M., Rowe, B. P., Stephens, G. A., and Williams, G. M. (1981): Sodium and angiotensin in the pathogenesis of experimental renovascular hypertension. *Am. J. Physiol.*, 240:H788–H792.

88. Campbell, W. A., and Pettinger, W. A. (1975): Sodium chloride suppression of renin release in the

unanesthetized rat. *Endocrinology,* 97:1394–1397.

89. Gross, F. (1971): The renin-angiotensin system and hypertension. *Ann. Intern Med.,* 75:777–787.

90. Margolius, H. S., Geller, R., DeJong, W., Pisano, J. J., and Sjoerdsma, A. (1972): Altered urinary kallikrein excretion in rats with hypertension. *Circ. Res.,* 30:358–362.

91. Douglass, B. H., Langford, H. G., and McCaa, R. E. (1979): Response to mineralocorticoid hypertensive animals to an angiotensin I converting enzyme inhibitor. *Proc. Soc. Exp. Biol. Med.,* 161:86–87.

92. Miyamori, I., Brown, M. J., and Dollery, C. T. (1980): Single dose captopril administration in DOCA/salt rats: Reduction of hypotensive effect of indomethacin. *Clin. Exp. Hypertension,* 2:935–945.

93. Tikkanen, I., Fyhrquist, F., Tikkanen, T., and Miettinen, A. (1980): Efficacy of captopril in experimental low renin hypertension. *Eur. J. Pharmacol.,* 68:197–200.

94. Page, I. H. (1939): Production of persistent arterial hypertension by cellophane perinephritis. *J.A.M.A.,* 113:2046.

95. Campbell, D. J., Skinner, S. L., and Day, A. J. (1973): Cellophane perinephritis hypertension and its reversal in rabbits. *Circ. Res.,* 33:105–112.

96. Vollmer, R. R., Boccagno, J. A., Steinbacher, T. E., Horovitz, Z. P., and Murthy, V. S. (1981): Antihypertensive activity of captopril (SQ 14,225), an orally active inhibitor of angiotensin converting enzyme in conscious two-kidney perinephritic dogs. *J. Pharmacol. Exp. Ther.,* 216:225–231.

97. Vollmer, R. R., Boccagno, J. A., Harris, D. N., and Murthy, V. S. (1978): Hypotension induced by inhibition of angiotensin-converting enzyme in pentobarbital-anesthetized dogs. *Eur. J. Pharmacol.,* 51:39–45.

98. Harris, D. N., Heran, C. L., Goldenberg, H. J., High, J. P., Laffan, R. J., Rubin, B., Antonaccio, M. J., and Goldberg, M. E. (1978): Effect of SQ 14,225 on orally active inhibitor of angiotensin converting enzyme on blood pressure, heart rate and plasma renin activity of conscious normotensive dogs. *Eur. J. Pharmacol.,* 51:345–349.

99. Murthy, V. S., Waldron, T. L., and Goldberg, M. E. (1978): Inhibition of angiotensin-converting enzyme by SQ 14,225 in anesthetized dogs: Hemodynamic and renal vascular effects. *Proc. Soc. Exp. Biol. Med.,* 157:121–124.

100. Jandhyala, B. S., Washington, G. F., and Lokhandwata, M. F. (1978): Influence of inhibition of angiotensin I converting enzyme with SQ 14,225 on the arterial blood pressure of mongrel dogs. *Res. Commun. Chem. Pathol. Pharmacol.,* 22:257–265.

101. Satoh, S., Fujisawa, S., Tanaka, R., and Nakai, K. (1980): Hypotensive effect of captopril, an angiotensin converting enzyme inhibitor, in pentobarbital anesthetized dogs. *Jpn. J. Pharmacol.,* 30:112–115.

102. Hall, J. E., Guyton, A. C., Smith, M. J., and Coleman, T. G. (1979): Chronic blockade of angiotensin II formation during sodium deprivation. *Am. J. Physiol.,* 237:F425–F432.

103. McCaa, R. E., Hall, J. E., and McCaa, C. S. (1978): The effects of angiotensin I-converting enzyme in-

hibitors in arterial blood pressure and urinary sodium excretion. *Circ. Res. [Suppl. I],* 43:I-32–I-39.

104. Williams, G. H., and Hollenberg, N. K. (1977): Accentuated vascular and endocrine response to SQ 14,225 in hypertension. *N. Engl. J. Med.,* 297:184–188.

105. Swartz, S. L., Williams, G. H., Hollenberg, N. K., Moore, T. J., and Dluhy, R. G. (1979): Converting enzyme inhibition in essential hypertension: The hypotensive response does not reflect only reduction angiotensin II formation. *Hypertension,* 1:106–111.

106. Vinci, J. M., Horwitz, D., Zusman, R. M., Pisano, J. J., Catt, K. J., and Keiser, H. R. (1979): The effect of converting enzyme inhibition with SQ 20,881 on plasma and urinary kinins, prostaglandin E and angiotensin II in hypertensive man. *Hypertension,* 1:416–426.

107. Johnston, C. I., McGrath, B. P., Millar, J. A., and Matthews, P. G. (1979): Long-term effects of captopril (SQ 14,225) on blood pressure and hormone levels in essential hypertension. *Lancet,* 2:493–495.

108. Levinsky, N. G. (1979): The renal kallikrein-kinin system. *Circ. Res.,* 44:441–451.

109. Mimran, A., Targhetta, R., and Laroche, B. (1980): The antihypertensive effect of captopril, evidence for and influence of kinins. *Hypertension,* 2:732–737.

110. Overlack, A., Stumpe, K. O., Kuhnert, M., Kolloch, R., Rossel, C., Heck, I., and Kruck, F. (1981): Evidence for participation of kinins in the antihypertensive effect of converting enzyme inhibition. *Klin. Wochenschr.,* 59:69–74.

111. Carretero, O. A., Miyazaki, S., and Scicli, A. G. (1981): Role of kinins in the acute antihypertensive effect of the converting enzyme inhibitor, captopril. *Hypertension,* 3:18–22.

112. Celio, M. R., and Inagami, T. (1981): Angiotensin II immunoreactivity co-exists with renin in the juxtaglomerular granular cells of the kidney. *Proc. Natl. Acad. Sci. U.S.A.,* 78:3897–3900.

113. Thurau, K. and Mason, J. (1974): The intra-renal function of the juxtaglomerular apparatus. In: *MTP (Medical and Technical Publishing Co.) International Review of Science, Physiology Series I, Kidney and Urinary Tract Physiology, Vol 6,* edited by K. Thurau, pp. 357–389. University Park Press, Baltimore.

114. Leckie, B., Gavras, H., McGregor, J., and McElwec, C. (1972): The conversion of angiotensin I to angiotensin II by rabbit glomeruli. *J. Endocrinol.,* 55:229–230.

115. Granger, P., Dahlheim, H., and Thurau, K. (1972): Enzyme activities of the single juxtaglomerular apparatus in the rat kidney. *Kidney Int.,* 2:78–88.

116. Kimbrough, H. M., Vaughan, E. D., Carey, R. M., and Ayers, C. R. (1977): Effect of intrarenal angiotensin II blockade on renal function in conscious dogs. *Circ. Res.,* 40:174–178.

117. Meggs, L. G., and Hollenberg, N. K. (1980): Converting enzyme inhibition and the kidney. *Hypertension,* 2:551–557.

118. Wong, P. C., and Zimmerman, B. G. (1980): Role of extrarenal and intrarenal converting enzyme inhibition in renal vasodilator response to intravenous captopril. *Life Sci.,* 27:1291–1297.

119. Wong, P. C., and Zimmerman, B. G. (1980): Mechanism of captopril-induced renal vasodilatation in anesthetized dogs after nonhypotensive hemorrhage. *J. Pharmacol. Exp. Ther.*, 215:104–109.

120. Jandhyala, B. S., Nandiwada, P., and Buckley, J. P. (1979): Studies on the mechanism of the hypotensive action of SQ 14,225, an angiotensin-converting enzyme inhibitor in anesthetized dogs. *Res. Commun. Chem. Pathol. Pharmacol.*, 25:429–446.

121. Zimmerman, B. G., Mommsen, C., and Kraft, E. (1980): Renal vasodilatation caused by captopril in conscious normotensive and Goldblatt hypertensive dogs. *Proc. Soc. Exp. Biol. Med.*, 164:459–465.

122. Satoh, S., Fujisawa, S., Tanaka, R., and Nakai, K. (1980): Effect of captopril, a converting enzyme inhibitor, on renal vascular resistance in pentobarbital anesthetized dogs. *Jpn. J. Pharmacol.*, 30:515–519.

123. Abe, K., Miura, K., Inanishi, M., Yokimura, K., Komori, T., Okahara, T., and Yamamoto, K. (1980): Effects of an orally active converting enzyme inhibitor (YS-980) on renal function in dogs. *J. Pharmacol. Exp. Ther.*, 214:166–170.

124. Mullane, K., and Moncada, S. (1980): Prostacyclin mediates the potentiated hypotensive effect of bradykinin following captopril treatment. *Eur. J. Pharmacol.*, 66:355–365.

125. Ayers, C. R., Vaughan, E. D., Yancey, M. R., Bing, K. T., Johnson, C. C., and Morton, C. (1974): Effect of 1-sarcosine-8-alanine angiotensin II and converting enzyme inhibitor on renin release in dog acute renovascular hypertension. *Circ. Res. [Suppl. I]*, 34–35:27–33.

126. Bunag, R. D., Page, I. H., and McCubbin, J. W. (1967): Inhibition of renin release by vasopressin and angiotensin. *Cardiovasc. Res.*, 1:67–73.

127. Blair-West, J. R., Coghlan, R. P., Denton, D. A., Funder, J. W., Scoggins, B. A., and Wright, R. D. (1971): Inhibition of renin secretion by systemic and intrarenal angiotensin infusion. *Am. J. Physiol.*, 220:1309–1315.

128. Shade, R. E., Davis, J. O., Johnson, J. A., Gotshall, R. W., and Spielman, W. S. (1973): Mechanism of action of angiotensin II and antidiuretic hormone on renin secretion. *Am. J. Physiol.*, 224:926–929.

129. Vander, A. J., and Geelhoed, G. W. (1965): Inhibition of renin secretion by angiotensin III. *Proc. Soc. Exp. Biol. Med.*, 120:399–403.

130. Schiffrin, E. L., Gutkowska, J., and Genest, J. (1981): Mechanism of captopril-induced renin release in conscious rats. *Proc. Soc. Exp. Biol. Med.*, 167:327–332.

131. Abe, K., Itoh, M., Satoh, T., Haruyama, T., Imai, Y., Goto, T., Satoh, K., Otsuka, Y., and Yoshinaga, K. (1980): Indomethacin (Ind) inhibits an enhanced renin release following captopril (SQ 14,225) administration. *Life Sci.*, 26:561–565.

132. Hatton, R., and Clough, D. P. (1982): Captopril interferes with neurogenic vasoconstriction in the pithed rat by angiotensin-dependent mechanism. *J. Cardiovasc. Pharmacol.*, 4:116–123.

133. Collis, M. G., and Keddio, J. C. (1981): Captopril attenuates adrenergic vasoconstriction in rat mesenteric arteries by angiotensin-dependent and independent mechanism. *Clin. Sci.*, 61:281–286.

134. Clough, D. P., Hatton, R., and Matthewman, S. C. (1981): Effect of angiotensin converting enzyme inhibitor on neurogenic vasoconstriction in the pithed rat. *Br. J. Pharmacol.*, 73:296P.

135. Antonaccio, M. J., and Kerwin, L. (1980): Evidence for prejunctional inhibition of norepinephrine release by captopril in spontaneously hypertensive rats. *Eur. J. Pharmacol.*, 68:209–212.

136. Antonaccio, M. J., and Kerwin, L. (1980): Pre- and postjunctional inhibition of vascular sympathetic function by captopril in spontaneously hypertensive rats. *Hypertension*, 3:I-54–I-62.

137. DeJonge, A., Wiffert, B., Kalkman, H. O., Van Meel, J. C. A., Thoolen, J. M. C. M., Timmermans, P. B. M. W. M., and van Zwieten, P. A. (1981): Captopril impairs the vascular smooth muscle contraction mediated by postsynaptic α_2-adrenoceptor in the pithed rat. *Eur. J. Pharmacol.*, 74:385–386.

138. Weare, J. A., Stewart, T. A., Gafford, J. T., and Erdos, E. G. (1981): Inhibition of human converting enzyme in vitro by a novel tripeptide analog. *Hypertension [Suppl. I]*, 3:I-50–I-54.

139. Meyer, R. F., Nicolaides, E. D., Tinney, J. F., Lunney, E. A., Holmes, A., Hoefle, M. L., Smith, R. D., Essenburg, A. D., and Kaplan, H. R. (1981): Novel synthesis of (S)-1-[5-(benzoylamine)-1,4-dioxo-6-phenylhexyl]-L-proline and analogues: Potent angiotensin converting enzyme inhibitors. *J. Med. Chem.*, 24:964–969.

140. Burnier, M., Turinc, G. A., Porchet, M., Brunner, D. B., Blasucci, D., Vukovich, R. A., Niess, E. S., Gavras, H., and Brunner, H. R. (1981): A new converting enzyme inhibitor administered orally to healthy volunteers (abstract). Presented at the eighth scientific meeting of the International Society for Hypertension, Milan, Italy, May 31–June 3, 1981.

141. Galardy, R. E. (1980): Inhibition of angiotensin converting enzyme with N^α-phosphonyl-L-alanyl-L-proline and N^α-phosphonyl-L-valyl-L-tryptphan. *Biochem. Biophys. Res. Commun.*, 97:94–99.

142. Iso, T., Yamuchi, H., Suda, H., Nakajima, N., Nishimura, K., Takada, T., Horiuchi, M., Nakata, K., and Iwao, J. (1980): Pharmacological studies on SA446. *Jpn. J. Pharmacol. [Suppl.]*, 30:136P.

143. Lai, F. M., Chan, P. S., Cervoni, P., Tanikella, T., Shepherd, C., Herzlinger, H., Quirk, G., and Ronsberg, M. A. (1982): Antihypertensive activity of [S-(R,S)-1-[3-(acetylthio)-3-benzoyl-2-methylpropionyl]-L-proline (CL 242,817), an inhibitor of angiotensin converting enzyme. *Fed. Proc.*, 41:1647.

144. Textor, S., Brunner, H. R., and Gavras, H. (1981): Converting enzyme inhibition during chronic angiotensin II infusion in rats, evidence against a nonangiotensin mechanism. *Hypertension*, 3:269–276.

145. Johnson, C. A., and Wakerlin, G. E. (1940): Antiserum for renin. *Proc. Soc. Exp. Biol. Med.*, 44:277–281.

146. Lamfrom, H., Haas, E., and Goldblatt, H. (1954): Studies on antirenin. *Am. J. Physiol.*, 177:55–64.

147. Helmer, O. M. (1958): Studies on renin antibodies. *Circulation*, 17:648–652.

148. Wakerlin, G. E. (1958): Antibodies to renin as a

proof of the pathogenesis of sustained renal hypertension. *Circulation,* 17:653–657.

149. Deodhar, S. D., Haas, E., and Goldblatt, H. (1964): Production of antirenin to homologous renin and its effect on experimental renal hypertension. *J. Exp. Med.,* 119:425–432.

150. Romero, J. L., Hoobler, S. W., Kozak, T. J., and Warzynski, R. J. (1973): Effect of antirenin on blood pressure of rabbits with experimental renal hypertension. *Am. J. Physiol.,* 225:810–817.

151. Dzau, V. J., Kopelman, R. I., Barger, A. C., and Haber, E. (1980): Renin-specific antibody for study of cardiovascular homeostasis. *Science,* 207:1091–1093.

152. Tigerstedt, R., and Bergman, P. G. (1898): Niere und Kreislauf. *Scand. Arch. Physiol.,* 8:223.

153. Page, I. H., and Helmer, O. M. (1940): Angiotonin-activator, renin and angiotonin-inhibitor, and the mechanism of angiotonin tachyphylaxis in normal, hypertensive and nephrectomized animals. *J. Exp. Med.,* 71:495–519.

154. Bumpus, F. M. (1965): Biochemical aspects of the renin-angiotensin system. *Trans. N.Y. Acad. Sci.,* 27:445–449.

155. Veyrat, R., de Champlain, J., Boucher, R., and Genest, J. (1964): Measurement of human arterial renin activity in some physiological and pathological states. *Can. Med. Assoc. J.,* 90:215–220.

156. Smeby, R. R., Sen, S., and Bumpus, F. M. (1967): A naturally occurring renin inhibitor. *Circ. Res.* [*Suppl. II*], 20–21:II-129–II-134.

157. Sen, S., Smeby, R. R., and Bumpus, F. M. (1967): Isolation of a phospholipid renin inhibitor from kidney. *Biochemistry,* 6:1572–1581.

158. Antonello, A., Baggio, B., Favaro, S., Corsini, A., Todesco, S., and Borsatti, A. (1973): Effect on blood pressure of intravenous administration of a phospholipid renin preinhibitor and its active form in renal hypertensive rats. *Pfluegers Arch.,* 341:113–120.

159. Sen, S., Smeby, R. R., and Bumpus, F. M. (1968): Antihypertensive effect of an isolated phospholipid. *Am. J. Physiol.,* 214:337–341.

160. Sen, S., Smeby, R. R., and Bumpus, F. M. (1969): Plasma renin activity in hypertensive rats after treatment with renin preinhibitor. *Am. J. Physiol.,* 216:499–503.

161. Ostrovsky, D., Sen, S., Smeby, R. R., and Bumpus, F. M. (1967): Chemical assay of phospholipid renin preinhibitor in urine and human blood. *Circ. Res.,* 21:497–505.

162. Osmond, D. H., Smeby, R. R., and Bumpus, F. M. (1969): Quantitative studies of renin preinhibitor and total phospholipids in organs and in plasma and erythrocytes of control, nephrectomized and very old rats. *J. Lab. Clin. Med.,* 73:795–808.

163. Osmond, D. H., Lewis, L. A., Smeby, R. R., and Bumpus, F. M. (1969): Renin "preinhibitor" in blood of anephric patients, in a case of hypobetalipoproteinemia and evidence of its major association with plasma alpha proteins. *J. Lab. Clin. Med.,* 73:809–818.

164. Baggio, B., Favaro, S., Antonello, A., and Borsatti, A. (1976): Preliminary studies on a rat kidney phospholipase A_2 activating a renin preinhibitor. *Res. Exp. Med.,* 169:77,81.

165. Baggio, B., Favaro, J., Antonello, A., Cannella, G., Todesco, J., and Borsatti, A. (1975): A possible role of the kidney in activating a renin preinhibitor. *Res. Exp. Med.,* 166:201–207.

166. Osmond, D. H., McFadzean, P. A. and Ross, L. J. (1973): Plasma phospholipase A_2-activity in nephrectomized rats and the question of renin inhibition. *Proc. Soc. Exp. Biol. Med.,* 144:969–973.

167. Poulsen, K. (1971): No evidence of active renin inhibitors in plasma. The kinetics of the reaction between renin and substrate in nonpretreated plasma. *Scand. J. Clin. Lab. Invest.,* 27:37–46.

168. Tinker, D. O., Schwartz, H.-J., Osmond, D. H., and Ross, L. J. (1973): Dog kidney phospholipids and the question of renin inhibition. *Can. J. Biochem.,* 51:863–875.

169. Turcotte, J. G., Boyd, R. E., Quinn, J. G., and Smeby, R. R. (1973): Isolation and renin inhibitory activity of phosphoglyceride from shark kidney. *J. Med. Chem.,* 16:166–168.

170. Būnag, R. D., and Walaszek, E. J. (1973): *In vitro* inhibition by synthetic phospholipids of pressor responses to renin. *Eur. J. Pharmacol.,* 23:191–196.

171. Hiwada, K., Kokubu, T., and Yamamura, Y. (1971): Inhibition of renin by sodium deoxycholate. *Biochem. Pharmacol.,* 20:914–916.

172. Rakhit, S. (1971): On the structure of the renin inhibitor from hog kidney. *Can. J. Biochem.,* 49:1012–1014.

173. Rakhit, S., Bagli, J. F., and Deghenghi, R. (1969): Phospholipids. Part 1. Synthesis of phosphotidylethanolamines. *Can. J. Chem.,* 47:2906–2910.

174. Pfeiffer, F. R., Hoke, S. C., Miao, C. K., Tedeschi, R. E., Pasternak, J., Hahn, R., Erickson, R. W., Lecin, H. W., Burton, C. A., and Weisbach, J. A. (1971): Lysophosphatidylethanolamine and 2-desoxylysophosphatidylethanolamine derivatives. 1. Potential renin inhibitors. *J. Med. Chem.,* 14:493–498.

175. Pfeiffer, F. R., Miao, C. K., Hoke, S. C., and Weisbach, J. A. (1972): Potential renin inhibitors. 2. Ethanolamine and ethylamine derivatives of phospholipids. *J. Med. Chem.,* 15:58–60.

176. Miyazaki, M., Hosoki, K., and Yamamoto, K. (1976): Renin inhibition by synthetic phosphatidyl- and phosphorylethanolamines. *Jpn. Circ. J.,* 40:901–910.

177. Miyazaki, M., and Yamamoto, K. (1977): Synthetic phosphatidylethanolamines as renin inhibitors. *Proc. Soc. Exp. Biol. Med.,* 155:468–473.

178. Hosoki, K., Miyazaki, M., and Yamamoto, K. (1977): Renin inhibitory effect of 2-[4-(4'-chlorophenoxy)phenoxyacetylamino] - ethyl - phosphoryl-ethanolamine (PE-104) *in vitro* and *in vivo*. *J. Pharmacol. Exp. Ther.,* 203:485–492.

179. Turcotte, J. G., Yu, C., Lee, H., Pavanaram, S. K., Sen, S., and Smeby, R. R. (1975): Synthesis of lysophosphatidylethanolamine analogs that inhibit renin activity. *J. Med. Chem.,* 18:1184–1190.

180. Kinoshita, M., Aburaki, S., Hagiwara, A., and Imai, J. (1973): Absolute configuration of 4-amino-3-hydroxy-6-methylheptanoic acid present in pepstatin

A and stereospecific synthesis of all four isomers. *J. Antibiot.*, 26:249–251.

181. Morishima, H., Takita, T., and Umezawa, H. (1972): The chemical synthesis of pepstatin A. *J. Antibiot.*, 25:551–552.

182. Gross, F., Lazar, J., and Orth, H. (1972): Inhibition of the renin-angiotensinogen reaction by pepstatin. *Science*, 175:656.

183. Lazar, J., Orth, H., Mohring, J., and Gross, F. (1972): Effects of the renin inhibitor pepstatin on the blood pressure of intact and nephrectomized rats. *Naunyn Schmiedebergs Arch. Pharmacol.*, 275:114–118.

184. Miyazaki, M., Komori, T., Okunishi, H., and Todo, N. (1979): Inhibition of dog renin activity by pepstatin A. *Jpn. Circ. J.*, 43:818–823.

185. McKown, M. M., Workman, R. J., and Gregerman, R. I. (1974): Pepstatin inhibition of human renin. Kinetic studies and estimation of enzyme purity. *J. Biol. Chem.*, 24:7770–7774.

186. Orth, H., Hackenthal, E., Lazar, J., Miksche, U., and Gross, R. (1974): Kinetics of the inhibitory effect of pepstatin on the reaction of hog renin with rat plasma substrate. *Circ. Res.*, 35:52–55.

187. Guyene, T. T., Devaux, C., Menard, J., and Corvol, P. (1976): Inhibition of human plasma renin activity by pepstatin. *J. Clin. Endocrinol. Metab.*, 43:1301–1306.

188. Miller, R. P., Poper, C. J., Wilson, C. W., and DeVito, E. (1972): Renin inhibition by pepstatin. *Biochem. Pharmacol.*, 21:2941–2944.

189. Scholkens, B. A., and Jung, W. (1974): Renin inhibition by pepstatin in experimental hypertension. *Arch. Int. Pharmacodyn. Ther.*, 208:24–34.

190. Tonnaer, J. A. D. M., Van Put, J. J., and DeJong, W. (1981): Intracerebroventricular infusions of N-acetyl-pepstatin attenuates the development of hypertension in the spontaneously hypertensive rat. *Eur. J. Pharmacol.*, 74:113–114.

191. Evin, G., Gardes, J., Kreft, C., Castro, B., Corvol, P., and Menard, J. (1978): Soluble pepstatins: A new approach to blockade *in vivo* of the renin-angiotensin system. *Clin. Sci. Mol. Med.*, 55:167s–169s.

192. Gardes, J., Evin, G., Castro, B., Corvol, P., and Menard, J. (1980): Synthesis and renin inhibitory properties of a new soluble pepstatin derivative. *J. Cardiovasc. Pharmacol.*, 2:687–698.

193. Miyazaki, M., Okuwishi, H., Komori, T., and Yamamoto, K. (1978): Renin inhibitory effects of N-acetyl-pepstatin. *Jpn. J. Pharmacol.*, 28:171–174.

194. Corvol, P., deVaux, C., and Menard, J. (1973): Pepstatin, an inhibitor for renin purification by affinity chromotography. *F.E.B.S. Lett.*, 34:189–192.

195. Overturf, M., Leonard, M., and Kirkendall, W. M.

(1974): Purification of human renin and inhibition of its activity by pepstatin. *Biochem. Pharmacol.*, 23:671–683.

196. Murakami, K., Inagami, T., Michelakis, A. M., and Cohen, S. (1973): An affinity column for renin. *Biochem. Biophys. Res. Commun.*, 54:482–487.

197. Skeggs, L. T., Jr., Kahn, J. R., Lentz, K. E., and Shumway, N. P. (1957): The preparation, purification and amino acid sequence of a polypeptide renin substrate. *J. Exp. Med.*, 106:439–453.

198. Skeggs, L. T., Jr., Lentz, K. E., Kahn, J. R., and Shumway, N. P. (1958): The synthesis of a tetradecapeptide renin substrate. *J. Exp. Med.*, 108:283–297.

199. Tewksbury, D. A., Dart, R. A., and Travis, J. (1979): Studies on the characterization of human angiotensinogen. *Circulation [Suppl. II]*, 59–60:132.

200. Kokubu, T., Ueda, E., Fujimoto, S., Hiwada, K., Kato, A., Akutsu, H., and Yamamura, Y. (1968): Peptide inhibitors of the renin-angiotensin system. *Nature*, 217:456–457.

201. Kokubu, T., Hwada, K., Ito, T., Ueda, E., Yamamura, Y., Mizoguchi, T., and Shigezane, K. (1973): Peptide inhibitors of renin-angiotensinogen reaction system. *Biochem. Pharmacol.*, 22:3217–3223.

202. Parry, M. J., Russell, A. B., and Szelke, M. (1972): Bio-isosteres of a peptide renin inhibitor. In: *Chemistry and Biology Peptides, Proc. 3rd Am. Peptide Symp.*, edited by J. Meienhofer, pp. 541–544. Ann Arbor Science Publishers Inc., Ann Arbor.

203. Parikh, I., and Cuatrecasas, P. (1977): Substrate analog competative inhibitors of human renin. *Biochem. Biophys. Res. Commun.*, 54:1356–1361.

204. Poulsen, K., Burton, J., and Haber, E. (1973): Competitive inhibitors of renin. *Biochemistry*, 12:3877–3882.

205. Shigezane, K., and Mizoguchi, T. (1973): Synthesis of antirenin active peptides. III. C-terminal carbinol analogues of peptides related to the partial structure of angiotensinogen as renin inhibitor. *Chem. Pharmacol. Bull.*, 21:972–980.

206. Burton, J., Poulsen, K., and Haber, E. (1975): Competative inhibitors of renin. Inhibitors effective at physiological pH. *Biochemistry*, 14:3892–3898.

207. Poulsen, K., Haber, E., and Burton, J. (1976): On the specificity of human renin: Studies with peptide inhibitors. *Biochim. Biophys. Acta*, 452:533–537.

208. Cody, R. J., Burton, J., Evin, G., Poulsen, K., Herd, J. A., and Haber, E. (1980): A substrate analog inhibitor of renin that is effective *in vivo*. *Biochem. Biophys. Res. Commun.*, 97:230–235.

209. Burton, J., Cody, R. J., Jr., Herd, J. A., and Haber, E. (1980): Specific inhibition of renin by an angiotensinogen analog: Studies in sodium depletion and renin-dependent hypertension. *Proc. Natl. Acad. Sci. U.S.A.*, 77:5476–5479.

Note added in proof: Recent publications from two laboratories have described new substrate analog renin inhibitors with substantially improved potency. Szelke et al. (*Nature*, 299:555–557, 1982) synthesized a series of compounds containing a reduced peptide bond at the scissile 10–11 bond, one of which also contained D-His at position 6. This compound, H-77, is a potent inhibitor of canine renin ($IC_{50} = 24$ nm) but less active against human and rat renins ($IC_{50} = 1$ μM and 0.6 μM, respectively) (Szelke et al., *Hypertension* 4 (suppl. II): II-59-II-69, 1982). Boger et al. (*Nature*, 303:81–84, 1983) reported on a series of statine containing compounds which are thought to be transition state analogs. The most active of these, Iva-His-Pro-Phe-His-Sta-Ile-Phe-NH$_2$, had an IC_{50} against human plasma renin of 1.9 nM and was only slightly less active against dog plasma renin activity.

Cardiovascular Pharmacology, Second Edition,
edited by Michael Antonaccio.
Raven Press, New York © 1984.

Central Transmitters: Physiology, Pharmacology, and Effects on the Circulation

Michael J. Antonaccio

Bristol-Myers Pharmaceutical Research and Development Division, Evansville, Indiana 47721

GENERAL ORGANIZATION OF CENTRAL NEURAL CONTROL

A very brief and, of necessity, incomplete description of the general organization of the central nervous system (CNS) with regard to the regulation of blood pressure and heart rate is given here. For a more complete and detailed review, the reader is referred to several excellent articles (1–8).

Lower Brainstem (Pons and Medulla)

Although originally thought of as the "vasomotor center" containing both vasodepressor and vasoconstrictor centers, the brainstem must now be considered as the most caudal link in a series of longitudinal systems in the brain, extending from as high as the cortex, that can control and integrate any number of efferent and afferent inputs for appropriate cardiovascular regulation. The medulla consists of a meshwork of interconnected and largely unspecific neurons described as the "reticular formation." The medulla not only organizes patterns of somatic motor and autonomic systems but also is responsible for the maintenance of normal levels of blood pressure and heart rate. Although there are certain areas in the brainstem that largely mediate pressor or depressor responses (and have therefore been labeled "centers") involving principally sympathetic excitation or inhibi-

tion of spinal sympathetic preganglionic neurons, these areas can also mediate opposing responses. They contain complex networks of interneurons that interact by inhibiting and exciting each other, thus causing any variety of mixed responses in the systemic circulation (3).

The medulla contains the nucleus of origin of cardiac vagal inhibitory fibers, most of which originate from the nucleus ambiguus (9). The nucleus ambiguus, in turn, receives a secondary excitatory neuron from the nucleus tractus solitarius (NTS), passing first through the medulla oblongata centralis (MOC). The NTS itself receives a large portion of the primary afferent fibers of the systemic baroreceptors and chemoreceptors and can act in at least three ways to regulate cardiovascular function (3): (a) It relays baroreceptor and chemoreceptor activity to other brainstem areas to modulate spinal preganglionic neurons. (b) It relays baroreceptor and chemoreceptor activity rostrally to such areas as the hypothalamus to regulate complex patterns of cardiovascular integration such as those occurring in the "defense reaction." (c) It participates in the regulation of body fluids and electrolytes through the control of antidiuretic and other hormones. Within the nucleus itself, carotid sinus afferent fibers can be inhibited presynaptically by hypothalamic stimulation. The NTS is heavily innervated by several types of nerve terminals with afferent neurotransmitters, and the possible role of these fibers in cardiovascular regulation will be discussed later.

The paramedian reticular nucleus (PRN) is a subnucleus of the medial reticular formation of the medulla and, unlike the NTS, does not have significant adrenergic innervation (3). This nucleus is also important in cardiovascular regulation, because it, too, receives afferent fibers from carotid sinus and aortic baroreceptors and is an area of interaction between baroreceptor and other inputs. Both vasodepressor and vasopressor responses can be obtained from stimulation of different neuronal groups from this nucleus.

The PRN also appears to mediate a powerful pressor response elicited by electrical stimulation of a cerebellar nucleus called the fastigial nucleus (10,11). The fastigial nucleus appears to receive inputs from the vestibular apparatus, which can occur on assumption of an upright posture. Thus, impulses for the orthostatic circulatory reflex are conveyed from the vestibular organs along the vestibular nerve to the fastigial nucleus in the cerebellum. The fastigial nucleus is then responsible for the increased sympathetic outflow that maintains blood pressure and increases heart rate when going from a supine position to a standing position.

In the dorsolateral pons, the nucleus parabrachialis (NPB) appears to play a significant role in cardiovascular control (12). It is heavily connected with other areas in the brainstem that control circulatory function, including the amygdala, hypothalamus, NTS, and medullary reticular formation and nucleus ambiguus. Electrical stimulation of the NPB results in increases in blood pressure and heart rate, effects unrelated to any effects on the NTS. The cardiovascular pattern observed after NPB stimulation is different from that occurring during the defense reaction (*vide infra*) and is quite powerful, suggesting that the NPB may play an important role in central cardiovascular control.

Electrical stimulation of the trigeminal complex in rabbits can cause hypotension and bradycardia, a pattern that has been named the trigeminal depressor response (13). The bradycardia is a consequence of both vagal activation and sympathetic activity to the heart, whereas the hypotension is mainly due to inhibition of sympathetic activity. Although functionally similar to baroreceptor activation, the trigeminal depressor response differs in its anatomical organization, because lesions of the NTS do not affect it. It has been suggested that this complex may serve to link the somatic and autonomic nervous system.

Hypothalamus

The hypothalamus region is one of the most important brain areas for controlling cardiovascular responses, because it can integrate inputs that involve somatic, endocrine, and autonomic functions, as well as emotional states. Stimulation of various areas of the hypothalamus can cause either vasopressor or vasodepressor responses, increases or decreases in heart rate, and interactions with baroreceptors. Much of the work involving the hypothalamus has centered on the defense reaction. Stimulation of the posterior hypothalamus produces changes throughout the organism that are strikingly similar to those occurring naturally during a "fight-or-flight" situation (4). From the circulatory standpoint, blood pressure, heart rate, muscular blood flow, and cardiac output are increased, whereas the baroreceptor reflexes are inhibited. Lesions of the posterior hypothalamus decrease blood pressure.

Both increases and decreases in blood pressure have been observed after stimulation of the anterior hypothalamus. In a study by Gauthier et al. (14), pressor sites were restricted to the ventral portion of the hypothalamus, and depressor responses to the dorsal area, suggesting a functional division of this area. Nathan and Reis (15) found that bilateral lesions of the anterior hypothalamus in rats resulted in hypertension, tachycardia, hyperthermia, and increased motor activity. These effects were prevented by bilateral adrenalectomy, adrenal demedullation, or adrenal denervation performed prior to lesioning. Thus, it appeared that the hypertension was due to a neurally mediated increase in peripheral resistance caused by the release of adrenal medullary catecholamines. This hypertension differed from that caused by bilateral lesions of the NTS, which result in central deafferentation of baroreceptors, because the pressure rise is mediated through an increased discharge of spinal preganglionic neurons resulting from the removal of an inhibitory drive from NTS neurons. Adrenalectomy has no effect on the development of "NTS hypertension." Although lesions of the anterior hypothalamus have consistently been reported to increase blood pressure, this may, in fact, be due to excitation of neurons in this area caused by irritation of ions deposited at the lesion sites by the lesioning electrodes (14).

Brody et al. (16) have established that electrical or chemical activation of tissue in the anterior hypothalamus encompassing the most anterior and ventral portion of the third ventricle, the AV3V area, results in a highly integrated cardiovascular pattern: hypertension that is a consequence of the net effects of vasoconstriction in mesenteric and renal vascular beds, and vasodilation in the hindquarters. In addition, this region is also partially responsible for the pressor response to peripherally, as well as centrally, administered angiotensin.

Lesions of the AV3V area prevent the pressor responses to central hypertonic saline and carbachol. In addition, lesions of the AV3V area prevent the development of several forms of hypertension, including two-kidney renal, DOCA-salt, and Dahl-strain salt-sensitive hypertension. Lesions of the AV3V also attenuate hypertension produced by lesions of the NTS and sectioning of the sinoaortic nerves. Interestingly, hypertension in spontaneously hypertensive rats (SHR) is neither decreased nor prevented from developing by AV3V lesions. The area of the AV3V is heavily innervated with noradrenergic and dopaminergic fibers. It will be important to determine if a causal relation exists between these fibers and changes occurring with AV3V manipulation.

It is again emphasized that, like the brainstem, the hypothalamus is not a "center" unto itself, but rather acts as a relay station to help produce and integrate longitudinally oriented patterns of effects. For instance, stimulation of the anterior hypothalamus causes sympathetic cholinergic vasodilation, an important physiological response that occurs in anticipation of exercise, as, for example, during the defense reaction. However, the sympathetic vasodilator neurons have their origin in the motor cortex, pass caudally to the hypothalamus, turn dorsally to the collicular area, make an abrupt turn ventrally, and pass through the ventrolateral portion of the medulla to the lateral horn of the spinal cord (17). Thus, although stimulation of one area may cause a particular response, the response itself should be considered in the context of the whole brain.

Limbic System and Cortex

The limbic system has a close anatomical and functional relationship with the hypothalamus and cortex. It seems to be particularly concerned with motivation and the expression of fear and rage, and it exerts a control over the autonomic system that is superimposed on that of the hypothalamus (4,18).

The cortex is especially involved in conditioned and learned cardiovascular responses. As mentioned previously, it is also responsible for anticipatory vasomotor adjustments such as vasodilation in skeletal muscles in situations of challenge. It has also been shown that the cortex can alter baroreceptor responses (5).

More definitive roles of the limbic and cortex areas in the regulation of circulatory responses must await further experimentation.

Many other areas of the brain can cause circulatory changes when stimulated electrically or by chemical activation. However, the normal physiological role of these areas remains unknown. The difficulty in attempting to ascribe a particular function to a particular

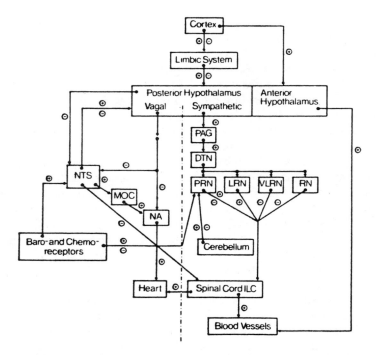

FIG. 1. Schematic representation of some of the CNS structures believed to play roles in the control of blood pressure and heart rate. The positive and negative signs indicate activation or inhibition of pathways, respectively, regardless of whether or not they are activating or inhibiting pathways in and of themselves. For example, activation of nucleus ambiguus (NA) is shown as positive, but it leads to a decrease in heart rate. PAG, periaqueductal gray; DTN, dorsal tegmental nucleus; LRN, lateral reticular nucleus; VLRN, ventrolateral reticular nucleus; RN, reticular nucleus; NTS, nucleus tractus solitarius; MOC, medulla oblongata centralis; NA, nucleus ambiguus; ILC, intermediolateral cell column.

area may be better perceived in Fig. 1, which shows only a few of the known interconnections of brain and muscle related to cardiovascular control.

CENTRAL TRANSMITTERS INVOLVED IN AUTONOMIC FUNCTIONS

The autonomic nervous system (ANS) plays a major role in the regulation of the circulation. Our knowledge of the pharmacology of the peripheral components of the ANS has built up gradually since the turn of the century. However, the neurochemistry of the central components of the ANS has been studied seriously for only a relatively short period of time.

Our knowledge of central neurotransmitters is still limited to acetylcholine, epinephrine,

norepinephrine, dopamine, serotonin, and a few other compounds. Among these it seems likely that γ-aminobutyric acid (GABA), histamine, glutamic acid, and other amino acids and peptides will all be proved to have central neurotransmitter roles. However, all of these putative transmitters together account for only a very small percentage of the neurons in the CNS. Many central neurons, both autonomic and somatic, probably utilize transmitter chemicals that have not yet been identified.

There is now a great deal of evidence that norepinephrine is an important neurotransmitter in central pathways subserving a cardiovascular function (19). There is also accumulating evidence that central serotonergic and epinephrine-containing nerves participate in circulatory control (17) and that central adrenergic tracts may contribute to central cardiovascular control. It should be stressed that most of the studies on central noradrenergic nerves were carried out before it was realized that epinephrine might also be involved. Hence, the experimental methods have generally not differentiated between epinephrine and norepinephrine. Therefore, most of the studies purporting to show involvement of noradrenergic neurons in effect merely demonstrate involvement of "catecholaminergic" nerves.

Central Pathways of Putative Transmitters

The intermediolateral cell column in the spinal cord is the origin of preganglionic sympathetic neurons. Descending projections from various areas of the brain and from various cell bodies containing different neurotransmitters that impinge on the intermediolateral cells are shown in Fig. 2. This figure shows only a few of the potential central systems that may alter cardiovascular function, and

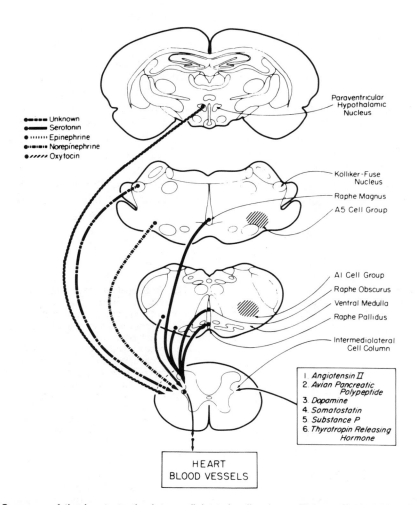

FIG. 2. Summary of the inputs to the intermediolateral cell column. The serotonergic inputs arise from the raphe pallidus, raphe obscurus, raphe magnus, and ventral medulla. The epinephrine input appears to arise from the region of the A_1 cell group. The norepinephrine input arises from the A_5 cell group. Other inputs come from the Kölliker-Fuse nucleus and paraventricular hypothalamic nucleus. (From Loewy and Neil, ref. 20, with permission.)

it is meant to be illustrative rather than comprehensive.

Noradrenergic fibers probably project to the spinal cord from the A_1, A_2, A_5, and other cell groups, whereas epinephrine fibers arise from A_1 and dopamine fibers from A_{11} and A_{13}. The serotonin input arises from the raphe nuclei and ventral medulla regions of B_1 and B_3. Several potential polypeptide pathways have also been suggested, but their cells of origin are unknown [see Loewy and Neil (20) for a review].

Mechanism of Baroreceptor Reflexes

The baroreceptor reflex arc is illustrated schematically in Fig. 3. This reflex is a homeostatic mechanism that serves to regulate arterial pressure through a negative-feedback loop that acts to minimize any change in pressure and return arterial pressure back toward its setpoint (2). This negative-feedback mechanism depends on the presence of inhibitory neurons between the afferent and efferent limbs of the reflex (Fig. 3). The afferent neurons arise from the carotid sinus and aortic arch and make their primary synapse in the NTS. The efferent limb effectively begins with bulbospinal neurons having their cell bodies in the brainstem in various "vasomotor" areas (VMC) and terminating in the intermediolateral cell columns of the spinal cord. Hence, the bulbospinal neurons synapse directly (or indirectly through short interneurons) with the sympathetic preganglionic neurons that pass out in the thoracolumbar outflow of the peripheral autonomic system (Fig. 3). The pathway between the NTS and the vasopressor areas (or VMC) is polysynaptic, and it is within this polysynaptic pathway that the inhibitory neurons are located. There is increasing evidence for modulation of baroreceptor reflex function from connections with higher centers, both ascending and descending (3). Activity in afferent fibers from arterial baroreceptors stimulated by a rise in pressure provides a major source of inhibition of central vasomotor tone and hence of peripheral sympathetic vasoconstrictor activity. Deafferentation of the arterial baroreceptors eliminates

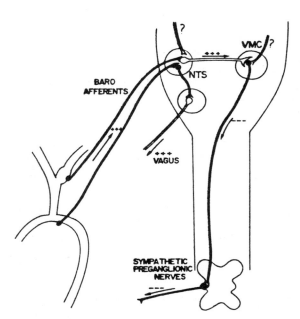

FIG. 3. Simplified schematic representation of baroreflex connections showing afferent nerves from arterial baroreceptors making their primary synapse in the nucleus of the tractus solitarius (NTS), inhibitory neurons from the NTS to the vasomotor center (VMC), descending facilitory bulbospinal vasomotor neurons, and sympathetic preganglionic nerves. Connections from the NTS to the vagal nuclei and efferent vagal fibers are also shown. Facilitory neurons are black, and inhibitory neurons are white. The half-black/half-white neurons connecting with the NTS and the VMC represent suprabulbar fibers that could be either inhibitory or facilitory. The plus and minus signs indicate the reciprocal relationship between afferent traffic and efferent sympathetic activity. The pluses indicate increases in activity and the minuses decreases. (From Chalmers, ref. 19, with permission.)

this inhibition and hence causes an increase in sympathetic activity and an increase in pressure, accompanied by tachycardia (2,19,21).

Potential Neurotransmitters of Baroreceptor and Chemoreceptor Afferents in the NTS

Catecholamines

Fluorescence microscopy has shown that the NTS is densely innervated with catecholaminergic fibers and that a cluster of catecholaminergic cells, designated the A_2 group, contributes to this innervation (22,23). This has led to the suggestion that catecholamines might normally be involved in centrally induced reflex bradycardia. Much evidence from early studies supported such a role. Electrolytic lesions of the NTS caused fulminating neurogenic hypertension and abolished baroreceptor reflexes (24,25). More selective lesions destroying only A_2 neurons in the NTS produced only a transient hypertension, with marked lability of blood pressure and inhibition of baroreflexes (26). Destruction of catecholaminergic nerve terminals by microinjection of 6-hydroxydopamine (6-OHDA) into the NTS similarly caused a transient hypertension, with lability of blood pressure and a decrease in baroreceptor sensitivity (27).

Pharmacological evidence has also supported a role for central catecholamines in reflex control mechanisms. Direct injection of α stimulants including epinephrine, norepinephrine, α-methylnorepinephrine, clonidine, and tyramine decreased blood pressure and/or heart rate when injected directly into the NTS. The order of potency of these α stimulants and the lack of effect of phenylephrine suggested that the receptor type involved was $α_2$ in nature. Moreover, $α_2$ receptor blockers were more effective in blocking these effects than were $α_1$ blockers (28). Finally, α blockers are also effective in reducing the effect of carotid sinus nerve stimulation when centrally administered. Thus, catecholaminergic neurons probably play a role in baroreceptor function.

However, catecholamines probably are not the primary transmitters of baroreceptor afferent fibers; rather, they probably have an indirect modulatory effect on these primary afferents. Several authors have found that there are several inputs to the NTS that are not catecholaminergic, including axons from hypothalamic nuclei, the fastigial nucleus, and the Kölliker-Fuse nucleus (29,30). In addition, some catecholaminergic neurons are located in the first presynaptic side of serial synapses, indicating a presynaptic modulation by catecholamines on synaptic transmission in the NTS. Similarly, severe central catecholamine depletion does not inhibit baroreceptor function (29).

In addition to A_2 neurons, A_1 neurons in the ventrolateral medulla are also catecholaminergic. Recently, lesions of this A_1 group have also been shown to result in hypertension and loss of the baroreceptor-vasoconstriction reflex in rabbits (31,32). It was suggested that this results from destruction of A_1 noradrenergic nerves that normally participate in baroreflex control of heart rate.

Catecholamines and suprabulbar effects on baroreflex function

Experiments in the rabbit have shown that sinoaortic denervation produces a selective increase in norepinephrine turnover in the hypothalamus and the thoracolumbar cord, measured by the rate of disappearance of intracisternally administered tritiated norepinephrine (33). The increase in hypothalamic norepinephrine turnover in this situation is consistent with the concept that baroreflex function is not mediated purely at medullary levels, but in fact utilizes neural loops involving higher centers. The selective increase in norepinephrine turnover in the thoracolumbar cord (there is no significant change in turnover rate in cervical segments) is consistent with an increase in the activity of bulbospinal noradrenergic nerves terminating in the lateral sympathetic horn. It should be noted that there are no monoaminergic cell bodies in the spinal cord, so that changes in norepinephrine metabolism in this region reflect changes in activity in the nerve endings of descending bulbospinal noradrenergic tracts. The observation that sinoaortic denervation accelerates norepinephrine turnover in the thoracolumbar cord has been supported by the finding that the activity of tyrosine hydroxylase, the rate-limiting enzyme in catecholamine biosynthesis, is also selectively increased in this region (33).

On the basis of these experiments, it was suggested that bulbospinal catecholaminergic nerves did, in fact, mediate baroreceptor reflexes and that at least some bulbospinal vasomotor neurons utilized catecholamines as neurotransmitters (33). This suggestion has been strengthened by the finding that destruction of central catecholaminergic nerves, using intracisternal administration of 6-OHDA, does in fact prevent and reverse the hypertension produced by sinoaortic denervation in the rabbit (34). Doba and Reis (24,25) have made similar observations in a different model of neurogenic hypertension, produced by central deafferentation of the baroreflexes using stereotactic lesions of the NTS in the rat. These workers have found that intracisternal 6-OHDA prevents the dramatic increase in pressure seen after this mode of baroreceptor deafferentation. However, other possibilities are discussed later.

It has also been shown (24) that destruction of catecholaminergic nerves in the NTS, by local stereotactic injection of 6-OHDA into this nucleus, produces an increase in blood pressure lasting about 10 days. These authors have therefore suggested that whereas bulbospinal noradrenergic nervous activity appears to facilitate an increase in pressure, the activity of catecholaminergic nerves synapsing in the NTS appears to depress arterial pressure (24). This suggestion is further supported by experiments in which local injection of norepinephrine into the NTS decreased arterial pressure in rats (35). The simplest explanation for this phenomenon might be that there are catecholaminergic nerves terminating in the NTS (originating either from high centers such as the hypothalamus, or elsewhere in the brainstem)

and synapsing with the inhibitory neurons drawn in Fig. 3. These inhibitory neurons might well be α-adrenoceptive neurons, as discussed later.

α Receptors and baroreceptor facilitation

Early studies with clonidine, a peripheral as well as central α stimulant, indicated that the drug could enhance reflex bradycardia (36–38). The enhancement was due to increased vagal activity, because it was abolished by atropine or vagotomy and persisted after sympathetic blockade by adrenergic neuron blockers or β receptor blockade. The enhancement of reflex bradycardia was due to an α stimulant effect, because it was blocked by α receptor antagonists. Moreover, the effect was mainly central in origin, because it occurred after direct central injection of clonidine and at much lower doses than those required intravenously. Although clonidine can cause an increase in impulse traffic in the aortic nerve and thereby exert its effects through a peripheral mechanism, the central actions appear to be of overwhelming importance [see Robson and Antonaccio (39) for a review]. The enhancement of reflex vagal bradycardia can be demonstrated for a large number of α agonists, including clonidine, xylazine, L-DOPA, naphazoline, phenylephrine, and oxymetazoline, and appears therefore to be a typical response to activation of central α receptors.

The site of action for the facilitation of the cardioinhibitory reflex appears to be localized in the medulla. It is suggested that α stimulation specifically at the NTS is what causes the facilitation of reflexes, because destruction of the NTS prevents the facilitation of reflex bradycardia, although the lowering of heart rate per se by the drug is not affected (40). In addition, lesions of the vagal centers of the brain also prevent the enhancement of reflex bradycardia. Thus, it seems that carotid sinus and aortic depressor nerve afferent fibers terminate in the NTS. Second-order neurons from the NTS then project to the vagal centers to activate the peripheral vagal component of the reflex. Stimulation of the NTS by α agonists enhances the vagal component of this reflex. Also, α blockers abolish the effects of carotid sinus nerve stimulation and of α stimulants (41). A diagrammatic representation is shown in Fig. 4.

The pharmacological effects of central α stimulation described earlier raise the possibility that catecholaminergic neurons might normally be involved in modulating reflex vagal bradycardia. However, the involvement of central cholinergic, glutaminergic, and substance P synapses in vagal cardioinhibitory responses has also been demonstrated (*vide infra*), and perhaps it is these neurons that transmit the impulses within the reflex loop (42). Thus, the information available at present allows the following considerations: The baroreceptor reflex chain in the CNS is probably not primarily catecholaminergic. However, α receptor activation, either through endogenous or exogenous means, facilitates reflex activity of the noradrenergic reflex loop either directly or indirectly by activation of a coupled catecholaminergic pathway(s) (42).

Paradoxically, the α stimulants such as clonidine, xylazine, and L-DOPA, although capable of enhancing reflex vagal bradycardia, also inhibit the carotid sinus reflex to a marked degree. In addition, carotid sinus debuffering does not alter the ability of clonidine and L-DOPA to enhance reflexes, whereas aortic nerve denervation prevents this effect (43). Enhancement by clonidine of the cardioinhibitory reflex initiated by aortic baroreceptor activation (but depression of the carotid sinus reflex) suggests that central modulations of these reflexes may differ.

Substance P

Substance P is an undecapeptide found in ganglia, spinal cord, and several areas of the

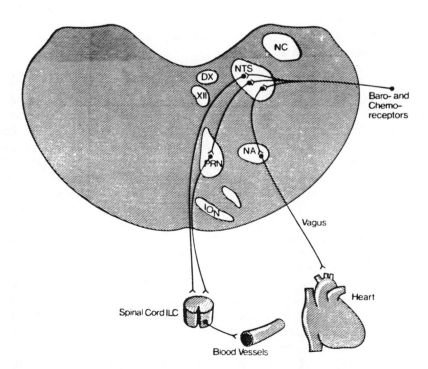

FIG. 4. Schematic representation of the medullary pathways involved in baroreceptor chemoreceptor reflexes. Pathway from NTS activates inhibitory fibers from the NA (vagal). All other fibers from the NTS are inhibitory. Notation the same as in Fig. 1. NC, cuneate nucleus; ION, inferior olivary nucleus; DX, nucleus of 10th cranial nerve; XII, nucleus of 12th cranial nerve.

brain (44,45). Anatomical, morphological, biochemical, and pharmacological evidence has been obtained to support the role of substance P as the neurotransmitter of baroreceptor afferent fibers. First, substance P is excitatory to nerve cells when applied iontophoretically (46). Using an immunohistochemical technique to localize substance P in the CNS, several authors have shown that the nodose and petrosal ganglia, containing the sensory cell bodies of baroreceptor and chemoreceptor afferent fibers, have very high levels of substance-P-immunoreactive (SP-I) material in both rats and cats. There was a nonuniform distribution of SP-I in the various regions of the NTS where baroreceptor and chemoreceptor fibers terminate. In these commissural and intermediate areas of the NTS, SP-I levels were significantly higher than in the caudal and rostral regions, the latter areas apparently playing no role in reflex activity. Moreover, chronic denervation of cranial nerves IX and X resulted in significant reductions in SP-I in the intermediate and commissural parts of the NTS (47).

In support of a neurotransmitter role for substance P in baroreflex and chemoreflex control, it has also been demonstrated that local application of either substance P or the nonpeptide capsaicin (which releases substance P from primary afferent fibers) to the region of the NTS results in hypotension and bradycardia (global administration of substance P into the brain produces hypertension and tachycardia) (48). Only in those areas of the NTS that responded to electrical activation of the baroreflex did microinjections of substance P produce similar cardiovascular effects. Such sites were located in the intermediate and commissural regions of the NTS that, as described earlier, contain the terminations of baroreceptor and chemoreceptor fibers and the highest levels of SP-I. Substance P nerve terminals, probably from cranial nerves IX and X, also form synapses with catecholaminergic cell bodies in the NTS that, as described earlier, may also play a modulating role on baroreflexes. However, it must be remembered

that destruction of central noradrenergic neurons by 6-OHDA, or depletion by reserpine plus α-methyl-p-tyrosine, does not affect the function of the baroreceptor reflex. Thus, it has been suggested that substance P is the primary neurotransmitter or neuromodulator released by afferents at the first synapse of the baroreceptor and chemoreceptor reflexes in the NTS (47,48).

On the other hand, Talman and Reis provide evidence contrary to such a role (49). In rats, they found that if there was careful control of the rate and volume of delivery of substance P injectates into the NTS, it never produced a fall in either blood pressure or heart rate, whereas L-glutamate always did. They suggested that previous studies demonstrating central actions of substance P when applied to the NTS were a consequence of local distortion, having demonstrated that microinjection of any substance into the NTS in sufficient volume invariably produced hypotension and bradycardia. Thus, the role of substance P in central cardiovascular control mechanisms remains undefined.

L-glutamate

L-glutamate is one of the most abundant amino acids in the brain, and on the basis of evidence derived primarily from microiontophoretic studies, it has been proposed to be an excitatory neurotransmitter in the CNS (50). Several lines of evidence suggest that L-glutamate may be (as was claimed earlier for substance P) the neurotransmitter of baroreceptor afferent nerve fibers. Two weeks after removal of the right nodose ganglion in rats, there was about a 40% reduction in high-affinity L-glutamate uptake in both the ipsilateral and contralateral NTS (51). Local unilateral injection of either L-glutamate or its rigid analogue kainic acid into the NTS resulted in dose-dependent reductions in blood pressure and heart rate (52). These effects were strictly limited to the intermediate third of the NTS, where baroreceptor afferent fibers terminate. Moreover, microinjection of the glutamate antagonist glutamic acid diethylester will block the cardiovascular consequences of central L-glutamate administration, as well as baroreceptor activation (53).

Further studies by Talman et al. have provided further evidence that L-glutamine is important in baroreflex control mechanisms. Whereas low doses of kainic acid were once again shown by these authors to reduce blood pressure and heart rate when unilaterally injected into the intermediate NTS of rats, bilateral injections of higher doses of kainic acid produced baroreflex blockade and neurogenic hypertension (54). These authors suggested that the baroreflexlike reductions in blood pressure and heart rate evoked by low doses of kainic acid injected into the NTS resulted from excitation of intrinsic NTS neurons that mediate baroreflexes. At the higher doses, kainic acid produced functional blockade of baroreflexes because of depolarization of NTS neurons. Because bilateral lesions of the NTS produced the same type and degree of hypertension as high doses of kainic acid, these effects seem to be entirely a consequence of impaired function of intrinsic neurons of the NTS.

Central administration of L-glutamate into the fastigial nucleus in dogs produced a pressor response, as did electrical stimulation of this nucleus (55). Partial unilateral lesions of the fastigial nucleus also partially reduced the L-glutamate pressor response. When injected into the cisterna magna in dogs, both L-glutamate and kainic acid produced dose-dependent increases in blood pressure and reductions in heart rate because of sympathetic activation, kainic acid being some 1,000 times as potent as glutamic acid (56). Finally, kainic acid applied to the ventral surfaces of the medulla in cats caused a biphasic effect on blood pressure: namely, an increase followed by a profound and prolonged decrease (57).

Although it is difficult to ascribe any physiological role for glutamate based on these latter studies, one can readily point to the similarities of the general pressor responses produced by substance P and glutamate when globally administered in the brain, as opposed to the hypotension and bradycardia produced by both substances when applied only to the intermediate NTS. Similarly, the anatomical distributions of substance P and glutamate are strikingly parallel. The very close similarities among the pharmacology, distributions, and proposed functions of substance P and L-glutamate raise the question whether or not these two substances play similar roles in baroreflexes, either in separate or identical neurons.

PUTATIVE CENTRAL NEUROTRANSMITTERS AND EFFECTS ON THE CIRCULATION

Catecholamines and Central α, Dopamine, and β Receptors

Effects on Blood Pressure and Heart Rate

α Receptors

Direct α receptor stimulation of most areas of the brain involved in cardiovascular regulation causes hypotension and bradycardia. Thus, the α stimulants norepinephrine, epinephrine, dopamine, α-methylnorepinephrine, clonidine, phenylephrine, and various others have been demonstrated to cause decreases in blood pressure and/or heart rate when injected into the anterior hypothalamus, medulla, or NTS, when applied onto the ventral surface of the medulla, and when given into the ventricular system or perfused through the vertebral artery (58–68). These effects are accompanied by decreases in cardiac, renal, and splanchnic nerve discharges that probably are responsible for the circulatory changes (58,69). Furthermore, these effects can be blocked by α receptor blockers, suggesting the presence of inhibitory α receptors in many areas of the brain that have been demonstrated to cause substantial cardiovascular changes.

In addition to the hypotension and bradycardia caused by direct central administration of dopamine, norepinephrine, and epinephrine, precursors to the synthesis of these compounds also decrease blood pressure and heart rate. The synthesis of catecholamines in the brain is controlled by the first enzyme in the biosynthetic pathway: tyrosine hydroxylase. Administration of excess tyrosine in the diet, by intravenous or intraperitoneal injection, or directly into the brain causes substantial reductions in blood pressure and heart rate in normotensive, DOCA-salt-hypertensive, spontaneously hypertensive, and two-kidney, one-clip renal-hypertensive rats (70–72). In contrast, the amino acids leucine, isoleucine, valine, alanine, aspartate, and arginine are without effect in SHR (70). Tyrosine's central cardiovascular actions are apparently due to its ability to increase central catecholaminergic activity, with concomitant release of norepinephrine and/or epinephrine, because MOPEG-SO$_4$ levels also rise after tyrosine (72). An alternative suggestion was made by Edwards, who showed that the production of tyramine and octopamine, but not catecholamine metabolites, was increased by tyrosine administration (73). He suggested that this increased production of tyramine and octopamine, both indirectly acting amines, might be responsible for the antihypertensive effects of tyrosine.

Another precursor to the catecholamines that is formed from L-tyrosine is L-DOPA. Administration of L-DOPA, either directly into the CNS or intravenously after extracerebral decarboxylase inhibition with MK-486 to prevent peripheral catecholamine formation, results in marked decreases in blood pressure and heart rate (74–78). In addition, the carotid sinus reflex and reflex responses elicited in preganglionic white rami and postganglionic renal nerves are also markedly depressed (79–83). Moreover, L-DOPA decreases spontaneous sympathetic nerve discharges in cardiac, renal, and splanchnic nerves, and this probably is responsible for the depression of blood pressure and heart rate (69,83,84). The location of the site of action of L-DOPA has been placed at either the medulla or spinal cord, because midcollicular decerebration in rats or transection of the upper border of the medulla-pons in dogs does not alter the central effects

of L-DOPA (85,86). Spinal transection abolishes them.

It is certain that L-DOPA must be decarboxylated in the brain to dopamine and/or norepinephrine, because central decarboxylation prevents the hypotensive and bradycardic actions of L-DOPA. However, whether L-DOPA acts through dopamine or norepinephrine or both is unclear. Both dopamine and norepinephrine caused hypotension, bradycardia, and reductions in sympathetic nerve activity when injected directly into the brain or ventricular system in rats, cats, and dogs (69,87,88). Biochemical studies in animals (85,89,90) and humans (91) have indicated that dopamine is the major catecholamine formed after the administration of L-DOPA. Nonetheless, it has been demonstrated that in rats and cats, the hypotensive effects of L-DOPA may be due to norepinephrine—perhaps by displacement by dopamine—because inhibition of dopamine-beta-hydroxylase prevents the effects of L-DOPA (74,92). In dogs, however, dopamine-β-hydroxylase inhibition has no effect on the cardiovascular actions of L-DOPA. This would suggest that dopamine itself is the metabolite responsible. However, neither dopamine nor α receptor blockade in the brain alters the hypotensive effect of L-DOPA, whereas serotonin receptor blockade attenuates it (93). Depletion of serotonin stores with parachlorophenylalanine (*vide infra*) is also effective in inhibiting the actions of L-DOPA. Similarly, both L-DOPA and 5-hydroxytryptophan (5HTP), the serotonin precursor, were found to depress sympathetic preganglionic reflexes. The close resemblance of the centrally mediated cardiovascular effects of L-DOPA and 5HTP (*vide infra*) may therefore indicate a common reliance on serotonergic stimulation.

Because α stimulants of various structural types are capable of reducing blood pressure and heart rate when they reach appropriate central structures, it seems clear that, indeed, α stimulation is responsible for the effect. However, there are now considered to be α_1 and α_2 receptors both peripherally and centrally. Recently, a good case has been made for the suggestion that the central hypotensive α-adrenoreceptors are of the α_2 type. The reader is referred to other publications for more complete discussion of this point (67,68).

Unlike other areas of the brain, the posterior hypothalamus most typically responds to norepinephrine by causing a pressor response. Electrical stimulation of the posterior hypothalamus elicits a rise in blood pressure along with a host of other somatic and autonomic effects, all of which together have been termed the "defense reaction." Evidence has accumulated to indicate that the hypothalamic pressor response may be due to the release of catecholamines (most likely norepinephrine) from the hypothalamus. The evidence is biochemical, anatomical, morphological, and pharmacological. The posterior hypothalamus contains very high concentrations of norepinephrine located in adrenergic nerve terminals that originate mainly from cell bodies located in the pontine locus ceruleus (94,95). Stimulation of the locus ceruleus causes a pressor response that is reduced by hypothalamic lesions (96). Direct electrical stimulation of various hypothalamic nuclei causes large rises in blood pressure and enhances the release of catecholamines from the hypothalamus (97). This pressor effect is enhanced by superfusion of the hypothalamus with desipramine (DMI). Presumably, DMI inhibits the reuptake of released norepinephrine into nerve endings and thereby enhances the effects of electrical stimulation (98). Perfusion of the hypothalamus with bretylium, which inhibits the release of norepinephrine from nerve endings, reduces the effects of hypothalamic nerve stimulation on blood pressure (99). Destruction of catecholaminergic nerve endings in the hypothalamus by prior pretreatment with 6-OHDA does not affect resting blood pressure but reduces the rise in pressure elicited by electrical stimulation (99). Furthermore, superfusion of the hypothalamus with norepinephrine or epinephrine causes marked rises in blood pressure that are also enhanced by DMI.

The pressor response caused by hypothalamic activation appears to be due to α receptor activation, because it is inhibited by central α receptor blockade; in addition, superfusion of the posterior hypothalamus with the α receptor stimulant, clonidine, enhances pressor responses to hypothalamic stimulation (100). Interestingly, α receptor stimulation in the NTS of the medulla diminishes the pressor responses to electrical stimulation of the hypothalamus, whereas α receptor blockade of the NTS enhances them (100). Thus, at least two adrenergic systems can influence responses to hypothalamic stimulation: one located in the posterior hypothalamus to promote rises in blood pressure and the other located in the caudal medulla to inhibit them. It is emphasized here that the pressor effects of catecholamines seem to be highly localized for the posterior hypothalamus, because injections of norepinephrine or other α stimulants into the anterior hypothalamus or other areas of the brain lead to hypotension and bradycardia. The involvement of central α and β receptors in the regulation of blood pressure will be discussed more completely later.

Dopamine receptors

The cardiovascular effects of dopamine are very complicated. Dopamine and other dopamine receptor stimulants may affect blood pressure (a) by causing direct vasodilation by stimulation of dopamine receptors in the peripheral vasculature, (b) by inhibiting the release of norepinephrine by stimulation of presynaptic dopamine receptors on peripheral and central noradrenergic nerve terminals, and (c) by directly stimulating central dopamine presynaptic and postsynaptic receptors. This is further complicated by the level of anesthesia and whether or not a particular agent gets into the brain when peripherally administered.

In anesthetized cats and rats, central administration of dopamine or dopamine receptor stimulants reduces blood pressure by direct activation of dopamine receptors, because this effect is selectively blocked by dopamine receptor antagonists (69,101,102). In anesthetized dogs, central dopamine has little or no effect on blood pressure. In contrast, central dopamine administration causes hypertension and tachycardia in conscious cats and dogs, an effect that is unaltered by β or α receptor blockade (103,104). Thus, the importance of anesthesia is clear in attempting to elucidate the role of central receptors in cardiovascular control (*vide infra*).

The antihypertensive effects of other dopamine stimulants, including pergolide, lergotrile, and *N,N*-di-*n*-propyldopamine, are largely peripheral in origin, although the bradycardia may have a central component (105–107); see Cavero and Lefevre-Borg (108) for a review.

β Receptors

Unlike the consistent effects (hypotension and bradycardia) observed in all species after intracerebroventricular injections of α agonists, circulatory effects observed after either central β receptor stimulation or blockade have been rather inconsistent. In general, central β receptor stimulation with agonists such as isoproterenol and salbutamol causes increases in heart rate in cats, rabbits, mice, and dogs (60,109,110), although bradycardia has also been reported to occur after central isoproterenol administration in cats and dogs (60). The tachycardia probably is not due to peripheral leakage of the β stimulant, because it is abolished by peripheral ganglion blockade or adrenergic neuron blockade. Furthermore, central β receptor blockade prevents the tachycardia caused by central β receptor stimulation (60).

The blood pressure effects caused by central β stimulation are not clearly defined. Both pressor and depressor effects have been noted in the same species by the same investigators, and in other species by different investigators (60). The great degree of variability may be due to the existence of two or more types of β receptors in brain, inefficient absorption or distribution to the required structure, differential metabolism, or simply nonspecific effects.

Although central administration of β blockers has been shown to cause hypotension, it is still not certain whether or not this effect is due to β blockade, because the dextro isomers, which are essentially devoid of β blocking properties, have also been reported to decrease blood pressure (111). The *l*-isomers but not *d,l*-isomers of propranolol and practolol reduce preganglionic sympathetic nerve activity and may thereby decrease blood pressure (112,113). However, sotalol, a β blocker with antihypertensive actions, is devoid of this effect.

Although many workers have sought to implicate "central resetting of baroreceptors" in the central hypotensive action of β blockers, the evidence for this is not substantial. Experiments in which baroreceptor function was tested following intracerebroventricular administration of propranolol in conscious rabbits failed to demonstrate any central effects on baroreceptor function, as judged by the heart rate responses to changes in arterial pressure produced using inflatable balloons around the aorta and venae cavae (114). However, it is important to note that the rapid leakage of β blocking agents across the blood-brain barrier in some species can cause significant degrees of peripheral β-adrenoceptive blockade (114).

Central Catecholamine Depletion with 6-OHDA

Administration of 6-OHDA into the CSF in normal rabbits produces a biphasic response similar to that seen with intravenous 6-OHDA. There is an initial transient increase in pressure, lasting about 5 min; this is seen only in unanesthetized animals and probably is due to release of the catecholamine transmitter (115). This is followed by a fall in pressure lasting a few hours (34,115,116), attributable to direct action of 6-OHDA on central inhibitory α-adrenoceptive neurons (116) leading to withdrawal of peripheral α-adrenergic vasoconstrictor tone (34,116). Permanent destruction of central catecholaminergic nerves by

6-OHDA has no permanent effects on resting arterial pressure in normal animals (34,116). Yet ablation of the peripheral components of the autonomic system by combined chemical sympathectomy and adrenalectomy lowers arterial pressure in animals (117,118).

However, intracisternal administration of 6-OHDA in the rabbit causes a permanent 30% reduction in heart rate (24,34,116). This bradycardia has been shown to be mediated peripherally mainly through increased vagal activity, because it can be blocked by intravenous atropine (24,34). It is also in part due to withdrawal of sympathetic drive, because it can be reduced by pretreatment with intravenous propranolol (34). Thus, it seems that intracisternal 6-OHDA destroys central catecholaminergic nerves that normally inhibit the vagus and thus causes a bradycardia by central vagal disinhibition. The 6-OHDA also destroys bulbospinal catecholaminergic nerves that normally facilitate cardic sympathetic drive, once again contributing to the bradycardia. Because there are few, if any, descending long aminergic tracts in the brain, it seems likely that the inhibitory fibers acting on the vagal nuclei are located within the brainstem itself, although they could possibly originate in the hypothalamus. These inhibitory fibers do not terminate on the NTS, the primary central baroreceptor reflex synapse, because NTS lesions do not cause bradycardia (25). Therefore, this inhibitory catecholaminergic tract probably terminates on a secondary synapse beyond the NTS.

Although destruction of central catecholaminergic nerves does not affect blood pressure in normotensive animals, there is evidence to indicate that activation of central catecholaminergic cell bodies and tracts can affect blood pressure and heart rate. Inhibition of sympathetic activity was obtained by stimulation in the ventrolateral medulla, where a group of catecholamine-containing cell bodies projecting to the spinal cord is situated (82). Both spontaneous sympathetic activity and supraspinal and spinal somatosympathetic reflex discharges were depressed. Pharmacological

evidence also supports this suggestion, as described earlier.

Prostaglandins and Bradykinin

Prostaglandin E_1 (PGE_1) and PGE_2 both caused increases in blood pressure and heart rate when centrally administered either by carotid or vertebral artery perfusion or when injected intracerebroventricularly in rats, cats, dogs, and goats (119–122). This effect was apparently a consequence of increasing central sympathetic outflow.

PGI_2 (prostacyclin), on the other hand, caused a dose-related decrease in blood pressure in conscious rats (121). However, high doses were required, and it was not clearly demonstrated that this powerful direct vasodilator did not leak into the periphery to cause its effects. PGF_2 has been reported either to increase blood pressure in rats or to have no effect (121,123).

Bradykinin causes a consistent increase in blood pressure in conscious rats when injected directly either into the ventricular system of the brain or into the septum (120,121,124–126). This pressor effect is apparently mediated by the release of pressor prostaglandins in the brain, because inhibition of prostaglandin synthesis by indomethacin prevents the bradykinin pressor response (120,126). Correa and Graeff (124) showed that the increase in blood pressure following intraseptal administration of bradykinin could be blocked by α blockers but not blockers of histamine, serotonin, cholinergic, opioid, or α receptors, thus suggesting an indirect stimulation of central α receptors as the final pathway, perhaps through the posterior hypothalamus.

Prostaglandins are normally found in the brain. However, inhibition of central prostaglandin synthesis has no effect on blood pressure (121,126), suggesting that prostaglandins do not normally play a physiological role in central blood pressure regulation. Furthermore, I am not aware of studies indicating that bradykinin is found in the brain. This fact, plus the high doses of bradykinin required to demonstrate an effect, also make it improbable that bradykinin plays a significant role in the normal central regulation of the circulation.

Cyclic Nucleotides

Cyclic AMP is found in high concentrations in various areas of the brain. It has been proposed as the second messenger of many neurotransmitters in the brain, including norepinephrine, histamine, and others. Therefore, it is possible that cyclic AMP plays a role in the central regulation of blood pressure as well (127).

Direct central administration of dibutyryl cyclic AMP, an analogue of cyclic AMP that is capable of penetrating cells, causes increases in blood pressure and heart rate in cats and rats that are due to an increase in sympathetic nervous activity (128–131). This effect is apparently suprabulbar, because administration of dibutyryl cyclic AMP has no effect when administered into the cisterna magna, but it is quite active after injection into the lateral or third ventricle. Moreover, the pathway(s) activated by dibutyryl cyclic AMP are catecholaminergic, because phentolamine or 6-OHDA pretreatment reduced the response, whereas 5,6-dihydroxytryptamine was without effect (130).

A number of drugs known to increase cyclic AMP levels by activating adenyl cyclase, including TRH, tetracosactide, the β stimulant NAB365, histamine, and ATP, all increased blood pressure after injection into the lateral ventricle in cats (128). Similarly, inhibitors of phosphodiesterase that prevent degradation of cyclic AMP, including theophylline, RO7/2956, papaverine, aminophylline, and RA642, all increased blood pressure and heart rate when centrally administered to cats and rats (131,132). Moreover, activators of adenyl cyclase via the catalytic subunit of the receptor-enzyme complex, including sodium fluoride and guanylyl-imido-diphosphate, caused marked increases in blood pressure when centrally administered. Finally, activators of

phosphodiesterase, such as imidazole, exert centrally mediated hypotensive effects (133).

In contrast, central administration of cyclic GMP either decreased blood pressure and heart rate or antagonized the pressor effect of cyclic AMP (133).

Based on the foregoing results, it has been suggested that cyclic nucleotides are a common final biochemical endpoint for the explanation of actions of various neurotransmitters having central cardiovascular effects. Obviously, much more information is needed before any firm conclusions can be drawn.

GABA

The last few years have seen renewed interest in the potential role of GABA in central regulation of blood pressure and heart rate. As has often been the case for other neurotransmitter systems, this has largely been the result of the development of new powerful tools that can be used to pharmacologically manipulate the GABAergic neuron and receptor.

The first report relating GABA to cardiovascular changes was by Takahashi et al. (134), who found that GABA caused a fall of blood pressure in rabbits when injected intravenously and that its effect was the most powerful among γ-amino acids. In a later report (135), these authors discussed the mechanism and site of action of GABA with remarkable prescience. In experiments performed in rabbits, dogs, and cats, they reached the following conclusions: (a) GABA caused centrally mediated reductions in blood pressure and heart rate, because GABA had no direct vascular or ganglionic blocking properties, but its effects were themselves prevented by sympathetic denervation or ganglion blockade. (b) The vagus, aortic depressor, and carotid sinus nerves were not necessary for the antihypertensive and bradycardic actions of GABA. (c) The region of the CNS responsible for the effect of GABA was caudal to the cerebrum and probably in the medulla.

Bhargava et al. (136,137) found that although GABA probably had a minor peripheral hypotensive action in dogs, the compound caused bradycardia and hypotension of central origin in both dogs and cats. Furthermore, pressor responses to both bilateral carotid artery occlusion and direct electrical stimulation of medullary vasomotor neurons were inhibited by large intraventricular doses (1 mg/kg) of GABA, further supporting central vasomotor depression by GABA. These authors were the first to explicitly implicate inhibition of central sympathetic neuronal activity as being responsible for both the bradycardia and reductions in blood pressure observed after GABA.

Hedwall et al. (138) examined the effects of several ω-amino acids on blood pressure, catecholamine stores, and the pressor response to physostigmine in the two-kidney one-clip renal-hypertensive rat. Orally administered GABA (300 mg/kg daily for 4 days) was without effect on blood pressure. However, intraperitoneal administration of GABA (1,000 mg/kg daily for 4 days) caused reductions in blood pressure similar to those caused by the same treatment schedule with α-methyldopa (300 mg/kg p.o.). This treatment with GABA had no effect on either cardiac or brain norepinephrine concentrations or on pressor responses to physostigmine, suggesting a central mechanism of action.

Guertzenstein (139) applied several substances to the ventral surfaces of the brainstem in anesthetized cats. Fairly high concentrations of GABA, as well as glycine, carbachol, and physostigmine, caused a fall in arterial blood pressure. In a difficult-to-interpret study, 20 μg of GABA "injected into the spinal cord" in anesthetized dogs caused a marked but transient reduction in blood pressure and abolished the reflex depressor response to sciatic nerve stimulation (140).

In a study of the effects of several amino acids on colonic temperature, arterial blood pressure, and behavior in conscious normotensive rats, Sgaragli and Pavan (141) found that intracisternal administrations of taurine, glycine, alanine, and GABA (80 mmoles/kg) all caused reductions in blood pressure. Taurine

was found to have the most pronounced effect and glycine the most prolonged, whereas alanine and GABA caused the least and shortest reduction in blood pressure.

Philippu et al. (142) superfused the hypothalamus in anesthetized cats with GABA to determine its effects on the release of catecholamines and the rise in blood pressure elicited by electrical stimulation of the posterior area of the hypothalamus. They found that GABA reduced blood pressure when injected into the third ventricle, but not when superfused into the posterior hypothalamus.

Because of the difficulties of working with large doses of GABA administered directly into the CNS, muscimol was used as a postsynaptic GABA agonist tool for further probing the potential role of GABA in the central regulation of blood pressure, and an attempt was made to systematically examine the central effects of GABA, glycine, and muscimol on blood pressure, heart rate, and renal sympathetic nervous discharge in anesthetized cats. It was demonstrated that both GABA and muscimol decreased blood pressure and heart rate, with parallel reductions in renal sympathetic nervous discharge, the latter effect being the first definitive proof for the central sympathetic inhibitory mechanism of GABA on blood pressure and heart rate. The hemodynamic as well as the sympathetic nerve effects were reversed by bicuculline, a reasonably specific GABA receptor antagonist (143). Furthermore, muscimol was found to be about 1,000 times as potent as GABA, thus eliminating the need for high doses of GABA previously required. Although central glycine also reduced blood pressure and heart rate, its effects were small in comparison with GABA and required very large doses. In a subsequent study (144), it was demonstrated that (a) the effects of muscimol were totally through a central mechanism, (b) its effects were due to specific postsynaptic GABA stimulation, because they were reversed by bicuculline but not strychnine, and (c) baroreceptors were not necessary for the effect. An example of the effects of muscimol is shown in Fig. 5.

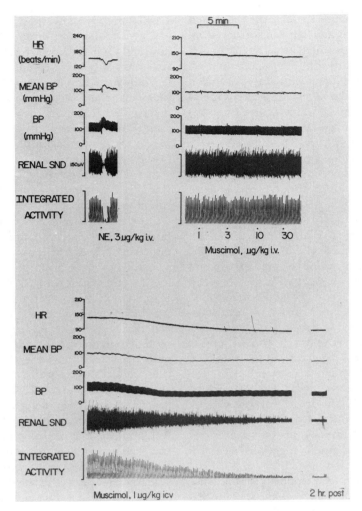

FIG. 5. Effects of muscimol on blood pressure (BP), heart rate (HR), and renal sympathetic nervous discharge (RENAL SND) in an anesthetized cat. Intravenous muscimol in doses as high as 30 μg/kg had no effect, whereas only 1 μg/kg given into the third ventricle had profound and long-lasting effects. (From Antonaccio et al., ref. 144, with permission.)

Several other studies have demonstrated the central hypotensive action of muscimol and GABA in anesthetized cats. A 10% solution of GABA applied to the exposed surface of the medulla oblongata in anesthetized cats reduced blood pressure by about 30% (145,146). Sweet et al. (147,148) showed that muscimol reduced both blood pressure and heart rate only when administered centrally; however, these authors observed only small changes af-

ter GABA. Similarly, Williford et al. (149) and Gillis et al. (150) also reported that muscimol reduced blood pressure and heart rate only when centrally administered. They further showed that pretreatment with the GABA receptor antagonist bicuculline, at a dose that had no effect by itself, prevented the effects of muscimol.

The pharmacological and anatomical specificity of the cardiovascular effects produced by central GABA receptor modulation has also been demonstrated. Clonidine is an antihypertensive agent whose central effects are mediated by α receptor stimulation. Muscimol administration after clonidine had no antagonistic effect, but rather caused further reductions in blood pressure and heart rate. Similarly, bicuculline did not prevent the reductions in blood pressure and heart rate caused by clonidine. Conversely, the reductions in blood pressure and heart rate initially observed after GABA antagonists were reversed by muscimol, but not by piperoxane, an α receptor antagonist that reversed the cardiovascular effects of clonidine (150). Finally, clonidine decreases blood pressure and heart rate at a locus in the caudal medulla, whereas muscimol acts at the anterior medulla (151).

Other GABA Agonists

Given the results with GABA and muscimol, one would anticipate that all postsynaptic GABA receptor stimulants would decrease blood pressure, heart rate, and renal sympathetic nervous discharge by centrally mediated reductions in sympathetic outflow, if GABA receptors indeed play any role in central cardiovascular regulation. Thus far, this seems to be the case. In addition to muscimol and GABA itself, the GABA agonists THIP (152), imidazole-4-acetic acid (153), isoguvacine (151), and kojic amine (147,148) all reduced blood pressure, heart rate, and renal sympathetic nervous discharge (the latter not measured for kojic amine) in anesthetized cats by a central mechanism. Moreover, the observed reductions in blood pressure were reasonably correlated with the ability of the GABA agonists to bind to postsynaptic GABA receptors *in vitro*, suggesting a cause-and-effect relationship (154).

Baclofen, β-(4-chlorophenyl)-GABA, represents a special problem when dealing with GABA receptor agonists. Despite its close structural similarity to GABA, baclofen is not usually considered to be a GABA receptor agonist, because its effects are not blocked by

GABA antagonists (155,156). It does not displace ^{3}H-GABA in receptor binding studies (157), nor does its pharmacological profile mimic that of GABA (158). However, recently it has been shown that baclofen can displace low-affinity but not high-affinity ^{3}H-GABA binding (159). Furthermore, studies by Bowery et al. (155,156) demonstrated that baclofen decreased neurotransmitter release in brain and periphery by acting at a bicuculline-insensitive novel GABA receptor. Thus, baclofen may be a weak GABA mimetic acting at a heretofore unidentified GABA receptor.

In anesthesized cats, central administration of baclofen caused marked reductions in blood pressure and heart rate (147,148). Similarly, in anesthetized and conscious rats, low doses of baclofen given intravenously caused reductions in blood pressure and heart rate (160,161). However, after higher doses of baclofen, the predominant effects were pronounced and long-lasting increases in blood pressure and heart rate. The hypertension and tachycardia were of central origin and were mediated by the sympathetic nervous system, because they were prevented by spinal cord section and sympatholytic agents (161,162). Persson (162) showed that the locus of action for baclofen is the NTS, because local application of a very small dose of baclofen (50 ng) into this area caused a consistent pressor response. Furthermore, the reflex heart rate reduction to norepinephrine was prevented by intravenous as well as NTS administration of baclofen. The cardiovascular effects of baclofen are consistent and interesting, but their relationship to GABA receptor involvement is not yet established.

Site of Action of Hypotensive Effect

The central site of action of GABA agonists to decrease blood pressure appears to be unique both anatomically and pharmacologically. Williford et al. (149) monitored changes in blood pressure during administration of muscimol into either the left lateral ventricle (restricting the drug to the lateral and third ventricles by cannulating the cerebral aqueduct) or the fourth ventricle. They found that muscimol had no effect on blood pressure when restricted to the lateral and third ventricles; in contrast, administration of muscimol into the fourth ventricle caused reductions in blood pressure that were comparable to those observed when the same dose was administered into the entire ventricular system. Snyder and Antonaccio (151) found that when muscimol was prevented from reaching the fourth ventricle by collecting the perfusate at the caudal end of the cerebral aqueduct, the largest dose produced a reduction of blood pressure that was less than 15%. Thus, these results are all consistent with a primary site of action for GABA agonists at the level of the fourth ventricle. However, unlike clonidine, L-DOPA, and other hypotensive agents, GABA agonists act at the anterior portion, as opposed to the caudal portion, of the medulla. Administration of muscimol into the caudal region of the fourth ventricle failed to alter blood pressure, heart rate, or renal sympathetic nerve discharge, whereas localization of muscimol to the anterior region of the fourth ventricle produced large reductions in blood pressure and heart rate (151).

Interestingly, pretreatment or simultaneous infusion with bicuculline into the cerebral aqueduct had no effect on blood pressure but prevented the hypotensive effects of muscimol (149,151).

GABA Antagonists

Bicuculline, an isoquinoline alkaloid, is the most widely used GABA receptor antagonist. It was first introduced by Curtis et al. (163), who convincingly demonstrated that bicuculline antagonized only the inhibitory spinal effects of GABA and "GABA-like" amino acids, but was without any effect on glycine and "glycine-like" amino acids (164). Later biochemical experiments provided strong confirmatory evidence that bicuculline was indeed a competitive GABA receptor antagonist and

displaced ^{3}H-GABA from postsynaptic membranes from rat brain.

Picrotoxin was also initially thought to be a GABA receptor antagonist. Like bicuculline, it is a convulsant and an antagonist of GABA at a number of inhibitory synapses (165). However, unlike bicuculline, picrotoxin is a noncompetitive antagonist in vivo and does not bind to GABA receptors in vitro. Rather, it appears to act in a manner not yet defined at the level of the GABA receptor regulator, chloride ionophore (157).

The effects of picrotoxin on blood pressure were widely studied and described through 1977 (166–172). Even its location of action has been tentatively established (171,172). However, virtually no attempts were made in these studies to relate the effects of picrotoxin to its ability to block the effects of GABA. With respect to bicuculline, virtually no cardiovascular studies were performed with it prior to 1977.

In an early study, it was demonstrated that both picrotoxin and bicuculline could reverse the cardiovascular effects of both muscimol and GABA, and it was suggested that its effects were the result of GABA receptor antagonism (143). Similar results were obtained in a later study (144).

DiMicco et al. (171–174) showed that both picrotoxin and bicuculline produced a biphasic response: first a decrease in blood pressure followed by an increase, effects that were prevented by spinal transection. Localizing the drugs to the third and lateral ventricles resulted only in increases in blood pressure (173), whereas perfusion of the fourth ventricle by cannulation of the cerebral aqueduct had no effect on blood pressure but counteracted or prevented the effects of muscimol (149,151).

Thus, unlike GABA agonists, which decrease blood pressure and renal sympathetic nervous discharge by stimulation of GABA receptors in the anterior medulla, GABA antagonists have the opposite effect, but at a site in the forebrain. Therefore, it seems apparent that there is a tonically active GABA system in forebrain that normally inhibits sympathetic outflow to blood vessels (150).

In addition to effects on central sympathetic activation, both bicuculline and picrotoxin cause release of large amounts of vasopressin and marked hypertension when applied to the rostral, but not caudal, ventral surface of the medulla (175). Therefore, GABA may also have a tonic inhibitory influence on vasopressin release in the brain.

Heart Rate Effects of GABA Agonists and Antagonists

Stimulation of central GABA receptors with muscimol results in bradycardia that apparently is totally mediated by a reduction in sympathetic tone to the heart. We have observed no differences in heart rate reductions after muscimol in groups of cats with vagi intact, in comparison with those with vagi bilaterally sectioned (143,144). Similarly, vagotomy had no effect on the bradycardia caused by muscimol, whereas stellate ganglionectomy prevented any decrease in heart rate without altering the reduction in blood pressure (149). Moreover, direct injection of muscimol into the nucleus amibiguus, the site thought to contain the cell bodies of preganglionic vagal fibers projecting to the heart, had no effect on heart rate in anesthetized cats (176).

Although muscimol had no effect on heart rate when placed directly into the nucleus ambiguus, it had very dramatic effects when parasympathetic output was first activated. Gillis et al. (150) showed that the reflex vagal bradycardia caused by the pressor response to phenylephrine was abolished by microinjections of 10 to 50 μg of muscimol into the nucleus ambiguus, an effect that was itself abolished by the GABA receptor antagonist bicuculline. Furthermore, GABA receptor antagonists can cause marked bradycardia by themselves.

Administration of bicuculline directly into the nucleus ambiguus resulted in bradycardia,

an effect that was antagonized by muscimol. Similarly, microinjections of the GABA synthesis inhibitor isoniazid into the nucleus ambiguus also caused bradycardia, an effect reversed by muscimol infusion into the nucleus ambiguus (173). Finally, picrotoxin and bicuculline acted at a brainstem location to block inhibitory modulation of reflex vagal bradycardia (177). All these data are consistent with the interpretation that there is a tonically active GABA system in the medulla that inhibits vagal outflow (150). Furthermore, this system is probably maximally active, because muscimol has no further effect, whereas picrotoxin and bicuculline have very dramatic effects on heart rate.

These pharmacological results are also consistent with anatomical and biochemical data. The GABA content and binding in the nucleus ambiguus were 2.5 to 3 times higher than those of surrounding reticular tissue (178). Although GABA contents of left and right nucleus ambiguus were comparable, GABA binding was usually greater in right than in left nucleus ambiguus (178). Moreover, intracranial sectioning of the right vagal trunk reduced the symmetry of GABA binding. Because the asymmetry in GABA binding in the nucleus ambiguus is coupled with the asymmetry in the vagal-reflex-induced response, these data are also consistent with the suggestion that tonic and reflex vagal activity may be determined by the density of GABA receptors.

Reflexes and Other Effects

Agents that modulate central GABA function have profound effects on vascular and cardiac reflex mechanisms. As mentioned earlier, local administration of muscimol into the nucleus ambiguus can totally abolish reflex vagal bradycardia caused by the pressor response to phenylephrine (176), whereas bicuculline enhances the reflex bradycardia caused by phenylephrine (150). Infusion of the GABA agonist imidazole-4-acetic acid into the lateral ventricle in anesthetized cats completely abolishes the reflex reduction in heart rate caused by norepinephrine, whereas intravenous administration is without effect (153). Conversely, the GABA receptor antagonists picrotoxin and bicuculline produce a dose-related blockade of inhibition of reflex vagal bradycardia elicited by stimulation of the lateral hypothalamus or branches of the brachial plexus in spinal cats (177). These data support the contention that increases in vagal tone, which appear to be under inhibition by a GABA input under normal conditions (*vide supra*), can be strongly and consistently modified by interference with GABA function, probably at a site in the nucleus ambiguus.

The effects of GABA agonists on the reflex response to bilateral carotid artery occlusion are not consistent. Muscimol and GABA were shown to cause either no effect or an inhibition of pressor and tachycardia responses to bilateral carotid occlusion (136,143,147,148,150). In addition, muscimol decreased the reflex vasodilation in hindlimb caused by the pressor response to norepinephrine (147,148). The GABA agonist imidazole-4-acetic acid had no important inhibitory effect on the response to bilateral carotid artery occlusion, despite causing marked reductions in blood pressure, heart rate, and renal sympathetic nervous discharge (153). Similarly, isoguvacine at 1 μg/kg/min into the lateral ventricle in anesthetized cats had no inhibitory effect on the pressor response to bilateral carotid occlusion, despite a 40% reduction in blood pressure. Thus, no clear-cut general conclusions can be made with respect to central GABA stimulation on reflex pressor responses to bilateral carotid occlusion.

Other Reflexes

Intrathecal injection of GABA reduced the vasomotor response to spinal compression in cats (136). Injection of GABA into the spinal cord in cats or application of cotton swabs soaked with GABA to the spinal cord at L1–2 segments did not change blood pressure, but

abolished the depressed portion of the response to sciatic nerve stimulation (140). In cats, GABA inhibited the reflex increase in blood pressure to sciatic nerve stimulation when administered to the fourth ventricle (179).

Taylor et al. (180) found that bicuculline and the GABA synthesis inhibitor thiosemicarbazide caused almost total blockade of inhibition of the somatosympathetic-reflex-induced potentials (evoked by somatic or renal nerve stimulation) resulting from stimulation of the medial medullary depressor region in cats. In contrast, neither bicuculline nor thiosemicarbazide had any effect on baroreceptor-induced inhibition of the somatosympathetic reflex.

In a recent study, Lalley (181) found that baclofen converted depressor responses evoked by stimulation of afferent fibers in the carotid sinus, aortic, and cervical vagus nerves to pressor responses. It was found that this reversal could itself be reversed by bicuculline or picrotoxin, but not by the glycine antagonists strychnine and pentylenetetrazol.

Electrically Evoked Pressor Responses

In an early study, Bhargava et al. (136) showed in one dog that GABA at 100 mg/kg intravenously decreased the pressor response to electrical stimulation of pressor sites in the medulla. In cats, intraventricular administration of muscimol caused marked inhibition of depressor responses elicited by electrical stimulation of the diencephalon (144). The inhibition apparently was a result of a reduction in centrally emanating sympathetic discharge to vasoconstrictor nerves and could be reversed by bicuculline.

GABA–Benzodiazepine Interactions

In the last few years there has been a remarkably rapid growth in the literature concerning the interactions between benzodiazepines and GABA agonists and/or receptors of the brain. In 1977, several articles appeared that demonstrated the existence of specific high-affinity benzodiazepine receptors in brain (182,183). Using indirect biochemical techniques, Costa et al. (184,185) implicated GABA in the mediation of the actions of benzodiazepines but did not provide any mechanism.

Because diazepam potentiated presynaptic inhibition in cat spinal cord, and because GABA is probably the transmitter mediating such an effect, Haefely (186,187) speculated that benzodiazepines generally act by modulating GABA synaptic transmission. In 1978, several investigators showed that GABA and GABA mimetics increased the affinity of benzodiazepines for their binding sites in rat brain (188–192), an effect subsequently confirmed and elaborated (193–198). Furthermore, the enhancement of benzodiazepine binding by GABA was prevented by bicuculline (192). The stimulation of diazepam binding by GABA receptor activation appears to be relevant to drug mechanism. Choi et al. (199) showed that chlordiazepoxide potentiated GABAergic synaptic potentials in spinal cord cell cultures, as well as those induced by exogenously applied GABA. Both direct and systemic applications of several benzodiazepines were found to potentiate the inhibitory response in the dorsal raphe nucleus produced by GABA without having any effect by themselves (200). Doses of diazepam that did not change spontaneous firing rates markedly enhanced GABA-mediated inhibition in rat cerebellum and in tissue cultures of rat hypothalamus (201,202). These effects were antagonized by picrotoxin and were not observed with glycine- or norepinephrine-induced inhibitions. Finally, both muscimol and THIP markedly potentiated the anticonflict effects of benzodiazepines in cats (203).

Thus, there is a basis for assuming that benzodiazepines, perhaps through an effect on GABA receptor binding, might also affect central cardiovascular control mechanisms.

As a class, the benzodiazepines have very little effect on blood pressure and heart rate (204). However, the benzodiazepines are very effective in inhibiting cardiovascular responses evoked by either direct or indirect central activation. Schalleck et al. (205) were the first to demonstrate that the benzodiazepines could inhibit the pressor response to hypothalamic stimulation without altering responses to peripheral sympathetic nerve stimulation or to epinephrine. These studies were confirmed and expanded by many others (204).

Although most early studies focused on the hypothalamic effects of the benzodiazepines on cardiovascular responses, other and more caudal specific central effects of diazepam have been demonstrated. In addition to the inhibition of posterior hypothalamic responses by diazepam, marked inhibitions of both pressor and positive chronotropic responses to stimulation of rostral periaqueductal gray and dorsal tegmentum were observed (206). In a later publication it was shown that pretreatment of cats with bicuculline could prevent the inhibition of electrically evoked pressor responses from diencephalon, suggesting very strongly that diazepam effects were GABA-mediated (207). Furthermore, centrally administered muscimol was also found to inhibit evoked pressor responses by preventing activation of sympathetic outflow, an effect that was totally reversed by bicuculline.

Because the benzodiazepines appear to have little effect on blood pressure or on medullary structures that control spontaneous sympathetic tone, these drugs would not be expected to be useful in controlling established hypertension; however, because these drugs prevent systemic hemodynamic changes induced by environment and by classic conditioning procedures (208,209), they may prove to be effective in attenuating the development of hypertension. This is an area of GABA research that is virtually untouched and should prove a fertile source of exciting information in the future.

Serotonin

Serotonin (5-hydroxytryptamine, 5HT) is an amine that is found in high concentrations in the brain but that does not readily cross the blood-brain barrier. Therefore, either the precursor tryptophan or 5-hydroxytryptophan (5HTP) must be administered peripherally in order for *de novo* synthesis of 5HT to occur centrally. Alternatively, preformed 5HT must be delivered directly into the brain. Although there is a large literature on the cardiovascular effects of drugs that affect 5HT function, the results are often confused; see Kuhn et al. (210) for an in-depth review.

Effects on Blood Pressure and Heart Rate

Virtually every study has found that tryptophan, given in reasonable doses, has little or no effect on blood pressure or heart rate in rats, cats, and dogs. However, very large doses of tryptophan alone (225 mg/kg) or in combination with a monoamine oxidase (MAO) inhibitor to prevent catabolism of newly formed 5HT have been shown to cause significant reductions in blood pressure (70).

In contrast to tryptophan, 5HTP either alone or in combination with a MAO inhibitor causes hypotension and bradycardia in every species studied. Systemically administered 5HTP increases brain 5HT, mainly by selective neuronal accumulation (211,212), an effect enhanced by inhibition of MAO. Intravenous injections of large amounts of 5HTP in non-MAO-inhibited dogs will cause increases in arterial pressure and heart rate, followed by decreases (213,214). The increases in pressure and heart rate are due to direct stimulatory effects of serotonin formed in the periphery from 5HTP on smooth muscle and heart (215,216) or by indirect release of norepinephrine. In contrast to large doses of 5HTP alone, small doses of 5HTP, extracerebral decarboxylase inhibition followed by 5HTP, or direct central administration of 5HTP will cause only reductions in blood pressure and heart rate (87,217–219). These effects probably are due to the formation of 5HT, because doses of 5HTP that were normally ineffective caused decreases in blood pressure and heart rate in MAO-inhibited dogs (217,218), suggesting that the effects were mediated by 5HT, be-

cause this substance (not 5HTP) is susceptible to oxidative deamination. The effects were central in origin, because inhibition of central and peripheral decarboxylase with RO 4-4602 prevented or greatly delayed the hypotensive actions of 5HTP, whereas selective extracerebral decarboxylase inhibition with MK-486 enhanced the hypotensive actions of 5HTP. In addition, extracerebral decarboxylase inhibition with MK-486 enhanced the bradycardia caused by small doses of 5HTP and converted the positive chronotropic effects of high doses of 5HTP into a negative effect, indicating that a centrally mediated bradycardia was normally opposed by a peripheral stimulant action (218). Others showed that 5HTP also decreased blood pressure and heart rate in cats after extracerebral decarboxylase inhibition; these effects were prevented by RO 4-4602 and enhanced by MAO inhibition (219,220). Similar hypotensive and bradycardic actions of 5HTP were also reported in unanesthetized dogs when the drug was administered into the lateral ventricle (87). Fuller et al. (221) found that fluoxetine, a selective inhibitor of 5HT uptake, reduced blood pressure in DOCA-salt-hypertensive rats, but not in SHR. However, the combination of 5HT and fluoxetine caused marked reductions in blood pressure in both models of hypertension.

The hypotensive and bradycardic actions of 5HTP probably are mediated through a reduction in centrally emanating sympathetic outflow, because intravenous 5HTP in MK-486-treated cats resulted in large and dose-related reductions in efferent sympathetic activity of cardiac, renal, and splanchnic nerves (219).

It would seem logical to conclude that the central cardiovascular effects of 5HTP are a result of its conversion to 5HT, with subsequent stimulation of central 5HT receptors. Evidence that the hypotension caused by 5HTP and 5HT was mediated by stimulation of serotonergic receptors was provided by the ability of methysergide and yohimbine, 5HT antagonists, to attenuate the response to 5HTP (218). Receptor blockade with haloperidol, which is capable of blocking both central α and dopamine receptors, failed to reduce the cardiovascular effects of 5HTP (218).

Furthermore, 5HT and other serotonergic receptor stimulants, including 5-methoxy-*N,N*-dimethyltryptamine, quipazine, and 5-methoxytryptamine-β-methyl-carboxylate, as well as the 5HT-releasing agent fenfluramine, all decreased blood pressure either in normotensive cats or in hypertensive rats (222–224). In addition, these effects were prevented by the 5HT antagonists metergoline and cyproheptadine.

Although the evidence is quite consistent that central activation of 5HT receptors causes a reduction in blood pressure, a curious exception appears to occur in the rat. Thus, although 5HTP and several serotonin receptor stimulants decrease blood pressure in the rat, 5HT and the 5HT agonist 2,5-dimethoxy-4-methylamphetamine increase it [see Kuhn et al. (210) for a review]. Lambert et al. (225) have suggested that the rise in blood pressure caused by 5HT in rats may be a result of hypoxia or hypercapnia. This unusual selective discrepancy is further discussed later with respect to the physiological role of 5HT in central regulation of hemodynamics.

Central Site of Action of 5HT: Relation to Endogenous Mechanisms

The anatomical areas responsible for the effects of 5HT receptor stimulation on blood pressure are not presently known. Injection of 5HT or 5HTP directly into the lateral ventricles in dogs and cats lowers blood pressure, probably at a site below the midcollicular level. Tadepalli et al. (226) demonstrated that when 5HTP was injected into either the lateral cerebral ventricle or third ventricle in cats but was prevented from reaching structures caudal to the third ventricle by cerebral aqueduct cannulation, 5HTP had no effect on blood pressure, heart rate, or sympathetic nerve activity. These authors concluded that stimulation of caudal brainstem or spinal cord centers by 5HT was responsible for its cardiovascular

effects. In this regard, Franz et al. (227) have shown that 5HTP produces marked dose-dependent depression of both spinal reflex and intraspinal pathways. Selective 5HT (but not norepinephrine) uptake inhibitors enhanced the depression produced by 5HTP, whereas prevention of 5HT synthesis by RO 4–4602 completely prevented it.

As mentioned earlier, normotensive rats present a unique exception in that they respond to central 5HT with a rise in blood pressure. Lambert et al. (225) confined this effect to the third ventricle. Direct application of 5HT to the anterior hypothalamus/preoptic area also raised blood pressure in rats (228). Similarly, direct application of 5HT to the NTS in rats caused a dose-dependent increase in blood pressure, an effect enhanced by fluoxetine and reduced by the serotonin antagonists metergoline and α-bromolysergic acid (229).

Electrical Stimulation

Anatomical and electrophysiological studies indicate a functional association between serotonergic neurons and brain areas normally associated with the regulation of cardiovascular functions. The serotonin-containing neurons arise from cell bodies in the nuclei of the raphe system in the medulla (22,210,230). Fibers extend rostrally to the pontine reticular formation, to the periaqueductal gray matter, and into the fields of Forel of the posterior hypothalamus, brain areas that can give rise to dramatic cardiovascular changes (230–232). The highest levels of serotonin are found in the basal and posterior hypothalamus (233).

Fibers also extend caudally to impinge on the intermediolateral cell columns of the thoracolumbar spinal cord, from which preganglionic sympathetic nerves originate.

Raphe neurons in the cat medulla with cardiac-related activity have recently been identified in the generation of naturally occurring rhythmic discharges of sympathetic nerves (234). The predominant effect (24 of 27 instances) of electrical stimulation of raphe stimulation was a decrease in sympathetic nerve discharge. Similarly, electrical stimulation with the nucleus raphe pallidus (B_1) and obscurus (B_2) also inhibited sympathetic discharge in cats, an effect abolished by discrete lesions placed in the dorsal portion of the dorsolateral funiculus, where there is a high density of 5HT-containing neurons. Furthermore, the inhibitory influences are exerted as far as the spinal level and can depress spontaneous as well as evoked activity of sympathetic nerves [see Kuhn et al. (210) for a review].

Once again, however, the results are not completely consistent. Adair et al. (235) found that B_1 stimulation caused both depressor and pressor activity, with depressor responses being predominant. Stimulation of the anterior region of B_2 caused primarily depressor responses, whereas stimulation of the posterior region of B_2 caused pressor responses. Similarly, stimulation of B_3 (nucleus raphe magnus) was divided into anterior pressor and posterior depressor areas.

In rats and cats, stimulation of nuclei of the ascending 5HT systems—namely dorsal (B_7) and median (B_8) raphe—consistently leads to increases in blood pressure.

5HT Depletors and Receptor Antagonists

Depletors

Parachlorophenylalanine (PCPA) has been extensively used to selectively reduce brain 5HT levels, because it is a potent inhibitor of tryptophan hydroxylase, the rate-limiting enzyme involved in the formation of 5HT.

In dogs, cats, and rabbits, PCPA caused little effect on blood pressure or heart rate. In both normotensive rats and SHR, there is general consensus, but not total agreement, that PCPA causes an increase in blood pressure. This is obviously consistent with the decreases in blood pressure caused by 5HTP, but not the increases caused by 5HT in this species.

5,6-Dihydroxytryptamine (DHT) and 5,7-DHT are neurotoxins that selectively destroy serotonergic neurons. In nine studies using these agents, blood pressure in normotensive rats, SHR, cats, and rabbits was either unchanged or decreased [see Kuhn et al. (210) for a review].

Thus, the foregoing experiments with depletors of central 5HT stores provide little consistency in their effects and little aid in deciding the role of central 5HT neurons in blood pressure regulation. However, it should be remembered that the actions of PCPA are not entirely specific, because it can compete with transport mechanisms for tryptophan, phenylalanine, and other amino acids. PCPA also inhibits phenylalanine hydroxylase and thus leads to increased levels of phenylalanine and abnormal metabolites of this amino acid. PCPA itself is decarboxylated in brain to parachlorophenethylamine, a substance that is itself claimed to have pharmacological effects (236). Furthermore, PCPA (and 5,6-DHT) can cause significant reductions in brain catecholamine levels (237,238). Finally, because 5HT levels are not totally depleted after PCPA treatment, it is possible that the residual or newly formed serotonin could maintain effective function in serotonergic systems (236).

Antagonists

Studies with 5HT antagonists on blood pressure control are more consistent than those with depletors, but they are also difficult to interpret. The 5HT antagonist methysergide, but not cyproheptadine or cinanserin, was shown to reduce blood pressure in SHR (223,239). Similarly, methysergide also reduced blood pressure, heart rate, and sympathetic nerve activity in dogs and cats (240, 241). In addition, the 5HT antagonists metergoline, cyproheptadine, and cinanserin reduced blood pressure, heart rate, and sympathetic nerve activity in anesthetized cats, effects blocked by PCPA (242).

Can one make any sense of these data on blood pressure with drugs that affect 5HT function? Perhaps the best attempt has been that of McCall and Humphrey (242). These authors have suggested that 5HT neurons act to enhance sympathetic outflow from the brain. 5HT receptor antagonists act to inhibit sympathetic outflow (decrease blood pressure) by acting postsynaptically to antagonize the excitatory effect of synaptically released 5HT on central sympathetic neurons. 5HT and other serotonin receptor stimulants would variably affect blood pressure, depending on where they had their primary site of action. Therefore, if serotonin receptor stimulants acted primarily on serotonergic cell bodies, the result would be inhibition of 5HT cell firing and decreases (disfacilitation) in sympathetic outflow and blood pressure. Conversely, if the major site and/or action of serotonin receptor stimulants was on postsynaptic neurons, the result would be increases (facilitation) in sympathetic outflow and blood pressure (Fig. 6). Of course, this hypothesis would also have to accommodate species differences, as well as the unexplainable findings with PCPA and the serotonergic neurotoxins. However, it provides a reasonable framework of explanation that has already gone far beyond previous hypotheses to explain the actions of central 5HT manipulation on circulatory control.

Reflexes and Other Effects

It is apparent that central serotonergic fibers participate in arterial baroreceptor reflexes (243). Sinoaortic denervation in the rabbit produces a selective 25% increase in serotonin (5HT) and 5-hydroxyindoleacetic acid (5-HIAA) stores in both the hypothalamus and the thoracolumbar segments of the spinal cord (243). Furthermore, 5HTP has been shown to reduce markedly the reflex responses to bilateral carotid artery occlusion and to suppress evoked sympathetic reflexes in spinal cord (82,83,217,218). This clearly suggests that serotonergic nerves contribute to baroreflexes, and this possibility has been pursued using intracisternal injections of 5,6-DHT to deplete serotonergic stores and destroy serotonergic nerve endings. Injection of 5,6-DHT produces a highly selective destruction of serotonergic bulbospinal tracts, with little effect on serotonergic tracts elsewhere in the CNS, and it completely prevents the increase in pressure normally seen after section of the carotid sinus and aortic nerves.

In other studies, 5HTP depressed bradycardia reflexly induced by norepinephrine or epinephrine, an effect blocked by prevention of central 5HTP conversion to 5HT (244,245). Conversely, depletion of central 5HT with either PCPA or 5,6-DHT enhanced reflex-induced bradycardia. In the same vein, central administration of the serotonin antagonist methysergide enhanced reflex vagal bradycardia in cats (246).

In cats, 5HTP depressed the carotid occlu-

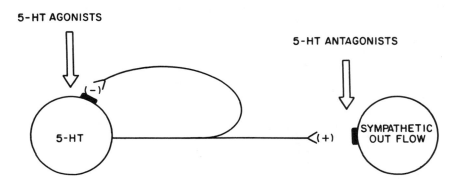

FIG. 6. Model depicting a possible interaction between serotonergic and central sympathetic neurons. Serotonin receptor agonists are shown as stimulating inhibitory presynaptic serotonergic receptors, thereby decreasing a postulated facilitory effect of 5HT neurons on sympathetic outflow. Serotonin receptor antagonists are shown as blocking the postsynaptic 5HT receptors that are facilitory to sympathetic outflow. Thus, both 5HT agonists and antagonists can decrease sympathetic nervous activity and blood pressure. (Adapted from McCall and Humphrey, ref. 242.)

sion response at a site different from that acting to reduce blood pressure. It was concluded that brainstem serotonergic mechanisms that require the integrity of neural pathways connecting subcollicular and supracollicular areas of the brain are responsible for inhibition of the carotid occlusion reflex (226).

Thus, cardiovascular reflexes are generally depressed by central 5HT stimulation and enhanced by its blockade or depletion.

L-tryptophan or 5HTP administered to MAO-inhibited dogs also receiving MK-486 decreased ventricular vulnerability to fibrillation by 50%, presumably by reducing central sympathetic activity (247). Similarly, the central 5HT receptor agonists melatonin, MK-212, and 5-methoxytryptophan produced significant increases in the vulnerable-period threshold in dogs, effects that were blocked by metergoline (248).

An attempt at a summary of the effects of central 5HT manipulation on circulatory function is presented in Table 1. Obviously, this is an oversimplification; it is intended to give a consensus view.

Opiates

Nonpeptides

Morphine and morphinomimetic narcotic analgesic agents including fentanyl and dextromoramide preferentially reduce blood pressure and heart rate in dogs, cats, and rats.

These effects are a result of a reduction in centrally emanating sympathetic nerve activity, as well as an increase in vagal activity. These effects are a consequence of activation of specific opiate receptors, because the opiate receptor antagonists naloxone and nalophrine can prevent or reverse the hypotensive, bradycardic, and sympathoinhibitory effects of narcotic analgesics.

The main site of the hypotensive action of the opiates appears to be at the level of the medulla oblongata. Intravertebral artery injection of fentanyl was much more effective than intravenous administration (249). Furthermore, mid-pontine transection in bilaterally vagotomized dogs did not alter the hypotensive effects of fentanyl and dextromoramide, whereas transection of the spinal cord at C-1 abolished the effect. Moreover, injection of narcotic analgesics into the cerebral ventricle in dogs reduced blood pressure and heart rate at doses much higher than those required when injected intracisternally or by vertebral artery. Finally, perfusion of the fourth ventricle, but not the lateral or third ventricle, by fentanyl caused naloxone-reversible hypotension and bradycardia (250).

In contrast to the reported site of action of many centrally active cardiovascular agents, the NTS appears to play no role in the central actions of the narcotic analgesics. Direct bilateral injection of fentanyl into the NTS had no direct effect on blood pressure or heart rate, although it facilitated barorecep-

TABLE 1. *Effects of central serotonergic manipulation on blood pressure of normotensive and hypertensive animals*

Drug	Normotensive	Hypertensive
Tryptophan	NC[a]	NT
5-Hydroxytryptophan	↓	NT
5-Hydroxytryptamine (5HT)	↓ (↑ in rats)	↓
5HT antagonists	↓	↓
PCPA	NC or ↑	↑, ↓, NC
Dihydroxytryptamines	NC or ↓	↓
B$_7$ or B$_8$ stimulation	↑	NT
B$_1$ or B$_3$ stimulation	↑ or ↓	NT

[a] NC, no change; NT, not tested.
Adapted from Kuhn et al. (210).

tor transmission (251). In dogs with bilateral lesions of the NTS and treated with a β-adrenoceptor blocking agent, fentanyl caused marked hypotension and bradycardia, thereby ruling out the NTS as a site of action (252). In other studies, direct injection of small doses of fentanyl into the nucleus ambiguus caused marked vagal bradycardia without decreasing blood pressure (253).

Therefore, whereas it is clear that narcotic analgesics can produce a specific opiate-receptor-mediated reduction in blood pressure by decreasing sympathetic nerve activity, and a vagal bradycardia by activating vagal outflow, the exact sites of action are unknown. Also, the physiological significances of such findings are moot, because the narcotic receptor antagonists have little or no effect on blood pressure or heart rate, suggesting that ongoing opiate-receptor-mediated tone is not important in regulating these parameters.

The narcotic analgesics can sometimes produce a transient hypertension, either before or after the more predominant and usual hypotension. However, the pressor response to the opiates apparently is mediated by release of catecholamines from the adrenal gland and probably is nonspecific, because it is not prevented by narcotic antagonists in the same animals in which the depressor response is completely blocked (254).

Peptides

The central cardiovascular effects of endogenous or synthetic opiate peptides are confusing and particularly contradictory. They have variously been reported to increase, decrease, or have biphasic effects on blood pressure and heart rate, depending on the species, peptide, anesthesia, and site of administration used.

In general, opiate peptides, including methionine and leucine enkephalin, α- and β-endorphin, and D-Ala²-met-enkephalinamide, all increase blood pressure and heart rate in rats, especially in conscious animals when centrally administered. Bellet et al. (255) have suggested

that the depressor responses to opiate peptides occur mainly at high doses and are associated with the respiratory depression observed with these high doses. All of the cardiovascular effects of the opiate peptides are blocked by opiate receptor antagonists and therefore are due to specific opiate receptor stimulation.

In conscious cats, D-Ala²-met-enkephalinamide administered intracerebroventricularly caused dose-related increases in blood pressure and heart rate and reduced baroreceptor reflex sensitivity (256). In anesthetized cats, as in rats, met-enkephalin reduced blood pressure when applied to the ventral surface of the brainstem (257). However, the reduction in blood pressure was associated with respiratory depression, supporting the suggestion that depressor effects of opiate peptides are a consequence of such depression.

In anesthetized dogs, intracisternal injection of methionine enkephalin did nothing to blood pressure, probably as a consequence of its rapid metabolic destruction, whereas β-endorphin, D-Ala²-met-enkephalin, and D-Ala²-met-enkephalinamide produced predominant reductions in blood pressure, heart rate, and sympathetic nerve activity (258). These effects were all blocked by naloxone. Direct injection of D-Ala²-met-enkephalinamide into the nucleus ambiguus in dogs caused marked vagal bradycardia. As far as can be determined, there have been no studies on the central cardiovascular effects of opiate peptides in conscious dogs.

Histamine

Histamine is found in relatively large quantities in the central nervous system, including areas known to be important in cardiovascular control mechanisms, such as the hypothalamus and median forebrain bundle. However, its involvement in such control mechanisms remains unclear.

Intraventricular injection of histamine in cats and rats causes increases in blood pressure and heart rate due to a centrally mediated increase in sympathetic nerve activity (259–

263). Both the pressor and tachycardic effects of histamine are prevented by H_1 receptor blockade with mepyramine or diphenhydramine, whereas H_2 receptor blockade with metiamide is without effect on the histamine response. However, both H_1 receptor stimulants (e.g., 2-methylhistamine) and H_2 receptor stimulants (e.g., dimaprit and 4-methylhistamine) produce pressor responses that are not blocked by H_2 receptor antagonists, suggesting a nonspecific effect of these latter agents in the brain.

Imidazole-4-acetic acid, a metabolite of histamine, causes marked reductions in blood pressure, heart rate, and sympathetic nerve activity when centrally (but not peripherally) administered (153). Clonidine is another imidazole compound that decreases blood pressure, heart rate, and sympathetic nerve activity. The effects of both imidazole-4-acetic acid and clonidine have been claimed to be blocked by the H_2 receptor antagonist metiamide, leading Pakkari et al. (264) to suggest that there may be a central "imidazole receptor" that is activated by the former agents. However, metiamide is also a central GABA receptor antagonist that causes marked increases in blood pressure (265). In addition, imidazole-4-acetic acid is a GABA receptor stimulant that also displaces ^3H-GABA from brain neurons and whose effects are blocked by the GABA receptor antagonist bicuculline. Therefore, imidazole-4-acetic acid probably acts by stimulating central GABA receptors, and histamine by stimulating central H_1 receptors (153). The prevention or reversal of central clonidine effects by metiamide probably is nonspecific, and the actions of clonidine are almost certainly due to stimulation of central α_2 receptors (vide supra).

Acetylcholine

Like serotonin, norepinephrine, and other catecholamines, acetylcholine (ACh) is an amine found in the brain and periphery, but it does not readily cross the blood-brain barrier. However, its biosynthetic and metabolic pathways are quite different from those of typical biogenic amines such as norepinephrine and serotonin.

ACh is synthesized in cholinergic neurons by active transport of choline into nerve terminals, where it is acetylated with acetyl coenzyme A by the enzyme choline acetyltransferase (choline acetylase). The ACh is then sequestered within synaptic vesicles until release is required. Following release, the ACh is very rapidly destroyed by acetylcholinesterase. In contrast with other aminergic systems, little or no ACh is taken back up into the nerve terminal for storage and release. The rapid extraneuronal enzymatic destruction of ACh accounts for the profound enhancement of cholinergic responses by acetylcholinesterase inhibitors, whereas inhibition of norepinephrine and serotonin metabolism has little or no enhancing action, because uptake processes are more important.

The foregoing describes the effects of cholinergic manipulation on cardiovascular function. Detailed reviews are available (266–268).

Effects on Blood Pressure and Heart Rate

As with most other studies involving the effects of drugs on central cardiovascular control, studies with agents affecting central cholinergic mechanisms are confounded by possible peripheral effects, species differences, routes and sites of administration, state of anesthesia, and the additional complication of muscarinic and nicotinic cholinergic receptors.

Direct Muscarinic Stimulation

In general, muscarinic cholinergic stimulation of the brain leads to an increase in blood pressure, with inconsistent effects on heart rate. Although Brezenoff et al. (268) initially reported that injection of muscarinic agents into the hypothalamus caused a decrease in blood pressure, this was deemed to be due to a methodological problem and was not an accurate reflection of typical results. In either anesthetized or conscious rats, central administrations of ACh, carbachol, bethanechol, and oxotremorine all increased blood pressure. Blockade of central receptors with atropine, but not hexamethonium, prevented the increase in blood pressure, as did spinal cord transection. These results clearly indicate that central muscarinic receptor activation leads to a sympathetically mediated increase in blood pressure in the rat. The precise site(s) involved in this mechanism is unknown; however, microinjection of carbachol into the posterior and ventral hypothalamic nuclei, supramamillary nucleus, and pars medialis of the medial mamillary nucleus increased blood pressure, whereas injection into the dorsomedial and premamillary hypothalamus areas decreased blood pressure [see Brezenoff and Giuliano (268) for a review].

In conscious cats, central administration of muscarinic receptor stimulants such as ACh and carbachol resulted in a pressor response that was abolished by central muscarinic receptor blockade with atropine. However, in anesthetized cats, carbachol and oxotremorine decreased blood pressure, apparently by acting on muscarinic receptors in the brainstem. Brezenoff and Giuliano have argued persuasively that decreases in blood pressure observed after central muscarinic stimulation are due to anesthesia and that the "normal" response is pressor in conscious animals (268).

In unanesthetized dogs, central muscarinic stimulation with ACh, carbachol, oxotremorine, and methacholine caused a rise in blood pressure that was abolished by atropine. As noted earlier for cats, hypotension is sometimes observed after central muscarinic stimulation in anesthetized dogs.

Direct Nicotinic Stimulation

In conscious rats, central administration of nicotine has essentially no effect on blood pressure (269), whereas it causes an initial brief pressor response followed by a prolonged hypotension in anesthetized rats (270).

In conscious cats, central nicotinic receptor stimulation with nicotine, tetramethylammonium chloride, or DMPP generally results in a pressor response. The occasional depressor response observed after central nicotine administration in anesthetized cats is probably due to the anesthesia, because the pressor response to intracerebroventricular nicotine can be reversed to a depressor response after choralose anesthesia in the same animals.

Superfusion of the posterior hypothalamic area with arecoline, nicotine, or DMPP enhanced the pressor response to hypothalamic stimulation, whereas muscarinic stimulation with oxotremorine or AHR 602 inhibited it.

In dogs, central nicotine administration increased blood pressure by increasing sympathetic nervous activity.

Inhibitors of Cholinesterase

As early as 1867, physostigmine was shown by von Bezold and Gotz (271) to increase blood pressure and heart rate, although these authors knew nothing of the drug's ability to inhibit cholinesterase. They also pointed out the central component to physostigmine's action, because spinal cord transection reduced its effects. Since that time, the cardiovascular effects of several cholinesterase inhibitors have been studied. Inhibitors that readily pass the blood-brain barrier or that are administered centrally generally increase blood pressure in rats, cats, and dogs, including physostigmine, sarin, diisopropylfluorphosphate, paraoxon, neostigmine, edrophonium, and echothiophate. However, quaternary cholinesterase inhibitors generally decrease blood pressure when injected intravenously, because they activate peripheral cholinergic receptors only.

The onset and duration of the pressor response to cholinesterase inhibitors are substantially earlier and longer than those observed after direct receptor stimulants, supporting the suggestion that these agents act by allowing ACh to accumulate after preventing its normal destruction. Further support for this hypothesis comes from several studies indicating that depletion of ACh stores reduces the pressor response to cholinesterase inhibitors.

The central receptor responsible for the

pressor response to cholinesterase inhibitors is muscarinic, because atropine both prevents and reverses their pressor effects, whereas the nicotinic receptor blocker mecamylamine is without influence. Furthermore, the pressor response to cholinesterase inhibitors is a consequence of stimulating sympathetic outflow. Blockade of peripheral sympathetic activity by α receptor blockers (yohimbine, dibenamine, phentolamine, tolazoline), neuron blockade (bretylium, 2,6-xylyl ether bromide), catecholamine depletion (reserpine), or spinal cord transection prevents the pressor response otherwise observed after central cholinesterase inhibition.

Although direct injection of cholinesterase inhibitors into the posterior hypothalamus raises blood pressure, the hypothalamus is not necessary for the response, because decerebration or transection of the brain caudal to the hypothalamus does not reduce the pressor effect.

Inhibition of ACh Synthesis

Hemicholinium-3 (HC-3) inhibits the synthesis of ACh by blocking the high-affinity transport of choline into intraneuronal sites of cholinergic nerve terminals. Intracerebroventricular (i.c.v.) injection of HC-3 into normotensive rats does not affect blood pressure. In contrast, significant decreases in blood pressure are observed in SHR and DOCA-salt- and renal-hypertensive rats after i.c.v. injection of HC-3, an effect that is related to reduction of central ACh levels.

In addition, HC-3 administered i.c.v. causes a reduction in the pressor response to physostigmine that is directly proportional to the reduction in ACh levels. Direct injection of HC-3 into the posterior hypothalamus also inhibits the pressor response to both physostigmine and neostigmine injected at the same site.

Reflexes and Other Effects

Central administration of physostigmine in the rat or neostigmine in the cat enhances reflex bradycardia induced by an increase in blood pressure and inhibits reflex tachycardia caused by a reduction in blood pressure. Central blockade of muscarinic receptors or reduction in central ACh stores prevents these reflex effects.

Similarly, both physostigmine and neostigmine potentiate the pressor response to bilateral carotid occlusion in rats, an effect blocked both by atropine and by HC-3 pretreatment given centrally.

In summary, central activation of muscarinic and nicotinic receptors leads to a rise in blood pressure, although reductions in blood pressure may occur in anesthetized animals. The lack of any effect on blood pressure after central muscarinic or nicotinic receptor blockade or depletion of ACh stores suggests that normal ongoing cholinergic tone plays little or no role in the central regulation of blood pressure in the normotensive animal. However, reductions in blood pressure after central HC-3 or muscarinic blockade in hypertensive animals suggest that an overactive central cholinergic pathway may play a role in initiating or maintaining the hypertension.

REFERENCES

1. Hilton, S. M. (1966): Hypothalamic regulation of the cardiovascular system. *Br. Med. Bull.*, 22:243–248.
2. Korner, P. I. (1971): Integrative neural cardiovascular control. *Physiol. Rev.*, 51:312–367.
3. Reis, D. J. (1972): Central neural mechanisms governing the circulation with particular reference to the lower brainstem and cerebellum. In: *Neural and Psychological Mechanisms in Cardiovascular Disease*, edited by A. Zanchetti, pp. 255–280. Casa Editrice, Milan.
4. Koizumi, K., and Brooks, C. M. (1972): The integration of autonomic system reactions. *Ergeb. Physiol.*, 67:1–68.
5. Smith, O. A. (1974): Reflex and central mechanisms involved in the control of the heart and circulation. *Annu. Rev. Physiol.*, 36:93–123.
6. Sato, A. (editor) (1975): *Brain Research, Vol. 87.* Elsevier, Amsterdam.
7. Elliott, J. M. (1979): The central noradrenergic control of blood pressure and heart rate. *Clin. Exp. Pharmacol. Physiol.*, 6:569–579.
8. Manning, J. W. (1980): Central integration of cardiovascular control. *Fed. Proc.*, 39:2485–2486.
9. Thomas, M. R., and Calaresu, F. R. (1974): Local-

ization and function of medullary sites mediating vagal bradycardia in the cat. *Am. J. Physiol.,* 226:1344–1349.

10. Miura, M., and Reis, D. J. (1970): A blood pressure response from fastigial nucleus and its relay pathway in brainstem. *Am. J. Physiol.,* 219:1330–1336.

11. Mirua, M., and Reis, D. J. (1971): The paramedian reticular nucleus: A site of inhibitory interaction between projections from fastigial nucleus and carotid sinus nerve acting on blood pressure. *J. Physiol. (Lond.),* 216:441–460.

12. Mraovitch, S., Kumada, M., and Reis, D. J. (1982): Role of the nucleus parabrachialis in cardiovascular regulation in cat. *Brain Res.,* 232:57–75.

13. Kumada, M., Dampney, R. A. L., and Reis, D. J. (1975): The trigeminal depressor response: A cardiovascular reflex originating from the trigeminal system. *Brain Res.,* 92:485–489.

14. Gauthier, P., Reis, D. J., and Nathan, M. A. (1981): Arterial hypertension elicited either by lesions or by electrical stimulations of the rostral hypothalamus in the rat. *Brain Res.,* 211:91–105.

15. Nathan, M. A., and Reis, D. J. (1975): Fulminating arterial hypertension with pulmonary edema from release of adrenomedullary catecholamines after lesions of the anterior hypothalamus in the rat. *Circ. Res.,* 37:226–235.

16. Brody, M. J., Haywood, J. R., and Touw, K. B. (1980): Neural mechanisms in hypertension. *Annu. Rev. Physiol.,* 42:441–453.

17. Uvnas, B.: Sympathetic vasodilator system and blood flow. *Physiol. Rev., [Suppl. 4],* 40:69–76.

18. Kaada, B. R. (1951): Somato-motor, autonomic, and electrocorticographic responses to electrical stimulation of "rhinencephalic" and other structures in primates, cats, and dogs. *Acta Physiol. Scand. [Suppl. 83],* 24:1–285.

19. Chalmers, J. P. (1975): Brain amines and models of experimental hypertension. *Circ. Res.,* 36:469–481.

20. Loewy, A. D., and Neil, J. J. (1981): The role of descending monoaminergic systems in central control of blood pressure. *Fed. Proc.,* 40:2778–2785.

21. Heymans, C., and Neil, E. (1958): *Reflexogenic Areas of the Cardiovascular System.* Churchill, London.

22. Dahlstrom, A., and Fuxe, K. (1965): Evidence for the existence of monoamine neurones in the central nervous system: II. Experimentally induced changes in the intraneuronal amine levels of bulbospinal neurone systems. *Acta Physiol. Scand. [Suppl. 247],* 64:1–37.

23. Fuxe, K. (1965): Distribution of monoamine terminals in the central nervous system. *Acta Physiol. Scand. [Suppl. 247],* 64:38–85.

24. Doba, N., and Reis, D. J. (1974): Role of central and peripheral adrenergic mechanisms in neurogenic hypertension produced by brainstem lesion in rats. *Circ. Res.,* 34:293–301.

25. Doba, N., and Reis, D. J. (1973): Acute fulminating neurogenic hypertension produced by brainstem lesions in the rat. *Circ. Res.,* 32:584–593.

26. Talman, W. T., Snyder, D. S., and Reis, D. J. (1980): Chronic lability of arterial pressure produced by de-

struction of A_2 catecholaminergic neurons in rat brainstem. *Circ. Res.,* 46:842–853.

27. Synder, D. W., Nathan, M. A., and Reis, D. J. (1978): Chronic lability of arterial pressures produced by selective destruction of the catecholamine innervation of the nucleus tractus solitarii in the rat. *Circ. Res.,* 43:662–671.

28. Kubo, T., and Misu, Y. (1981): Pharmacological characterization of the α-adrenoceptors responsible for a decrease of blood pressure in the nucleus tractus solitarii of the rat. *Naunyn Schmiedebergs Arch. Pharmacol.,* 317:120–125.

29. Chiba, T., and Kato, M. (1978): Synaptic structures and quantification of catecholaminergic axons in the nucleus tractus solitarius of the rat: Possible modulatory roles of catecholamines in baroreceptor reflexes. *Brain Res.,* 151:323–338.

30. Ross, C. A., Ruggiero, D. A., and Reis, D. J. (1981): Afferent projections to cardiovascular portions of the nucleus of the tractus solitarius in the rat. *Brain Res.,* 223:402–408.

31. Blessing, W. W., West, M. J., and Chalmers, J. P. (1981): Hypertension, bradycardia, and pulmonary edema in the conscious rabbit after brainstem lesions coinciding with the A_1 group of catecholamine neurons. *Circ. Res.,* 49:949–958.

32. West, M. J., Blessing, W. W., and Chalmers, J. (1981): Arterial baroreceptor reflex function in the conscious rabbit after brainstem lesions coinciding with the A_1 group of catecholamine neurons. *Circ. Res.,* 49:959–970.

33. Chalmers, J. P., and Wurtman, R. J. (1971): Participation of central noradrenergic neurones in arterial baroreceptor reflexes in the rabbit. *Circ. Res.,* 28:480–491.

34. Chalmers, J. P., and Reid, J. L. (1972): Participation of central noradrenergic neurones in arterial baroreceptor reflexes in the rabbit. *Circ. Res.,* 31:789–804.

35. DeJong, W. (1974): Noradrenaline: Central inhibitory control of blood pressure and heart rate. *Eur. J. Pharmacol.,* 29:179–181.

36. Robson, R. D., and Kaplan, H. R. (1969): An involvement of ST-155 [2-(2,6-dichlorophenylamino)-2-imidazoline hydrochloride, Catapres] in cholinergic mechanisms. *Eur. J. Pharmacol.,* 5:328–337.

37. Nayler, W., and Stone, J. (1970): An effect of ST-155 (clonidine), 2-(2,6-dichlorophenylamino)-2-imidazoline hydrochloride, Catapres, on relationship between blood pressure and heart rate in dogs. *Eur. J. Pharmacol.,* 10:161–167.

38. Kobinger, W., and Walland, A. (1972): Facilitation of vagal reflex bradycardia by an injection of clonidine on central alpha-receptors. *Eur. J. Pharmacol.,* 19:210–217.

39. Robson, R. D., and Antonaccio, M. J. (1976): Modification of cardiovascular reflexes by clonidine in dogs. In: *New Antihypertensive Drugs,* edited by A. Scriabine and C. Sweet, pp. 461–479. University Park Press, Baltimore.

40. Antonaccio, M. J., and Halley, J. (1977): Clonidine hypotension: Lack of effect of bilateral lesions of the nucleus solitary tract in anesthetized cats. *Neuropharmacology,* 16:431–433.

41. Haeusler, G. (1973): Effects of alpha-adrenolytics

on central cardiovascular control. *Naunyn Schmiedebergs Arch. Pharmacol.*, 277:R27.

42. Kobinger, W., and Walland, A. (1973): Modulating effect of central adrenergic neurones on a vagally mediated cardioinhibitory reflex. *Eur. J. Pharmacol.*, 22:344–350.

43. Antonaccio, M. J., Robson, R. D., and Burrell, R. (1975): Effects of clonidine on baroreceptor function in anesthetized dogs. *Eur. J. Pharmacol.*, 30:6–14.

44. Lundberg, J. M., Hokfelt, T., Fahrenkrug, J., Nilsson, G., and Terenius, L. (1979): Peptides in the carotid body (glomus caroticum): VIP-, enkephalin-, and substance P-like immunoreactivity. *Acta Physiol. Scand.*, 107:279–281.

45. Ljungdahl, A., Hokfelt, T., and Nilsson, G. (1978): Distribution of substance P-like immunoreactivity in the central nervous system of the rat. I. Cell bodies and nerve terminals. *Neuroscience*, 3:861–943.

46. Guyenet, P. G., and Aghajanian, G. K. (1977): Excitation of neurons in the locus coeruleus by substance P and related peptides. *Brain Res.*, 136:178–184.

47. Gillis, R. A., Helke, C. J., Hamilton, B. L., Norman, W. P., and Jacobowitz, D. M. (1980): Evidence that substance P is a neurotransmitter of baro- and chemoreceptor afferents in nucleus tractus solitarius. *Brain Res.*, 181:476–481.

48. Haeusler, G., and Osterwalder, R. (1980): Evidence suggesting a transmitter or neuromodulatory role for substance P at the first synapse of the baroreceptor reflex. *Naunyn Schmiedebergs Arch. Pharmacol.*, 314:111–121.

49. Talman, W. T., and Reis, D. J. (1981): Baroreflex actions of substance P microinjected into the nucleus tractus solitarii in rat: A consequence of local distortion. *Brain Res.*, 220:402–407.

50. Curtis, D. R., and Johnston, G. A. R. (1974): Amino acid transmitters in the central nervous system. *Ergeb. Physiol.*, 69:97–188.

51. Perrone, M. H. (1981): Biochemical evidence that L-glutamate is a neurotransmitter of primary vagal afferent nerve fibers. *Brain Res.*, 230:283–293.

52. Talman, W. T., Perrone, M. H., and Reis, D. J. (1980): Evidence for L-glutamate as the neurotransmitter of baroreceptor afferent nerve fibers. *Science*, 209:813–815.

53. Talman, W. T., Perrone, M. H., Scher, P., Kwo, S., and Reis, D. J. (1981): Antagonism of the baroreceptor reflex by glutamate diethyl ester, an antagonist to L-glutamate. *Brain Res.*, 217:186–191.

54. Talman, W. T., Perrone, M. H., and Reis, D. J. (1981): Acute hypertension after the local injection of kainic acid into the nucleus tractus solitarii of rats. *Circ. Res.*, 48:292-298.

55. Dormer, D. J., Foreman, R. D., and Stone, H. L. (1977): Glutamate induced fastigial pressor response in the dog. *Neuroscience*, 2:577–584.

56. Chelly, J., Kouyoumdjian, J. C., Mouille, P., Huchet, A. M., and Schmitt, H. (1979): Effects of L-glutamic acid and kainic acid on central cardiovascular control. *Eur. J. Pharmacol.*, 60:91–94.

57. McAllen, R. M., Neill, J. J., and Loewy, A. D. (1982): Effects of kainic acid applied to the ventral surface of the medulla oblongata on vasomotor tone, the baroreceptor reflex, and hypothalamic autonomic responses. *Brain Res.*, 238:65–76.

58. Schmitt, H., Schmitt, H., and Fenard, S. (1971): Evidence for an alpha-sympathomimetic component in the effects of catapresan on vasomotor centres: Antagonism by piperoxane. *Eur. J. Pharmacol.*, 14:98–100.

59. Van Zwieten, P. A. (1973): The central action of antihypertensive drugs mediated via central alpha-receptors. *J. Pharm. Pharmacol.*, 25:89–95.

60. Day, M. D., and Roach, A. G. (1974): Central adrenoreceptors and the control of arterial blood pressure. *Clin. Exp. Pharm. Physiol.*, 1:347–360.

61. Struyker-Boudier, H. A. J., Smeets, G. W. M., Brouwer, G. M., and Van Rossum, J. M. (1974): Hypothalamic alpha-adrenergic receptors in cardiovascular regulation. *Neuropharmacology*, 13:837–846.

62. Struyker-Boudier, H., Smeets, G., Brouwer, G., and Van Rossum, J. (1974): Central and peripheral activity of imidazoline derivatives. *Life Sci.*, 15:887–899.

63. Nijkamp, F. P., and DeJong, W. (1975): Alpha-methylnoradrenaline induced hypotension and bradycardia after administration into the area of the nucleus tractus solitarii. *Eur. J. Pharmacol.*, 32:361–364.

64. Struyker-Boudier, H. A. J., and Bekers, A. D. (1975): Adrenaline-induced cardiovascular changes after intrahypothalamic administration to rats. *Eur. J. Pharmacol.*, 31:153–155.

65. Borkowski, K. R., and Finch, L. (1978): Cardiovascular responses to intraventricular adrenaline in spontaneous hypertensive rats. *Eur. J. Pharmacol.*, 47:281–290.

66. Van Zwieten, P. A. (1980): Pharmacology of centrally acting hypotensive drugs. *Br. J. Clin. Pharmacol.*, 10:135–205.

67. Timmermans, P. B. M. W. M., and Van Zwieten, P. A. (1981): Correlations between central hypotensive and peripheral hypertensive effects of structurally dissimilar alpha-adrenoreceptor agonists. *Life Sci.*, 28:653–660.

68. De Jonge, A., Timmermans, P. B. M. W. M., and Van Zwieten, P. A. (1982): Quantitative aspects of alpha-adrenergic effects induced by clonidine like imidazolidines. II. Central and peripheral bradycardic activities. *J. Pharmacol. Exp. Ther.*, 222:712–719.

69. Baum, T., and Shropshire, A. T. (1974): Reduction of sympathetic outflow by central administration of L-DOPA, dopamine, and norepinephrine. *Neuropharmacology*, 12:49–56.

70. Sved, A. F., Fernstrom, J. D., and Wurtman, R. J. (1979): Tyrosine administration reduces blood pressure and enhances brain norepinephrine release in spontaneously hypertensive rats. *Proc. Natl. Acad. Sci. U.S.A.*, 76:3511–3514.

71. Bresnahan, M. R., Halzinikolaou, P., Brunner, H. R., and Gavras, H. (1980): Effects of tyrosine infusion in normotensive and hypertensive rats. *Ann. J. Physiol.*, 239:H206–H211.

72. Yamori, Y., Fujiwara, M., Horie, R., and Lovenberg, W. (1980): The hypotensive effect of centrally administered tyrosine. *Eur. J. Pharmacol.*, 68:201–204.

73. Edwards, D. J. (1982): Possible role of octopamine and tyramine in the antihypertensive and antidepressant effects of tyrosine. *Life Sci.*, 30:1427–1434.

74. Henning, M., and Rubenson, A. (1970): Evidence for a centrally mediated hypotensive effect of L-DOPA in the rat. *J. Pharm. Pharmacol.*, 22:241–243.

75. Watanabe, A. M., Parks, L. C., and Kopin, I. J. (1971): Modification of the cardiovascular effects of L-DOPA by decarboxylase inhibitors. *J. Clin. Invest.*, 50:1322–1328.

76. Robson, R. D. (1971): Modification of the cardiovascular effects of L-DOPA in anesthetized dogs by inhibitors of enzymes involved in catecholamine metabolism. *Circ. Res.*, 29:662–670.

77. Minsker, D. H., Scriabine, A., Strokes, A. L., Stone, C. A., and Torchiana, M. L. (1971): Effects of L-DOPA alone and in combination with dopa decarboxylase inhibitors on the arterial pressure and heart rate of dogs. *Experientia*, 27:529–531.

78. Osborne, M. W., Wenger, J. J., and Willems, W. (1971): The cardiovascular pharmacology of L(-)-DOPA: Peripheral and central actions. *J. Pharmacol. Exp. Ther.*, 178:517–528.

79. Antonaccio, M. J., Robson, R. D., and Burrell, R. (1974): The effects of L-DOPA and alpha-methyldopa on reflexes and sympathetic nerve function. *Eur. J. Pharmacol.*, 25:9–18.

80. Hare, B. D., Neumayr, R. J., and Franz, D. N. (1972): Opposite effects of L-DOPA and 5-HTP on spinal sympathetic reflexes. *Nature*, 239:336–337.

81. Schmitt, H., Schmitt, H., and Fenard, S. (1972): New evidence for an alpha-adrenergic component in the sympathetic centres: Centrally mediated decrease in sympathetic tone and its antagonism by piperoxane and yohimbine. *Eur. J. Pharmacol.*, 17:293–296.

82. Neumayr, R. J., Hare, B. D., and Franz, D. N. (1974): Evidence for bulbospinal control of sympathetic preganglionic neurons by monoaminergic pathways. *Life Sci.*, 14:793–806.

83. Coote, J. H., and Macleod, V. H. (1974): The influence of bulbospinal monoaminergic pathways on sympathetic nerve activity. *J. Physiol. (Lond.)*, 241:453–475.

84. Watanabe, A. M., Judy, W. V., and Cardon, P. V. (1974): Effect of L-DOPA on blood pressure and sympathetic nerve activity after decarboxylase inhibition in cats. *J. Pharmacol. Exp. Ther.*, 188:107–113.

85. Henning, M., Rubenson, A., and Trolin, G. (1972): On the localization of the hypotensive effect of L-DOPA. *J. Pharm. Pharmacol.*, 24:447–451.

86. Schmitt, H., Schmitt, H., and Fenard, S. (1973): Localization of the site of the central sympathoinhibitory action of L-DOPA in dogs and cats. *Eur. J. Pharmacol.*, 22:212–216.

87. McCubbin, J. W., Kaneko, Y., and Page, I. H. (1960): Ability of serotonin and norepinephrine to mimic the central effects of reserpine on vasomotor activity. *Circ. Res.*, 8:849–858.

88. Bloch, R., Bousquet, P., Feldman, J., Velly, J., and Schwartz, J. (1974): Action hypotensive de la clonidine appliquee sur la surface ventrale du bulbe rachi-

dien: Analogie avec la dopamine. *Therapie*, 29:251–259.

89. Butcher, L., Engel, J., and Fuxe, K. (1970): L-DOPA-induced changes in central monoamine neurons after peripheral decarboxylase inhibition. *J. Pharm. Pharmacol.*, 22:313–316.

90. Nakamura, K., Mizogami, S., and Nakamura, K. (1975): Difference in hypotensive response to L-DOPA and a decarboxylase inhibitor in various forms of hypertensive rats. *Jpn. J. Pharmacol.*, 25:85–92.

91. Davidson, L., Lloyd, K., Dankova, J., and Hornykiewicz, O. (1971): L-DOPA treatment in Parkinson's disease: Effect on dopamine and related substances in discrete brain regions. *Experientia*, 27:1048–1049.

92. Torchiana, M. L., Lotti, V. J., Clark, C. M., and Stone, C. A. (1973): Comparison of centrally mediated hypotensive action of methyldopa and DOPA in cats. *Arch. Int. Pharmacodyn. Ther.*, 205:103–113.

93. Antonaccio, M. J., and Robson, R. D. (1974): L-DOPA hypotension: Evidence for mediation through 5-HT release. *Arch. Int. Pharmacodyn. Ther.*, 212:89–102.

94. Ungerstedt, U. (1971): Stereotaxic mapping of the monoamine pathways in the rat brain. *Acta Physiol. Scand. [Suppl. 367]* 1–48.

95. Palkovits, M., Brownstein, M., Saavedra, J. M., and Axelrod, J., Jr. (1974): Norepinephrine and dopamine content of hypothalamic nuclei of the rat. *Brain Res.* 77:137–149.

96. Przuntek, H., and Philippu, A. (1973): Reduced pressor responses to stimulation of the locus caeruleus after lesion of the posterior hypothalamus. *Naunyn Schmidedbergs Arch. Pharmacol.*, 276:119–122.

97. Philippu. A., Heyd, G., and Burger, A. (1970): Release of noradrenaline from the hypothalamus *in vivo. Eur. J. Pharmacol.*, 9:52–58.

98. Philippu, A., Przuntek, H., Heyd, G., and Burger, A. (1971): Central effects of sympathomimetic amines on the blood pressure. *Eur. J. Pharmacol.*, 15:200–208.

99. Przuntek, H., Guimaraes, S., and Philippu, A. (1971): Importance of adrenergic neurons of the brain for the rise of blood pressure evoked by hypothalamic stimulation. *Naunyn Schmiedebergs Arch. Pharmacol.*, 271:311–319.

100. Philippu, A., Demmeler, R., and Roensberg, G. (1974): Effects of centrally-applied drugs on pressor responses to hypothalamic stimulation. *Naunyn Schmiedebergs Arch. Pharmacol.*, 282:389–400.

101. Dutta, S. N., Guha, D., and Pradhan, S. N. (1975): Cardiovascular effects of central microinjections of apomorphine in cats. *Arch. Int. Pharmacodyn. Ther.*, 315:259–265.

102. Heise, A. (1976): Hypotensive action by central alpha-adrenergic and dopaminergic receptor stimulation. In: *New Antihypertensive Drugs*, edited by A. Scriabine and C. S. Sweet, pp. 135–145. Spectrum Publications, New York.

103. Day, M. D., and Roach, A. G. (1976): Cardiovascular effects of dopamine after central administration

into conscious cats. *Br. J. Pharmacol.*, 58:505–515.

104. Lang, W. J., and Woodman, O. L. (1979): Cardiovascular responses produced by the injection of dopamine into the cerebral ventricles of the unanesthetized dog. *Br. J. Pharmacol.*, 66:235–240.

105. Yen, T. T., Stamm, N. B., and Clemens, J. A. (1979): Pergolide: A potent dopaminergic antihypertensive. *Life Sci.*, 25:209–216.

106. Sved, A. F., and Fernstrom, J. D. (1979): Reduction in blood pressure in normal and spontaneously hypertensive rats by lergotrile mesylate. *J. Pharm. Pharmacol.*, 31:814–817.

107. Cavero, I., Lefevre-Borg, F., and Gomeni, R. (1981): Heart rate lowering effects of *N,N*-di-*n*-propyl-dopamine in rats: Evidence for stimulation of central dopamine receptors leading to inhibition of sympathetic tone and enhancement of parasympathetic outflow. *J. Pharmacol. Exp. Ther.*, 219:510–519.

108. Cavero, I., and Lefevre-Borg, F. (1981): Functional and pharmacological role of cardiovascular dopamine receptors. In: *New Trends in Arterial Hypertension*, edited by M. Worcel, pp. 87–99. Elsevier/North Holland, Armsterdam.

109. Bhargava, K. P., Mishra, N., and Tangri, K. K. (1972): An analysis of central adrenoceptors for control of cardiovascular function. *Br. J. Pharmacol.*, 45:596–602.

110. Burden, D. T., and Parks, M. W. (1975): An investigation of the tachycardia produced by intracerebroventricular injections of isoprenaline in mice. *Br. J. Pharmacol.*, 53:341–347.

111. Kelliher, G. J., and Buckley, J. P. (1970): Central hypotensive activity of *dl*- and *d*-propranolol. *J. Pharm. Sci.*, 59:1276–1280.

112. Roberts, J., and Kelliher, G. (1973): Effect of practolol and sotalol on adrenergic nervous activity. *Fed. Proc.*, 32:780.

113. Lewis, P. J., and Haeusler, G. (1975): Reduction in sympathetic nervous activity as a mechanism for hypotensive effect of propranolol. *Nature*, 256:440.

114. Chalmers, J. P. (1976): Neuropharmacology of central mechanisms regulating pressure. In: *Central Actions of Drugs in the Regulation of the Circulation*, edited by J. L. Reid and D. S. Davies, pp. 36–60. Pitman Medical Press, London.

115. Lewis, P. J., Rawlins, M. D., and Reid, J. L. (1972): Acute thermoregulatory and cardiovascular effects of 6-hydroxydopamine administered centrally in rabbits and cats. *Br. J. Pharmacol.*, 44:559 (abstract).

116. Haeusler, G., Gerold, M., and Theonen, T. (1972): Cardiovascular effects of 6-hyroxydopamine injected into a lateral brain ventricle of the rat. *Naunyn Schmiedebergs Arch. Pharmacol.*, 274:211–228.

117. De Champlain, J., and Van Amerigen, M. R. (1972): Regulation of blood pressure by sympathetic nerve fibers and adrenal medulla in normotensive and hypertensive rats. *Circ. Res.*, 31:617–628.

118. Korner, P. I., and White, S. W. (1966): Circulatory control in hypoxia by the sympathetic nerves and adrenal medulla. *J. Physiol. (Lond.)*, 184:272–290.

119. Leskell, L. G. (1976): Influence of prostaglandin E$_1$ on cerebral mechanisms involved in the control of fluid balance. *Acta Physiol. Scand.*, 98:85–93.

120. Kondo, K., Okuno, T., Konishi, K., Saruta, T., and Kato, E. (1979): Central and peripheral effects of bradykinin and prostaglandin E$_2$ on blood pressure in conscious rats. *Naunyn Schmiedebergs Arch. Pharmacol.*, 308:111–115.

121. Kondo, K., Okuno, T., Saruta, T., and Kato, E. (1979): Effects of intracerebroventricular administration of prostaglandins I$_2$, E$_2$, F$_2$, and indomethacin on blood pressure in the rat. *Prostaglandins*, 17:769–774.

122. Hoffman, W. E., and Valigura, T. J. (1979): Independence of cardiovascular and hyperthermic effects of central prostaglandin E$_2$. *Brain Res.*, 173:160–163.

123. Karppanen, H., Siren, A., and Eskeli-Kaivosoja, A. (1979): Central cardiovascular and thermal effects of prostaglandin F$_2$ in rats. *Prostaglandins*, 17:385–394.

124. Correa, F. M. A., and Graeff, F. G. (1974): Central mechanisms of the hypertensive action of intraventricular bradykinin in the unanesthetized rat. *Neuropharmacology*, 13:65–75.

125. Correa, F. M. A., and Graeff, F. G. (1976): On the mechanism of the hypertensive action of intraseptal bradykinin in the rat. *Neuropharmacology*, 15:713–717.

126. Takahashi, H., and Bunag, R. D. (1981): Centrally induced cardiovascular and sympathetic nerve responses to bradykinin in rats. *J. Pharmacol. Exp. Ther.*, 216:192–197.

127. Bloom, F. E. (1975): The role of cyclic nucleotides in central synaptic function. *Rev. Physiol. Biochem. Pharmacol.*, 74:1–32.

128. Delbarre, B., Senon, D., and Schmitt, H. (1977): Cyclic 3′5′-adenosine monophosphate and central circulatory control in cats and dogs. *Clin. Exp. Pharmacol. Physiol.*, 4:341–348.

129. White, H. S., and Isom, G. E. (1978): Central effects of $N^6,O^{2'}$-dibutyryl adenosine 3′5′-cyclic monophosphate on blood pressure. *Proc. West. Pharmacol. Soc.*, 21:253–256.

130. White, H. S., Sriver, P. S., and Isom, G. E. (1979): Studies on the central pressor activity of dibutyryl cyclic AMP. *Eur. J. Pharmacol.*, 57:107–113.

131. Clipsham, P. J., Hamilton, T. C., Hunt, A. A. E., and Poyser, R. H. (1980): Cyclic nucleotides and central cardiovascular control in the conscious cat. *Eur. J. Pharmacol.*, 65:193–200.

132. Kobinger, W., Walland, A., and Kadatz, R. (1976): Stimulation of sympathetic cardiovascular centres by RA 642, a new pyrimido-pyrimidine derivative. *Naunyn Schmiedebergs Arch. Pharmacol.*, 292:105–111.

133. Schuhmacher, P., and Walland, A. (1980): Central blood pressure effects of guanylyl-imideo-diphosphate and cyclic guanosine monophosphate. *Naunyn Schmiedebergs Arch. Pharmacol.*, 312:31–35.

134. Takahashi, H., Tiba, M., Ino, M., and Takayasu, T. (1955): The effect of γ-aminobutyric acid on blood pressure. *Jpn. J. Physiol.*, 5:334–339.

135. Takahashi, H., Tiba, M., Yamazaki, T., and Noguchi, F. (1958): On the site of action of γ-aminobutyric acid on blood pressure. *Jpn. J. Physiol.*, 8:378–390.

136. Bhargava, K. P., Bhattacharya, S. S., and Srimal,

R. C. (1964): Central cardiovascular actions of γ-aminobutyric acid. *Br. J. Pharmacol.*, 23:383–390.

137. Bhattacharya, S. S., Kishor, K., Saxena, P. N., and Bhargava, K. P. (1964): A neuropharmacological study of gamma-aminobutyric acid (GABA). *Arch. Int. Pharmacodyn. Ther.*, 150:295–305.

138. Hedwall, P. R., Maitre, L., and Brunner, H. (1968): Influence of ω-amino acids on blood pressure, catecholamine stores, and the pressor response to physostigmine in the rat. *J. Pharm. Pharmacol.*, 20:737–743.

139. Guertzenstein, P. G. (1973): Blood pressure effects obtained by drugs applied to the ventral surface of the brainstem. *J. Physiol. (Lond.)*, 229:395–408.

140. Seetha Devi, K., and Reddy, L. R. K. (1972): Effect of gamma-amino-butyric acid on spinal vascular reflex mechanism. *Indian J. Physiol. Pharmacol.*, 16:309–313.

141. Sgaragli, G., and Pavan, F. (1972): Effects of amino acid compounds injected into cerebrospinal fluid spaces, on colonic temperature, arterial blood pressure and behaviour of the rat. *Neuropharmacology*, 11:45–56.

142. Philippu, A., Przuntek, H., and Roensberg, W. (1973): Superfusion of the hypothalamus with gamma-aminobutyric acid. *Naunyn Schmiedebergs Arch Pharmacol.*, 276:137–143.

143. Antonaccio, M. J., and Taylor, D. G. (1977): Involvement of central GABA receptors in the regulation of blood pressure and heart rate of anesthetized cats. *Eur. J. Pharmacol.*, 46:283–287.

144. Antonaccio, M. J., Kerwin, L., and Taylor, D. G. (1978): Reductions in blood pressure, heart rate, and renal sympathetic nerve discharge in cats after the central administration of muscimol, a GABA agonist. *Neuropharmacology*, 17:783–791.

145. Srimal, R. C., Gulati, K., and Dhawan, B. H. (1977): On the mechanism of central hypotensive action of clonidine. *Can. J. Physiol. Pharmacol.*, 55:1007–1014.

146. Bousquet, P., Feldman, J., Bloch, R., and Schwartz, J. (1978): Ventromedullary hypotensive action of muscimol. *C. R. Soc. Biol. (Paris)*, 172:770–773.

147. Sweet, C. W., Wenger, H. C., and Gross, D. M. (1979): Central antihypertensive properties of muscimol and related γ-aminobutyric acid agonists and the interaction of muscimol with baroreceptor reflexes. *Can. J. Physiol. Pharmacol.*, 57:600–605.

148. Sweet, C. S., Wenger, H. C., Taylor, D. A., and Gross, D. M. (1980): Central antihypertensive properties of muscimol and related structures. *Brain Res. Bull. [Suppl. 2]*, 5:491–496.

149. Williford, D. J., Hamilton, B. L., Dias Souza, J., Williams, T. P., DiMicco, J. A., and Gillis, R. A. (1980): Central nervous system mechanisms involving GABA influence arterial pressure and heart rate in the cat. *Circ. Res.*, 47:80–86.

150. Gillis, R. A., DiMicco, J. A., Williford, D. J., Hamilton, B. L., and Gale, K. N. (1980): Importance of CNS GABAergic mechanisms in the regulation of cardiovascular function. *Brain Res. Bull. [Suppl. 2]*, 5:303–315.

151. Snyder, D. W., and Antonaccio, M. J. (1980): Central sites involved in the hypotensive effects of muscimol. *Brain Res. Bull. [Suppl. 2]*, 5:317–323.

152. Snyder, D. W., Macklem, L. J., and Severini, W. H. (1980): Central cardiovascular effects of the GABA-mimetic agent, THIP. *Neurosciences*, 6:755.

153. Antonaccio, M. J., and Snyder, D. W. (1981): Reductions in blood pressure, heart rate, and renal sympathetic nervous discharge after imidazole-4-acetic acid: Mediation through central GABA receptor stimulation. *J. Pharmacol. Exp. Ther.*

154. Antonaccio, M. J. (1982): GABA and inhibition of autonomic outflow: A central transmitter role? In: *Trends in Autonomic Pharmacology, Vol. 2,* edited by S. Kalsner, pp. 217–236. Urban and Schwarzenberg, Baltimore.

155. Bowery, N. G., Doble, A., Hill, D. R., Hudson, A. L., Shaw, J., and Turnbull, M. J. (1980): β-chlorophenyl GABA (baclofen) is a selective ligand for a novel GABA receptor on nerve terminal. *Brain Res. Bull. [Suppl. 2]*, 5:497–502.

156. Bowery, N. G., Hill, D. R., Hudson, A. L., Doble, A., Middlemias, D. N., Shaw, J., and Turnbull, M. (1980): Baclofen decreases neurotransmitter release in the mammalian CNS by an action at a novel GABA receptor. *Nature*, 283:92–94.

157. Olsen, R. W., Ticku, M. K., Greenlee, D., and Van Ness, P. T. (1979): GABA receptor and ionophore binding sites: Interaction with various drugs. In: *GABA Neurotransmitters*, edited by P. Krogsgaard-Larsen, J. Scheel-Kruger, and H. Kofold, pp. 165–178. Munksgaard, Copenhagen.

158. Naik, S. R., Guidotti, A., and Costa, E. (1976): Central GABA receptor antagonists: Comparison of muscimol and baclofen. *Neuropharmacology*, 15:479–484.

159. Waddington, J. L., and Cross, A. J. (1980): GABA-ergic properties of baclofen *in vivo* and *in vitro*. *Brain Res. Bull. [Suppl. 2]*, 5:503–505.

160. Persson, B., and Henning, M. (1980): Central cardiovascular and biochemical effects of baclofen in the conscious rat. *J. Pharm. Pharmacol.*, 32:417–422.

161. Chahl, L. A., and Walker, S. B. (1980): The effect of baclofen on the cardiovascular system of the rat. *Br. J. Pharmacol.*, 69:631–637.

162. Persson, B. (1980): GABA-ergic mechanisms in blood pressure control. *Acta Physiol. Scand. [Suppl. 491]* 1–54.

163. Curtis, D. R., Duggan, A. W., Felix, D., and Johnston, D. A. R. (1970): Bicuculline and central GABA receptors. *Nature*, 228:676–677.

164. Curtis, D. R., Duggan, A. W., Felix, D., and Johnston, D. A. R. (1971): Bicuculline, an antagonist of GABA and synaptic inhibition in the spinal cord of the cat. *Brain Res.*, 32:69–96.

165. Takeuchi, A., and Takeuchi, N. (1969): A study of the action of picrotoxin on the inhibitory neuromuscular junction of the crayfish. *J. Physiol. (Lond.)*, 205:377–391.

166. Shore, N. N., and Melville, K. I. (1965): Intraventricular injections of picrotoxin following central adrenergic blockade with phenoxybenzamine and dichloroisoproterenol. *Int. J. Neuropharmacol.*, 4:149–156.

167. Polosa, C., Lake Teare, J., and Wyszogrodski, I. (1972): Slow rhythms of sympathetic discharge induced by convulsant drugs. *Can. J. Physiol. Pharmacol.*, 50:188–194.

168. Polosa, C., Rosenberg, P., Mannard, A., Wolkove, N., and Wyszogrodski, I. (1969): Oscillatory behavior of the sympathetic system induced by picrotoxin. *Can. J. Physiol. Pharmacol.*, 47:815–826.

169. Lee, T. M., Yang, K. L., Keo, J. S., and Choi, C. Y. (1972): Importance of sympathetic mechanism on cardiac arrhythmias induced by picrotoxin. *Exp. Neurol.*, 36:389–398.

170. Bircher, R. P., Kanai, T., and Wang, S. C. (1963): Mechanisms of cardiac arrhythmias and blood pressure changes induced in dogs by pentylenetetrozal, picrotoxin, and digitoxin. *J. Pharmacol. Exp. Ther.*, 141:6–14.

171. DiMicco, J. A., Hamilton, B. L., and Gillis, R. A. (1977): Central nervous system sites involved in the cardiovascular effects of picrotoxin. *J. Pharmacol. Exp. Ther.*, 203:64–71.

172. DiMicco, J. A., Prestel, T., Pearle, D. L., and Gillis, R. A. (1977): Mechanism of cardiovascular changes produced in cats by activation of the central nervous system with picrotoxin. *Circ. Res.*, 4:446–451.

173. DiMicco, J. A., Gale, K., Hamilton, B., and Gillis, R. A. (1979): GABA receptor control of parasympathetic outflow to heart: Characterization and brainstem localization. *Science*, 204:1106–1109.

174. DiMicco, J. A., and Gillis, R. A. (1979): Neurocardiovascular effects produced by bicuculline in the cat. *J. Pharmacol. Exp. Ther.*, 210:1–6.

175. Feldberg, W., and Rocha e Silva, M. Jr. (1978): Vasopressin release produced in anaesthetized cats by antagonists of γ-aminobutyric acid and glycine. *Br. J. Pharmacol.*, 62:99–106.

176. Williford, D. J., Hamilton, B. L., and Gillis, R. A. (1980): Evidence that a GABA-ergic mechanism at nucleus ambiguus influences reflex induced vagal activity. *Brain Res.*, 193:584–588.

177. Barman, S. M., and Gebber, G. L. (1979): Picrotoxin and bicuculline sensitive inhibition of cardiac vagal reflexes. *J. Pharmacol. Exp. Ther.*, 209:67–72.

178. Gale, K., Hamilton, B. L., Brown, S. C., Norman, W. P., Dias Souza, J., and Gillis, R. A. (1980): GABA and specific GABA binding sites in brain nuclei associated with vagal outflow. *Brain Res. Bull. [Suppl. 2]*, 5:325–328.

179. Georgiev, V. P., Doda, M., and Hyorgy, L. (1978): The effects of intraventriculatory administered GABA and picrotoxin and their interactions on somato-vegetative reflexes in cats. *Arch. Int. Pharmacodyn. Ther.*, 23:139–147.

180. Taylor, D. G., Taylor, F. A., and Antonaccio, M. J. (1982): Pharmacological studies on sympathoinhibition produced by the medial medullary depressor region: Proposed γ-aminobutyric acid involvement in inhibition of somatosympathetic reflexes. *J. Pharmacol. Exp. Ther.*, 222:517–525.

181. Lalley, P. M. (1980): Inhibition of depressor cardiovascular reflexes by a derivative of γ-aminobutyric acid (GABA) and by general anesthetics with suspected GABA-mimetic effects. *J. Pharmacol. Exp. Ther.*, 215:418–425.

182. Bosmann, H. B., Fenney, D. P., Case, K. R., DiStefano, P., and Averill, K. (1978): Diazepam receptor specific binding of ^{3}H-flunitrazepam to rat brain subfractions. *F.E.B.S. Lett.*, 87:199.

183. Mohler, H., and Okada, T. (1977): Benzodiazepine receptor: Demonstration in the central nervous system. *Science*, 198:849–851.

184. Costa, E., Guidotti, A., and Mao, S. C. (1976): A GABA hypothesis for the action of benzodiazepines. In: *GABA in Nervous System Function*, edited by E. Roberts, T. N. Chase, and D. B. Tower, pp. 413–426. Raven Press, New York.

185. Costa, E., Guidotti, A., Mao, C. C., and Suria, A. (1975): New concepts on the mechanism of action of benzodiazepines. *Life Sci.*, 17:167–186.

186. Haefely, W., Kulcsar, A., Mohler, H., Pieri, L., Polc, P., and Schaffner, R. (1975): Possible involvement of GABA in the central actions of benzodiazepines. In: *Mechanism of Action in Benzodiazepines*, edited by E. Costa and P. Greengard, pp. 131–151. Raven Press, New York.

187. Haefely, W., Polc, P., Schaffner, R., Keller, H. H., Pieri, L., and Mohler, H. (1979): Facilitation of GABA-ergic transmission by drugs. In: *GABA Neurotransmitters*, edited by P. Krogsgaard-Larsen, J. Scheel-Kruger, and H. Kofod, pp. 357–375. Munksgaard, Copenhagen.

188. Briley, M. S., and Langer, S. Z. (1978): Influence of GABA receptor agonists and antagonists on the binding of ^{3}H-diazepam to the benzodiazepine receptor. *Eur. J. Pharmacol.*, 52:129–132.

189. Martin, I. L., and Candy, J. M. (1978): Facilitation of benzodiazepine binding by sodium chloride and GABA. *Neuropharmacology*, 17:993–998.

190. Gallagher, D. W., Thomas, J. W., and Tallman, J. F. (1978): Effect of GABA-ergic drugs on benzodiazepine binding site sensitivity in rat cerebral cortex. *Biochem. Pharmacol.*, 27:2745–2749.

191. Wastek, G. J., Speth, S. C., Reisine, T. D., and Yamamura, H. I. (1978): The effect of γ-aminobutyric acid on ^{3}H-flunitrazepam binding. *Eur. J. Pharmacol.*, 50:445–447.

192. Tallman, J. F. (1980): Interactions between GABA and benzodiazepines. *Brain Res. Bull. [Suppl. 2]*, 5:829–832.

193. Chiu, T. H., and Rosenberg, H. C. (1979): GABA-receptor mediated modulation of H^3-diazepam binding in rat cortex. *Eur. J. Pharmacol.*, 56:337–345.

194. Gavish, M., and Snyder, S. H. (1980): Soluble benzodiazepine receptors: GABA-ergic regulation. *Life Sci.*, 26:579–582.

195. Karobath, M., and Lippitsch, M. (1979): THIP and isoguvacine are partial agonists of GABA-stimulated benzodiazepine receptor binding. *Eur. J. Pharmacol.*, 58:485–488.

196. Karobath, M., and Sperk, G. (1979): Stimulation of benzodiazepine receptor binding by γ-aminobutyric acid. *Proc. Natl. Acad. Sci. U.S.A.*, 76:1004–1006.

197. Massotti, M., and Guidotti, A. (1980): Endogenous regulators of benzodiazepine recognition sites. *Life Sci.*, 27:847–854.

198. Speth, R. C., Bresolin, N., and Yamamura, H. I. (1979): Acute diazepam administration produces

rapid increases in brain benzodiazepine receptor density. *Eur. J. Pharmacol.,* 59:159–160.

199. Choi, D. W., Farb, D. H., and Fischbach, G. D. (1977): Chlordiazepoxide selectivity augments GABA action in spinal cord cell cultures. *Nature,* 269:342–344.

200. Gallager, D. W. (1978): Benzodiazepines: Potentiation of a GABA inhibitory response in the dorsal raphe nucleus. *Eur. J. Pharmacol.,* 49:133–143.

201. Geller, H. M., Hoffer, B. J., and Taylor, D. A. (1980): Electrophysiological actions of benzodiazepines. *Fed. Proc.,* 39:3016–3023.

202. Geller, H. M., Taylor, D. A., and Hoffer, B. J.: Benzodiazepines and central inhibitory mechanisms. *Naunyn Schmiedebergs Arch. Pharmacol.,* 304:81–88.

203. Cananzi, A. R., Costa, E., and Guidotti, A. (1980): Potentiation by intraventricular muscimol of the anticonflict effect of benzodiazepines. *Brain Res.,* 196:447–453.

204. Antonaccio, M. J. (1979): Cardiovascular pharmacology of anxiolytics. In: *Anxiolytics,* edited by S. Fielding and L. Harbans, pp. 197–209. Futura Publishing, Mount Kisco, N.Y.

205. Schalleck, W., Zabransky, F., and Kuehn, A. (1964): Effects of benzodiazepines on central nervous system of cat. *Arch. Int. Pharmacodyn. Ther.,* 149:467–483.

206. Antonaccio, M. J., and Halley, J. (1975): Inhibition of centrally evoked pressor responses by diazepam: Evidence for an exclusively supramedullary action. *Neuropharmacology,* 14:649–657.

207. Antonaccio, M. J., Kerwin, L., and Taylor, D. G. (1978): Effects of central GABA receptor agonism and antagonism on evoked diencephalic cardiovascular responses. *Neuropharmacology,* 17:597–603.

208. Benson, J., Herd, J. A., Morse, W. H., and Kelleher, R. T. (1970): Hypotensive effects of chlordiazepoxide, amobarbital, and chlorpromazine on behaviorally induced elevated arterial blood pressure in the squirrel monkey. *J. Pharmacol. Exp. Ther.,* 173:399–406.

209. Bergamaschi, M., and Longoni, A. M. (1973): Cardiovascular events in anxiety: Experimental studies in the conscious dog. *Am. Heart J.,* 86:385–394.

210. Kuhn, D. M., Wolf, W. A., and Lovenberg, W. (1980): Review of the role of the central serotonergic neuronal system in blood pressure regulation. *Hypertension,* 2:243–255.

211. Fuxe, K., Butcher, L. L., and Engel, J. (1971): DL-5-hydroxytryptophan induced changes in central monoamine neurons after peripheral decarboxylase inhibition. *J. Pharm. Pharmacol.,* 23:420–424.

212. Corrodi, H., Fuxe, K., and Hokfelt, T. (1967): Replenishment by 5-hydroxytryptophan of the amine stores in the central 5-hydroxytryptamine neurons after depletion induced by reserpine or by an inhibitor of monoamine synthesis. *J. Pharm. Pharmacol.,* 19:433–438.

213. Bogdanski, D. F., Weissbach, H., and Udenfriend, S. (1958): Pharmacological studies with serotonin precursor, 5-hydroxytryptophan. *J. Pharmacol. Exp. Ther.,* 122:182–194.

214. Dunkley, B., Sanghvi, I., Friedman, E., and Gershon, S. (1972): Comparison of behavioural and cardiovascular effects of L-DOPA and 5-HTP in conscious dogs. *Psychopharmacologia,* 26:161–172.

215. McGregor, D. D., and Smirk, F. H. (1970): Vascular responses to 5-hydroxytryptamine in genetic and renal hypertensive rats. *Am. J. Physiol.,* 219:687–690.

216. Antonaccio, M. J., and Cavaliere, T. (1974): A comparison of the effects of some inotropic and chronotropic agents on isolated atria from normotensive (NTR) and spontaneously hypertensive (SHR) rats. *Arch. Int. Pharmacodyn. Ther.,* 209:273–282.

217. Antonaccio, M. J., and Robson, R. D. (1973): Cardiovascular effects of 5-hydroxytryptophan in anesthetized dogs. *J. Pharm. Pharmacol.,* 25:495–497.

218. Antonaccio, M. J., and Robson, R. D. (1975): Centrally mediated cardiovascular effects of 5-hydroxytryptophan in MAO-inhibited dogs: Modification by autonomic antagonists. *Arch. Int. Pharmacodyn. Ther.,* 213:200–210.

219. Baum, T., and Shropshire, A. T. (1975): Inhibition of efferent sympathetic nerve activity by 5-hydroxytryptophan and centrally administered 5-hydroxytryptamine. *Neuropharmacology,* 14:227–233.

220. Florez, J., and Armijo, J. A. (1974): Effect of central inhibition of the *l*-amino acid decarboxylase on the hypotensive action of 5-HT precursors in cats. *Eur. J. Pharmacol.,* 26:108–110.

221. Fuller, R. W., Holland, D. R., Yen, T. T., Bemis, K. G., and Stamm, N. B. (1979): Antihypertensive effects of fluoxetine and L-5-hydroxytryptophan in rats. *Life Sci.,* 25:1237–1242.

222. Fuller, R. W., Yen, T. T., and Stamm, N. B. (1981): Lowering of blood pressure by direct and indirect-acting serotonin agonists in spontaneously hypertensive rats. *Clin. Exp. Hypertension,* 3:497–508.

223. Antonaccio, M. J., and Kerwin, L. (1981): On the effect and mechanism of action of the antihypertensive agent, TR 3369 (5-methoxytryptamine-β-methylcarboxylate) in SHR. *J. Cardiovasc. Pharmacol.,* 3:1306–1311.

224. Nava-Felix, P., and Hong, E. (1979): Nature of the central serotonin receptors mediating hypotension. *J. Cardiovasc. Pharmacol.,* 1:461–466.

225. Lambert, G. A., Friedman, E., Buchweitz, E., and Gershon, S. (1978): Involvement of 5-hydroxytryptamine in the central control of respiration, blood pressure and heart rate in the anaesthetized rat. *Neuropharmacology,* 17:807–813.

226. Tadepalli, A. S., Mills, E., and Schanberg, S. M. (1977): Central depression of carotid baroreceptor pressor responses, arterial pressure, and heart rate by 5-hydroxytryptophan influence of supracollicular areas of the brain. *J. Pharmacol. Exp. Ther.,* 202:310–319.

227. Franz, D. N., Madsen, P. W., Peterson, R. G., and Sangda, C. (1982): Functional roles of monoaminergic pathways to sympathetic preganglionic neurons. *Clin. Exp. Hypertension.* A4:543–562.

228. Smits, J. F., and Struyker-Boudier, H. A. (1976): Intrahypothalamic serotonin and cardiovascular control in rats. *Brain Res.,* 111:422–427.

229. Wolf, W. A., Kuhn, D. M., and Lovenberg, W. (1981): Blood pressure responses to local application of serotonergic agents in the nucleus tractus solitarii. *Eur. J. Pharmacol.,* 69:291–299.

230. Bobillier, P., Petitjean, F., Salvert, D., Ligier, M., and Seguin, S. (1975): Differential projections of the nucleus raphe dorsalis and nucleus raphe centralis as revealed by autoradiography. *Brain Res.,* 85:205–210.

231. Chu, N., and Bloom, F. E. (1974): The catecholamine-containing neurons in the cat dorsolateral pontine tegmentum: Distribution of the cell bodies and some axonal projections. *Brain Res.,* 66:1–21.

232. Antonaccio, M. J., and Halley, J. (1975): Inhibition of centrally evoked pressor responses by diazepam: Evidence for an exclusively supramedullary action. *Neuropharmacology,* 14:649–658.

233. Saavedra, J. M., Palkovits, M., Brownstein, M. J., and Axelrod, J. (1974): Serotonin distribution in the nuclei of the rat hypothalamus and preoptic region. *Brain Res.,* 77:157–165.

234. Morrison, S. F., and Gebber, G. L. (1982): Classification of raphe neurons with cardiac related activity. *Am. J. Physiol.,* 12:R49–R59.

235. Adair, J. R., Hamilton, B. L., Scappaticci, K. A., Helke, C. J., and Gillis, R. A. (1977): Cardiovascular responses to electrical stimulation of the medullary raphe area of the cat. *Brain Res.,* 128:141–151.

236. Chase, T. N., and Murphy, D. L. (1973): Serotonin and central nervous system function. *Annu. Rev. Pharmacol.,* 33:181–197.

237. Koe, B. K., and Weissman, A. (1966): *p*-Chlorophenylalanine: A specific depletor of brain serotonin. *J. Pharmacol. Exp. Ther.,* 154:499–516.

238. Wing, L. M. H., and Chalmers, J. P. (1973): Participation of central serotonergic neurones in the control of the circulation in the rabbit: A study using 5,6-dihydroxytryptamine in experimental neurogenic and renal hypertension. *Circ. Res.,* 35:504–513.

239. Antonaccio, M. J., and Cote, D. (1976): Centrally mediated antihypertensive and bradycardic effects of methylsergide in spontaneously hypertensive rats. *Eur. J. Pharmacol.,* 36:451–454.

240. Antonaccio, M. J., Kelly, E., and Halley, J. (1975): Centrally mediated hypotension and bradycardia by methysergide in anesthetized dogs. *Eur. J. Pharmacol.,* 33:107–117.

241. Antonaccio, M. J., and Taylor, D. G. (1977): Reduction in blood pressure, sympathetic nerve discharge, and centrally evoked pressor responses by methysergide in anesthetized cats. *Eur. J. Pharmacol.,* 42:331–338.

242. McCall, R. B., and Humphrey, S. J. (1982): Involvement of serotonin in the central regulation of blood pressure: Evidence for a facilitating effect on sympathetic nerve activity. *J. Pharmacol. Exp. Ther.,* 222:94–102.

243. Wing, L. M. H., and Chalmers, J. P. (1974): Effects of *p*-chlorophenylalanine on blood pressure and heart rate in normal rabbits and with neurogenic hypertension. *Clin. Exp. Pharmacol. Physiol.,* 1:219–229.

244. Lin, M. T., and Chern, S. I. (1979): Effect of brain 5-hydroxytryptamine alterations on reflex bradycardia in rats. *Am. J. Physiol.,* 236:R302–R306.

245. Tadepalli, A. S. (1980): Inhibition of reflex vagal bradycardia by a central action of 5-hydroxytryptophan. *Br. J. Pharmacol.,* 69:647–650.

246. Tadepalli, A. S., Ho, K. W., and Buckley, J. P. (1979): Enhancement of reflex vagal bradycardia following intracerebroventricular administration of methysergide in cats. *Eur. J. Pharmacol.,* 59:85–93.

247. Rabinowitz, S. H., and Lown, B. (1978): Central neurochemical factors related to serotonin metabolism and cardiac ventricular vulnerability for repetitive electrical activity. *Am. J. Cardiol.,* 41:516–522.

248. Blatt, C. M., Rabinowitz, S. H., and Lown, B. (1979): Central serotonergic agents raise the repetitive extrasystole threshold of the vulnerable period of the canine ventricular myocardium. *Circ. Res.,* 44:723–730.

249. Laubie, M., Schmitt, H., Canellas, J., Roquebert, J., and Demichel, P. (1974): Centrally mediated bradycardia and hypotension induced by narcotic analgesics: Dextromoramide and fentanyl. *Eur. J. Pharmacol.,* 28:66–75.

250. Freye, E., and Arndt, J. O. (1979): Perfusion of the fourth cerebral ventricle with fentanyl induces naloxone-reversible bradycardia, hypotension, and EEG synchronisation in conscious dogs. *Naunyn Schmiedebergs Arch. Pharmacol.,* 307:123–128.

251. Laubie, M., and Schmitt, H. (1979): Vagal bradycardia produced by microinjections of morphine-like drugs into the nucleus ambiguus in anesthetized dogs. *Eur. J. Pharmacol.,* 59:287–290.

252. Laubie, M., Schmitt, H., and Droinllat, M. (1977): Central sites and mechanisms of the hypotensive and bradycardic effects of the narcotic analgesic agent, fentanyl. *Naunyn Schmiedebergs Arch. Pharmacol.,* 296:255–261.

253. Laubie, M., Schmitt, H., and Vincent, M. (1979): Vagal bradycardia produced by microinjections of morphine-like drugs into the nucleus ambiguus in anaesthetized dogs. *Eur. J. Pharmacol.,* 59:287–291.

254. Wallenstein, M. C. (1979): Biphasic effects of morphine on cardiovascular system of the cat. *Eur. J. Pharmacol.,* 59:253–260.

255. Bellet, M., Teglozi, J. L., and Meyer, P. (1981): Central hypotensive effect of diprenorphine in normotensive rat and SHR. *Arch. Int. Pharmacodyn. Ther.,* 252:147–151.

256. Yukimura, T., Stock, G., Stumpf, H., Unger, T., and Gauten, D. (1981): Effects of [*O*-Ala²]-methionine-enkephalin on blood pressure, heart rate, and baroreceptor reflex sensitivity in conscious cats. *Hypertension,* 3:528–533.

257. Florez, J., and Mediavilla, A. (1977): Respiratory and cardiovascular effects of met-enkephalin applied to the ventral surface of the brain stem. *Brain Res.,* 138:585–590.

258. Laubie, M., Schmitt, H., Vincent, M., and Remond, G. (1977): Central cardiovascular effects of morphinomimetic peptides in dogs. *Eur. J. Pharmacol.,* 46:67–71.

259. Trendelenburg, U. (1957): Stimulation of sympathetic centers by histamine. *Circ. Res.,* 5:105–110.

260. White, T. (1961): Some effects of histamine and two histamine metabolites on the cats brain. *J. Physiol. (Lond.),* 159:198–202.

261. Finch, L., and Hicks, P. E. (1976): Central hypertensive action of histamine in conscious normotensive cats. *Eur. J. Pharmacol.*, 36:262–266.

262. Finch, L., and Hicks, P. E. (1976): The cardiovascular effects of intravenously administered histamine in the anaesthetized rat. *Naunyn Schmiedebergs Arch. Pharmacol.*, 293:151–157.

263. Finch, L., and Hicks, P. E. (1977): Involvement of hypothalamic histamine receptors in the central cardiovascular actions of histamine. *Neuropharmacology*, 16:211–218.

264. Pakkari, I., Karppanen, H., and Pakkari, P. (1979): Histaminergic and related mechanisms in the central control of blood pressure. *Acta Med. Scand. [Suppl. 625]*:81–85.

265. Antonaccio, M. J., Asaad, M., and Baccagno, J. (1981): Centrally mediated pressor response to metiamide as a result of GABA-receptor antagonism. *Eur. J. Pharmacol.*, 72:369–372.

266. Philippu, A. (1981): Involvement of cholinergic systems of the brain in the central regulation of cardiovascular functions. *J. Auton. Pharmacol.*, 1:321–330.

267. Brezenoff, H. E., and Coram, W. (1982): The role of brain acetylcholine in cardiovascular regulation and hypertension: A mini-review and therapeutic implications. *Drug Dev. Res.*, 2:251–258.

268. Brezenoff, H. E., and Giuliano, R. (1982): Cardiovascular control by cholinergic mechanisms in the central nervous system. *Annu. Rev. Pharmacol. Toxicol.*, 22:341–381.

269. Hoffman, W. E. (1979): Central cholinergic receptors in cardiovascular and antidiuretic effects in rats. *Clin. Exp. Pharmacol. Physiol.*, 6:373–380.

270. Kubo, T., and Misu, Y. (1981): Cardiovascular responses to intracisternal administration of nicotine in rats. *Can. J. Physiol. Pharmacol.*, 59:615–617.

271. von Bezold, A., and Gotz, E. (1967): Ueber einige physiologische Wirkungen des Calabar-Giftes. *Zentralbl. Med. Wissenschaften*, 5:241–244.

Cardiovascular Pharmacology, Second Edition,
edited by Michael Antonaccio.
Raven Press, New York © 1984.

Prejunctional Receptors and the Cardiovascular System: Pharmacological and Therapeutic Relevance

Salomon Z. Langer and J. Michael Armstrong

Department of Biology, Synthelabo, 75013 Paris, France

The norepinephrine that is released from sympathetic postganglionic nerve terminals by nerve impulses evokes a response from the postjunctional cell by acting on specific receptor sites present on the effector cell membrane. The magnitude of the response thus produced depends chiefly on the concentration of norepinephrine in the biophase of the effector tissue receptor. Therefore, factors that alter the concentration of norepinephrine in the junction between nerve terminal varicosity and the effector cell receptor have great influence on the magnitude of the response produced. Until recently, studies of these factors were confined to the processes of norepinephrine synthesis, the effect of the frequency of nerve traffic, the exocytotic process of release, and the elimination of the amine from the neuroeffector junction by neuronal and extraneuronal uptake mechanisms and by enzymatic degradation. In addition to these mechanisms, studies in the last decade have revealed a new receptor-mediated pathway by which the amount of neurotransmitter released per impulse can be regulated. A general assumption is that the receptor sites involved are present on the nerve terminals. Although there is no direct proof that the receptors lie on the terminal varicosities, there is evidence that the mechanism alters the exocytotic release of norepinephrine. Therefore, it is likely that the neuronal receptors influencing this process are located on or near the prejunctional membranes

close to the site of transmitter release. Several types of prejunctional receptors have been identified. Their characterization has been accomplished by means of pharmacological techniques using agonists to modify norepinephrine output and employing specific antagonists to block this effect. Although the direction of the response most frequently observed is inhibition of norepinephrine release, facilitation of electrically evoked transmitter output has also been found. Stimulation of prejunctional receptors has been observed in the case of substances released locally within the neuroeffector junctions and by hormonal substances formed at a distance from the junction and brought to the site of action by the circulation. Some receptors appear to be vestigial, because although they can be activated by exogenously administered agents, no endogenous substance appears readily available for interaction with them in physiological conditions. The presynaptic receptor types present may differ among sympathetic nerves. Therefore, their influences on the cardiovascular system will depend on the tissue innervated and the type of the prejunctional receptor present. Hypotheses have also been forwarded to explain the involvement of prejunctional receptors in the pathogenesis of disease and whether or not changes in their state result from disease once developed. An exciting possibility is that prejunctional release-modulating receptors may be target sites for drugs and therefore play an important role in the treatment of disease.

The purpose of this chapter is to highlight the physiological and pharmacological relevance of prejunctional receptors on peripheral sympathetic nerves for the release of transmitter within the cardiovascular system. The wider implications of these mechanisms in both the peripheral and central nervous systems have been reviewed recently by Langer (1).

HISTORICAL BACKGROUND

The discovery that sympathetic nerves contain receptors on or near the membrane of the terminal varicosities is a recent event. Sympathetic nerves were formerly considered to be concerned only with the synthesis, storage, output, and subsequent inactivation of the transmitter norepinephrine. Mechanisms that served to control the release of transmitter locally at the vicinity of the nerve ending were slow to be discovered, most of the important developments taking place during the last 15 years. The historical events leading to their discovery have been recounted by Langer (2) and Gillespie (3).

An early observation was that phenoxybenzamine, an α-adrenoceptor blocking agent, greatly increased the amount of norepinephrine appearing in the venous effluent arising from the cat spleen when its sympathetic nerves were stimulated electrically. This effect was attributed to blockade of postjunctional α-adrenoceptors that normally mediate the response of the tissue. It was supposed that α-adrenoceptors acted as a site of loss for molecules of noradrenergic transmitter and that blockade of these postsynaptic α-adrenoceptors by phenoxybenzamine elevated overflow of norepinephrine during nerve stimulation.

An alternative explanation for phenoxybenzamine's activity on norepinephrine overflow was suggested when the drug was shown to inhibit the neuronal and extraneuronal uptake mechanisms that are the principal means by which noradrenergic transmitter is inacti-

vated. However, this second hypothesis did not hold when put to the test. Cocaine and desimipramine, which did not block α-adrenoceptors but were potent inhibitors of neuronal uptake, did not by themselves augment the stimulation-evoked release of the neurotransmitter. It was found that extraneuronal uptake of norepinephrine could be inhibited by phenoxybenzamine, but this effect could not account for the size of the increase in release of transmitter by nerve stimulation. It seemed more likely that the effect of phenoxybenzamine on release was associated with blockade of α-adrenoceptors, because other α-adrenoceptor antagonists, such as phentolamine, also produced an increase in stimulation-evoked release of neurotransmitter in concentrations that did not inhibit neuronal or extraneuronal uptake of norepinephrine. Additional evidence supporting the view that a real increase in transmitter output occurs was provided by means of measurement of concomitant release of dopamine β-hydroxylase. This enzyme is stored with the transmitter norepinephrine in storage vesicles within the nerve, and the two are released simultaneously into the junctional cleft during nerve stimulation. Dopamine β-hydroxylase is a molecule of large molecular weight and is not subject to elimination by neuronal or extraneuronal uptake, nor to metabolism in the same manner as norepinephrine. Measurement of dopamine β-hydroxylase, therefore, provided a direct means of assessing transmitter output. Using this technique, De Potter et al. (4) and Cubeddu et al. (5) showed that increased enzyme output and therefore transmitter release from the perfused spleen occurred in the presence of phenoxybenzamine or phentolamine.

Concentrations of α-adrenoceptor blocking agents that increased norepinephrine release were of the same order as those needed for blockade of postjunctional α-adrenoceptors. Evidence such as this led Häggendahl (6) and Hedqvist (7) to suggest that the amount of transmitter output might be controlled transsynaptically by the response of the effector cells. The main point of the transsynaptic hypothesis was that α-adrenoceptor antagonists increase transmitter output by reducing the tissue response. This view was abandoned when it was shown that α antagonists effectively increased transmitter overflow from guinea pig atria (8,9), rabbit heart (10), and cat heart (11) in which the tissue response was mediated by adrenoceptors of the β type. In these tissues, α-adrenoceptor blocking agents do not antagonize postsynaptic responses evoked by nerve stimulation, and according to the transsynaptic theory they should not increase transmitter release. Nevertheless, an increase in norepinephrine output was observed in the presence of α-adrenoceptor antagonists, and this effect led to an increase in the end-organ response.

Although it was recognized that α-adrenoceptors were essential components of the increase in transmitter release produced by phenoxybenzamine, the theory was subsequently reformulated to locate them on the nerve terminal (2). According to the new proposal, prejunctional α-adrenoceptors are stimulated by the released norepinephrine to diminish the subsequent output of the transmitter by a mechanism of negative feedback. The new theory holds that when sympathetic nerves are stimulated, norepinephrine is released into the junctional cleft, where the transmitter concentration increases to a threshold level for stimulation of the neuronal α-adrenoceptors. The latter leads to reduction in further transmitter release. This concept of presynaptic regulation gained support from studies showing that α-adrenoceptor agonists inhibited norepinephrine release evoked during nerve stimulation, and an increase in release could be elicited by α-adrenoceptor blocking agents. In tissues in which α-adrenoceptor antagonists by themselves augmented release, the negative-feedback mechanism is considered to be operative under the experimental conditions used, and when these results are also obtained *in vivo*, they support the physiological relevance of this negative-feedback mechanism. In most organs and tissues, the presynaptic mechanism appears to operate most effectively when the

nerves are stimulated at frequencies in the low or intermediate range. The term *autoreceptor* is used for those neuronal receptors that are acted on by the nerve's own transmitter to modulate release. In the peripheral cardiovascular system, the principal autoreceptor is an α-adrenoceptor. Receptors of other agonist types (e.g., dopamine, acetylcholine, 5-hydroxytryptamine) may also be present on sympathetic nerve terminals, but they are acted on only by transmitters released by adjacent nerve terminals or by other locally produced or blood-borne substances to modulate neurotransmission. This has been shown to be the case in tissues of the central nervous system as well as the peripheral nervous system (1).

Since the formulation of this hypothesis, important advances have been made in pharmacological differentiation between the prejunctional α-adrenoceptors from those located postjunctionally and in recognizing the existence in some peripheral noradrenergic nerves of β-adrenoceptors that mediate facilitation of release. The classification of receptor subtypes has moved from the original scheme based on the receptor's anatomic location to one of characterization using pharmacological techniques that involve the use of selective agonists and antagonists on each receptor subtype.

PREJUNCTIONAL α-ADRENOCEPTORS AND REGULATION OF ADRENERGIC TRANSMITTER RELEASE

A representative diagram of the mechanism by which norepinephrine released in response to nerve stimulation acts at prejunctional α-adrenoceptors to inhibit the further release of transmitter is shown in Fig. 1. In tissues such as cat spleen and nictitating membrane, the postjunctional response is also mediated by an α-adrenoceptor. Therefore, α blocking agents will augment the evoked release of transmitter, but at the same time inhibit the mechanical response to nerve stimulation, because they block both prejunctional and

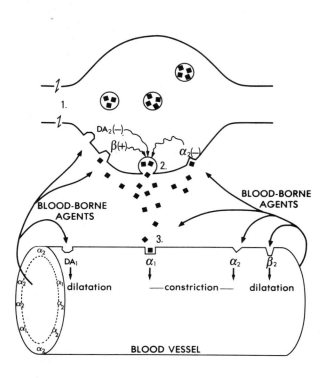

FIG. 1. The major receptor types for catecholamines that are found in blood vessels. A noradrenergic varicosity of a postganglionic sympathetic neuron innervating vascular smooth muscle. The possible sites of action of blood-borne agents are indicated by long solid lines. The modulatory effects (positive or negative) resulting from the activity of agonists at prejunctional sites are shown by wavy lines. Electrical stimulation of the nerve (1) leads to the exocytotic release (2) of norepinephrine (*squares*) that crosses the junctional cleft to occupy (3) vascular α_1-adrenoceptors (*square indent*) that mediate vasoconstriction. At the same time, neuronally released norepinephrine may act at prejunctional α_2-adrenoceptors to inhibit, and perhaps at β-adrenoceptors to enhance, the quantity of the transmitter subsequently released per impulse. Vasoactive agents brought via the circulation may act at prejunctional dopamine receptors (DA$_2$) to inhibit the evoked release of transmitter and at extrajunctional DA$_1$ receptors to produce vasodilatation and hypotension. These dopamine receptor subtypes may be of pharmacological rather than physiological importance. Stimulation of extrajunctional β_2-adrenoceptors also leads to vasodilatation. Postjunctional α_2-adrenoceptors appear not to be innervated, but when stimulated by exogenously administered agonists mediate vasoconstriction.

postjunctional receptor sites simultaneously.

However, agents are now available that are selective for either one or the other site. Such compounds are selective not because of the anatomic location of the receptor but because of a greater or lesser affinity that they have for the receptor site. α-Adrenoceptors have now been classified into α_1 and α_2 subtypes (2), a scheme that has been extended by others (12,13), and to which additional subdivisions have been proposed (14).

The selectivities of some agonists and antagonists at α_1- and α_2-adrenoceptors are shown in Table 1. An antagonist selective for the α_2 subtype can be expected to increase transmitter output during nerve stimulation without reducing the effector-organ response when the latter response is mediated by α_1-adrenoceptors. The converse may also be expected. In the same tissue, an antagonist selective for α_1-adrenoceptors should be expected to block

the end-organ response to nerve stimulation without augmenting transmitter release. The situation is much less complicated in tissues with β-adrenoceptor-mediated effector-cell responses, such as occur in the heart. Augmentation of the postsynaptic response is expected to accompany an increase in transmitter release in the case of an antagonist selective for α_2-adrenoceptors or a nonselective α_1- and α_2-adrenoceptor antagonist. A blocking agent highly selective for α_1-adrenoceptors, like prazosin, is likely to have little or no effect on either transmitter output or cardiac tissue response during sympathetic nerve stimulation. Although α_1-adrenoceptors have been identified in the heart, there is no evidence as yet to suggest that these are innervated or that they play a physiological role.

Some of the predictions given earlier have been tested experimentally. The positive chronotropic responses to accelerans nerve stimu-

TABLE 1. *Preferential selectivity of some representative agonists and antagonists for α-adrenoceptor subtypes*

Agonists			Antagonists		
α_1	α_2	$\alpha_1 + \alpha_2$	α_1	α_2	$\alpha_1 + \alpha_2$
Amidephrine	BHT 920[a]	Norepinephrine	Corynanthine	Rauwolscine	Tolazoline
Cirazoline	Guanabenz	Epinephrine	Labetalol	Yohimbine	Phentolamine
Methoxamine	Clonidine		Prazosin	RS 21361[e]	
Phenylephrine	M-7[b]			WY 26703[f]	
	UK 14304[c]			RX 781094[g]	
	BHT 933[d]				

[a] 2-amino-6-allyl-4,5,7,8-tetrahydro-6*H*-thiazolo-[4,5-*d*]-azepine.
[b] 2-(*N,N*-dimethylamino-5,6-dihydroxy-1,2,3,4-tetrahydro-naphthalene.
[c] 5-bromo-6-[2-imidazolinylamino]-quinoxaline.
[d] 2-amino-6-ethyl-4,5,7,8-tetrahydro-6*H*-oxazolo-[5,4-*d*]-azepin-dihydrochloride.
[e] 2-(1-ethyl-2-imidazolyl-ethyl)-1,4-benzodioxan.
[f] *N*-methyl-*N*-(1,3,4,6,7,11b-α-hexahydro-2*H*-benzo-[a]-quinolizin-2-β-yl)butanesulphonamide hydrochloride.
[g] 2-[2-(1,4-benzodioxanyl)]-2-imidazoline.

lation in guinea pig atria are potentiated in the presence of phentolamine in concentrations that also substantially increase neurotransmitter release (15). In anesthetized dogs, α-adrenoceptor blockade potentiates chronotropic responses evoked by cardiac nerve stimulation (16–19). In spinal dogs, the α-adrenoceptor agonist clonidine decreases both tachycardia and the accompanying norepinephrine that overflows into the coronary sinus during cardioaccelerans nerve stimulation. Clonidine's effects were blocked by phentolamine (16). Taken together, these findings support the view that the negative-feedback mechanism mediated by prejunctional α-adrenoceptors plays a physiological role in both *in vitro* and *in vivo* conditions.

The effectiveness of α-adrenoceptor antagonists in enhancing transmitter release is dependent on there being sufficient concentration of noradrenergic transmitter in the synaptic cleft to stimulate prejunctional α-adrenoceptors. In tissues depleted of norepinephrine by administration of reserpine, phenoxybenzamine fails to enhance the stimulation-evoked release of dopamine β-hydroxylase (DBH), the presence of which is unaffected by reserpine. This is because without norepinephrine to activate the negative-feedback mechanism,

inhibition of transmitter release, as indicated by DBH output, does not occur.

The evidence in favor of the presynaptic location of inhibitory α-adrenoceptors that regulate noradrenergic neurotransmission can be summarized as follows:

1. Changes in norepinephrine release produced by α-adrenoceptor agonists or antagonists are independent of the type of postjunctional adrenoceptor mediating the response of the effector tissue.

2. Enhanced transmitter release caused by α-adrenoceptor blocking agents such as phentolamine can still be obtained after atrophy of the postjunctional effector cell (20).

3. α-Adrenoceptor blockade increases potassium-induced ³H-norepinephrine release from newly formed nerve endings in culture and in the absence of postjunctional tissue.

4. A decrease in specific binding of an α-adrenoceptor ligand occurs after destruction of nerve endings by chemical sympathectomy in rat heart.

A major feature of the negative-feedback mechanism mediated by α-adrenoceptors is that it operates only for the calcium-dependent component of transmitter release: that evoked by electrical nerve stimulation or potassium depolarization. On the other hand, the calcium-independent release of norepinephrine from nerves by tyramine is not altered by α-adrenoceptor agonists or antagonists. Therefore, it is likely that agonists at prejunctional receptors may act by reducing the availability of calcium for the process of excitation-secretion coupling that is involved in exocytosis. Little is known of the biochemical mechanisms occurring after the prejunctional α-adrenoceptors have been activated. However, transmitter output may be linked to decreases in cyclic AMP levels or activation of the sodium-potassium-ATPase system.

Another characteristic of the negative-feedback mechanism is that it is most effective in inhibiting norepinephrine output when nerves are stimulated at low and intermediate frequencies. It is less effective at high frequencies of nerve activity. The negative-feedback mechanism becomes operational only when sufficient norepinephrine builds up in the synaptic cleft to allow its activity at neuronal receptors. Therefore, α-adrenoceptor antagonists increase release only during trains of stimulus pulses in which the pulse intervals are sufficiently close together to allow norepinephrine to build up to a sufficient concentration in the synaptic cleft. The importance of this latter point has been emphasized in a recent debate (21–23).

Differences between the Release-Regulating Prejunctional α-Adrenoceptors and the Postjunctional α-Adrenoceptors Mediating the Response of the Effector Tissue

Before the discovery of presynaptic, release-modulating α-adrenoceptors, it was generally believed that the α-adrenoceptors represented a homogeneous population. Considerable evidence has now been accumulated to support the view that the α-adrenoceptors that mediate changes of norepinephrine output differ from those that are located postjunctionally within the synapse and that are stimulated by noradrenergic transmitter once released. The terminology and subclassification of α-

adrenoceptors have been reviewed recently by Starke and Langer (24,25). The two receptor subtypes differ in their pharmacological characteristics. The principal criterion for the subclassification of α-adrenoceptors, as with other receptor subtypes, is the relative order of potency with which agonists and antagonists interact at the two receptor subtypes (Table 2). It was originally reported that the two subtypes of receptors were located anatomically in different areas, the α_2-adrenoceptors predominating prejunctionally, whereas the α_1 subtype was the principal postjunctional receptor. Thus, Dubocovich and Langer (26) and Cubeddu et al. (5) reported that phenoxybenzamine was 30 to 100 times more potent at postjunctional α receptors than at prejunctional α receptors. In contrast, phentolamine showed little difference in antagonist potency at the two sites, indicating a lack of selectivity. Starke et al. (27) reported that yohimbine preferentially blocked prejunctional receptors, indicating a selectivity for α_2-adrenoceptors. Agonists can also be placed on a scale of selectivity that extends from those exhibiting high affinity for α_1-adrenoceptors to those with high affinity for α_2-adrenoceptors. Whereas the neurotransmitter norepinephrine has the same affinity for both α_1- and α_2-adrenoceptors, agents such as guanabenz, M-7, UK 14304, BH-T 920, and BH-T 933 are preferential agonists at α_2-adrenoceptors, whereas cirazoline, methoxamine, and phenylephrine are selective α_1-adrenoceptor agonists (28). In the case of some agonists, such as clonidine, the situation is further complicated because in particular experimental conditions they can behave as α-adrenoceptor antagonists rather than agonists (29,30). This phenomenon is a characteristic of "partial agonists." Agents of this kind stimulate receptors to produce a tissue response when added alone, but they antagonize the effects of full agonists when added before the agonists. Partial agonism by clonidine has recently been invoked to account for the rebound hypertension and tachycardia that occur on its acute withdrawal during long-term therapy (31). The explanation forwarded is as follows. During clonidine admin-

TABLE 2. *Relative orders of selectivity of agonists and antagonists for α_1- and α_2-adrenoceptors*[a]

Relative order of agonist selectivity	Relative order of antagonist selectivity
$(\alpha_2 \rightarrow \alpha_1)$	$(\alpha_2 \rightarrow \alpha_1)$
guanabenz > tramazoline > clonidine > α-methyl-norepinephrine > oxymetazoline > naphazoline = epinephrine = norepinephrine > phenylephrine > methoxamine = amidephrine	RX 781094 > rauwolscine > yohimbine > piperoxan > tolazoline $\gg$ phentolamine > phenoxybenzamine $\gg$ WB 4101 [b] $\gg$ labetalol = prazosin

[a] Selectivity determined in peripheral noradrenergically innervated tissues of several species.
[b] 2-(2,6-dimethoxyphenoxyethylaminomethyl)-1,4-benzodioxan.

istration, stimulation of central α_2-adrenoceptors lowers peripheral sympathetic activity and thereby reduces the amount of noradrenergic transmitter available to stimulate prejunctional autoreceptors on cardiovascular sympathetic nerves. In these conditions, endogenous norepinephrine levels in the synaptic cleft are reduced as clonidine acts at prejunctional sites to inhibit the output of the transmitter. After clonidine administration is stopped, the concentration of clonidine in the brain falls, and this allows peripheral sympathetic activity to increase. There follows a greater output of norepinephrine. In this situation there may be subsensitivity of α_2-adrenoceptors, and in addition, residual clonidine competes with endogenous transmitter for the autoreceptor. This is manifest as tachycardia and an increase in blood pressure.

In the case of blood vessels *in vivo,* the situation is further complicated, because α-adrenoceptors present postjunctionally in arteries, and veins appear to be a heterogeneous mixture of the two α_1 and α_2 subtypes (32,33). Stimulation of either α-adrenoceptor subtype can produce vasoconstriction. Quantification of the activity of agonists and antagonists has been made more difficult by the lack of suitable vascular *in vitro* preparations containing postjunctional α_2-adrenoceptors. So far, the only preparation of practical use is the canine saphenous vein (34,35). α_2-Adrenoceptors in arterial tissue appear to become uncoupled from their contractile process once bathed in physiological salt solutions. This may be related to changes in the acid–base balance under these conditions (14). To date, the only

reported functional α_2-adrenoceptors in arterial tissue *in vitro* are in isolated cerebral arteries of the dog (36) and the cat (37,38). Cerebral arteries appear to be richly innervated with sympathetic noradrenergic nerves, but when these are stimulated electrically, vasoconstriction does not occur (39–41). These observations are in accord with the postulate of Langer et al. (42,43) that vascular smooth-muscle α_2-adrenoceptors are not innervated. Rather, they may be better placed close to the intima, in the inner layers of the media, to be activated by circulating catecholamines.

Pharmacological differentiation of α-adrenoceptors has important implications because it is a prerequisite for the discovery of agents that stimulate or block each subtype with a high degree of affinity and selectivity. The presence of α_2- and α_1-adrenoceptors postsynaptically in arterial beds in the rat and the dog has been used to explain the paradoxical results obtained with prazosin. This agent is a selective α_1-adrenoceptor antagonist; it effectively inhibits the pressor effects of phenylephrine (α_1-selective agonist) but attenuates much less effectively the pressor responses produced by the nonselective agonist norepinephrine on intravenous administration (43). Prazosin, in low doses, has also been shown to markedly attenuate pressor responses evoked by sympathetic nerve stimulation in the perfused hindlimb of the dog, while leaving little affected the same responses caused by injections of norepinephrine. The greater effectiveness of prazosin in blocking endogenously released norepinephrine relative to inhibition of exogenous amines may be due to high concentrations of α_1-adrenoceptors postjunctionally in the adventitial-medial region acted on by the released transmitter, whereas postjunctional α_2-adrenoceptors may be chiefly beyond the reach of the neuronal norepinephrine. In this case, exogenously administered norepinephrine may be resistant to prazosin blockade because it acts mainly at extrasynaptic α_2-adrenoceptors. The latter may be more evenly distributed throughout the medial smooth muscle or concentrated toward the intima, and the α_1 subtype may be confined to the adventitial-medial border, where the sympathetic nerve terminals are located (Fig. 1). An alternative explanation is that innervated blood vessels contain receptors of the α_1 type, and noninnervated vessels contain α_2 receptors (14). In support of the latter suggestion is the finding of functional α_2-adrenoceptors in the smooth muscle in cerebral arteries in the cat, with a dense sympathetic innervation, although it appears to be nonfunctional (37,39).

The loss of function that postjunctional arterial α_2 receptors undergo *in vitro* emphasizes the need to support the results of ligand-binding studies with those of functional studies so that further subdivision of receptor recognition sites by binding studies will actually reflect differences in physiologically relevant receptor populations.

Physiological Significance of the Negative-Feedback Mechanism Mediated by α-Adrenoceptors

Changes in the output of noradrenergic neurotransmitter from sympathetic nerve endings is only of physiological significance when associated with a corresponding alteration in the response of the effector tissue during nerve stimulation. If the negative-feedback mechanism mediated by α-adrenoceptors normally operates to regulate norepinephrine release, then α-adrenoceptor blocking agents should increase transmitter release as well as the size of the end-organ response. Demonstration of this is difficult in the case of tissues in which

both the prejunctional and postjunctional receptors are α-adrenoceptors. Nevertheless, yohimbine has been shown to increase transmitter release and at the same time augment the contractions evoked by electrical sympathetic nerve stimulation in the pulmonary artery. Synthesis and use of antagonists with even greater selectivity should allow further clarification of the physiological role of the negative-feedback mechanism mediated by presynaptic α-adrenoceptors. A means of avoiding the problem posed by the presence of both prejunctional and postjunctional α-adrenoceptors is to use tissues in which the postjunctional receptor is of another type. In the case of guinea pig atria, the postjunctional receptors are of the β-adrenoceptor type. Electrical stimulation of the cardiac nerves in this preparation in the presence of phentolamine increases the evoked tachycardia and the output of transmitter. With human tissue, too, there is evidence that a negative-feedback mechanism mediated by prejunctional α-adrenoceptors is operating during nerve stimulation. Human peripheral arteries and veins taken post-mortem liberate noradrenergic transmitter in quantities that can be decreased by α-adrenoceptor agonists and increased by α-adrenoceptor antagonists (44).

PREJUNCTIONAL FACILITORY β-ADRENOCEPTORS AND NORADRENERGIC TRANSMISSION

Evidence for the presence of presynaptic β-adrenoceptors on sympathetic nerves was obtained from experiments in which small concentrations of isoproterenol facilitated release of norepinephrine during low-frequency nerve stimulation in guinea pig atria, cat thoracic aorta, calf muscle, perfused cat spleen, and rat pineal gland and portal vein. These findings lent support to an earlier proposal by Langer et al. (45) concerning a β-adrenoceptor-mediated prejunctional facilitatory feedback mechanism regulating the norepinephrine released by nerve stimulation. A representation of this mechanism is shown in Fig. 2.

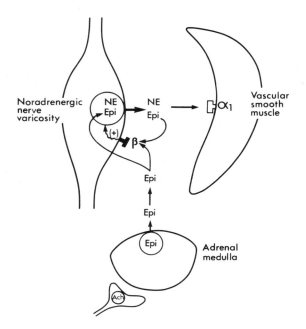

FIG. 2. The possible interaction of circulating epinephrine (Epi) with prejunctional β-adrenoceptors of a terminal noradrenergic nerve varicosity. Action potentials in preganglionic sympathetic nerves innervating the adrenal medulla release acetylcholine (Ach), which then activates nicotinic cholinoceptors to release epinephrine (Epi) from chromaffin cells. Blood-borne epinephrine may then act directly on prejunctional neuronal β-adrenoceptors or be stored with norepinephrine (NE) in vesicles to be subsequently released as a cotransmitter on nerve stimulation. The effect of prejunctional β-adrenoceptor stimulation by the neuronally released or circulating epinephrine (*wavy line*) is to enhance the output of transmitter from the terminal and increase its concentration at α_1-adrenoceptors postjunctionally. This leads to greater smooth-muscle contraction, vasoconstriction, and possibly hypertension.

Isoproterenol also increases the stimulation-evoked release of norepinephrine in anesthetized dogs, and this effect is blocked by the β-adrenoceptor blocking agent sotalol. Prejunctional facilitory receptors of this type have been reported to be present in the human oviduct and in human vasoconstrictor nerves. This facilitory mechanism is not present in all postganglionic sympathetic nerves, and even when present it may not always be under tonic stimulation from the norepinephrine released from nerves. Propranolol antagonizes isoprenaline-induced facilitation of norepinephrine release. By itself, propranolol has been shown to decrease release from isolated guinea pig atria, cat spleen, perfused calf muscle of the cat, and isolated portal vein in spontaneously hypertensive rats. On the other hand, propranolol alone does not reduce the stimulation-evoked release of ³H-norepinephrine from human omental arteries and veins. Conclusions concerning the presence of prejunctional β-adrenoceptors and their possible physiological role should be made only when selective β-adrenoceptor antagonists are used in concentrations corresponding to blockade of β-adrenoceptors, not to their nonspecific

membrane-stabilizing effects that prevail at higher concentrations.

In anesthetized dogs, isoproterenol infusion increases the release of norepinephrine evoked by cardioaccelerans stimulation, whereas sotalol reduces the release at stimulation frequencies within the range 1 to 5 Hz.

Prejunctional β-adrenoceptors, like α-adrenoceptors, are stereoselective for agonists and antagonists. Facilitation of transmitter release was observed with (−)-isoproterenol but not with (+)-isoproterenol. The (−)-isomer of isoproterenol was the active enantiomer responsible for augmenting release of transmitter from isolated portal veins of spontaneously hypertensive rats.

At present, there is more evidence to favor the view that prejunctional receptors are of the β_2 subtype rather than the β_1 subtype. Whereas Dahlöf et al. (46) and Rand et al. (47) successfully blocked prejunctional facilitory receptors with the β_1-selective antagonist metoprolol in atria of rats and guinea pigs and vasomotor nerves, Stjärne and Brundin (48) and Majewski et al. (49) concluded that the receptors in human vasoconstrictor nerves were of the β_2 type, because terbutaline and salbutamol were highly effective in augmenting transmitter output, and the β_1-selective agonist H 110/38 was ineffective. Prejunctional β-adrenoceptors are particularly sensitive to stimulation by exogenously administered epinephrine. It has been proposed (31,47) that circulating epinephrine, perhaps liberated during stressful situations, may be accumulated within sympathetic nerves (Fig. 2). This surrogate transmitter might subsequently be liberated by nerve activity and activate the facilitatory mechanism, thereby liberating greater quantities of transmitter. There is experimental evidence to support this view. Epinephrine is a substrate for the neuronal uptake process and thus can be accumulated by noradrenergic nerves. When peripheral nerve terminals are labeled with epinephrine, propranolol becomes more effective in reducing transmitter release during nerve stimulation. In these circumstances, epinephrine released from nerves could participate in the positive-feedback mechanism to enhance the effectiveness of sympathetic nerve function. Antagonists at prejunctional β-adrenoceptors may oppose this mechanism. Enhanced release of norepinephrine in resistance blood vessels may predispose to hypertensive disease, and it is possible that blockade of prejunctional β-adrenoceptors by antagonists could contribute to the antihypertensive effects of β blocking agents.

Classification of prejunctional β-adrenoceptors awaits rigorous examination of the affinity of agonists and antagonists wherever such receptors are found. It should not be ruled out that species differences may occur and that the β_1-β_2 classification accepted for postjunctional receptors may not be appropriate for those that are located on the nerves and that modulate norepinephrine release.

PREJUNCTIONAL INHIBITORY DOPAMINE RECEPTORS

Prejunctional receptors stimulated by dopamine and mediating inhibition of noradrenergic transmitter release from peripheral nerves have been identified using both *in vitro* and *in vivo* conditions. These receptors are also stimulated by N,N-di-n-propyldopamine (DPDA), apomorphine, and the ergolines bromocriptine, pergolide, and LY 141865 (50–52). The reduction in the output of norepinephrine thus produced is accompanied by a reduction in the size of the end-organ responses during nerve stimulation. Stimulation of prejunctional dopamine receptors is unaffected by α-adrenoceptor antagonists in concentrations that block prejunctional α_2-adrenoceptors. Neuronal dopamine receptors are effectively blocked by chlorpromazine, pimozide, metoclopramide, haloperidol, or sulpiride in concentrations that do not block α_2-adrenoceptors. Such results strongly support the view that prejunctional dopamine receptors are different from prejunctional α_2-adrenoceptors, even though their stimulation leads to the same response (i.e., a reduction in transmitter output).

A further difference between prejunctional dopamine receptors and α_2-adrenoceptors is that the presynaptic dopamine receptors do not appear to be continuously stimulated during transmitter release. This conclusion is reached because dopamine receptor antagonists by themselves, unlike α_2-adrenoceptor antagonists, do not enhance transmitter release (53–55). Dopamine-sensitive sites are also to be found postjunctionally in blood vessels, and their stimulation leads to vasodilatation. Receptors for dopamine present in sympathetic ganglia, in nerve terminals, and postjunctionally in blood vessels are likely to be of clinical significance (56). Agonists and antagonists differ in their affinity for the two sites, and this gives rise to the notion that they represent two distinct classes of receptors (57). Recent experimental evidence supports this view. (S)-sulpiride preferentially blocks prejunctional dopamine receptors in the heart and nictitating membrane in the anesthetized dog, and bulbocapnine selectively blocks the postjunctional dopamine receptors in the mesenteric artery in the same species (58).

The contributions of prejunctional and

postjunctional dopamine receptors to the cardiovascular effects of dopaminelike agents depend on the selectivity of the agent used. However, in general, prejunctional DA_2 receptors appear to be involved in the hypotension and bradycardia produced by infusions of DPDA, and the renal vasodilating effects of this agent appear to be mediated also by postjunctional vascular DA_1 receptors.

Although classification of dopamine receptors, as with other receptor systems, is best accomplished by pharmacological means rather than by an anatomic system, the presynaptic dopamine receptors that inhibit norepinephrine release are of the DA_2 subtype, whereas the postsynaptic vascular dopamine receptors that mediate vasodilatation are of the DA_1 subtype. The concentrations of these peripheral dopamine receptor subtypes at important cardiovascular sites make them targets for the development of drugs with agonist properties at these dopamine receptor subtypes. Such agents may turn out to be novel antihypertensive drugs.

PROSTAGLANDIN AND OTHER PREJUNCTIONAL RECEPTORS

Modulation of noradrenergic transmitter output by prostaglandins has been demonstrated using many cardiovascular tissues and organs (59). Little is known of the receptor sites that mediate prostaglandin-induced modulation of norepinephrine release from nerves during stimulation. This is because competitive antagonists for these sites are not readily available. Prostaglandins are produced to varying extents by all cell types thus far studied, including sympathetic nerves and the tissues that they innervate. Prostaglandins can be released during arterial perfusion when evoked by a variety of stimuli, including nerve stimulation. It is theoretically possible that neuronal prostaglandins released with the noradrenergic transmitter may act at nerve terminals to modulate the subsequent output of norepinephrine. Prostaglandins formed postjunctionally need to cross the synaptic cleft

to alter transmitter output (i.e., a transsynaptic process of regulation). Overall, the available evidence points to the effector tissue as the primary source of release of prostaglandins, because similar quantities of prostaglandinlike substances are released after the nerve supply has been destroyed. Competitive antagonists for these agents are not readily available, and therefore most investigators make use of aspirinlike drugs to inhibit endogenous prostaglandin formation, thereby allowing an indirect assessment of their physiological role on norepinephrine release.

Prostaglandin E_2 (PGE$_2$) has been the prostanoid most studied. This is because PGE$_2$-like material was shown to be released on sympathetic nerve stimulation. When added exogenously, PGE$_2$ inhibited norepinephrine output and in so doing mimicked the effects of arachidonic acid, its endogenous precursor. Transmitter release was often increased, although to a small extent, when prostaglandin synthesis was inhibited. This was not always the case, and a notable exception is the cat spleen (60). Hedqvist and associates (61) proposed that prostaglandins of the E series may counteract the effect of sympathetic nerve function in some blood vessels by reducing noradrenergic transmitter released by nerve stimulation. On closer examination, it appeared that a reduction in the stimulation-evoked overflow was a consequence of a reduction in the amount of transmitter released per impulse and was mediated by decreases in the availability of calcium. Like other prejunctional inhibitory mechanisms, the effect appeared most prominent at low frequencies of stimulation. The major challenge to the hypothesis that PGE$_2$ is the primary endogenous regulator of transmitter release is that in blood vessels, prostacyclin (PGI$_2$), not PGE$_2$, is the major product of arachidonic acid metabolism. Therefore, prostacyclin may play the regulatory role previously attributed to PGE$_2$. However, prostacyclin and its principal product of metabolic degradation, 6-oxo-PGF$_{1\alpha}$, are much less active than PGE$_2$ in modulating norepinephrine released by nerve stimulation, and there is little evidence that PGI_2 acts to regulate sympathetic noradrenergic neurotransmission *in vivo,* as reviewed by Armstrong (59).

Muscarinic cholinoceptor agonists inhibit noradrenergic neurotransmission in the heart in rabbits, chickens, and guinea pigs (62). This effect is blocked by atropine and other muscarinic receptor antagonists. It appears that the inhibitory effect of agonists at muscarinic cholinoceptor sites is secondary to a decrease in the availability of calcium for the excitation-secretion coupling process for the release of norepinephrine. Acetylcholine can also be shown to decrease the stimulation-evoked release of norepinephrine from blood vessel tissues in animals and humans through stimulation of prejunctional inhibitory muscarinic cholinoceptors (63,64).

Presynaptic muscarinic receptors may play a physiological role in the regulation of neuro-transmission in the heart (see Fig. 3). Stimulation of the vagus nerves reduces the output of norepinephrine evoked by the simultaneous stimulation of postganglionic sympathetic nerves of the dog and rabbit (65). It is thought that acetylcholine released during nerve stimulation acts on prejunctional inhibitory muscarinic cholinoceptors on the noradrenergic nerve terminals (Fig. 3) (64).

Adenosine and adenine nucleotides have been found to inhibit noradrenergic neurotransmission in several tissues in rats, rabbits, and dogs (66). The inhibitory activity of adenosine is more pronounced at low frequencies of stimulation. Such observations have led to the suggestion that purine nucleotides (e.g., ATP) released with noradrenergic transmitter may be rapidly transformed to adenosine, which subsequently acts on P_1 purinergic receptor sites to attenuate transmitter output (67). The prejunctional inhibitory effects of

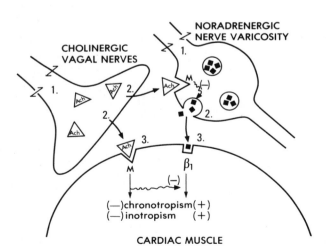

FIG. 3. Inhibition by acetylcholine (Ach) of the release and activity of noradrenergic transmitter in the heart. A postganglionic cholinergic vagal nerve terminal is shown in close proximity to a noradrenergic varicosity and cardiac striated muscle. The sites of release and subsequent activity of acetylcholine and norepinephrine are shown by solid lines. The inhibitory effects of acetylcholine are shown by the wavy lines. Electrical stimulation of these nerves (1) leads to the release of their respective transmitters (2), which then traverse the junctional cleft to stimulate postjunctional receptors (3). The norepinephrine released activates postjunctional β-adrenoceptors to produce positive inotropic and chronotropic responses. Acetylcholine, when liberated from the vagus, can act at muscarinic receptors on the noradrenergic nerve terminal to inhibit transmitter release and on postjunctional cells to depress cardiac activity (negative chronotropic and inotropic actions). The latter effect also counteracts the stimulatory effects of norepinephrine postjunctionally. Other receptor mechanisms (not shown) operating prejunctionally on sympathetic noradrenergic nerves (e.g., DA_2 and β- or α_2-adrenoceptors) can modulate norepinephrine output and modify cardiac function.

adenosine do not appear to be mediated through prostaglandin mechanisms or by way of prejunctional α-adrenoceptors.

Theophylline blocks the inhibitory activity of adenosine on neurotransmission and by itself increases the stimulation-evoked release of the transmitter. Therefore, it is possible that the augmented release of norepinephrine observed with theophylline and other methylxanthines could reflect antagonism of adenosine originating either prejunctionally or postjunctionally, rather than inhibition of phosphodiesterase, which is the traditional explanation. As with prostaglandin modulation of neurotransmission, it is possible that adenosine is generated postsynaptically and therefore may be involved in a transsynaptic regulatory mechanism for the release of transmitter in the peripheral nervous system.

Facilitory prejunctional angiotensin II receptors have been described in peripheral noradrenergic nerve terminals of several tissues in the dog and rabbit. The activity of angiotensin on sympathetic nerve function might be complicated when accompanied by prostaglandin release. When the latter is PGE_2, the angiotensin-induced facilitation may be opposed by prostaglandin-evoked inhibition of transmitter release (68).

There is some evidence that endorphin and enkephalinlike substances are present in the brain and can be released into the circulation from the adrenal medulla (69). These may affect the neural control of blood pressure by altering noradrenergic transmitter output.

POSSIBLE THERAPEUTIC IMPLICATIONS

Pharmacological studies of receptor-mediated events with the use of selective agonists and antagonists are essential for receptor populations to be differentiated one from another. This is the rationale underlying the search for agents that selectively interact with receptor subtypes, because it is generally recognized that selectivity of drug action is a characteristic of successful therapeutic agents. Such selec-

tivity can be achieved when physiological differentiation in tissues has been demonstrated. There is historical precedence to indicate that novel molecules can be synthesized that can interact with receptor subtypes, and with high specificity. Pharmacological exploitation of such knowledge has already led to the development of therapeutic agents acting at postjunctional receptor sites. In recent times, this is true of postjunctional histamine receptors and β-adrenoceptors. By analogy, prejunctional receptors can be considered as potential targets for the development of selective agonists and antagonists. Such agents might be expected to modulate the output of noradrenergic transmitter both centrally and peripherally.

It is likely that prejunctional receptors are involved in the mechanisms of action of a number of known therapeutic agents:

1. Clonidine is a clinically useful antihypertensive agent. When administered to humans and animals, clonidine lowers arterial blood pressure and heart rate. These actions result from its high affinity for adrenoceptors of the α_2 subtype. Lowering of arterial blood pressure occurs after passage of clonidine into the central nervous system and within the cardiovascular regulatory centers in the medulla, where it stimulates α_2-adrenoceptors. This effect leads to a reduction in the frequency of impulse traffic passing down efferent sympathetic nerves and thereby reduces the output of noradrenergic transmitter. Although its primary therapeutic effect may be due to an action within the brain, stimulation of peripheral prejunctional α_2-adrenoceptors located on sympathetic nerves may also contribute to the overall activity of clonidine, particularly its bradycardic action. This may become more important when one considers that inhibition of peripheral sympathetic nerve function by stimulation of autoreceptors is maximal when the frequency of nerve impulse flow is low. A reduction of noradrenergic transmitter from cardiac nerves may result from the stimulation of α_2-adrenoceptors situated both centrally

and peripherally. Sedation is an unwanted effect associated with clonidine therapy in the early stages of administration, and this, too, appears to be due to stimulation of central α_2-adrenoceptors.

2. The antihypertensive effects of α-methyldopa are attributable to the activity of its principal metabolite α-methylnorepinephrine within the central nervous system. α-Methylnorepinephrine is a preferential agonist at α_2-adrenoceptors. Stimulation of these receptors within the central nervous system leads to a reduction in sympathetic nerve activity, as also occurs with clonidine. In the periphery, activation of α_2-adrenoceptors by α-methylnorepinephrine formed from α-methyldopa leads to a reduction in the output of noradrenergic transmitter, and this effect may also contribute to the antihypertensive action.

3. Prazosin is a selective antagonist at α_1-adrenoceptors, and this activity undoubtedly plays a role in the mechanism of its antihypertensive activity (70). A major therapeutic advantage of this agent is absence of the tachycardia in association with the lowering of blood pressure. Increased heart rate is an unwanted effect of nonselective α-adrenoceptor blocking agents that limits their use in humans. The selectivity of prazosin for α_1-adrenoceptors may explain why plasma renin levels are not elevated at dose levels that decrease blood pressure. A lack of α_2-adrenoceptor blocking activity in therapeutic doses may also explain the absence of tachycardia, although other mechanisms like changes in baroreceptor sensitivity and absence of right atrial pressure increases might also be involved. The high concentration of α_1-adrenoceptors within the junctional cleft of sympathetic nerves in blood vessels may explain the high potency with which prazosin blocks the effects of sympathetic nerve stimulation and its high degree of effectiveness in lowering peripheral arterial resistance and blood pressure.

4. β-Adrenoceptor blocking agents are now among the first-line drugs used to treat hypertension. At present, no single explanation is universally accepted to explain their effectiveness. Although the principal pharmacological property shared in common by these compounds is blockade of postjunctional cardiac β-adrenoceptors, it is possible that blockade of prejunctional facilitory β-adrenoceptors may contribute to their antihypertensive activity. This effect in blood vessels could lead to a reduction in the release of noradrenergic transmitter and thereby lower peripheral vascular resistance.

Stimulation of some prejunctional receptors by drugs may also account for some of their unwanted side effects. For example, rebound hypertension and tachycardia are known to occur after acute withdrawal of clonidine from chronic administration. The rebound syndrome is associated with increased catecholamine secretion that could indicate increased activity of the sympathetic nervous system. Although this effect is imperfectly understood, it may be due to the development of subsensitivity of α_2-adrenoceptors either centrally or peripherally following chronic administration of clonidine.

Stimulation of α_2-adrenoceptors by clonidine may lead to sedation and dry mouth. In chicks, induction of sleep by clonidine can be antagonized by selective α_2-adrenoceptor antagonists, but not by prazosin. The sedative effect of clonidine is mediated by receptors within the central nervous system. In the periphery, clonidine reduces submaxillary salivation elicited by electrical stimulation of parasympathetic nerves in the cat. It is probable that this effect is mediated by stimulation of α_2-adrenoceptors on cholinergic nerves. Such an effect of clonidine would lead to reduced output of the cholinergic transmitter during nerve activity.

The orthostatic hypotension observed after treatment with L-DOPA and dopamine receptor agonists such as bromocryptine could be related to activation of presynaptic inhibitory dopamine receptors on peripheral noradrenergic nerve endings.

SUMMARY

There is now good evidence to suggest that receptors are present on the terminal membranes of nerves within the central and peripheral nervous systems. Stimulation of prejunctional receptors initiates calcium-dependent mechanisms that modulate the subsequent output of transmitter released by nerve action potentials. *Autoreceptors* is the term used to describe prejunctional sites stimulated by the neuron's own transmitter. In the case of prejunctional adrenoceptors, these have been classified as belonging to the α_2 subtype because they are stimulated preferentially by clonidine and guanabenz and blocked by yohimbine. New antagonists with even greater selectivity are currently being developed (e.g., RX 781094, WY 26703, RS 21361), and the use of these agents assists in the classification of α-adrenoceptor subtypes. Pharmacological differentiation allows them to be distinguished from the α_1 subtype that usually lie postjunctionally in the neuronal cleft. α_1-Adrenoceptors are stimulated preferentially by phenylephrine and blocked by prazosin and corynanthine.

Selective α_2-adrenoceptor blocking agents antagonize the effects of exogenously administered agonists, and at the level of autoreceptors these antagonists by themselves augment transmitter release by antagonizing the effects of the endogenously released transmitter.

In addition to α_2-adrenoceptors, several other receptor types may be present on nerve endings and when stimulated may modulate transmitter release. They may be acted on by blood-borne agents or substances formed locally or in some cases in response to the release of transmitter and its effect postjunctionally. Prejunctional mechanisms that inhibit transmitter release are activated by (a) α_2-adrenoceptor agonists, (b) muscarinic cholinergic agonists, (c) dopaminelike agents, (d) adenosine, (e) prostaglandins, and (f) opiate receptor agonists. Prejunctional receptor-mediated mechanisms involved in facilitation of the stimulation-evoked release of norepinephrine include β-adrenoceptor agonists and angiotensin II.

Agents that stimulate or block such receptors involved in the modulation of norepinephrine release can have significant effects in the regulation of the cardiovascular system and in the treatment of cardiovascular disease.

Further studies on the pharmacological characteristics of prejunctional receptors may lead to the development of therapeutic agents with greater selectivity of action and fewer unwanted side effects.

REFERENCES

1. Langer, S. Z. (1981): Presynaptic regulation of the release of catecholamines. *Pharmacol. Rev.*, 32:337–362.
2. Langer, S. Z. (1974): Presynaptic regulation of catecholamine release. *Biochem. Pharmacol.*, 23:1793–1800.
3. Gillespie, J. S. (1980): Presynaptic receptors in the autonomic nervous system. In: *Adrenergic Activators and Inhibitors*, edited by L. Szekeres, pp. 353–425. Springer-Verlag, Berlin.
4. De Potter, W. P., Chubb, I. W., Put, A., and De Shaepdryver, A. F. (1971): Facilitation of the release of noradrenaline and dopamine-β-hydroxylase at low stimulation frequencies by α-blocking agents. *Arch. Int. Pharmacodyn. Ther.*, 193:191–197.
5. Cubeddu, L. X., Barnes, E. M., Langer, S. Z., and Weiner, N. (1975): Release of norepinephrine and dopamine-β-hydroxylase by nerve stimulation. I. Role of neuronal and extraneuronal uptake and of alpha presynaptic receptors. *J. Pharmacol. Exp. Ther.*, 190:431–450.
6. Häggendahl, J. (1970): Some further aspects on the release of the adrenergic transmitter. In: *New Aspects of Storage and Release Mechanisms of Catecholamines*, edited by H. J. Schümann and G. Kroneberg, pp. 100–109. Springer-Verlag, Berlin.
7. Hedqvist, P. (1970): Studies on the effect of prostaglandins E_1 and E_2 on the sympathetic neuromuscular transmission in some animal tissues. *Acta. Physiol. Scand.*, 345:1–40.
8. Langer, S. Z., Adler, E., Enero, M. A., and Stefano, F. J. E. (1971): The role of the alpha receptor in regulating noradrenaline overflow by nerve stimulation. In: *Proceedings of the XXVth International Congress of Physiological Sciences*, p. 335. German Physiological Society, Munich.
9. McCulloch, M. W., Rand, M. J., and Story, D. F. (1972): Inhibition of ^{3}H-noradrenaline release from sympathetic nerves of guinea-pig atria by a presynaptic adrenoceptor mechanism. *Br. J. Pharmacol.*, 46:523–524P.
10. Starke, K. (1971): Influence of α-receptor stimulants on noradrenaline release. *Naturwissenschaften*, 58:420.
11. Farah, M. B., and Langer, S. Z. (1974): Protection by phentolamine against the effects of phenoxybenzamine on transmitter release elicited by nerve stimulation in the perfused cat heart. *Br. J. Pharmacol.*, 52:549–557.
12. Berthelsen, S., and Pettinger, W. (1977): A functional basis for classification of α-adrenergic receptors. *Life Sci.*, 21:595–606.

13. Wickberg, J. E. S. (1979): The pharmacological classification of adrenergic α_1 and α_2 receptors and their mechanisms of action. *Acta. Physiol. Scand.*, 468:1–99.

14. McGrath, J. C. (1982): Evidence for more than one type of postjunctional α-adrenoceptor. *Biochem. Pharmacol.*, 31:467–484.

15. Langer, S. Z., Adler-Graschinsky, E., and Giorgi, O. (1977): Physiological significance of the alpha-adrenoceptor mediated negative feed-back mechanism that regulates noradrenaline release during nerve stimulation. *Nature*, 265:648–650.

16. Cavero, I., Dennis, T., Lefèvre-Borg, F., Perrot, P., Roach, A. G., and Scatton, B. (1979): Effect of clonidine, prazosin and phentolamine on heart rate and coronary sinus catecholamine output during cardioaccelerator nerve stimulation in spinal dogs. *Br. J. Pharmacol.*, 67:283–292.

17. Lokhandwala, M. F., and Buckley, J. P. (1976): Effect of presynaptic α-adrenoceptor blockade on responses to cardiac nerve stimulation in anaesthetized dogs. *Eur. J. Pharmacol.*, 40:183–186.

18. Yamaguchi, N., De Champlain, J., and Nadeau, R. A. (1977): Regulation of norepinephrine release from cardiac sympathetic fibers in the dog by presynaptic alpha and beta receptors. *Circ. Res.*, 41:108–117.

19. Shepperson, N. B., Duval, N., Massingham, R., and Langer, S. Z. (1981): Pre- and postsynaptic alpha adrenoceptor selectivity studies with yohimbine and its two diasterioisomers, rauwolsine and corynanthine in the anaesthetised dog. *J. Pharmacol. Exp. Ther.*, 219:540–546.

20. Filinger, E. J., Langer, S. Z., Perec, C. J., and Stefano, F. J. E. (1978): Evidence for the presynaptic location of the alpha-adrenoceptors which regulate noradrenaline release in the rat submaxillary gland. *Naunyn Schmiedebergs Arch. Pharmacol.*, 304:21–26.

21. Angus, J., and Korner, P. I. (1980): Evidence against presynaptic α-adrenoceptor modulation of cardiac sympathetic transmission. *Nature*, 286:288–291.

22. Story, D. F., McCulloch, M. W., Rand, M. J., and Stanford-Starr, C. A. (1981): Conditions required for the inhibitory feedback loop in noradrenergic transmission. *Nature*, 293:62–65.

23. Langer, S. Z. (1981): Presence and physiological role of presynaptic inhibitory α_2-adrenoceptors in guinea-pig atria. *Nature*, 294:671–672.

24. Starke, K., and Langer, S. Z. (1979): A note on terminology for presynaptic receptors. In: *Presynaptic Receptors*, edited by S. Z. Langer, K. Starke, and M. L. Dubocovich, pp. 1–3. Pergamon Press, London.

25. Starke, K. (1981): α-Adrenoceptor subclassification. *Rev. Physiol. Biochem. Pharmacol.*, 88:199–236.

26. Dubocovich, M. L., and Langer, S. Z. (1974): Negative feed-back regulation of noradrenaline release by nerve stimulation in the perfused cat's spleen: Differences in potency of phenoxybenzamine in blocking pre- and post-synaptic adrenergic receptors. *J. Physiol. (Lond.)*, 237:505–519.

27. Starke, K., Borowski, E., and Endo, T. (1975): Preferential blockade of presynaptic α-adrenoceptors by yohimbine. *Eur. J. Pharmacol.*, 34:385–388.

28. Armstrong, J. M., Lefèvre-Borg, F., Scatton, B., and Cavero, I. (1982): Urethane inhibits cardiovascular responses mediated by the stimulation of alpha-2-adrenoceptors in the rat. *J. Pharmacol. Exp. Ther.*, 223:524–535.

29. Medgett, I. C., McCulloch, M. W., and Rand, M. J. (1978): Partial agonist action of clonidine on prejunctional and postjunctional α-adrenoceptors. *Naunyn Schmiedebergs Arch. Pharmacol.*, 304:215–221.

30. Medgett, I. C., and Rand, M. J. (1981): Dual effects of clonidine on rat prejunctional α-adrenoceptors. *Clin. Exp. Pharm. Physiol.*, 8:503–507.

31. Rand, M. J., Majewski, H., Medgett, I. C., McCulloch, M. W., and Story, D. F. (1980): Prejunctional receptors modulating autonomic neuroeffector transmission. *Circ. Res. [Suppl. 1]*, 46:I-70–I-76.

32. Drew, G. M., and Whiting, S. B. (1979): Evidence for two distinct types of postsynaptic α-adrenoceptor in vascular smooth muscle in vivo. *Br. J. Pharmacol.*, 67:207–215.

33. Docherty, J. R., and McGrath, J. C. (1980): A comparison of pre- and post-junctional potencies of several alpha-adrenoceptor agonists in the cardiovascular system and anococcygeus of the rat. *Naunyn Schmiedebergs Arch. Pharmacol.*, 312:107–116.

34. de Mey, J., and Vanhoutte, P. M. (1981): Uneven distribution of postjunctional alpha-1 and alpha-2-like adrenoceptors in canine arterial and venous smooth muscle. *Circ. Res.*, 48:875–884.

35. Shepperson, N. B., and Langer, S. Z. (1981): The effects of the 2-amino-tetrahydronaphthalene derivative M7, a selective α_2-adrenoceptor agonist in vitro. *Naunyn Schmiedebergs Arch. Pharmacol.*, 318:10–13.

36. Sakakibara, Y., Fujiwara, M., and Muramatsu, I. (1982): Pharmacological characterisation of the alpha-adrenoceptors of the dog basilar artery. *Naunyn Schmiedebergs Arch. Pharmacol.*, 319:1–7.

37. Skärby, T., Anderson, K.-E., and Edvinsson, L. (1981): Characterisation of the postsynaptic α-adrenoceptor in isolated feline cerebral arteries. *Acta Physiol. Scand.*, 220:216–222.

38. Medgett, I., and Langer, S. Z. (1983): Characterisation of smooth muscle α-adrenoceptors and of responses to electrical stimulation in the cat isolated perfused middle cerebral artery. *Naunyn Schmiedebergs Arch. Pharmacol.*, 323:24–32.

39. Lee, T. J.-F., Hume, W. R., Su, C., and Bevan, J. A. (1978): Neurogenic vasodilatation of cat cerebral arteries. *Circ. Res.*, 42:535–542.

40. Duckles, S. P. (1979): Neurogenic dilator and constrictor responses of pial arteries in vitro: Differences between dogs and sheep. *Circ. Res.*, 44:482–490.

41. Lee, T. J.-F., Kinkead, L. R., and Sarwinski, S. (1982): Norepinephrine and acetylcholine transmitter mechanisms in large cerebral arteries of the pig. *J. Cereb. Blood Flow Metab.*, 2(4):439–450.

42. Langer, S. Z., Shepperson, N. B., and Massingham, R. (1981): Preferential noradrenergic innervation of α_1-adrenergic receptors in vascular smooth muscle. *Hypertension [Suppl. I]*, 3:112–118.

43. Langer, S. Z., Massingham, R., and Shepperson, N. B. (1980): Presence of postsynaptic α_2-adrenoceptors of predominantly extrasynaptic location in the vascular smooth muscle of the dog hind limb. *Clin. Sci.*, 59:225s–228s.

44. Moulds, R. F. W., Rittinghausen, R., and Shaw, J. (1980): Prejunctional receptors in human digital arteries. *Circ. Res., [Suppl. I]*, 46:I-80–I-82.
45. Langer, S. Z., Adler-Graschinsky, E., and Enero, M. A. (1974): Positive feedback mechanism for the regulation of noradrenaline released by nerve stimulation. In: *Satellite Symposium: XXVIth International Congress of Physiological Sciences*, p. 81. Israel Physiological and Pharmacological Society, Jerusalem.
46. Dahlöf, C., Ljung, B., and Ablad, B. (1978): Relative potency of β-adrenoceptor agonists on neuronal transmitter release in isolated rat portal vein. In: *Recent Advances in the Pharmacology of Adrenoceptors*, edited by E. Szabadi, C. M. Bradshaw, and P. Bevan, pp. 355–356. Elsevier, Amsterdam.
47. Rand, M. J., McCulloch, M. W., and Story, D. F. (1980): Catecholamine receptors on nerve terminals. In: *Adrenergic Activators and Inhibitors*, edited by L. Szekeres, pp. 223–266. Springer-Verlag, Berlin.
48. Stjärne, K., and Brundin, J. (1976): β_2-Adrenoceptors facilitating noradrenaline secretion from human vasoconstrictor nerves. *Acta. Physiol. Scand.*, 94:88–93.
49. Majewski, H., Tung, L. H., and Rand, M. J. (1982): Adrenaline activation of prejunctional beta-adrenoceptors and hypertension. *J. Cardiovasc. Pharmacol.*, 4:99–106.
50. Tsuruta, K., Frey, E. A., Grewe, C. W., Cote, T. E., Eskay, R. L., and Kebabian, J. W. (1981): Evidence that LY-141865 specifically stimulates the D-2 dopamine receptor. *Nature*, 292:463–466.
51. Cavero, I., Lefèvre-Borg, F., and Gomeni, R. (1981): Blood pressure lowering effects of *N,N*-di-*n*-propyldopamine in rats: Evidence for stimulation of peripheral dopamine receptors leading to inhibition of sympathetic vasculature. *J. Pharmacol. Exp. Ther.*, 218:515–524.
52. Massingham, R., Dubocovich, M. L., and Langer, S. Z. (1980): The role of presynaptic receptors in the cardiovascular actions of *N,N*-di-*n*-propyldopamine in the cat and dog. *Naunyn Schmiedebergs Arch. Pharmacol.*, 314:17–28.
53. Enero, M. A., and Langer, S. Z. (1975): Inhibition by dopamine of ^{3}H-noradrenaline release elicited by nerve stimulation in the isolated cat's nictitating membrane. *Naunyn Schmiedebergs Arch. Pharmacol.*, 289:179–203.
54. Dubocovich, M. L., and Langer, S. Z. (1980): Dopamine and alpha-adrenoceptor agonists inhibit neurotransmission in the cat spleen through different presynaptic receptors. *J. Pharmacol. Exp. Ther.*, 212:144–152.
55. Kalsner, S., and Chan, C. C. (1980): Inhibition by dopamine of the stimulation induced efflux of ^{3}H-noradrenaline in renal arteries: Limitations of the unitary hypothesis of presynaptic regulation of transmitter release. *Can. J. Physiol. Pharmacol.*, 58:504–512.
56. Clark, B. J., and Menninger, K. (1980): Peripheral dopamine receptors. *Circ. Res. [Suppl. I]*, 46:I-59–I-63.
57. Goldberg, L. I., and Kohli, J. D. (1980): Agonists and antagonists of peripheral pre- and post-synaptic dopamine receptors: Clinical implications. In: *Apomorphine and Other Dopaminomimetics, Vol. 1, Basic Pharmacology*, edited by G. L. Gessa and G. U. Corsini, pp. 273–284. Raven Press, New York.
58. Shepperson, N. B., Duval, N., Massingham, R., and Langer, S. Z. (1982): Differential blocking effects of several dopamine receptor antagonists for peripheral pre- and post-synaptic dopamine receptors in the anesthetised dog. *J. Pharmacol. Exp. Ther.*, 221:753–761.
59. Armstrong, J. M. (1980): Prostaglandins: Pre- and post-junctional modulation of adrenergic nerve function. In: *Cardiovascular Pharmacology of the Prostaglandins*, edited by A. G. Herman, P. M. Vanhoutte, H. Denolin, and A. Goosens, pp. 51–64. Raven Press, New York.
60. Dubocovich, M. L., and Langer, S. Z. (1975): Evidence against a physiological role of prostaglandins in the regulation of noradrenaline release in the cat spleen. *J. Physiol. (Lond.)*, 251:737–762.
61. Hedqvist, P. (1974): Effect of prostaglandins and prostaglandin synthesis inhibitors on norepinephrine release from vascular tissue. In: *Prostaglandin Synthesis Inhibitors*, edited by H. J. Robinson and J. R. Vane, pp. 303–309. Raven Press, New York.
62. Muscholl, E. (1980): Peripheral muscarinic control of norepinephrine release in the cardiovascular system. *Am. J. Physiol.*, 239:H713–H720.
63. Rorie, D. K., Rusch, N. J., Shepherd, J. T., Vanhoutte, P. M., and Tyce, G. M. (1981): Prejunctional inhibition of norepinephrine release caused by acetylcholine in the human saphenous vein. *Circ. Res.*, 49:337–341.
64. Vanhoutte, P. M., and Levy, M. N. (1980): Prejunctional cholinergic modulation of adrenergic neurotransmission in the cardiovascular system. *Am. J. Physiol.*, 238:H275–H281.
65. Löffelholz, K., and Muscholl, E. (1970): Inhibition by parasympathetic nerve stimulation of the release of the adrenergic transmitter. *Naunyn Schmiedebergs Arch. Pharmacol.*, 267:181–184.
66. Burnstock, G. (1980): Purinergic receptors in the heart. *Circ. Res. [Suppl. I]*, 46:I-175–I-182.
67. De Mey, J., Burnstock, G., and Vanhoutte, P. M. (1979): Modulation of the evoked release of noradrenaline in canine saphenous vein via presynaptic receptors for adenosine but not ATP. *Eur. J. Pharmacol.*, 55:401–405.
68. Antonaccio, M. J., and Kerwin, L. (1981): Pre- and post-junctional inhibition of vascular sympathetic function by captopril in SHR. *Hypertension*, 3:I-54–I-62.
69. Lang, R. E., Bruckner, U. B., Kempf, B., Rascher, W., Sturm, V., Unger, T., Speck, G., and Ganten, D. (1982): Opioid peptides and blood pressure regulation. *Clin. Exp. Hypertens.*, A4:249–269.
70. Cavero, I., and Roach, A. G. (1981): The pharmacology of prazosin, a novel antihypertensive agent. *Life Sci.*, 27:1525–1540.

Cardiovascular Pharmacology, Second Edition,
edited by Michael Antonaccio.
Raven Press, New York © 1984.

Vascular Changes in Hypertension

R. Clinton Webb

Department of Physiology, University of Michigan Medical School, Ann Arbor, Michigan 48109

Hypertension, which is probably the most common of all cardiovascular diseases, is recognized as a major health problem. Depending on the criteria used to define hypertension and the age of individuals used in the analysis, current estimates indicate that 23 to 60 million persons in the United States have elevated arterial pressure (1). It is likely that approximately one-third of these individuals are not aware of their high blood pressure, because hypertension is an asymptomatic disorder prior to the onset of cardiovascular complications (1). Furthermore, it is likely that approximately 50% of the individuals who are diagnosed are not treated (1).

Hemodynamically, blood pressure is a reflection of the amount of blood pumped by the heart (cardiac output) and the ease with which the blood flows through the peripheral vasculature (vascular resistance). The elevated arterial pressure of chronic hypertension is caused by an increase in total peripheral vascular resistance. Consequently, hypertension is the result of vascular change. The primary goal of this chapter is to focus on the research that characterizes this vascular change. As background, it is important to recognize that hypertension is a disease of regulation. Something has happened to impair the function of one or more of the controlling systems that normally regulate vascular resistance. These systems include (a) the autonomic nervous system, which expresses the activity of reflex neurogenic arcs and of the central nervous system, (b) the kidney, which functions in salt

and water metabolism and in the production of regulatory hormones with either pressor or depressor actions, (c) the adrenal cortex, which produces steroid hormones that help regulate sodium stores in the body, and (d) the blood vessel wall, which regulates its activity through the production of local hormones such as prostaglandins and kinins. In hypertension, alterations in these neurogenic, humoral, and local factors affect the small blood vessels in such a way that total peripheral vascular resistance is increased. Other factors, which can be broadly classified as genetic and environmental influences, contribute as risk factors associated with hypertension. These include obesity, physical inactivity, pregnancy, oral contraception in women, race, high dietary salt intake, familial history, stress, and increasing age (1).

Usually it is difficult to determine the primary event that initiates the overall process leading to elevated arterial pressure. This is particularly true of the most frequent types of the disease: clinical, essential hypertension and experimental, spontaneous hypertension in the rat. Even when the initiating factor is known, such as renal ischemia or mineralocorticoid excess, the sequence of changes leading from the primary event to increased total peripheral vascular resistance is not known (Fig. 1). However, it is apparent that regardless of the state of cardiac output, hypertension would not occur if mechanisms controlling blood vessel resistance were normal. This is ample evidence to suggest that characteriza-

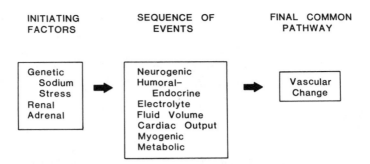

INITIATING FACTORS — SEQUENCE OF EVENTS — FINAL COMMON PATHWAY

Genetic
Sodium
Stress
Renal
Adrenal

Neurogenic
Humoral–
    Endocrine
Electrolyte
Fluid Volume
Cardiac Output
Myogenic
Metabolic

Vascular
Change

FIG. 1. Various aspects of the pathophysiology of hypertension. The pathophysiology of hypertension can be separated into three components. The importance of the vascular change is indicated by the fact that it is the "final common pathway" responsible for pressure elevation. In considering the cause of the vascular change, it is useful to differentiate the "initiating factors" from the "sequence of events" that leads from this starting point to the vascular change. (From Bohr (2). Reproduced by permission.)

tion of structural and functional changes in the vasculature will provide an important aspect to understanding the hypertensive process. Readers interested in more detailed discussions of the current state of hypertension research and clinical aspects of hypertension are referred to several recent publications (1–11).

STRUCTURAL CHANGES IN THE VASCULATURE

Morphological studies have demonstrated that the vasculature undergoes dramatic modifications when exposed to elevated arterial pressure. From a historical perspective, the description of morphological changes preceded the concept of hypertension (12). However, many of these changes characterize the malignant phase of hypertension, and it is unlikely that they are important components contributing to elevated vascular resistance during the developmental phase of the disease. For example, in malignant or established forms of essential hypertension, large renal arteries show atherosclerotic changes consisting of intimal thickening, with splitting of the internal elastic lamina (13). These large arteries do not show histological changes in the early stages. Similarly, focal lesions (elastosis, regenerative intimal thickening, subintimal fatty thickening, etc.) in small arteries and

arterioles are probably the consequence of elevated blood pressure rather than a vascular change that contributes to increased peripheral vascular resistance.

Two types of structural changes that occur in hypertension can have hemodynamic consequence, because they alter the background on which vasoconstrictor influences operate: (a) increased vascular wall thickness and (b) rarefaction of resistance vessels. The importance of these structural changes to elevated blood pressure is demonstrated by the observation that vascular beds in hypertensive animals show higher flow resistance under conditions of maximal vasodilation induced either pharmacologically or by reactive hyperemia (14–21). Because all active wall tension generated by vascular smooth muscle is presumed to be removed, the difference in resistance between hypertensive and normotensive animals occurs because of structural changes in the vascular bed.

Increased Vascular Wall Thickness

Folkow et al. (11,19,22–26) have provided clinical and experimental evidence that increased vascular wall thickness may account for the increased peripheral resistance and enhanced vascular reactivity seen in hypertension. These investigators have hypothesized that media hypertrophy of resistance vessels increases the bulk of wall tissue so that it encroaches on the lumen even when the blood vessel is relaxed. This increase in wall mass in relation to the lumen also results in a steeper resistance curve when the smooth muscle contracts in response to vasoactive stimuli. In studies of forearm and hand vessels of hypertensive and normotensive subjects (24,25) they found that resting vascular tone was normal in hypertensive patients, but vascular resistance was increased at maximal vasodilation. Threshold sensitivity to norepinephrine was not altered in hypertensive patients, but the change in vascular resistance produced by increasing doses resulted in a steeper resistance curve than that in normotensive subjects. Similar studies by Conway (15) and Sivertsson (16) have confirmed these observations.

A change in vascular wall thickness in relation to the lumen also characterizes the vasculature of spontaneously hypertensive rats (SHR) of the Okamoto-Aoki strain (19,22,26). Dose–response curves for vasoconstrictor agents were studied in isolated hindquarters of SHR and normotensive control rats perfused at constant flow. It was observed that (a) vascular resistance was higher in SHR under conditions of maximal vasodilation, (b) threshold sensitivities to vasoconstrictor agents were similar in SHR and normotensive rats, and (c) dose–response curves of vascular resistance to norepinephrine were steeper and the maximal response attained was greater in SHR than in control rats. Folkow and associates showed that these experimental results are similar to those predicted by a mathematical model in which 30% media hypertrophy is assumed (Fig. 2). They believe that the structural change in the vasculature could maintain elevated vascular resistance and increased blood pressure even at normal levels of vascular smooth-muscle tone.

An increase in wall mass in relation to lumen diameter may also account for the compromised response of blood vessels in hypertensive patients to external subatmospheric pressure. Hartling et al. (20) measured the rate of radioactive xenon washout from the anterior tibial muscle in hypertensive and normotensive subjects during reactive hyperemia before and after an increase in vascular transmural pressure (brought about by application of subatmospheric pressure to the leg). At ambient pressure, the washout was not different between the hypertensive and normotensive subjects, whereas an increase in transmural pressure augmented the rate of labeled xenon washout in normotensive subjects almost twice as much as in hypertensive subjects. This suggests that the resistance vessels of hypertensive patients are less distensible than those in normotensive subjects, supporting the concept that structural changes take place in hypertension.

From a morphological standpoint, the increased media thickness of resistance vessels in hypertension could result from any of the following: (a) smooth-muscle cell hypertrophy, (b) smooth-muscle cell hyperplasia, and/or (c) increased amount of paracellular matrix.

Smooth-Muscle Cell Hypertrophy

Friedman et al. (27) observed that smooth-muscle cell volume and surface area are increased in the tail artery and superior epigastric artery in rats made hypertensive with deoxycorticosterone acetate (DOCA), suggesting cellular hypertrophy. Mallov (28) observed that the aortas in DOCA-hypertensive rats and two-kidney/one-clip (2K-1C) renal-hypertensive rats contained greater quantities of smooth muscle per unit of wet tissue than did those of normotensive rats. Wolinsky et al. (29) observed increased media thickness, with no change in cellular DNA content, in aortas from 2K-1C renal-hypertensive rats. Smooth-muscle cell hypertrophy has also been reported in blood vessels from SHR (30) and from dogs made hypertensive by unilateral nephrectomy and cellophane wrap of the remaining kidney (31). Recently, Greenberg et al. (30) concluded that the cell hypertrophy that occurs in portal veins in SHR is initiated by a circulating humoral factor. The basis for this conclusion was that Wistar-Kyoto

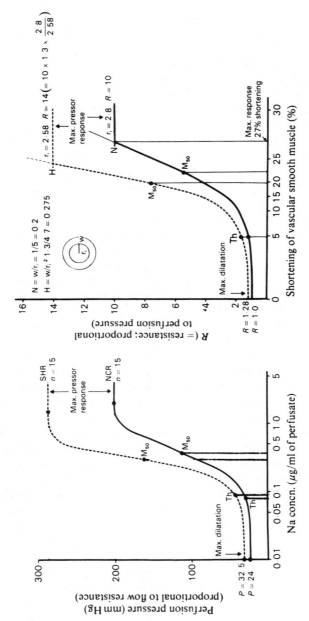

FIG. 2. Increased wall thickness accounts for increased vascular resistance and enhanced vascular reactivity in hypertension. The experimental results (*left panel*) are based on resistance changes induced by norepinephrine (NA) in the hindquarter vascular beds of spontaneously hypertensive (SHR) and normotensive control rats (NCR). The *right panel* represents mathematically deduced "resistance curves" for two hypothetical resistance vessels (H and N), where H differs from N only in the respect that its media thickness is increased by 30% compared to N. (From Folkow (22); for details, see this volume. Reproduced by permission.)

(WKY) normotensive rats parabiosed to SHR developed hypertension, and portal veins from these hypertensive WKY rats contained enlarged smooth-muscle cells.

Smooth-Muscle Cell Hyperplasia

The uptake of tritiated thymidine by vascular tissue in hypertensive animals is greater than that in control animals, suggesting cellular proliferation; the models of hypertension studied include DOCA-hypertensive rats (32,33), one-kidney/one-clip (1K-1C) renal-hypertensive rats (34,35), and rats (36) and rabbits (37) made hypertensive by aortic coarctation. Bevan et al. (38) reported an increased content of DNA in aortas from aortic-coarctation-induced hypertensive rabbits as compared with those from controls. Mitotic figures have been observed in smooth-muscle cells composing interlobar arteries in the kidney in aortic-coarctation-induced hypertensive rats (12,36) and in duodenal arteries in rats with 1K-1C renal hypertension (39). Mulvany et al. (40) measured the morphological properties of resistance vessels in mesenteric vascular beds of SHR and normotensive rats. They observed that relaxed blood vessels in SHR had a 16% smaller lumen diameter and a 49% thicker media at a given transmural pressure than did those of normotensive rats. Histologically, the smooth-muscle cells were arranged in four circumferential layers in SHR vessels and in three layers in normotensive vessels. Warshaw et al. (41) also observed greater numbers of smooth-muscle cells in mesenteric resistance vessels in SHR. Increased numbers of smooth-muscle cells have also been reported for larger vessels in SHR, such as the renal artery (42).

Increased Amount of Paracellular Matrix

There is a marked increase in the amount of paracellular matrix in blood vessels from hypertensive patients and animals [see Rojo-Ortega and Hatt (12) for a review]. Palaty et al. (43) demonstrated an increased content of acid mucopolysaccharides in the tail artery in DOCA-hypertensive rats. Crane (44,45) demonstrated an increase in the synthesis of mucopolysaccharides in arteries from rats with aortic-coarctation-induced hypertension. This increase in acidic groups may provide for an increased amount of sodium binding in the vascular wall that results in the osmotic trapping of water. Tobian et al. (46–49) have presented extensive evidence supporting the concept that extra water, which accumulates in blood vessels in hypertensive animals, increases vascular wall stiffness. This greater wall stiffness reduces the average caliber of the arterioles and thus increases resistance to blood flow.

Rarefaction of Resistance Vessels

A second type of structural alteration that has been proposed to contribute to increased vascular resistance in hypertension is rarefaction of resistance vessels. Hutchins and Darnell (50) observed a 50% reduction in the number of resistance vessels (12–25 μm) in the cremaster muscle in SHR as compared with normotensive rats. Arteriolar rarefaction has also been reported in the mesenteric (51), cutaneous (52), and skeletal muscular vasculatures (53) in SHR and in the conjunctiva in hypertensive patients (54). Hutchins and Darnell (50) postulated that a reduction in the number of arterioles reflects a long-term autoregulatory reaction to overperfusion by elevated arterial pressure. This hypothesis was supported by experiments on SHR that were treated with the β_2 agonist salbutamol to prevent the development of hypertension (55). In these pharmacologically protected rats there was no decrease in the number of small arterioles. Arteriolar rarefaction does not occur in the cerebral cortex in rats made hypertensive with DOCA, although the number of capillaries per unit area of cortex is decreased in hypertensive rats as compared with that in control animals (56).

Recently, Chen et al. (57) used quantitative stereological techniques to examine neural and vasodilator effects on vessel length and surface area per unit volume in cremaster muscles in SHR and normotensive rats. The lengths and surface areas of small arterioles and capillaries per unit volume of muscle were reduced in SHR as compared with those in control rats. Cutting the hypogastric nerve or treating the preparation with nitroprusside resulted in larger percentage increases in vessel length and surface area in SHR than in normotensive rats. These investigators concluded that there are fewer terminal arterioles and capillaries in the cremaster muscle in SHR, and under resting conditions greater percentages (but similar absolute numbers) of these vessels are closed to flow.

Hallback et al. (58) presented evidence they interpreted as indicating that rarefaction of resistance vessels does not contribute to the increased vascular reactivity characteristic of hypertension. They compared dose–response curves of vascular resistance to norepinephrine in hindquarter vascular beds in SHR and normotensive rats to those obtained from vascular beds rarefied by partial plugging of precapillary resistance vessels with microspheres. They reported that a 35% reduction in the number of arterioles (50 μm) did not alter the hindquarter pressor response to norepinephrine in a manner similar to that seen in hindquarters in SHR. Thus, they concluded that the major structural change that contributes to increased vascular reactivity in hypertension is the increased wall thickness in relation to lumen diameter.

Importance of Transmural Pressure

Regardless of the type of structural alteration (increased media thickness or arteriolar rarefaction) that occurs in the vasculature in hypertensive animals, the change in morphology probably is not primary, but an adaptive change in response to the elevation in arterial pressure (22). For example, Warshaw et al. (41) observed that the amount of cellular hyperplasia that occurred in mesenteric resistance arteries in SHR was linearly related to blood pressure. Treatment of SHR with antihypertensive drug therapy resulted in parallel changes in smooth-muscle cell content and systolic blood pressure. Similarly, Henrichs et al. (42) observed that the hyperplasia that occurred in renal arteries in SHR was reversed by antihypertensive treatment with captopril. Lundgren et al. (23) observed that increased media thickness occurred in the hindlimb vasculature after development of a sustained increase in arterial blood pressure in 2K-1C renal-hypertensive rats. Reversibility of the structural alteration required 2 to 3 weeks following removal of the clip from the renal artery, whereas arterial blood pressure returned to normal 1 day after clip removal. Rorive et al. (35) observed an immediate fall in blood pressure in 1K-1C renal-hypertensive rats following removal of the clip from the renal artery; however, the DNA content in the aorta, mesenteric artery, and tail artery remained significantly higher than that in controls 3 weeks after normalization of blood pressure. Folkow et al. (59) observed that aortic obstruction lowered the blood pressure in hindquarter vascular beds in SHR. This hemodynamic effect (reduction in arterial pressure) was immediate, whereas reversibility of structural changes required 2 to 3 weeks. Berecek and Bohr (14) demonstrated that structural changes that occurred in DOCA-hypertensive pigs were related to the pressure within the vasculature. They observed that hindlimb vascular resistance after maximal vasodilation with papaverine was greater in hindlimbs with normal circulation in both normotensive and hypertensive pigs than in the contralateral hindlimbs that had been protected from systemic arterial pressure by iliac artery ligation. Arteriolar rarefaction is not evident in SHR at 3 weeks of age, and the development of this structural change is reversed in 6-week-old SHR when the blood pressure is controlled by treatment with propranolol (60). The increased water content of the aorta, which may reflect increased paracellular matrix, falls within 1 week after reversal of hypertension, whereas the sodium content remains elevated

(61). Thus, it appears that the dominant stimulus for structural changes in the vasculature in hypertensive animals is the increase in the local transmural pressure.

Interestingly, the structural changes that occur in hypertension may play a protective role in certain regional circulations. In SHR, there is an increased cerebral vascular resistance at maximal vasodilation, as well as an increased media thickness in intracerebral vessels. This structural alteration renders these rats less susceptible to disruption of the blood-brain barrier by an acute hypertensive crisis (62,63).

Importance of Neural and Humoral Influences

Although most experimental studies have suggested that structural changes are secondary to the increase in arterial pressure, a number of recent publications have suggested that other factors may contribute to morphological alterations in the vasculature in hypertensive animals. Cerebral and mesenteric arteries in stroke-prone SHR exhibit structural changes indicative of hypertrophy prior to an increase in intracerebral pressure or to an increase in mean arterial pressure (64). Hart et al. (65) observed that the increased wall thickness in cerebral arteries in stroke-prone SHR requires an intact sympathetic nerve supply for full development. Reserpine, but not captopril, prevents the increase in DNA content in vascular smooth muscle in 1K-1C renal-hypertensive rats (34). Both agents lower blood pressure, suggesting that transmural pressure is not the only determinant of structural vascular changes in hypertension. Bell and Overbeck (66) suggested that neural or humoral influences may play an important role in determining structural changes in the vasculature in rats made hypertensive by aortic coarctation. These investigators observed elevated resistance in vascular beds below the aortic obstruction that were not exposed to elevated levels of blood pressure. The major component of elevated resistance was related to

neural influences, because nerve section dramatically reduced hindlimb resistance in these rats. However, a significant portion of elevated resistance persisted after maximal vasodilation with nitroprusside, suggesting that structural changes had occurred in vascular beds that were exposed to normal pressure. Structural changes also occur on the low-pressure side of the circulation. Using the isogravimetric technique, Nilsson and Folkow (67) observed decreased venous wall compliance in perfused hindquarter in SHR following maximal vasodilation as compared with that in hindquarters in normotensive rats. Veins from 2K-1C renal-hypertensive rats have increased wall contents of water and sodium as compared with veins from control rats (30,61), and veins from 2K-1C renal-hypertensive rats and SHR undergo hypertrophy (68–72). Because venous pressure is not elevated in these animals, it has been suggested that other factors may produce structural changes in the vasculature.

FUNCTIONAL CHANGES IN THE VASCULATURE

Because the structural changes that occur in hypertension are primarily adaptive phenomena in response to the increase in arterial pressure, other mechanisms must be considered to account for the genesis of elevated arterial blood pressure. The following evidence is cited in support of the concept that functional changes in the blood vessels contribute to the altered state of the vasculature in hypertension: (a) There is increased sensitivity to vasoactive stimuli in isolated vascular preparations from hypertensive animals. (b) The magnitudes of the changes in sensitivity in vascular preparations from hypertensive animals are qualitatively and quantitatively different for each agonist. (c) Functional vascular changes often precede or accompany the development of high blood pressure. (d) The changes in vascular sensitivity occur in the absence of increased wall stress in hypertension. The studies that have attempted to characterize mechanisms for functional vascular changes have been complicated by the marked individualities of these changes observed under different conditions. The following factors contribute to the variations in experimental results: (a) the primary cause of the hypertension, (b) the time course of the hypertension, (c) the animal species, (d) the age and sex of the animal, (e) the technique used to evaluate a functional change, and (f) the anatomical location of the vascular bed.

Increased Sensitivity to Vasoconstrictor Stimuli

Many investigators have observed that isolated vascular preparations from hypertensive animals show increased sensitivity to vasoactive stimuli (14,73–111). This functional change in the vasculature usually is measured as a reduced threshold for a constrictor response or as a reduction in the effective dose that produces a half-maximal constrictor response (ED_{50}). These changes in sensitivity cannot be explained on the basis of structural alterations in the vasculature.

It seems reasonable to suggest a causal relationship between increased vascular sensitivity and the initiation and maintenance of hypertension; however, few studies have presented evidence to support this concept. This gap in our knowledge is due mainly to a lack of understanding of the complicated interactions between the systems that regulate vascular resistance in the intact animal and the observations of increased sensitivity to vasoactive stimuli in isolated vascular preparations. Two recent studies clearly implicate changes in vascular sensitivity as contributing components to hypertension. Berecek et al. (103) observed that Brattleboro rats, homozygous for diabetes insipidus, did not become hypertensive with DOCA unless given vasopressin replacement therapy. More important, restoration of hypertension by vasopressin therapy in these animals was associated with an induction of increased renal vascular sensitivity, and this induction occurred rapidly, preceding the rise in arterial pressure (Fig. 3). Vanhoutte et al.

(98,105) have demonstrated increased vascular sensitivity to serotonin in the renal vascular bed in SHR. Ketanserin, a sertonergic receptor antagonist, causes dose-related reductions in arterial blood pressure in SHR (Fig. 4). The reductions in arterial blood pressure are larger and occur at lower doses in SHR than in normotensive rats. The unique features of these studies in establishing a role for increased vascular sensitivity in hypertension are different: (a) The study by Berecek et al. (103) showed a temporal relationship between changes in vascular sensitivity that require a neurohumoral "trigger" to initiate the sequence. (b) The studies by Vanhoutte et al. (98,105) demonstrated that a specific receptor antagonist lowers blood pressure in an animal model that evidences increased vascular sensitivity to the appropriate agonist.

The increased vascular sensitivity to some vasoactive stimuli may be masked in the hypertensive animal by compensatory mechanisms that take place in the vasculature or in the intact organism. For example, increased activity of the neuronal uptake mechanism may partially mask the increased sensitivity to norepinephrine in vascular preparations isolated from SHR. Collis and Vanhoutte (98) observed that isolated perfused kidneys from SHR were more sensitive to injected norepinephrine than were those from normotensive rats. Constrictor responses to renal nerve stimulation were normal in SHR kidneys; however, blockade of the neuronal pump with cocaine potentiated constrictor responses to renal nerve stimulation to a greater extent in SHR than in control kidneys. These observations suggest that a more efficient uptake of norepinephrine by nerve endings in the blood vessel wall may mask the true sensitivity of vascular smooth-muscle cells in SHR. Other investigators have substantiated these observations and performed further studies demonstrating that the cocaine-sensitive uptake of radiolabeled norepinephrine is enhanced in blood vessels from SHR (73,77–80,104, 112,113).

The observations of many investigators in-

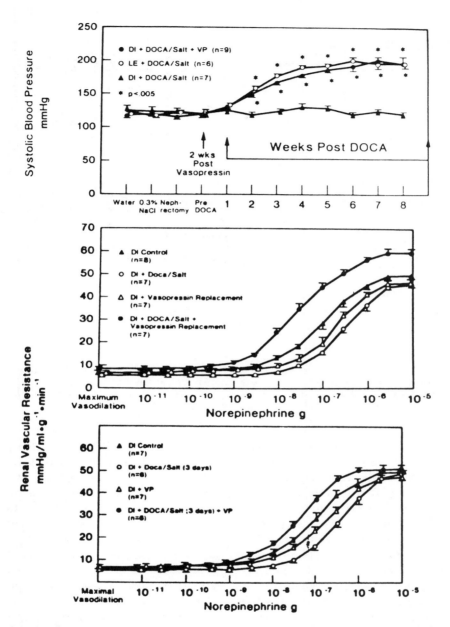

FIG. 3. Blood pressure and renal vascular reactivity in DOCA hypertensive rats with hereditary diabetes insipidus. *Top panel:* Systolic blood pressures in diabetes insipidus (DI) rats that lacked vasopressin (VP) (△, DI + DOCA-salt), in DI rats replaced with VP (● DI + DOCA-salt + VP) and in normal Long-Evans (LE) rats (○ LE + DOCA-salt) after treatment with DOCA (100 mg/kg) + unilateral nephrectomy + 0.3% NaCl. Values are mean ± SEM. Asterisks indicate responses significantly different from pre-DOCA measurements. *Middle panel:* Dose-response curves to norepinephrine in isolated perfused kidneys from untreated DI rats (▲ D1 control), DI rats treated with VP alone (△ DI + VP replacement), DI rats treated with DOCA-salt alone (○ DI + DOCA-salt) and DI rats treated with both VP and DOCA (● D1+ DOCA-salt + vasopressin replacement). Kidneys were perfused 6–10 weeks post-DOCA. Values are mean ± SEM. *Bottom panel:* Dose-response curves to norepinephrine in isolated perfused kidneys from untreated DI rats (▲ DI control), D1 rats treated with DOCA-salt alone (○ DI + DOCA-salt), DI rats treated with DOCA-salt and VP (● DI + DOCA-salt + VP) and DI rats treated with vasopressin alone (△ DI + VP). Kidneys were perfused 3 days post DOCA. Values are the mean ± SEM. (From Berecek et al. (103). Reproduced by permission.)

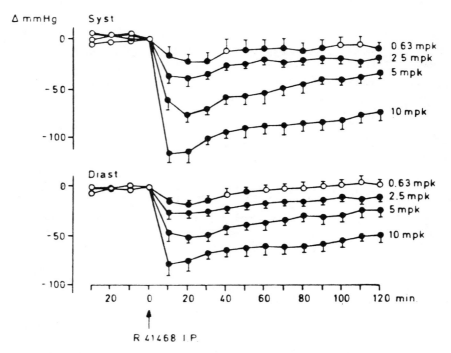

FIG. 4. Effect of increasing doses of ketanserin (R41468) on systolic (Syst.) and diastolic (Diast.) blood pressures in spontaneously hypertensive rats. Ketanserin was given i.p. Values are the mean ± SEM for 6 rats. Closed symbols indicate that the values obtained in the presence of ketanserin are significantly different from control (p < 0.05); mpk = mg/kg. (From Van Nueten et al. (105). Reproduced by permission.)

dicate that the sensitivity of vascular smooth muscle in hypertension is most variable. For example, microvessels from the mesenteric vasculature in SHR are more sensitive to norepinephrine than those from normotensive rats (77,78), whereas microvessels in the cremaster muscle in SHR do not differ from those of controls in terms of sensitivity to the catecholamine (114). Isolated carotid arteries from SHR are more sensitive to stimulation by strontium or lanthanum than are those from 2K-1C renal-hypertensive or DOCA-hypertensive rats (94). Increased sensitivity to epinephrine and KCl is much more prominent in isolated femoral arteries from DOCA-hypertensive rats and 2K-1C renal-hypertensive rats than in femoral arteries from SHR (106). The changes in vascular sensitivity to norepinephrine vary in different strains of genetic-hypertensive rats. Dose–response curves for norepinephrine in renal vascular beds of stroke-prone SHR and stroke-resistant SHR

are shifted to the left of control values, indicating increased vascular sensitivity (107). The shift is greater in stroke-prone rats than in the stroke-resistant strain. Furthermore, the degree of the change in sensitivity to norepinephrine in SHR is related to the sex of the animal. Collis and Vanhoutte (98) observed that the magnitude of the shift to the left in dose–response curves to norepinephrine was greater in renal vascular beds in male SHR than in female SHR. As a generalization, it appears that in some types of hypertension, some vascular beds display an increased sensitivity in response to certain constrictor agonists. Conversely, it is certain that not all vascular smooth muscle in all types of hypertension is abnormal in its sensitivity.

Altered Sensitivity to Various Agonists

There is a unique feature of the increased vasoconstrictor sensitivity observed in vascular beds in hypertensive animals: Vascular sensitivity to some agonists is augmented to a greater degree than for other agonists. McGregor and Smirk (115) observed that isolated perfused mesenteric vascular beds of SHR and renal-hypertensive rats constricted to a greater degree than did those from normotensive rats when treated with norepinephrine or serotonin. Following injection of 0.5 mg of norepinephrine into the perfusates of mesenteric vasculatures from normotensive, SHR, and renal-hypertensive rats, they observed pressor responses of 35, 44, and 50 mm Hg, respectively. This enhanced pressor response to norepinephrine in the hypertensive rats was exceeded by the enhanced response that occurred when 10 mg of serotonin was in-

jected into the mesenteric beds: normotensive rats, 15 mm Hg; SHR, 112 mm Hg; renal-hypertensive rats, 94 mm Hg. From these observations they suggested that altered pressor responsiveness could not be due to a structural change and that a differential augmentation of responsiveness by the two agonists demonstrates a functional alteration in smooth muscle of resistance vessels in hypertensive animals. Collis and Vanhoutte (98), studying the renal vasculature of SHR, observed that responses to serotonin were potentiated to a greater degree than were responses to norepinephrine, angiotensin II, or barium (Fig. 5). Other laboratories have also demonstrated a greater enhancement of vascular responses to serotonin in hypertension (82,84,89,115–118).

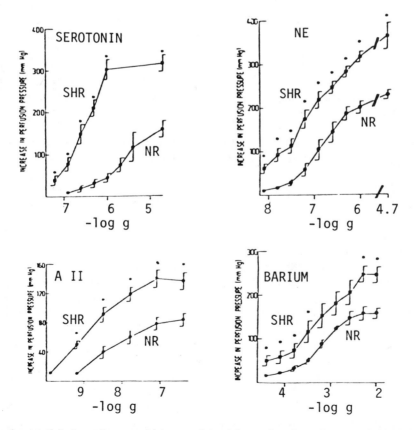

FIG. 5. Vascular reactivity to various constrictor agonists of the perfused renal vascular bed in spontaneously hypertensive rats (SHR) and in normotensive controls (NR). The augmentation of the reactivity in response to serotonin in the SHR is greater than that of the response to norepinephrine (NE), angiotensin II (AII) or barium. Values are the mean ± SEM. (From Collis and Vanhoutte (98). Reproduced by permission.)

Added insight into the significance of the exaggerated potentiation of serotonin responses in hypertension has been obtained through the use of methysergide, a serotonergic antagonist that displays partial agonist properties in certain vascular beds (119). Webb and Bohr (84) observed that isolated aortic strips from DOCA-hypertensive rats were only minimally more sensitive to norepinephrine than those from normotensive rats, whereas aortic strips from hypertensive rats evidenced enormous increases in sensitivity to serotonin and especially to methysergide (Fig. 6). Methysergide added to the muscle bath during a serotonin contraction of the normotensive aortic strips produced a relaxation that reflected the antagonistic action of the drug on serotonin receptors. When this relationship was studied in aortic strips from DOCA-hypertensive rats, there was no relaxation. These results suggest an alteration in the receptors that mediate responses to serotonergic agonists and antagonists in hypertension.

It has also been shown that the increased vascular sensitivity to epinephrine in hypertension is much greater than that to potassium (106). Comparison of vascular responses to norepinephrine and to calcium has also yielded differential sensitivities in hypertensive preparations. It has been observed that the response to calcium of potassium-depolarized vascular smooth muscle is not different, whereas smooth-muscle sensitivity to calcium is greater in hypertensive animals when norepinephrine is used as the activating agent. Similarly, the vasoconstrictor effect of barium is less than that of norepinephrine (97). It has been proposed that contractions caused by these cation manipulations may reflect a change in the contractile components of the vascular smooth muscle and not involve an earlier event of the contractile sequence that is initiated by norepinephrine (97). This possibility leads to the suggestion that it is this earlier event in the contractile sequence, perhaps the initial membrane excitation, that is altered in vascular smooth muscle in hypertensive animals.

Increased Vascular Sensitivity Precedes the Rise in Arterial Pressure

Many investigators have observed a temporal dissociation between functional vascular changes and the development of high arterial pressure, suggesting that these changes play a role in the elevation of resistance in hypertension. The following paragraphs summarize observations on the three major forms of experimental hypertension:

Renal Hypertension

Ogden et al. (120) observed that vascular responsiveness to pitressin increases before the rise in arterial pressure in 1K-1C renal-hypertensive rabbits. Similarly, McQueen (121) showed that pressor responsiveness to norepinephrine in the isolated hindquarters of rats is also increased at an early time after the induction of 1K-1C renal hypertension, 2K-1C renal hypertension, and renoprival hypertension. Increased vascular sensitivity to norepinephrine in microvessels of the cheek pouch in hamsters occurs rapidly following figure-of-eight ligature of the kidneys (109). The mesenteric vascular bed in 2K-1C renal-hypertensive rats develops a progressive blood-pressure-related increased sensitivity to norepinephrine and angiotensin II. Whereas blood pressure and vascular sensitivity to these agonists were near maximum in 2 weeks, structural changes in the vascular bed had reached only about one-quarter of their maximum at that time (108). Lundgren et al. (23) observed that the development of high arterial pressure was faster than the development of structural changes in 2K-1C renal-hypertensive rats. Greenberg (85) observed increased sensitivity to serotonin, angiotensin II, prostaglandin H_2, and prostaglandin B_2 in various arteries and veins isolated from 2K-1C renal-hypertensive dogs at 24 hr after the clipping procedure (when blood pressure was not significantly elevated). He suggested that immediately following the clipping of the renal artery, circulating humoral factors or neural

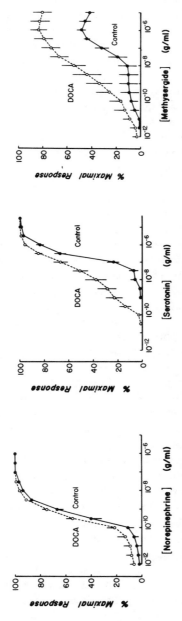

FIG. 6. Vascular sensitivity to norepinephrine, serotonin, and methysergide in DOCA hypertensive rats. Cumulative addition of norepinephrine (*left panel*), serotonin (*middle panel*) or methysergide (*right panel*) to the muscle bath produced contraction in aortic strip preparations from DOCA hypertensive and control normotensive rats. Arterial preparation from DOCA hypertensive rats were more sensitive to all three agonists; the change in sensitivity to serotonin and methysergide exceeded that to norepinephrine. Values are the mean ± SEM. (From Webb and Bohr (84). Reproduced by permission.)

factors are released from, or activated by, the constricted kidney. These factors act on the vascular smooth muscle to modify the receptor activation mechanism for some vasoactive agents.

Mineralocorticoid-Induced Hypertension

Berecek et al. (110) observed that renal vascular sensitivity to vasopressin and norepinephrine increases in DOCA-treated rats before the arterial pressure rises. Systemic vascular sensitivity to angiotensin II and norepinephrine is greater in DOCA-hypertensive pigs than in normotensive pigs. These changes in vascular sensitivity were found to occur at a time when mean arterial pressure was starting to rise (111). Increased sensitivity to serotonin and methysergide in aortic strips from DOCA-hypertensive rats parallels the development of high arterial pressure (82).

Genetic Hypertension

Increased vascular sensitivity to norepinephrine was observed in SHR as young as 3 weeks of age (99). At this stage of development, there was little or no difference in systolic blood pressure between SHR and normotensive rats. Shibata et al. (122) demonstrated that abnormal vascular sensitivity to nonphysiological cations preceded the development of hypertension in SHR. Increased vascular reactivity was found in SHR that were 12 to 14 weeks old (123), whereas structural narrowing of the resistance vessels was not evident until the rats were 20 weeks old.

Increased Vascular Sensitivity Occurs in the Absence of Elevated Wall Stress

The increased vascular sensitivity that occurs in hypertension is not secondary to an increase in wall stress. Abel and Hermsmeyer (76) transplanted tail artery segments from 2-week-old SHR and WKY into innervated and denervated anterior eye chambers in the same or the opposite strain. Seven weeks later

they observed that the transplants that had reinnervated developed vascular sensitivity traits characteristic of the host strain (i.e., ED_{50} values for norepinephrine were lower in tail artery segments from SHR implanted into SHR eye chambers than in SHR segments implanted into WKY). These results suggest that neural influences control the development of increased vascular sensitivity in SHR. These changes occurred in the absence of an increase in wall stress, because the transplants were not connected to the vasculature of the host anterior eye chamber and therefore were not subject to the elevated blood pressure.

Bohr et al. (14,100,102) studied changes in vascular sensitivity in hindlimbs of hypertensive animals that were protected from high arterial pressure by chronic occlusion of the iliac artery. This procedure decreases wall stress, because the arterial pressure in the occluded leg is approximately half that in the contralateral unoccluded leg. It was observed that the increased vascular sensitivity associated with hypertension could not be reversed or prevented by lowering blood pressure in one leg in DOCA-hypertensive pigs and rats, SHR, and 2K-1C renal-hypertensive rats. Threshold doses of vasoactive agonists (norepinephrine, epinephrine, KCl) required to produce constrictor responses remained significantly lower in vascular preparations from hypertensive animals than in those from normotensive animals. These studies suggest that changes in vascular sensitivity are independent of elevated wall stress and hence may be related to the pathogenesis of hypertension.

Observations that increased sensitivity to vasoactive agents occurs on the venous side of the circulation further support the hypothesis that this functional abnormality is unrelated to increased wall stress in hypertension. Greenberg (85) observed that mesenteric, gracilis, pulmonary, and dorsal metatarsal veins isolated from 2K-1C renal-hypertensive dogs are more sensitive to several constrictor agents than those isolated from normotensive dogs. Other investigators have documented that the reactivity of venous smooth muscle to norepinephrine and other constrictor agonists is increased in hypertensive animals (71,87,90,91,93,101).

CELLULAR MECHANISMS FOR FUNCTIONAL VASCULAR CHANGES

Because the vasculature in hypertensive animals displays altered sensitivity to exogenous stimuli, it is reasonable to characterize mechanisms that may account for these functional changes. The component of the vascular smooth-muscle cell that is most likely responsible for changes in vascular sensitivity in hypertension is the cell membrane. Other cellular changes that have been considered include abnormalities in (a) agonist–receptor interactions, (b) the relaxation system, (c) cyclic nucleotides and related enzymes, and (d) prostaglandin metabolism.

Altered Cellular Membrane Properties

Both teleological and mechanistic arguments can be made to support the hypothesis that changes in cell membrane properties are responsible for altered vascular smooth-muscle function in hypertension. Teleologically, the cell membrane is the structure that is most likely to sense environmental changes for which altered cellular activity may be required. Mechanistically, the environmental change can induce a chemical or morphological alteration in the membrane whereby cellular function is regulated. The following paragraphs document experimental evidence suggesting that the cell membrane plays an important role in chronic cellular dysfunction in hypertension.

Spontaneous Contractions of Vascular Smooth Muscle

The occurrence of spontaneous rhythmic contractions in isolated vascular smooth muscle from hypertensive animals is increased (84,106,124–128). These phasic contractions are variable in magnitude, frequency, and sta-

bility. Investigations by Bohr and Sitrin (124) and Holloway and Bohr (106) demonstrated that these spontaneous contractions are dependent on extracellular calcium concentration (Fig. 7). Isolated femoral artery strips from SHR, DOCA-hypertensive rats, and 2K-1C renal-hypertensive rats exhibited marked increases in the magnitude of spontaneous contractions when the concentration of calcium in the muscle bath was increased from 1.6 mM to 3.2 mM. This increased sensitivity to extracellular calcium in hypertensive vessels is not related to the presence of spontaneous contractions, because femoral artery strips from normotensive rats that exhibited myogenic phasic activity did not contract when the concentration of calcium in the bath was increased. The spontaneous rhythmic contractions of vascular segments from hypertensive animals are not the result of increased passive tension applied to the preparations, nor are they altered by pharmacological blockade of α-adrenergic or β-adrenergic receptors.

A recent study by Moreland et al. (83) suggested that the increased occurrence of spontaneous contractions in mesenteric arteries isolated from DOCA-hypertensive rats may be related to an increased number of membrane channels for calcium ion. These investigators placed DOCA-hypertensive rats on a protein-deficient diet and observed that spontaneous contractions in response to elevated calcium were decreased in arteries from these rats, as compared with those from DOCA-hypertensive rats maintained on a normal diet. Because a major action of the mineralocorticoid is to stimulate the synthesis of transport proteins (129,130), these investigators concluded that vascular smooth muscle from DOCA-hypertensive rats may contain an increased number of membrane channels for calcium.

The frequency of spontaneous contractions in portal veins from SHR is increased, as compared with that in portal veins from normotensive WKY rats (30,71). Normotensive WKY rats parabiosed to SHR develop hypertension, and the frequency of spontaneous contractions in portal veins from the hypertensive WKY

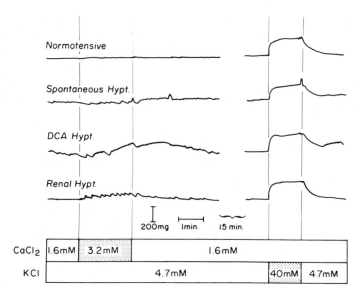

FIG. 7. Spontaneous rhythmic contractions in vascular smooth muscle from hypertensive animals. Spontaneous rhythmic contractions were observed in isolated femoral artery strips from the three types of hypertensive rats shown, but were not seen in arterial strips from normotensive rats. Femoral artery strips from DOCA and renal hypertensive rats contracted in response to 3.2 mM $CaCl_2$, but strips from normotensive rats and SHR did not. All arterial strips responded to 40 mM KCl. (From Holloway and Bohr (106). Reproduced by permission.)

rats is increased as compared with the controls (30). As noted earlier, these results suggest that a circulating factor may be responsible for vascular changes in SHR.

Increased Membrane Permeability to Calcium

Infusion of calcium ions into intact limbs and isolated vascular beds, at rates that do not alter systemic levels of calcium, causes increased vascular resistance (131–133). Similar studies on 1K-1C renal-hypertensive dogs have shown that changes in vascular resistance to calcium in the forelimb are not different from those in control dogs (132). Similarly, vasoconstrictor responses to calcium in isolated, innervated hindquarters of SHR do not differ from those for normotensive controls (131). In contrast, intravenous infusion of calcium (7–8 mg/kg body weight) into hypertensive patients increases peripheral vascular resistance; vascular resistance in normotensive patients is not altered by infusion of calcium

(134). Hinke (135) observed that contractile responses of isolated perfused segments of tail artery from DOCA-hypertensive and normotensive rats were abolished when calcium was removed from the perfusate. When calcium was restored at various concentrations (0–1.2 mM), less calcium was required to reestablish contraction in the hypertensive arteries. Similar studies by Holloway et al. (127) showed that contractile responses to epinephrine in isolated femoral artery strips from DOCA-hypertensive rats and control rats were abolished in calcium-free solutions. When the bath concentration of calcium was increased to 1.6 mM, the rate of force development in arterial strips from hypertensive animals was more rapid than in controls. These latter studies have been interpreted to reflect a faster rate of entry of ionized calcium into vascular smooth-muscle cells in hypertensive animals because of increased membrane permeability.

Measurements of calcium flux in vascular smooth muscle from hypertensive animals also suggest that there may be a leak of calcium ions through the cell membrane. The efflux of radiolabeled calcium from aortic strips of SHR is faster than that from aortic strips of normotensive rats (136–138). Noon et al. (139) concluded that smooth-muscle cell membranes in aortas in SHR were leaky to calcium, based on observations that aortic strips from SHR relaxed when placed in calcium-free solution; aortic strips from normotensive rats were unaffected by manipulations of calcium concentration in the bathing medium. Suzuki et al. (140) and Fitzpatrick and Szentivanyi (141) demonstrated that following calcium depletion, elevations in the concentration of calcium in the bathing medium produced an increase in tone in aortic strips from SHR. Because aortas from normotensive rats did not develop tone in response to calcium, both groups concluded that smooth-muscle cells in aortas of SHR have increased permeability to calcium. Pederson et al. (142,143) reached similar conclusions based on experiments showing that aortic strips from SHR relax faster than those from normotensive rats when treated with the calcium-channel blocker nifedipine.

Additional evidence that probably reflects altered permeability of the cell membrane in hypertension has been developed by the use of nonphysiological cations and potassium. Lanthanum, which in normal vascular smooth muscle blocks the movement of calcium through the cell membrane and causes relaxation, produces contraction of vascular smooth muscle from SHR (Fig. 8) (94, 100,122,144). Similarly, manganese and strontium cause contraction of vascular smooth muscle from SHR, but not in that from normotensive rats (94). Holloway and Bohr (106) have shown that femoral artery strips from 2K-1C renal-hypertensive and DOCA-hypertensive rats are more sensitive to potassium than are controls. Contractile responses to depolarizing concentrations of potassium in aortic strips from SHR are more sensitive to inhibition by calcium-channel blockers (verapamil, diltiazem) than those for normo-

tensive rats (140,145). Because contractile responses to potassium are dependent on an influx of extracellular calcium (146), these changes in vascular smooth muscle in hypertensive rats may reflect greater than normal permeability of the cell membrane to calcium.

Decreased Membrane Stability to Calcium

Deficient calcium binding to the cell membrane in vascular smooth muscle may account for a greater membrane lability in normal calcium concentrations and a greater sensitivity of the smooth muscle to various vasoactive agents. Holloway and Bohr (106) and Hansen and Bohr (100) observed that vascular smooth muscle from SHR, DOCA-hypertensive rats, and 2K-1C renal-hypertensive rats required a higher calcium concentration to depress a contractile response than did that from normotensive controls (Fig. 9). This change in responsiveness to calcium is more evident in arterial segments that develop myogenic tone. Winquist et al. (147) observed that helical strips of basilar artery from control normotensive and DOCA-hypertensive pigs developed a maintained contraction spontaneously following application of resting force, whereas helical strips of renal, tail, and femoral arteries did not. Renal, tail, and femoral arteries were contracted in response to 40-mM KCl. Increasing the bath concentration of calcium from 1.6 mM to 2.1 mM and then to 4.1 mM caused progressive increases in the force of contraction in response to potassium in renal, tail, and femoral arteries from control pigs. Further increases in calcium (6.1–20.1 mM) elicited dose-dependent decreases in the level of contraction. The magnitude of relaxation was in the order of tail > femoral > renal. Basilar artery strips relaxed dose-dependently to small increases in extracellular calcium, with the threshold at 1.7 mM and a 50% relaxation at 7.6 mM. The relaxant dose–response curve to calcium was shifted significantly upward and to the right in all arteries from DOCA-hypertensive pigs. These results suggest that vascular smooth muscle with intrin-

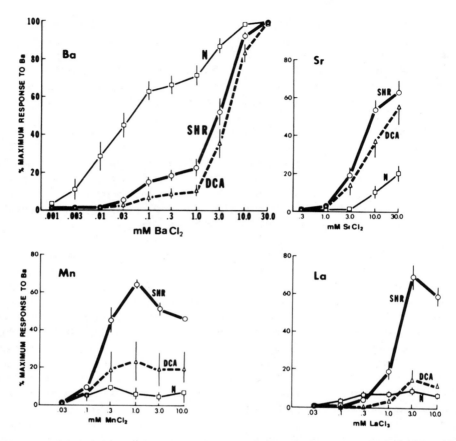

FIG. 8. Dose-response curves to barium, strontium, manganese, and lanthanum. Carotid artery strips from SHR, DOCA hypertensive rats and normotensive rats were made to contract in response to the cumulative addition of barium, strontium, manganese, or lanthanum. Values are means ± SEM. (From Bohr (94). Reproduced by permission.)

sic tone is more sensitive to the stabilizing influence of calcium and that calcium-induced relaxation is attenuated in all vessels of DOCA-hypertensive pigs.

The mechanism by which calcium stabilizes the excitable membrane is believed to result from a decrease in the conductance of major ions across the cell membrane (148,149). Conversely, a reduction in the external concentration of the cation produces a partial depolarization of the cell membrane (150), an increase in potassium efflux (149,151), and a transient contraction in some smooth-muscle preparations (151). Presumably, the binding of calcium to specific loci in the membrane reduces

membrane permeability to monovalent ions, and therefore, by altering the membrane potential, calcium influences its own ability to permeate the membrane or to be released from intracellular stores. In hypertension, it has been postulated that the plasma membrane of vascular smooth-muscle cells has fewer calcium-binding sites or that the affinity for calcium at the existing sites is low (106). Jones et al. (148,149) have shown that the plasma membrane of aortic smooth muscle from SHR and DOCA-hypertensive rats is leakier to potassium. This leakiness is reduced by increasing the concentration of calcium in the bathing medium, and the response to calcium is atten-

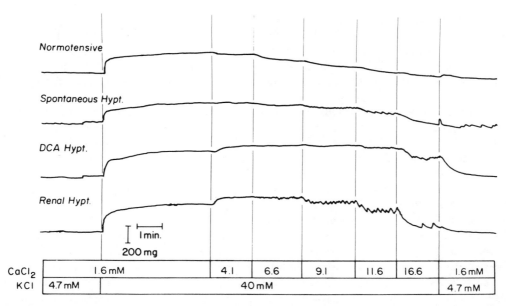

FIG. 9. Membrane stabilizing effect of calcium in vascular smooth muscle from hypertensive rats. The membrane stabilizing effect of calcium was evaluated in femoral artery strips from hypertensive and normotensive rats. The arterial strips were contracted with 40 mM KCl. The femoral artery strips from SHR, DOCA hypertensive rats and renal hypertensive rats required a higher calcium concentration to depress contractile responses compared to normotensive vascular tissue. (From Holloway and Bohr (106). Reproduced by permission.)

uated in aortas from hypertensive animals. Several investigators (152,153) have shown that calcium binding by cell membrane fragments isolated from vascular smooth muscle of hypertensive animals is significantly depressed as compared with normotensive controls. Thus, a basic feature of vascular smooth muscle from hypertensive animals may be increased membrane permeability (*vide infra*) and less than normal membrane stability.

Increased Membrane Permeability to Monovalent Ions

Extensive evidence indicates that the cell membrane of vascular smooth muscle from hypertensive animals is more permeable to monovalent ions. Jones et al. (148,149,154–162) have consistently demonstrated that the fluxes of radiolabeled potassium, sodium, and chloride are increased in isolated vascular strips from hypertensive animals, as compared with those in normotensive controls. Jones

and Hart (148) demonstrated that increases in the turnover rate of radiolabeled potassium in aortic strips from DOCA-treated rats preceded the development of high blood pressure. Garitz and Jones (158) observed increased turnover of radiolabeled potassium and chloride in aortas and femoral arteries isolated from rats made hypertensive by infusion of aldosterone. Increases in monovalent ion turnover were evident at 1 week after the start of aldosterone infusion, well before a significant rise in blood pressure had occurred. Additionally, the magnitude of the change in turnover rate was related to the dose of aldosterone infused, as was the magnitude of the blood pressure response to the mineralocorticoid. Treatment with various combinations of antihypertensive drugs reduces blood pressure in DOCA-treated rats and reduces the rate of turnover of radiolabeled potassium in aortic smooth muscle (156,159). Jones (160) observed that the turnover of radiolabeled potassium in aortic strips from 1K-1C renal-hypertensive rats was unchanged at 10 to 12 weeks after surgery, whereas at 12 to 20 weeks after surgery a significant elevation was observed. Friedman et al. (163–167) have also consistently demonstrated that the passive permeability of the cell membrane to sodium and potassium is increased in vascular smooth muscle from SHR and mineralocorticoid-hypertensive rats.

Because the membrane permeability to ions and the concentration gradients are major determinants of the membrane potential, the foregoing observations have been interpreted as an indication that the membrane potential of vascular smooth muscle from hypertensive animals may be decreased to a greater extent when acted on by vasoactive agents. Indeed, the passive movement of monovalent ions through receptor-operated ionic channels is changed in vascular smooth muscle from hypertensive animals. Jones et al. (159) observed that norepinephrine, serotonin, angiotensin II, and vasopressin induced an increased turnover of radiolabeled potassium in vascular smooth muscle from DOCA-hypertensive and normotensive rats (Fig. 10); the magnitude of the increase for each agonist was greater in aortic

strips from DOCA-hypertensive rats. Interestingly, the dose–response relationship for serotonin in potassium turnover in aortas from DOCA-treated rats was shifted more to the left of control values than was that for norepinephrine (Fig. 11). These results confirm the observations that vascular smooth muscle from hypertensive animals shows an unusual change in sensitivity to serotonin as compared with other vasoactive agents (*vide supra*).

Membrane Potential and the Electrogenic Sodium Pump

Another membrane abnormality that may alter vascular responsiveness is a change in the activity of electrogenic transport of sodium and potassium. Hermsmeyer (74,75) reported that vascular smooth-muscle cells from SHR have less negative membrane potentials than those from normotensive rats at 15°C but not at 37°C. He postulated that at physiological temperature, the components of the membrane potential contributed by ionic gradients and by electrogenic ion transport mechanisms differ in SHR and normotensive rats. The smaller ionic gradient in SHR, created by in-

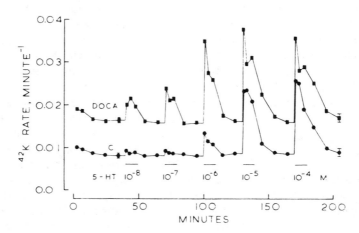

FIG. 10. Effects of serotonin (5-HT) on the potassium efflux (^{42}K rate, minute^{-1}) from aortic strips isolated from DOCA hypertensive and control normotensive rats. Aortic strips from hypertensive and normotensive rats were loaded with radioactive potassium. The rate of efflux of radioactive potassium was measured in normal solution in the presence and absence of different concentrations of serotonin (indicated by horizontal bars). The magnitude of the increase in rate of efflux was greater in aortic strips from hypertensive rats at low doses of serotonin. (From Jones et al. (159). Reproduced by permission.)

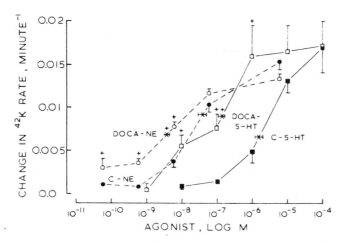

FIG. 11. Dose-response effects of norepinephrine (NE) and serotonin (5-HT) on the potassium efflux (^{42}K rate, minute^{-1}) from aortic strips isolated from DOCA hypertensive and control normotensive rats. ED$_{50}$ values are indicated by X. Responses for DOCA rats which are significantly different from the corresponding control are identified by (+). Values are mean ± SEM. (From Jones *et al.* (159). Reproduced by permission.)

creased membrane permeability, is compensated in the unstimulated state by a larger contribution of the electrogenic pump (Fig. 12).

Similar conclusions regarding increased active ion transport in vascular smooth muscle from hypertensive animals have been made based on the following techniques: (a) potassium-induced relaxation, (b) ion flux measurements, (c) measurement of sodium-potassium adenosine triphosphatase (ATPase) activity, and (d) potentiation of vascular responsiveness following blockade with ouabain. Relaxation in response to potassium is greater in tail arteries isolated from SHR, 1K-1C renal-hypertensive rabbits, and DOCA-hypertensive pigs than in respective arteries from normotensive animals (168–170) (Fig. 13). This potassium-induced relaxation is known to reflect the electrogenic pumping of sodium and potassium

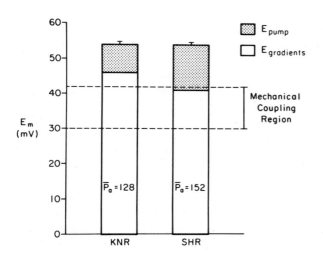

FIG. 12. Electrogenesis of the membrane potential in vascular smooth muscle from spontaneously hypertensive (SHR) and normotensive rats (KNR). The values represent the magnitude of membrane potential of cells in the tail artery; minus signs indicating intracellular negativity have been omitted. The components of the membrane potential contributed by ionic gradients ($E_{gradients}$) and electrogenic ion transport (E_{pump}) mechanisms differed in KNR and SHR. The small ionic gradient in SHR is compensated at normal potassium concentration and in the unstimulated state by a larger contribution of the electrogenic pump. During depolarization, the electrogenic component is inactivated by the increased passive movement of ions through the membrane. The dotted lines indicate the region in which contractile activation occurs. (From Hermsmeyer (75). Reproduced by permission.)

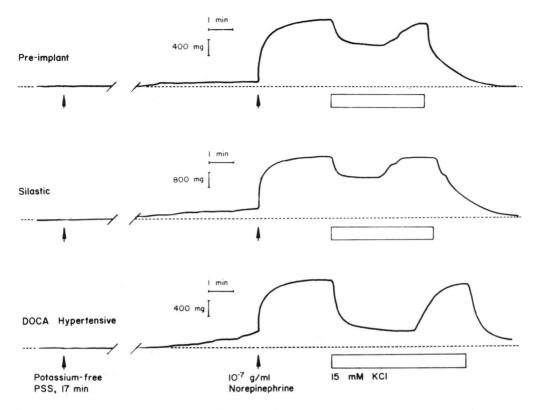

FIG. 13. Potassium-induced relaxation in vascular smooth muscle from DOCA hypertensive pigs. Helical strips of tail arteries from DOCA hypertensive and normotensive pigs (Pre-implant and Silastic) relaxed in response to potassium (15.0 mM) after contraction induced by norepinephrine (10^{-7} g/ml) in potassium-free solution. Tail artery strips from DOCA hypertensive pigs consistently showed greater relaxation in response to potassium than those from normotensive pigs. Following the increase in mechanical response which occurred after several minutes of relaxation, the strips were returned to normal solution (5.0 mM potassium). (From Webb (169). Reproduced by permission.)

by sodium-potassium ATPase (169). Jones et al. (155,157,160,161) have shown that ouabain and potassium-free solution slow the washout of radiolabeled sodium from vascular smooth muscle of DOCA-hypertensive and normotensive rats. The rate constant for sodium washout in both cases was higher for vascular tissues from the hypertensive rats. Friedman et al. (163,164,166,167) have also observed that the active exchange of cellular sodium for potassium is increased in tail arteries of SHR and DOCA-hypertensive rats. Several investigators (172–177) have observed that ouabain-sensitive uptake of radioactive rubidium is greater in vascular smooth muscle of hyper-

tensive animals. The models of hypertension include SHR, DOCA-hypertensive rats, aortic-coarctation-induced hypertensive rats, one-kidney figure-of-eight-ligature hypertensive rats, Dahl salt-sensitive hypertensive rats, 2K-1C renal-hypertensive rats, and 1K-1C renal-hypertensive rats. Allen and Seidel (178) reported that the activity of sodium-potassium ATPase in microsomal fractions from aortas of SHR was increased [28 moles inorganic phosphate (Pi)/mg protein/hr] as compared with that in aortic microsomal fractions of normotensive rats (18 moles Pi/mg protein/hr). Gothberg et al. (179) have shown that ouabain produces a leftward shift in the vascular resistance dose–response curves to norepinephrine in the hindquarters of SHR and normotensive rats. The shift in the curve produced by ouabain was greater in SHR than in normotensive rats. Similar results were obtained when barium and vasopressin were used as the vasoconstrictor agonists. Webb and Bohr (180) observed that calcium-induced relaxation was inhibited to a greater degree by ouabain in tail arteries of SHR than in tail arteries from WKY.

The development of altered membrane electrogenesis in vascular smooth muscle in SHR appears to be due to a trophic influence of the sympathetic nervous system. Abel and Hermsmeyer (76) transplanted tail artery segments from 2-week-old SHR and WKY into innervated and denervated anterior eye chambers of the same or opposite strain. At 7 weeks after surgery the transplants had reinnervated and developed membrane properties of the host strain, interconverting between SHR and WKY characteristics in cross-transplantations. There was no interconversion of membrane-potential properties in cross-transplants of SHR and WKY following sympathetic denervation of the anterior eye chamber by removal of the superior cervical ganglion in the host animal (Fig. 14).

In contrast to these studies, Overbeck et al. (181,182) and Overbeck and Clark (183) have suggested that diminished vasodilator responses to potassium in 1K-1C renal-hypertensive dogs and essential-hypertensive patients may be attributable to depression of the activity of the electrogenic sodium pump. Haddy et al. (184–187) have presented extensive evidence suggesting that ouabain-sensitive uptake of radioactive rubidium is depressed in vascular smooth muscle from animals with several different forms of experimental hypertension. Recent observations by Pamnani et al. (187) provide evidence that these observations of suppressed electrogenic sodium pump activity in vascular tissues of hypertensive animals may be apparent only because of the presence of a humoral factor that inhibits pump activity. These investigators observed that ouabain-sensitive rubidium uptake was depressed in tail artery segments from DOCA-hypertensive rats when the measurements were made on arteries immediately removed from the animals. Interposition of an incubation period of 4.5 hr between the time of re-

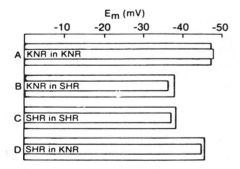 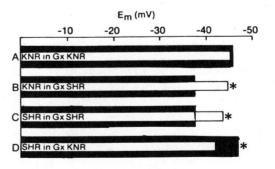

FIG. 14. Membrane properties in tail artery transplants. *Left panel:* Interconversion of membrane properties in reinnervated transplants is shown by membrane potential measurement (E_m) at 16°C. The outer bars represent values in host tail arteries, whereas the inner open bars are values in tail artery transplants. Tail artery transplants showed E_m values characteristic of the host strain whether transplants were from the same or the opposite strain (SHR = spontaneously hypertensive rat; KNR = normotensive rat). *Right panel:* Failure of interconversion by ganglionectomy (Gx) before transplantation is shown by membrane potential measurements at 16°C. Outer dark bars are tail artery hosts and inner light bars are denervated tail artery transplants. In cross-transplants, ganglionectomy prevented the donor-to-host conversion of E_m found in innervated transplants. Asterisks indicate transplants significantly different from host tail arteries. (From Abel and Hermsmeyer (76). Reproduced by permission.)

moval of the artery and the measurement of rubidium uptake revealed increased electrogenic pump activity. These findings suggest the washout of a humoral factor present in the blood of the hypertensive animals that may suppress pump activity. Recent studies (185) suggest that this humoral inhibitor of the electrogenic sodium pump originates in the region of the anteroventral third ventricle of the brain.

The mechanism that provides for an increase in electrogenic pumping of sodium and potassium in vascular smooth muscle in hypertensive animals is unknown. It may be that there are increased numbers of pump sites in the membrane or increased activity of existing sites. A recent study by Hagen et al. (170) suggests that there are similar numbers of membrane sites in aortas of 1K-1C renal-hypertensive rabbits and normotensive rabbits but that the affinity of these sites for ouabain is increased in the former (Fig. 15). Regardless of the precise chemical nature, it is likely that smooth-muscle cells in hypertensive animals depolarize to a greater extent during application of vasoactive agents that alter membrane conductance because the electrogenic component is inactivated by the increased passive movement of ions through the cell membrane (74,75).

Sodium-Calcium Exchange Mechanism

Blaustein (188,189) has presented a hypothesis suggesting that an altered sodium-calcium exchange mechanism may contribute to altered vascular responsiveness in hypertension. The basis for this hypothesis is that the electrochemical gradient for sodium across the cell membrane plays an important role in the regulation of cellular calcium concentration. The stoichiometry of this countertransport system is proposed to be three sodium ions to one calcium ion. Thus, a 10% increase in intracellular sodium would be expected to cause a 33% increase in intracellular calcium. Because increased membrane permeability to

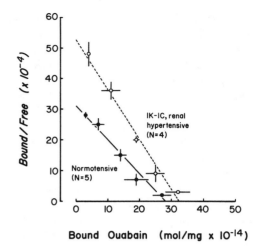

FIG. 15. Ouabain binding in aortae from 1K-1C, renal hypertensive rabbits. Aortic strips from normotensive and 1K-1C, renal hypertensive rabbits were incubated in varying concentrations of tritiated ouabain and the tissue content was determined following an efflux period. As determined by Scatchard analysis, there was no significant difference between aortae from normotensive and hypertensive rabbits in the maximal binding capacity (x-intercept), suggesting that the number of pump sites is similar. The affinity of the binding sites for ouabain (indicated by the slope of the Scothard plot) in aortic strips from hypertensive rabbits was greater than that for strips from normotensive rabbits. (From Hagen et al. (170). Reproduced by permission.)

sodium exists in vascular smooth muscle in hypertensive animals, this mechanism may alter the operating point of the cell. The increase in intracellular calcium may be sufficient to induce contraction or to alter the magnitude of a contractile response induced by a vasoconstrictor agonist.

Although this hypothesis of altered sodium-calcium exchange is attractive, it has been difficult to substantiate because the techniques for determination of intracellular sodium do not allow sufficient accuracy to measure small changes in concentration (i.e., 10% or less). For example, Jones et al. (159–161) reported that the cellular concentrations of sodium are similar in aortic smooth muscle in normotensive and hypertensive rats (11–12 mmoles/liter cell water).

Agonist–Receptor Interactions in Hypertension

Altered sensitivity to vasoactive drugs in hypertension could derive from changes in the binding of the agonist to receptor sites on the vascular smooth-muscle cell membrane. Relatively few studies have been performed that characterize membrane receptors on vascular tissue from hypertensive animals. Additionally, the new classifications of adrenergic (α_1 and α_2) and serotonergic (5HT-1 and 5HT-2) receptors have not been adequately tested to arrive at a clear understanding of receptor interactions in the hypertensive state. The following paragraphs summarize the experimental observations suggesting that agonist–receptor interactions may be altered in hypertension.

α-Adrenergic Receptors

Strecker et al. (190) and Clineschmidt et al. (191) determined the affinity of α-adrenergic receptors for norepinephrine in aortic strips from SHR and normotensive rats. Dissociation constants for phenoxybenzamine and phentolamine reacting with α-adrenergic receptors in the aortas of SHR were similar to values determined for aortas from normotensive rats. Thus, it was concluded that the α-adrenergic receptors mediating aortic contraction were similar in SHR and normotensive rats. Strecker et al. (190) also observed that antihypertensive therapy (hydralazine, chlorothiazide, reserpine) did not alter the affinity of α-adrenergic receptors in either SHR or normotensive rats. In temporal arteries from essential-hypertensive and normotensive humans, the α-adrenergic receptors were also shown not to be different, based on the similarity of vascular responsiveness to phenylephrine before and after blockade of the receptors with phentolamine (192). More recently, Johnson and Webb (193) observed that tail artery strips from SHR were more sensitive to clonidine (an α_2 agonist) than were those

from WKY (Fig. 16). Yohimbine was a competitive antagonist against clonidine. The competitive antagonistic properties of yohimbine (determined by Schild plot) were more pronounced in tail artery strips from SHR than in those from WKY. These results demonstrate that the sensitivity of α_2-adrenergic receptors to clonidine is greater in tail arteries from SHR and that the affinity of the receptors for yohimbine is greater in SHR.

β-Adrenergic Receptors

The function of β-adrenergic receptors has been shown to be either increased or decreased in experimental hypertension. Aortic smooth muscle from renal-hypertensive rats shows reduced relaxation following treatment with isoproterenol, as compared with that from normotensive rats (194). Activation of β-adrenergic receptors in SHR aortas results in either a greater (195) or lesser (194,196,197) response as compared with controls. Deragon et al. (198) observed increased responsiveness to β-adrenergic stimulation in perfused hindlimbs of SHR. Woodcock et al. (199) observed reduced numbers of β-adrenergic receptors in membranes isolated from mesenteric arteries of DOCA-hypertensive rats, as compared with those isolated from mesenteric arteries of normotensive rats. The affinities of the receptors for various β-adrenergic agonists were unchanged in membranes from hypertensive mesenteric arteries. Limas and Limas (200) reported reduced concentrations of β-adrenergic receptors in aortas and inferior venae cavae of SHR as compared with those in similar vessels of normotensive rats.

Serotonergic Receptors

Recent studies (82,84,92,201) suggest that the receptors that mediate constrictor responses to serotonin may be altered in hypertension. In addition to the increased sensitivity to this agonist (*vide supra*), vascular preparations from SHR exhibit delayed tachyphylaxis

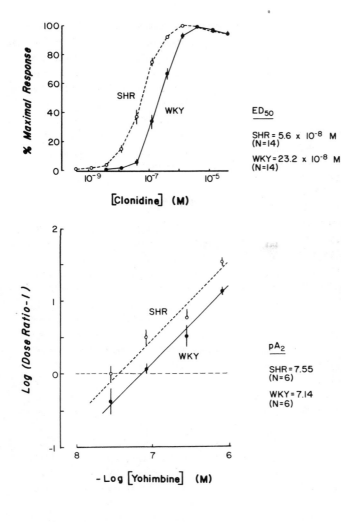

FIG. 16. Vascular responses to clonidine in spontaneously hypertensive rats. *Top panel:* Dose-response to clonidine. Tail artery strips from SHR and WKY were made to contract in response to the cumulative addition of clonidine to the muscle bath. Tail arteries from SHR were more sensitive to clonidine than those from WKY as indicated by the reduced ED_{50} value. *Bottom panel:* Schild plot for yohimbine antagonism of vascular reponses to clonidine. The competitive antagonistic properties were more pronounced in tail artery strips from SHR than in those from WKY. Values are the mean ± SEM. (From Johnson and Webb, *unpublished observations.*)

to serotonin as compared with that in normotensive rats (92,202,208). Ketanserin, a 5HT-2 receptor antagonist, causes dose-related reductions in arterial blood pressure in SHR (105,201) and in essential-hypertensive patients (201,204). This blood-pressure-lowering effect of ketanserin does not appear to be due to inhibition of α_2-adrenergic receptors (105,201), although a recent study by Kaulkman et al. (209) suggests that a portion of the antihypertensive action may be the result of blockade of α_1-adrenergic receptors. Higher doses of the antagonist are required to achieve smaller reductions in aortic pressure in nor-

motensive animals and subjects. Isolated vascular-strip preparations from SHR and DOCA-hypertensive rats were more sensitive to the partial agonistic properties of methysergide than were those from normotensive rats (82,84). Aortic strips from DOCA-hypertensive rats showed the greatest change in sensitivity to methysergide, whereas tail arteries from these animals showed the least change in sensitivity; mesenteric arteries were intermediate in terms of change in sensitivity. The agonistic action of methysergide in DOCA-hypertensive rats paralleled the development of high arterial pressure, and a low-sodium diet abated the high pressure in DOCA-treated rats and reduced vascular sensitivity to methysergide.

Relaxation System

Relaxation or vasodilation is an active response of the vasculature. Thus, it has been proposed that the elevated vascular resistance characteristic of hypertension results from abnormalities in the cellular processes causing vasodilation. The experimental evidence documenting diminished vasodilation is not convincing, whereas several investigators have observed abnormalities in the subcellular membrane systems that may decrease the intracellular concentration of activator calcium.

Diminished Vasodilation

Aortic-strip preparations from SHR and renal-hypertensive rats do not relax to a variety of vasodilators as well as do those from normotensive vessels (Table 1). These observations have been supported by experimental data from several investigators using a variety of vascular preparations. However, several studies have shown no difference in the ability of vascular preparations from hypertensive animals to relax as compared with their respective controls. Indeed, some vascular preparations from hypertensive animals are more sensitive to isoproterenol, nitroprusside, and acetylcholine than are their normotensive controls.

Decreased Subcellular Uptake of Calcium

Several investigators (138,152,153,219–230) have observed that microsomal and plasma membrane fractions of vascular smooth muscle from hypertensive animals show reduced calcium-accumulating ability as compared with those from normotensive control animals. Kwan et al. (229) have shown that reduced ATP-dependent calcium uptake by plasma membrane fractions precedes the de-velopment of hypertension in SHR, and the impaired uptake process is reversed in DOCA-treated rats on withdrawal of the mineralocorticoid. Impaired uptake of activator calcium by these membrane fractions may affect the relaxation process in hypertensive blood vessels.

Cyclic Nucleotides and Related Enzymes

It is likely that cyclic nucleotides serve as second messengers in various biochemical events in vascular smooth muscle. Consequently, several investigators have suggested that abnormalities in vascular cyclic nucleotides may contribute to altered vascular responsiveness in hypertension. Four major hypotheses have been generated: (a) increased ratio of cyclic GMP/cyclic AMP; (b) decreased basal adenylate cyclase; (c) reduced stimulation of adenylate cyclase; (d) altered cyclic-AMP-dependent protein kinase activity.

Increased Ratio of Cyclic GMP/Cyclic AMP

Amer et al. (231–237) presented extensive evidence suggesting that the ratio of cyclic GMP/cyclic AMP reflects the tone of vascular smooth muscle. They observed that this ratio was elevated in vascular preparations from animals with several different forms of experimental hypertension: SHR, DOCA-hypertensive rats, and rats with stress-induced hypertension and neurogenic-induced hypertension. In each model of hypertension, alterations in adenylate and guanylate cyclases and cyclic AMP and cyclic GMP phosphodiesterases were associated with the altered cyclic nucleotide levels.

Decreased Basal Adenylate Cyclase

Studies by Ramanathan and Shibata (238) suggested that unstimulated levels of adenylate cyclase are lower in aortas from SHR than in normotensive controls. Adenylate cy-

TABLE 1. *Vasodilators in hypertension*

Reference	Preparation	Agonist	Results (compared with controls)
Shibata and Cheng (205)	Thoracic aortic strips (SHR)	Isoproterenol, acetylcholine, Mg^{++}, Mn^{++}	Decreased % relaxation
	Thoracic aortic strips (renal hypertensive rats)	Isoproterenol	Decreased % relaxation
Cohen and Berkowitz (194)	Thoracic aortic strips (SHR and renal hypertensive rats)	cAMP, cGMP, isoproterenol, nitroglycerin, adenosine	Decreased % relaxation
Antonaccio et al. (206)	Aortic strips (SHR)	Nitroglycerin	Decreased % relaxation
Triner et al. (196)	Thoracic aortic strips (SHR)	Isoproterenol	Decreased % relaxation
Hutchins et al. (207)	Cremaster microvessels (SHR)	Isoproterenol	Decreased max. % diameter increase
Bell et al. (66)	Blood-perfused hindlimb (aortic coarctation rats)	Nitroprusside	Impaired maximal vasodilation
Godfraind and Dieu (197)	Thoracic aortic ring (SHR)	Isoproterenol	Decreased relaxation
Hamed and Lokhandwala (208)	Blood-perfused hindlimb (DOCA hypertensive dog)	Acetylcholine, histamine	Impaired vasodilation
Katovich et al. (209)	Tail skin temperature (renal encapsulation-hypertensive rats)	Isoproterenol	Impaired vasodilation
Shibata and Cheng (205)	Thoracic aortic strip (SHR)	Nitroglycerin, papaverine	No difference in % relaxation
	Abdominal aortic strip (SHR)	Isoproterenol, acetylcholine, Mg^{++}, Mn^{++}, nitroglycerin, papaverine	No difference in % relaxation
	Abdominal aortic strip (renal hypertensive rats)	Isoproterenol	No difference in % relaxation
Deragon et al. (198)	Krebs-perfused hindlimb (SHR)	Nitroprusside	No difference in sensitivity

Reference	Vasodilator	Result
Fink and Brody (210–212)	Blood-perfused renal vasculature (Dahl-salt sensitive rats)	Acetylcholine	No difference in max. vasodilation
	Blood-perfused renal vasculature (SHR)	Acetylcholine	No difference in sensitivity
	Blood-perfused renal vasculature (one kidney, figure-of-eight hypertensive rats and two kidney, figure-of-eight hypertensive rats)	Acetylcholine	No difference in sensitivity or max. vasodilation
Castro-Tavares (213)	Saphenous vein strips (perinephretic hypertensive dog)	Nitroprusside isoproterenol	No difference in sensitivity or % relaxation
Folkow et al. (25)	Forearm resistance vessels (human essential hypertension)	Vasodilator metabolites	No difference in ability to relax
Brody et al. (214)	Blood-perfused hindlimb (1K-1C, renal hypertensive dog)	Histamine, nitroglycerin	No difference in vasodilation
Kamikawa et al. (215)	Krebs-perfused mesenteric bed (SHR)	Adenosine, ATP	No difference in vasodilation
Dadkar et al. (216)	Krebs-perfused mesenteric bed (DOCA hypertensive rats, 2K-1C, renal hypertensive rats)	Isoproterenol, papaverine, adenosine	No difference in vasodilation
Spector et al. (195)	Thoracic aortic strips (SHR)	Isoproterenol	Increased % relaxation
Deragon et al. (198)	Krebs-perfused hindlimb (SHR)	Isoproterenol	Increased sensitivity
Hutchins et al. (207)	Cremaster microvessels (SHR)	Isoproterenol	Decreased threshold dose
Hollenberg et al. (217)	Intact renal vascular bed (human essential hypertension)	Acetylcholine	Increased sensitivity
Cohen et al. (81)	Blood-perfused renal vasculature (DOCA hypertensive rat)	Nitroprusside	Increased sensitivity
	Tail artery strip (DOCA hypertensive rat)	Nitroprusside	Increased % relaxation
Dadkar et al. (216)	Krebs-perfused mesenteric bed (SHR)	Isoproterenol, papaverine, adenosine	Increased % relaxation
Castro-Tavares (213)	Mesenteric artery (perinephretic hypertensive dog)	Nitroprusside, isoproterenol	Increased sensitivity and increased % relaxation

Modified from Cohen et al. (81). By permission.

clase activity was stimulated to similar levels as in controls by epinephrine, glucagon, and sodium flouride. Basal cyclic AMP levels were reduced in SHR.

Reduced Stimulation of Adenylate Cyclase

Several investigators (196,239) observed that the basal levels of cyclic AMP in aortas of SHR did not differ from those in normotensive controls. Treatment with isoproterenol resulted in increased cyclic AMP formation, and higher doses of isoproterenol were required to produce the same level of nucleotide formation in SHR aortas as in controls. Adenylate cyclase activity in blood vessels of SHR was higher than that in controls following treatment with sodium fluoride. These studies have been interpreted to indicate that higher adenylate cyclase activity following sodium fluoride stimulation reflects a compensatory mechanism for the deficiency of the enzyme to respond to β-adrenergic stimulation.

Altered Cyclic-AMP-Dependent Protein Kinase Activity

Cyclic-AMP-induced phosphorylation of microsomal membranes and cyclic-AMP-dependent protein kinase activity in vascular smooth muscle in SHR are reduced as compared with those in normotensive controls (138,220,240). Additionally, Bhalla et al. (138,220) observed an increase in phosphoprotein phosphatase activity in the soluble fraction of vascular smooth muscle of SHR. Calcium uptake by the microsomal fractions from SHR was reduced as compared with that in microsomes from normotensive rats. These investigators suggested that alterations in the phosphorylation–dephosphorylation reaction may account for reduced calcium uptake in membrane fractions from vascular tissues of SHR. This change in membrane function appears to be specific to the arterial side of the circulation, and the change precedes the development of hypertension (138,220).

Prostaglandin Metabolism

Prostaglandins and related compounds (endoperoxides, thromboxanes) are synthesized in the vascular wall, and it has been proposed that these agents participate in the regulation of contractile events in vascular smooth muscle (241–243). In addition to having direct actions on the vasculature, various prostaglandins are synthesized in response to vasoconstrictor hormones (angiotensin II and norepinephrine) that may serve to attenuate or augment the response of the vasculature. To date, there is no general agreement as to the role of prostaglandins in hypertension. The following paragraphs review some recent evidence demonstrating the variability of experimental findings concerning the synthesis of prostaglandins and the responsiveness of the vasculature to these agents in the hypertensive state.

Vascular Responses to Prostaglandins and Arachidonate

In general, constrictor responses to various prostaglandins are augmented in the vasculature in hypertensive animals (85,101,244,245), whereas vasodilator responses to arachidonate, prostaglandin E_2, and prostacyclin can be unchanged, increased, or decreased in the vasculature in hypertensive animals (246–249). The results of different studies are highly variable. For example, Dusting et al. (246,247) reported that depressor effects of arachidonic acid were greater and more prolonged in SHR than in WKY. Lukacsko et al. (248) observed that intraarterial injections of arachidonic acid caused dose-dependent decreases in mean arterial pressure in SHR and WKY; the hypotensive response in SHR was less at low doses of the prostaglandin precursor, whereas decreases in blood pressure at high doses did not differ between SHR and WKY. Laborit and Valette (249) observed that administration of arachidonic acid to DOCA-hypertensive rats increased blood pressure by 25 to 37%.

Lockette et al. (250) reported that sodium arachidonate (1 mg/ml) produced contraction in isolated aortic strips from DOCA-hypertensive rats (approximately 50% of the maximum response to norepinephrine), but not in aortic strips from normotensive rats.

Blood Pressure and Cyclooxygenase Blockade

If altered prostaglandin production plays a role in hypertension, chronic blockade of cyclooxygenase should alter blood pressure. Consequently, numerous investigators have attempted to produce changes in pressor mechanisms by administration of cyclooxygenase inhibitors. Again, the results from different studies are highly variable. Colina-Chourio et al. (251) observed that daily administration of indomethacin elevated the mean arterial blood pressure in rabbits by approximately 15 mm Hg. Administration of indomethacin to normal subjects and to patients with idiopathic hypotension causes blood pressure to rise significantly (252,253). In anesthetized dogs, indomethacin causes a marked increase in vascular resistance in the kidney and a smaller increase in limb vascular

resistance (254). Cyclooxygenase blockade has been reported to aggravate hypertension in humans (255,256), SHR (257,258), DOCA-hypertensive rats (259), and 1K-1C renal-hypertensive rats (260). Romero and Strong (261) observed that the blood pressure response to indomethacin depended on the level of renal function in 2K-1C and 1K-1C renal-hypertensive rabbits. In hypertensive rabbits with severe impairment of renal circulation, administration of indomethacin caused renal insufficiency and elevated blood pressure associated with either volume expansion or increased plasma renin activity. Cyclooxygenase blockade has also been shown to lower blood pressure in dogs (262) and rats with renal hypertension and in rats with DOCA hypertension (264).

Prostaglandin Synthesis

Most investigators have observed increased production of prostacyclin in isolated arterial smooth muscle from hypertensive animals (265–268). This increased production of prostacyclin appears to be associated with increased cyclooxygenase activity. Skidgel and

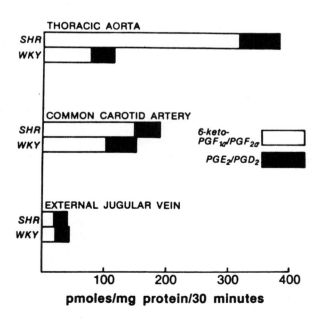

FIG. 17. Cyclooxygenase activity in blood vessels from SHR and WKY. Cyclooxygenase activity was determined by incubating vessel hemogenates (250 mg) with $[1-^{14}C]$-arachidonic acid for 30 min at 24°C in the absence of added cofactors. (From Skidgel and Printz (266). Reproduced by permission.)

Printz (266) observed that conversions of prostaglandin H_2 to 6-keto prostaglandin $F_1\alpha$ were similar in arteries and veins from SHR and WKY. In contrast, cyclooxygenase activity was increased in aortas and carotid arteries from SHR as compared with those from WKY, whereas no difference was observed in the external jugular vein (Fig. 17). These investigators concluded that enhanced cyclooxygenase activity is responsible for increased production of prostacyclin in SHR, because prostacyclin synthetase activity was the same in vessels from SHR and WKY.

SUMMARY

This chapter has focused on the assessment of vascular changes that contribute to increased total peripheral resistance in hypertension (Fig. 18). Structural changes (increased media thickness and microvessel rarefaction) in the vasculature clearly contribute to elevated vascular resistance in hypertension. Most experimental evidence suggests that these structural changes are adaptive processes in response to increased wall stress. Recent studies suggest that humoral and neural influences may contribute to morphological alterations in the vasculature in hypertensive animals.

Studies evaluating functional changes in vascular smooth muscle in hypertension have been carried out in many laboratories. Although the results of these studies are more variable than those documenting structural adaptations, it seems that increased sensitivity to vasoconstrictor stimuli characterizes the hypertensive process. This increased vascular sensitivity precedes or parallels the development of high blood pressure, and it occurs in the absence of elevated wall stress. Increased sensitivity to some agonists (e.g., serotonin and methysergide) is augmented to a greater degree than that to other agonists. The variability in responsiveness of the vasculature to vasodilator agents suggests that impaired relaxation is not an important functional change in hypertension.

The increased sensitivity of vascular smooth muscle in hypertension is probably due to changes in one or more of the following cellular processes: (a) cell membrane permeability, (b) agonist–receptor interactions, (c) subcellular membranes regulating intracellular calcium, (d) cyclic nucleotides and related enzymes, and (e) prostaglandin metabolism. The

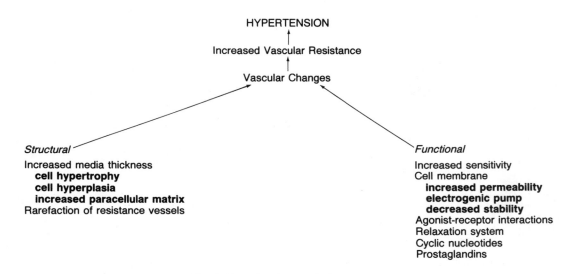

FIG. 18. Vascular changes in hypertension.

fact that these cellular processes are interrelated complicates our effort to understand the functional changes in the vasculature in hypertensive animals and humans. For example, certain prostaglandins elevate the levels of cyclic nucleotides in vascular smooth muscle, presumably through stimulation of the appropriate cyclase. The cyclic nucleotides participate in the regulation of intracellular calcium concentration through phosphorylation–dephosphorylation reactions at membrane sites. Calcium ions are known to alter the activity of enzymes controlling cyclic nucleotide synthesis and degradation and to alter membrane permeability to monovalent ions through a stabilizing influence. Membrane permeability to monovalent ions affects cellular electrogenesis, and the activities of several enzymes depend on a high intracellular concentration of potassium. Based on the experimental evidence, it appears that the cell membrane is the cellular component that is most likely responsible for changes in vascular sensitivity in hypertension. This membrane abnormality is the product of impaired function of one or more of the controlling systems that normally regulate vascular resistance.

ACKNOWLEDGMENTS

This work was supported by grants from the Michigan Heart Association and the National Institutes of Health (HL-27020 and HL-18575). Dr. Webb is a recipient of a Research Career Development Award from the National Institutes of Health (HL-00813).

REFERENCES

1. Hypertension Task Force (1979): *Report of the Hypertension Task Force, Vols. 1–9.* NIH publication no. 79–1623. Department of Health, Education, and Welfare, U.S. Public Health Service, National Institutes of Health.
2. Bohr, D. F. (1981): What makes the pressure go up? A hypothesis. *Hypertension [Suppl. II]*, 3:160–165.
3. Genest, J., Kouiw, E., and Kuchel, D. (editors) (1977): *Hypertension, Physiology and Treatment.* McGraw-Hill, New York.
4. Laragh, J. H. (editor) (1975): *Hypertension Mechanisms.* Yorke Medical Books, New York.
5. Sokabe, H. (1979): Proceedings of the third international symposium on the spontaneously hypertensive rat and related studies. *Jpn. Heart J. [Suppl. I]*, 20:1–373.
6. Bevan, J. A., Godfraind, T., Maxwell, R. A., and Vanhoutte, P. M. (editors) (1980): *Vascular Neuroeffector Mechanisms.* Raven Press, New York.
7. Davis, J. O., Laragh, J. H., and Selwyn, A. (editors) (1977): *Hypertension: Mechanisms, Diagnosis and Management.* HP Publishing, New York.
8. Yamori, Y., Lovenberg, W., and Freis, E. D. (editors) (1979): *Prophylactic Approach to Hypertensive Diseases.* Raven Press, New York.
9. Abboud, F. M. (1982): The sympathetic system in hypertension. *Hypertension [Suppl. II]*, 4:208–225.
10. DeQuattro, V., Campese, V., and Antonaccio, M. J. (1977): Hypertension: Etiology, pathology and control. In: *Cardiovascular Pharmacology,* edited by M. Antonaccio, pp. 185–268. Raven Press, New York.
11. Folkow, B. (1982): Physiological aspects of primary hypertension. *Physiol. Rev.,* 62:347–428.
12. Rojo-Ortega, J. M., and Hatt, P.-V. (1977): Histopathology of cardiovascular lesions in hypertension. In: *Hypertension, Physiology and Treatment,* edited by J. Genest, E. Kouiw and D. Kuchel, pp. 910–944. McGraw-Hill, New York.
13. Hepinstall, R. H. (1974): *Pathology of the Kidney,* pp. 150–155. Little, Brown, Boston.
14. Berecek, K. H., and Bohr, D. F. (1977): Structural and functional changes in vascular resistance and reactivity in the deoxycorticosterone acetate (DOCA)-hypertensive pig. *Circ. Res., [Suppl. I],* 40:146–152.
15. Conway, J. (1963): A vascular abnormality in hypertension—a study of blood flow in the forearm. *Circulation,* 27:520–529.
16. Sivertsson, R. (1970): Hemodynamic importance of structural vascular changes in essential hypertension. *Acta Physiol. Scand. [Suppl. 343],* 79:1–56.
17. Weiss, L. (1974): Aspects of the relation between functional and structural cardiovascular factors in primary hypertension. *Acta Physiol. Scand. [Suppl. 409],* 83:1–58.
18. Angus, J. A., West, M. J., and Korner, P. I. (1976): Assessment of autonomic and non-autonomic components of resting hindlimb vascular resistance and reactivity to pressor substances in renal hypertensive rabbits. *Clin. Sci. Mol. Med.,* 51:57s–59s.
19. Folkow, B., Gothberg, G., Lundin, S., and Rickstein, S. E. (1977): Structural resetting of the renal vascular bed in spontaneously hypertensive rats (SHR). *Acta Physiol. Scand.,* 100:270–272.
20. Hartling, O., Svendsen, T. L., Nielson, P. E., and Trap-Jensen, J. (1978): The distensibility of resistance vessels of skeletal muscle in hypertensive patients. *Acta Physiol. Scand.,* 103:430–436.
21. Amery, A., Bossaert, H., and Verstraete, M. (1969): Muscle blood flows in normal and hypertensive subjects. Influence of age, exercise and body position. *Am. Heart J.,* 78:211–216.
22. Folkow, B. (1978): Cardiovascular structural adap-

tation: Its role in the initiation and maintenance of hypertension. *Clin. Sci. Mol. Med.,* 55:3s–22s.

23. Lundgren, Y., Hallback, M., Weiss, L., and Folkow, B. (1974): Rate and extent of adaptive cardiovascular changes in rats during experimental renal hypertension. *Acta Physiol. Scand.,* 91:103–115.

24. Folkow, B., Hallback, M., Lundgren, Y., Sivertsson, R., and Weiss, L. (1972): The importance of adaptive changes in vascular design for the establishment and maintenance of primary hypertension as studied in man and in the spontaneously hypertensive rat. In: *Spontaneous Hypertension. Its Pathogenesis and Complications,* edited by K. Okamoto, et al. pp. 103–104. Springer-Verlag, New York.

25. Folkow, B., Gimby, G., and Thulesius, O. (1958): Adaptive structural changes of the vascular walls in hypertension and their relation to the control of the peripheral resistance. *Acta Physiol. Scand.,* 44:255–272.

26. Folkow, B., Hallback, M., Lundgren, Y., and Weiss, L. (1970): Background of increased flow resistance and vascular reactivity in spontaneously hypertensive rats. *Acta Physiol. Scand.,* 80:93–106.

27. Friedman, S. M., Nakashima, M., and Mar, M. A. (1971): Morphological assessment of vasoconstriction and vascular hypertrophy in sustained hypertension in the rat. *Microvasc. Res.,* 3:416–425.

28. Mallov, S. (1965): Effect of hypertension and sodium chloride on the reactivity of rat aortic strips in vitro. In: *Electrolytes and Cardiovascular Diseases,* edited by E. Bajusz, pp. 356–362. S. Karger, Basel.

29. Wolinsky, H., Goldfischer, S., Schiller, B., and Kasak, L. E. (1974): Modification of the effects of hypertension on lysosomes and connective tissue in the rat aorta. *Circ. Res.,* 35:233–241.

30. Greenberg, S., Gaines, K., and Sweatt, D. (1981): Evidence for circulating factors as a cause of venous hypertrophy in spontaneously hypertensive rats. *Am. J. Physiol.,* 241:H421–H430.

31. Azevedo, I., Castro-Tavares, J., and Garrett, J. (1981): Ultrastructural changes in blood vessels of perinephritic hypertensive dogs. *Blood Vessels,* 18:110–119.

32. Crane, W. A. J., and Dutta, L. P. (1963): The utilization of tritiated thymidine for deoxyribonucleic acid synthesis by the lesions of experimental hypertension in rats. *J. Pathol. Bacteriol.,* 86:83–97.

33. Crane, W. A. J., and Ingle, D. J. (1964): Tritiated thymidine uptake in rat hypertension. *Arch. Pathol.,* 78:209–216.

34. Foidart, J. M., Rorive, G. L., Nusgens, B. V., Corlier, P. J., and Lapiere, C. M. (1979): Early biochemical changes in the arterial wall of renal hypertensive rats. In: *Prophylactic Approach to Hypertensive Diseases,* edited by Y. Yamori, pp. 241–248. Raven Press, New York.

35. Rorive, G. L., Carlier, P. J., and Foidart, J. M. (1980): Hyperplasia of rat arteries smooth muscle cells associated with development and reversal of renal hypertension. *Clin. Sci.,* 59:335s–338s.

36. Fernandez, D., and Crane, W. A. J. (1970): New cell formation in rats with accelerated hypertension due to partial aortic constriction. *J. Pathol. Bacteriol.,* 100:307–315.

37. Bevan, R. D. (1976): An autoradiographic and pathological study of cellular proliferation in rabbit arteries correlated with an increase in arterial pressure. *Blood Vessels,* 13:100–128.

38. Bevan, R. D., Eggena, P., Hume, W. R., Morthens, E. V., and Bevan, J. A. (1980): Transient and persistent changes in rabbit blood vessels associated with maintained elevation in arterial pressure. *Hypertension,* 2:63–72.

39. Aikawa, M., and Koletsky, S. (1970): Arteriosclerosis of the mesenteric arteries of rats with renal hypertension. *Am. J. Pathol.,* 61:293–322.

40. Mulvany, M. J., Hansen, P. K., and Aalkjaer, C. (1978): Direct evidence that the greater contractility of resistance vessels in spontaneously hypertensive rats is associated with a narrow lumen, a thickened media, and an increased number of smooth muscle cell layers. *Circ. Res.,* 43:854–864.

41. Warshaw, D. M., Mulvany, M. J., and Halpern, W. (1979): Mechanical and morphological properties of arterial resistance vessels in young and old spontaneously hypertensive rats. *Circ. Res.,* 45:280–289.

42. Henrichs, K. J., Unger, T., Berecek, K. H., and Ganten, D. (1980): Is arterial media hypertrophy in spontaneously hypertensive rats a consequence or a cause for hypertension? *Clin. Sci.,* 59:331s–333s.

43. Palaty, V., Gustafson, B., and Friedman, S. M. (1969): Sodium binding in the arterial wall. *Can. J. Physiol. Pharmacol.,* 47:763–770.

44. Crane, W. A. J. (1962): Sites of mucopolysaccharide synthesis in the lesions of experimental hypertension in rats. *J. Pathol. Bacteriol.,* 83:183–193.

45. Crane, W. A. J. (1962): Sulfated utilization and mucopolysaccharide synthesis by the mesenteric arteries of rats with experimental hypertension. *J. Pathol. Bacteriol.,* 84:113–122.

46. Tobian, L., Olson, R., and Chesley, G. (1969): Water content of arteriolar wall in renovascular hypertension. *Am. J. Physiol.,* 216:22–24.

47. Tobian, L., and White, L. (1956): The electrolytes of arterial wall in experimental renal hypertension. *Circ. Res.,* 4:671–675.

48. Tobian, L., and Binion, J. T. (1952): Tissue cations and water in arterial hypertension. *Circulation,* 5:754–758.

49. Tobian, L., Janecek, J., Tomboulian, A., and Ferreira, D. (1961): Sodium and potassium in the walls of arterioles in experimental renal hypertension. *J. Clin. Invest.,* 40:1922–1925.

50. Hutchins, P. M., and Darnell, A. E. (1974): Observation of a decreased number of small arterioles in spontaneously hypertensive rats. *Circ. Res. [Suppl. I],* 34–35:164–165.

51. Henrich, H., Hertel, R., and Assmann, R. (1978): Structural differences in the mesentery microcirculation between the normotensives and SHR's. *Pfluegers Arch.,* 375:153–159.

52. Haack, D. W., Schaffer, J. J., and Simpson, J. G. (1979): Microvascular patterns in the skins of spontaneously hypertensive rats, normotensive Wistar-Kyoto rats and normal Wistar rats. *Proc. Soc. Exp. Biol. Med.,* 164:453–458.

53. Henrich, H., and Hertel, R. (1979): Hemodynamics

and "rarefication" of the microvasculature in spontaneously hypertensive rats. *Bibl. Anat.,* 18:184–186.

54. Harper, R. N., Moore, M. A., Morr, M. C., Watts, L. E., and Hutchins, P. M. (1979): Arteriolar rarefaction in the conjunctiva of human essential hypertensives. *Microvasc. Res.,* 16:369–372.

55. Dusseau, J. W., and Hutchins, P. M. (1979): Stimulation of arterial number by salbutamol in spontaneously hypertensive rats. *Am. J. Physiol.,* 236:H134–H140.

56. Webb, D. R. (1982): Analysis of cerebral arterial vasculature in the DOCA/NaCl hypertensive rat. Doctoral dissertation, Department of Anatomy, University of Michigan.

57. Chen, I. I. H., Prewitt, R. L., and Dowell, R. F. (1981): Microvascular rarefaction in spontaneously hypertensive rat cremaster muscle. *Am. J. Physiol.,* 241:H306–H310.

58. Hallback, M., Gothberg, G., Lundin, S., Rickstein, S. E., and Folkow, B. (1976): Hemodynamic consequences of resistance vessel rarefaction and of changes in the smooth muscle sensitivity. *Acta Physiol. Scand.,* 97:233–240.

59. Folkow, B., Gurevich, M., Hallback, M., Lundgren, Y., and Weiss, L. (1971): The hemodynamic consequences of regional hypotension in spontaneously hypertensive and normotensive rats. *Acta Physiol. Scand.,* 83:532–541.

60. Hutchins, P. M. (1979): Arteriolar rarefaction in hypertension. *Bibl. Anat.,* 18:166–168.

61. Pamnani, M. B., and Overbeck, H. W. (1976): Abnormal ion and water composition of veins and normotensive arteries in coarctation hypertension in rats. *Circ. Res.,* 38:375–378.

62. Mueller, S. M., and Heistad, D. D. (1980): Effect of chronic hypertension on the blood brain barrier. *Hypertension,* 2:809–812.

63. Johansson, B. (1974): Blood brain barrier dysfunction in acute arterial hypertension after papaverine induced vasodilation. *Acta Neurol. Scand.,* 50:573–580.

64. Nordborg, C., and Johansson, B. B. (1979): The ratio between thickness of media and internal radius in cerebral, mesenteric and renal arterial vessels in spontaneously hypertensive rats. *Clin. Sci.,* 57:27s–29s.

65. Hart, M. N., Heisted, D. D., and Brody, M. J. (1980): Effect of chronic hypertension and sympathetic denervation on wall/lumen ratio of cerebral vessels. *Hypertension,* 2:419–423.

66. Bell, D. R., and Overbeck, H. W. (1979): Increased resistance and impaired maximal vasodilation in normotensive vascular beds of rats with coarctation hypertension. *Hypertension,* 1:78–85.

67. Nilsson, H., and Folkow, B. (1980): Structurally reduced compliance of the venous capacitance vessels in spontaneously hypertensive rats. *Acta Physiol. Scand.,* 110:215–217.

68. Greenberg, S., Palmer, E. C., and Wilborn, W. M. (1978): Pressure-independent hypertrophy of veins and pulmonary arteries of spontaneously hypertensive rats. *Clin. Sci. Mol. Med.,* 55:31s–36s.

69. Mulvany, M. J., Ljung, B., Stoltze, M., and Kjellstedt, A. (1980): Contractile and morphological

properties of the portal vein in spontaneously hypertensive and Wistar-Kyoto rats. *Blood Vessels,* 17:202–215.

70. Simon, G. (1978): Venous changes in renal hypertensive rats: The role of humoral factors. *Blood Vessels,* 15:311–321.

71. Greenberg, S. (1980): Venous function in hypertension. *Trends Pharmaceut. Sci.,* 1:121–125.

72. Greenberg, S., and Bohr, D. F. (1975): Venous smooth muscle in hypertension. Enhanced contractility of portal veins from spontaneously hypertensive rats. *Circ. Res. [Suppl. I],* 36–37:208–215.

73. Webb, R. C., Vanhoutte, P. M., and Bohr, D. F. (1981): Adrenergic neurotransmission in vascular smooth muscle from spontaneously hypertensive rats. *Hypertension,* 3:93–103.

74. Hermsmeyer, K. (1976): Electrogenesis of increased norepinephrine sensitivity of arterial vascular muscle in hypertension. *Circ. Res.,* 38:362–367.

75. Hermsmeyer, K. (1976): Cellular basis for increased sensitivity of vascular smooth muscle in spontaneously hypertensive rats. *Circ. Res. [Suppl. I],* 38:53–57.

76. Abel, P. W., and Hermsmeyer, K. (1981): Sympathetic cross-innervation of SHR and genetic controls suggests a trophic influence on vascular muscle membranes. *Circ. Res.,* 49:1311–1318.

77. Mulvany, M. J., Aalkjaer, C., and Christensen, J. (1980): Changes in noradrenaline sensitivity and morphology of arterial resistance vessels during development of high blood pressure in spontaneously hypertensive rats. *Hypertension,* 2:664–671.

78. Whall, C. W., Myers, M. M., and Halpern, W. (1980): Norepinephrine sensitivity, tension development and neuronal uptake in resistance arteries from spontaneously hypertensive and normotensive rats. *Blood Vessels,* 17:1–15.

79. Webb, R. C., and Vanhoutte, P. M. (1979): Sensitivity to noradrenaline in isolated tail arteries from spontaneously hypertensive rats. *Clin. Sci.,* 57:31s–33s.

80. Webb, R. C., and Vanhoutte, P. M. (1982): Cocaine and contractile responses of vascular smooth muscle from spontaneously hypertensive rats. *Arch. Int. Pharmacodyn. Ther.,* 253:241–256.

81. Cohen, D. M., Webb, R. C., and Bohr, D. F. (1982): Nitroprusside induced vascular relaxation in DOCA hypertensive rats. *Hypertension,* 4:13–19.

82. Webb, R. C. (1982): Increased vascular sensitivity to serotonin and methysergide in hypertension in rats. *Clin. Sci.,* 63:73–75.

83. Moreland, R. S., Webb, R. C., and Bohr, D. F. (1982): Vascular changes in DOCA hypertension: Influence of a low protein diet. *Hypertension [Suppl. III],* 4:99–107.

84. Webb, R. C., and Bohr, D. F. (1983): The membrane of the vascular smooth muscle cell in experimental hypertension and its response to serotonin. In: *Smooth Muscle Contractions,* edited by N. Stephens, *(in press).* Marcel Dekker, New York.

85. Greenberg, S. (1981): Properties of intestinal and cutaneous arteries and veins in two-kidney one-clip Goldblatt hypertension. *Am. J. Physiol.,* 241:H525–H540.

86. Bohlen, H. G. (1979): Arteriolar closure mediated by hyperresponsiveness to norepinephrine in hypertensive rats. *Am. J. Physiol.,* 236:H157–H164.

87. Bevan, J. A., Bevan, R. D., Chang, P. C., Pegram, B. L., Purdy, R. E., and Su, C. (1975): Analysis of changes in reactivity of rabbit arteries and veins two weeks after induction of hypertension by coarctation of the abdominal aorta. *Circ. Res.,* 37:183–190.

88. Berecek, K. H., Rascher, W., and Gross, F. (1979): Vascular reactivity in the pathogenesis of spontaneous hypertension. *Clin. Sci.,* 57:51s–53s.

89. Berecek, K. H., Schwertschlag, U., and Gross, F. (1980): Alterations in renal vascular resistance and reactivity in spontaneous hypertension of rats. *Am. J. Physiol.,* 238:H287–H293.

90. Bevan, J. A., Bevan, R. D., Pegram, B. L., Purdy, R. E., and Su, C. (1974): Increased responsiveness of veins to adrenergic stimulation in experimental hypertension. *Blood Vessels,* 11:241–244.

91. Couture, R., and Regoli, D. (1980): Vascular reactivity to angiotensin and noradrenaline in rats maintained on a sodium free diet or made hypertensive with deosoxycorticosterone acetate and salt (DOCA/salt). *Clin. Exp. Hypertension,* 2:25–43.

92. Collis, M. G., and Vanhoutte, P. M. (1978): Increased renal vascular reactivity to angiotensin II but not to nerve stimulation or exogenous norepinephrine in renal hypertensive rats. *Circ. Res.,* 43:544–552.

93. Bevan, J. A., Bevan, R. D., Chang, P. C., Pegram, B. L., Purdy, R. E., and Su, C. (1976): Changes in the contractile response of arteries and veins from hypertensive rabbits to sympathetic nerve activity: Assessment of some postsynaptic influences. *Blood Vessels,* 13:167–180.

94. Bohr, D. F. (1974): Reactivity of vascular smooth muscle from normal and hypertensive rats: Effect of several cations. *Fed. Proc.,* 33:127–132.

95. Schomig, A., Dietz, R., Rascher, W., and Schmidt, J. (1979): Sympathetic vascular tone in spontaneously hypertensive rats. *Jpn. Heart J. [Suppl. I],* 20:113–115.

96. Phelan, E. L., Young, P. L., Jones, D. R., and Simpson, F. D. (1979): Developmental aspects of vascular reactivity: Relationship to genetic hypertension in the New Zealand strain of rats. *Jpn. Heart J. [Suppl. I],* 20:210–212.

97. Lais, L. T., and Brody, M. J. (1975): Mechanism of vascular hyperresponsiveness in the spontaneously hypertensive rat. *Circ. Res. [Suppl. I],* 36–37:216–222.

98. Collis, M. G., and Vanhoutte, P. M. (1977): Vascular reactivity of isolated perfused kidneys from male and female spontaneously hypertensive rats. *Circ. Res.,* 41:759–767.

99. Lais, L. T., and Brody, M. J. (1978): Vasoconstrictor hyperresponsiveness: An early pathogenic mechanism in the spontaneously hypertensive rat. *Eur. J. Pharmacol.,* 47:177–189.

100. Hansen, T. R., and Bohr, D. F. (1975): Hypertension, transmural pressure and vascular smooth muscle response in rats. *Circ. Res.,* 36:590–598.

101. Altura, B. M., Carella, A., and Altura, B. T. (1980):

Magnesium ions control prostaglandin reactivity of venous smooth muscle from spontaneously hypertensive rats. *Prostaglandins and Medicine,* 4:255–261.

102. Berecek, K. H., and Bohr, D. F. (1976): Bases for increased vascular reactivity in experimental hypertension. In: *Vascular Neuroeffector Mechanisms,* edited by J. A. Bevan, T. Godfraind, R. A. Maxwell, and P. M. Vanhoutte, pp. 199–204. Karger, Basel.

103. Berecek, K. H., Murray, R. D., Gross, F., and Brody, M. J. (1982): Vasopressin and vascular reactivity in the development of DOCA hypertension in rats with hereditary diabetes insipidus. *Hypertension,* 4:3–12.

104. Collis, M. J., and Vanhoutte, P. M. (1978): Neuronal and vascular reactivity in isolated perfused kidneys during the development of spontaneous hypertension. *Clin. Sci. Mol. Med.,* 55:233s–235s.

105. Van Neuten, J. M., Janssen, P. A. J., Van Beek, J., Xhonneux, R., Verbeuren, T. J., and Vanhoutte, P. M. (1981): Vascular effects of ketanserin (R41468), a novel antagonist of 5-HT2 serotonergic receptors. *J. Pharmacol. Exp. Ther.,* 218:217–230.

106. Holloway, E. T., and Bohr, D. F. (1973): Reactivity of vascular smooth muscle in hypertensive rats. *Circ. Res.,* 33:678–685.

107. Nagoaka, A., Toyoda, S., and Iwatsuka, H. (1978): Increased renal vascular reactivity to norepinephrine in stroke-prone spontaneously hypertensive rat (SHR). *Life Sci.,* 23:1159–1166.

108. Collis, M. G., and Alps, B. J. (1975): Vascular reactivity to noradrenaline, potassium chloride and angiotensin II in the rat perfused mesenteric vasculature during the development of renal hypertension. *Cardiovasc. Res.,* 9:118–126.

109. Click, R. I., Gilmore, J. P., and Joyner, W. L. (1979): Differential response of hamster cheek pouch microvessels to vasoactive stimuli during the early development of hypertension. *Circ. Res.,* 44:512–517.

110. Berecek, K. H., Stocker, M., and Gross, F. (1980): Changes in renal vascular reactivity at various stages of deoxycorticosterone hypertension in rats. *Circ. Res.,* 46:619–624.

111. Berecek, K. H., and Bohr, D. F. (1978): Whole body vascular reactivity during the development of deoxycorticosterone acetate hypertension in the pig. *Circ. Res.,* 42:764–771.

112. Zsoter, T. T., Sirko, S., Wolchinsky, C., Kadar, D., and Endrenyi, L. (1981): Adrenergic activity in arteries of spontaneously hypertensive rats. *Can. J. Physiol. Pharmacol.,* 59:1104–1107.

113. Zsoter, T. T., Wolchinsky, C., Lawrin, M., and Sirko, S. (1982): Norepinephrine release in arteries of spontaneously hypertensive rats. *Clin. Exp. Hypertension,* 4:431–444.

114. Wiegman, D. L., Joshua, I. G., Morff, R. J., Harris, P. D., and Miller, F. N. (1979): Microvascular responses to norepinephrine in renovascular and spontaneously hypertensive rats. *Am. J. Physiol.,* 236:H545–H548.

115. McGregor, D. D., and Smirk, F. H. (1970): Vascular responses to 5-hydroxytryptamine in genetic and renal hypertensive rats. *Am. J. Physiol.,* 219:687–690.

116. Haeusler, G., and Finch, L. (1972): Vascular reactiv-

ity to 5-hydroxytryptamine and hypertension in the rat. *Arch. Exp. Pathol. Pharmacol.*, 272:101–116.

117. Shibata, S., and Cheng, J. B. (1979): Responses to 5-hydroxytryptamine, NE, and KCl in the perfused hindquarters of the SHR and renal hypertensive rat. *Jpn. Heart J. [Suppl. I]*, 20:213–215.

118. Cheng, J. B., and Shibata, S. (1980): Pressor response to 5-hydroxytryptamine, norepinephrine and KCl in the perfused hindquarter preparation from the spontaneously hypertensive rat. *J. Pharmacol. Exp. Ther.*, 214:488–495.

119. Apperley, E., Feniuk, W., Humphrey, P. P. A., and Levy, G. P. (1980): Evidence for two types of excitatory receptors for 5-hydroxytryptamine in dog isolated vaculature. *Br. J. Pharmacol.*, 68:215–224.

120. Ogden, E., Brown, L. T., and Page, E. W. (1940): The increased sensitivity of arterial muscle in the pre-hypertensive phase of experimental renal hypertension. *Am. J. Physiol.*, 129:560–564.

121. McQueen, E. G. (1956): Vascular reactivity in experimental renal and renoprival hypertension. *Clin. Sci.*, 15:523–532.

122. Shibata, S., Kurahasi, K., and Kuchii, M. (1973): Possible etiology of contractile impairment of vascular smooth muscle from spontaneously hypertensive rats. *J. Pharmacol. Exp. Ther.*, 185:406–417.

123. Finch, L., and Haeusler, G. (1974): Vascular resistance and reactivity in hypertensive rats. *Blood Vessels*, 11:145–158.

124. Bohr, D. F., and Sitrin, M. (1970): Regulation of vascular smooth muscle. Changes in experimental hypertension. *Circ. Res. [Suppl. I]*, 26–27:83–90.

125. Field, F. P., Janis, R. A., and Triggle, D. J. (1972): Aortic reactivity of rats with genetic and experimental hypertension. *Can. J. Physiol. Pharmacol.*, 59:1072–1079.

126. Spector, S., Fleisch, J. H., Maling, H. M., and Brodie, B. B. (1969): Vascular smooth muscle reactivity in normotensive and hypertensive rats. *Science*, 166:1300–1301.

127. Holloway, E. T., Sitrin, M. D., and Bohr, D. F. (1972): Calcium dependence of vascular smooth muscle from normotensive and hypertensive rats. In: *Hypertension—1972*, edited by J. Genest and E. Kouiw, pp. 400–408. Springer-Verlag, Berlin.

128. Brann, L. R., Root, D. T., and Halpern, W. (1980): Intrinsic tone and contractile responsiveness of a small cerebral artery in SHR and WKY rats. *Fed. Proc.*, 39:1191.

129. Sharp, G. W. G., and Leaf, A. (1973): Effect of aldosterone and its mechanism of action on sodium transport. In: *Handbook of Physiology, Sec. 8, Renal Physiology*, edited by J. Orloff and J. W. Berliner, pp. 815–830. American Physiological Society, Bethesda.

130. Sharp, G. W. G., and Leaf, A. (1966): Mechanism of action of aldosterone. *Physiol. Rev.*, 46:593–633.

131. Overbeck, H. W. (1972): Vascular responsiveness to Ca^{++} in hypertensive rats. *Clin. Res.*, 20:771.

132. Overbeck, H. W. (1972): Vascular responses to cations, osmolality and angiotensin in renal hypertensive dogs. *Am. J. Physiol.*, 223:1358–1364.

133. Haddy, F. J., Scott, J. B., Florio, M., Daugherty, R. M., and Huizenga, J. N. (1963): Local vascular effects of hypokolemia, alkalosis, hypercalcemia and hypomagnesemia. *Am. J. Physiol.*, 204:202–212.

134. Vlachakis, N. D., Frederics, R., Velasquez, M., Alexander, N., Singer, F., and Maronde, R. F. (1982): Sympathetic system function and vascular reactivity in hypercalcemic patients. *Hypertension*, 4:452–458.

135. Hinke, J. A. M. (1966): Effect of Ca^{++} upon contractility of small arteries from DOCA-hypertensive rats. *Circ. Res. [Suppl. I]*, 18–19:23–34.

136. Zsoter, T. T., Wolchinsky, C., Henein, N. F., and Ho, L. C. (1977): Calcium kinetics in the aorta of spontaneously hypertensive rats. *Cardiovasc. Res.*, 11:353–357.

137. Zsoter, T. T., and Wolchinsky, C. (1978): Effect of antihypertensives on calcium kinetics in the aorta of spontaneously hypertensive rats. *Arch. Int. Pharmacodyn. Ther.*, 234:287–293.

138. Bhalla, R. C., Webb, R. C., Singh, D., Ashley, T., and Brock, T. (1978): Calcium fluxes, calcium binding and adenosine cyclic $3'5'$-monophosphate-dependent protein kinase activity in the aorta of spontaneously hypertensive and Kyoto Wistar normotensive rats. *Mol. Pharmacol.*, 14:468–477.

139. Noon, J. P., Rice, P. J., and Baldessarini, P. J. (1978): Calcium leakage as a cause of the high resting tension in vascular smooth muscle from the spontaneously hypertensive rat. *Proc. Natl. Acad. Sci. U.S.A.*, 75:1605–1607.

140. Suzuki, A., Yanagawa, T., and Tajiri, T. (1979): Effects of some smooth muscle relaxants on the tonus and on the actions of contractile agents in isolated aorta of SHRSP. *Jpn. Heart J. [Suppl. I]*, 20:219–221.

141. Fitzpatrick, D. F., and Szentivanyi, A. (1980): The relationship between increased myogenic tone and hyporesponsiveness in vascular smooth muscle of spontaneously hypertensive rats. *Clin. Exp. Hypertension*, 2:1023–1037.

142. Pederson, O. L. (1979): Role of extracellular calcium in isometric contractions of the SHR aorta. Influence of age and antihypertensive treatment. *Arch. Int. Pharmacodyn. Ther.*, 239:208–220.

143. Pederson, O. L., Mikkelsen, F., and Anderson, K. E. (1978): Effects of extracellular calcium on potassium and noradrenaline induced contractions in the aorta of spontaneously hypertensive rats—increased sensitivity to nifedipine. *Acta Pharmacol. Toxicol.*, 43:137–144.

144. Goldberg, M. T., and Triggle, C. R. (1977): An analysis of the action of lanthanum on aortic tissue from normotensive and spontaneously hypertensive rats. *Can. J. Physiol. Pharmacol.*, 55:1084–1090.

145. Mochizuki, A., Aoki, K., Kondo, S., Mizuno, T., and Hotta, K. (1979): Specificity of tension development and calcium flux of the arterial smooth muscle in SHR. *Jpn. Heart J. [Suppl. I]*, 20:225–227.

146. Van Breemen, C., Farinas, B. R., Gerba, P., and McNaughten, E. D. (1972): Excitation-contraction coupling in rabbit aorta studied by the lanthanum method for measuring cellular calcium influx. *Circ. Res.*, 30:44–54.

147. Winquist, R. J., Webb, R. C., and Bohr, D. F. (1982): Vascular smooth muscle in hypertension. *Fed. Proc.*, 41:2387–2893.

148. Jones, A. W., and Hart, G. (1975): Altered ion transport in aortic smooth muscle during deoxycorticosterone acetate hypertension in the rat. *Circ. Res.*, 37:333–341.

149. Jones, A. W. (1974): Altered ion transport in large and small arteries from spontaneously hypertensive rats and the influence of calcium. *Circ. Res. [Suppl. I]*, 34:117–122.

150. Burnstock, G., and Straub, R. (1958): A method for studying the effects of ions and drugs on the resting and action potentials in smooth muscle with external electrodes. *J. Physiol. (Lond.)*, 40:156–167.

151. Hurwitz, L., Tinsley, B., and Battle, F. (1960): Dissociation of contraction and potassium efflux in smooth muscle. *Am. J. Physiol.*, 107:107–111.

152. Wei, J.-W., Janis, R. A., and Daniel, E. E. (1977): Alterations in calcium transport and binding by the plasma membrane of mesenteric arteries from spontaneously hypertensive rats. *Blood Vessels,* 14:55–64.

153. Wei, J.-W., Janis, R. A., and Daniel, E. E. (1976): Calcium accumulation and enzymatic activities of subcellular fractions from aortas and ventricles of genetically hypertensive rats. *Circ. Res.,* 39:133–140.

154. Jones, A. W. (1974): Reactivity of ion fluxes in rat aorta during hypertension and circulatory control. *Fed. Proc.,* 33:133–137.

155. Jones, A. W., and Miller, L. A. (1978): Ion transport in tonic and phasic vascular smooth muscle and changes during deoxycorticosterone hypertension. *Blood Vessels,* 15:83–92.

156. Jones, A. W., Sander, P. D., and Kampschmidt, D. L. (1977): The effect of norepinephreine in aortic ^{42}K turnover during deoxycoricosterone acetate hypertension and antihypertensive therapy in the rat. *Circ. Res.,* 41:256–260.

157. Jones, A. W. (1981): Kinetics of active sodium transport in aortas from control and deoxycorticosterone hypertensive rats. *Hypertension,* 3:631–640.

158. Garitz, E. T., and Jones, A. W. (1982): Aldosterone infusion into the rat and dose-dependent changes in blood pressure and arterial ionic transport. *Hypertension,* 4:374–381.

159. Jones, A. W., Heidlage, J. F., Maeyer, R., Day, B., and Freeland, A. (1981): Non-specific supersensitivity of aortic ^{42}K effluxes during DOCA hypertension in the rat, and the effects of anti-hypertensive therapy. In: *New Trends in Arterial Hypertension,* edited by M. Worcel et al., pp. 163–173. Elsevier/North Holland, Amsterdam.

160. Jones, A. W. (1982): Ionic dysfunction and hypertension. *Adv. Microcirc.,* 11:134–159.

161. Jones, A. W., Dutta, P., Garwitz, E. T., Heidlage, J. F., and Warden, D. H. (1981): Altered active and passive transport in vascular smooth muscle during experimental hypertension. In: *International Symposium on Cell Membrane in Function and Dysfunction of Vascular Tissue,* edited by T. Godfraind and P. Meyer, pp. 192–208. Elsevier/North Holland, Amsterdam.

162. Jones, A. W. (1973): Altered ion transport in vascular smooth muscle from spontaneously hypertensive rats and influences of aldosterone, norepinephrine and angiotensin. *Circ. Res.,* 33:563–572.

163. Friedman, S. M., and Friedman, C. L. (1976): Cell permeability, sodium transport and the hypertensive process in the rat. *Circ. Res.,* 39:433–441.

164. Friedman, S. M., Nakashima, M., and Friedman, C. L. (1975): Cell Na and K in the rat tail artery during the development of hypertension induced by deoxycorticosterone acetate. *Proc. Soc. Exp. Biol. Med.,* 150:171–176.

165. Friedman, S. M., McIndoe, R. A., and Spiekemann, G. (1982): Ion-selective electrode studies of cell Na components in vascular smooth muscle of WKY and SHR. *Am. J. Physiol.,* 242:H751–H759.

166. Friedman, S. M. (1979): Evidence for enhanced Na transport in the tail artery of the spontaneously hypertensive rat. *Hypertension,* 1:572–582.

167. Friedman, S. M., and Nakashima, M. (1978): Evidence for enhanced transport in hypertension induced by DOCA in the rat. *Can. J. Physiol. Pharmacol.,* 56:1029–1035.

168. Webb, R. C., and Bohr, D. F. (1979): Potassium relaxation of vascular smooth muscle from spontaneously hypertensive rats. *Blood Vessels,* 16:71–79.

169. Webb, R. C. (1982): Potassium relaxation of vascular smooth muscle from DOCA hypertensive pigs. *Hypertension,* 4:609–619.

170. Hagen, E. C., Johnson, J. C., and Webb, R. C. (1982): Ouabain binding and potassium relaxation in aortae from renal hypertensive rabbits. *Am. J. Physiol.,* 12:H896–H902.

171. Webb, R. C., and Bohr, D. F. (1978): Potassium-induced relaxation as an indicator of Na-K ATPase activity in vascular smooth muscle. *Blood Vessels,* 15:198–207.

172. Overbeck, H. W., Bell, D. R., Grissette, D. E., and Brock, T. A. (1982): Function of the sodium pump in arterial smooth muscle in experimental hypertension: Role of pressure. *Hypertension,* 4:394–399.

173. Brock, T. A., Smith, J. B., and Overbeck, H. W. (1982): Relationship of vascular sodium-potassium pump activity to intracellular sodium in hypertensive rats. *Hypertension [Suppl. II],* 4:43–48.

174. Overbeck, H. W., Ku, D. D., and Rapp, J. R. (1981): Sodium pump activity in arteries of Dahl salt-sensitive rats. *Hypertension,* 3:306–312.

175. Overbeck, H. W., and Grissette, D. E. (1982): Sodium pump activity in arteries of rats with Goldblatt hypertension. *Hypertension,* 4:132–139.

176. Pamnani, M. B., Clough, D. L., Huot, S. J., and Haddy, F. J. (1980): Vascular Na^+-K^+ pump activity in Dahl S and R rats. *Proc. Soc. Exp. Biol. Med.,* 165:440–444.

177. Pamnani, M. B., Clough, D. L., and Haddy, F. J. (1979): Na^+-K^+ pump activity in tail arteries of spontaneously hypertensive rats. *Jpn. Heart J. [Suppl.],* 1:228–130.

178. Allen, J. C., and Seidel, C. (1977): EGTA stimulated and ouabain inhibited ATPase of vascular smooth muscle. In: *Excitation-Contraction Coupling in Smooth Muscle,* edited by R. Casteels, T. Godfraind, and J. C. Ruegg, pp. 211–218. Elsevier/North Holland, Amsterdam.

179. Gothberg, G., Jandhyala, B., and Folkow, B. (1980): Studies on the role of sodium-potassium-activated ATPase as determinant of vascular reactivity in Wis-

tar-Kyoto and spontaneously hypertensive rats. *Clin. Sci.,* 59:187s–189s.

180. Webb, R. C., and Bohr, D. F. (1980): Vascular reactivity in hypertension: Altered effects of ouabain. *Experientia,* 36:220–222.

181. Overbeck, H. W., Dersfield, R. S., Pamnani, M. B., and Sozen, T. (1974): Attenuated vasodilator responses to potassium in essential hypertensive men. *J. Clin. Invest.,* 53:678–686.

182. Overbeck, H. W., Pamnani, M. B., Alkers, T., Brody, T. M., and Haddy, F. J. (1976): Depressed function of an ouabain-sensitive sodium-potassium pump in blood vessels from renal hypertensive dogs. *Circ. Res. [Suppl. II],* 38:48–52.

183. Overbeck, H. W., and Clark, D. W. J. (1975): Vasodilator responses to K$^+$ in genetic hypertensive and in renal hypertensive rats. *J. Lab. Clin. Med.,* 86:973–983.

184. Haddy, F., Pamnani, M., and Clough, D. (1978): The sodium-potassium pump in volume expanded hypertension. *Clin. Exp. Hypertension,* 1:295–336.

185. Pamnani, M., Huot, S., Buggy, J., Clough, D., and Haddy, F. (1981): Demonstration of a humoral inhibitor of the Na$^+$-K$^+$ pump in some models of experimental hypertension. *Hypertension [Suppl. II],* 3:96–101.

186. Haddy, F. J., Pamnani, M., Clough, D., and Huot, S. (1982): Role of a humoral sodium-potassium pump inhibitor in experimental low renin hypertension. *Life Sci.,* 30:571–575.

187. Pamnani, M. B., Clough, D. L., Huot, S. L., and Haddy, F. J. (1981): Sodium-potassium pump activity in experimental hypertension. In: *Vasodilation,* edited by P. M. Vanhoutte and I. Leusen, pp. 391–403. Raven Press, New York.

188. Blaustein, M. P. (1977): Sodium ions, calcium ions, blood pressure regulation and hypertension: A reassessment and an hypothesis. *Am. J. Physiol.,* 232:C165–C173.

189. Blaustein, M. P. (1981): What is the link between vascular smooth muscle sodium pumps and hypertension? *Clin. Exp. Hypertension,* 3:173–178.

190. Strecker, R. B., Hubbard, W. C., and Michelakis, A. M. (1975): Dissociation constant of the norepinephrine-receptor complex in normotensive and hypertensive rats. *Circ. Res.,* 37:658–663.

191. Clineschmidt, B. V., Geller, R. G., Govier, W. C., and Sjoerdsma, A. (1970): Reactivity to norepinephrine and nature of the alpha-adrenergic receptor in vascular smooth muscle of genetically hypertensive rats. *Eur. J. Pharmacol.,* 10:45–50.

192. Horowitz, D., Clineschmidt, J. M., Van Buren, J. M., and Ommaya, A. K. (1974): Temporal arteries from hypertensive and normotensive man: Reactivity to norepinephrine and characteristics of alpha-adrenergic receptors. *Circ. Res. [Suppl. I],* 34–35:109–115.

193. Johnson, J. C., and Webb, R. C. (1981): Postjunctional alpha-2 adrenergic receptors in vascular smooth muscle from spontaneously hypertensive rats (SHR). *Physiologist,* 24:73.

194. Cohen, M. L., and Berkowitz, B. A. (1976): Decreased vascular relaxation in hypertension. *J. Pharmacol. Exp. Ther.,* 196:396–406.

195. Spector, S., Fleisch, J. H., Maling, H. M., and Brodie, B. B. (1969): Vascular smooth muscle reactivity in normotensive and hypertensive rats. *Science,* 166:1300–1301.

196. Triner, L., Vulliemoz, Y., Veosky, M., and Manger, W. M. (1975): Cyclic adenosine monophosphate and vascular reactivity in spontaneously hypertensive rats. *Biochem. Pharmacol.,* 24:743–745.

197. Godfraind, T., and Dieu, D. (1978): Influence of aging on the isoprenaline relaxation of aortae from normal and hypertensive rats. *Arch. Int. Pharmacodyn. Ther.,* 236:300–302.

198. Deragon, G., Regoli, D., and Rioux, F. (1978): The effects of vasodilators in the perfused hindlimbs of spontaneously hypertensive and normotensive rats. *Can. J. Physiol. Pharmacol.,* 56:624–629.

199. Woodcock, E. A., Olsson, C. A., and Johnston, C. I. (1980): Reduced vascular beta-adrenergic receptors in deoxycorticosterone-salt hypertensive rats. *Biochem. Pharmacol.,* 29:1465–1468.

200. Limas, C. J., and Limas, C. (1979): Decreased number of beta-adrenergic receptors in hypertensive vessels. *Biochem. Biophys. Acta,* 582:533–536.

201. Vanhoutte, P. M., Van Neuten, J. M., Symuens, J., and Janssen, P. A. J. (1983): Antihypertensive properties of ketanserin (R41468). *Fed. Proc.,* 42:182–185.

202. DeMey, C., and Vanhoutte, P. M. (1981): Effects of age and spontaneous hypertension on the tachyphylaxis to 5-hydroxytryptamine and angiotensin II in the isolated rat kidney. *Hypertension,* 3:718–724.

203. Collis, M. G., and Vanhoutte, P. M. (1981): Tachyphylaxis to 5-hydroxytryptamine in perfused kidneys from spontaneously hypertensive rats. *J. Cardiovasc. Pharmacol.,* 3:229–235.

204. DeCree, J., Leempoels, J., Geukens, H., DeCrock, W., and Verhaegen, H. (1981): The antihypertensive effects of ketanserin (R41468), a novel 5-hydroxytryptamine-blocking agent, in patients with essential hypertension. *Clin. Sci.,* 61:473s–476s.

205. Shibata, S., and Cheng, J. B. (1978): Vascular relaxation in hypertensive rats. In: *Mechanisms of Vasodilation,* edited by P. M. Vanhoutte and I. Leusen, pp. 181–186. Karger, Basel.

206. Antonaccio, M. J., Caveliere, T., and Cote, D. (1980). Ontogenesis of hypertension and responsiveness to antihypertensive agents in spontaneously hypertensive rats. *Blood Vessels,* 17:78–85.

207. Hutchins, P. M., Greene, A. W., and Rains, T. D. (1975): Effect of isoproterenol on the blood vessels of the spontaneously hypertensive rat. *Microvasc. Res.,* 9:101–105.

208. Hamed, A. T., and Lokhandwala, M. F. (1981): Control of hindlimb vascular resistance and vascular responsiveness in DOCA-salt hypertensive dogs. *Clin. Exp. Hypertension,* 3:85–101.

209. Kaulkman, H. O., Timmermans, P. B. M. W. M., and Van Zweiten, P. A. (1982): Characterization of the antihypertensive properties of ketanserin (R-41468) in rats. *J. Pharmacol. Exp. Ther.,* 222:227–231.

210. Katovich, M. J., Fregly, M. J., and Barney, C. C. (1978): Reduced responsiveness to beta-adrenergic

stimulation in renal hypertensive rats. *Proc. Soc. Exp. Biol. Med.,* 158:363–369.

211. Fink, G. D., and Brody, M. J. (1979): Renal vascular resistance and reactivity in two forms of genetic hypertension in the rat. *Jpn. Heart J.* [*Suppl. I*], 20:71–73.

212. Fink, G. D., and Brody, M. J. (1980): Impaired neurogenic control of renal vasculature in renal hypertensive rats. *Am. J. Physiol.,* 238:H770–H775.

213. Fink, G. D., and Brody, M. J. (1979): Renal vascular resistance and reactivity in the spontaneously hypertensive rat. *Am. J. Physiol.,* 237:F128–F132.

214. Castro-Tavares, J. (1980): Sensitivity of vascular smooth muscle from hypertensive dogs to vasodilator drugs. *Blood Vessels,* 17:146–147.

215. Brody, M. J., Dorr, L. D., and Shaffer, R. A. (1970): Reflex vasodilation and sympathetic transmission in the renal hypertensive dog. *Am. J. Physiol.,* 219:1746–1750.

216. Kamikawa, Y., Cline, W. H., and Su, C. (1980): Diminished purinergic modulation of the vascular adrenergic neurotransmission in spontaneously hypertensive rats. *Eur. J. Pharmacol.,* 66:347–353.

217. Dadkar, N. K., Aroska, V. A., and Dohodwalla, A. N. (1980): Peripheral vascular smooth muscle relaxation in normotensive and hypertensive rats. *J. Pharm. Pharmacol.,* 32:74–76.

218. Hollenberg, N. K., and Adams, D. F. (1976): The renal circulation in hypertensive disease. *Am. J. Med.,* 60:773–784.

219. Twietmeyer, T. A., Bhalla, R. C., and Maynard, J. A. (1978): Acid and alkaline phosphatase activities and calcium transport in aortic smooth muscle from DOCA hypertensive rats. *J. Mol. Cell. Cardiol.,* 10:646–654.

220. Bhalla, R. C., Sharma, R. V., and Webb, R. C. (1979): Possible role of cyclic AMP and calcium in the pathogenesis of hypertension. *Jpn. Heart J.* [*Suppl. I*], 20:222–224.

221. Aoki, K., Ikeda, N., Yamashita, K., Tazumi, K., Sato, I., and Hotta, K. (1974): Cardiovascular contraction in spontaneously hypertensive rat: Ca⁺⁺ interaction of myofibrils and subcellular membrane of heart and arterial muscle. *Jpn. Circ. J.,* 38:1115–1121.

222. Aoki, K., Yamashita, K., Tomita, N., Tazumi, K., and Hotta, K. (1974): ATPase activity and Ca⁺⁺ binding activity of subcellular membrane of arterial smooth muscle in spontaneously hypertensive rat. *Jpn. Heart J.,* 15:180–181.

223. Moore, L., Hurwitz, L., Davenport, G. R., and London, E. J. (1975): Energy-dependent calcium uptake activity of microsomes from the aorta of normal and hypertensive rats. *Biochim. Biophys. Acta,* 413:432–451.

224. Muchlin, P. S., RamaSastry, B. V., Boerth, R. G., Surber, M. J., and Landon, E. J. (1978): Dithiothreitol-induced alterations of blood pressure, vascular reactivity, and aortic microsomal calcium uptake in spontaneously hypertensive rats. *J. Pharmacol. Exp. Ther.,* 207:331–339.

225. Chaturvedi, A. K., Landon, E. J., and RamaSastry, B. V. (1978): Influence of 6-(*N,N*-diethylamino) hexyl-3,4,5-trimethoxybenzoate on the responsive-

ness of aortae to norepinephrine and calcium movements in microsomes from spontaneously hypertensive and normotensive rats. *Pharmacology,* 17:315–322.

226. Webb, R. C., and Bhalla, R. C. (1976): Altered calcium sequestration by subcellular fractions of vascular smooth muscle from spontaneously hypertensive rats. *J. Mol. Cell. Cardiol.,* 8:651–660.

227. Orlov, S. N., and Postnov, Y. V. (1980): Calcium accumulation and calcium binding by the cell membranes of cardiomyocytes and smooth muscle of aorta in spontaneously hypertensive rats. *Clin. Sci.,* 59:207s–209s.

228. Kwan, C.-Y., Belbeck, L., and Daniel, E. E. (1980): Abnormal biochemistry of vascular smooth muscle plasma membrane isolated from hypertensive rats. *Mol. Pharmacol.,* 17:137–140.

229. Kwan, C.-Y., Belbeck, L., and Daniel, E. E. (1979): Abnormal biochemistry of vascular smooth muscle plasma membrane as an important factor in the initiation and maintenance of hypertension in rats. *Blood Vessels,* 16:259–268.

230. Kwan, C.-Y., Belbeck, L., and Daniel, E. E. (1980): Characteristics of arterial plasma membrane in renovascular hypertension in rats. *Blood Vessels,* 17:131–140.

231. Amer, M. S. (1973): Cyclic adenosine monophosphate and hypertension in rats. *Science,* 179:807–809.

232. Amer, M. S. (1975): Cyclic nucleotides in disease; on the biochemical etiology of hypertension. *Life Sci.,* 17:1021–1038.

233. Amer, M. S., Doba, N., and Reis, D. J. (1975): Changes in cyclic nucleotide metabolism in aorta and heart of hypertensive rats, possible trigger mechanism of hypertension. *Proc. Natl. Acad. Sci. U.S.A.,* 72:2135–2139.

234. Amer, M. S. (1975): Possible involvement of the cyclic nucleotide system in hypertension. In: *Cyclic Nucleotides in Disease,* edited by B. Weiss, pp. 133–156. University Park Press, Baltimore.

235. Amer, M. S., Gomoll, A. W., Perhach, J. L., Ferguson, H. D., and McKinney, G. R. (1974): Aberrations of cyclic nucleotide metabolism in hearts and vessels of hypertensive rats. *Proc. Natl. Acad. Sci. U.S.A.,* 71:4930–4931.

236. Reis, D. J., Doba, N., and Amer, M. S. (1973): The central neural regulation by baroreceptors of peripheral catecholaminergic mechanisms. In: *Frontiers in Catecholamine Research,* edited by E. Usdin and S. Snyder, pp. 883–889. Pergamon Press, New York.

237. Reis, D. J., Nathan, M. A., Doba, N., and Amer, M. S. (1976): Two models of arterial hypertension in rat produced by lesions of inhibitory areas of brain. In: *The Nervous System in Arterial Hypertension,* edited by S. Julius and M. D. Esler, pp. 119–150. Charles C Thomas, Springfield, Ill.

238. Ramanathan, S., and Shibata, S. (1974): Cyclic AMP blood vessels of spontaneously hypertensive rat. *Blood Vessels,* 2:312–318.

239. Klenerova, K., Albrecht, I., and Hynie, S. (1975): The activity of adenylate cyclase and phosphodiesterase in hearts and aortas of spontaneously hyper-

tensive rats. *Pharmacol. Res. Commun.*, 7:453–462.

240. Bhalla, R. C., Sharma, R. V., and Ramanathan, S. (1980): Possible role of phosphorylation-dephosphorylation in the regulation of calcium metabolism in cardiovascular tissues of SHR. *Hypertension*, 2:207–214.

241. McGiff, J. C., and Quilley, J. (1981): Prostaglandins, hypertension and the cardiovascular system. In: *Prostaglandins and Cardiovascular Disease*, edited by R. J. Hegyeli, pp. 101–107. Raven Press, New York.

242. Nasjletti, A., and Malik, K. U. (1982): Interrelations between prostaglandins and vasoconstrictor hormones: Contribution to blood pressure regulation. *Fed. Proc.*, 41:2394–2399.

243. McGiff, J. C., and Quilley, J. (1980): Prostaglandins, kinins, and the regulation of blood pressure. *Clin. Exp. Hypertension*, 2:729–740.

244. Greenberg, S. (1976): Evidence for enhanced venous smooth muscle turnover of prostaglandin-like substance in portal veins from spontaneously hypertensive rats. *Prostaglandins*, 11:163–177.

245. Ellis, E., and Hutchins, P. (1974): Cardiovascular responses to prostaglandin F$_{2alpha}$ in spontaneously hypertensive rats. *Prostaglandins*, 7:345–353.

246. Dusting, G. J., DiNicolantonio, R., Drysdale, T., and Doyle, A. E. (1981): Vasodepressor effects of arachidonic acid and prostacyclin (PGI$_2$) in hypertensive rats. *Clin. Sci.*, 61:315s–318s.

247. Dusting, G. J., Davies, W., Drysdale, T., and Doyle, A. E. (1981): Increased conversion of arachidonic acid to vasodilator prostanoids in spontaneously hypertensive rats. *Clin. Exp. Pharmacol. Physiol.*, 8:435–440.

248. Lukacsko, P., Messina, E. J., and Kaley, G. (1980): Reduced hypotensive action of arachidonic acid in the spontaneously hypertensive rat. *Hypertension*, 2:657–663.

249. Laborit, H., and Valette, N. (1974): Action de l'acide arachidonique sur l'hypertension arterielle experimentale du rat. *Agressologie*, 14:387–393.

250. Lockette, W. E., Webb, R. C., and Bohr, D. F. (1981): A change in responsiveness to sodium arachidonate in aortae from deoxycorticosterone acetate (DOCA) hypertensive rats. *Physiologist*, 24:5.

251. Colina-Chourio, J., McGiff, J. C., and Nasjletti, A. (1979): Effect of indomethacin on blood pressure in the normotensive unanesthetized rabbit: Possible relation to prostaglandin synthesis inhibition. *Clin. Sci.*, 57:359–365.

252. Nowak, J., and Wennmalm, A. (1978): Influence of indomethacin and prostaglandin E, on total and regional blood flow in man. *Acta Physiol. Scand.*, 102:484–491.

253. Davies, I. B., Bannister, R., Hensby, C., and Sever, P. S. (1980): The pressor actions of noradrenaline and angiotensin II in chronic autonomic failure treated with indomethacin. *Br. J. Clin. Pharmacol.*, 10:223–229.

254. Lonign, A. J., Itskovitz, H. D., Growshaw, K., and McGiff, J. C. (1973): Dependency of renal blood flow on prostaglandin synthesis in the dog. *Circ. Res.*, 32:712–717.

255. Patak, R. B., Mookerjee, C., Bentzel, P., Hyseut,

P., Babe, M., and Lee, J. (1975): Antagonism of the effects of furosemide by indomethacin in normal and hypertensive rats. *Clin. Exp. Hypertension*, 1:381–391.

256. Martin, K., Zipser, R., and Horton, R. (1981): Effect of prostaglandin inhibition on the hypertensive action of sodium retaining steroids. *Hypertension*, 3:622–628.

257. Chrysant, S. B., Townsend, S. M., and Morgan, P. R. (1978): The effects of salt and meclofenamate administration on the hypertension of spontaneously hypertensive rats. *Clin. Exp. Hypertension*, 1:381–391.

258. Chrysant, S. G., Mandal, A. K., and Nordquist, J. A. (1980): Renal function and organic changes induced by salt and prostaglandin inhibition in spontaneously hypertensive rats. *Nephron*, 25:151–155.

259. Rugsley, D. J., Mullins, R., and Beilin, L. J. (1976): Renal prostaglandin synthesis in hypertension induced by deoxycorticosterone and sodium chloride in the rat. *Clin. Sci. Mol. Med.*, [Suppl. 3], 51:253s–256s.

260. Pugsley, D. J., Beilin, L. J., and Petro, R. P. (1975): Renal prostaglandin synthesis in the Goldblatt hypertensive rat. *Circ. Res.* [Suppl. 1], 36:81–88.

261. Romero, J. C., and Strong, C. G. (1977): The effect of indomethacin blockade on prostaglandin synthesis on blood pressure of normal rabbits and rabbits with renovascular hypertension. *Circ. Res.*, 40:35–41.

262. Yun, J., Kelly, G., and Bartter, F. C. (1979): Effect of indomethacin on renal function and plasma renin activity in dogs with chronic renovascular hypertension. *Nephron*, 24:278–282.

263. McQueen, D., and Bell, K. (1976): The effects of prostaglandin E, and sodium meclofenamate on blood pressure in renal hypertensive rats. *Eur. J. Pharmacol.*, 37:223–235.

264. Rioux, F., and Regoli, D. (1975): In vitro production of prostaglandins by isolated aorta strips of normotensive and hypertensive rats. *Can. J. Physiol. Pharmacol.*, 53:673–677.

265. Botha, J. H., Leary, W. P., and Asmal, A. C. (1980): Enhanced release of a "prostacyclin-like" substance from aortic strips of spontaneously hypertensive rats. *Prostaglandins*, 19:285–289.

266. Skidgel, R. A., and Printz, M. P. (1980): Vascular PG synthesis in hypertensive and normotensive rats. In: *Advances in Prostaglandin and Thromboxane Research, Vol. 7*, edited by S. Samuelsson, P. W. Ramwell, and R. Paoletti, pp. 803–805. Raven Press, New York.

267. Okuma, M., Yamori, Y., Ohta, K., and Uchino, H. (1979): Production of prostacyclin-like substance in stroke-prone and stroke-resistant spontaneously hypertensive rats. *Prostaglandins*, 17:1–7.

268. Pace-Asciak, C. R., and Carrara, M. C. (1980): Ontogeny of aortic PGI$_2$ formation in the developing spontaneously hypertensive rat—correlation with elevations in blood pressure. In: *Advances in Prostaglandin and Thromboxane Research, Vol. 7*, edited by B. Samuelson, P. W. Ramwell, and R. Paoletti, pp. 797–801. Raven Press, New York.

Cardiovascular Pharmacology, Second Edition,
edited by Michael Antonaccio.
Raven Press, New York © 1984.

Antihypertensive Drugs

Alexander Scriabine and David G. Taylor

Miles Institute for Preclinical Pharmacology, New Haven, Connecticut 06509

During the last two decades, significant advances have been made in the treatment of hypertension. These advances were made possible by new and highly effective antihypertensive drugs that were developed in the laboratories of pharmaceutical companies. The development of these drugs was not based on a better understanding of the pathogenesis of essential hypertension; our knowledge of the cause or causes of this disease remains remarkably poor. The antihypertensive drugs were found to modify physiological mechanisms of blood pressure control. In some instances, new drugs led to identification of previously unknown mechanisms of cardiovascular regulation, e.g., presynaptic control of norepinephrine release.

In accordance with their mechanisms of action, the available antihypertensive drugs can be classified as follows: (a) diuretics, (b) drugs that interfere with the renin-angiotensin system, (c) drugs that interfere with the sympathetic control of arterial pressure, and (d) smooth-muscle relaxants.

The size limitations for this chapter do not permit adequate coverage of all drugs with antihypertensive activity. For more detailed information on the pharmacology of antihypertensive drugs, readers are referred to a recent book on this subject (1). The major sites of antihypertensive actions of drugs are shown in Fig. 1, and the major mechanisms are listed in Table 1.

DIURETICS

Diuretics are commonly used in the initial therapy for hypertension. However, a higher diuretic efficacy does not imply higher antihypertensive efficacy. Loop diuretics (diuretics with the major site of action in the ascending limb of Henle's loop) are more effective than thiazides as diuretics, but not as antihypertensives. Thiazides are therefore preferred to loop diuretics in therapy for hypertension (2,3). The generic names, chemical structures, and clinical doses for some thiazide diuretics and related compounds are given in Table 2. The major pharmacological differences among these compounds involve their durations of action. Polythiazide, methyclothiazide, and chlorthalidone have the longest durations of action, which can exceed 24 hr.

Their longer durations of action are attributed to greater binding to plasma proteins and/or to greater lipophilicity and consequently greater tubular reabsorption (4). All known diuretics increase plasma renin activity, and consequently they increase the formation of angiotensin II and aldosterone; this tends to limit their antihypertensive effects. Therefore, combined use of diuretics with antihypertensives known to lower plasma renin activity (e.g., methyldopa, clonidine) is justified.

Most diuretics act by inhibiting tubular reabsorption of ions and water rather than by

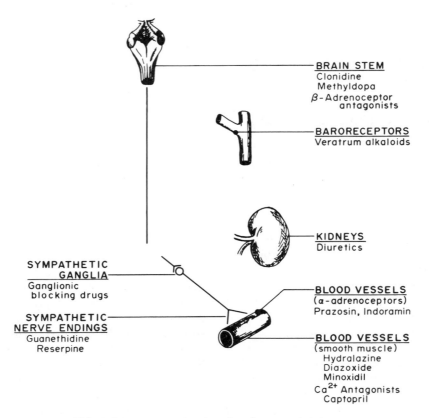

FIG. 1. Primary sites of action of antihypertensive drugs.

increasing glomerular filtration. There are at least four sites of action for diuretics in the renal tubules: proximal tubules, the ascending limb of Henle's loop, and lower and upper segments of distal tubules. The site of action of a diuretic is of clinical significance, because the saluretic effects of two diuretics are more likely to be additive if the drugs act at different tubular sites. Also, if a patient does not respond to one diuretic, he may respond to another diuretic acting at a different tubular site. The biochemical mechanisms involved in the inhibition of tubular transport of sodium and chloride by diuretics remain obscure, although some renal enzymes have been found to be inhibited by diuretics. The saluretic effect of acetazolamide is considered to be the consequence of inhibition of carbonic anhydrase. Thiazides also inhibit carbonic anhydrase, but their *in vitro* carbonic anhydrase inhibitory

activity is not correlated with their *in vivo* saluretic effects (3). Furosemide, ethacrynic acid, and organomercurial diuretics inhibit Na^+-K^+-dependent ATPase *in vitro*, but no clear correlation between their ATPase inhibitory activity and saluretic activity has been established. Thiazides inhibit glycolysis *in vitro* (5), and chlorothiazide has been found to inhibit utilization of glucose in the dog aorta (6).

Various investigators have suggested that prostaglandins may mediate or modulate the renal effects of diuretics (7,8). Some diuretics inhibit 9-ketoreductase (9KR) or 15-hydroxy-prostaglandin dehydrogenase and can therefore be expected to increase the availability of prostaglandins (9,10). Indomethacin or other inhibitors of cyclooxygenase reduce, but do not abolish, the effects of saluretics. The involvement of prostaglandins in the pharma-

TABLE 1. *Proposed major mechanisms of action*

	Sympathetic control					Renin-angiotensin system inhibition	Vasodilator action	Buffer nerve enhancement
	Central α receptor activation	Ganglion blockade	Decrease NE release	α-Adrenoceptor blockade	β-Adrenoceptor blockade			
Captopril			X			X		
Veratrum alkaloids								X
Methyldopa	X		X					
Clonidine	X		X					X
Guanfacine	X		X					X
Guanabenz	X		X					
Trimethaphan camsylate		X						
Reserpine			X					
Guanethidine			X					
Prazosin				X				
Indoramin				X				
Propranolol	X				X	X		X
Labetalol				X	X			
Sodium nitroprusside							X	
Diazoxide							X	
Minoxidil							X	
Hydralazine							X	
Nifedipine							X	

TABLE 2. *Thiazides and thiazidelike diuretics commonly used in hypertension*

Generic Name	Structure	Daily Dose mg
Hydrochlorothiazide		25-200
Chlorothiazide		500-2000
Polythiazide		1-4
Methyclothiazide		2.5-10
Chlorthalidone		25-50 or 100 every second day
Metolazone		5-10

cological effects of diuretics may also be relevant to their antihypertensive activity. The acute antihypertensive effect of a new diuretic, 2-aminoethyl-4-(1,1-dimethylethyl)-6-10-iodophenol hydrochloride (MK-447) is reduced by indomethacin (11). The antihypertensive activity of diuretics was first shown in humans (12) and subsequently demonstrated in various animal models (13,14). An initial diuretic-induced decrease in plasma volume and subsequent reduction in vascular Na^+ content are the likely mechanisms of antihypertensive action. According to Friedman and Friedman (15), an increase in the sodium pool or in the "net Na^+ pumping activity" is likely to lead to hypertrophy of the vascular smooth-muscle cells and to vasoconstriction. Blaustein

(16) suggested that an increase in ionized intracellular Na^+ may increase Ca^{2+} influx and decrease Ca^{2+} efflux out of vascular smooth-muscle cells, leading to vasoconstriction and to elevation of arterial pressure.

The major side effects of thiazide diuretics are hypokalemia, hyperuricemia, and a shift in the glucose tolerance curve toward a diabetic type. The loop diuretics furosemide, ethacrynic acid, and bumetanide produce the same side effects, but in addition they are more likely to produce severe electrolyte imbalance and dehydration than are thiazides. They can also produce a usually reversible loss of hearing. Serum lipid concentrations, primarily of β-lipoproteins, were reported to be elevated in patients receiving diuretics (17).

Diuretics alone cannot be expected to lower arterial pressure in more than 50% of hypertensive patients, but up to 80% of patients will respond to combined therapy with diuretics and drugs that interfere with the renin-angiotensin system or the sympathetic nervous system.

DRUGS AFFECTING THE RENIN-ANGIOTENSIN SYSTEM

Captopril

The involvement of the renin-angiotensin system in the pathogenesis of hypertension and control of arterial pressure has been suggested by various investigators over the last 80 years (18–20), but attempts to control hypertension by inhibitors of angiotensin II formation or by competitive antagonists of angiotensin II at vascular receptors have not been made until recently (21). Teprotide was the first inhibitor of the converting enzyme that was shown to lower arterial pressure in humans by intravenous (but not oral) administration (22). The first orally active inhibitor of the enzyme was captopril (Fig. 2). It was designed to bind to the active site of the converting enzyme in a manner similar to that of angiotensin I (20,23).

Because angiotensin-converting enzyme is identical with kininase II, the enzyme controlling the breakdown of bradykinin, captopril is capable of enhancing the vasodilator effect of bradykinin. Bradykinin enhancement could conceivably contribute to the mechanism of antihypertensive action of captopril (24,25), although, contrary to this view, Textor et al. (26) found that continuous infusion of angiotensin II blocked the antihypertensive effects of captopril, even when bradykinin responsiveness was enhanced 10-fold in rats. Furthermore, at therapeutic doses, captopril pro-

duces little elevation of plasma bradykinin in humans (27). Some investigators have suggested that bradykinin-induced increases in the formation and release of prostaglandins contribute partially to the captopril antihypertensive effects (28,29); however, this idea has not been supported by other studies in spontaneously hypertensive rats (30,31).

In animals and humans, captopril inhibits the pressor effects of angiotensin I, but the pressor effects of angiotensin II are either unchanged or enhanced by captopril (20,32). In normotensive animals, the effect of captopril on the arterial pressure depends on the state of the salt balance. Greater effects are observed in sodium-depleted animals than in sodium-replete animals (20,33,34). In renin-dependent experimental renal hypertension (two-kidney renal-hypertensive rats) the onset of the antihypertensive action of captopril is immediate, but in one-kidney, one-clip renal hypertension a marked effect is not obtained until several days of therapy (20–23,30–35).

In spontaneously hypertensive rats, captopril has been shown to effectively lower arterial pressure (36). A recent report by Antonaccio and Kerwin (37) provides clues concerning the mechanism of action of captopril in this low-renin hypertensive model. In these studies, acute and chronic treatment with captopril quite selectively decreased the pressor responses, but not the cardiac responses, evoked by sympathetic outflow stimulation. The inhibitory effects of captopril were reversed by intravenous administration of angiotensin II plus indomethacin, but not nephrectomy. It was suggested that the reduced pressor responses and, quite possibly, the blood pressure levels produced by captopril were the results of decreased angiotensin-II-facilitated release of norepinephrine occurring at the prejunctional vascular sympathetic neuronal site.

In all species studied, the antihypertensive effect of captopril is associated with a reduction in total calculated peripheral vascular resistance, with either no effect or an increase in cardiac output. In hypertensive patients, peripheral resistance reductions are enhanced

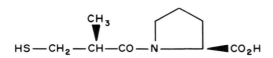

FIG. 2. Chemical structure of captopril.

with chronic captopril treatment (38). Renal vascular resistance is consistently decreased by captopril (32). Plasma renin activity is usually increased by captopril in animals as well as humans. This increase is likely due to abolition of the negative-feedback mechanism involving the inhibitory effect of angiotensin II on the juxtaglomerular apparatus and renin release. As a consequence of inhibition of the conversion of angiotensin I to angiotensin II, captopril reduces the aldosterone levels in animals and humans (39–41). In sodium-depleted rats and dogs, captopril increases sodium and water excretion.

Captopril-induced lowering of arterial pressure is not associated with reflex tachycardia. It has been suggested that captopril inhibits reflex tachycardia by removing the angiotensin-II-induced facilitation of sympathetic transmission. Captopril may also cause reflex vagal stimulation by enhancing the effects of bradykinin or by increasing the release of prostaglandins (42).

Captopril was studied in humans at doses ranging from 25 to 1,000 mg/day and was found active in most forms of human hypertension, with the exception of primary aldosteronism. Captopril was effective even in patients with renal failure (43–47). The side effects of captopril include fever, maculopapular rash, itch, disturbance of taste, proteinuria, and occasional leukopenia. Decreases in white cell counts have been observed in approximately 0.5% of patients during the first 3 months of therapy.

Absorption of orally administered captopril in humans is rapid and extensive; 75% of the radioactivity after a single oral dose of ^{14}C-captopril has been recovered in the urine within 48 hr (20). The metabolites of captopril include disulfides and endogenous sulfhydryl compounds, e.g., cysteine.

DRUGS INTERFERING WITH THE SYMPATHETIC NERVOUS SYSTEM

Drugs can reduce sympathetic tone by acting at the following sites: (a) afferent pathways, increasing the sensitivity of peripheral receptors to pressor stimuli; (b) central nervous system, controlling sympathetic activity and consequently arterial pressure; (c) sympathetic ganglia, reducing the transmission of impulses; (d) sympathetic nerve endings, reducing the release of norepinephrine; (e) vascular α-adrenoceptors, blocking the vasoconstrictor effect of norepinephrine; (f) cardiac β-adrenoceptors, blocking cardiac stimulant effects of sympathetic stimulation.

Veratrum Alkaloids

Veratrum alkaloids increase the sensitivity of peripheral pressure or stretch receptors and increase traffic in the afferent receptors, leading to a reduction in sympathetic tone and an increase in vagal tone. The side effects of nausea and vomiting have made veratrum alkaloids obsolete in the treatment of hypertension. Attempts to separate the emetic and antihypertensive effects of veratrum alkaloids have failed. This failure is attributed to the similarity of receptors mediating the antihypertensive effects and the emetic effects of veratrum alkaloids. Other side effects of veratrum alkaloids include substernal distress, blurring of vision, mental confusion, and cardiac arrhythmias. Severe hypotension and bradycardia, which can develop following intravenous administration of veratrum alkaloids, usually are due to vagal hyperactivity and can be antagonized by atropine.

Absorption of orally administered veratrum alkaloids is poor. Consistent antihypertensive effects are obtained with parenteral preparations of veratrum alkaloids: cryptenamine, protoveratrines A and B. Parenteral use of veratrum alkaloids can still be justified in hypertensive emergencies, e.g., toxemia of pregnancy, when other less toxic antihypertensive drugs produce no satisfactory response.

Methyldopa

The chemical name of methyldopa is L-α-3,4-dihydroxyphenylalanine. Its structure is

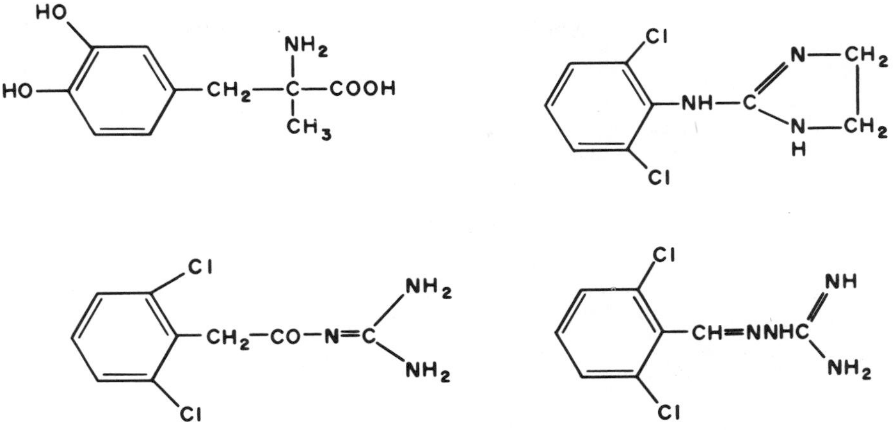

FIG. 3. Chemical structures of some centrally acting adrenoceptor agonists with antihypertensive activity: *Top left,* methyldopa; *top right,* clonidine; *bottom left,* guanfacine; *bottom right,* guanabenz.

shown in Fig. 3. The D isomer of methyldopa has no antihypertensive activity.

Most investigators agree that methyldopa lowers arterial pressure in patients with hypertension by reducing sympathetic tone. The precise mechanism of this effect is still a subject of controversy. Initially, the antihypertensive activity of methyldopa was attributed to the inhibition of aromatic amino acid decarboxylase (Fig. 4). Inhibition of this enzyme by methyldopa and other derivatives of phenylalanine was described by Sourkes (48). However, soon after the discovery of the antihypertensive action of methyldopa, it became apparent that the methyldopa-induced inhibition of decarboxylase does not correlate quantitatively with its antihypertensive activity. Although methyldopa reduces norepinephrine levels in various tissues, this depletion is not likely to result from inhibition of decarboxylase, because norepinephrine stores remain depleted for several days after dopamine levels return to normal.

Subsequently, an alternative "false-transmitter" hypothesis for the mechanism of the antihypertensive action of methyldopa was proposed. This was based on observations that methyldopa can form α-methyldopamine and α-methylnorepinephrine *in vitro* and *in vivo* (49). α-Methylnorepinephrine formed in the sympathetic nerve endings was believed to be used instead of norepinephrine as a false transmitter. It was assumed that α-methylnorepinephrine is a weaker vasoconstrictor, and therefore replacement of norepinephrine with α-methylnorepinephrine should lead to a reduction in sympathetic tone and consequently to a lowering of arterial pressure in hypertensive patients. The evidence against the false-transmitter hypothesis included observations that norepinephrine and α-methylnorepinephrine are equally potent as pressor agents in cats and rats and that there is no correlation between the time course of the hypotensive effect and the norepinephrine-replacing effect of methyldopa.

Still another hypothesis on the mechanism of the antihypertensive action of methyldopa was suggested by Holtz et al. (50), who proposed that α-methyldopamine, a relatively weaker α-adrenoceptor stimulant, is synthesized from methyldopa largely in the liver and reaches the α-adrenoceptors via the bloodstream to compete with endogenous norepinephrine at the receptor sites. This competition was thought to lead to a reduction in the sympathetic tone. In addition, α-methyldopamine forms a condensation product with β-hydroxyphenylacetaldehyde, which can be formed by oxidative deamination of tyramine

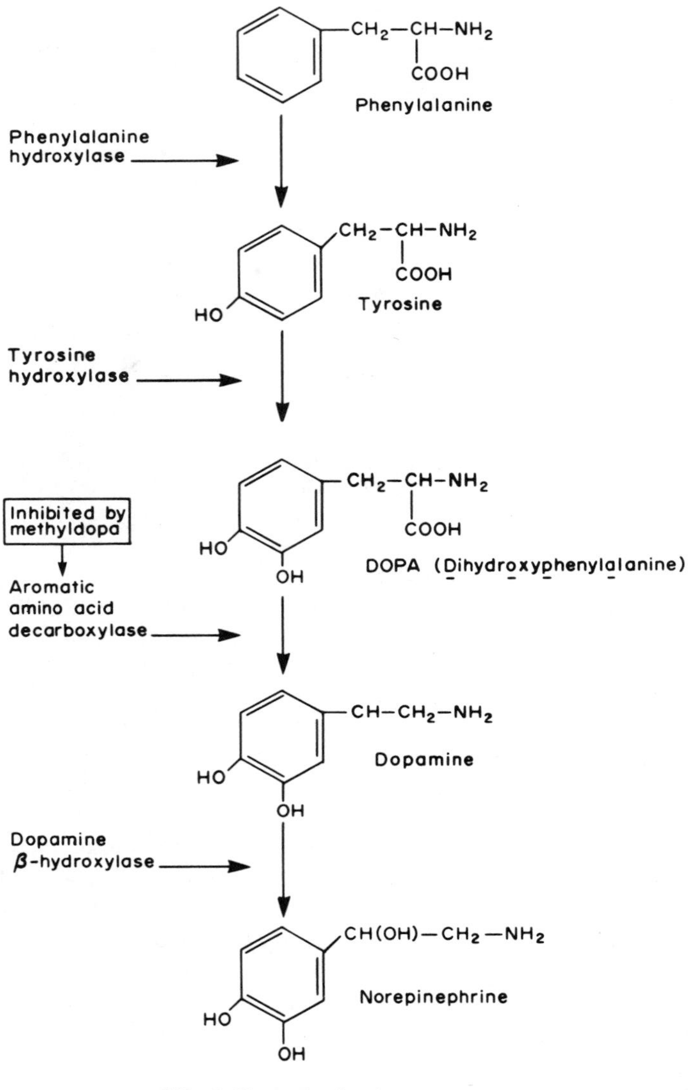

FIG. 4. Biosynthesis of norepinephrine.

by monoamine oxidase (MAO). This condensation product is 3-methyl-3'-deoxytetrahydropapaveroline, which is an effective β-adrenergic stimulant and may conceivably mediate the antihypertensive action of methyldopa. Further experimental evidence will be required before acceptance of this hypothesis.

The currently popular hypothesis involves the central nervous system (CNS) as the site of action for methyldopa. The idea was first proposed by Henning (51) and was based on

the observation that during slow infusion into the vertebral artery in the cat methyldopa produces gradual decreases in arterial pressure and brain norepinephrine levels, whereas cardiac norepinephrine levels remain unaffected; the D isomer of methyldopa has no hypotensive effect even by intravertebral administration. Further work by Henning revealed that the hypotensive effect of methyldopa in rats is inhibited by central, but not peripheral, inhibitors of decarboxylase. These findings suggest that the site of hypotensive action of methyldopa is likely to be central and that α-methylnorepinephrine may mediate the antihypertensive effect of methyldopa.

Methyldopa lowers arterial pressure in hypertensive animals. In spontaneously hypertensive rats of the Okamoto-Aoki strain, methyldopa is effective at 30 mg/kg p.o. and higher doses. In normotensive animals, methyldopa produces hypotension only at exceedingly high doses. The antihypertensive effects of methyldopa are associated with a reduction in the peripheral vascular resistance (52), with arterial and venous vasodilatation (53), and with a reduction in plasma renin activity (54).

Absorption of orally administered methyldopa can vary from 26 to 74% of the dose given (55). The peak plasma levels of methyldopa occur at 3 to 6 hr after oral treatment. Eighty to 90% of the oral dose is eliminated within 48 hr. The major urinary metabolites are methyldopa mono-*O*-sulfide and 3-methoxy methyldopa. The elimination of methyldopa is biphasic; the half-life of the first phase is approximately 2 hr and that of the second phase 7 to 16 hr.

Methyldopa is used in mild, moderate, or severe hypertension. Its use in mild hypertension is limited to patients resistant to thiazide diuretics. In moderate hypertension, methyldopa is often used in combination with thiazides. In severe hypertension, methyldopa alone may not control arterial pressure, and addition of an adrenergic neuron blocking drug, e.g., guanethidine, may be required.

The side effects of methyldopa include sedation, hepatotoxicity, positive Coombs' test, fever, and allergic skin reactions. "Rebound" hypertension, after withdrawal of methyldopa, was reported by two groups of investigators (56,57).

Clonidine

Clonidine is 2-(2,6-dichlorophenylamino)-2-imidazoline hydrochloride. Its chemical structure is shown in Fig. 3. Clonidine is an α-adrenoceptor stimulant and was therefore expected to produce vasoconstriction and to elevate arterial pressure. Its antihypertensive activity was discovered in humans while the drug was being evaluated for nasal decongestant activity. The mechanism of its antihypertensive action intrigued many investigators, and elucidation of the mechanism of antihypertensive action of clonidine led to the establishment of a new concept in autonomic pharmacology: a "feedback inhibition" of transmitter release by the transmitter itself or by drugs that mimic the effects of the transmitter. In the case of sympathetic nerve endings, norepinephrine, the transmitter, was shown to inhibit its own release by stimulation of presynaptic α-adrenoceptors, also known as α_2-adrenoceptors. These adrenoceptors are blocked preferentially by yohimbine, whereas postsynaptic (α_1) adrenoceptors are preferentially blocked by prazosin. Clonidine was shown to stimulate preferentially the presynaptic α-adrenoceptors and therefore to inhibit release of the transmitter. The site of antihypertensive activity of clonidine is believed to be primarily central. Interaction of clonidine with central adrenoceptors leads to reduction in the sympathetic tone. However, it is still controversial whether the antihypertensive effect of clonidine is primarily due to stimulation of central presynaptic or postsynaptic adrenoceptors (58,59).

In addition to the reduction in sympathetic tone, clonidine was shown to enhance vagal reflexes, e.g., cardiac slowing and reflex vasodilatation initiated by vasoconstriction. The enhancement of vagal tone is likely to play a contributory role in the mechanism of the antihypertensive action of clonidine.

Because of the complexity of the mechanism of the antihypertensive action of clonidine, the hemodynamic effects of clonidine are also complex and depend on the dose, route, and rate of administration. By rapid intravenous administration, clonidine, at a sufficiently high dose (e.g., 30 μg/kg), will initially increase arterial pressure and peripheral vascular resistance and lower cardiac output. After the initial pressor phase, clonidine will tend to lower arterial pressure, with peripheral vascular resistance returning to control or even below control levels. Cardiac output also returns to control levels while arterial pressure is still lowered.

In dogs, clonidine decreases cardiac output. The total peripheral vascular resistance is increased by clonidine initially, but it returns to control values during the hypotensive response (60).

Clonidine has sedative effects that are attributed to its α-adrenoceptor stimulant activity. Also, it has analgesic properties and antagonizes morphine withdrawal effects. The intraocular pressure is decreased by clonidine (61); this effect is probably mediated centrally.

The increase in blood glucose after clonidine was attributed to stimulation of α-adrenoceptors at the β cells of the pancreas and consequent reduction of insulin release (62). Clonidine inhibits the secretion of vasopressin and produces diuresis in rats (58). Salivary and gastric secretions (volume and acidity) are reduced by clonidine.

All species, including humans, degrade clonidine to the same metabolites, but to different extents. Degradation is greatest in the dog. The most important metabolites are p-hydroxyclonidine and dichlorophenylguanidine. Clonidine is almost completely absorbed after oral administration. Maximal blood levels of clonidine are reached within 1 hr after oral dosing. The drug is excreted predominantly in the urine; oral doses are excreted in 72 hr. The half-life of clonidine in humans is 7 to 13 hr.

Clonidine is effective in therapy for mild to severe hypertension (63,64). The drug was also used successfully in combination with diuretics (65) or prazosin (66). The major undesirable effect of clonidine is the withdrawal reaction following discontinuation of the therapy (67,68). The withdrawal reaction consists of a sudden rise in arterial pressure, nervousness, agitation, headache, and an increase in heart rate. The reaction is known to occur with other centrally acting antihypertensive agents, e.g., methyldopa, although the inci-

dence of the withdrawal reaction with clonidine appears to be higher. Other side effects of clonidine include dry mouth, drowsiness, sedation, and occasional orthostatic hypotension. The clinical dose of clonidine should be adjusted according to the patient response. It is recommended to start therapy with 0.1 mg. The total daily dose should not exceed 1 mg, although doses up to 2.4 mg/day have been given to humans.

Guanfacine

Guanfacine is N-amidino-2-(2,6-dichlorophenyl)acetamide hydrochloride (Fig. 3). Its mechanism of antihypertensive action is in some respects similar to that of clonidine. Guanfacine stimulates central α-adrenoceptors and inhibits sympathetic tone. In addition, guanfacine, like clonidine, interferes with the release of norepinephrine at sympathetic nerve endings and enhances vagally mediated reflexes (69,70). These effects of guanfacine are mediated by α-adrenoceptors and are antagonized by α-adrenoceptor antagonists.

Guanfacine differs from clonidine quantitatively as well as qualitatively. The relative potency of guanfacine is lower than that of clonidine. In humans, 7 to 10 times higher doses of guanfacine are required to produce the same antihypertensive effect as with clonidine. At the equivalent antihypertensive doses, the sedative effect of guanfacine is less pronounced in animals. The site of action of guanfacine in the CNS may differ from that for clonidine. Clonidine applied to the ventral surface of the medulla oblongata in cats lowers arterial pressure, but guanfacine is ineffective under the same experimental conditions (69). The turnover rate of dopamine in the rat brain is slowed by clonidine, but unaffected by guanfacine (71).

Guanfacine is rapidly and almost completely absorbed following oral administration. Its half-life in humans following oral doses is 21 hr, twice as long as that of clonidine. There is no evidence for a first-pass effect, and the oral bioavailability is 100%. The drug is primarily (80%) eliminated by urinary excretion. The principal metabolites in humans, rats, and dogs are the glucuronide and sulfate of 3-hydroxyguanfacine and the oxidized mercapturic acid derivatives of guanfacine (72).

Extensive clinical studies have been published on guanfacine (70,73,74). The results indicate that guanfacine is as effective as clonidine in the treatment of moderate to severe hypertension. The major side effects include occasional "withdrawal syndrome," dryness of mouth, sedation, orthostatic hypotension, and constipation. The incidence of side effects tends to diminish with chronic therapy.

Guanabenz

Guanabenz is the generic name for 2,6-dichlorobenzylidene aminoguanidine acetate (Fig. 3). Like clonidine and guanfacine, guanabenz is a centrally acting α-adrenoceptor stimulant. Guanabenz reduces sympathetic nerve activity (75,76) and central norepinephrine turnover (77) and displaces clonidine from binding sites in the rat cerebral cortex (78).

Unlike clonidine, guanabenz has no effect on baroreceptors. Following intravenous administration to animals, guanabenz produces a pressor effect that, according to Baum et al. (79), is not easily antagonized by α-adrenoceptor antagonists. The mechanism of the acute pressor effect of guanabenz may therefore be different from that of clonidine. According to Roller (80), the pressor effect of guanabenz may be similar to that of guanethidine and may involve the uptake of guanabenz into the neuronal storage sites and displacement of norepinephrine from these sites. Guanabenz lowers arterial pressure in various hypertensive models: renal-hypertensive, DOCA-hypertensive, and spontaneously hypertensive rats and renal-hypertensive dogs (81).

Extensive clinical studies have demonstrated the efficacy of guanabenz in the treatment of essential hypertension, either alone or in combination with thiazide diuretics (82–

86). The absence of any sodium or water retention with the drug is considered an important clinical advantage of guanabenz. Like clonidine or methyldopa, guanabenz lowers plasma renin activity in rats and humans. Guanabenz is used clinically at total daily doses up to 64 mg and divided doses up to 16 mg. The ideal regimen is not yet determined. The most common side effects of guanabenz are dry mouth, sedation, dizziness, weakness, and tiredness. According to one report (87), guanabenz produces a "withdrawal syndrome" consisting of nervousness, palpitation, diaphoresis, and insomnia.

Ganglionic Blocking Drugs

The side effects of ganglionic blocking drugs include inhibition of gastric and salivary secretion, impotence, postural hypotension, and inhibition of vasomotor reflexes. In view of the availability of other antihypertensive drugs with lesser side effects, the use of ganglionic blocking drugs in the treatment of hypertension cannot be further recommended, and most have been withdrawn from the market. The remaining important indication for ganglionic blockade is "controlled hypotension" to reduce bleeding in surgery. Blood loss is reduced by ganglionic blocking drugs as a result of reduction in cardiac output as well as reduction in arterial pressure. Vessel surgery is facilitated by decreased vessel tension (88).

The ganglionic blocking drug of choice for "controlled hypotension" is trimethaphan camsylate. The duration of action of trimethaphan is short, and the drug is given primarily by infusion. Its pharmacology was described by Randall et al. (89). In addition to ganglionic blocking action, trimethaphan has histamine-releasing effects (90), direct vasodilator effects (91), and neuromuscular blocking effects (92).

Reserpine

Reserpine, an alkaloid from *Rauwolfia serpentina* (93), is still widely used, particularly in combination with other antihypertensive drugs. Reserpine depletes the transmitters from adrenergic, dopaminergic, and serotonergic neurons (94). Depletion of peripheral adrenergic nerve endings of norepinephrine is believed to be primarily responsible for the antihypertensive action of reserpine (95). Depletion of monoamine-containing CNS neurons may also contribute to the antihypertensive action of the drug. Reserpine depletes monoamines by inhibiting their storage; it is believed to attach itself irreversibly to the carrier sites at the membrane of the storage granules.

Reserpine lowers arterial pressure in normotensive animals, but it is more active in hypertensive animals (96,97). The onset of the antihypertensive action of reserpine is slow, the effect being seen at 2 to 3 hr following parenteral administration, with the maximal effect at 12 to 18 hr. Cardiac output and peripheral vascular resistance usually are reduced by reserpine. After prolonged therapy, cardiac output returns to control levels, but peripheral resistance remains reduced.

Reserpine has pronounced sedative and tranquilizing effects. This depressive reaction is its major side effect. A single dose of reserpine releases ACTH. Repeated administration of reserpine depletes the pituitary ACTH stores and abolishes the release of ACTH in response to stressful stimuli (98). Reserpine is also known to inhibit the release of thyroxine (99), gonadotropin, and ovarian estrogen (100,101). The release of prolactin is increased by reserpine, apparently because of depression of dopamine release (102). The increase in prolactin release led to the suspicion (supported by retrospective studies) of possible association between reserpine intake and breast cancer in women (103,104). The carcinogenic activity of reserpine was not confirmed by further studies (105).

Reserpine is well absorbed following oral administration. The peak plasma levels are achieved at 2 to 3 hr after an oral dose (106). The plasma concentration of ^{3}H-reserpine was found to decline, with two biological half-lives

of 4.5 and 271 hr (107). The major metabolites of reserpine, methylreserpate and trimethoxybenzoic acid, are products of hydrolytic cleavage. Trimethoxybenzoic acid forms glucuronide as well as sulfate conjugates (108). Animal studies indicate that reserpine metabolites are excreted predominantly in the urine (109–111). In humans, the major portion of radioactivity after ^{3}H-reserpine was found in feces (107).

In the treatment of essential hypertension, reserpine is used preferably in combination with thiazide diuretics. Such combinations are considered effective in almost all cases of mild hypertension and in most patients with moderate hypertension (112). The side effects of reserpine severely limit its usefulness. Reserpine can produce depression, impotence, weight gain, fluid retention, peptic ulcers, gastrointestinal hemorrhage, diarrhea, and nasal congestion. The reserpine-induced depression is antagonized by tricyclic antidepressants.

ADRENERGIC NEURON BLOCKING AGENTS

Adrenergic neuron blocking agents act at the sympathetic nerve terminals to prevent release of the transmitter, without inhibiting the interaction of the transmitter with the receptors. At the parasympathetic nerve endings they produce only slight and transient blockade of transmitter release; they largely lack, therefore, the side effects associated with blockade of the parasympathetic nervous system. The first and the most widely used adrenergic neuron blocking agent is guanethidine. Other drugs with similar pharmacological profiles include bethanidine (113), guanisoquin (114), debrisoquine (115), and guanacline (116).

Guanethidine

Guanethidine (Fig. 5) inhibits the release and uptake of norepinephrine by the nerve terminals. The consequence of this effect is

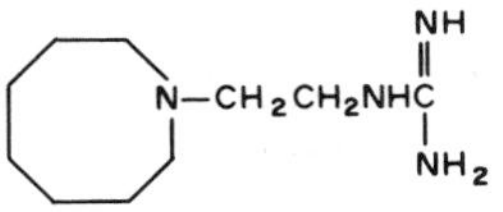

FIG. 5. Guanethidine.

depletion of norepinephrine stores in the sympathetic nerve terminals. After guanethidine, the vasoconstrictor nerves do not provide reflex compensation to the erect position. The hypotensive response to the drug is therefore largely orthostatic.

Guanethidine is taken up by adrenergic neurons and stored by the same process and in the same granules as norepinephrine. Subsequently, the drug is released from the granules by nerve stimulation. It acts, therefore, also as a false transmitter. Guanethidine produces a transient sympathomimetic effect that is usually seen following intravenous administration of the drug. This effect is attributed to the release of catecholamines from the adrenergic nerve endings (117). Guanethidine also has direct vasodilator action on vascular smooth muscle. This effect can be demonstrated in animals after pretreatment with reserpine (118). Reserpine converts the usual positive inotropic effect of guanethidine to a negative inotropic effect (119). At the neuromuscular junction, guanethidine exerts a postjunctional blocking action similar to that of d-tubocurarine (120). Guanethidine also has a delayed depressant effect on the contractile response of skeletal muscle to direct stimulation (121). This delayed effect is different from the acute curare-like action and probably is responsible for the occasional muscle weakness observed in patients receiving guanethidine.

In humans, guanethidine acutely decreases heart rate and lowers cardiac output, with little or no effect on peripheral vascular resistance (122,123). Chronic therapy with guanethidine leads to reductions in peripheral vascular resistance and in heart rate, with little or no effect on cardiac output (124,125).

Guanethidine is excreted slowly; 36% of a dose is recovered from the urine in 72 hr following oral administration and 72% follow-

ing intravenous administration (126). Two metabolites of guanethidine have been identified as 2-(6-carboxyhexylamino)ethylguanidine and guanethidine-N-oxide (126). Both metabolites have antihypertensive activity, but in animals they are only 1/30 as potent as guanethidine (127). According to McMartin et al. (126), 90% of radioactivity was accounted for as guanethidine and the two metabolites following administration of labeled guanethidine to patients.

Guanethidine is used in the treatment of severe hypertension. The starting dosage is 12.5 to 25 mg once a day; this can be slowly increased to 150 or even 400 mg/day. The side effects include orthostatic hypotension (which can lead to dizziness or syncope), Na^+ and water retention, failure of ejaculation without loss of potency, diarrhea, tenderness in the region of the parotid glands, and muscle weakness. The antihypertensive effect of guanethidine can be antagonized by tricyclic antidepressants, amphetamine, or ephedrine.

α-ADRENOCEPTOR ANTAGONISTS

Attempts to use older α-adrenoceptor antagonists, e.g., phenoxybenzamine or phentolamine, were disappointing in the treatment of hypertension. Tachycardia, which was attributed to a reflex increase in sympathetic activity, and rapidly developing tolerance limited the effectiveness of these drugs. Combinations of α and β antagonists have had varying degrees of success in the treatment of hypertension (128–130). Interest in the use of α-adrenoceptor antagonists in hypertension was revived with the discoveries of prazosin (131) and indoramin (132). These drugs are selective postsynaptic α-adrenoceptor antagonists. The relative ineffectiveness of older α-adrenoceptor antagonists may have been due to their presynaptic action, because blockade of presynaptic α-adrenoceptors can be expected to lead to greater release of norepinephrine from the sympathetic nerve endings and, therefore, oppose their antihypertensive actions.

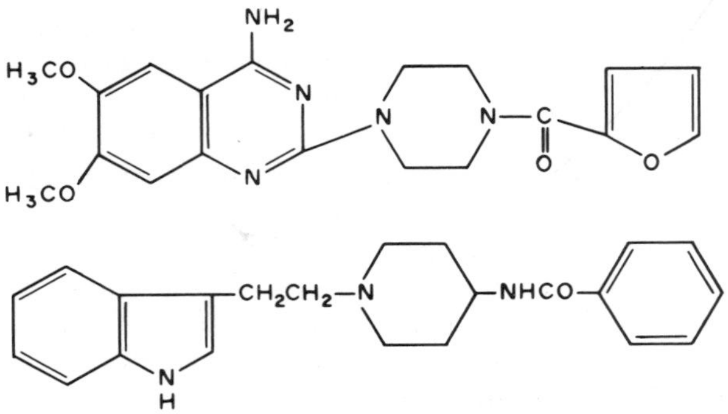

FIG. 6. Chemical structures of selective α_1-adrenoceptor antagonists with antihypertensive activity: *top,* prazosin; *bottom,* indoramin.

Prazosin

The antihypertensive activity of prazosin (Fig. 6) was discovered during a search for novel vasodilator drugs (131,133). It was noted in early pharmacological studies that prazosin has α-adrenoceptor antagonist activity that is not associated with tachycardia. The selectivity of prazosin for postsynaptic adrenoceptors was observed in rabbit pulmonary artery (134), pithed rat (135), and isolated rat vas deferens (136), and at the cardiac sympathetic nerve endings of the dog, prazosin also inhibits presynaptic adrenoceptors (137,138). Unlike phentolamine, prazosin does not antagonize the vasoconstrictor effects of 5-hydroxytryptamine (5HT) (139). In anesthetized dogs, prazosin lowers arterial pressure and peripheral vascular resistance, whereas cardiac output and left ventricular maximum *dp/dt* are increased (133,140).

In patients with essential hypertension, prazosin either increases or does not change cardiac output (141,142). Prazosin dilates veins as well as arteries, and venous pooling is believed to precede prazosin-induced arterial vasodilation. A consistent decrease in peripheral vascular resistance, even after long-term therapy, differentiates prazosin from other antihypertensive agents (e.g., methyldopa, clonidine). In hypertensive patients, prazosin either reduces or causes no change in plasma renin activity (141–143).

Prazosin is well absorbed when taken orally, rapidly distributed in the tissues, and exten-

sively metabolized. The plasma half-life of prazosin in humans is estimated at 2.4 hr. The major metabolites of prazosin are 6-*O*-demethylprazosin and 7-*O*-demethylprazosin; they are excreted as glucuronide conjugates.

Comparative clinical studies have indicated that prazosin at 3.5 to 7.5 mg/day is comparable in antihypertensive activity to methyldopa at 750 mg/day or propranolol at 120 to 160 mg/day (144). Prazosin is used successfully in combination with thiazide diuretics or with β-adrenoceptor antagonists (145,146).

The major side effect of prazosin is the "first-dose phenomenon"—severe initial hypotension associated with syncope. This effect is believed to be due to selective blockade of visceral sympathetic activity (147). Patients on a low-sodium diet (100 mM) appear to be more likely to develop this phenomenon (148). The syncope can be largely avoided if the initial dose of prazosin is kept low (0.5–1 mg) and the drug is given before retiring. It is recommended that the initial dosage of prazosin be maintained for 2 weeks, then followed by gradually increasing dosage (149,150). Other side effects of prazosin include increased frequency of urination, an anticholinergic effect, and an increase in the frequency of anginal attacks (151–153).

Indoramin

Indoramin, 3-[2-(4-benzamidopiperidilyl)-ethyl]indole (Fig. 6) is primarily a postsynaptic α_1-adrenoceptor antagonist useful in the treatment of hypertension (132,154). In anesthetized animals, indoramin lowers arterial pressure and reduces heart rate. On isolated rabbit aorta, indoramin is a potent α_1 antagonist with a pA_2 value of 7.4. It is also a potent H_1 receptor antagonist on guinea pig ileum, with a pA_2 value of 8.2. In addition to peripheral α_1-adrenoceptor antagonism, indoramin has a central component of antihypertensive action. At 5 mg/kg i.v. indoramin was found to decrease spontaneous activity recorded in the splanchnic, cardiac, and renal nerves (155–157).

Clinical studies with indoramin in patients with essential hypertension at dosages ranging from 20 to 150 mg/day demonstrated its antihypertensive activity, with sedation being the major side effect (158,159).

β-ADRENOCEPTOR ANTAGONISTS

β-Adrenoceptor antagonists are now well accepted in therapy for hypertension and are recommended even as the first-step approach (160,161). The major reason for their acceptance is their relative freedom from side effects, particularly orthostatic hypotension and sexual disturbances. Alone, β-adrenoceptor antagonists do not produce satisfactory lowering of arterial pressure in the majority of patients. In combination with diuretics, however, they control arterial pressure in over 80% of patients. β-Adrenoceptor antagonists are known to antagonize certain side effects of thiazide diuretics, e.g., the increase in plasma renin activity and hypokalemia; these are additional benefits of combined therapy.

The mechanism of antihypertensive action of β-adrenoceptor antagonists is still controversial. Various hypotheses have been critically reviewed (160). β-Adrenoceptor antagonists have been suggested to lower arterial pressure by various mechanisms: a centrally induced reduction in sympathetic nerve activity, a decrease in cardiac output, resetting of baroreceptors, a reduction in renin release, presynaptic inhibition of sympathetic transmission at the peripheral sympathetic nerve endings, a decrease in enzymatic activity in the sympathetic ganglia, or "restoration" of

vascular relaxant activity. The central action leading to reduction in sympathetic tone and/ or the peripheral presynaptic inhibition at sympathetic nerve endings are the more likely mechanisms of the antihypertensive action of β-adrenoceptor antagonists.

More recently, Tackett et al. (162) demonstrated that propranolol produces a dose-dependent increase in cerebrospinal fluid norepinephrine and that propranolol-induced hypotension is antagonized by intracisternally administered phentolamine. These investigators concluded that propranolol and probably other β-adrenoceptor antagonists release norepinephrine centrally and that their antihypertensive effect is mediated by stimulation of central α-adrenoceptors and a consequent decrease in sympathetic tone.

There are at present approximately 100 β-adrenoceptor antagonists available for sale in various countries or in various stages of evaluation in animal and clinical studies. The scope of this chapter does not permit a comprehensive review of all of them. The discussion will therefore be limited to β-adrenoceptor antagonists approved for sale in the United States and to a few additional drugs with distinctly different pharmacological profiles.

β-Adrenoceptor antagonists differ from one another in potency, cardioselectivity, intrinsic sympathomimetic activity (ISA), membrane-stabilizing action (MSA), lipophilicity, duration of action, tissue distribution, and metabolism. There are at least two types of β-adrenoceptors: β_1 cardiac and β_2 vascular. The nonselective β-adrenoceptor antagonists and β_1-selective antagonists are antihypertensive. β_2-selective antagonists (e.g., butoxamine) have no antihypertensive activity.

Table 3 summarizes the pharmacological differences between the β-adrenoceptor antagonists to be discussed next. The "yes" and "no" statements represent relative judgments and refer to activities at therapeutic doses or slightly higher than therapeutic doses.

Propranolol

The chemical name for propranolol is 1-isopropylamino-3-(1-naphthyloxy)propan-2-ol

TABLE 3. *Characterization of β-adrenoceptor antagonists*

Generic Name	Chemical Structure	β_1 (cardiac) Selectivity	ISA Intrinsic Sympathomimetic Activity	MSA Membrane Stabilizing Action
Propranolol	$OCH_2CHCH_2NHCH(CH_3)_2$ OH (naphthalene ring)	No	No	Yes
Metoprolol	OH $OCH_2CHCH_2NHCH(CH_3)_2$ $CH_2CH_2OCH_3$	Yes	No	No
Nadolol	OH OH OH $O-CH_2-CH-CH_2NHC(CH_3)_3$	No	No	No

TABLE 3. (continued)

Generic Name	Chemical Structure	β_1(cardiac) Selectivity	ISA Intrinsic Sympathomimetic Activity	MSA Membrane Stabilizing Action
Pindolol	$OCH_2CHCH_2NHCH(CH_3)_2$, OH (indole ring)	No	Yes	Weak
Timolol	$OCH_2CHCH_2NHC(CH_3)_3$, OH (morpholine–thiadiazole ring)	No	No	Weak
Acebutolol	$O-CH_2-CH-CH_2-NH-CH$ ... OH, CH_3, CH_3, $CO-CH_3$, $HN-CO-CH_2-CH_2-CH_3$	Yes	Yes	Yes
Labetalol	$CHCH_2NHCH-CH_2CH_2$, OH, CH_3, H_2NOC, HO (phenyl ring)	No	Weak	Yes

hydrochloride. Propranolol is the most widely used β antagonist. It is marketed as the racemic mixture of two isomers. The β-adrenoceptor antagonist activity resides in the (+)-isomer.

Propranolol has no intrinsic sympathomimetic activity and is nonselective with respect to its effects at β_1-adrenoceptors in comparison to β_2-adrenoceptors. The β_2-adrenoceptor antagonist activity of propranolol leads to increased bronchial tone; this effect is clinically significant in asthmatic patients. Propranolol and other non-β_1-selective antagonists are therefore contraindicated in patients with bronchial asthma.

Following acute intravenous administration to animals or humans, propranolol reduces heart rate, cardiac output, mean arterial pressure, and left ventricular work (161). Left ventricular maximum dp/dt, velocity of fiber shortening, and coronary, renal, and splanchnic blood flows are also reduced by propranolol. Propranolol-induced cardiac slowing is maintained with chronic oral administration, whereas peripheral vascular resistance is first elevated but subsequently becomes reduced (163). Plasma renin activity is consistently reduced by propranolol. It is currently controversial whether or not reduction in plasma renin activity determines the antihypertensive activity of propranolol (164,165).

Propranolol produces membrane stabilization, which is unspecific in nature and results in local anesthesia as well as cardiac depression. Membrane stabilization is observed at concentrations higher than those required for β-adrenoceptor blocking activity.

In humans, propranolol is rapidly and completely absorbed from the gastrointestinal tract. Peak plasma levels are obtained at 90 to 120 min after oral administration of the drug. The plasma half-life of propranolol is about 3.9 hr. The metabolic pathway of propranolol in humans is similar to that in dogs or rats. A total of 16 metabolites of propranolol have been identified. The major metabolites are N-desisopropylpropranolol; 4-hydroxypropranolol, and naphthoxylacetic acid.

The average dosage of propranolol in the treatment of hypertension is 100 to 320 mg daily in four divided doses. If a satisfactory response is not obtained, a thiazide diuretic or a vasodilator is added (166,167). A slow-release preparation of propranolol was shown to control arterial pressure when given once daily (168).

The side effects of propranolol (bradycardia, A-V heart block, and cardiac failure) are dependent on the sympathetic tone and are more severe in patients with high sympathetic activity. In patients with asthma, propranolol can produce severe bronchospasms. α-Adrenergic vasoconstriction can be enhanced by propranolol and can lead to cold extremities or Raynaud's phenomenon. Propranolol can enhance hypoglycemia and produce fatigue, gastrointestinal disturbances, vivid dreams, and hallucinations.

Metoprolol

Metoprolol was the second β-adrenoceptor antagonist approved for clinical use in the United States. It differs from propranolol primarily in relative selectivity for β_1-adrenoceptors and in the absence of membrane-stabilizing action. As a consequence of its selectivity for β_1-adrenoceptors, metoprolol has relatively little effect on bronchial smooth muscle. As a β_1-adrenoceptor antagonist, metoprolol is equipotent with propranolol. The pressor effect of epinephrine is enhanced by propranolol to a greater extent than by metoprolol. This is explained by the relative inability of metoprolol to block β_2-adrenoceptors in vascular smooth muscle. The differences between propranolol and metoprolol have also been demonstrated clinically. Metoprolol reduces skin temperature to a lesser extent than does propranolol (169). An important difference between metoprolol and propranolol is that propranolol-treated patients respond to vascular hypoglycemia with a marked increase in arterial pressure and bradycardia. This effect is not seen with metoprolol. In diabetic patients, a change from propranolol to metoprolol can lead to an improvement in glucose tolerance. Unlike nonselective β antagonists, metoprolol does not prolong the duration of the hypoglycemic response to insulin (170–172). Metoprolol is less effective than propranolol as an inhibitor of FFA release (173). The capacity of healthy human subjects to perform physical exercise is reduced less by metoprolol than by propranolol, possibly because of lesser reduction in the skeletal-muscle blood flow (174).

Metoprolol is completely absorbed when given by the oral route in humans, dogs, and rats. The bioavailability of metoprolol in humans is higher than in the two animal species and can reach 70% if the drug is given together with a meal. The half-life of metoprolol is 3 to 4 hr in humans and 1.5 hr in dogs. Metoprolol is extensively metabolized; the major metabolic pathways include O-demethylation, followed by oxidation, oxidative deamination, and aliphatic hydroxylation. Some of the metoprolol metabolites have β_1-adrenoceptor antagonist activity, but they are considerably less potent than metoprolol (175,176).

As an antihypertensive in humans, metoprolol is at least as effective as nonselective β-adrenoceptor antagonists. At daily doses of 150 to 300 mg, metoprolol is as effective as hydrochlorothiazide at 50 to 100 mg. The reported side effects of metoprolol are mild and include shortness of breath, heartburn, nausea, tiredness, and depression. Their incidence is not significantly different from that reported for placebo. Sudden withdrawal of metoprolol can cause malaise, palpitations, headache, and tremor (177). Slow withdrawal of metoprolol is recommended over a 10-day period.

Nadolol

Nadolol is a 2,3-*cis*-1,2,3,4-tetrahydro-5-[(2-hydroxy-3-*tert*-butylamino)propoxy]-2,3-naphthalenediol. It is not cardioselective and has no ISA and no MSA (Table 3). The duration of the β-adrenoceptor blocking action of nadolol in dogs is four to five times longer

than that of propranolol (178). Unlike propranolol, nadolol increases renal blood flow in dogs and humans (179,180).

Only 20 to 34% of an oral dose of nadolol is absorbed in humans (181). Unlike other β-adrenoceptor antagonists, nadolol is not metabolized. Its half-life is 16 to 17 hr (182).

As an antihypertensive, nadolol at 40 to 240 mg once a day is as effective as propranolol in the treatment of hypertension (183). It is conceivable that the renal vasodilator effects and the absence of MSA represent clinical advantages of the drug. The side effects of nadolol are typical for a nonselective β-adrenoceptor antagonist.

Pindolol

Pindolol, 4-(2-hydroxy-3-isopropylaminopropoxy)indole, is not cardioselective; it has only a weak MSA, but a relatively strong ISA (Table 3). In spite of the strong ISA component in humans, pindolol produces no tachycardia at clinical doses (184,185). The strong ISA component is probably responsible for a relatively lesser bradycardia with pindolol than with most other β-adrenoceptor antagonists (186). The ISA may also tend to antagonize cardiac conduction disturbances associated with β-adrenoceptor blockade (187,188), and bronchoconstriction, leading to lesser impairment in pulmonary function than with propranolol (189).

Pindolol is rapidly and nearly completely absorbed from the gastrointestinal tract. Unlike other β antagonists, pindolol has only a slight (13%) first-pass effect. Sixty percent of pindolol is metabolized in the liver, and 40% is excreted unchanged by the kidney (190). The plasma half-life of pindolol in humans is 3 to 4 hr. The usual clinical dosage of pindolol is 10 to 30 mg/day. The side effects of pindolol are similar to those of other β-adrenoceptor antagonists, but peripheral circulatory problems are less common with pindolol than with propranolol (191). Commonly seen CNS effects are insomnia and vivid dreams.

Timolol

Timolol is the (−)-isomer of 3-(3-*tert*-butylamino-2-hydroxypropoxy)-4-morpholino-1,2,5-thiadiazole. Timolol is not cardioselective, has no ISA, and is considerably less negative-inotropic than propranolol (192). As a β-adrenoceptor antagonist, timolol is 5 to 10 times more potent than propranolol (192). In comparison with propranolol, timolol is less lipophilic, has less effect on the CNS, and has lesser affinity for central 5HT receptors. The absence of a local anesthetic action makes timolol particularly useful in therapy for glaucoma (193–196).

Timolol is rapidly absorbed and metabolized. The plasma half-life of timolol in humans is 5.5 hr. The major metabolites have been identified as 1-*tert*-butylamino[4-(*N*-2-hydroxyethylglycolamido)-1,2,5-thiadiazol-3-yloxy]-2-propanol and 1-*tert*-butylamino-3-[4-(2-hydroxyethylamino)-1,2,5-thiadiazol-3-yloxy]-2-propanol. These metabolites have no or only weak β-adrenoceptor antagonist activity.

Clinical studies indicate that timolol and propranolol have comparable antihypertensive activities when timolol is used at 30 mg/day and propranolol at 120 mg/day (197). Hemodynamic studies with both drugs in humans suggest that the left ventricular ejection rate index after an initial decrease returns to control levels during timolol therapy but not during propranolol therapy (198). The reported side effects of timolol include tiredness, dizziness, increase in body weight, and occasional increases in serum urea and creatinine.

In a recent double-blind study in Norway (199), timolol was shown to prolong life and to reduce the reinfarction rate among patients who survived myocardial infarction. This study justified the use of timolol in patients with myocardial infarction.

Acebutolol

Acebutolol is cardioselective and has ISA and MSA. As a β_1-adrenoceptor antagonist, acebutolol is one-fifth to one-tenth as potent as propranolol (200,201). The ISA is seen with acebutolol only at doses two to three times higher than those required for β-adrenoceptor antagonism.

After acute intravenous administration, the plasma half-life of acebutolol is 3.1 hr. The major metabolite is diacetolol: *RS*-1-(2-acetyl-4-acetylamidophenoxy)-2-hydroxy-3-isopropylamino propane (202–205). The plasma levels of diacetolol following subacute or chronic administration of acebutolol exceed those of acebutolol by two to three times. Diacetolol has β-adrenoceptor antagonist activity similar to that of acebutolol, but little or no MSA.

Acebutolol is active in the treatment of hypertension in 200- to 800-mg doses. Acebutolol is usually given two or three times a day, but an adequate effect can be obtained with a single dose of the drug (206,207). Like other β-adrenoceptor antagonists, acebutolol is contraindicated in patients with bradycardia or A-V conduction disorders.

Labetalol

Labetalol differs from most β-adrenoceptor antagonists by exhibiting α-adrenoceptor antagonist properties as well. Chemically, labetalol is 2-hydroxy-5-[1-hydroxy-2-(1-methyl-3-phenylpropyl)aminoethyl]benzamide hydrochloride. It exists as a mixture of four stereoisomers. Labetalol is more potent as a β-adrenoceptor antagonist than as an α-adrenoceptor antagonist. β_1-Adrenoceptors and β_2-adrenoceptors are blocked to similar extents by labetalol. Labetalol elevates transmitter outflow at the sympathetic nerve endings by blocking uptake, rather than through an action at presynaptic α-adrenoceptors (208–210). Labetalol has weak ISA at β_1- and β_2-adrenoceptors (211). It also has MSA (212).

Labetalol releases norepinephrine in certain tissues (213). The effectiveness of labetalol in antagonizing the effects of sympathetic stimulation depends on the balance of α- and β-

adrenoceptor antagonist activities, as well as on its effects on norepinephrine uptake and release.

Like propranolol, labetalol reduces heart rate, cardiac contractile force, and cardiac output (208). It has no effect on peripheral vascular resistance at low doses, but it decreases peripheral resistance at high doses. Labetalol lowers arterial pressure in most antihypertensive models, including spontaneously hypertensive rats, renal-hypertensive dogs, and DOCA-hypertensive rats. Larger doses of labetalol are required to lower arterial pressure in rats as compared with dogs.

In humans, labetalol reduces blood pressure without any significant effect on resting heart rate or on cardiac output (214,215). In hypertensive patients, labetalol is effective at daily doses ranging from 75 to 3,200 mg (216). No tolerance to the drug has been observed in patients receiving the drug for over 6 years (217).

Peak plasma concentrations of labetalol are observed in humans at 1 to 2 hr after a single oral dose. Labetalol experiences considerable first-pass metabolism. The drug is well absorbed when given orally, but it is converted to inactive metabolites, primarily glucuronides, in the gastrointestinal tract and liver (218). The plasma half-life of the drug in humans is 4 hr.

At higher doses, labetalol can produce postural hypotension typical for α-adrenoceptor antagonists (216,219). Heart failure and asthma are uncommon with labetalol. Tiredness, dizziness, upper gastrointestinal symptoms, sexual problems, and scalp tingling have been reported in patients receiving labetalol.

DIRECTLY ACTING SMOOTH-MUSCLE RELAXANTS

Sodium Nitroprusside

Sodium nitroprusside is an organic salt, $Na_2Fe(CN)_5NO\cdot2H_2O$, with a hydrated molecular weight of 297.95. Nitroprusside is readily soluble in water, but it decomposes in light when in solution. Because nitroprusside is not absorbed from the gastrointestinal tract, it must be given by systemic infusion.

Nitroprusside exerts a vasodilatory effect on both the arterial and venous sides of the vasculature. Infusion of sodium nitroprusside at 1 to 100 μg/kg/min produces a uniform fall in systolic and diastolic blood pressure. The onset of action is usually rapid (<60 sec) and well maintained, but some attenuation has been reported in dogs (220). Recovery of blood pressure is rapid following cessation of drug infusion (221). This most likely is the result of rapid cellular degradation of nitroprusside. Because of this rapid degradation, the magnitude of the hypotensive response to nitroprusside can be controlled easily by varying the rate of infusion. Tolerance to repeated nitroprusside infusions occurs rarely (222).

The fall in blood pressure is accompanied by reflex changes in heart rate. The magnitude and direction of change are variable in the anesthetized animal and most likely are affected by the level of anesthesia (220). In conscious animals, nitroprusside produces dose-related tachycardia (223,224). Heart rate increases usually are attenuated, but not abolished, by β-adrenoceptor antagonists. This suggests that the tachycardia is the result of not only sympathetic activation but also parasympathetic withdrawal.

Total peripheral vascular resistance and central venous pressure are decreased during nitroprusside infusion. Blood flow is initially elevated by nitroprusside in coronary, mesenteric, femoral, and renal vascular beds. On continuous infusion, blood flow tends to normalize in all but the renal vascular bed (220). Increases in renal flow do not appear to augment renal function, as determined by p-aminohippuric acid and inulin clearance (225). Coronary flow may decrease during episodes of marked hypotension (226).

Left ventricular end-diastolic pressure and peak systolic pressure are reduced and left ventricular maximum dp/dt and cardiac output are increased by nitroprusside. These changes in cardiac function are results of the pronounced dilatation of venous and arterial vasculature as well as concomitant reflex changes in neural outflow to the heart (220). Cardiac work usually is reduced by nitroprusside (227).

The vasodilatory effects of nitroprusside do not involve α- or β-adrenoceptors (228) or inhibition of norepinephrine release (229). Also, nitroprusside will relax aortic strips that have been contracted by angiotensin II or vasopressin; it does not affect contractions induced by potassium (228) or ouabain (227). Nitroprusside produces hyperpolarization of up to 12 mV in rabbit pulmonary artery (230) and decreases membrane resistance (R_m) to about 60% of control (230). The hyperpolarization coupled with a decreased R_m suggests that nitroprusside is altering potassium conductance. However, $^{42}K^+$ efflux from norepinephrine-stimulated aorta is decreased by nitroprusside (231).

Nitroprusside does not increase vascular smooth-muscle cAMP, but does elevate levels of cGMP (231). An analogue of cGMP, 8-bromo-cGMP also relaxes rat aorta (232). Agents that prevent the release of the NO moiety by nitroprusside prevent not only the relaxant effects but also the increases in cGMP in isolated coronary artery (233). Cyanide is an intermediate degradation product of nitroprusside that is rapidly metabolized to thiocyanate. Cyanide can abolish nitroprusside-induced elevations of cGMP (234) and the relaxant effects on vascular smooth muscle (235–237).

Diazoxide

Diazoxide, 7-chloro-1,2,4-benzothiadiazine-3-methyl-1,1-dioxide, is chemically related to chlorothiazide and other benzothiadiazines (Fig. 7).

At intravenous doses of 2 to 10 mg/kg, diazoxide reduces blood pressure for periods of 0.5 to 4 hr. The hypotensive effects are not antagonized by agents that interfere with sympathetic, parasympathetic, or ganglionic transmission (238). Following oral administration, diazoxide at a dose of 5 mg/kg lowers arterial pressure in hypertensive dogs. Maximal antihypertensive effects require at least 2 to 5 days to develop. Oral antihypertensive efficacy is also observed in DOCA-hypertensive (239) and renal-hypertensive (238) rats.

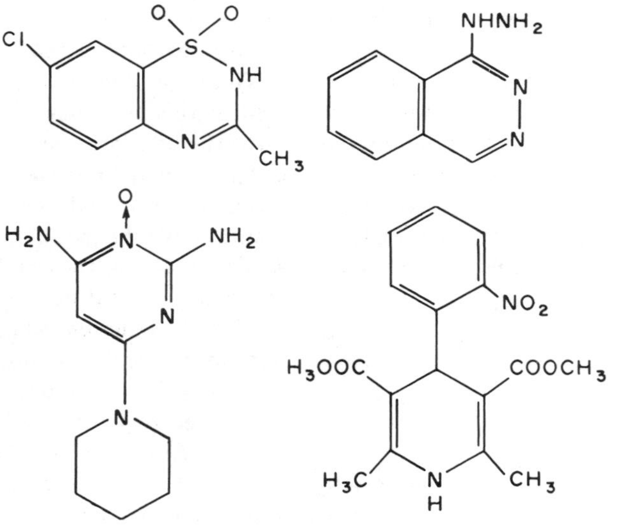

FIG. 7. Chemical structures of some directly acting smooth-muscle relaxants: *Top left,* diazoxide; *top right,* hydralazine; *bottom left,* minoxidil; *bottom right,* nifedipine.

Total peripheral vascular resistance is decreased during diazoxide-induced hypotension; cardiac output and stroke volume are increased. Blood flow is increased in coronary vascular beds and decreased in renal and splanchnic vascular beds (240). Following intraarterial administration, diazoxide elicits increases in femoral, renal, and coronary blood flow in dogs (238). Diazoxide produces little or no change in venous tone at doses that induce arterial dilatation (241).

In humans, heart rate and left ventricular maximum dp/dt are increased during diazoxide-induced hypotension. Left ventricular systolic and end-diastolic pressures are decreased by diazoxide. It has been found that β blockade attenuates the elevations in heart rate and left ventricular dp/dt, but augments the diazoxide-induced reduction in left ventricular systolic pressure (242). Right atrial pressure usually is elevated by diazoxide (243).

Most studies on its mechanism of action suggest that the major effect of diazoxide is mediated through a direct action on arterial smooth muscle. However, a portion of the vasodilatory effects may be attributed to α-adrenergic receptor inhibition (239,244–246) or quite possibly to β-adrenergic receptor activation (247). Diazoxide competitively blocks Ca^{2+}- and Ba^{2+}-induced contractions of aortic strips (248–250). Furthermore, inhibition appears to reside in the membrane-potential-dependent channel involved in the excitation-contraction coupling (251). Alternatively, diazoxide may produce dilatation by increasing levels of cAMP (252).

Although diazoxide is chemically related to the diuretic agent chlorothiazide, it possesses no diuretic activity. Diazoxide causes Na^+ and water retention that can be related to changes in vascular resistance (253). Diazoxide elevates plasma renin activity (254,255). Plasma renin elevations are correlated to the decreases in arterial pressure, plasma Na^+, or $U_{Na}V$. Diazoxide stimulates renin secretion following direct application in isolated perfused rat kidneys (257).

Hyperglycemia is observed during diazoxide therapy. This effect is attenuated by propranolol (258) and chlorisondamine (259,260). Diazoxide-induced hyperglycemia occurs also in alloxan-diabetic rats (261) and is related inversely to plasma K^+ levels (262). The propensity of diazoxide to cause hyperglycemia and Na^+ and fluid retention has restricted the clinical use of diazoxide to acute life-threatening hypertensive emergencies.

Minoxidil

Minoxidil, 2,4-diamino-6-piperidinopyrimidine-3-oxide, is a white, crystalline solid with a molecular weight of 209.25 (Fig. 7). Dose-dependent reductions in blood pressure are produced by minoxidil in normotensive animals and in a number of hypertensive animal models. The effective oral dose range is between 0.15 and 150 mg/kg. A single oral dose has been shown to lower arterial pressure for 48 to 72 hr (263). In conscious dogs, minoxidil lowers blood pressure for up to 30 days during repeated administration without tolerance development (264). Total peripheral vascular resistance is decreased by minoxidil (263, 265,266).

Radioactive microsphere distribution studies in dogs reveal that minoxidil markedly increases blood flow to the myocardium. Increases of lesser magnitude are observed in flow distribution to skin, muscle, pancreas, and the gastrointestinal tract; flow distribution is unchanged in kidneys, spleen, liver, and brain (267). Calculated vascular resistance is decreased by minoxidil in all vascular beds.

Heart rate and cardiac output are elevated during minoxidil-induced decreases in arterial pressure (263). The tachycardia is not prevented by β blockade with propranolol and α blockade with phenoxybenzamine (268). Furthermore, the tachycardia is not reversed by elevating blood pressure to pretreatment levels by administration of angiotensin II. Thus, the tachycardia may result not only from reflex adjustment to blood pressure reduction but also from a direct positive chronotropic action of minoxidil.

Hypotensive responses are not affected by β blockade, anticholinergic and antihistaminic agents, ganglionic blockade, or spinal anesthesia. In perfused dog hindlimb, minoxidil fails to affect responses to norepinephrine, acetylcholine, glyceryl trinitrate, or histamine (263). Chronic administration of minoxidil at antihypertensive doses to spontaneously hypertensive rats did not change the *in vitro* sensitivity (EC_{50}) and maximal contractile tension of mesenteric artery or portal veins to prostaglandins D_2, E_2, $F_{2\alpha}$, B_2, or A_2, norepinephrine, angiotensin II, $CaCl_2$, or KCl. In this same study, minoxidil increased the extensibility of mesenteric artery and portal vein (269). It has been proposed that minoxidil interferes in some way with calcium mobilization in vascular smooth muscle (270–272). However, the calcium chelator EGTA produces minimal effects on the extensibility of portal veins (273). Thus, it is suggested that the vasodilatation produced by minoxidil results from a specific action of minoxidil on vascular smooth muscle, not from a general depressant action (269). The specific cellular mechanism of action remains to be defined.

Minoxidil effectively reduces arterial pressure in patients with essential or renal hypertension. Stroke volume, heart rate, and cardiac output are elevated by minoxidil (274). Plasma renin activity is raised and sodium and water excretions are reduced during therapy; β blockade and diuretics effectively overcome these side effects. The major limitation to therapy is the high incidence of hypertrichosis produced by minoxidil (264).

Hydralazine

Hydralazine, 1-hydrazinophthalazine (Fig. 7), lowers arterial pressure in many experimental hypertensive models and is clinically effective (275–277). Certain structural requirements are necessary for maximal antihypertensive efficacy and duration of action (278,279).

Hydralazine-induced reductions in blood pressure are principally the result of arterial vasodilatation and decreased total peripheral resistance and are not due to a decrease in venous tone (277,280–284). Heart rate and cardiac output are increased by hydralazine. These increases may result from either a reflex adjustment to venous pressure elevation (285) or a direct action of hydralazine on the myocardium (286). The cardiac effects are antagonized by propranolol (286).

In anesthetized dogs, blood flow is elevated by hydralazine in splanchnic, renal, carotid, femoral, and coronary arteries (285,287–289). Studies have shown that the renal vasculature is most sensitive to hydralazine (285). The renovascular effects of low doses of hydralazine are antagonized by the prostaglandin synthesis inhibitors indomethacin and diclofenac sodium (285).

Contractile responses elicited in vascular smooth muscle by norepinephrine, epinephrine, angiotensin, vasopressin, serotonin, histamine, prostaglandins D_2, $F_{2\alpha}$, B_2, and A_2, barium chloride, and potassium chloride are depressed by hydralazine (287,290–293). Hydralazine causes a 4-mV hyperpolarization in rat caudal artery contracted by phenylephrine. This hyperpolarization can be partially attenuated by the addition of 2-chloroadenosine (294). In spontaneously hypertensive rats, hydralazine decreases the passive stiffness of both mesenteric arteries and portal veins, suggesting that hydralazine affects connective tissue and smooth-muscle elements in blood vessels (269).

Hydralazine interferes with calcium entry or calcium release from intracellular stores in vascular smooth muscle that are depolarized by potassium cloride (293,295,296). In teniae coli, the relaxant effects of hydralazine are not related to changes in tissue levels of cyclic GMP (297). It has been suggested that hydralazine intereferes with cellular metabolic pathways needed for maintenance of muscle tone and responsiveness to agonists (287,291).

The clinical antihypertensive effects of hydralazine are enhanced by the addition of drugs that antagonize adrenergic transmission (e.g., β-adrenoceptor antagonists, reserpine, guanethidine, methyldopa, and clonidine) or a diuretic (298,299). Hydralazine given alone or in combination with venodilators has proved useful in the treatment of congestive heart failure (300–304).

Nifedipine

New vasodilators termed "Ca^{2+}-entry blockers," "Ca^{2+} antagonists," or "slow channel blockers" are being tested in the treatment of hypertension. Although a number of chemically and structurally different agents are considered Ca^{2+}-entry blockers (305), nifedipine (Fig. 7) has been studied most extensively in the treatment of hypertension.

Nifedipine has been reported to lower blood pressure in experimental models of hypertension (306,307). Nifedipine is efficacious in mild to moderate essential hypertensive patients (308–311), as well as in patients exhibiting severe hypertension (312,313). Following oral administration, the antihypertensive responses are rapid in onset (30–60 min), with a duration of 3 hr. Interestingly, nifedipine demonstrates no hypotensive activity in normotensive subjects (308,310). This disparity, as will be discussed later, may be related to differences in the handling of Ca^{2+} in blood vessels of hypertensives (314,315).

The antihypertensive effects of nifedipine are the result, most likely, of direct vasodilatation and reduced vascular resistance (308, 310,316,317). Usually the vasodepressor responses are accompanied by compensatory increases in heart rate and stroke volume and therefore cardiac output. Plasma norepinephrine levels and plasma renin activity are increased by nifedipine. The increase in plasma renin activity and tachycardia are blunted by concomitant administration of propranolol. Long-term therapy with nifedipine produced no change in one study (311) and a slight increase in another study (318) of sodium and plasma fluid volume. Sodium and volume retentions were controlled by the addition of diuretic therapy (311). Combined therapy with nifedipine plus propranolol slightly enhanced the antihypertensive response (308,318). The addition of methyldopa to nifedipine in severely hypertensive patients increased the magnitude of the antihypertensive response and also reduced the fluctuations in blood pressure observed between doses; sodium and water retentions were not a problem with this combination therapy (313).

In addition to sodium and volume retentions, other side effects include headache, flushing, and nausea. The incidence of angina pectoris is relatively low, most likely as a result of the marked coronary vasodilatating actions of nifedipine (316).

Nifedipine inhibits KCl-induced contractions of vascular smooth-muscle strips (319). KCl-induced contractions are dependent on the transmembrane influx of extracellular Ca^{2+} ions (320). Norepinephrine-induced contractions of vascular smooth muscle from a number of different beds are dependent on Ca^{2+} released from intracellular stores, as well as the transmembrane influx of extracellular Ca^{2+} (320–322). Concentrations of nifedipine that completely antagonize KCl-induced contractions exhibit very little inhibitory effect on norepinephrine-induced contractions. Lederballe-Pedersen (314) has demonstrated an age-dependent change in norepinephrine-induced contractions of aortas from spontaneously hypertensive rats, which exhibited more dependence on extracellular sources of Ca^{2+}. Ca^{2+} entry evoked by norepinephrine is also elevated in mesenteric vessels of adult spontaneously hypertensive rats (315). The ability of nifedipine to relax norepinephrine-contracted aortas was significantly greater in spontaneously hypertensive rats (314). KCl-induced contraction in these studies showed no difference in tissues taken from spontaneously hypertensive and normotensive rats, thereby suggesting an alteration in the receptor-operated channel (320) in spontaneously hypertensive rats. These observations might be extended to the clinic, suggesting possibly that the efficacy of nifedipine in hypertensive patients in comparison with normotensive patients is related to an altered transmembrane

Ca^{2+} flux in the blood vessels of hypertensive patients.

NEW ANTIHYPERTENSIVE DRUGS IN DEVELOPMENT

In addition to the drugs described earlier, many new antihypertensive agents are in various stages of development and are likely to be marketed within the next few years. Many of them represent improvements over existing products in respect to their pharmacological or toxicological properties. Some of these new drugs will be described briefly.

Trimazosin

Trimazosin is 2-hydroxy-2-methylpropyl-4-(4-amino-6,7,8-trimethoxy-2-quinazolinyl)-1-piperazine carboxylate hydrochloride. This quinazoline derivative is chemically and pharmacologically related to prazosin (323). Its major mechanism of antihypertensive action is a competitive and selective blockade of postsynaptic α-adrenoceptors. Trimazosin differs from prazosin pharmacologically in its ability to reduce arterial pressure in spinal animals. This suggests an additional peripheral vasodilator mechanism possibly unrelated to α-adrenoceptor blockade. In dogs, trimazosin at 1 mg/kg/min for 7 min attenuated the pressor effects caused by occlusion of carotid arteries but not by norepinephrine (324). It is presently unclear whether or not this observation can be interpreted as an evidence for an additional site of antihypertensive action of trimazosin. Trimazosin is active as an antihypertensive agent in humans (325).

Urapidil

Urapidil, 6-3-[4-(O-methoxyphenyl)piperazinyl]propylamino-1,3-dimethyluracil, combines clonidinelike inhibition of sympathetic tone with a prazosinlike postsynaptic α-adrenoceptor blockade (326). The combination of these two effects is attractive and may lead to better control of arterial pressure. Success-

ful preliminary clinical studies with urapidil have been published (327,328).

Prizidilol Hydrochloride

Prizidilol hydrochloride, dl-3-[2-(3-t-butylamino-2-hydroxypropyl)phenyl]-6-hydrazanino pyridazine, is a β-adrenoceptor antagonist with precapillary vasodilator properties (329,330). The combination of the two activities should be considered attractive. Peripheral vasodilatation is likely to improve blood supply to various organs as well as to the skeletal muscle, whereas the reflex tachycardia common with vasodilators is likely to be antagonized by the β-adrenoceptor antagonist component of the prizidilol action. The concept of combining these two properties in one drug is not new and was previously attempted by others (331).

MK-421

Successful development of captopril stimulated attempts by various pharmaceutical companies to develop new converting enzyme inhibitors with improved pharmacological or toxicological profiles. An example of such a development is MK-421, N-[(S)-1-carboxy-3-phenylpropyl]-ala-L-pro. In addition to higher potency, MK-421 has no SH group in its molecule and is therefore believed less likely to produce hematological side effects (332,333). MK-421 is probably a pro-drug and will have to be deesterified to have full in vivo activity.

CONCLUSIONS

With the available drugs, even severe hypertension can be controlled in almost all patients. From the point of view of efficacy, little further improvement is needed, but further reduction of side effects and a longer duration of action still represent achievable goals in the development of new antihypertensive drugs.

A widely used approach to therapy for hypertension involves "stepped care." The first

TABLE 4. *Hemodynamic effects of commonly used antihypertensive drugs*

Drugs		Total Peripheral Resistance — acute	Total Peripheral Resistance — chronic	Heart Rate	Myocardial Contractility	Cardiac Output	Coronary Blood Flow	Renal Vascular Resistance	Sodium Excretion	Plasma Renin Activity
Diuretics	Hydrochlorothiazide	↑	↓	↑		↑	↑	↑	→	←
	Furosemide	↑ →	↑ ↓	↑		↑	↑	→	→	←
Converting Enzyme Inhibitor	Captopril	→	↓	↑	↑	↑	→	→	↑	← *
Centrally Acting Antihypertensives	Methyldopa	→	→	→	↑	→	←	→	→	→
	Clonidine	←	→	→	↑	→	↑ ↓	→	↑	→
Catecholamine Depletor	Reserpine	↑	→	→	←	→	?	↑	→	←
Adrenergic Neuron Blocker	Guanethidine	↑	→	← →	←	↑	?	↑	→	?
α Adrenoceptor Antagonist	Prazosin	→	→	↑	←	↑	↑	←	→	←
β Adrenoceptor Antagonists	Propranolol	←	←	→	←	↑	→	→	→	→
	Nadolol	←		→	←	↑	→	→	→	→
	Metoprolol	↑ ←		→	←	↑	→	→	→	→
	Labetalol	↑ ←		↑ →	←	↑	←	←	↑	←
Direct Vasodilators	Diazoxide	→	**	←	←	←	←	↑ →	→	←
	Minoxidil	→	→	←	←	←	←	↑ →	→	←
	Hydralazine	→	→	←	←	←	←	↑ →	→	←
	Sodium Nitroprusside	→	**	←	←	←	↑	→	→	←
	Nifedipine	→	→	←	←	←	→	←	↑	←

* Angiotensin II levels are decreased by captopril
** Not used chronically

↑ Increase
↓ Decrease
→ No change
↑↓ Two arrows indicate that changes in both directions were observed

step is either a thiazide diuretic or a β-adreno-ceptor antagonist. If a diuretic is used as the first step, a β-adrenoceptor antagonist is added as the second step. Instead of a β-adrenoceptor antagonist, methyldopa, clonidine, or prazosin can be used. A directly acting smooth-muscle relaxant, e.g., hydralazine, can be added to the therapy as the third step. In resistant patients with severe hypertension, guanethidine is often used as the fourth step. The introduction of converting enzyme inhibitors and of Ca^{2+}-entry blocking drugs is certain to modify the currently used therapeutic approaches. With further advances in our knowledge of the pathogenesis of essential hypertension, new drugs that will conceivably correct the causes of the disease are likely to be introduced.

The antihypertensive drugs discussed in this chapter differ substantially in their sites and mechanisms of action. They also differ in their hemodynamic effects, which are summarized in Table 4. Particularly noteworthy are the differences in the effects of antihypertensive drugs on cardiac output, heart rate, plasma renin activity, and Na^+ and water retention. These differences justify combined therapy for hypertension with two or even three antihypertensive drugs.

REFERENCES

1. Scriabine, A. (editor) (1980): *Pharmacology of Antihypertensive Drugs.* Raven Press, New York.
2. Beyer, K. H., Jr., Baer, J. E., Russo, H. F., and Noll, R. (1958): Electrolyte excretion as influenced by chlorothiazide. *Science,* 127:146–147.
3. Beyer, K. H., and Baer, J. E. (1961): Physiological basis for the action of newer diuretic agents. *Pharmacol. Rev.,* 13:517–562.
4. Scriabine, A., Schreiber, E. C., Yu, M., and Wiseman, E. H. (1962): Renal clearance of polythiazide. *Proc. Soc. Exp. Biol. Med.,* 110:872–875.
5. Baer, J. E., and Beyer, K. H. (1972): Subcellular pharmacology of natriuretic and potassium-sparing drugs. In: *Progress in Biochemical Pharmacology. Vol. 7: Drugs Affecting Kidney Function and Metabolism,* edited by K. D. G. Edwards, pp. 59–93. Karger, Basel.
6. Weller, J. M., and Borodny, M. (1976): Effects of chlorothiazide on glucose content and lactic acid production of aorta. *Proc. Soc. Exp. Biol. Med.,* 153:483–485.
7. Kover, G., and Tost, H. (1977): The effect of indomethacin on kidney function: Indomethacin and furosemide antagonism. *Pfluegers Arch.,* 372:215–220.
8. Scriabine, A., Watson, L. S., Fanelli, G. M., Jr., Shum, W. K., Blaine, E. N., Russo, H. F., and Bohidar, N. R. (1980): Studies on the interaction of indomethacin with various diuretics. In: *Prostaglandins in Cardiovascular and Renal Function,* edited by A. Scriabine, A. M. Lefer, and F. A. Kuehl, Jr., pp. 471–483. Spectrum Publications, New York.
9. Stone, K. J., and Hart, M. (1976): Inhibition of renal PGE_2-9-ketoreductase by diuretics. *Prostaglandins,* 12:197–207.
10. Kuehl, F. A., Jr., Oien, H. G., and Ham, E. A. (1980): Prostaglandin E-related action of drugs regulating renal function. In: *Prostaglandins in Cardiovascular and Renal Function,* edited by A. Scriabine, A. M. Lefer, and F. A. Kuehl, Jr., pp. 31–46. Spectrum Publications, New York.
11. Scriabine, A., Watson, L. S., Russo, H., Ludden, C. T., Sweet, C. S., Fanelli, G. M., Jr., Bohidar, N., and Stone, C. A. (1979): Diuretic and antihypertensive effects of 2-aminoethyl-4-(1,1-dimethylethyl)-6-iodophenol hydrochloride (MK447). *J. Pharmacol. Exp. Ther.,* 208:148–154.
12. Fries, E. D., Wanko, A., Wilson, I. M., and Parrish, A. E. (1958): Treatment of essential hypertension with chlorothiazide (Diuril). *J.A.M.A.,* 166:137–140.
13. Scriabine, A., Korol, B., Kondratas, B., Yu, M., P'an, S. Y., and Schneider, S. A. (1961): Pharmacological studies with polythiazide, a new diuretic and antihypertensive agent. *Proc. Soc. Exp. Biol. Med.,* 107:869–872.
14. Kohler, C., Berkowitz, B., and Spector, S. (1977): The effect of guanethidine and hydrocholothiazide on blood pressure and vascular tyrosine hydroxylase activity in the spontaneously hypertensive rat. *Eur. J. Pharmacol.,* 42:161–170.
15. Friedman, S. M., and Friedman, C. L. (1978): Cell permeability, sodium transport and the hypertensive process in the rat. *Circ. Res. [Suppl. 1],* 26–27:141–146.
16. Blaustein, M. P. (1977): Sodium ions, calcium ions, blood pressure regulation and hypertension: A reassessment and a hypothesis. *Am. J. Physiol.,* 232:C165–C173.
17. Ames, R. P., and Hill, P. (1978): Raised serum lipid concentration during diuretic treatment of hypertension. A study of predictive indexes. *Clin. Sci. Mol. Med.,* 55:311s–314s.
18. Tigerstedt, R., and Bergman, P. G. (1898): Niere und Kreislauf. *Scand. Arch. Physiol.,* 8:223–271.
19. Laragh, J. H. (1960): The role of aldosterone in man. Evidence for regulation of electrolyte balance and arterial pressure by a renal-adrenal system which may be involved in malignant hypertension. *J.A.M.A.,* 174:293–295.
20. Horovitz, Z. P. (editor) (1981): *Angiotensin Converting Enzyme Inhibitors: Mechanisms of Action and Clinical Implications.* Urban and Schwarzenberg, Baltimore.
21. Cushman, D. E., Cheung, H. S., Sabo, E. F., and Ondetti, M. A. (1978): Design of new antihyperten-

sive drugs: Potent and specific inhibitors of angiotensin-converting enzyme. *Prog. Cardiovasc. Dis.,* 21:176–182.

22. Case, D. R., Wallace, J. M., Keim, H. J., Weber, M. A., Drayer, J. I., White, R. P., Sealey, J. E., and Laragh, J. H. (1976): Estimating renin participation in hypertension: Superiority of converting enzyme inhibition over saralasin. *Am. J. Med.,* 61:790–796.

23. Heald, A. F., and Ita, C. E. (1977): Distribution in rats of an inhibitor of angiotensin-converting enzyme, SQ 14,225, as studied by whole body autoradiography and liquid scintillation counting. *Pharmacologist,* 19:129.

24. Thurston, H., Bing, R. F., Marks, E. S., and Swales, J. D. (1980): Response of chronic renovascular hypertension to surgical correction of prolonged blockade by two inhibitors in rat. *Clin. Sci.,* 58:15–20.

25. Marks, E. S., Bing, R. F., Thurston, H., and Swales, J. D. (1980): Vasodepressor property of the converting enzyme inhibitor captopril (SQ 14,225): The role of factors other than renin-angiotensin blockade in the rat. *Clin. Sci.,* 58:1–6.

26. Textor, S. C., Brunner, H. R., and Gavras, H. (1981): Converting enzyme inhibition during chronic angiotensin II infusion in rats. Evidence against a nonangiotensin mechanism. *Hypertension,* 3:269–276.

27. Johnston, C. I., Yasujima, M., and Clappison, B. H. (1981): The kallikrein-kinin system and angiotensin converting enzyme inhibition in hypertension. In: *Angiotensin Converting Enzyme Inhibitors: Mechanisms of Action and Clinical Implications,* edited by Z. P. Horovitz, pp. 123–139. Urban and Schwarzenberg, Baltimore.

28. Swartz, S. L., Crantz, F. R., Moore, T. J., Dluhy, R. G., Hollenberg, N. K., and Williams, G. H. (1979): Prostaglandin changes associated with the hypotensive response to captopril (SQ 14,225) in normotensive males. *Clin. Res.,* 27:595H.

29. Crantz, F. R., Swartz, S. L., Hollenberg, N. K., Moore, T. J., Bluhy, R. G., Levine, L., and Williams, G. H. (1979): Role of prostaglandins in the hypotensive response to captopril in essential hypertension. *Clin. Res.,* 27:592A.

30. Antonaccio, M. J., Harris, D., Goldenberg, H., High, J. P., and Rubin, B. (1979): The effects of captopril, propranolol and indomethacin on blood pressure and plasma renin activity in spontaneously hypertensive and normotensive rats. *Proc. Soc. Exp. Biol. Med.,* 162:429–433.

31. Antonaccio, M. J., Asaad, M., Rubin, B., and Horovitz, Z. P. (1981): Captopril: Factors involved in its mechanism of action. In: *Angiotensin Converting Enzyme Inhibitors: Mechanisms of Action and Clinical Implications,* edited by Z. P. Horovitz, pp. 161–180. Urban and Schwarzenberg, Baltimore.

32. Murthy, V. S., Waldron, T. L., and Goldberg, M. E. (1978): Inhibition of angiotensin converting enzyme by SQ 14,225 in anesthetized dogs: Hemodynamic and renal vascular effects. *Proc. Soc. Exp. Biol. Med.,* 157:121–124.

33. Bengis, R. G., Coleman, T. G., Young, D. B., and McCaa, R. E. (1978): Long term blockade of angio-

tensin formation in various normotensive and hypertensive rat models using converting enzyme inhibitor (SQ 14,225). *Circ. Res.* [*Suppl. I*], 43:145–153.

34. McCaa, R. E., Hall, J. E., and McCaa, C. S. (1978): The effects of angiotensin I-converting enzyme inhibitors on arterial blood pressure and urinary sodium excretion. Role of the renal renin-angiotensin and kallikrein-kinin systems. *Circ. Res.* [*Suppl. I*], 43:132–139.

35. Rubin, B., Antonaccio, M. J., and Horovitz, Z. P. (1978): Captopril (SQ 14,225)(D-3-mercapto-2-methylpropanoyl-L-proline): A novel orally active inhibitor of angiotensin-converting enzyme and antihypertensive agent. *Prog. Cardiovasc. Dis.,* 21: 183–194.

36. Antonaccio, M. J., Rubin, B., and Horovitz, Z. P. (1980): Effects of captopril in animal models of hypertension. *Clin. Exp. Hypertension,* 2:613–637.

37. Antonaccio, M. J., and Kerwin, L. (1981): Pre- and postjunctional inhibition of vascular sympathetic function by captopril in SHR. Implication of vascular angiotensin II in hypertension and antihypertensive actions of captopril. *Hypertension* [*Suppl. I*], 3:I-54–I-62.

38. Fagard, R., Lijnen, P., and Amery, A. (1981): Hemodynamic effects of long-term captopril therapy in hypertensive man. In: *Angiotensin Converting Enzyme Inhibitors: Mechanisms of Action and Clinical Implications,* edited by Z. P. Horovitz, pp. 255–262, Urban and Schwarzenberg, Baltimore.

39. Brunner, H. R., Gavras, H., Waeber, B., Kershaw, G. R., Turini, G. A., Vukovich, R. A., and McKinstry, D. N. (1979): Oral angiotensin-converting enzyme inhibitor in long-term treatment of hypertensive patients. *Ann. Intern. Med.,* 90:19–23.

40. McKinstry, D. N., Willard, D. A., and Vukovich, R. A. (1979): Antihypertensive and hormonal effects of the converting enzyme inhibitor, captopril, alone or combined with hydrochlorothiazide. *Clin. Pharmacol. Ther.,* 25:237.

41. McCaa, R. E., McCaa, C. S., Bengis, R. G., and Guyton, A. C. (1979): Role of aldosterone in experimental hypertension. *J. Endocrinol.,* 81:69P–78P.

42. Murthy, V. S., and Waldron, T. L. (1979): Modification of chronotropic effects on bradykinin (BK) by captopril (C) and indomethacin (I) in conscious rabbits. *Fed. Proc.,* 38:738.

43. Atlas, S. A., Case, D. B., Sealey, J. E., McKinstry, D. N., and Laragh, J. H. (1978): Blunted aldosterone secretion, natriuresis and potassium retention during chronic aldosterone blockade in hypertensive patients. *Clin. Res.,* 26:361A.

44. Atlas, S. A., Case, D. B., Sealey, J. E., Sullivan, P. M., and Laragh, J. H. (1978): Involvement of the renin-angiotensin-aldosterone axis in the antihypertensive action of captopril (SQ 14,225). *Circulation* [*Suppl. II*], 57:II-143.

45. Bravo, E. L., and Tarazi, R. C. (1979): Converting enzyme inhibition with an orally active compound in hypertensive man. *Hypertension,* 1:39–46.

46. Brunner, H. R., Gavras, H., Turini, G. A., Waeber, B., and Wauters, J. P. (1978): Long-term angiotensin blockade in hypertensive patients with chronic renal failure. *Clin. Res.,* 26:459A.

47. Oates, J. A., Gillespie, L., Udenfriend, S., and Sjoerdsma, A. (1960): Decarboxylase inhibition and blood pressure reduction by α-methyl-3,4-dihydroxy-dl-phenylalanine. *Science,* 131:1890–1891.

48. Sourkes, T. L. (1954): Inhibition of dihydroxyphenylalanine decarboxylase by derivatives of phenylalanine. *Arch. Biochem. Biophys.,* 51:444–456.

49. Carlsson, A., and Lindqvist, M. (1962): In vivo decarboxylation of α-methyl metatyrosine. *Acta Physiol. Scand.,* 54:87–94.

50. Holtz, P., Stock, K., and Westerman, E. (1964): Pharmakologie des Tetrahydropapaverolins und seine Entstehung aus Dopamin. *Naunyn Schmiedebergs Arch. Pharmacol.,* 248:387–405.

51. Henning, M. (1969): Studies on the mode of action of α-methyldopa. *Acta Physiol. Scand.* [*Suppl. 322*], 75:1–37.

52. Onesti, G., Brest, A. N., Novack, P., Kasparian, H., and Moyer, J. H. (1964): Pharmacodynamic effects of alpha-methyldopa in hypertensive subjects. *Am. Heart J.,* 67:32–38.

53. Mohammed, S., Gaffney, T. E., Yard, A. C., and Gomez, H. (1968): Effect of methyldopa, reserpine and guanethidine on hindleg vascular resistance. *J. Pharmacol. Exp. Ther.,* 160:300–307.

54. Mohammed, S., Fasola, A. F., Privitera, P. J., Lipicky, R. J., Martz, B. L., and Gaffney, T. E. (1969): Effect of methyldopa on plasma renin activity in man. *Circ. Res.,* 25:543–548.

55. Sjoerdsma, A., Vendsalu, A., and Engelman, K. (1963): Studies on the metabolism and mechanism of action of methyldopa. *Circulation,* 28:492–502.

56. Burden, A. C., and Alexander, C. P. T. (1976): Rebound hypertension after acute methyldopa withdrawal. *Br. Med. J.,* 2:1056–1057.

57. Frewin, D. B., and Penhall, R. K. (1977): Rebound hypertension after sudden discontinuation of methyldopa therapy. *Med. J. Aust.,* 1:659.

58. Hoefke, W., and Kobinger, W. (1966): Pharmakologische Wirkungen des 2-(2,6-Dichlophenylamino)-2-imidazolinhydrochlorids, einer neuen, antihypertensiven Substanz. *Arzneim. Forsch.,* 16:1038–1050.

59. Kobinger, W. (1967): Uber den Wirkungsmechnismus einer neuen antihypertensiven Substanz mit Imidazolinstruktur. *Naunyn Schmiedebergs Arch. Pharmacol.,* 258:48–58.

60. Kobinger, W., and Walland, A. (1967): Kreislaufuntersuchungen mit 2-(2,6-Dichlorphenylamino)-2-imidazolin-hydrochlorid. *Arzneim. Forsch.,* 17:292–300.

61. Allen, R. C., and Langham, M. E. (1976): The intraocular pressure response of conscious rabbits to clonidine. *Invest. Ophthalmol.,* 15:815–823.

62. Senft, G., Sitt, R., Losert, W., Schultz, G., and Hoffmann, M. (1968): Hemmung der Insulininkretion durch α-Receptoren stimulierende Substanzen. *Naunyn Schmiedebergs Arch. Pharmacol.,* 260:309–323.

63. Elkeles, R. S., Goldby, F. S., and Oliver, D. O. (1970): A double blind study of Catapres, a new hypotensive agent. In: *Catapres in Hypertension,* edited by M. E. Conolly, pp. 139–144. Butterworth, London.

64. Raftos, J., Bauer, G. E., Lewis, R. G., Stokes, G. S., Mitchell, A. S., Yound, A. A., and MacLachlan, I. (1973): Clonidine in the treatment of severe hypertension. *Med. J. Aust.,* 1:786–793.

65. Mroczek, W. J., Davidov, M., and Finnerty, F. A., Jr. (1972): Prolonged treatment with clonidine: Comparative antihypertensive effects alone and with a diuretic agent. *Am. J. Cardiol.,* 30:536–541.

66. Kirkendall, W. M., Hammond, J. J., Thomas, J. C., Overturf, M. L., and Zama, A. (1978): Effect of prazosin and clonidine on blood pressure, pulse, plasma renin activity, aldosterone and cholesterol. *Clin. Res.,* 26:119A.

67. Geyskes, G. G., Boer, P., and Dorhout Mees, E. J. (1979): Clonidine withdrawal mechanism and frequency of rebound hypertension. *Br. J. Clin. Pharmacol.,* 7:55–62.

68. Goldberg, A. D., Wilkinson, P. R., and Raftery, E. B. (1976): The over-shoot phenomenon of withdrawal of clonidine therapy. *Postgrad. Med. J.* [*Suppl. 7*], 52:128–134.

69. Scholtysik, G., Lauener, H., Eichenberger, E., Burki, H., Salzmann, R., Muller-Schweinitzer, E., and Waite, R., (1975): Pharmacological actions of the antihypertensive agent N-amidino-2(2,6-dichlorophenyl)acetamide hydrochloride (BS 100-141). *Arzneim. Forsch.,* 25:1483–1491.

70. Scholtysik, G., Jerie, P., and Picard, C. W. (1980): Guanfacine. In: *Pharmacology of Antihypertensive Drugs,* edited by A. Scriabine, pp. 79–98. Raven Press, New York.

71. Saameli, K., Scholtysik, G., and Waite, R. (1975): Pharmacology of BS 100-141, a centrally acting antihypertensive drug. *Clin. Exp. Pharmacol. Physiol.* [*Suppl.*], 2:207–212.

72. Kiechel, J. R. (1980): Pharmacokinetics and metabolism of guanfacine in man: A review. *Br. J. Clin. Pharmacol.,* 10:255–325.

73. Jaeaettelae, A. (1976): Clinical efficacy of BS 100-141 in essential hypertension. A single-blind pilot study. *Eur. J. Clin. Pharmacol.,* 10:69–72.

74. Kirch, W., and Distler, A. (1978): Antihypertensive effect of N-amidino-2(2,6-dichlorophenyl)acetamide hydrochloride. A double-blind cross-over trial versus clonidine. *Int. J. Clin. Pharmacol.,* 16:132–135.

75. Baum, T., and Shropshire, A. T. (1970): Inhibition of spontaneous sympapathetic nerve activity by the antihypertensive agent Wy-8678. *Neuropharmacology,* 9:503–506.

76. Baum, T., and Shropshire, A. T. (1976): Studies on the centrally mediated hypotensive activity of guanabenz. *Eur. J. Pharmacol.,* 37:31–44.

77. Fuller, R. W., Snoddy, H. D., and Marshall, W. S. (1977): Lowering of rat brain 3-methoxy-4-hydroxy phenylethylene glycol sulphate (MOPEG sulphate) concentration by 2,6-dichlorobenzylidene amino-guanidine. *J. Pharm. Pharmacol.,* 29:375–376.

78. Jarrott, B., Louis, W. J., and Summers, R. L. (1979): The effect of a series of clonidine anlogues on [³H]clonidine binding in rat cerebral cortex. *Biochem. Pharmacol.,* 28:141–144.

79. Baum, T., Shropshire, A. T., Rowles, G., Van Pelt, R., Fernandez, S. P., Eckfeld, D. K., and Gluckman, M. I. (1970): General pharmacologic actions of the

antihypertensive agent 2,6-dichlorobenzylidene aminoguanidine acetate (Wy-8678). *J. Pharmacol. Exp. Ther.*, 171:276–287.

80. Roller, L. (1976): Sympathomimetic and adrenergic neurone blocking actions of compounds in an isolated arterial preparation. *Aust. J. Pharm. Sci.*, 5:35–40.

81. Baum, T., Eckfeld, D. K., Metz, N., Dinish, J. L., Rowles, G., Van Pelt, R., Gluckman, M. I., and Bruce, W. F. (1969): 2,6-Dichlorobenzylidene amino guanidine acetate (Wy-8678), a new hypotensive agent. *Experientia*, 25:1066–1067.

82. Bosanac, P., Dubb, J., Walker, B., Goldberg, M., and Agus, Z. S. (1976): Renal effects of guanabenz: A new antihypertensive. *J. Clin. Pharmacol.*, 16:631–636.

83. McMahon, F. G., Ryan, J. R., Jain, A. K., Vargas, R., and Vanov, S. K. (1977): Guanabenz in essential hypertension. *Clin. Pharmacol. Ther.*, 21:272–277.

84. Shah, R. S., Walker, B. R., Vanov, S. K., and Helfant, R. H. (1976): Guanabenz effects on blood pressure and noninvasive parameters of cardiac performance in patients with hypertension. *Clin. Pharmacol. Ther.*, 19:732–737.

85. Walker, B. R., Shah, R. S., Ramanathan, K. B., Vanov, S. K., and Helfant, R. H. (1977): Guanabenz and methyldopa on hypertension and cardiac performance. *Clin. Pharmacol. Ther.*, 22:868–874.

86. Vanov, S., and Vergis, J. (1975): Guanabenz in essential hypertension. *Clin. Pharmacol. Ther.*, 17:245–246.

87. Ram, C. V. S., Holland, O. B., Fairchild, C., and Gomez-Sanchez, C. E. (1979): Withdrawal syndrome following cessation of guanabenz therapy. *J. Clin. Pharmacol.*, 19:148–150.

88. Boba, A., and Converse, J. G. (1967): Ganglionic blockade in management of acute massive hemorrhage: A 10-year reappraisal. *Anesth. Analg. (Clere.)*, 46:211–223.

89. Randall, L. O., Peterson, W. G., and Lehman, G. (1949): The ganglionic blocking action of thiophanium derivatives. *J. Pharmacol. Exp. Ther.*, 97:48–57.

90. Mitchell, R., Newman, P. J., Macgillivnay, D., and Clark, B. B. (1951): Evaluation of histamine liberator activity, illustrated by a thiophanium compound, RO 2-2222. *Fed. Proc.*, 10:325.

91. McCubbin, J. W., and Page, I. H. (1952): Nature of the hypotensive action of a thiophanium derivative (RO 2-2222) in dogs. *J. Pharmacol. Exp. Ther.*, 105:437–442.

92. Deacock, A. R., and Davis, T. D. W. (1958): The influence of certain ganglion blocking agents on neuromuscular transmission. *Br. J. Anaesth.*, 30:217–225.

93. Dorfman, L., Furlenmeier, A., Huebner, C. F., Lucas, R., MacHullamy, H. B., Mueller, J. M., Schlittler, E., Schwyzer, R., and St. Andre, A. F. (1954): Die Konstitution des Reserpins. *Helv. Chim. Acta.*, 37:59–75.

94. Shore, P. A. (1972): Transport and storage of biogenic amines. *Annu. Rev. Pharmacol.*, 12:209–226.

95. Gaffney, T. E., Chidsey, C. A., and Braunwald, E. (1963): Study of the relationship between the neurotransmitter store and adrenergic nerve block induced by reserpine and guanethidine. *Circ. Res.*, 12:264–268.

96. Ebinhara, A., and Martz, B. L. (1970): Comparative effects of currently available antihypertensive agents on spontaneously and renal hypertensive rats. *Am. J. Med. Sci.*, 259:257–261.

97. Ganett, R. L., Canver, O., Jr., and Douglas, B. H. (1967): Effects of reserpine on blood pressure and vascular electrolytes in hypertension. *Eur. J. Pharmacol.*, 2:236–238.

98. Westermann, E. O., Maickel, R. P., and Brodie, B. B. (1962): On the mechanism of pituitary-adrenal stimulation by reserpine. *J. Pharmacol. Exp. Ther.*, 138:208–217.

99. Harrison, T. S. (1961): Some factors influencing thyrotropin release in the rabbit. *Endocrinology*, 68:466–478.

100. Cranston, E. M. (1958): Effects of tranquilizers and other agents on sexual cycle of mice. *Proc. Soc. Exp. Biol. Med.*, 98:320–322.

101. Mayer, G., Meunier, J. M., and Thevenot-Duluc, A. J. (1960): Prolongation de la grossesse par retards de nidation obtenus chez la ratte par administration de reserpine. *Ann. Endocrinol. (Paris)*, 21:1–13.

102. MacLeod, R. M., and Lehmeyer, J. E. (1974): Studies on the mechanism of the dopamine-mediated inhibition of prolactin secretion. *Endocrinology*, 94:1077–1085.

103. Armstrong, B., Stevens, N., and Doll, R. (1979): Retrospective study of the association between use of rauwolfia derivatives and breast cancer in English women. *Lancet*, 2:672–675.

104. Armstrong, B., Skegg, D., White, G., and Doll, R. (1976): Rauwolfia derivatives and breast cancer in women. *Lancet*, 2:8–11.

105. Laska, E. M., Siegel, C., Meisner, M., Fischer, S., and Wanderling, J. (1975): Matched-pairs study of reserpine use and breast cancer. *Lancet*, 2:296–300.

106. Tripp, S. L., Williams, E., Wagner, W. E., Jr., and Lukas, G. (1975): A specific assay for subnanogram concentrations of reserpine in human plasma. *Life Sci.*, 16:1167–1178.

107. Maas, A. R., Jenkins, B., Shen, Y., and Tannenbaum, P. (1969): Studies on absorptin, excretion and metabolism of ^{3}H-reserpine in man. *Clin. Pharmacol. Ther.*, 10:366–371.

108. Stitzel, R. E. (1976): The biological fate of reserpine. *Pharmacol. Rev.*, 28:179–205.

109. Domino, E. F. (1962): Human pharmacology of tranquilizing drugs. *Clin. Pharmacol. Ther.*, 3:599–664.

110. Sheppard, H., Lucas, R. C., and Tsien, W. H. (1955): The metabolism of reserpine-C^{14}. *Arch. Int. Pharmacodyn. Ther.*, 103:256–269.

111. Sheppard H., and Tsien, W. H. (1955): Metabolism of reserpine-C^{14}. II. Species differences as studied in vitro. *Proc. Soc. Exp. Biol. Med.*, 90:437–446.

112. Smith, W. M., Thurm, R. H., and Brown, L. A. (1969): Comparative evaluation of Rauwolfia whole root and reserpine. *Clin. Pharmacol. Ther.*, 10:338–343.

113. Boura, A. L. A., Copp, F. C., Green, A. F., Hodson, H. F., Ruffel, G. K., Sim, M. F., and Walton, E.

(1961): Adrenergic neurone blocking agents related to choline 2,6-xylyl ether bromide (T.M.10), bretylium, and guanethidine. *Nature*, 191:1312–1313.

114. Scriabine, A., Booher, K. D., Perera, J. N., McShane, W. K., Constantine, J. W., Koch, R. C., and Miknius, S. (1965): Pharmacological studies with guanisoquin. *J. Pharmacol. Exp. Ther.*, 147:277–287.

115. Moe, R. A., Bates, H. M., Palkoski, Z. M., and Banziger, R. (1964): Cardiovascular effects of 3,4-dihydro-2(*H*)isoquinoline carboxamidine (Declinax). *Curr. Ther. Res.*, 6:299–318.

116. Kroneberg, G., Schlossmann, K., and Stoepel, K. (1967): Pharmacology of *N*-(2-guanidinoethyl)-4-methyl-1,2,3,6-tetrahydropyridine, a new antihypertensive agent. *Arzneim. Forsch.*, 17:199–207.

117. Harrison, D. C., Chidsey, C. A., Goldman, R., and Braunwald, E. (1963): Relationships between the release and tissue depletion of norepinephrine from the heart by guanethidine and reserpine. *Circ. Res.*, 12:256–263.

118. Abboud, F. M., Eckstein, J. W., and Pereda, S. A. (1961): Acute hemodynamic responses to intravenous and intra-arterial guanethidine. *Am. J. Physiol.*, 201:462–466.

119. Gaffney, T. E., Braunwald, E., and Cooper, T. (1962): Analysis of the acute circulatory effects of guanethidine and bretylium. *Circ. Res.*, 10:83–88.

120. Rand, M. J., and Wilson, J. (1967): The actions of some adrenergic neurone blocking drugs at cholinergic junctions. *Eur. J. Pharmacol.*, 1:210–221.

121. Chang, C. C., Chen, T. F., and Cheng, H. C. (1967): On the mechanism of neuromuscular blocking action of bretylium and guanethidine. *J. Pharmacol. Exp. Ther.*, 158:89–98.

122. Cohn, J. N., Liptak, T. E., and Fries, E. D. (1963): Hemodynamic effects of guanethidine in man. *Circ. Res.*, 12:298–307.

123. Richardson, D. W., Wyso, E. M., Magee, J. H., and Cavell, G. C. (1960): Circulatory effects of guanethidine. *Circulation*, 22:184–190.

124. Chamberlain, D. A., and Howard, J. (1964): Guanethidine and methyldopa: A haemodynamic study. *Br. Heart J.*, 26:528–536.

125. Villarreal, H., Exaire, J. E., Rubio, V., and Davila, H. (1964): Effect of guanethidine and bretylium tosylate on systemic and renal hemodynamics in essential hypertension. *Am. J. Cardiol.*, 14:633–640.

126. McMartin, C., Rondel, R. K., Vinter, J., Allan, B. R., Humberstone, P. M., Leishman, A. W. D., Sandler, G., and Thirkettle, J. L. (1970): The fate of guanethidine in two hypertensive patients. *Clin. Pharmacol. Ther.*, 11:423–431.

127. Maitre, L., Staehelin, M., and Brunner, H. (1971): Antihypertensive and noradrenaline-depleting effects of guanethidine metabolites. *J. Pharm. Pharmacol.*, 23:327–331.

128. Berlin, L. J., and Juel-Jensen, B. E. (1972): Alpha and beta adrenergic blockade in hypertension. *Lancet*, 1:979–982.

129. Majid, P. A., Meeran, M. K., Benaim, M. E., Sharma, B., and Taylor, S. H. (1974): Alpha- and beta-adrenergic receptor blockade in the treatment of hypertension. *Br. Heart J.*, 36:588–596.

130. Vladrakis, N. D., and Mendlowitz, M. (1976): An approach to the treatment of essential hypertension. *Am. Heart J.*, 92:750–757.

131. Scriabine, A., Constantine, J. W., Hess, J. J., and McShane, W. K. (1968): Pharmacological studies with some new antihypertensive aminoquinazolines. *Experientia*, 24:1150–1151.

132. Alps, B. J., Johnson, E. S., and Wilson, A. B. (1970): Cardiovascular actions of Wy-21901, a new hypotensive and antiarrhythmic agent. *Br. J. Pharmacol.*, 40:151P–152P.

133. Constantine, J. W., McShane, W. K., Scriabine, A., and Hess, H. J. (1973): Analysis of the hypotensive action of prazosin. In: *Hypertension: Mechanism and Management*, edited by G. Onesti, K. E. Kim, and J. H. Moyer, pp. 429–444. Grune & Stratton, New York.

134. Cambridge, D., Davey, M. J., and Massingham, R. (1977): Prazosin: A selective antagonist of post synaptic alpha-adrenoceptors. *Br. J. Pharmacol.*, 59:514P–515P.

135. Hua, A. S. P., and Moulds, R. F. W. (1978): The effect of prazosin on pre- and postsynaptic α-receptors in the pithed rat. *Clin. Exp. Pharmacol. Physiol.*, 5:525–528.

136. Doxey, J. C., Smith, C. F. C., and Walker, J. M. (1977): Selectivity of blocking agents for pre- and postsynaptic α-adrenoceptors. *Br. J. Pharmacol.*, 60:91–96.

137. Constantine, J. E., Weeks, R. A., and McShane, W. K. (1978): Prazosin and presynaptic α-receptors in the cardioaccelerator nerve of the dog. *Eur. J. Pharmacol.*, 50:51–60.

138. Roach, A. G., Lefevre, F., and Cavero, I. (1978): Effects of prazosin and phentolamine on cardiac presynaptic α-adrenoceptors in the cat, dog and rat. *Clin. Exp. Hypertension*, 1:87–101.

139. Lefevre-Borg, F., Roach, A. G., and Cavero, I. (1979): Comparison of cardiovascular actions of dihydralazine, phentolamine and prazosin in spontaneously hypertensive rats. *J. Cardiovasc. Pharmacol.*, 1:19–29.

140. Komarek, J., and Cartheuser, C. F. (1977): Dihydralazine versus Prazosin. Der haemodhynamische Effect der Modellsubstanzen. *Z. Kardiol.*, 66:706–711.

141. Koshy, M. C., Mickley, D., Bourgoignie, J., and Blaufox, M. D. (1977): Physiologic evaluation of a new antihypertensive agent: Prazosin HCl. *Circulation*, 55:533–537.

142. Hayes, J. M., Graham, R. M., O'Connell, B. P., Speers, E., and Humphrey, T. J. (1976): Effect of prazosin on plasma renin activity. *Aust. N.Z. J. Med.*, 6:90.

143. Bolli, P., Wood, A. J., Phelan, E. L., Lee, D. R., and Simpson, F. O. (1975): Prazosin: Preliminary clinical and pharmacological observations. *Clin. Sci. Mol. Med.*, 48:177S–179S.

144. Stokes, G. S., and Weber, M. A. (1974): Prazosin: Preliminary report and comparative studies with other antihypertensive agents. *Br. Med. J.*, 2:298–300.

145. Guevara, J., Collet-Velasco, H., and Velasco, M. (1976): Antihypertensive effect of prazosin alone and its combination with polythiazide in patients with

essential hypertension. *Curr. Ther. Res.*, 20:751–756.

146. Marshall, A. J., Barritt, D. W., Pocock, J., and Heaton, S. T. (1977): Evaluation of beta blockade, bendrofluazide, and prazosin in severe hypertension. *Lancet*, 1:271–274.

147. Moulds, R. F. W., and Jauernig, R. A. (1977): Mechanism of prazosin collapse. *Lancet*, 1:200–201.

148. Stokes, G. S., Graham, R. M., Gain, J. M., and Davis, P. R. (1977): Influence of dosage and dietary sodium on the first-dose effects of prazosin. *Br. Med. J.*, 1:1507–1508.

149. Graham, R. M., Thornell, I. R., Gain, J. M., Bagnoli, C., Oates, H. F., and Stokes, G. S. (1976): Prazosin: The first-dose phenomenon. *Br. Med. J.*, 2:1293–1294.

150. Turner, A. S. (1976): Prazosin in hypertension. *Br. Med. J.*, 2:1257–1258.

151. Lowenstein, J., and Steele, J. M. (1978): Prazosin. *Am. Heart J.*, 95:262–265.

152. Pitts, N. E. (1975): The clinical evaluation of prazosin, a new antihypertensive agent. *Postgrad. Med.*, 117–127.

153. Stokes, G. S., and Oates, H. F. (1978): Prazosin: New alpha-adrenergic blocking agent in treatment of hypertension. *Cardiovasc. Med.*, 3:41–57.

154. Archibald, J. L., Alps, B. J., Cavalla, J. F., and Jackson, J. L. (1971): Synthesis and hypotensive activity of benzamidopiperidylethylindoles. *J. Med. Chem.*, 14:1054–1059.

155. Alps, B. J., Hill, M., Johnson, E. S., and Wilson, A. B. (1972): Quantitative analysis on isolated organs of the autonomic blocking properties of indoramin. *Br. J. Pharmacol.*, 44:52–62.

156. Baum, T., and Shropshire, A. T. (1975): Central and peripheral contribution to the antihypertensive action of indoramin. *Eur. J. Pharmacol.*, 32:30–38.

157. Archibald, J. L. (1980): Indoramin. In: *Pharmacology of Antihypertensive Drugs*, edited by A. Scriabine, pp. 161–177. Raven Press, New York.

158. Lewis, P. J., George, C. F., and Dollery, C. T. (1973): Clinical evaluation of indoramin, a new antihypertensive agent. *Eur. J. Clin. Pharmacol.*, 6:211–216.

159. Rosendorff, C. (1976): Comparison of indoramin and methyldopa in hypertension. *S. Afr. Med. J.*, 50:764–768.

160. Scriabine, A. (1979): β-Adrenoceptor blocking drugs in hypertension. *Annu. Rev. Pharmacol. Toxicol.*, 19:269–284.

161. Meier, M., Orwin, J., Rogg, H., and Brunner, H. (1980): β-Adrenoceptor antagonists in hypertension. In: *Pharmacology of Antihypertensive Drugs*, edited by A. Scriabine, pp. 179–194. Raven Press, New York.

162. Tackett, R. L., Webb, J. G., and Privitera, P. J. (1981): Cerebroventricular propranolol elevates cerebrospinal fluid norepinephrine and lowers arterial pressure. *Science*, 213:911–913.

163. Conway, J. (1975): Beta adrenergic blockade and hypertension. In: *Modern Trends in Cardiology, Vol. 3*, edited by M. Oliver, pp. 376–404. Butterworth, London.

164. Buhler, F. R., Laragh, J. H., Baer, L., Vaughan,

E. D., and Brunner, H. R. (1972): Propranolol inhibition of renin secretion. *N. Engl. J. Med.*, 287:1209–1214.

165. Hansson, L., and Zweifler, A. J. (1974): The effect of propranolol and plasma renin activity and blood pressure in mild essential hypertension. *Acta Med. Scand.*, 195:397–401.

166. Baber, N. S., and Dawes, P. M. (1979): Beta adrenoceptor blocking drugs and diuretics in hypertension. *Br. J. Clin. Pharmacol.*, 7:404–405.

167. Hansson, L., Olander, R., Aberg, H., Malmcroma, R., and Westerlund, A. (1971): Treatment of hypertension with propranolol and hydralazine. *Acta Med. Scand.*, 190:531–534.

168. Douglas-Jones, A. P. (1979): Comparison of a once daily long-acting formulation of propranolol with conventional propranolol given twice daily in patients with mild to moderate hypertension. *J. Int. Med. Res.*, 7:221–223.

169. McSorley, P. D., and Warren, D. J. (1978): Effects of propranolol and metoprolol on the peripheral circulation. *Br. Med. J.*, 2:1598–1600.

170. Davidsson, N. M., Corrall, R. J. M., Shaw, T. R. D., and French, E. B. (1977): Observations in man of hypoglycaemia during selective and non-selective beta-blockade. *Scott. Med. J.*, 22:69–76.

171. Lager, I., Blohme, G., and Smith, U. (1979): Effect of cardioselective and non-selective beta-blockade on the hypoglycemic response in insulin-dependent diabetics. *Lancet*, 1:458–462.

172. Waal-Manning, H. J. (1976): Metabolic effects of beta-adrenoceptor blockers. *Drugs [Suppl. 1]*, 11:121–126.

173. William-Olsson, T., Fellenius, E., Smith, U., and Bjorntorp, P. (1979): Differences in metabolic responses to beta-adrenergic stimulation after propranolol or metoprolol administration. *Acta Med. Scand.*, 205:201–206.

174. Waal-Manning, H. J. (1976): Experience with beta adrenoceptor blockers in hypertension. *Drugs [Suppl. 1]*, 11:164–171.

175. Borg, K. O., Carlsson, E., Hoffmann, K.-J., Jonsson, T. -E., Thorin, H., and Wallin, B. (1975): Metabolism of metoprolol-(^{3}H) in man, the dog and the rat. *Acta Pharmacol. Toxicol. [Suppl. V]*, 36:125–135.

176. Regårdh, C. -G., Borg, K. O., Johansson, R., Johnsson, G., and Palmer, L. (1974): Pharmacokinetic studies on the selective β_1-receptor antagonist metoprolol in man. *Pharmacokinet. Biopharm.*, 2:347–364.

177. Lederballe-Pedersen, O. (1976): Comparison of metoprolol and hydrochlorothiazide as antihypertensive agents. *Eur. J. Clin. Pharmacol.*, 10:381–385.

178. Lee, R. J., Evans, D. B., Baky, S. J., and Laffan, R. J. (1975): Pharmacology of nadolol (SQ 11725), a β-adrenergic antagonist lacking direct myocardial depression. *Eur. J. Pharmacol.*, 33:371–382.

179. Duchin, K., Antonaccio, M., and Steinbacher, T. (1978): Novel effects of nadolol, a new beta-adrenoceptor antagonist on renal function: Comparison with propranolol. *Circulation [Suppl. II]*, 57-58:183.

180. Hollenberg, N. K., Adams, D. F., McKinstry,

D. N., Williams, G. H., Borucki, L. J., and Sullivan, J. M. (1979): Beta-blockers and the kidney: The effect of nadolol and propranolol on the renal circulation. *Br. J. Clin. Pharmacol.* [*Suppl. 2*], 7:219–226.

181. Dreyfuss, J., Shaw, J. M., and Ross, J. J., Jr. (1978): Absorption of the β-adrenergic-blocking agent, nadolol, by mice, rats, rabbits, hamsters, dogs, monkeys, and man: An unusual species difference. *Xenobiotica,* 8:503–508.

182. Dreyfuss, J., Griffith, D. L., Singhvi, S. M., Shaw, J. M., Ross, J. J., Jr., Vukovich, R. A., and Willard, D. A. (1979): Pharmacokinetics of nadolol, a β-receptor antagonist: Administration of therapeutic single and multiple dosage regimens to hypertensive patients. *J. Clin. Pharmacol.,* 19:712–720.

183. El-Mehairy, M. M., Shaker, A., Ramadan, M., Harnza, S., and Tardos, S. S. (1979): Long-term treatment of essential hypertension using nadolol and hydrochlorothiazide combined. *Br. J. Clin. Pharmacol.* [*Suppl. 2*], 7:199–203.

184. Clark, B. J. (1977): Pharmacology of beta-adrenoceptor blocking agents. *Curr. Med. Res. Opin.* [*Suppl. 5*], 4:6–23.

185. Thorpe, P. (1971): Prindolol in hypertension. *Med. J. Aust.,* 58:1242.

186. Louis, W. J., McNeil, M. B., and Drummer, O. H. (1977): How safe are beta-blocking drugs? *Med. J. Aust.* [*Spec. Suppl.*], 2:20–24.

187. Duchene-Marullaz, P., Boucher, M., Delaigue, R., Kantelip, J. P., and Gueorguev, G. (1978): Action comparee de beta-bloquants adrenergiques sur l'automatisme cardiaque et la conduction auriculoventriculaire du chien non narcose. *Nouv. Presse Med.,* 7:2689–2696.

188. Giudicelli, J. F., Lhoste, F., and Boissier, J. R. (1975): β-Adrenergic blockade and atrio-ventricular conduction impairment. *Eur. J. Pharmacol.,* 31: 216–225.

189. Oh, V. M. S., Kaye, C. M., Warrington, S. J., Taylor, E. A., and Wadsworth, J. (1978): Studies of cardioselectivity and partial agonist activity in β-adrenoceptor blockade comparing effects on heart rate and peak expiratory flow rate during exercise. *Br. J. Clin. Pharmacol.,* 5:107–120.

190. Meier, J. (1977): Pindolol: A pharmacokinetic comparison with other beta-adrenoceptor blocking agents. *Curr. Med. Res. Opin.* [*Suppl. 5*], 4:31–38.

191. Morgan, T. O., Sabto, J., Anavekar, S. N., and Louis, W. J. (1974): A comparison of beta adrenergic blocking drugs in the treatment of hypertension. *Postgrad. Med. J.,* 50:253–259.

192. Scriabine, A., Torchiana, M. L., Stavorski, J. M., Ludden, C. T., Minsker, D. H., and Stone, C. A. (1973): Some cardiovascular effects of timolol, a new β-adrenergic blocking agent. *Arch. Int. Pharmacodyn. Ther.,* 205:76–93.

193. Vareilles, P., Silverstone, D., Plazonnet, B., Le-Douarec, J. C., Sears, M. L., and Stone, C. A. (1977): Comparison of the effects of timolol and other adrenergic agents on intraocular pressure in the rabbit. *Invest. Ophthalmol. Visual Sci.,* 16:987–996.

194. Katz, I. M., Hubbard, W. A., Getson, A. J., and Gould, A. L. (1976): Intraocular pressure decrease in normal volunteers following timolol ophthalmic solution. *Invest. Ophthalmol.,* 15:489–492.

195. Ritch, R., Harget, N. A., and Podos, S. M. (1978): The effect of 1.5% timolol maleate on intraocular pressure. *Acta Ophthalmol.,* 56:6–10.

196. Sonntag, J. R., Brindley, G. O., and Shields, M. B. (1978): Effect of timolol therapy on outflow facility. *Invest. Ophthalmol.,* 17:293–296.

197. Lohmoller, G., and Frohlich, E. D. (1975): A comparison of timolol and propranolol in essential hypertension. *Am. Heart J.,* 89:437–442.

198. Dunn, F. G., de Carvalho, J. G. R., and Frohlich, E. D. (1978): Hemodynamic, reflexive and metabolic alterations induced by acute and chronic timolol therapy in hypertensive man. *Circulation,* 57:140–144.

199. Norwegian Multicenter Study Group (1981): Timolol-induced reduction in mortality and reinfarction in patients surviving acute myocardial infarction. *N. Engl. J. Med.,* 304:801–807.

200. Basil, B., Jordan, R., Loveless, A. H., and Maxwell, D. R. (1973): Beta-adrenoceptor blocking activity and cardioselectivity of M&B 17803A. *Br. J. Pharmacol.,* 48:198–211.

201. Levy, B. (1973): The selective β-receptor blocking properties of DL-1-(2-acetyl-4-*n*-butyramidophenoxy)-2-hydroxy-3-isopropyl amino propane hydrochloride (M&B 17803A) in the anaesthetised dog. *J. Pharmacol. Exp. Ther.,* 86:134–144.

202. Maxwell, D. R., and Collins, R. F. (1973): Acebutolol (Sectral): I. Review of the Pharmacology and pharmacokinetics. *Clin. Trials J.* [*Suppl. 3*], 11:9–18.

203. Collins, R. F. (1975): Pharmacokinetics of acebutolol. *Nouv. Presse Med.,* 4:3223–3228.

204. Meffin, P. J., Winkle, R. A., Peters, F. A., and Harrison, D. C. (1978): Dose-dependent acebutolol disposition after oral administration. *Clin. Pharmacol. Ther.* 24:542–547.

205. Winkle, R. A., Meffin, P. J., Ricks, W. B., and Harrison, D. C. (1977): Acebutolol metabolite plasma concentrations during chronic oral therapy. *Br. J. Clin. Pharmacol.,* 4:519–522.

206. Ashton, W. L. (1977): An open, multicentre study of acebutolol given as a single daily dose, in the management of hypertension. *Curr. Med. Res. Opin.,* 5:279–283.

207. Baker, P. G., and Goulton, J. (1979): A multicentre study of a one daily dosage of acebutolol in the treatment of hypertension in general practice. *J. Int. Med. Res.,* 7:201–214.

208. Brittain, R. T., and Levy, G. P. (1976): A review of the animal pharmacology of labetalol, a combined α- and β-adrenoceptor blocking drug. *Br. J. Pharmacol.* [*Suppl.*], 3:681–694.

209. Blakely, A. G. H., and Summers, R. J. (1977): The effects of labetalol (AH 5158) on adrenergic transmission in the cat spleen. *Br. J. Pharmacol.,* 59:643–650.

210. Levy, G. P., and Richards, D. A. (1980): Labetalol. In: *Pharmacology of Antihypertensive Drugs,* edited by A. Scriabine, pp. 325–347. Raven Press, New York.

211. Carey, B., and Whalley, E. I. (1979): Labetalol possesses β-adrenoceptor agonist action on the isolated rat uterus. *J. Pharm. Pharmacol.*, 31:791–792.

212. Farmer, J. B., Kennedy, I., Levy, G. P., and Marshall, R. J. (1972): Pharmacology of AH 5158; a drug which blocks both α- and β-adrenoceptors. *Br. J. Pharmacol.*, 45:660–675.

213. Doggrell, S. A., and Paton, D. M. (1978): Effect of labetalol on the accumulation and release of noradrenaline in rat ventricle. *Eur. J. Pharmacol.*, 51:303–307.

214. Koch, G. (1977): Acute haemodynamic effects of an alpha and beta receptor blocking agent (AH 5158) on the systemic and pulmonary circulation at rest and during exercise in hypertensive patients. *Am. Heart J.*, 93:585–591.

215. Pritchard, B. N. C., Thompson, F. D., Boakes, A. J., and Joekes, A. M. (1975): Some haemodynamic effects of compound AH 5158 compared with propranolol, propranolol plus hydrallazine and diazoxide: The use of AH 5158 in the treatment of hypertension. *Clin. Sci. Mol. Med.*, 48:97s.

216. Pritchard, B. N. C., and Boakes, A. J. (1976): Labetalol in long term treatment of hypertension. *Br. J. Clin. Pharmacol. [Suppl.]*, 3:743–750.

217. Pritchard, B. N. C., Boakes, A. J., and Hernandez, R. (1979): Long term treatment of hypertension. *Br. J. Clin. Pharmacol. [Suppl.]*, 8:171S–178S.

218. Hopkins, R., Martin, L. E., and Bland, R. A. (1976): The metabolism of labetalol in animals and man. *Biochem. Soc. Trans.*, 4:726–729.

219. Dargie, H. J., Dollery, C. T., and Daniel, J. (1976): Labetalol in resistant hypertension. *Br. J. Clin. Pharmacol.*, *[Suppl.]*, 3:751–755.

220. Pagani, M., Vatner, S. F., and Braunwald, E. (1978): Hemodynamic effects of intravenous sodium nitroprusside in the conscious dog. *Circulation*, 57:144–151.

221. Kreye, V. A. W., and Marquard, E. (1979): Comparison of sodium nitroprusside and isoprenaline aerosols in histamine-induced bronchial asthma of the guinea pig. *Naunyn Schmiedebergs Arch. Pharmacol.*, 306:203–207.

222. Tuzel, I. H. (1974): Sodium nitroprusside. A review of its clinical effectiveness as a hypotensive agent. *J. Clin. Pharmacol.*, 14:494–503.

223. Adams, A. P., Clarke, T. N. S., Edmonds-Seal, J., Foex, P., Prys-Roberts, C., and Roberts, J. G. (1974): The effects of sodium nitroprusside on myocardial contractility and haemodynamics. *Br. J. Anaesth.*, 46:807–817.

224. Kyncl, J. (1971): Circulatory effects of sodium nitroprusside. *Naunyn Schmiedebergs Arch. Pharmacol.*, 269:390–391.

225. Bastron, R. D., and Kaloyanides, G. J. (1972): Effect of sodium nitroprusside on function in the isolated intact dog kidney. *J. Pharmacol. Exp. Ther.*, 181:244–249.

226. Ross, G., and Cole, P. V. (1973): Cardiovascular actions of sodium nitroprusside in dogs. *Anaesthesia*, 28:400–406.

227. Kreye, V. A. W. (1980): Sodium nitroprusside: Approaches towards the elucidation of its mode of action. *Trends Pharmacol. Sci.*, 1:384–388.

228. Kreye, V. A. W., Baron, G. D., Luth, J. B., and Schmidt-Gayk, H. (1975): Mode of action of sodium nitroprusside on vascular smooth muscle. *Naunyn Schmiedebergs Arch. Pharmacol.*, 288:381–402.

229. Verhaege, R. H., and Shephard, J. T. (1976): Effect of nitroprusside on smooth muscle and adrenergic nerve terminals in isolated blood vessels. *J. Pharmacol. Exp. Ther.*, 199:269–277.

230. Ito, Y., Suzuki, H., and Kuriyama, H. (1978): Effects of sodium nitroprusside on smooth muscle cells of rabbit pulmonary artery and portal vein. *J. Pharmacol. Exp. Ther.*, 207:1022–1031.

231. Kreye, V. A. W., Kern, R., and Schleich, I. (1977): [36]Chloride efflux from noradrenaline-stimulated rabbit aorta inhibited by sodium nitroprusside and nitroglycerine. In: *Excitation-Contraction Coupling in Smooth Muscle*, edited by R. Casteels, T. Godfraind, and J. D. Ruegg, pp. 145–150. Elsevier/North Holland, New York.

232. Schultz, G., Schultz, K. D., Bohme, E., and Kreye, V. A. W. (1978): The possible role of cyclic GMP in the actions of hormones and drugs on smooth muscle tone: Effects of exogenous cyclic GMP derivatives. *Adv. Pharmacol. Ther.*, 3:113–122.

233. Gruetter, C. A., Barry, B. K., McNamarra, D. B., Gruetter, D. Y., Kadowitz, P. T., and Ignarro, L. J. (1979): Relaxation of bovine coronary artery and activation of coronary arterial guanylate cyclase by nitric oxide, nitroprusside and a carcinogenic nitrosoamine. *J. Cyclic Nucleotide Res.*, 5:211–224.

234. Smith, R. P., Kruszyna, R., and Kruszyna, H. (1981): Cyanide reverses nitroprusside relaxation of rabbit aortic stips and decreases the c-GMP content. *Fed. Proc.*, 40:690.

235. Grayling, W. G., Miller, E. D., Jr., and Peach, M. J. (1978): Sodium cyanide antagonism of the vasodilator action of sodium nitroprusside in the isolated rabbit aortic strip. *Anesthesiology*, 49:21–25.

236. Kreye, V. A. W. (1977): Inhibition of nitroprusside-induced relaxation of isolated vascular smooth muscle by cyanide. Cause of clinical tachyphylaxis? *Naunyn Schmiedebergs Arch. Pharmacol. [Suppl. II]*, 297:R30.

237. Tremblay, N. A. G., Davies, D. W., Volgyesi, G., Kadar, D., and Steward, D. J. (1977): Sodium nitroprusside: Factors which attenuate its action. Studies with the isolated gracilis muscle of the dog. *Can. Anaesth. Soc. J.*, 24:641–650.

238. Rubin, A. A., Roth, F. E., Taylor, R. M., and Rosenkilde, H. (1962): Pharmacology of diazoxide, and antihypertensive, nondiuretic benzothiadiazine. *J. Pharmacol. Exp. Ther.*, 136:344–352.

239. Hamilton, T. C., and Robson, D. (1975): Evidence for the involvement of a α-adrenoceptor blockade in the antihypertensive action of diazoxide in the renal hypertensive rat. *Eur. J. Pharmacol.*, 32:273–278.

240. Nayler, W. G., McInnes, I., Swann, J. B., Race, D., Carlson, V., and Lowe, T. E. (1968): Some effects of the hypotensive drug, diazoxide, on the cardiovascular system. *Am. Heart J.*, 75:223–232.

241. Thirlwell, M. P., and Zsoter, T. T. (1972): The effect

of diazoxide on the veins. *Am. Heart J.*, 83:512–517.

242. Limbourg, P., Fiegel, P., Justin, H., and Lang, K. F. (1975): Effect of diazoxide on left ventricular performance in hypertension. *Eur. J. Clin. Pharmacol.*, 8:387–392.

243. Rubin, A. A., Zitowitz, L., and Hausler, L. (1963): Acute circulatory effects of diazoxide and sodium nitrate. *J. Pharmacol. Exp. Ther.*, 140:46–51.

244. Dhasmana, K. M., Fokker, W. A. B., and Spilker, B. A. (1972): Peripheral cardiovascular effects, in the pithed rat, of compounds used in the treatment of hypertension. *Br. J. Pharmacol.*, 46:508–510.

245. Neuvonen, P. J. (1971): Influence of diuretics and diazoxide on ions and vascular reactivity in normotensive and spontaneously hypertensive rats. *Ann. Med. Exptl. Biol. Fenn.*, 49:109–119.

246. Schmitt, H., and Fenard, S. (1969): Modifications par le diazoxide de la reponse electrique des nerfs sympathiques a des hypertension aigues. *Therapie*, 24:523–530.

247. Taylor, J., and Green, R. D. (1970): Evidence for an antagonistic action of diazoxide at alpha-adrenergic receptors in rabbit aorta. *Eur. J. Pharmacol.*, 12:385–387.

248. Wohl, A. J., Hausler, L. M., and Roth, F. E. (1967): Studies on the mechanism of antihypertensive action of diazoxide in vitro vascular pharmacodynamics. *J. Pharmacol. Exp. Ther.*, 158:531–539.

249. Wohl, A. J., Hausler, L. M., and Roth, F. E. (1968): Mechanism of the antihypertensive effect of diazoxide: In vitro vascular studies in the hypertensive rat. *J. Pharmacol. Exp. Ther.*, 162:109–114.

250. Wohl, A. J., Hausler, L. M., and Roth, F. E. (1968): The role of calcium in the mechanism of the antihypertensive action of diazoxide. *Life Sci.*, 7:381–387.

251. Rhodes, H. J., and Sutter, M. C. (1971): The action of diazoxide on isolated vascular smooth muscle electrophysiology and contraction. *Can. J. Physiol. Pharmacol.*, 49:276–287.

252. Maxwell, G. M. (1971): Effects of diazoxide and dipyridamole derivative on cardiac nucleotide content. *Nature*, 233:250.

253. Pohl, J. E. F., Thurston, H., and Swales, J. D. (1972): The antidiuretic action of diazoxide. *Clin. Sci.*, 42:145–152.

254. Küchel, O., Fishman, L. M., Liddle, G. W., and Michelakis, A. (1967): Effect of diazoxide on plasma renin activity in hypertensive patients. *Ann. Intern. Med.*, 67:791–799.

255. Winer, N., Chokstri, D. S., Yoon, M. S., and Freedman, A. D. (1969): Adrenergic receptor mediation of renin secretion. *J. Clin. Endocrinol. Metab.*, 29:1168–1175.

256. Baer, L., Goodwin, F. J., and Laragh, J. H. (1969): Diazoxide-induced renin release in man; dissociation from plasma and extracellular fluid volume changes. *J. Clin. Endocrinol. Metab.*, 29:1107–1109.

257. Vandongen, R., and Greenwood, D. M. (1975): The stimulation of renin secretion by diazoxide in the isolated rat kidney. *Eur. J. Pharmacol.*, 33:197–200.

258. Sponer, G., Schelling, P., Ganten, D., and Gross, F. (1978): Effect of beta-adrenoceptor blockade on the cardiovascular and hyperglycemic actions of diazoxide. *Naunyn Schmiedebergs Arch. Pharmacol.*, 303:15–20.

259. Tabachnick, I. I. A., Gulbenkian, A., and Seidman, F. (1965): Further studies on the metabolic effects of diazoxide. *J. Pharmacol. Exp. Ther.*, 150:455–462.

260. Tabachnick, I. I. A., and Gulbenkian, A. (1968): Mechanism of diazoxide hyperglycemia in animals. *Ann. N.Y. Acad. Sci.*, 150:204–218.

261. Losert, W., Senft, G., Sitt, R., and Schultz, G. (1966): Die Beteiligung des Insulins an der Diazoxid-Hyperglykamie. *Naunyn Schmiedebergs Arch. Pharmacol.*, 253:388–394.

262. Kaess, H., Senft, G., Losert, W., Sitt, R., and Schultz, G. (1966): Mechanismus der gesteigerten glykogenolytischen Wirkung des Diazoxids im Kalium-Mangel. *Naunyn Schmiedebergs Arch. Pharmacol.*, 253:395–401.

263. DuCharme, D. W., Freyburger, W. A., Graham, B. E., and Carlson, R. G. (1973): Pharmacologic properties of minoxidil: A new hypotensive agent. *J. Pharmacol. Exp. Ther.*, 184:662–670.

264. DuCharme, D. W., and Green, G. R. (1980): Minoxidil. In: *Pharmacology of Antihypertensive Drugs*, edited by A. Scriabine, pp. 415–421. Raven Press, New York.

265. Pettinger, W. A., and Keeton, K. (1975): Altered renin release and propranolol potentiation of vasodilatory drug hypotension. *J. Clin. Invest.*, 55:236–243.

266. Weir, E. K., Chidsey, C. A., Weil, J. V., and Grover, R. F. (1976): Minoxidil reduces pulmonary vascular resistance in dogs and cattle. *J. Lab. Clin. Med.*, 88:885–894.

267. Humphrey, S. J., Wilson, E., and Zins, G. R. (1974): Whole body tissue blood flow in conscious dogs treated with minoxidil. *Fed. Proc.*, 33:583.

268. Wendling, M. G., DeGraaf, G. L., and DuCharme, D. W. (1979): The effects of sympatholytics, angiotensin and vasopressin on the cardiovascular response to minoxidil or hydralazine in conscious dogs. *Clin. Exp. Hypertension*, 1:521–537.

269. Greenberg, S. (1980): Studies on the effect of chronic oral administration of minoxidil and hydralazine on vascular function in spontaneously hypertensive rats. *J. Pharmacol. Exp. Ther.*, 215:279–286.

270. Bonaccorsi, A., Franco, R., Garattini, S., and Chidsey, C. (1973): Mechanism of vasodilator activity of the antihypertensive minoxidil. *Circulation* [Suppl. IV], 48:45.

271. Limas, C. J., and Cohn, J. N. (1973): Stimulation by vasodilators of the (Na^+K^+)-ATPase of vascular smooth muscle. *Fed. Proc.*, 32:406.

272. Limas, C. J., and Cohn, J. N. (1974): Stimulation of vascular smooth muscle sodium, potassium-adenosinetriphosphatase by vasodilators. *Circ. Res.*, 35:601–607.

273. Greenberg, S., and Bohr, D. (1975): Venous smooth muscle in hypertension. Enhanced contractility of portal veins from spontaneous hypertensive rats. *Circ. Res.* [Suppl. 1], 36:I208–I214.

274. Gilmore, E., Weil, J., and Chidsey, C. A. (1970): Treatment of essential hypertension with a new vaso-

dilator in combination with beta-adrenergic blockade. *N. Engl. J. Med.,* 282:521–527.

275. Gross, F., Druey, J., and Meier, R. (1950): Eine neue Gruppe blutdrucksenkender Substanzen von besonderem Wirkungscharakter. *Experientia,* 6:19–21.

276. Gross, F. (1977): Drugs acting on arteriolar smooth muscle (vasodilator drugs). In: *Antihypertensive Agents,* edited by F. Gross, pp. 399–418. Springer-Verlag, New York.

277. Koch-Weser, J. (1974): Vasodilator drugs in the treatment of hypertension. *Arch. Intern. Med.,* 133:1017–1027.

278. Francis, J. E. (1976): Antihypertensives acting by a peripheral mechanism. *ACS Symposium Series,* 27:55–79.

279. Druey, J., and Tripod, J. (1967): Hydralazines. In: *Antihypertensive Agents,* edited by E. Schlittler, pp. 223–262. Academic Press, New York.

280. Ablad, B., and Mellander, J. (1963): Comparative effects of hydralazine, sodium nitrite and acetylcholine on resistance and capacitance blood vessels and capillary filtration in skeletal muscle in the cat. *Acta Physiol. Scand.,* 58:319–329.

281. Baum, T., Shropshire, A. T., and Varner, L. L. (1972): Contributions of central nervous system to the actions of several antihypertensive agents (methyldopa, hydralazine and guanethidine). *J. Pharmacol. Exp. Ther.,* 182:135–144.

282. Craver, B. N., Barrett, N., Cameron, A., and Yonkman, F. F. (1951): The activities of 1-hydrazinophthalazine (Ba 5968), a hypotensive agent. *J. Am. Pharm. Assoc. Sci. Ed.,* 40:559–564.

283. Freis, E. D., Rose, J. C., Higgins, T. F., Finnerty, F. A., Jr., Kelley, R. T., and Partenope, E. A. (1973): The hemodynamic effects of hypotensive drugs in man. IV. 1-Hydrazinophthalazine. *Circulation,* 8:199–204.

284. Mellander, S., and Johansson, B. (1968): Control of resistance, exchange, and capacitance functions in the peripheral circulation. *Pharmacol. Rev.,* 20:117–196.

285. Spokas, E. G., and Wang, H. (1980): Regional blood flow and cardiac responses to hydralazine. *J. Pharmacol. Exp. Ther.,* 212:294–303.

286. Khatri, I., Uremura, N., Notargiacomo, A., and Freis, E. (1977): Direct and reflex cardiostimulatory effects of hydralazine. *Am. J. Cardiol.,* 40:38–42.

287. Oblad, B. (1963): A study of mechanism of the hemodynamic effects of hydralazine in man. *Acta Pharmacol. Toxicol. [Suppl. 1],* 29:1–53.

288. Marks, P. A., Reynell, P. C., and Bradley, S. E. (1955): Hemodynamic effects of 1-hydrazinophthalazine in the dog, with special reference to circulating splanchnic blood volume. *Am. J. Physiol.,* 183:144–148.

289. Stein, D. H., and Hecht, H. H. (1955): Cardiovascular and renal responses to the combination of hexamethonium and 1-hydrazinophthalazine (Apresoline) in hypertensive subjects. *J. Clin. Invest.,* 34:867–874.

290. Kirpekar, S. M., and Lewis, J. J. (1958): Effects of reserpine and hydralazine on isolated strips of carotid arteries. *J. Pharm. Pharmacol.,* 10:255–259.

291. Kirpekar, S. M., and Lewis, J. J. (1958): Antagonism of the actions of hydralazine, reserpine, potassium cyanide, sodium azide and anoxia on arterial smooth muscle. *J. Pharm. Pharmacol.,* 10:307–314.

292. Schroeder, H. A. (1959): The pharmacology of hydralazine. In: *Hypertension,* edited by H. Moyer, pp. 332–344. W. B. Saunders, Philadelphia.

293. Pedersen, O. L., Mikkelsen, E., and Anderson, K. E. (1979): Comparison of the in vitro effects of prazosin, nifedipine, and dihydralazine in isolated human mesenteric and crural vessels. *Arch. Int. Pharmacodyn. Ther.,* 241:224–234.

294. Trapani, A., Abel, P., Matsuki, N., Worcel, M., and Hermsmeyer, K. (1980): Hydralazine vasodilation produced by membrane hyperpolarization. *Blood Vessels,* 17:164.

295. McLean, A. J., Barron, K., DuSouich, P., Haegele, K. D., McNay, J. L., Carrier, O., and Briggs, A. (1978): Interaction of hydralazine and hydrazone derivatives with contractile mechanisms in rabbit aortic smooth muscle. *J. Pharmacol. Exp. Ther.,* 205:418–425.

296. McLean, A. J., DuSouich, P., Barron, K. W., and Briggs, A. H. (1978): Interaction of hydralazine with tension development and mechanisms of calcium accumulation in K^+-stimulated rabbit aortic strips. *J. Pharmacol. Exp. Ther.,* 207:40–48.

297. Diamond, J., and Janis, R. A. (1980): Effects of hydralazine and verapamil on phosphorylase activity and guanosine cyclic 3′,5′-monophosphate levels in guinea-pig taenia coli. *Br. J. Pharmacol.,* 68:275–282.

298. Hansson, L., Olander, R., Aberg, H., Malmcrona, R., and Westerlund, A. (1971): Treatment of hypertension with propranolol and hydralazine. *Acta Med. Scand.,* 190:531–534.

299. Newsome, C. K. (1961): Combined therapy in the treatment of hypertension. Reserpine, hydralazine, hydrochlorothiazide. *Southwest. Med.,* 42:558–567.

300. Franciosa, J. A., Pierpont, G., and Cohn, J. N. (1977): Hemodynamic improvement after oral hydralazine in left ventricular failure. A comparison with nitroprusside infusion in 16 patients. *Ann. Intern. Med.,* 86:388–393.

301. Chatterjee, K., Parmley, W. W., Massie, B., Greenberg, B., Werner, J., Klausner, S., and Norman, A. (1976): Oral hydralazine therapy for chronic refractory heart failure. *Circulation,* 54:879–883.

302. Massie, B., Chatterjee, K., Werner, J., Greenberg, B., Hart, R., and Parmley, W. W. (1977): Hemodynamic advantage of combined administration of hydralazine orally and nitrates nonparenterally in the vasodilator therapy of chronic heart failure. *Am. J. Cardiol.,* 40:794–801.

303. Mehta, J., Pepine, C. J., and Conti, C. R. (1978): Hemodynamic effects of hydralazine and hydralazine plus glyceryl trinitrate paste in heart failure. *Br. Heart J.,* 40:845–850.

304. Ginks, W. R., and Redwood, D. R. (1980): Haemodynamic effects of hydralazine at rest and during exercise in patients with chronic heart disease. *Br. Heart J.,* 44:259–264.

305. Triggle, D. J., and Swamy, V. C. (1980): Pharmacol-

ogy of agents that affect calcium-agonists and antagonists. *Chest,* 78:174–179.

306. Hiwatari, M., Satoh, K., and Taira, N. (1979): Antihypertensive effect of nifedipine on conscious renal-hypertensive dogs. *Arzneim. Forsch./Drug. Res.,* 29:256–260.

307. Garthoff, B., and Kazda, S. (1981): Calcium antagonist nifedipine normalizes high blood pressure and prevents mortality in salt-loaded DS substrain of Dahl rats. *Eur. J. Pharmacol.,* 74:111–112.

308. Aoki, K., Kondo, S., Mochizuki, A., Yoshida, T., Kato, S., Kato, K., and Takikawa, K. (1978): Antihypertensive effect of cardiovascular Ca^{2+}-antagonist in hypertensive patients in the absence and presence of beta-adrenergic blockade. *Am. Heart J.,* 96:218–226.

309. Guazzi, M., Olivari, M. T., Polese, A., Fiorentini, C., Magrini, F., and Moruzzi, P. (1977): Nifedipine, a new antihypertensive with rapid action. *Clin. Pharmacol. Ther.,* 22:528–532.

310. Lederballe-Pedersen, O., Christensen, N. J., and Ramsch, K. D. (1980): Comparison of acute effects of nifedipine in normotensive and hypertensive man. *J. Cardiovasc. Pharmacol.,* 2:357–366.

311. Olivari, M. T., Bartorelli, C., Polese, A., Fiorentini, C., Moruzzi, P., and Guazzi, M. D. (1979): Treatment of hypertension with nifedipine, a calcium antagonistic agent. *Circulation,* 59:1056–1062.

312. Kuwajima, I., Ueda, K., Kamata, C., Matsushita, S., Kuramoto, K., Murakami, M., and Hada, Y. (1978): A study in the effects of nifedipine in hypertensive crises and severe hypertension. *Jpn. Heart J.,* 19:455–467.

313. Guazzi, M. D., Fiorentini, C., Olivari, M. T., Bartorelli, A., Necchi, G., and Polese, A. (1980): Short- and long-term efficacy of a calcium-antagonistic agent (nifedipine) combined with methyldopa in the treatment of severe hypertension. *Circulation,* 61:913–919.

314. Lederballe-Pedersen, O. (1979): Role of extracellular calcium in isometric contractions of the SHR aorta. Influence of age and antihypertensive treatment. *Arch. Int. Pharmacodyn. Ther.,* 239:208–220.

315. Mulvany, M. J., and Nyborg, N. (1980): An increased calcium sensitivity of mesenteric resistance vessels in young and adult spontaneously hypertensive rats. *Br. J. Pharmacol.,* 71:585–596.

316. Vater, W., Kroneberg, G., Hoffmeister, F., Saller, H., Meng, K., Oberdorf, A., Puls, W., Schlossmann, K., and Stoepel, K. (1972): Pharmacology of 4-(2-nitrophenyl)-2,6-dimethyl-1,4-dihydropyridine-3,5-dicarboxylic acid dimethyl ester (nifedipine, BAY a 1040). *Arzneim. Forsch.,* 22:1–14.

317. Robinson, B. F., Dobbs, R. J., and Kelsey, C. R. (1980): Effects of nifedipine on resistance vessels, arteries and veins in man. *Br. J. Clin. Pharmacol.,* 10:433–438.

318. Lederballe-Pedersen, O., Christensen, C. K., Mikkelsen, E., and Ramsch, K. D. (1980): Relationship between the antihypertensive effect and steady-state plasma concentration of nifedipine given along or in combination with a beta-adrenoceptor blocking agent. *Eur. J. Clin. Pharmacol.,* 18:287–293.

319. Fleckenstein, A. (1977): Specific pharmacology of calcium in myocardium, cardiac pacemakers, and

vascular smooth muscle. *Annu. Rev. Pharmacol. Toxicol.,* 17:149–166.

320. Bolton, T. B. (1979): Mechanisms of action of transmitters and other substances on smooth muscle. *Physiol. Rev.,* 59:606–718.

321. Bevan, J. A., Garstka, W., Su, C., and Su, M. O. (1973): The bimodal basis of the contractile response of the rabbit ear artery to norepinephrine and other agonists. *Eur. J. Pharmacol.,* 22:47–53.

322. Van Breemen, C., and Siegel, B. (1980): The mechanism of α-adrenergic activation of the dog coronary artery. *Circ. Res.,* 46:426–429.

323. Constantine, J. W., and Hess, H. -J. (1981): The cardiovascular effects of trimazosin. *Eur. J. Pharmacol.,* 74:227–238.

324. Macho, P., and Vatner, S. F. (1981): Effects and mechanism of action on coronary and left ventricular dynamics in conscious dogs. *J. Pharmacol. Exp. Ther.,* 217:333–339.

325. De Guice, D., Mendlowitz, M., Russo, C., Vlachakis, N. D., and Antram, S. (1973): The effect of trimazosin in essential hypertension. *Curr. Ther. Res.,* 15:339–348.

326. Schoetensack, W., Bischler, P., Dittmann, E. C., and Steinijans, V. (1977): Tieresperimentelle Untersuchungen über den Einflug des Antihypertensivums Urapidil auf den Kreislauf und die Kreislaufregulation. *Arzneim. Forsch.,* 27:1908–1919.

327. Bruckschen, E. G., and Haerlin, R. (1980): Hockdrucktherapie mit Ebrantil®. *Therapiewoche,* 30:7850–7851.

328. Haerlin, R., Bruckschen, E. G., and Henze, F. (1981): Antihypertensive Therapie with Ebrantil® Retard Kapseln Ergebnisse einer Multicenterstudie. *Therapiewoche,* 31:7930–7939.

329. Collier, J. G., and Pitcher, D. W. (1980): Investigation of a combined arteriolar dilator and adrenoceptor antagonist (SK&F92657) in the peripheral vessels of man. *Br. J. Clin. Pharmacol.,* 10:567–571.

330. Edmonstone, W. M., Mangliani, K. K., Bell, A. J., McLeod, M., Milton-Thompson, G. J., and Burland, W. L. (1981): Cardiovascular effects in man of intravenous prizidolol hydrochloride (SK&F92657); a new antihypertensive agent. *Br. J. Clin. Pharmacol.,* 12:567–572.

331. Baldwin, J. S., Lumma, W. C., Lundell, C. F., Ponticello, G. S., Raab, A. W., Engelhardt, E. L., Hirschmann, R. C., Sweet, C. S., and Scriabine, A. (1979): Symbiotic approach to drug design: Antihypertensive β-adrenergic blocking agents. *J. Med. Chem.,* 22:1284–1290.

332. Gross, D. M., Sweet, C. S., Ulm, E. H., Backlund, E. P., Morris, A. A., Weitz, D., Bohn, D. L., Wenger, H. C., Vassil, T. C., and Stone, C. A. (1981): Effect of *N*-[(*S*)-1-carboxy-3-phenylporopyl]-L-Ala-L-Pro and its ethyl ester (MK-421) on angiotensin converting enzyme in vitro and angiotensin I pressor responses in vivo. *J. Pharmacol. Exp. Ther.,* 216:552–557.

333. Sweet, C. S., Gross, D. M., Arbegast, P. T., Gaul, S. L., Britt, P. M., Ludden, C. T., Weitz, D., and Stone, C. A. (1981): Antihypertensive activity of *N*-[(*S*)-1-(ethoxycarbonyl)-3-phenylpropyl]-L-Pro (MK-421), an orally active converting enzyme inhibitor. *J. Pharmacol. Exp. Ther.,* 216:558–566.

Cardiovascular Pharmacology, Second Edition,
edited by Michael Antonaccio.
Raven Press, New York © 1984.

Angina Pectoris and Chronic Congestive Heart Failure: Pathophysiology and Therapy

Gary S. Francis and Jay N. Cohn

Cardiovascular Division, Department of Medicine, University of Minnesota Medical School; and Veterans Administration Medical Center, Minneapolis, Minnesota 55417

Coronary artery disease (CAD) is the most common single cause of death in the United States today, accounting for more than 700,000 deaths per year (1). Although usually only symptomatic patients are brought to the attention of a physician, one can assume that the number of CAD cases in the asymptomatic, healthy population of middle-aged men is much higher than previously anticipated, with an incidence of approximately 5 to 6% (2). Complications of coronary artery disease include angina pectoris, myocardial infarction, and sudden death. Men who develop angina pectoris can expect to have a 25% chance of having a myocardial infarction within 5 years of the onset of symptoms. Among those who survive infarction (for which the immediate overall mortality is approximately 33%) (4), the average survivor will face a 50% incidence of angina pectoris, a 10-fold increase in the risk of congestive heart failure, a four-fold increase in risk of sudden death, a 6% annual recurrence rate of infarction, and a 4% annual mortality (5). It has been estimated that the annual cost to the nation of cardiovascular disease in 1975 was more than $40 billion (6). Clearly, CAD is a problem of great magnitude in this country today. This chapter presents a brief and, out of necessity, incomplete description of the pathophysiology and treatment of two complications of CAD (angina pectoris and congestive heart failure).

ANGINA PECTORIS

Historical Perspective on the Pathophysiology of Angina Pectoris

Angina pectoris, although not clearly defined until 1772 by William Heberden (7), undoubtedly involved humans throughout history (8). Heberden described it as "a disorder which comes on by walking . . . goes off almost immediately upon stopping" and characterized it as a "strangling . . . painful and most disagreeable sensation in the breast." Although Heberden's description of angina remains a time-honored classic, it is of interest that he demonstrated no knowledge of the pathophysiology of the event and did not appreciate the connection between angina pectoris and the heart. That ischemia of the myocardium due to diseased coronary arteries was the cause of angina was first proposed by Allan Burns (9) in 1809. This idea was not generally accepted, however, because many persons who never had angina were found at autopsy to have severely diseased coronary arteries. Spasm of the ventricular muscle was suggested as a cause of angina by Nothnagel (10) in 1867, after he was struck by the fact that clinical signs of peripheral constriction accompanied anginal attacks. He suggested that a systemic "vasomotor storm" was occurring that might cause peripheral arteriolar spasm, causing a rise in blood pressure and "difficulty for the heart to pump blood out," leading to cardiac distension and angina. William Osler (11), in reviewing the causes of angina in 1910, listed coronary artery spasm among a number of possible mechanisms. Osler's views became widely accepted, despite the absence of experimental validation. Careful studies by Herrick (12) published in 1912 described the clinical and pathologic features of acute coronary thrombosis, although these classic reports antedated the use of the electrocardiogram. In 1918, Smith (13), at the suggestion of Herrick, recorded electrocardiograms of dogs after ligating one of the coronary arteries. He observed for the first time the acute elevation of the ST segment and T waves we now associate with transmural ischemic injury. Pardee (14) later reported the electrocardiographic findings in a patient during the acute phase of an inferior infarction, EKG features later to be recognized as the hallmark of myocardial injury. By 1924, Danielopolu (15) suggested the theory that angina is a result of an imbalance between the work of the heart and its blood supply, and that provides the basis of our current understanding of this important pathophysiologic event.

The idea that angina is largely due to inadequate perfusion of the myocardium is based on the careful and widely referenced autopsy studies of Blumgart et al. (16), who reported that in the absence of valvular disease, angina was almost always associated with severe two- and three-vessel coronary obstruction. Keefer and Resnick (17) had already suggested that coronary arteries with fixed occlusive lesions would be unlikely to have active vasomotion, indicating that angina is more likely due to an increase in myocardial oxygen demand rather than a dynamic change in oxygen supply. This idea was largely supported by Roughgarden and Newman (18), who concluded that even spontaneous angina usually was preceded by increases in blood pressure and heart rate. As late as 1971, many influential physicians subscribed to the belief that conditions tending to precipitate ischemic pain

usually were associated with circulatory changes that increased myocardial oxygen consumption (19). The diagnosis of coronary artery spasm was considered a "resort of the diagnostically destitute" (20). A distinct exception to this thinking was proposed by Prinzmetal et al. (21), who suggested that some patients may have angina at rest associated with transient ST-segment elevation on the electrocardiogram in the distribution of a single large coronary artery. Prinzmetal postulated that the clinical manifestations of the syndrome resulted from increased tonus of the coronary vessel wall superimposed on a large diseased artery with a lumen narrowed by atherosclerotic plaque. This idea of increased vasomotor tone was largely ignored, for following the advent of selective coronary arteriography (22), angiographers were unable to document coronary artery spasm, probably because of the routine practice of administering nitrate coronary dilators just prior to coronary arteriography and the unwillingness to make coronary injections during attacks of angina. Coronary artery spasm was not actually proved until 1973, when Oliva et al. (23) demonstrated angiographically recurrent right coronary artery spasm in a patient in whom ST-segment elevation was documented simultaneously. Oliva's work was soon confirmed by a number of investigators (24–26), and Maseri et al. (27) suggested that coronary artery spasm eventually culminates in myocardial infarction in some patients. Even angina occurring during exercise was documented to be due to coronary artery spasm in some cases (28,29), although this was considered not to be a frequent cause of exertional angina. Careful quantitative studies by Brown et al. (30) demonstrated the ability of atheromatous coronary artery stenosis to change the luminal diameter significantly as the result of active coronary vasomotion in patients with variant or classic anginal syndrome. It is now clear that circulatory changes that increase myocardial oxygen consumption (i.e., increases in blood pressure and/or heart rate) and coronary vasomotor activity both contribute as important mechanisms in the pathophysiology of ischemic heart disease, particularly in the setting of atherosclerotic coronary artery disease. It is only through an understanding of these mechanisms that rational therapy for patients can be achieved.

Control of Myocardial Oxygen Consumption

Ischemia is the condition of oxygen deprivation accompanied by inadequate removal of metabolites consequent to reduced perfusion. Myocardial ischemia is difficult to define in absolute terms, because the blood flow requirement to the myocardium varies under different conditions. Under basal physiologic conditions, regional flow of 60 to 90 ml/min per 100 g of myocardium is generally required. When the work of the heart or its metabolic requirements are reduced, viability can be maintained by perfusion at much lower rates. The stress of exercise or tachycardia will increase perfusion requirements. The balance between oxygen supply and demand is then largely a product of the determinants of myocardial oxygen consumption ($M\dot{V}O_2$). $M\dot{V}O_2$ is calculated by an application of the Fick principle as the product of coronary blood flow per minute and the coronary arteriovenous difference. In humans, catheterization of the coronary sinus and measurement of coronary blood flow by inert-gas washout methods permit reasonably accurate steady-state assessment of $M\dot{V}O_2$ expressed per 100 g of tissue (31). In the normal resting human subject, values for $M\dot{V}O_2$ average about 8.5 ml O_2 per 100 g of left ventricle (32). Coronary blood flow and $M\dot{V}O_2$ can increase severalfold during exercise. There are at least six determinants of $M\dot{V}O_2$:

1. Basal metabolism;
2. Activation metabolism;
3. Intracardiac systolic pressure and myocardial wall stress (or tension);
4. Myocardial fiber shortening and cardiac work;
5. Inotropic state;
6. Frequency of contraction.

Four of these play major roles in the beat-to-beat demand for oxygen. For simplicity, the discussion of $M\dot{V}O_2$ is restricted to the left ventricle, which is responsible for a major fraction of the heart's total $M\dot{V}O_2$.

Basal Metabolism

The resting energy of the heart reflects primarily ATP-utilizing processes, such as cell membrane activity and protein synthesis, that are not directly related to contraction. It averages about 1.5 to 2 ml/100 g/min, or about 20% of total $M\dot{V}O_2$, and appears to be relatively stable under most conditions, including acute pharmacologic interventions (33).

Activation Metabolism

The O_2 cost of activation of contraction has not been accurately measured, but it appears to include both electrical activation and the release and reuptake of Ca^{2+} by the sarcoplasmic reticulum. The cost of electrical activation is small, constituting 0.5% of the $M\dot{V}O_2$ at a normal heart rate (34). The sarcotubular Ca^{2+} pump uses substantial energy during inotropic stimulation of heart muscle, but the overall cost of activation metabolism is considered small when related to other determinants of $M\dot{V}O_2$.

Intracardiac Systolic Pressure and Myocardial Wall Stress (or Tension)

Because left ventricular wall tension varies directly in proportion to intraventricular volume and pressure, an increase in either will augment wall tension and thereby increase $M\dot{V}O_2$. The relation between peak wall stress and $M\dot{V}O_2$ is almost linear (35), and a fivefold or sixfold increase in $M\dot{V}O_2$ can be produced during isovolumic pressure development, suggesting that the development of wall tension is more important in O_2 cost than the actual ejection of blood. Afterloading conditions, or the load against which the heart must build up tension prior to ejection, therefore constitute a major component of myocardial oxygen demand. Fortunately, afterload, which is a major element of the total impedance to ejection, is relatively accessible to pharmacologic intervention.

Myocardial Fiber Shortening and Cardiac Work

There appears to be an increment of $M\dot{V}O_2$ during shortening beyond that associated with tension alone (36). It is estimated that in the normal heart this shortening component could account for as much as 17% of the total $M\dot{V}O_2$. Although it is relatively small, an analysis of its relative contribution over a wide range of loading conditions and at different inotropic states has not been performed in the intact heart.

Inotropic State

A variety of positive inotropic stimuli, including paired electrical stimulation, norepinephrine, calcium, and digitalis, consistently increase the $M\dot{V}O_2$ as much as 100%, even when mean arterial pressure, stroke volume, and myocardial wall tension are kept constant or decrease. The increase in $M\dot{V}O_2$ is generally proportional to the speed of myocardial contraction (37). The inotropic state, although difficult to measure in the intact human heart, plays a major role in determining $M\dot{V}O_2$. All drugs that increase the inotropic state tend to increase $M\dot{V}O_2$. However, in the failing heart, wall tension may fall with inotropic therapy because of decreased cardiac volume brought about by more efficient performance; the net effect of such a pharmacologic intervention may be a fall in $M\dot{V}O_2$. Therefore, the net effect of inotropic stimuli on $M\dot{V}O_2$ will depend on the basal efficiency of myocardial performance. In the nonfailing heart, inotropic stimuli will always increase $M\dot{V}O_2$.

Frequency of Contraction

The $M\dot{V}O_2$ varies markedly with heart rate. Changing the rate from 100 to 200 beats per minute, even when wall stress is held constant, will more than double $M\dot{V}O_2$ (38). It is evident, therefore, that the heart rate is a very important determinant of $M\dot{V}O_2$. This has important therapeutic implications, because many cardiovascular drugs are known to alter heart rate.

Thus, many factors influence $M\dot{V}O_2$, and each must be considered when assessing the effectiveness of a therapeutic intervention designed to diminish or prevent ischemic chest pain.

Regulation of Myocardial Oxygen Delivery

Three mechanisms theoretically available for increasing myocardial oxygen supply during periods of increased demand are blood flow through the coronary vascular bed, the oxygen content of arterial blood, and the amount of oxygen extracted from the blood by the heart. However, only one of these factors, coronary blood flow, is of major importance in most patients with ischemic heart disease. The critical factors that regulate blood flow within the myocardium include the diastolic pressure, the duration of diastole, and the multiple sites of resistance to blood flow.

Whenever aortic diastolic pressure is diminished, the capacity to perfuse the coronary arteries is compromised. However, the absolute level of aortic diastolic pressure is not the perfusing pressure of the myocardium; the intramyocardial diastolic pressure must be subtracted from the aortic diastolic pressure to calculate the net driving pressure. Under normal circumstances the left ventricular diastolic pressure is low enough to be of little importance. However, when the myocardium fails, or even during episodes of spontaneous angina, the left ventricular diastolic pressure may be greatly increased, reducing the pressure gradient between the aorta and the coronary arteries and markedly diminishing blood flow to the coronary vascular bed.

Resistance to myocardial blood flow occurs primarily during systole when the myocardium develops tension that compresses the perforating coronary arteries. The major physiologic resistance vessels of the myocardium are the arterioles, which, when maximally dilated, can accomodate blood flow four to five times the normal value. Control of the arteriolar resistance is primarily local, the major stimulus to dilatation being ischemia. Changes in arteriolar resistance are primarily through autoregulation by local metabolites, although α and β receptor stimulation may play some role. In the presence of ischemic heart disease, the coronary collateral system is also an important site offering changes in resistance to coronary flow. Of course, in patients with fixed obstructive coronary lesions, resistance in the large involved epicardial vessels also limits blood flow. Exertional angina may be caused not only by the inability of partially occluded arteries to meet the increased myocardial oxygen demand but also by a fall in flow beyond the stenosis. In the presence of partially obstructed fixed lesions of the coronary arteries, dilatation of the vessels downstream from a lesion brought on by exercise may enlarge the volume of the distal vascular bed, thus creating a demand for more blood to maintain the distal pressure. As the distal pressure falls because of exercise-induced vasodilatation, flow to subendocardial layers to the heart also falls. This sequence of events may account for angina during exercise. Coronary artery spasm, when it occurs, also involves these large epicardial vessels, but the mechanism and extent of this problem are currently unresolved. The regulation of myocardial oxygen delivery is therefore dependent on multiple variables, only some of which are amenable to pharmacologic intervention.

The Medical Approach to Treatment of Angina Pectoris

The traditional first step in medical therapy is treatment of coexisting problems that tend to increase $M\dot{V}O_2$. This concept was constructed before much information was available indicating that coronary artery spasm was common and before it was known that dis-

eased coronary vessels could dilate. It was generally conceded that the salutary clinical benefits derived from drug therapy in the treatment of angina pectoris resulted principally from the actions of these interventions on myocardial oxygen consumption rather than on coronary blood flow (39). More current data suggest that these agents, specifically the vasodilators, have an important influence on coronary blood flow (40). It is primarily by increasing the caliber of large epicardial coronary arteries and thereby reducing the severity of the stenosis that nitrates relieve ischemia (40), although peripheral effects related to reduced $M\dot{V}O_2$ are also important.

Modern medical treatment of angina pectoris requires knowledge of agents that alter both $M\dot{V}O_2$ and delivery of myocardial oxygen. It is by optimizing the balance between demand and flow that symptoms are usually relieved. Angina therapy in the past was based on a model of myocardial perfusion that was oversimplified and misleading. New findings about the interactions of dynamic factors in angina pectoris, along with the arrival of new drugs that alter these factors, have made angina therapy more challenging than in the past. However, the concept of an imbalance between oxygen demand and delivery has remained intact (Fig. 1).

Nitroglycerin

Although each of the nitrates directly relaxes smooth muscle and produces coronary vasodilatation, their mechanisms are complex and, in certain respects, controversial. Nitroglycerin is said to reduce myocardial oxygen requirements by diminishing systolic wall tension through reduced systemic pressure (afterload) and reduced left ventricular diastolic pressure and cavity size (preload) (42). By reducing intraventricular diastolic pressure, it improves the transmural distribution of myocardial perfusion by reducing extrinsic diastolic compression of the subendocardial vessels. Although nitroglycerin does not appear to dilate the coronary arteriolar resistance bed, it does dilate collateral vessels and the un-

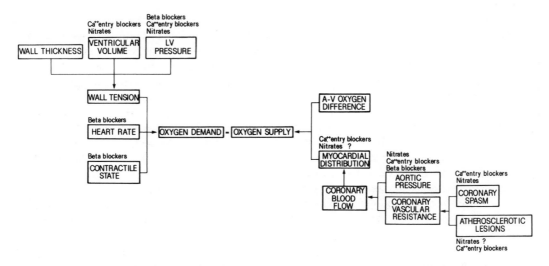

FIG. 1. Pathophysiology of myocardial ischemia: sites of action of antianginal agents.

diseased, as well as diseased, large coronary epicardial vessels (40). However, the principal effect was for some time believed to be mainly peripheral, supported by the observation of Ganz and Marcus (43) that intracoronary nitroglycerin failed to relieve pacing-induced angina. Because the size of the heart is related to the development of myocardial tension and $M\dot{V}O_2$, the reduction in ventricular volume caused by pooling of blood in the peripheral veins reduces myocardial oxygen requirements. The actions on the veins appear to dominate over the arterioles, because cardiac output and stroke volume are diminished except at high doses (44). Although the peripheral effects of nitroglycerin are important in reducing myocardial oxygen demand, recent information has focused attention on the ability of these agents to directly influence coronary blood flow. Whereas it has previously been believed that an increase in coronary arteriolar diameter brought on by nitroglycerin would improve oxygen delivery to the myocardium, vasodilatation distal to a fixed occlusive lesion may actually reduce pressure and flow to the subendocardium (41). More direct evidence now indicates that a primary action of nitroglycerin is to increase the caliber of large epicardial coronary arteries and thereby reduce the severity of the stenosis (40). That

the more direct effects on coronary arteries play a major role is supported by the recent demonstration of a striking improvement in ischemic left ventricular compliance abnormalities after low-dose intracoronary nitroglycerin (40).

The sublingual form of nitroglycerin is highly effective in both the prevention and amelioration of angina pectoris, but its duration of action is usually less than 20 min. More recently, the use of intravenous nitroglycerin has gained widespread popularity for patients hospitalized with unstable angina, in doses ranging from 10 to 300 μg/min. The larger parenteral doses tend to decrease systemic vascular resistance, as well as increase venous capacitance, and are usually titrated against systolic blood pressure (45). The short duration of action of sublingual nitroglycerin and the requirement for hospitalization when using intravenous nitroglycerin have resulted in the widespread use of oral nitrates for chronic control of angina pectoris.

Oral Nitrates

For years the efficacy of orally administered nitrates in the treatment of angina pectoris was questioned because of the demonstration in animals that nitrates undergo extensive first-pass metabolism (46). Eventually, however, data emerged indicating that the hemodynamic effects of oral isosorbide dinitrate, the oral nitrate prototype, persist for 4 to 6 hr in patients with heart failure (47,48). Substantial amounts of the drug do enter the systemic circulation, and high concentrations of isosorbide dinitrate have been found in systemic venous blood after oral administration in humans (49,50). Several studies have shown that oral isosorbide dinitrate administered in large doses improves exercise performance in patients with angina pectoris (51–53). However, tolerance to the circulatory effects of nitrates has been reported to develop rapidly (54,55). In fact, chronic sustained therapy with isosorbide dinitrate may result in some attenuation of the antianginal effect, and there may be some attenuation of the favorable effect on ST-segment changes during exercise, as well as on the reduction of standing blood pressure (56). However, this attenuation of pharmacologic effect with chronic nitrate therapy does not pose a major clinical problem.

The pharmacokinetic disposition of plasma isosorbide dinitrate has been found to show a biexponential characteristic, with elimination half-lives of approximately 1.5 hr and 4 hr for the alpha and beta phases, respectively (57). Tolerance to the antianginal and circulatory effects is only partial, however, and sustained benefit from oral nitrates has been demonstrated clinically in most patients, which is supported by many years of favorable clinical experience with these drugs. Because the duration of effects is considerably reduced during sustained therapy, however, current studies suggest that oral isosorbide dinitrate should be prescribed in doses of 15 to 30 mg every 2 to 3 hr for continued beneficial effects (56). Clearly, such frequent dosing poses a major practical problem for most patients. Such problems have prompted the search for longer-acting delivery systems.

Topical Nitrates

Nitroglycerin applied to the skin in ointment form enters the circulation in a manner that bypasses the gastrointestinal tract and portal circulation. It has been administered percutaneously for circulatory disorders since 1944 (58), and in 1955 Davis et al. (59) reported that topical nitroglycerin had favorable effects in patients with angina pectoris. This finding was later confirmed by Reicheck et al. (60), who demonstrated at least a 3-hr increase in exercise capacity in patients with angina pectoris. Subsequent studies have shown that patients with angina pectoris, myocardial infarction, and congestive heart failure experience the maximum hemodynamic effects of nitroglycerin ointment at 60 to 90 min following application, and these effects persist for 4 to 6 hr (61–63). One to two inches of nitroglycerin ointment applied over the chest or flank (3- $\times$ 3-inch area) will increase plasma levels of nitroglycerin to 3.1 $\pm$ 3 ng/ml at 60 min, and this will persist for 240 min (64). Two inches applied to two separate skin sites will produce plasma levels of 8.9 $\pm$ 4 ng/ml at 60 min, also persisting for 240 min. Although the measurement of nitroglycerin levels is not standardized and not readily available, these data suggest that there is a good relationship between the dose of nitroglycerin ointment and its bioavailability. From a practical standpoint, the ointment is messy and often unpleasant for both patients and nursing personnel. Recently, several pharmaceutical companies have begun to market topical therapeutic systems that are marked improvements esthetically and appear capable of administering a more precise dose of nitroglycerin at a prescribed rate over an extended period of time. Some of these systems use a nitroglycerin reservoir sandwiched between an impenetrable backing and a membrane that controls the rate of flow of drug to the skin. The drug passes through the membrane by thermodynamic activity, seeking an area of lower concentration. An integral adhesive holds the reservoir to the skin. The system is designed to provide a uniform rate of flow of nitroglycerin through the skin for 24 hr. These devices have become extremely popular among both patients and physicians and should be explored to provide more imaginative ways to deliver other medications.

β Blockers

Many patients continue to have frequent angina pectoris despite the prophylactic use of nitrates. In recent years there has been considerable enthusiasm for the use of β-adrenergic blockers to prevent anginal attacks. These agents act by diminishing the effects of sympathetic activity, thus affecting several of the hemodynamic determinants of MVO_2 at rest and during exercise. They are generally used in combination with oral or topical nitrates, whereas sublingual nitroglycerin is used almost exclusively to abort the acute anginal attack. There is currently a wide variety of β blockers available, the choice being based largely on their relative "selectivity" and duration of action (Table 1). Nonselective β blockers, such as propranolol, timolol and pindolol, tend to block both β_1 and β_2 receptors. The blocking of the β_2 receptor is undesirable for some patients, because it can lead to exacerbation of bronchial airway disease (asthma or chronic obstructive lung disease) or peripheral vascular disease (by blocking the arterial β_2 receptor that presumably modulates vasodilatation). Some β blockers have relatively more intrinsic sympathomimetic activity (e.g., pindolol), but the precise biological importance of this characteristic is undefined. Some have relatively more membrane-stabilizing properties (e.g., propanolol), but this is of no clinical importance in the doses currently used.

All β blockers, with the possible exception of pindolol, tend to reduce the resting heart rate by 10 to 30%. Systolic blood pressure is usually lowered, and there may be a modest decline in cardiac output (again, pindolol, presumably because of its intrinsic sympathomimetic activity, tends not to reduce resting cardiac output). There may be a subclinical decrease in contractility, but usually this is not provocative of frank heart failure unless there is underlying severe left ventricular dysfunction. Contractility may be even less affected by agents with partial agonist activity. The net effect of these actions is a decrease in MVO_2 at rest and during exercise. This action reduces the disparity between oxygen supply and demand in most patients with symptomatic coronary artery disease. Although coronary blood flow may be reduced, this is overridden by the marked decline in MVO_2.

When β blockade is induced, the heart rate, blood pressure, cardiac output, and contractility rise less than predicted for a given exercise workload. Alderman et al. (65) have demonstrated that the extent of symptomatic improvement (reduction in anginal episodes) relates closely to the extent to which the heart rate is attenuated during exercise. Both the degree of β blockade and the response are dose-related, although doses may vary widely for various agents. Chronotropic blockade may still be present 24 hr following administration, whereas inotropic blockade seems to dissipate 12 hr after dosing, suggesting that different β receptor activities may modulate heart rate and inotropy.

Following abrupt cessation of β blocker therapy after chronic administration, exacerbation of angina pectoris and, in some cases, acute myocardial infarction have been reported (66). Two double-blind randomized trials confirmed the reality of a β blocker withdrawal syndrome (67,68). A "rebound" effect has not been well defined for β blocking drugs other than propranolol, although it seems prudent that discontinuation of such therapy should be done gradually and cautiously in patients with ischemic heart disease. It remains to be determined if β blockers with more partial agonist activity will demonstrate less rebound effect.

Although it is possible that nonselective β blockers may aggravate coronary artery spasm by blocking coronary arterial β_2 receptors and thereby leaving unopposed α vasoconstrictor activity, such a hypothesis has not been carefully documented. On the contrary, Guazzi et al. (69,70) have demonstrated in controlled studies that almost three-fourths of their subjects with Prinzmetal's variant angina had marked relief of attacks with propranolol at doses totaling 160 to 800 mg/day. The advisa-

TABLE 1. Dosages and pharmacology of β blocking drugs

Generic name	Comparative β blocking activity	Cardio-selectivity	Average i.v. dose (mg/kg body weight)	Average oral dose (mg/day)	$T_{1/2}$ (hr)	Active metabolite identified	Intrinsic sympathomimetic activity
Propranolol	1.0	−	0.15	80–320	2–3	Yes	0
Practolol	0.3	+	0.4	400–1200	5–13	No	++
Alprenolol	1.0	−	0.2	400	2–3	Yes	++
Pindolol	4.0	−	0.15	20–40	3–4	No	+++
Acebutolol	0.3	+	0.4	600–1200	2–3	Yes	+

TABLE 1. (Continued)

Generic name	Comparative β blocking activity	Cardio-selectivity	Average i.v. dose (mg/kg body weight)	Average oral dose (mg/day)	$T_{1/2}$ (hr)	Active metabolite identified	Intrinsic sympatho-mimetic activity
Metroprolol	1.0	+	0.15	100–450	3–4	No	0
Oxprenolol	1.0	–	0.2	160–300	1–2	No	++
Atenolol	0.5	+	–	50–100	5–7	No	0
Nadolol	1.0	–	–	40–240	16–18	No	0
Timolol	6.0	–	–	30	4–5	–	0

Metroprolol:
$CH_3-O-CH_2-CH_2-$ (phenyl) $-O-CH_2-CH(OH)-CH_2-NH-CH(CH_3)_2$

Oxprenolol:
(benzene ring) with $-O-CH_2-CH(OH)-CH_2-NH-CH(CH_3)_2$ and $-O-CH_2-CH=CH_2$

Atenolol:
$NH_2-CO-CH_2-$ (phenyl) $-O-CH_2-CH(OH)-CH_2-NH-CH(CH_3)_2$

Nadolol:
(naphthalene with two OH) $-O-CH_2-CH(OH)-CH_2-NH-C(CH_3)_3$

Timolol:
(morpholine)-(thiadiazole ring)$-O-CH_2-CH(OH)-CH-NH-C(CH_3)_3$

bility of β blockers for presumed coronary artery spasm is therefore somewhat unclear, and the decision to use them in this setting must be individualized for each patient.

The use of β blockers to control angina pectoris represents a major therapeutic breakthrough. The interested reader is referred to a recent monograph for a more comprehensive review of the subject (71).

Calcium-Entry Blockers

Drugs now classified as calcium-channel blockers or calcium-entry blockers have been in clinical use in Europe for more than 15 years. However, the sites of action of these drugs, their diverse pharmacologic effects, and their potential for clinical application are only now being appreciated (72,73). Because the process by which they inhibit calcium movement across the cell membrane is not entirely understood, and because of their individually variable effects on smooth muscle, pacemaker tissue, and myocardial tissue, these drugs defy simple grouping into a hemogeneous classification. They do share a common effect of reducing the transmembrane transport of extracellular calcium ions on which specialized tissues depend for contraction or impulse generation. Marked differences among the many agents suggest either that the blocking action of each of the drugs is relatively specific for different tissues or that other actions of these agents account for their heterogeneous effects. As of this writing, only verapamil, nifedipine, and diltiazem are currently being marketed in the United States. Because coronary vascular effects are prominent with each of these agents, it is quite reasonable that they are already receiving widespread use in the syndrome of angina pectoris.

Names such as calcium antagonist and calcium blocker, although widely used, are scientifically incorrect; the substances do not actually antagonize the cellular effects of the activator ion. In cardiac cells, under normal conditions, these drugs can inhibit the entry of calcium through the so-called slow channel; hence, the name slow-calcium-channel inhibitors has been proposed. For other tissues, in particular vascular smooth muscle, such evidence is lacking, although the effects of these drugs correlate best with reduction of the entry of calcium, whether or not this is initiated by a change in membrane potential. It is generally appreciated, however, that they relieve angina both by increasing coronary blood flow (through coronary smooth-muscle relaxation) and by reducing $M\dot{V}O_2$. The principal effects of each of the three most widely used of these drugs in the syndrome of angina pectoris will be considered separately, because their actions vary widely.

Verapamil

It has been reported that orally administered verapamil, a prototype slow-channel inhibitor, decreases angina frequency, nitroglycerin consumption, and the extent of ST-segment depression induced by treadmill stress, while increasing exercise capacity (74–79). Intravenously administered verapamil may prevent myocardial lactate production and reverse the ischemic regional and global left ventricular dysfunction produced by atrial pacing in patients with coronary artery disease (80,81). Although verapamil, by virtue of its negative chronotropic effects on the pacemaker cells of the heart, may intrinsically slow the activity of the sinoatrial node and heart rate, the effect at rest is largely overridden by its peripheral arteriolar vasodilatory action, which promotes a reflex increase in heart rate, the net result being that the resting heart rate does not change much (81). During exercise, however, there is about a 10% decrease in heart rate response following verapamil usage (as opposed to about a 25% decrease in heart rate induced by propranolol) (82). Likewise, verapamil induces a small decrease in mean arterial pressure at rest and during exercise, so that the rate-pressure product falls by about 15% during exercise (82). By comparison, the rate-pressure product falls by about 35% during exercise in patients treated with propranolol. Because verapamil and propranolol have comparable potencies in reducing the ischemic consequences of exercise stress in angina patients, in the case of verapamil additional mechanisms such as those involving myocardial metabolism or primary changes in perfusion must be involved. There is even some evidence to suggest that verapamil may be superior to propranolol as an antianginal agent in some patients (83). More important, the fact that these agents vitiate angina pectoris by different mechanisms indicates that the combination of a β blocker and verapamil may be synergistic.

Verapamil, unlike nifedipine and diltiazem, may have a more obvious negative inotropic propensity. Although reduction in myocardial contractility may be minimal or subclinical in patients with normal or moderately impaired left ventricular performance owing to its peripheral "unloading" effects, it can depress myocardial function substantially in patients with more compromised left ventricular function (84). Because the combination of significant negative inotropic and chronotropic effects may occur in patients treated with verapamil and a β blocker, this combination therapy should be used with caution (85). It has been suggested that verapamil not be used if the pulmonary capillary wedge pressure is in excess of 20 mm Hg or the ejection fraction is less than 30% (84).

The use of verapamil in unstable angina pectoris is less well documented, although it has been used successfully in such patients (72,86). Experimental work has indicated that verapamil pretreatment exerts beneficial effects on the mechanical performance of ischemic myocardium (87). Because patients with unstable angina frequently have marked and acute depression of myocardial performance, and because other calcium-channel blockers have far less negative inotropic effects, agents such as nifedipine and diltiazem may eventually find more widespread use in this syndrome.

Patients with Prinzmetal's variant angina are known to respond to verapamil (88), pre-sumably in relation to its potent vasodilator effect. Such therapy usually is given in conjunction with "long-acting" nitrates such as isosorbide dinitrate. Although more clinical experience is needed with this indication to put verapamil into perspective with other calcium-entry blockers known to be useful for coronary artery spasm, this action of the drug remains an attractive pharmacologic property.

Verapamil has well-documented antiarrhythmic properties by virtue of its ability to markedly suppress sinus and A-V nodal events (89). It is used widely for control of ventricular rate in atrial fibrillation and flutter and is probably the agent of choice for converting paroxysmal supraventricular tachycardia to normal sinus rhythm (90). Although it may potentially eliminate slow-current mechanisms in ischemic arrhythmias, it has generally not been useful in the control of ventricular ectopic activity.

Although the pharmacokinetics of verapamil are not well understood, the drug is almost (90%) completely absorbed when given orally. The usual intravenous dose, 5 to 10 mg given rapidly, corresponds to 10 to 20 times the oral dose needed to obtain comparable effects, suggesting that extensive first-pass metabolism occurs following oral administration (91). A typical starting dose might be 80 to 120 mg every 8 hr by mouth, up to a total of 480 mg/day. Chronic oral administration of verapamil increases the serum digoxin concentration, indicating that some caution is warranted when it is given in combination with digitalis (92). Studies have also indicated that verapamil may accumulate to a greater extent than predicted from its half-life (3–6 hr), because of reduction in hepatic clearance (93,94). The drug may improve glucose tolerance in patients with non-insulin-dependent diabetes mellitus (95). Major potential adverse effects are largely predictable and include aggravation of underlying sinoatrial and A-V nodal disease (heart block), left ventricular failure, and hypotension. Verapamil is contraindicated in sick-sinus syndrome or heart block (unless a pacemaker is in place), congestive heart failure, and hypotension.

Nifedipine

Nifedipine is a dihydropyridine derivative first synthesized in 1971 by Bossert and Vater for the West German firm Bayer. The drug has been widely used in Germany and Japan for variant angina and has recently been released for use in the United States for the treatment of both chronic stable angina and variant angina. It can be given intravenously, sublingually, or orally, although only the oral preparation is available in the United States. Like verapamil, nifedipine is a calcium-entry blocker and inhibits the influx of extracellular calcium ions through the cell membrane, effectively reducing the availability of intracellular free calcium necessary for activation of the contractile process. However, the structural dissimilarities and different pharmacologic effects suggest that the precise mechanisms and sites of action probably are quite different for verapamil and nifedipine. Although nifedipine has a negative inotropic action *in vitro* (96,97), this seems to be completely overridden by its potent peripheral arteriolar dilating effects *in vivo* (98). The direct negative chronotropic action of nifedipine is offset by the reflex increase in β-adrenergic tone, so that resting heart rate changes only slightly. In fact, the marked arteriolar dilatation usually more than offsets the negative inotropic effect with nifedipine. The drug has been used to treat left ventricular failure (99–101) and pulmonary edema (102), although such therapy can occasionally cause an exacerbation of congestive heart failure. Plasma norepinephrine levels increase following the use of nifedipine in normal and hypertensive patients (103) and also in patients with heart failure (104). The increase in β-adrenergic drive might also account for the obvious lack of negative inotropic action. Another distinct difference between verapamil and nifedipine is that nifedipine has virtually no important clinical effect on specialized conduction tissue,

and thereby lacks antiarrhythmic activity. It can therefore be used in patients with underlying sinus and A-V nodal disease, where verapamil is proscribed.

In addition to being highly effective in patients with Prinzmetal's variant angina (105), nifedipine is very useful in chronic stable angina pectoris (106). As with verapamil, exercise tolerance is significantly increased with nifedipine, and there is less ST-segment depression during exercise. The frequency of angina attacks is reduced by about 50% during chronic oral therapy. The heart-rate-blood-pressure product is slightly decreased at rest and at the onset of angina during exercise, but this alone cannot account for its protective effect. Like verapamil, nifedipine likely exerts a major influence by enhancing coronary blood flow (107). The drug may also normalize the pressure–volume relationship in the left ventricle during angina in some patients (108,109), accounting for additional antianginal effect. Because of its relative lack of negative inotropic effect, perhaps it can be more safely combined with a β blocker than can verapamil. Various combinations of nifedipine, a "long-acting" nitrate, and a β blocker are now widely used to control chronic angina pectoris, where singular use of one or more of these agents had previously proved unsuccessful.

Nifedipine has recently been reported to be superior to "conventional treatment" in patients hospitalized with unstable angina (110). It proved to be particularly beneficial in patients with ST-segment elevation during angina. This seems quite reasonable, because in most patients with unstable angina it is likely that a combination of both fixed obstruction and coronary spasm is important in limiting myocardial perfusion (27). The eventual role of this agent in the syndrome of unstable angina is still evolving; at this time it seems reasonable to add it to therapy for patients not responding to β blockers and nitrates.

Nifedipine is almost completely absorbed in the oral form (>90%), most of it within the first 60 min. It is strongly bound to serum proteins, which may account for its rather long-acting oral effects. Within 12 hr, 50 to 80% of a single dose is eliminated in the urine, the remainder being excreted in the feces. Compared with other calcium-entry blockers, it is the most potent pansystemic arteriolar dilator, which accounts for its side effects of flushing, hypotension, headache, reflex tachycardia, and peripheral edema. These side effects appear to occur more often with nifedipine than with verapamil and diltiazem. The usual starting dose is 10 mg every 8 hr, which can be gradually increased to a maximal dose of 90 mg/day.

Diltiazem

Diltiazem is a benzothiazepine, and therefore it has a chemical structure unlike that of verapamil or nifedipine (Fig. 2). It is a calcium-entry blocker that is intermediate in potency between verapamil and nifedipine. The vasodilating effects of diltiazem seem to be more selective for the coronary arteries; little effect is seen in peripheral vasculature responses except at higher doses. It is typically prescribed in doses of 30 to 60 mg four times per day. Although the drug has depressant electrophysiologic effects on specialized cardiac conduction tissue, they are less than those observed with verapamil (111). As with verapamil and nifedipine, chronic use of diltiazem decreases angina frequency and increases exercise time in patients with chronic stable angina (112). Exercise ST-segment changes are also blunted (113). The heart-rate-pressure product during maximal exercise is not markedly changed, suggesting that effects of the drug on afterload and heart rate are probably not solely responsible for its antianginal effects. Diltiazem is also highly effective and well tolerated for long-term prophylaxis and treatment of angina in patients with coronary spasm (114). Its relative selectivity of relaxation of the coronary vascular bed, compared with effects on peripheral or mesenteric vessels and cardiac muscle (115,116), and its striking absence of adverse effects make it an extraordinarily attractive agent for use in angina pectoris.

CONGESTIVE HEART FAILURE

Heart failure can be defined as the pathophysiologic state in which an abnormality of cardiac function is responsible for failure of the heart to pump blood at a rate commensurate with the requirements of the metabolizing tissues during stress or exercise. It occurs as a consequence of many forms of heart disease and is one of the most common serious disorders, afflicting about 4 million Americans (117). Although epidemiologic studies have suggested that hypertension plays the dominant causative role in the development of heart failure (118), these data were collected in the 1950s and 1960s and may not reflect the changes in disease patterns and improvements in the recognition and management of hypertension during the past two decades. Coronary

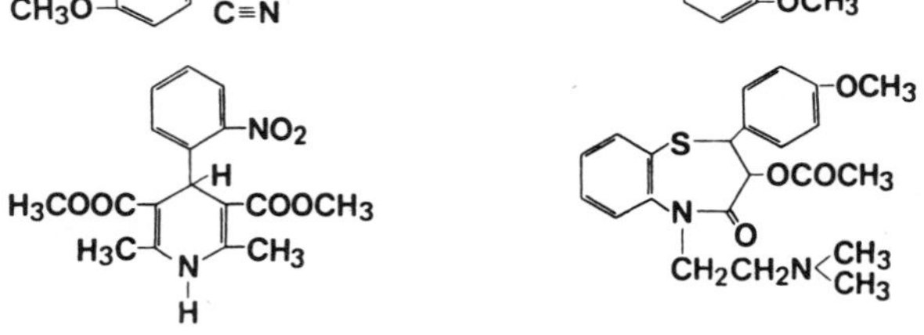

FIG. 2. Structural formulas of commonly used Ca^{2+}-entry blockers: *Top,* Verapamil; *bottom left,* Nifedipine; *bottom right,* Diltiazem.

artery disease, alcoholic and idiopathic cardiomyopathy, and valvular and congenital heart disease are clearly responsible for a substantial proportion of congestive heart failure seen by practicing physicians. Heart failure due to rheumatic heart disease and congenital heart disease is largely mechanical in nature and frequently requires surgical correction. Hypertension, rather than being viewed as a causative factor in heart failure, might better be viewed as a stress that decompensates an otherwise damaged left ventricle. Thus, the focus of this discussion is largely heart failure due to coronary artery disease or due to cardiomyopathy of a primary nature or cardiomyopathy due to chronic alcoholism. Although pharmacologic therapy is used in virtually all forms of heart failure, it is these groups of patients who are basically committed to a lifelong program of medical therapy once the diagnosis is established, though a few may benefit from cardiac transplantation.

Even though both are manifestations of ischemic heart disease, severe degrees of angina pectoris and chronic congestive heart failure rarely occur in the same patient (119). The patient with numerous attacks of angina usually has a normal-size heart as revealed by chest roentgenogram and a normal-size ventricular cavity with a well-contracting ventricle globally, although regional wall motion abnormalities may be evident angiographically. In contrast, the patient with chronic severe congestive heart failure either due to primary myocardial disease or consequent to healing of an acute myocardial infarction ("ischemic cardiomyopathy") (120,121) has a large cardiac silhouette as revealed by chest X-ray and a dilated, poorly contracting left ventricle revealed by angiography. Histologic examination of the coronary arteries may disclose no detectable differences in degrees of luminal narrowing among patients with isolated angina pectoris and those with chronic congestive heart failure following myocardial infarction (122). Of course, not all patients who develop acute myocardial infarction ultimately display clinical heart failure. Patients with chronic heart failure from ischemic heart

disease usually have large transmural myocardial scars (119). Why ischemic heart disease is manifested clinically in one patient by isolated angina pectoris and in another by recurrent infarction and heart failure is unclear, but the reason does not seem to reside in the degree of coronary artery narrowing, which is similar in both patients.

Despite the relative frequency and prognostic importance of congestive heart failure, there is no general agreement on diagnostic criteria. The major difficulty has been the absence of a reliable, noninvasive measure of myocardial performance that correlates directly with functional capacity (123). Patients with heart failure frequently complain of dyspnea and fatigue, but these symptoms are very nonspecific and lack predictive power, and the pathophysiologic basis is poorly understood. A ventricular gallop sound (S_3) is the most sensitive and specific physical finding in patients with heart failure, and the most informative clinical descriptor is cardiac size measured on a roentgenogram of the chest (124). Patients with more advanced failure and high left ventricular end-diastolic pressure (>20 mm Hg) tend to have the more classic findings of peripheral edema, neck vein distension, and hepatomegaly. It is generally agreed that patients who complain of fatigue and/or dyspnea at rest or with physical activity and who demonstrate cardiomegaly, a third heart sound, and some objective evidence of diminished left ventricular performance have the clinical syndrome of congestive heart failure. However, precise diagnostic criteria are elusive; there is a wide spectrum of signs and symptoms and marked heterogeneity in the population of patients with heart failure. Numerous ultrastructural, biochemical, bioenergetic, and autonomic nervous system abnormalities have been described in heart failure, but it is not known which, if any, of these abnormalities are causally related.

Pathophysiology

Congestive heart failure is frequently, but not always, caused by a defect in myocardial contraction. This eventually leads to an excessive hemodynamic burden, for which three principal compensatory mechanisms are recruited for maintenance of pump function: (a) the Frank-Starling mechanism, in which the sarcomeres lengthen to allow for optimal overlap between thick and thin myofilaments; this increase in "preload" acts to increase stroke volume, which then sustains cardiac performance; (b) myocardial hypertrophy, with or without dilatation, in which the mass of contractile tissue is augmented; (c) increased release of norepinephrine by the sympathetic nervous system that acts initially to augment myocardial contractility through myocardial β receptors. The precise signal that activates these different compensatory mechanisms is not fully understood. Initially, these mechanisms may be adequate to restore relatively normal pump performance. However, the potential for each of these compensatory mechanisms is limited, and the clinical syndrome of heart failure occurs most obviously when these systems are maximally activated. As cardiac output and regional distribution of blood flow are further curtailed, other vasoconstrictor forces, including the renin-angiotensin system and arginine vasopressin, are activated and may collectively contribute to heightened systemic vascular resistance, which further depresses myocardial performance (125), allowing for the operation of a vicious circle (Fig. 3). There is a reduction in oxygen consumption of exercising skeletal muscle that is proportional to the reduction in blood flow, which may be reduced in large measure because of "increased vascular stiffness" of arterioles in heart failure (126). This abnormal redistribution of flow during exercise and a marked decline in flow (or cardiac output) when impedance to ejection is augmented by heightened systemic vascular resistance are hallmarks of more advanced heart failure. Thus, it is the compensatory mechanisms that ultimately lead to the clinical expression of congestive heart failure.

The Basic Lesion

There is general agreement that in many forms of heart failure the myocardium fails

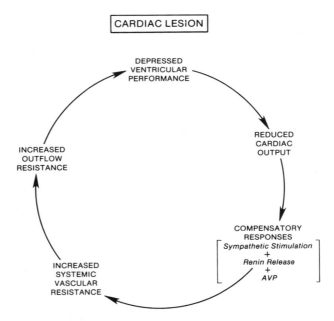

FIG. 3. Potential vicious cycle of congestive heart failure. Therapy focused on the neurohumoral response may lead to improved prognosis.

to generate an appropriate velocity of shortening for any given load. Papillary muscles removed from the right ventricles of cats in which hypertrophy and heart failure have developed following banding of the pulmonary artery demonstrate reduced maximum velocity of shortening (V_{max}) *in vitro* (127). The depression of contractility of the failing heart muscle appears to be related to an intrinsic defect of the muscle rather than to its operation at an abnormal position on a basically normal length–tension curve. Whereas the contractile state may be depressed, the cardiac index and stroke volume are often maintained in the resting state, albeit at elevated ventricular end-diastolic volumes and pressures, as muscle mass increases and the heart dilates. The elevations in ventricular pressure and volume in accordance with the Frank-Starling mechanism stretch sarcomeres to optimal levels, but this tends to promote pulmonary and systemic venous congestion and the formation of pulmonary and peripheral edema.

Myocardial Energy Production and Utilization

The depression of myocardial contractility probably is not due to a reduction of total myocardial high-energy stores. The concentrations of both adenosine triphosphate (ATP) and creatine phosphate (CP) have been found to be normal in the papillary muscles removed from failing hearts and hypertrophied hearts studied *in vitro* (128). However, it is possible that ATP is depleted in a small compartment vital for muscular contraction. Also, the activity of myofibrillar ATPase activity may be reduced, and this could explain many of the functional changes in failing heart muscle, such as depression of the force–velocity curve.

Excitation-Contraction Coupling

Studies in a number of *in vitro* systems have indicated that there is impairment of the delivery of Ca^{2+} for activation of the contractile process in heart failure. The uptake of Ca^{2+} by sarcolemma, the sarcoplasmic reticulum, and the mitochondria that is partly dependent on Ca^{2+}-activated ATPase could play a role in the development of myocardial failure. Experimental heart failure in the rabbit produced by aortic regurgitation appears to be associated with a significant alteration in the intracellular distribution of Ca^{2+} (129). Whereas total intracellular Ca^{2+} is normal, mitochondrial Ca^{2+} is greatly increased, and the rate and binding of Ca^{2+} to the sarcoplasmic reticulum are reduced. This may limit the quantity of Ca^{2+} available to initiate contraction. Although disturbances of Ca^{2+} transport frequently accompany heart failure, the nature of the abnormality of Ca^{2+} transport differs in various forms of heart failure.

β Receptor Activity

Recent studies on human myocardium removed from patients undergoing heart transplantation have indicated that there is decreased catecholamine sensitivity and β-adrenergic receptor density in failing human hearts (130). The reductions in β receptor density, adenylate cyclase, and contractile response to isoproterenol suggest that human myocardium has no "spare" receptors, a situation that places β-adrenergic receptor regulation in a crucial position for modulating the contractile state of the heart. The cause of this reduction in β receptor density is unknown, and it is unclear if it is simply due to a loss of functioning myocytes or is indicative of a generalized defect present with even less degrees of heart failure. This is currently an area of intense research interest, but the role of this alteration in initiating or sustaining heart failure is uncertain (131).

Autonomic Nervous System

The heart is rich in autonomic nerve supply, which, although not necessary for basal myocardial contractility, does provide an important mechanism for appropriately meeting physiologic demands. A derangement in sympathetic neurotransmitter metabolism in the hypertrophied and failing heart was first documented by Chidsey et al. (132), who reported the depletion of cardiac norepinephrine stores in congestive heart failure in patients who had their papillary muscles removed at surgery. Subsequently, it was shown that heart failure patients have a blunted reflex chronotropic response to both upright tilt and nitroglycerin-induced hypotension (133). Plasma norepinephrine levels are invariably elevated, however, and they generally relate to the severity of the heart failure (134). Patients with heart failure also exhibit a marked reduction in heart rate slowing for any given elevation of systemic arterial pressure, suggesting an abnormality of heart rate control by the parasympathetic nervous system. Although the precise mechanism responsible for the demonstrated impairment of autonomic nervous system function in heart failure is not clear, this disturbance may be of considerable functional importance in contributing to the overall pathogenesis of the syndrome.

Extracellular Fluid Accumulation

Edema formation, although occurring in less than half of patients with heart failure, is a cardinal manifestation of the syndrome. As central venous pressure rises, there is increased capillary venous pressure, with transudation of fluid into extravascular spaces. The effective arterial blood volume, as yet a poorly defined parameter, is eventually reduced in heart failure. Renal blood flow is reduced, and the ratio of glomerular filtration rate to renal plasma flow (filtration fraction) rises. Flow to the outer renal cortex, in particular, is reduced, and sodium and water are retained. The precise signal for sodium and water retention is unclear, but when perfusion pressure to the kidney is maintained experimentally, increased left atrial pressure alone fails to result in sodium retention. On the other hand, a reduction in cardiac output per se is not closely correlated with renal sodium retention

(135,136). There is also evidence that totally denervated and isolated kidneys can retain salt and water in the presence of heart failure (137), suggesting that the sympathetic nervous system is not an essential element serving this pathophysiologic event. There is experimental evidence, however, that anatomically described innervation of the renal tubules participates in the direct regulation of renal tubular sodium reabsorption (138). Patients with heart failure are well known to activate the renin-angiotensin system, especially when in a decompensated state, and this stimulates aldosterone production, further contributing to salt and water retention (139). Intracardiac volume receptors may be activated to produce increased antidiuretic hormone and other currently undefined humoral substances that might also contribute to edema formation. Therefore, there appears to be a complex and poorly understood sequence of events occurring in heart failure and leading in some cases to extracellular fluid accumulation. Hyponatremia, peripheral edema, and refractoriness to therapy may eventually ensue.

Medical Therapy for Advanced Congestive Heart Failure

Diuretics

There has been no major breakthrough in diuretic therapy since the introduction of the loop diuretics furosemide and ethacrynic acid about 15 years ago. Many physicians begin heart failure patients on a thiazide diuretic and add or change to a loop diuretic as signs and symptoms of extracellular fluid accumulation appear. The goal is not so much to induce diuresis alone but to achieve this result without reducing "preload" to the extent that cardiac output falls. This can be a most difficult task, as experienced clinicians are well aware.

In addition to reducing peripheral edema, successful diuretic therapy should serve to increase cardiac output by reducing systemic vascular resistance. Because the left ventricular end-diastolic dimension appears not to change substantially during diuresis in severe heart failure, it is probable that reduced "afterload" is operative when diuretic therapy improves stroke volume (140). The decrease in afterload or impedance to ejection could be due to withdrawal of elevated sympathetic tone or a reduction in vascular "stiffness," although neither of these mechanisms is well documented. Overly aggressive use of diuretics in heart failure may further reduce circulating effective volume, however, thus further reducing cardiac output and renal blood flow, resulting in worsening azotemia and other untoward consequences. Unfortunately, there is no simple and safe method to monitor the effects of diuretic therapy in heart failure.

Thiazides act on the distal convoluted tubule of the kidney to cause a maximal increase in sodium excretion of 5 to 8% of the filtered load. They are relatively ineffective in patients with glomerular filtration rates below 30 ml/min, and this limits their effectiveness in severe congestive heart failure. Their effects may be potentiated by spironolactone or triamterene, agents that act primarily on the distal tubule to inhibit potassium loss. The quinethazone derivative metolazone has a site of action and potency similar to those of chlorothiazide, but at the usual doses it does not reduce renal blood flow or glomerular filtration rate. Metolazone also has a longer duration of action (24–48 hr), is effective even in patients with markedly reduced glomerular filtration rates, and is particularly useful when added to a diuretic acting through a different mechanism, such as furosemide.

In more advanced heart failure, diuretics that are capable of increasing the fractional sodium excretion to more than 20% of the filtered load usually are employed. Furosemide and ethacrynic acid act to inhibit chloride transport in the ascending limb of the loop of Henle, thereby enhancing the excretion of sodium and water. They are powerful diuretics that also act to remove the gradient for passive water movement from the descending limb of Henle's loop and may somewhat reverse the shunting of renal blood flow away from the cortex of the kidney. For very refractory cases of extracellular fluid accumulation in heart failure, a combination of a thiazide (or metolazone) plus a loop diuretic plus a distal tubular diuretic is often used.

Digitalis

Despite its clinical use for some 200 years, controversy regarding the use of digitalis in congestive heart failure continues to thrive. Even today the precise mechanism of action remains elusive, although the inhibition of monovalent cation transport seems intimately involved (141). The drug appears to increase the cell content of exchangeable sodium, and this is accompanied by an increase in exchangeable Ca^{2+} available for contractile proteins, although this sodium pump inhibition hypothesis is by no means universally accepted (142).

The efficacy of digitalis in heart failure is no less controversial than its basic mechanism of inotropic action. There is little doubt that a substantial fraction of patients receiving chronic maintenance digitalis do not derive obvious benefit from use of the drug, while at the same time being subjected to an appreciable risk of toxicity (143). This is particularly true of patients in normal sinus rhythm. Much-needed information documenting the long-term effects of digoxin administration in chronic heart failure has recently been provided by Arnold et al. (144), clearly demonstrating the beneficial effects in a selected group of patients. These observations were subsequently confirmed by another group of investigators (145), who demonstrated that patients who responded to digoxin had more chronic and more severe heart failure, greater left ventricular dilatation and ejection fraction depression, and a third heart sound. Based on the available data, a case can be made to use digoxin doses sufficient to maintain levels in the range of 1.0 to 2.0 ng/ml. However, there are important gaps in our knowledge regarding the combined use of digitalis and vasodilators, in the special setting of heart failure complicating acute myocardial infarction, and the importance of digitalis as a first-line drug in the treatment of heart failure. There are no data available regarding the impact of digitalis therapy on the long-term prognosis for patients with heart failure.

Vasodilator Therapy

The importance of left ventricular outflow resistance or aortic impedance as a factor controlling left ventricular performance has long been recognized (146–148). The application of this physiologic principle into therapy for the failing left ventricle was reported in the early 1970s when the vasodilators phentolamine (148) and nitroprusside (149) were used to produce acute improvement in patients. These early studies have been followed by a number of investigations using a wide variety of vasodilator drugs, all of which produce similar functional responses (150–152). The use of vasodilator drugs has become increasingly popular (153,154), although more probing questions about which patients should be treated, drug tolerance, distribution of increased cardiac output, exercise capacity, and long-term efficacy are being posed (152).

Clinical application of vasodilator therapy for heart failure has emphasized the need for a measurement that can quantitate the total resistance opposing left ventricular ejection. This resistance has often been referred to as "afterload," but this term has its origin in isolated muscle studies and is defined as the amount of ventricular wall stress that builds up during shortening. It is only one of the factors opposing ventricular emptying. Systemic vascular resistance likewise is an incomplete descriptor of impedance to ejection, because it measures only small-vessel (arteriole) contributions meaned over a number of cardiac cycles. True impedance to ejection also takes into account large-vessel distensibility, blood vessel compliance, and blood viscosity and inertia (155). It is a dynamic phenomenon that traditionally is described by frequency-dependent moduli that require Fourier analy-

sis of high-fidelity pressure and flow signals that are not easily obtained in the clinical setting of heart failure (156). Because of these complexities, systemic vascular resistance is often used clinically in assessing "afterload" conditions, although a time-domain pulse wave analysis based on a modified Windkessel model can be used as a clinical alternative (157).

The variety of vasodilator drugs available has greatly expanded the therapeutic armamentarium for severe heart failure. However, these new advances in therapeutics also represent a challenge to the physician who must understand the pathophysiology of the heart failure and the mechanisms and primary sites of action of the drugs to apply therapy rationally. Some of these agents have balanced effects on both veins and arterioles (nitroprusside, prazosin), whereas others act more selectively on arterioles (hydralazine, minoxidil) or veins (nitrates). Some vasodilators act directly on the smooth muscle of the vessel (nitroprusside, hydralazine) to induce relaxation, whereas others act to block the postsynaptic α receptors (prazosin) or the vasoconstriction produced by enhanced renin-angiotensin activity (captopril). The mechanisms and sites of action of commonly used vasodilators are shown in Table 2. Relaxation of arterial vascular tone results in a decrease in impedance to left ventricular ejection. This reduced impedance results in enhanced left ventricular performance and thus a reduced end-systolic volume and larger ejection fraction. The net effect of this improved systolic function on stroke volume is highly dependent on concomitant changes in left ventricular end-diastolic volume. When drugs with little or no venodilator effect are employed, end-diastolic ventricular volume is not acutely altered, and the increased ejection fraction is translated into an increased stroke volume (158). When venodilator drugs are used, however, blood volume is acutely redistributed to the capacitance system, and ventricular filling is reduced. This reduced ventricular end-diastolic volume may therefore

TABLE 2. *Vasodilator therapy in congestive heart failure*

Drug	Route	Site of action	Mechanism of action	Dose [a]
Nitroprusside	Intravenous	Balanced (venodilator and arteriolar dilator)	Acts directly on smooth muscle	15–300 µg/min
Nitroglycerin	Intravenous, sublingual, topical	Mainly venodilator; arteriolar dilator in higher doses	Acts directly on smooth muscle	10–300 µg/min i.v., 1/150 grain sublingual, 1–4 inches topical
Isosorbide dinitrate	Oral	Mainly venodilator, arteriolar dilator in higher doses	Acts directly on smooth muscle	10–100 mg q. 3–4 hr
Hydralazine	Oral	Arteriolar dilator	Acts directly on smooth muscle	75–200 mg q. 8–12 hr
Minoxidil	Oral	Arteriolar dilator	Acts directly on smooth muscle	10–20 mg q. 12 hr
Prazosin	Oral	Balanced (venodilator and arteriolar dilator)	α_1 postsynaptic blocker	2–10 mg q. 6 hr
Captopril	Oral	Balanced (venodilator and arteriolar dilator)	Converting enzyme inhibitor (blocks formation of angiotensin II); other mechanisms likely, but poorly understood	6.25–25 mg q. 8 hr

[a] These doses are based on the personal experience of the authors and do not necessarily conform to doses recommended by the FDA or pharmaceutical companies.

limit the increase in stroke volume to some extent (159). The decrease in end-diastolic volume produced by a venodilator helps reduce pulmonary vascular congestion and alleviates symptoms of dyspnea. Thus, the net effect of the vasodilator therapy on hemodynamics depends importantly on the relative effects of the drug on the capacitance and resistance vessels.

Effects on heart rate may also be variable. The reflex tachycardia seen in normal individuals in response to arteriolar dilator drugs usually does not occur in patients with heart failure. Indeed, the heart rate frequently slows in response to some of the vasodilator drugs. Although the mechanism of this abnormal response is not entirely clear, it may be related to the very high basal sympathetic tone that heart failure patients display (134), as well as to the basic dysautonomia present in these patients (133). The improvements in stroke volume and cardiac output may offset the reflex sympathetic stimulation that otherwise normally accompanies the fall in systemic blood pressure.

In heart failure, vasoconstriction is most pronounced in the cutaneous, renal, and splanchnic circulations (160). Changes in regional blood flow induced by vasodilator drugs may result both from direct vascular effects of the drug and from reflex changes in neurohumoral vasoconstrictor activity. Although not all vasodilator drugs have been evaluated with regard to their effects on regional distribution of flow, some work has been published. Magorien et al. (161) reported that hydralazine significantly increased renal blood flow in patients with heart failure, whereas prazosin was shown not to affect renal blood flow or renal vascular resistance. Hydralazine was shown to increase renal blood flow by about 20% (acutely in the supine position) in patients with heart failure, whereas limb blood flow increased slightly less (162). Mean hepatic flow did not change. Isosorbide dinitrate alone was found not to alter regional blood flow in patients with heart failure (162), and experimental data have indicated that nitro-

glycerin increases renal, gastrointestinal, and cutaneous blood flow during exercise in a rat model of heart failure (163). Whether or not such acute responses persist in patients during chronic therapy remains to be determined.

During dynamic exercise in normal individuals, total systemic vascular resistance falls, there is sympathetic discharge to the heart, and cardiac output increases as a result of an increase in heart rate and, during more intense exercise, from an increase in stroke volume. Activation of the sympathetic nervous system leads to regional redistribution of flow favoring exercising muscles, with reduction of flow to the viscera and to nonexercising skeletal beds. In heart failure, the hemodynamic response to exercise is markedly altered (164). The effects of vasodilator drugs on the hemodynamic response to exercise appear less striking than one might have anticipated, because maximum cardiac output during exercise is only slightly affected by hydralazine or isosorbide dinitrate (165,166). At submaximal levels of exercise, however, improved cardiac output has been demonstrated with vasodilators (167), and chronic therapy has been shown to increase exercise tolerance (168). The precise mechanism by which chronic therapy improves exercise tolerance, whereas acute therapy does not, remains to be elucidated, but it may in part be a manifestation of improved peripheral utilization of oxygen (167).

Although vasodilator therapy alone or in various combinations acutely improves the hemodynamic state in patients with heart failure, the long-term results of such therapy are uncertain. Tolerance to certain vasodilator therapy may occur (169). Ischemic events may be provoked even in the absence of hypotension and tachycardia (170), and not all patients respond favorably to this type of therapy (171). Left ventricular metabolic function can deteriorate during vasodilator therapy in some patients with chronic ischemic heart failure (172), and rebound worsening of hemodynamics may occur following abrupt withdrawal of acute therapy (173). A large-scale Veterans

Administration cooperative study (V-HEFT, or vasodilator heart failure trial) is currently under way using a double-blind placebo-controlled technique that may answer numerous questions about which patients may benefit most from this type of treatment. Until this and other ongoing studies are completed, the use of vasodilator therapy in the management of congestive heart failure should be considered experimental.

Inotropic Therapy

Whereas vasodilator drugs act to enhance left ventricular performance primarily by altering peripheral loading conditions and have no intrinsic ability to stimulate contractility per se, the inotropic agents act directly on myocardial cells to increase the velocity of shortening and thereby improve pump function through a much more direct mechanism. The use of inotropic agents presumes that there is residual functioning myocardium; there is no evidence that these agents change the underlying basic lesion of heart failure, but only serve to augment the already depressed contractile system by increasing the amount of activating calcium available for contraction. All inotropic drugs also exert some peripheral vascular actions that make it difficult to assess the effects of a pure inotropic intervention. Changes in heart rate and reflex circulatory effects occur when these drugs are given to a patient with heart failure, making it difficult to separate secondary responses from the primary response to the inotropic stimulation (174). The exact mechanism by which these drugs increase the availability of activating Ca^{2+} varies for different inotropes and in some cases is poorly understood, but it is this common mechanism of action that allows them to be separated as a class despite their widely varying actions on failing circulation (Table 3).

A number of agents with the basic catecholamine structure increase contractility by stimulating β_1 receptors located on the surfaces of cardiac cells (175). Normally this re-

ceptor is endogenously activated by norepinephrine, which is synthesized and released by cardiac nerves; β_1 stimulation activates adenyl cyclase in the cell surface membrane, with subsequent increase in intracellular 3'5'-cyclic AMP. Protein kinases are then activated, with phosphorylation of multiple membrane systems that augment Ca^{2+} availability to the contractile system (176). The catecholamines currently available as drugs to treat heart failure are primarily intravenous in route, and their overall action relative to the circulation is affected by their stimulation of receptors other than cardiac receptors, such as α receptors in peripheral vessels producing vasoconstriction and β_2 receptors in peripheral vessels and lung airways stimulating vasodilatation and bronchodilatation. In addition to enhancement of myocardial contractility, the sinus node of the heart is stimulated, because this structure is also influenced by β_1 activity. Myocardial oxygen consumption is therefore greatly increased. Manipulation of the catecholamine molecule has yielded drugs with greater propensity to activate one receptor or another, thus allowing for their widely differing effects on heart rate and peripheral resistance.

Norepinephrine is the catecholamine endogenous to the circulation. However, stores of norepinephrine are depleted in the nerve endings of the myocardium in chronic heart failure, so that drugs that act to release norepinephrine stores, such as metaraminol, may be ineffective in this setting. Norepinephrine, given exogenously to patients with heart failure, may increase contractility and heart rate, but it also augments peripheral vascular resistance by stimulating peripheral α_1 receptors in the systemic vasculature. Although it is useful in severe hypotension accompanying heart failure, the excessive vasoconstriction it produces has prevented its widespread use outside the shock syndrome, where restoration of blood pressure is of prime importance.

Isoproterenol has lost favor as an inotropic drug because it produces excessive tachycardia and because its peripheral vasodilating effects

TABLE 3. *Nonglycoside inotropic agents used to treat congestive heart failure*

Drug	Receptor activity			Structure	Response	Dose
	Vascular		Cardiac			
	α_1	β_2	β_1			
Norepinephrine	++++	0	++	(structure)	Systemic vasoconstriction; increased contractility	4–16 μg/min
Isoproterenol	0	++++	++++	(structure)	Systemic vasodilation; increased contractility; increased heart rate	1–6 μg/min
Dopamine	++	++	++	(structure)	Vasodilation of renal and mesenteric vascular beds at low dose; systemic vasoconstriction at high dose; increased contractility; increased heart rate	2–10 μg/kg/min
Dobutamine	0	?+	+++	(structure)	Increased contractility; reflex vasodilation; increased heart rate at high dose	2.5–10 μg/kg/min i.v.

Drug	Mechanism	Structure	Ratings	Effect	Dosage
Amrinone[a]	Non-receptor-mediated (? phosphodiesterase inhibitor)			Increased contractility; decreased systemic vascular resistance	40 µg/kg/min i.v.; 2–3 mg/kg p.o. q. 8 hr
Pirbuterol[a]			0 +++ ?++	Increased contractility; decreased systemic vascular resistance	20–30 mg t.i.d. p.o.
Prenalterol[a]			0 0 +++	Increased contractility; increased heart rate	1–5 mg i.v.
MDL 17,043[a]	Non-receptor-mediated; phosphodiesterase inhibitor			Increased contractility; decreased systemic vascular resistance	0.03–0.1 mg/kg/min i.v.

[a] Oral form currently undergoing clinical trials.

(β_2) involve predominantly the skeletal muscle bed (177). The increase in cardiac output that it promotes is basically insufficient to keep up with the marked decrease in systemic vascular resistance that accompanies its use. Moreover, the excessive tachycardia greatly adds to its propensity to increase $M\dot{V}O_2$. Today its use is generally restricted to cases of sudden and severe heart block, where it can maintain heart rate prior to insertion of a temporary pacemaker.

Dopamine was introduced as an inotropic drug with lesser peripheral vascular and chronotropic properties (178). It has gained widespread use in the acute treatment of severe pump failure because it induces less vasoconstriction than norepinephrine and less tachycardia than isoproterenol (179). Peripheral vascular actions are present, however, and as the dose is increased, α-adrenergic vasoconstriction begins to predominate (180). In higher doses, the drug is much akin to norepinephrine. In low doses, a specific dopaminergic effect may ensue, resulting in renal and mesenteric vasodilatation. This is presumed to be due to selective stimulation of vascular dopaminergic receptors (181). The drug may promote sodium diuresis through this action, although the mechanism of this effect is difficult to separate from the effect on cardiac output (182). Today it is most commonly used to treat shock (183), particularly associated with acute myocardial infarction, and it is also used in conjunction with nitroprusside to treat patients with severe pump failure (184). When these two agents are used together, the increase in cardiac output is significantly greater than with either agent alone (185).

The presently available catecholamine derivative that comes closest to providing a specific inotropic effect is dobutamine (186). It lacks dopamine's direct vasodilator effect on the renal and mesenteric vasculature and also lacks the predominant vasoconstrictor (α-adrenergic) effects observed with higher doses of dopamine (187). Furthermore, dobutamine has been shown not to increase heart rate as much as other catecholamines, even when given in doses that produce a prominent increase in myocardial contractility (186). Although dobutamine is a powerful inotropic agent that markedly increases cardiac output, its lack of peripheral vasoconstrictor effects implies that any increase in blood pressure it produces is due to an increase in stroke volume rather than to augmented peripheral vascular resistance. It therefore is not an ideal agent in shock, where it is unlikely to raise perfusion pressure (188). Dobutamine is most widely used in patients with acutely decompensated heart failure without hypotension, where it is less likely than dopamine to produce increased left ventricular filling pressure, clinical evidence of pulmonary vascular congestion, tachycardia, and persistent elevation of vascular resistance (189). Its prolonged and continuous use is precluded by the development of drug tolerance, which may occur even within 48 to 72 hr (190).

A major problem to date with catecholamine derivatives is that they have required the intravenous route. Only recently have newer, orally active β_1- and β_2-stimulating catecholamines undergone clinical studies. Salbutamol, largely a β_2 agonist, is widely used in Europe to treat bronchospasm. It has recently been shown to have vasodilator and inotropic effects in patients with heart failure (191). Pirbuterol, primarily a β_2 stimulant, has also been shown to improve the hemodynamic perturbations of heart failure (192). Prenalterol appears to be a β_1 stimulator that augments contractility when given intravenously or orally (193). Butopamine, a β_1 receptor agonist structurally related to dobutamine, manifests substantial inotropy (194) and can be given orally. TA-064 is an oral catecholamine derivative that probably is converted to dopamine once ingested and has been used successfully to treat heart failure (195). Important questions in the use of the newer oral catecholamine agents will focus on long-term tolerance relative to initial efficacy. The development of tachyphylaxis, as well as the effects of the drugs on the natural course of heart failure, will greatly determine the chronic usefulness of such agents (196).

Recent interest has focused on a new class of inotropic agents, the prototype of which is amrinone (197). Although the mechanism of action of this drug is unknown, it does not affect the Na^+-K^+-stimulated ATPase or enzymes associated with β_1 stimulation. It may possibly act to block or inhibit phosphodiesterase activity (198), which would lead to an increase in $3'5'$-cyclic AMP and ultimately augmented cardiac contractility and reduced systemic vascular resistance. Oral inotropic agents that are structurally unrelated to amrinone, but are also believed to work by inhibiting phosphodiesterase, are the imidazoles AR-L115BS (199) and MDL 17,043 (200,201). Newer and more imaginative oral inotropic agents can be expected to be studied in the near future, as this is currently an area of intense research.

Despite promising initial clinical results with many of the new oral inotropic agents, there is open uncertainty about the long-term effects of these agents in patients with heart failure (202). Whether or not primary damage is continuing while inotropic therapy is being given is unknown. Despite this caveat, our ability to manage patients with congestive heart failure has clearly been enhanced (117), and, perhaps just as important, the search for newer and better therapy for heart failure may ultimately help us to better understand the disease process itself.

ACKNOWLEDGMENTS

The stimulation and excellent technical skills of the members of the Heart Failure Study Unit at the University of Minnesota are gratefully acknowledged. Sandy Thiesse provided secretarial services.

This work was supported by grants HL22977–03 and HL07184, NHLBI, NIH, and by a grant from the Veterans Administration Research Service.

REFERENCES

1. National Center for Health Statistics (1972): *Vital Statistics of the United States, 1968, Vol. 2, Part A, Mortality.*
2. Cohn, P. F. (1981): Asymptomatic coronary artery disease. *Mod. Concepts Cardiovasc. Dis.,* 50:55–60.
3. Kannel, W. B., and Feinleib, M. (1972): Natural history of angina pectoris in the Framingham study: prognosis and survival. *Am. J. Cardiol.,* 29:154–163.
4. Borow, K. M., Alpert, J. S., and Cohn, P. F. (1978): The natural history and treatment of coronary artery disease: a perspective. *Cardiovasc. Med.,* 3:87–102.
5. Kannel, W. B. (1976): Some lessons in cardiovascular epidemiology from Framingham. *Am. J. Cardiol.,* 37:269–282.
6. Kolata, G. B. (1975): Prevention of heart disease: clinical trials at what cost? *Science,* 190:764–765.
7. Heberden, W. (1772): Some account of a disorder of the breast. *M. Trans. Roy. Coll. Physicians (London),* 2:59–67.
8. White, P. D. (1974): The historical background of angina pectoris. *Mod. Concepts Cardiovasc. Dis.,* 43:109–112.
9. MacAlpin, R. N. (1980): Coronary arterial spasm: a historical perspective. *J. Hist. Med.,* 35:288–312.
10. Nothnagel, H. (1867): Angina pectoris vasomotoria. *Dt. Arch. Klin. Med.,* 3:309–322.
11. Osler, W. (1910): The Lumleian lectures on angina pectoris II. *Lancet,* 1:839–844.
12. Herrick, J. B. (1912): Clinical features of sudden obstruction of the coronary arteries. *J.A.M.A.,* 59:2015–2020.
13. Smith, F. M. (1918): The ligation of coronary arteries with electrocardiographic study. *Arch. Intern. Med.,* 22:8–27.
14. Pardee, H. E. B. (1920): An electrocardiographic sign of coronary artery obstruction. *Arch. Intern. Med.,* 26:244–257.
15. Danielopolu, D. (1924): The pathology and surgical treatment of angina pectoris. *Br. Med. J.,* 2:553–557.
16. Blumgart, H. L., Schlesinger, M. J., and Davis, D. (1940): Studies on the relation of the clinical manifestations of angina pectoris, coronary thrombosis and myocardial infarction to the pathologic findings. *Am. Heart J.,* 19:1–91.
17. Keefer, C. S., and Resnick, W. H. (1928): Angina pectoris: A syndrome caused by anoxemia of the myocardium. *Arch. Intern. Med.,* 41:769–807.
18. Roughgarden, J., and Newman, E. V. (1966): Circulatory changes during the pain of angina pectoris. *Am. J. Med.,* 41:935–946.
19. Epstein, S. E., Redwood, D. R., Goldstein, R. E., Beiser, G. D., Rosing, D. R., Glancy, D. L., Reis, R. L., and Stinson, E. B. (1971): Angina pectoris: pathophysiology, evaluation, and treatment. *Ann. Intern. Med.,* 75:263–296.
20. Daly, R. (1957): The autonomic nervous system in its relation to some forms of heart and lung disease. I. heart disease. *Br. Med. J.,* 2:173–179.
21. Prinzmetal, M., Ekmekci, A., Kennamer, R., Kwoc-

zynski, J., Shubin, H., and Toyoshima, H. (1960): Variant form of angina pectoris. Previously undelineated syndrome. *J.A.M.A.,* 174:102–108.

22. Sones, F. M., and Shirey, E. K. (1962): Cine coronary arteriography. *Mod. Concepts Cardiovasc. Dis.,* 31:735–738.

23. Oliva, P. B., Potts, D. E., and Pluss, R. G. (1973): Coronary arterial spasm in Prinzmetal angina. *N. Engl. J. Med.,* 288:745–750.

24. Yasue, H., Touyama, M., Shimantoto, M., Kato, H., Tanaka, S., and Akiyam, F. (1974): Role of the autonomic nervous system in the pathogenesis of Prinzmetal's variant form of angina. *Circulation,* 50:534–539.

25. Endo, M., Hirosawa, K., and Kaneko, N. (1976): Prinzmetal's variant angina: coronary arteriogram and left ventriculogram during angina attack induced by methacholine. *N. Engl. J. Med.,* 294:252–255.

26. Maseri, A., Pesola, A., Marzilli, M., Severi, S., L'Abbate, A., Denes, D. M., Parodi, O., Ballestra, A. M., Maltinti, G., and Biagini, A. (1977): Coronary vasospasm in angina pectoris. *Lancet,* 1:713–717.

27. Maseri, A., L'Abbate, A., Baroldi, G., Chierchia, S., Marzilla, M., Ballestra, A. M., Severi, S., Parodi, O., Biagini, A., Distante, A., and Pesola, A. (1978): Coronary vasospasm as a possible cause of myocardial infarction. A conclusion derived from the study of "preinfarction" angina. *N. Engl. J. Med.,* 299:1271–1277.

28. Yasue, H., Omote, S., Takizawa, A., Nagao, M., Wiwa, K., and Tanaka, S. (1979): Circadian variation of exercise capacity in patients with Prinzmetal's variant angina: role of exercise-induced coronary arterial spasm. *Circulation,* 59:938–948.

29. Specchia, G., DeServi, S., Falcone, C., Bramucci, E., Angoli, L., Mussini, A., Piero Marinomi, G., Montemartini, C., and Bobba, P. (1979): Coronary artery spasm as a cause of exercised-induced ST-segment elevation in patients with variant angina. *Circulation,* 59:948–954.

30. Brown, B. G., Bolson, E., Frimer, M., and Dodge, H. (1977): Quantitative coronary arteriography: estimation of dimensions, hemodynamic resistance, and atheroma mass of coronary artery lesions using the arteriogram and digital computation. *Circulation,* 55:329–337.

31. Klocke, F. J., Koberstein, R. C., Pittman, D. E., Bunnell, I. L., Greene, D. G., and Rosing, D. R. (1968): Effects of heterogeneous myocardial perfusion on coronary venous H_2 desaturation curves and calculations of coronary flow. *J. Clin. Invest.,* 47:2711–2724.

32. Bing, R. J. (1965): Cardiac metabolism. *Physiol. Rev.,* 45:171–213.

33. Klocke, F. J., Kaiser, G. A., Ross, J., Jr., and Braunwald, E. (1965): Mechanism of increase of myocardial oxygen uptake produced by catecholamines. *Am. J. Physiol.,* 209:913–918.

34. Klocke, F. J., Braunwald, E., and Ross, J., Jr. (1966): Oxygen cost of electrical activation of the heart. *Circ. Res.,* 18:357–365.

35. Graham, T. P., Jr., Covell, J. W., and Sonnenblick, E. H. (1968): The control of myocardial oxygen consumption: relative influence of contractile state and tension development. *J. Clin. Invest.,* 47:375–385.

36. Burns, J. W., and Covell, J. W. (1972): Myocardial oxygen consumption during isotonic and isovolumic contractions in the intact heart. *Am. J. Physiol.,* 223:1491–1497.

37. Sonnenblick, E. H., Ross, J., Jr., Covell, J. W., Kaiser, G., and Braunwald, E. (1965): Velocity of contraction as a determinant of myocardial consumption. *Am. J. Physiol.,* 209:919–927.

38. Boerth, R. C., Covell, J. W. Pool, P. E., and Ross, J., Jr. (1969): Increased myocardial oxygen consumption and contractile state associated with increased heart rate. *Circ. Res.,* 24:725–734.

39. Mason, D. T., Spann, J. F., Jr., Zelis, R., and Amsterdam, E. (1969): Physiologic approach to the treatment of angina pectoris. *N. Engl. J. Med.,* 281:1225–1228.

40. Brown, B. G., Bolson, E., Peterson, R. B., Pierce, C. D., and Dodge, H. T. (1981): The mechanism of nitroglycerin action: stenosis vasodilatation as a major component of the drug response. *Circulation,* 64:1089–1097.

41. Schwartz, J. S., Carlyle, P. F., and Cohn, J. N. (1979): Effect of dilation of the distal coronary bed on flow and resistance in severely stenotic coronary arteries in dogs. *Am. J. Cardiol.,* 43:219–224.

42. Burggraff, G. W., and Parker, J. O. (1974): Left ventricular volume changes after amyl nitrate and nitroglycerin in man, as measured by ultrasound. *Circulation,* 49:136–143.

43. Ganz, W., and Marcus, H. S. (1972): Failure of intracoronary nitroglycerin to alleviate pacing-induced angina. *Circulation,* 46:880–889.

44. Williams, J. F., Jr., Glick, G., and Braunwald, E. (1965): Studies on cardiac dimensions in intact unanesthetized man. V. Effects of nitroglycerin. *Circulation,* 32:767–771.

45. Hill, N. S., Antman, E. M., Green, L. H., and Alpert, J. S. (1981): Intravenous nitroglycerin: a review of pharmacology, indications, therapeutic effects and complications. *Chest,* 79:69–76.

46. Needleman, P., Lang, S., and Johnson, E. M., Jr. (1972): Organic nitrates: relationship between biotransformation and rational angina pectoris therapy. *J. Pharmacol. Exp. Ther.,* 181:489–497.

47. Sweatman, T., Strauss, G., Selzer, A., and Cohn, K. (1972): The long-acting hemodynamic effects of isosorbide dinitrate. *Am. J. Cardiol.,* 29:475–480.

48. Franciosa, J. A., Mikulic, E., Cohn, J. N., Jose, E., and Fabie, A. (1974): Hemodynamic effects of orally administered isosorbide dinitrate in patients with congestive heart failure. *Circulation,* 50:1020–1024.

49. Shane, S. J., Iazzeta, J. J., Chisholm, A. W., Berka, J. F., and Leung, D. (1978): Plasma concentrations of isosorbide dinitrate and its metabolites after chronic high oral dosage in man. *Br. J. Clin. Pharmacol.,* 6:37–41.

50. Thadani, U., Dark, A., Fung, H. L., and Parker, J. (1978): Comparison of plasma levels and circulatory effects of isosorbide dinitrate during acute and

chronic therapy. *Circulation* [Suppl. 11], 59–60:11–15.

51. Glancy, D. L., Ritcher, M. A., Ellis, E. V., and Johnson, W. (1977): Effect of swallowed isosorbide nitrate on blood pressure, heart rate, and exercise capacity in patients with coronary artery disease. *Am. J. Med.,* 62:39–46.

52. Markis, J. E., Gorlin, R., Mills, R. M., Williams, R. A., Schweitzer, P., and Ransil, B. J. (1979): Sustained effects of orally administered isosorbide dinitrate on exercise performance of patients with angina pectoris. *Am. J. Cardiol.,* 43:265–271.

53. Thadani, U., Fung, H. L., Darke, A. C., and Parker, J. (1980): Oral isosorbide dinitrate in the treatment of angina pectoris—dose-response relationship and duration of action during acute therapy. *Circulation,* 62:491–502.

54. Needleman, P., and Johnson, E. J., Jr. (1973): Mechanism of tolerance development to organic nitrates. *J. Pharmacol. Exp. Ther.,* 184:709–715.

55. Thadani, U., Manyari, D., Parker, J. O., Fung, H. L. (1980): Tolerances to the circulatory effects of oral isosorbide dinitrate—rate of development and cross tolerance to glyceryl trinitrate. *Circulation,* 61:526–535.

56. Thadani, U., Fung, H. L., Darke, A. C., and Parker, J. O. (1982): Oral isosorbide dinitrate in angina pectoris: comparison of duration of action and dose-response relation during acute and sustained therapy. *Am. J. Cardiol.,* 49:411–419.

57. Fung, H. L., McNiff, E. F., Ruggirello, D., and Parker, J. O. (1981): Kinetics of isosorbide dinitrate and relationship to pharmacological effects. *Br. J. Clin. Pharmacol.,* 11:579–590.

58. Lund, F. (1948): Percutaneous nitroglycerin treatment in cases of peripheral circulatory disorders, especially Raynaud's disease. *Acta Med. Scand.* [*Suppl.*], 206:196–206.

59. Davis, J. A., Wiesel, B. H., and Epstein, S. E. (1955): The treatment of angina pectoris with nitroglycerin ointment. *Am. J. Med. Sci.,* 230:259–263.

60. Reicheck, N., Goldstein, R. E., Redwood, D. R., and Epstein, S. E. (1974): Sustained effects of nitroglycerin ointment in patients with angina pectoris. *Circulation,* 50:348–352.

61. Parker, J. O., Augustine, R. J., Burton, J. R., West, R. O., and Armstrong, P. W. (1976): The effect of nitroglycerin ointment on the clinical and hemodynamic response to exercise. *Am. J. Cardiol.,* 38:162–166.

62. Armstrong, P. W., Mathew, M. T., Boroomand, K., and Parker, J. O. (1976): Nitroglycerin ointment in acute myocardial infarction. *Am. J. Cardiol.,* 38:74–78.

63. Franciosa, J. A., Blank, R., Cohn, J. N., and Mikulic, E. (1977): Hemodynamic effects of topical, oral and sublingual nitroglycerin in left ventricular failure. *Curr. Ther. Res.,* 22:231–245.

64. Armstrong, P. W., Armstrong, J. A., and Marks, G. S. (1980): Pharmaco-kinetic-hemodynamic studies of nitroglycerin ointment in congestive heart failure. *Am. J. Cardiol.,* 46:670–676.

65. Alderman, E. L., Davies, R. O., Crowley, J. J., Lopes, M. G., Brooker, J. Z., Friedman, J. P., Graham, A. F., Matlof, H. J., and Harrison, D. C. (1975): Dose response effectiveness of propranolol for the treatment of angina pectoris. *Circulation,* 51:964–975.

66. Alderman, E. L., Coltart, D. J., and Wettach, G. E. (1974): Coronary artery syndrome after sudden propranolol withdrawal. *Ann. Intern. Med.,* 81:925–927.

67. Miller, R. R., Olson, H. G., Amsterdam, E. A., and Mason, D. T. (1975): Propranolol withdrawal rebound phenomenon: exacerbation of coronary events after abrupt cessation of anti-anginal therapy. *N. Engl. J. Med.,* 293:416–418.

68. Frishman, W. H., Christodoulou, J., Weksler, B., Smithen, C., Killip, T., and Scheidt, S. (1978): Abrupt propranolol withdrawal in angina pectoris: effects on platelet aggregation and exercise tolerance. *Am. Heart J.,* 95:169–179.

69. Guazzi, M., Magrini, F., Fiorentini, C., and Polese, A. (1971): Clinical, elecrocardiographic, and hemodynamic effects of long term use of propranolol in Prinzmetal's variant angina pectoris. *Br. Heart J.,* 33:889–894.

70. Guazzi, M., Fiorentini, C., Polese, A., Magrini, F., and Olivari, M. T. (1975): Treatment of spontaneous angina pectoris with beta blocking agents: a clinical, electrocardiographic, and hemodynamic appraisal. *Br. Heart J.,* 37:1235–1245.

71. Frishman, W. H. (1980): *Clinical pharmacology of the Beta-adrenoreceptor Blocking Drugs.* Appleton-Century-Croft, New York.

72. Ellrodt, G., Chew, C. Y. C., and Singh, B. (1980): Therapeutic implications of slow-channel blockade in cardiocirculatory disorders. *Circulation,* 62:669–679.

73. Antman, E. M., Stone, P. H., Muller, J. E., and Braunwald, E. (1980): Calcium channel blocking agents in the treatment of cardiovascular disorders. Part I: basic and clinical electrophysiologic effects. *Ann. Intern. Med.,* 93:875–885.

74. Balasubramanian, V., Khana, P. K., Naryanan, G. R., and Hoon, R. S. (1976): Verapamil in ischemic heart disease—quantitative assessment by serial multistage treadmill exercise. *Postgrad. Med. J.,* 52:143–147.

75. Livesley, B., Catley, P. F., Campbell, R. C., and Oram, S. (1973): Double blind evaluation of verapamil, propranolol and isosorbide dinitrate against a placebo in the treatment of angina pectoris. *Br. Med. J.,* 1:375–378.

76. Andreasen, F., Boye, E., and Christoffersen, E. (1975): Assessment of verapamil in the treatment of angina pectoris. *Eur. J. Cardiol.,* 2:443–452.

77. Sandler, G., Clayton, G. A., and Thornicroft, S. (1968): Clinical evaluation of verapamil in angina pectoris. *Br. Med. J.,* 3:224–227.

78. BalaSubramanian, V., Lahiri, A., Paramasivan, R., and Raftery, E. B. (1980): Verapamil in chronic stable angina. *Lancet,* 1:841–844.

79. Leon, M. B., Rosing, D. R., Bonow, R. O., Lipson, L. C., and Epstein, S. E. (1981): Clinical efficacy of verapamil alone and combined with propranolol in treating patients with chronic stable angina pectoris. *Am. J. Cardiol.,* 48:131–139.

80. Ferlinz, J., and Turbow, M. E. (1980): Antianginal and myocardial metabolic properties of verapamil in coronary artery disease. *Am. J. Cardiol.,* 46:1019–1026.

81. Ferlinz, J., Easthope, J. L., Aronow, W. S. (1979): Effects of verapamil on myocardial performance in coronary disease. *Circulation,* 59:313–319.

82. Josephson, M. A., Hecht, H. S., Hopkins, J., Guerrero, J., and Singhi, B. (1982): Comparative effects of oral verapamil and propranolol on exercise-induced myocardial ischemia and energetics in patients with coronary artery disease: single-blind placebo crossover evaluation using radionuclide ventriculography. *Am. Heart J.,* 103:978–985.

83. Frishman, W. H., Klein, N. A., Strom, J. A., Willens, H., Lejemtel, T. H., Jentzer, J., Siegel, L., Klein, P., Kirschen, N., Silverman, R., Pollack, S., Doyle, R., Kirsten, E., and Sonnenblick, E. H. (1982): Superiority of verapamil to propranolol in stable angina pectoris: a double-blind, randomized crossover trial. *Circulation* [Suppl I], 65:51–59.

84. Chew, C. Y. C., Hecht, H. S., Collett, J. T., McAllister, R. G., and Singh, B. N. (1981): Influence of severity of ventricular dysfunction on hemodynamic responses to intravenously administered verapamil in ischemic heart disease. *Am. J. Cardiol.,* 47:917–922.

85. Packer, M., Meller, J., Medina, N., Yushak, M., Smith, H., Holt, J., Guererro, J., Todd, G. D., McAllister, R., and Gorlin, R. (1982): Hemodynamic consequences of combined beta-adrenergic and slow calcium channel blockade in man. *Circulation,* 65:660–668.

86. Parodi, O., Maseri, A., and Simonetti, I. (1979): Management of unstable angina at rest by verapamil: a double-blind cross-over study in coronary care unit. *Br. Heart J.,* 41:167–174.

87. Sherman, L. G., Liang, C., Boden, W. E., and Hood, W. B. (1981): The effect of verapamil on mechanical performance of acutely ischemic and reperfused myocardium in the conscious dog. *Circ. Res.,* 48:224–232.

88. Soleberg, L. E., Nissen, R. G., Vlietstra, R. E., and Callahan, J. A. (1978): Prinzmetal's variant angina-response to verapamil. *Mayo Clin. Proc.,* 53:256–259.

89. Yamaguchi, I., Obayashi, K., and Mandel, W. J. (1978): Electrophysiological effects of verapamil. *Cardiovasc. Res.,* 12:597–608.

90. Waxman, H. L., Myerburg, R. J., Appel, R., and Sung, R. J. (1981): Verapamil for control of ventricular rate in paroxysmal supraventricular tachycardia and atrial fibrillation or flutter. *Ann. Intern. Med.,* 94:1–6.

91. Krikler, D. M., and Spurrell, K. H. (1974): Verapamil in the treatment of paroxysmal supraventricular tachycardia. *Postgrad. Med.,* 50:447–453.

92. Schwartz, J. B., Keefe, D., Kates, R. E., Kirsten, E., and Harrison, D. (1982): Acute and chronic pharmacodynamic interaction of verapamil and digoxin in atrial fibrillation. *Circulation,* 65:1163–1170.

93. Kates, R. E., Keefe, D. L., Schwartz, J., Harapat, S., Kirsten, E. B., and Harrison, D. C. (1981): Verapamil disposition kinetics in chronic atrial fibrillation. *Clin. Pharmacol. Ther.,* 30:44–51.

94. Shand, D. G., Hammill, S. C., Aanonsen, L., and Pritchett, E. L. C. (1981): Reduced verapamil clearance during long-term oral administration. *Clin. Pharmacol. Ther.,* 30:701–703.

95. Anderson, D. E. H., and Rojdmark, S. (1981): Improvement of glucose tolerance by verapamil in patients with non-insulin dependent diabetes mellitus. *Acta. Med. Scand.,* 210:27–33.

96. Bayer, R., Rodenkirchen, R., and Kaufmann, R. (1977): The effects of nifedipine on contraction and monophasic action potential of isolated cat myocardium. *Naunyn Schmiedebergs Arch. Pharmacol.,* 301:29–37.

97. Chiba, S., Furukawa, Y., and Kobayashi, M. (1978): Effect of nifedipine on frequency-force relationship in isolated dog left ventricular muscle. *Jpn. J. Pharmacol.,* 28:783–785.

98. Low, R. I., Takeda, P., Mason, D. T., and DeMaria, A. N. (1982): The effects of calcium channel blocking agents on cardiovascular function. *Am. J. Cardiol.,* 49:547–553.

99. Matsumota, S., Ito, T., Sada, T., Takahashi, M., Su, K., Ueda, A., Okabe, F., Sato, M., Sekine, I., and Ito, Y. (1980): Hemodynamic effects of nifedipine in congestive heart failure. *Am. J. Cardiol.,* 46:476–479.

100. Matsui, S., Murakami, E., and Takekoshi, N. (1979): Hemodynamic effects of sublingual nifedipine in congestive heart failure. *Jpn. Circ. J.,* 43:1081–1088.

101. Cantelli, T., Camillo, P., and Naccavella, F. (1981): Comparison of acute haemodynamic effects of nifedipine and isosorbide dinitrate in patients with heart failure following acute myocardial infarction. *Int. J. Cardiol.,* 1:151–163.

102. Polese, A., Fiorentini, C., Olivari, M. T., and Guazzi, M. (1979): Clinical use of a calcium antagonist agent (nifedipine) in acute pulmonary edema. *Am. J. Med.,* 66:825–830.

103. Corea, L., Miele, N., Bentiroglio, M., Buschetti, E., Agabiti-Rosei, E., and Muiesan, G. (1979): Acute and chronic effects of nifedipine on plasma renin activity and plasma adrenaline and noradrenaline in controls and hypertensive patients. *Clin. Sci.,* 57:115–117.

104. Corea, L., Bentiroglio, M., Cosmi, F., and Alunni, G. (1981): Catecholamines plasma levels and haemodynamic changes induced by nifedipine in chronic severe heart failure. *Current Ther. Res.,* 30:698–707.

105. Antman, E., Muller, J., Goldberg, S., MacAlpin, R., Rubenfire, M., Tabatznik, B., Liang, C., Heupler, F., Achuff, S., Reichek, N., Geltman, E., Kerin, N., Neff, R., and Braunwald, E. (1980): Nifedipine therapy for coronary-artery spasm. *N. Engl. J. Med.,* 302:1269–1273.

106. Mueller, H. S., and Chahine, R. A. (1981): Interim report of multicenter double-blind, placebo-controlled studies of nifedipine in chronic stable angina. *Am. J. Med.,* 71:645–657.

107. Engel, H., and Lichtlen, P. R. (1981): Beneficial enhancement of coronary blood flow by nifedipine. Comparison with nitroglycerin and beta blocking agents. *Am. J. Med.,* 71:658–666.

108. Lorell, B. H., Turi, Z., and Grossman, W. (1981): Modification of left ventricular response to pacing tachycardia by nifedipine in patients with coronary artery disease. *Am. J. Med.,* 71:667–675.

109. Ludbrook, P. A., Tiefenbrunn, A. J., and Sobel, B. E. (1981): Influence of nifedipine on left ventricular systolic and diastolic function. *Am. J. Med.,* 71:683–692.

110. Gerstenblith, G., Ouyang, P., and Achuff, S. C. (1982): Nifedipine in unstable angina. A double-blind, randomized trial. *N. Engl. J. Med.,* 306:885–889.

111. Mitchell, L. B., Schroeder, J. S., and Mason, J. W. (1982): Comparative clinical electrophysiologic effects of dilitiazem, verapamil and nifedipine: a review. *Am. J. Cardiol.,* 49:629–635.

112. Hossack, K. F., Pool, P. E., Steele, P., Crawford, M. H., DeMaria, A. N., Cohen, L. S., and Ports, T. A. (1982): Effect of diltiazem in angina on effort: a multicenter trial. *Am. J. Cardiol.,* 49:567–572.

113. Pool, P. E., and Seagren, S. C. (1982): Long-term efficacy of diltiazem in chronic stable angina associated with atherosclerosis: effect on treadmill exercise. *Am. J. Cardiol.,* 49:573–577.

114. Schroeder, J. S., Lamb, I. H., Ginsburg, R., Bristow, M. R., and Hung, J. (1982): Diltiazem for long-term therapy of coronary artery spasm. *Am. J. Cardiol.,* 49:533–537.

115. Ginsberg, R., Bristow, M. R., and Schroder, J. S. (1981): Selective action of diltiazem in the isolated human heart. *Circulation,* [Suppl 11], 64:11–60.

116. Ginsberg, R., Bristow, M. B., Harrison, D. C., and Stinson, E. B. (1980): Studies with isolated human coronary arteries. *Chest* [Suppl. 1], 78:180–186.

117. Weber, K. T. (1982): New hope for the failing heart. *Am. J. Med.,* 72:665–671.

118. Kannel, W. B., Castelli, W. P., McNamara, P. M., and Kannel, W. B. (1972): Role of blood pressure in the development of congestive heart failure: the Framingham study. *N. Engl. J. Med.,* 285:1441–1446.

119. Roberts, W. C., Buja, L. M., Bulkley, B. H., and Ferrans, W. J. (1974): Congestive heart failure and angina pectoris. *Am. J. Cardiol.,* 34:870–872.

120. Burch, G. E., Tsui, C. Y., and Harb, J. M. (1972): Ischemic cardiomyopathy. *Am. Heart J.,* 83:340–350.

121. Gould, K. L., Lipscomb, K., Hamilton, G. W., and Kennedy, J. W. (1973): Left ventricular hypertrophy in coronary artery disease. A cardiomyopathy syndrome following myocardial infarction. *Am. J. Med.,* 55:595–601.

122. Roberts, W. C., and Buja, L. M. (1972): The frequency and significance of coronary arterial thrombi and other observations in fatal acute myocardial infarction. *Am. J. Med.,* 52:425–443.

123. Franciosa, J. A., Park, M., and Levine, T. B. (1981): Lack of correlation between exercise capacity and indexes of resting left ventricular performance in heart failure. *Am. J. Cardiol.,* 47:33–39.

124. Harlan, W. R., Oberman, A., Grimm, R., and Rosati, R. A. (1977): Chronic congestive heart failure in coronary artery disease: clinical criteria. *Ann. Intern. Med.,* 86:133–138.

125. Cohn, J. N., Levine, T. B., Francis, G. S., and Goldsmith, S. (1981): Neurohumoral control mechanisms in congestive heart failure. *Am. Heart J.,* 102:509–514.

126. Nellis, S. H., Flain, S. F., Zelis, R., and McCauley, K. M. (1980): Alpha-stimulation protects exercise increment in skeletal muscle oxygen consumption. *Am. J. Physiol.,* 238:331–339.

127. Spann, J. F., Jr., Buccino, R. A., Sonnenblick, E. H., and Braunwald, E. (1967): Contractile state of cardiac muscle obtained from cats with experimentally produced ventricular hypertrophy and heart failure. *Circ. Res.,* 21:341–354.

128. Pool, P. E., Spann, J. F., Jr., Buccino, R. A., Sonnenblick, E. H., and Braunwald, E. (1967): Myocardial high energy phosphate stores in cardiac hypertrophy and heart failure. *Circ. Res.,* 21:365–673.

129. Ito, Y., Suko, J., and Chidsey, C. A. (1974): Intracellular calcium and myocardial contractility. *J. Mol. Cell. Cardiol.,* 6:237–247.

130. Bristow, M. R., Ginsburg, R., and Minobe, W. (1982): Decreased catecholamine sensitivity and beta adrenergic receptor density in failing human hearts. *N. Engl. J. Med.,* 307:205–211.

131. Willerson, J. T. (1982): What is wrong with the failing heart. *N. Engl. J. Med.,* 307:243–245.

132. Chidsey, C. A., Braunwald, E., Morrow, A. G., and Mason, D. T. (1963): Myocardial norepinephrine concentration in man. Effects of reserpine and of congestive heart failure. *N. Engl. J. Med.,* 269:653–659.

133. Goldstein, R. E., Beiser, G. D., Stampfer, M., and Epstein, S. E. (1978): Impairment of autonomically mediated heart rate control in patients with cardiac dysfunction. *Circ. Res.,* 36:571–578.

134. Levine, T. B., Francis, G. S., and Goldsmith, S. R. (1982): Activity of the sympathetic nervous system and renin-angiotension system assessed by plasma hormone levels and their relation to hemodynamic abnormalities in congestive heart failure. *Am. J. Cardiol.,* 49:1659–1666.

135. Bennett, E. D., Brooks, W. H., Keddie, J., Lis, Y., and Wilson, A. (1977): Increased renal function in patients with acute left ventricular failure: a possible hemostatic mechanism. *Clin. Sci. Mol. Med.,* 52:43–50.

136. Migdal, S., Alexander, E. A., and Levinsky, W. G. (1977): Evidence that decreased cardiac output is not the stimulus to sodium retention during acute constriction of the vena cava. *J. Lab. Clin. Med.,* 89:809–816.

137. Goldberg, M. (1978): The kidney in heart failure. In: *Heart Failure,* edited by A. P. Fishman, pp. 261–271. Hemisphere, Washington.

138. DiBona, G. F. (1978): Neural control of renal tubular sodium reabsorption in the dog. *Fed. Proc.,* 37:1214–1217.

139. Dzau, V. J., Collucci, W. S., Hollenberg, N. K., and Williams, G. H. (1981): Relation of the renin-angiotensin-aldosterone system to clinical state in congestive heart failure. *Circulation,* 63:645–651.

140. Wilson, J. R., Reichek, N., and Dunkman, W. B. (1981): Effect of diuresis on the performance of the

failing left ventricle in man. *Am. J. Med.,* 70:234–239.

141. Hougen, T. J., and Smith, T. W. (1978): Inhibition of myocardial monovalent cation active transport by subtoxic doses of ouabain in the dog. *Circ. Res.,* 42:856–863.

142. Okita, G. T. (1977): Dissociation of Na⁺, K⁺-ATPase inhibition from digitalis inotropy. *Fed. Proc.,* 36:2225–2230.

143. Smith, T. W., and Braunwald, E. (1980): The management of heart failure. In: *Cardiovascular Diseases,* edited by E. Braunwald, p. 509. W. B. Saunders, New York.

144. Arnold, S. B., Byrd, R. C., Meister, W., Melmon, K., Cheitlin, M. D., Bristow, J. D., Pamley, W. W., and Chatterjee, K. (1980): Long-term digitalis therapy improves left ventricular function in heart failure. *N. Engl. J. Med.,* 303:1443–1448.

145. Lee, D. C. S., Johnson, R. A., Binghamm, J. B., Leahy, M., Dinsmore, R. E., Goroll, A. H., Strauss, H. W., and Haber, E. (1982): Heart failure in outpatients. A randomized trial of digoxin versus placebo. *N. Engl. J. Med.,* 306:699–705.

146. Imperial, E. S., Levy, M. N., and Zieske, H., Jr. (1961): Outflow resistance as an independent determinant of cardiac performance. *Circ. Res.,* 9:1148–1155.

147. Sonnenblick, E. H., and Downing, S. E. (1963): Afterload as a primary determinant of ventricular performance. *Am. J. Physiol.,* 204:604–610.

148. Majid, P. A., Sharma, B., and Taylor, S. H. (1971): Phentolamine for vasodilator treatment of severe heart failure. *Lancet,* 2:719–723.

149. Franciosa, J. A., Guiha, N. H., Limas, C. J., Rodriguera, E., and Cohn, J. N. (1972): Improved left ventricular function during nitroprusside infusion in acute myocardial infarction. *Lancet,* 1:650–657.

150. Mason, D. T. (1978): Symposium on vasodilator and inotropic therapy of heart failure. *Am. J. Med.,* 65:101–105.

151. Packer, M., Meller, J. (1978): Oral vasodilator therapy for chronic heart failure: a plea for caution. *Am. J. Cardiol.,* 42:686–689.

152. Zelis, R., Flaim, S. F., Moskowitz, R. M., and Nellis, S. H. (1979): How much can we expect from vasodilator therapy in congestive heart failure? *Circulation,* 59:1092–1097.

153. Cohn, J. N., and Franciosa, J. A. (1977): Vasodilator therapy of cardiac failure. *N. Engl. J. Med.,* 297:27–31, 254–258.

154. Chatterjee, K., and Parmley, W. W. (1977): The role of vasodilator therapy in heart failure. *Prog. Cardiovasc. Dis.,* 19:301–325.

155. O'Rourke, M. F., and Taylor, M. G. (1967): Input impedance of the systemic circulation. *Circ. Res.,* 20:365–380.

156. Milnor, W. R. (1975): Arterial impedance as ventricular afterload. *Circ. Res.,* 36:565–570.

157. Zobel, L. R., Finklstein, S. M., Carlyle, P. F., and Cohn, J. N. (1980): Pressure pulse contour analysis in determining the effect of vasodilator drugs on vascular hemodynamic impedance characteristics in dogs. *Am. Heart J.,* 100:81–88.

158. Franciosa, J. A., Pierpont, G., and Cohn, J. N.

(1977): Hemodynamic improvement after oral hydralazine in left ventricular failure. *Ann. Intern. Med.,* 86:388–393.

159. Franciosa, J. A., Blank, R. C., and Cohn, J. N. (1978): Nitrate effects on cardiac output and left ventricular outflow resistance in chronic congestive heart failure. *Am. J. Med.,* 64:207–213.

160. Zelis, R., and Longhurst, J. (1975): The circulation in congestive heart failure. In: *The Peripheral Circulations,* edited by R. Zelis, p. 283. Grune & Stratton, New York.

161. Magorien, R. D., Tritton, D. W., Desch, C. E., Bay, W. H., Univerferth, D. V., and Leier, C. V. (1981): Prazosin and hydralazine in congestive heart failure. Regional hemodynamic effects in relation to dose. *Ann. Intern. Med.,* 95:5–13.

162. Leier, C. V., Magorien, R. D., Desch, C. E., Thompson, M. J., and Univerferth, D. V. (1981): Hydralazine and isosorbide dinitrate: comparative central and regional hemodynamic effects when administered alone or in combination. *Circulation,* 63:102–109.

163. Flaim, S. F., Weitzel, R. L., and Zelis, R. (1981): Mechanism of action of nitroglycerin during exercise in a rat model of heart failure. Improvement of blood flow to the renal, splanchnic, and cutaneous beds. *Circ. Res.,* 49:458–468.

164. Moskowitz, R. M., Kinney, E. L., and Zelis, R. (1979): Hemodynamic and metabolic responses to upright exercise in patients with congestive heart failure. *Chest,* 76:640–646.

165. Franciosa, J. A., and Cohn, J. N. (1979): Immediate effects of hydralazine-isosorbide dinitrate combination on exercise capacity and exercise hemodynamics in patients with left ventricular failure. *Circulation,* 59:1085–1091.

166. Rubin, S. A., Chatterjee, K., and Ports, T. A. (1979): Influence of short-term oral hydralazine therapy on exercise hemodynamics in patients with severe chronic heart failure. *Am. J. Cardiol.,* 43:810–815.

167. Franciosa, J. A., and Cohn, J. N. (1979): Effect of isosorbide dinitrate on response to submaximal and maximal exercise in patients with congestive heart failure. *Am. J. Cardiol.,* 43:1009–1014.

168. Colucci, W. S., Wynne, J., Holman, B. L., and Braunwald, E. (1980): Long-term therapy of heart failure with prazosin: A randomized double-blind trial. *Am. J. Cardiol.,* 45:337–343.

169. Packer, M., Meller, J., Gorlin, R., and Herman, M. V. (1979): Hemodynamic and clinical tachyphylaxis to prazosin-mediated afterload reduction in severe chronic heart failure. *Circulation,* 59:531–539.

170. Packer, M., Meller, J., Medina, N., Yushak, M., and Gorlin, R. (1981): Provocation of myocardial ischemic events during initiation of vasodilator therapy for severe chronic heart failure. *Am. J. Cardiol.,* 48:939–946.

171. Walsh, W. F., and Greenberg, B. H. (1981): Results of long-term vasodilator therapy in patients with refractory congestive heart failure. *Circulation,* 64:499–505.

172. Rouleau, J. L., Chatterjee, K., Benge, W., Parmley, W. W., and Hiramatsu, B. (1982): Alterations in left ventricular function and coronary hemodynamics with captopril, hydralazine and prazosin in

chronic ischemic heart failure. *Circulation,* 65:671–678.

173. Packer, M., Meller, J., Medina, N., Gorlin, R., and Herman, M. V. (1979): Rebound hemodynamic events after the abrupt withdrawal of nitroprusside in patients with severe chronic heart failure. *N. Engl. J. Med.,* 301:1193–1197.

174. Cohn, J. N., and Franciosa, J. A. (1978): Selection of vasodilator, inotropic or combined therapy for the management of heart failure. *Am. J. Med.,* 65:181–188.

175. Wayne, A. R., Williams, A. T., and Lefkowitz, R. (1975): Identification of cardiac B-adrenergic receptors (−)³H-Alprenolol binding. *Proc. Natl. Acad. Sci. U.S.A.,* 72:1564–1568.

176. Katz, A. M., Tada, M., and Kirchberger, M. A. (1975): Control of calcium transport in the myocardium by the cyclic AMP-protein kinase system. *Adv. Cyclic Nucleotide Res.,* 5:453–472.

177. Barcroft, H., Kronzett, H. (1949): The actions of noradrenaline, adrenaline and isoprophylnoradrenaline on the arterial blood pressure, heart rate and muscle blood flow in man. *J. Physiol.,* 110:194.

178. MacCannell, K. F., McNay, J. L., Meyer, M. B., and Goldberg, L. I. (1966): Dopamine in the treatment of hypotension and shock. *N. Engl. J. Med.,* 275:1389–1400.

179. Goldberg, L. I. (1972): Cardiovascular and renal actions of dopamine: potential clinical applications. *Pharmacol. Rev.,* 24:1–29.

180. Goldberg, L. I. (1974): Dopamine—clinical use of an endogenous catecholamine. *N. Engl. J. Med.,* 291:701–710.

181. Goldberg, L. I., Volkman, P. H., and Kohli, J. D. (1978): A comparison of the vascular dopamine receptor with other dopamine receptors. *Annu. Rev. Pharmacol. Toxicol.,* 18:57–79.

182. Goldberg, L. I., McDonald, R. H., and Zimmerman, A. M. (1963): Sodium diuresis produced by dopamine in patients with congestive heart failure. *N. Engl. J. Med.,* 269:1060–1064.

183. Loeb, H. S., Winslow, E. B. J., Rahimtoola, S. H., Rosen, K. M., and Gunnar, R. M. (1971): Acute hemodynamic effects of dopamine in patients with shock. *Circulation,* 44:163–173.

184. Miller, R. R., Awan, N. A., Joye, J. A., Maxwell, K. S., DeMaria, A. N., Amsterdam, E. A., and Mason, D. T. (1977): Combined dopamine and nitroprusside therapy in congestive heart failure. *Circulation,* 55:881–884.

185. Stemple, D. R., Kleiman, J. H., and Harrison, D. C. (1978): Combined nitroprusside-dopamine therapy in severe chronic congestive heart failure. *Am. J. Cardiol.,* 42:267–275.

186. Akhtar, N., Mikulic, E., Cohn, J. N., and Chaudhry, M. H. (1975): Hemodynamic effect of dobutamine in patients with severe heart failure. *Am. J. Cardiol.,* 36:202–205.

187. Sonnenblick, E. H., Frishman, W. H., and LeJemtel, T. H. (1979): Dobutamine: a new synthetic cardiac active sympathetic amine. *N. Engl. J. Med.,* 300:17–22.

188. Francis, G. S., Sharma, B., and Hodges, M. (1982): Comparative hemodynamic effects of dopamine and dobutamine in patients with acute cardiogenic circulatory collapse. *Am. Heart J.,* 103:995–1000.

189. Loeb, H. S., Bredakis, J., and Gunnar, R. M. (1977): Superiority of dobutamine over dopamine for augmentation of cardiac output in patients with chronic low output failure. *Circulation,* 55:375–381.

190. Univerferth, D. V., Blanford, M., Kates, R. E., and Leier, C. V. (1980): Tolerance to dobutamine after a 72 hour continuous infusion. *Am. J. Med.,* 69:262–266.

191. Sharma, B., and Goodwin, J. F. (1978): Beneficial effects of salbutamol on cardiac function in severe congestive cardiomyopathy. Effect on systolic and diastolic function of the left ventricle. *Circulation,* 58:449–459.

192. Sharma, B., Hoback, J., Francis, G. S., Hodges, M., Asinger, R. W., Cohn, J. N., and Taylor, C. R. (1981): Pirbuterol: a new oral sympathomimetic amine for the treatment of congestive heart failure. *Am. Heart J.,* 102:533–541.

193. Klein, W., Brandt, D., Maurer, E. (1981): Hemodynamic assessment of prenalterol: a cardioselective beta agonist in patients with impaired left ventricular function. *Clin. Cardiol.,* 4:325–329.

194. Nelson, S., and Leier, C. V. (1981): Butopamine in normal human subjects. *Curr. Ther. Res.,* 30:405–411.

195. Kino, M., Hirota, Y., Yamamoto, S., Sawada, K., Moriguchi, M., Kotaka, M., Kuba, S., and Kawamura, K. (1982): Cardiovascular effects of a newly synthesized cardiotonic agent (TA-064) upon normal and diseased hearts in man. *Am. J. Cardiol.,* 49:1039 (abstract).

196. Colucci, W. S., Alexander, R. W., Williams, G. H., Rude, R. E., Holman, B. L., Konstam, M. A., Wynne, J., Mudge, G. H., and Braunwald, E. (1981): Decreased lymphocyte beta-adrenergic-receptor density in patients with heart failure and tolerance to the beta-adrenergic agonist pirbuterol. *N. Engl. J. Med.,* 305:185–190.

197. Benotti, J. R., Grossman, W., Braunwald, E., Davolas, D. D., and Alousi, A. A. (1978): Hemodynamic assessment of amrinone: a new inotropic agent. *N. Engl. J. Med.,* 299:1373–1377.

198. Levine, S. A., Jacoby, M., Sariano, J. A., and Schlondorff, D. (1981): The effects of amrinone in transport and cyclic AMP metabolism in toad urinary bladder. *J. Pharmacol. Exp. Ther.,* 216:220–224.

199. Verdouw, P. D., Hartog, A. M., and Rutterman, A. M. (1981): Systemic and regional myocardial response to AR-L115BS, a positive inotropic imidazopyridine, in the absence or in the presence of the bradycardic action of alinidine. *Basic Res. Cardiol.,* 76:328–343.

200. Dage, R. C., Roebel, L. E., and Hsieh, C. P. (1982): Cardiovascular properties of a new cardiotonic agent: MDL 17,043. *J. Cardiovasc. Pharmacol.,* 4:500–508.

201. Kariya, T., Wille, L. J., and Dage, R. C. (1982): Biochemical studies on the mechanism of cardiotonic activity of MDL 17,043. *J. Cardiovasc. Pharmacol.,* 4:509–514.

202. Siegel, L., Strom, J., and Fein, E. (1981): Long-term effect of oral amrinone in heart failure. Improvement in exercise performance despite declining left ventricular failure. *Am. J. Cardiol.,* 47:428 (abstract).

Cardiovascular Pharmacology, Second Edition,
edited by Michael Antonaccio.
Raven Press, New York © 1984.

Antiarrhythmic Drugs

Benedict R. Lucchesi and Eugene S. Patterson

Department of Pharmacology and the Upjohn Center for Clinical Pharmacology,
The University of Michigan Medical School, Ann Arbor, Michigan 48109

The ideal approach to treatment of cardiac rhythm disorders depends on proper identification of the arrhythmia, an understanding of the factors involved in the production of the arrhythmia, knowledge of the mechanisms of action of the wide variety of available pharmacologic agents, and an understanding of the clinical effects of the antiarrhythmic agents, particularly as they relate to the clinical setting in which they are employed. Because this text is not concerned with the problems of clinical diagnosis, we shall devote primary attention to the possible electrophysiologic mechanisms underlying the genesis of arrhythmias and the pharmacologic properties of drugs used in the control of abnormal cardiac rhythms.

NORMAL CARDIAC ACTION POTENTIAL

Two major types of electrical activity exist in cardiac cells. These two types of electrical activity are termed the "fast response" and "slow response" and are characteristic for the specialized electrical functions provided by the various cardiac conductile tissues.

The fast-response fibers of the heart are those cardiac fibers that conduct electrical activity at a relatively rapid rate (0.3–3 m/sec). This group includes working atrial and ventricular muscle fibers and fibers of the specialized conducting systems of atria and ventricles. The property of rapid conduction and other related electrophysiologic characteristics that will be described here are dependent on a transmembrane action potential with a rapid rate of depolarization known as the fast-response potential.

Under physiologic conditions, the transmembrane potential of working atrial and ventricular muscle fibers and fibers of the specialized atrial and ventricular conducting system is characterized by a resting membrane potential between -80 and -95 mV. On excitation, a rapid regenerative depolarization is activated at a threshold potential of about -70 mV and rapidly carries the transmembrane potential to a value of $+25$ to $+35$ mV. The rapid depolarization (phase 0 of the cardiac cell action potential) is dependent on rapid influx of sodium ions, carrying a strong positive inward current through specific membrane channels. These channels controlling sodium conductance of the membrane respond rapidly to a change in transmembrane potential, resulting in a rapid depolarization or fast response (Fig. 1). Sodium conductance of the membrane is then inactivated rapidly, and the inward sodium current ceases. In addition, in these fast-response fibers, a second inward positive current (depolarizing current) is activated when the fast depolarization phase has lowered the membrane potential to values less negative than -55 mV. This is a weaker current than the initial sodium current, and it is probably carried by calcium ions through a "slow" membrane channel that is distinct

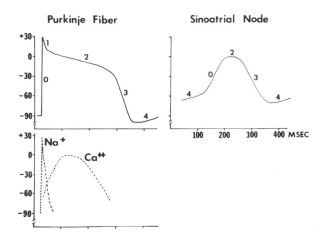

Purkinje Fiber   Sinoatrial Node

FIG. 1. Diagrammatic representation of the membrane action potential as recorded from a Purkinje fiber and the sinoatrial node. The membrane resting potential is −90 mV with respect to the exterior of the fiber. At the point of depolarization there is a rapid change (phase 0) to a more positive value. The phases of depolarization and repolarization are indicated by the numbers 0, 1, 2, 3, and 4. The sinoatrial node has a resting value of only −60 mV, and depolarization (phase 0) proceeds at a much slower rate. The lower graph shows the rates of influx of sodium and calcium during the Purkinje fiber action potential.

from the "fast" sodium channel. This slow current is not affected by tetrodotoxin or other inhibitors of sodium influx through the rapid-response channel. Because the slow membrane channels are activated slowly and the current density is low in comparison to the initial inward rapid sodium current, the slow current does not contribute significantly to the rapid depolarization (phase 0) of the normal cardiac action potential. However, inactivation of this secondary inward current is slow; the current still flows after the initial rapid depolarization is over and maintains the membrane in a depolarized state. Thus, the slow current is primarily responsible for the plateau phase (phases 2 and 3) of the action potential (Fig. 1).

Because of the nature of the voltage and time dependence of the mechanisms that control the fast sodium channels, fibers that generate action potentials by this fast-response mechanism have certain characteristic electrophysiologic properties. The large resting potential (−75 to −90 mV), the value of the threshold potential (−70 mV), the rapid rate of phase-0 upstroke velocity, and the large amplitude of depolarization (100–130 mV) result in relatively rapid conduction of the cardiac impulse. Fast responses have a large safety factor for conduction, so that propagation of the impulse usually is not blocked by minor electrical and anatomic impediments

to its spread. A normal response in these fibers can be elicited only when repolarization has restored the normal resting potential.

Slow cardiac fibers of the heart conduct electrical activity at a relatively slow rate (0.01–0.10 m/sec). This group includes the sinus and atrioventricular nodes, cardiac fibers of the atrioventricular ring, and mitral and tricuspid valve leaflets. The property of slow conduction is dependent on a transmembrane action potential with a slow rate of depolarization. This type of action potential has been termed the "slow response."

The electrophysiologic characteristics of the slow response are entirely different from those described for the fast-response fibers. The slow fibers have a low resting membrane potential between −70 and −60 mV, and on excitation a slow regenerative depolarization phase carries the transmembrane potential to a value of only 0 to +15 mV. This slow depolarization is not dependent on sodium influx through a rapid membrane channel but rather is due to a weak inward current, possibly carried by calcium through a slow membrane channel. This channel is also inactivated slowly, resulting in a prolonged phase of repolarization. There is no evidence for rapid channels in these fibers, and the depolarization phase is not affected by tetrodotoxin or other inhibitors of rapid sodium influx.

MECHANISMS FOR GENESIS OF CARDIAC ARRHYTHMIAS

Current theories of the electrophysiologic mechanisms thought to be responsible for the origin and perpetuation of cardiac arrhythmias have been derived primarily from experimental models. Of the many proposed mechanisms, the simplest approach is to consider abnormal rhythm formations as being due to either altered impulse formation (automaticity) or altered conduction or both acting simultaneously in the same location or different locations in the heart. The reader who would like to pursue this study in detail should consult one or more of the excellent publications in this area (1–4).

RHYTHM DISTURBANCES DUE TO ECTOPIC IMPULSE FORMATION

An impulse can be generated by an excitable membrane when its transmembrane potential is reduced (becomes less negative) from the normal resting potential to some critical level of potential that has been designated the "threshold potential" or the "critical firing potential." This change from the resting potential to the critical firing potential is achieved by a flow of positive charge into an area of resting membrane. At the time of excitation, the cell membrane suddenly becomes permeable to sodium. The intense inward sodium current carries sufficient positive charge into the cell to alter the transmembrane voltage to a value near the sodium equilibrium potential (transmembrane potential becomes positive). Figure 1 is a schematic representation of the transmembrane action potential of a Purkinje fiber and is represented as having five phases. The generation of the cardiac impulse is normally confined to specialized tissues in the heart that spontaneously depolarize during phase 4. Slow spontaneous depolarization proceeds to a threshold, at which an action potential is initiated and propagated through the cardiac conduction system to the myocardial cells. Cells capable of giving rise to slow diastolic depolarization have the property of automaticity (Fig. 2).

In the normal heart, automaticity is most prominent in the specialized cells of the sinoatrial node located in the right atrium. This region is commonly referred to as the "pace-

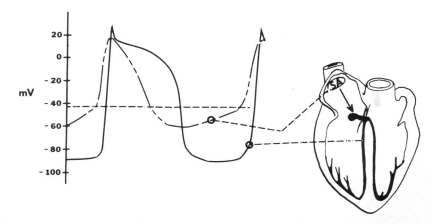

FIG. 2. Diagrammatic representation of the membrane action potential as recorded from the sinoatrial node (SA: *broken line*) and from a Purkinje fiber (*solid line*). The generation of the cardiac impulse is normally confined to the specialized cells in the sinoatrial node. Pacemaker cells possess the characteristic of spontaneous phase-4 depolarization (automaticity). When the slow spontaneous depolarization reaches the level of the threshold potential (*horizontal broken line*), an action potential is generated and propagated through the cardiac conduction system to the myocardial cells.

maker," for it is this area of the heart that gives rise to the normal rhythmic beat of the heart. The spontaneous electrical activity that can be recorded from the sinoatrial node serves as the impulse that ultimately depolarizes or excites all the cardiac cells and causes the heart to contract. The spontaneous electrical depolarization of the sinoatrial pacemaker cells is independent of the nervous system and can be demonstrated to proceed in the heart removed from the body and maintained with adequate oxygen and metabolic substrates. The specialized pacemaker cells of the sinoatrial node are innervated by both sympathetic and parasympathetic nerves. The sympathetic nerve fibers (adrenergic nerves) release the

catecholamine norepinephrine, which causes an increase in the rate of spontaneous diastolic depolarization in the sinoatrial nodal pacemaker cells and an increase in the heart rate. In contrast, the parasympathetic nerves (vagus nerve) to the sinoatrial node release the chemical neurotransmitter acetylcholine, which causes a decrease in the rate of pacemaker discharge and a slowing of the heart rate. The pacemaker cells of the sinoatrial node display the property of automaticity, which, although independent of the nervous system, can be modified by the influence of the sympathetic and parasympathetic nervous systems. The neuronal influences on the pacemaker cells help the beating heart to adjust its rate in

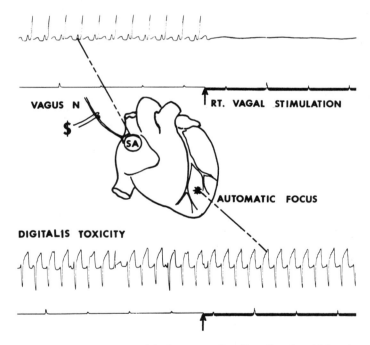

FIG. 3. Under special circumstances, automaticity in areas other than the sinoatrial node may dominate the rhythm of the heart. The electrocardiogram in the upper portion of the figure illustrates the normal sequence of events in which the cardiac pacemaker originates within the sinoatrial node and leads to activation of the atrial and ventricular fibers, thus giving rise to the electrocardiogram showing the P, QRS, and T-wave configuration. Stimulation of the right vagus nerve suppresses pacemaker activity within the sinoatrial node, leading to a loss of electrical activity from the heart as the subsidiary pacemakers fail to discharge during the brief period of vagal-induced sinoatrial arrest. Under certain conditions, such as in the presence of toxic doses of a digitalis glycoside (ouabain), the action of subsidiary pacemakers may be enhanced to the point where they dominate the cardiac rhythm (*lower panel*). Stimulation of the right vagus nerve is ineffective in terminating the ectopic ventricular pacemaker. Thus, the enhancement of automaticity in cardiac cells outside the sinoatrial node is an important mechanism for the genesis of cardiac arrhythmias.

24 HOURS POST MYOCARDIAL INFARCTION

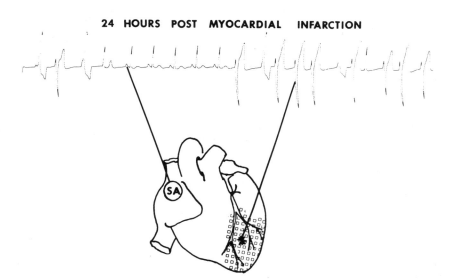

FIG. 4. Role of enhanced automaticity in the genesis of cardiac arrhythmias. Twenty-four hours after experimental infarction in the canine heart, multiple sites of pacemaker activity exist within the ventricle, simultaneously with pacemaker activity from the sinoatrial node. The objective in antiarrhythmic therapy is to suppress the ectopic pacemaker sites so that the sinoatrial node can once more control the cardiac rhythm.

an effort to regulate the cardiac output to meet the needs of the body.

Other specialized cells in the normal heart also possess the property of automaticity. Under circumstances where the normal pacemaker cells of the sinoatrial node fail to pace the heart, the subsidiary pacemaker cells serve the function of maintaining the heartbeat. The subsidiary pacemaker cells discharge at a slower rate than those of the sinoatrial node, and their rate of discharge is not as well modulated by the autonomic nervous system. Because the cardiac rhythm is dominated by the fastest pacemaker, the normal heart rhythm is controlled by the automaticity of the sinoatrial node. The subsidiary pacemakers influence the cardiac rhythm when the normal pacemaker is suppressed or when, because of pathologic changes or drugs, the rate of discharge is increased to the point where it can dominate the cardiac rhythm (Figs. 3 and 4). Automaticity of subsidiary pacemakers can occur as a result of myocardial cell damage due to infarction or can be due to digitalis toxicity or excessive amounts of catecholamines released from sympathetic nerve fibers

to the heart or circulating in the blood. Thus, the enhancement of automaticity in specialized cardiac cells can lead to cardiac arrhythmias. Cardiac cells other than those of the sinoatrial node that are capable of automaticity include (a) specialized atrial fibers, (b) atrioventricular nodal cells in the N-H region, (c) the bundle of His, and (d) Purkinje fibers.

Depression of automaticity in pacemaker fibers is a property common to all class I antiarrhythmic drugs. It is fortunate that most antiarrhythmic agents depress subsidiary pacemaker cells to a greater degree than those of the sinoatrial node, although toxic doses of some antiarrhythmic drug can suppress all cardiac pacemaker activity and result in arrest of the heartbeat.

The differential effects of antiarrhythmic drugs on automaticity in the various tissues of the heart are, in part, due to the different mechanisms involved in impulse formation in the various heart regions. Spontaneous diastolic depolarization in fast-response fibers begins immediately after repolarization, at a maximum diastolic potential of -75 to -90 mV. The inward current that depolarizes cells until threshold potential is attained results from a time- and voltage-dependent decrease in membrane potassium conductance and a coexisting steady inward sodium current. A second mechanism for spontaneous diastolic depolarization probably exists only in slow cardiac fibers. This spontaneous diastolic depolarization occurs at maximum diastolic potentials of -60 mV or less. The prototype for this second slow-fiber automaticity is the sinus node. The rapid-response fiber automaticity is very sensitive to class I antiarrhythmic agents, whereas the slow-response fiber automaticity is most sensitive to the class IV antiarrhythmic agents.

RHYTHM DISTURBANCES DUE TO ABNORMAL CONDUCTION

Premature beats or extrasystoles originate in ectopic foci in the atria, the ventricles, or the atrioventricular junctional tissue and may, in turn, initiate episodes of sustained tachyarrhythmias of either supraventricular or ventricular origin. Some of these ectopic rhythms are no doubt due to enhanced automaticity of specialized fibers in the intraatrial conduction tissue and the His-Purkinje system. Certain features of clinically encountered and experimentally induced arrhythmias suggest that ectopic rhythms may result from some mechanism other than enhanced automaticity of the specialized fibers. These abnormal mechanisms seem to be related to the phenomenon called reentrant activity or reentry, which is thought to result from nonuniformity of the cardiac tissues with respect to excitability and impulse conductivity.

To understand better the mechanisms involved in the origin and perpetuation of arrhythmias due to disturbances in conduction, it is necessary to consider the factors that determine normal conduction.

Conduction velocity is dependent on a number of interrelated factors that include (a) the maximal rate of depolarization during the rising phase of the action potential (maximal dV/dt of phase 0), (b) the magnitude of the depolarization (amplitude of the action potential), (c) the levels of threshold and membrane potentials, (d) the cable properties of the fibers (membrane resistance and capacitance), and (e) the fiber diameter. Two of the variables (maximal dV/dt during phase 0 and the amplitude of the action potential) are of singular importance in the determination of conduction velocity.

The conduction velocity of an impulse away from a given site will depend not only on the conduction velocity of the impulse as it approaches the given site but also on the ability of the given site to respond to the excitatory nature of the impulse. The most important determinant of the ability of a fiber to respond to an impulse or stimulus is the level of membrane potential at the moment of excitation. The relationship between fiber response and transmembrane potential has been determined by Weidmann (5) and Hoffman et al. (6) and has been shown to resemble a sigmoid curve. This relationship is depicted on the right side of Fig. 5, which illustrates the relationship between the maximum depolarization rate during phase 0 ($\dot{V}_{max}$) of the canine Purkinje fiber action potential in volts per second on the abscissa and the level of membrane potential (E_m) at the moment of fiber excitation in millivolts on the ordinate. The Purkinje

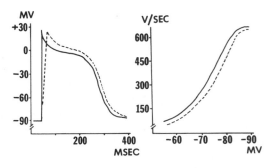

FIG. 5. Diagrammatic relationship between the transmembrane action potential **(left)** and fiber responsiveness **(right).** Membrane responsiveness is reduced by factors causing depolarization. For any given level of transmembrane potential, antiarrhythmic drugs will either reduce membrane responsiveness, as occurs with quinidine or procainamide, or improve membrane responsiveness, as is seen with lidocaine or diphenylhydantoin.

fiber action potential is shown to the left. The role of $\dot{V}_{max}$ or maximum upstroke velocity as a major determinant of conduction velocity has been demonstrated for heart muscle by the studies of Noble (7). From the relationship between upstroke velocity and conduction velocity, it can readily be seen how impulse conduction in a given fiber will be decreased if the membrane potential at the moment of excitation is reduced (8).

Figure 6 is a schematic representation of possible mechanisms for reentrant excitation due to unidirectional block and the development of a bigeminal or coupled ventricular rhythm. Under normal circumstances, impulse conduction from terminal branches of Purkinje fibers to ventricular muscle causes ventricular depolarization (Fig. 6A). Activation of ventricular myocardium is rapid and synchronous. Impairment of impulse conduction may result because of ischemic injury, which leads to depolarization in the involved fibers and establishes the essential conditions necessary for localized reentry of myocardial electrical activity, slowed conduction, and unidirectional block. Thus, as shown in Fig. 6B, the impulse in Purkinje fiber 2 fails to propagate beyond the injured zone because of a reduced membrane potential in the ischemically injured area. However, the same impulse spreading through a normal terminal branch and reaching the ventricle may enter the depolarized zone (Fig. 6C) from the opposite direction through ventricular tissue. The impulse conducts slowly through the damaged Purkinje fiber and exits the fiber only after the normal Purkinje fiber has regained the ability to conduct this impulse to again excite ventricular muscle. Because the ventricular muscle is excited shortly after the previous event (Fig. 6B), the two resulting ventricular depolarizations are related temporarily (coupled) and may account for the genesis of bigeminal rhythms. Antiarrhythmic drugs, by reducing the responsiveness of cardiac cell membranes to stimulation and thus reducing conduction velocity, abolish reentry by converting unidirectional block to bidirectional block, or by altering myocardial refractoriness may prevent the entry of electrical activity to normal or damaged myocardium.

ELECTROPHARMACOLOGY OF DRUGS USED FOR TREATMENT OF VENTRICULAR ARRHYTHMIAS

Actions of Class I Drugs

Quinidine is often regarded as the prototype of antiarrhythmic drugs, and along with the other agents listed in Table 1, it makes up the class I antiarrhythmic drugs.

The characteristic actions of the members of this class are that they interfere with myocardial cell depolarization, causing a reduction in the maximum rate of depolarization without producing a change in the resting membrane potential or significant prolongation of the action-potential duration (Fig. 5). The presumed mechanism by which class I antiarrhythmic drugs decrease phase 0 of the membrane action potential is believed to result from a reduction in the rate of entry of the depolarizing sodium current. Because the inward flow of sodium during membrane depolarization is reduced, the rate of rise of phase 0 of the membrane action potential is reduced, as is the absolute height or "overshoot" of the action potential. To obtain a propagated action potential, it is necessary to obtain a minimum rate of depolarization, the latter being dependent on the resting membrane potential and the availability of a sufficient number of active sodium carriers. Without attaining this minimal rate of depolarization, conduction of the premature beat is sufficiently poor that the premature beat fails to propagate to surrounding ventricular tissue. In the presence of class I drugs, therefore, the entry of the depolarizing current is reduced, and the process of repolarization must proceed for a longer time before an adequate rate of rise for phase 0 can be obtained in order to assure propagation of the impulse to neighboring cells. Thus, repolarization must continue for a longer time in the presence of a class I drug

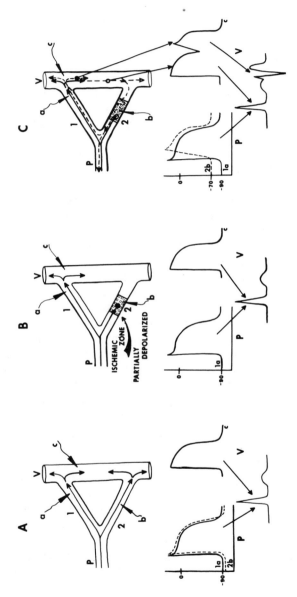

FIG. 6. Schematic representation of possible mechanisms for reentrant excitation due to unidirectional block and the development of a bigeminal or coupled ventricular rhythm. P: Purkinje fiber and its terminal branches 1 and 2 as they enter ventricular muscle. V: Microelectrode recordings from sites a, b, and c are shown below each of the diagrams along with the compound electrocardiogram. The demarcated segment in 2b of **B** and **C** represents a partially depolarized region in which unidirectional block exists.

Table 1. *Classification of antiarrhythmic drugs*

Class I	Class II	Class III	Class IV
Quinidine	Propranolol	Bretylium	Verapamil
Procainamide	Metoprolol	Amiodarone	Diltiazem
Disopyramide	Nadolol	Sotalol	Nifedipine
Phenytoin	Atenolol	Clofilium	
Mexiletine	Acebutolol	Pranolium	
Lidocaine	Sotalol[a]		
Aprindine			
Tocainide			
Ethmozin			
Propranolol[a]			
Pranolium[a]			

[a] Additional mechanism.

before a propagated event can occur. The result of this action is that class I drugs prolong the effective refractory period of fast-response cardiac fibers.

In summary, class I antiarrhythmic drugs are characterized by their ability to (a) restrict the rate of sodium entry during cardiac membrane depolarization, (b) decrease the rate of rise of phase 0 of the cardiac membrane action potential, (c) require that a greater (more negative) membrane potential be achieved before the membrane becomes excitable and can propagate to its neighbors, and (d) prolong the effective refractory period of fast-response fibers.

Class I antiarrhythmic drugs are characterized further by the fact that they possess local anesthetic actions on nerve and depress myocardial contractile force. Both actions are observed at concentrations greater than that needed to depress the rate of depolarization of phase 0 of the cardiac cell membrane action potential.

How can the electrophysiologic actions of the class I drugs be converted into a salutary effect? Electrophysiologic studies have presented evidence to suggest that slowed conduction in damaged or partially depolarized myocardial cells can contribute to the development of unidirectional block and reentrant cardiac rhythms (Fig. 6). The speed of impulse conduction is related to the rate of depolarization, which in turn is dependent on the level of the resting membrane potential. Antiarrhythmic drugs belonging to class I may convert unidirectional block into bidirectional block and abolish reentry by further depressing conduction through a partially depolarized region (Fig. 6). The beneficial effect would result from the depressant effects of the drugs on the inward sodium current and the production of conduction block.

As indicated earlier, cardiac rhythm disorders can arise from spontaneous impulses or altered automaticity. Two different automatic mechanisms are known to exist in heart tissue. One type of automaticity occurs at membrane potentials between -90 and -60 mV and is due to a time- and voltage-dependent decrease in outward potassium ion current. The second mechanism for the development of automaticity occurs when the membrane potential has been reduced to -65 mV or less. At this level of membrane potential, the fast inward current is inactivated, and the inward current is then dependent on the slow inward movement of calcium ions. This latter type of automaticity is enhanced by the presence of catecholamines.

The antiarrhythmic drugs in class I are known to suppress both normal Purkinje fiber and His-bundle automaticity, as well as abnormal automaticity resulting from myocardial damage that occurs at membrane potentials between -60 and -90 mV. Because the normal pacemaker activity in the sinoatrial node is more dependent on the slow inward calcium current, the antiarrhythmic drugs in class I can suppress spontaneous diastolic depolarization and automatic impulse formation that occur at membrane potentials between -60 and -90 mV at concentrations that do not suppress impulse formation in the sinoatrial node. The ability to "selectively" suppress abnormal automaticity permits the sinoatrial node to once again assume the role of the dominant pacemaker.

In summary, class I antiarrhythmic agents can exert an antiarrhythmic effect by virtue of their ability to depress myocardial conduction in damaged ventricular myocardium and, in addition, suppress abnormal ectopic pacemaker activity.

Actions of Class II Drugs

Drugs belonging to class II exert antisympathetic effects by competitive blockade of β-adrenergic receptors. It should also be noted that whereas all β-adrenergic receptor blocking drugs can modify or prevent stimulation of cardiac β-adrenergic receptors and can be classified as class II drugs, a few members of this group also possess class I actions. Thus, propranolol and acebutolol possess class I actions often referred to as "membrane-stabilizing" effects. β-adrenergic receptor antagonists also include drugs such as sotalol, metoprolol, atenolol, and nadolol.

Determining which of the actions of the β receptor blocking drugs can explain their antiarrhythmic effects has proved to be a complex problem. There is no doubt that adrenergic stimulation of the heart can lead to disorders of cardiac rhythm. It is also well known that all β receptor blocking drugs prevent catecholamine-induced alterations of the transmembrane action potential and that this action itself can lead to an antiarrhythmic effect. The arrhythmias associated with halothane or cyclopropane anesthesia have been attributed to the interaction of the anesthetic with catecholamines (9) and have been suppressed with propranolol (10,11). Similarly, catecholamine-induced arrhythmias in experimental animals are known to respond favorably to propranolol, but not to the non-β receptor blocking dextro isomer (12,13).

Davis and Temte (14) have described the effects of propranolol on Purkinje fiber preparations from canine hearts. Propranolol (3.0 mg/liter) decreased the rate of rise of phase 0 of the action potential, decreased the overshoot potential, and decreased membrane responsiveness. At somewhat lower concentrations (0.3 mg/liter) the drug increased the effective refractory period relative to the duration of the action potential. These actions of the drug are also those actions associated with class I antiarrhythmic agents. Most important was the observation that low concentrations (0.1 mg/liter) of propranolol, which had no effect on transmembrane potentials, blocked the usual increase in diastolic depolarization produced by epinephrine. This would suggest that this is a mechanism by which β receptor blocking agents may suppress or prevent ventricular arrhythmias induced by catecholamines. In addition, the direct effects of propranolol on membrane responsiveness and conduction, plus its direct depressant effects on spontaneous automaticity, may provide mechanisms by which propranolol counteracts ventricular arrhythmias that are not due to β-receptor-mediated events. Depending on the clinical circumstances in which the drug is used, either of the two actions of propranolol (β-adrenergic receptor blockade or direct membrane effects) can be important with respect to the mechanisms by which propranolol produces its antiarrhythmic action.

There is no doubt that many clinically encountered arrhythmias are influenced by endogenously released catecholamines, and all β receptor blocking agents would be effective in removing this component of the arrhythmia-generating mechanism. It is also a well-established fact that propranolol and other β receptor blocking agents are most effective as antiarrhythmic drugs when used for the management of supraventricular arrhythmias. For example, chronic atrial fibrillation and flutter are not usually converted to sinus rhythm, although the ventricular rate may be controlled. The mechanism is undoubtedly due to β receptor blockade, especially in the region of the atrioventricular node; this result can be achieved with all β receptor blocking agents at plasma concentrations that do not exert direct effects on the cardiac cells that usually are associated with class I antiarrhythmic drugs. On the other hand, propranolol is only partially effective in suppressing ventricular arrhythmias not caused by digitalis or exercise (15). Similarly, although propranolol may convert paroxysmal ventricular tachycardia to sinus rhythm, or prevent exercise-induced attacks, the rate of ventricular tachycardia is not slowed by propranolol given in β receptor blocking doses (16,17). Once again, one could attribute the effectiveness of propranolol in paroxysmal supraventricular tachycardia to its β blocking effects within the atrioventricular node; β receptor blockade would decrease the conduction velocity and increase the refractory period within the atrioventricular node and interrupt or make it less possible for a reciprocating mechanism to be established. This would be less likely to occur in ventricular tachycardia in the absence of plasma concentrations of propranolol that would be required to achieve direct membrane effects.

In summary, the class II antiarrhythmic drugs, primarily the β receptor blocking agents, are characterized by the fact that they inhibit catecholamine-induced stimulation of cardiac β-adrenergic receptors. In addition, some members of the group, propranolol in particular, produce electrophysiologic alterations in Purkinje fibers that resemble those observed with class I antiarrhythmic drugs. These latter effects have been referred to as direct membrane effects. Because the direct membrane effects occur at plasma concentrations above those needed to achieve β receptor blockade, they are considered to be of little significance in the antiarrhythmic effects of propranolol and related drugs; this conclusion is contrary to what one would reach on the basis of experimental and animal studies. The most likely reason for the controversy is that clinical studies have not resorted to dosages of propranolol that would result in direct membrane effects and that the greatest effectiveness of β blocking agents has been in the management of supraventricular tachyarrhythmias in which interference with sympathetic innervation to the region of the atrioventricular node would be expected to produce a beneficial effect. It was found that β receptor blockade alone was not as effective in reverting ventricular arrhythmias, premature ventricular beats, and ventricular tachycardia in which

digitalis or catecholamines were not involved. There is a need for further exploration of this subject, both in experimental animals and in humans with cardiac rhythm disorders other than supraventricular arrhythmias.

Actions of Class III Drugs

The members of class III include bretylium, amiodarone, and sotalol. The feature common to all three is that they prolong the duration of the action potential and the effective refractory period. The data are most complete for bretylium which has been examined in experimental animals as well as in humans.

When examined in canine Purkinje fibers, bretylium was found to possess electrophysiologic properties that differed markedly from those of other antiarrhythmic agents (18,19). Except at high concentrations, bretylium usually does not affect the resting potential, the rate of rise of phase 0 and the amplitude, membrane responsiveness, or conduction velocity. When examined in partially depolarized fibers, bretylium was reported to produce a transient hyperpolarization that was due to catecholamine release, because the response was not observed in Purkinje fiber preparations obtained from reserpine-pretreated dogs. Thus, bretylium does not resemble the members of class I or II in its electrophysiologic effects. Bretylium's primary electrophysiologic action is to prolong ventricular muscle and Purkinje fiber action potentials, thereby increasing the ventricular effective refractory period.

Amiodarone, a member of the class III antiarrhythmic agents, differs from bretylium in that it does not alter neuronal function by either releasing or blocking the release of the adrenergic neurotransmitter. It does resemble bretylium, however, in that it produces a significant prolongation of the intracellular cardiac action potential. This effect was observed in studies in which the drug was given both acutely (20) and chronically to animals prior to removal of the hearts for the purpose of conducting intracellular recordings (21).

In summary, the class III antiarrhythmic

drugs possess complex and unrelated pharmacologic properties, but they seem to share one common property, that of prolonging the duration of the membrane action potential without altering the phase of depolarization or the resting membrane potential. The prolongation of recovery, as well as that of the effective refractory period, is uniform in that it occurs both in ventricular muscle and in Purkinje fibers. It is most likely that the antiarrhythmic actions of class III compounds can be attributed to this singular electrophysiologic effect rather than to the secondary effects that involve alterations in responses of the heart to sympathetic innervation. The importance of the class III drugs is that bretylium, a quaternary ammonium drug, has been shown clinically to be effective in cases of intractable ventricular tachycardia and ventricular fibrillation. This observation alone deserves to be pursued further in the hope that it can lead to the development of an effective and safe antifibrillatory agent. The existence of such a drug would be of extreme value in patients who are at risk of sudden cardiac death and in whom the most common mechanism of death is ventricular fibrillation.

Actions of Class IV Drugs

The prototype drug of the class IV antiarrhythmic agents is verapamil. The members of this group are characterized by their ability to block the slow inward current in cardiac tissue, a current that is dependent on the inward movement of the calcium ion during phases 0–2 of the membrane action potential.

The most pronounced electrophysiologic effects of verapamil are exerted on cardiac fibers with slow-response action potentials. These slow-response fibers are found in the sinus node and atrioventricular node. Administration of verapamil slows conduction velocity and increases refractoriness in the atrioventricular node, thereby reducing the ability of the atrioventricular node to conduct supraventricular impulses to the ventricle. This action will terminate supraventricular tachycardias that utilize the atrioventricular node as a point of reentry and will reduce atrioventricular conduction of supraventricular impulses during atrial flutter or atrial fibrillation. Verapamil and other calcium antagonists do not exert marked electrophysiologic actions that depress conduction in fibers other than slow-response fibers of the sinus and atrioventricular node.

An attempt has been made to review the electropharmacology of the four classes of antiarrhythmic drugs and to relate these events to mechanisms suspected of being involved in the genesis of cardiac rhythm disorders. Although it is possible to classify the known antiarrhythmic agents according to their predominant electrophysiologic or pharmacologic action, there are many instances in which an agent can possess a multiple number of effects, each of which may exert a beneficial effect in controlling cardiac arrhythmias. Thus, whereas the grouping of antiarrhythmic drugs into four classes may be convenient, it may fall short of explaining the underlying mechanisms by which drugs exert their antiarrhythmic effects.

Assuming that we know the mechanisms for the development of cardiac arrhythmias, then it becomes possible to examine the electrophysiologic effects of drugs on cardiac cells and attempt to provide an electrophysiologic explanation for antiarrhythmic efficacy. Another difficulty occurs when one recognizes that most of our knowledge concerning the electrophysiologic effects of drugs on cardiac cells has been obtained from essentially "normal" heart muscle preparations. Thus, the challenge remains for the pharmacologist to reexamine the accepted concepts, but to do so in models that represent the pathophysiologic state as it would occur under clinical conditions. Much of the controversy surrounding the electrophysiologic mechanisms of antiarrhythmic drug actions may then be resolved. More important, such an approach may lead to the development of antiarrhythmic drugs that are specifically effective in clearly defined arrhythmias. Antiarrhythmic drug therapy may then be based on a scientific basis rather than on the empirical methods of today.

PHARMACOLOGIC BASIS FOR MANAGEMENT OF SUPRAVENTRICULAR TACHYARRHYTHMIAS

Most examples of paroxysmal supraventricular tachycardia (PSVT) have been presumed for many years to be the result of circus movement reentry or reciprocation within a portion of the atrioventricular conduction system. However, reentry has been observed in experimental animal studies to occur within the sinoatrial node (22), the atrium (23), the atrioventricular (A-V) node (24), and the His-Purkinje system (25). Of primary importance is the fact that similar sites for reentry or reciprocation have been suggested as occurring in humans (26–28). The potential reciprocating circuit is activated when it is penetrated by an extrasystole that can be supraventricular or ventricular in origin. A requisite for a re-

ciprocating tachycardia is the combination of two pathways with unequal conduction velocities and unidirectional block in one of the pathways, thus permitting the initiating impulse to set up a circus movement (Fig. 7). The presence of unidirectional block in one pathway and slow conduction in the second pathway provides sufficient time for the first pathway to recover from its refractory state and allow reentry of the impulse to the site of original block and return of the impulse, which may now reenter the second pathway in the form of an echo or circus movement tachycardia (Fig. 7). Variations in the velocity of conduction and the duration of refractoriness within the atria, sinus node, A-V node, or His-Purkinje system are frequent and can result in formation of multiple functional pathways. Because of the influences of the parasympathetic and sympathetic nervous systems, this functional dissociation of conduction and formation of dual pathways occurs most commonly in the A-V node.

In addition to the foregoing mechanisms of reentry as means of initiating and sustaining

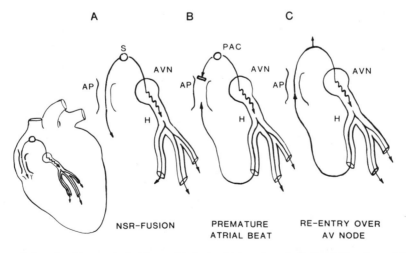

FIG. 7. A: Normal sinus beat is conducted from atria to ventricles along both the A-V node and the accessory pathway. Preexcitation occurs as the ventricles are excited prematurely through the accessory pathway and after a delay through the A-V node. **B:** Premature atrial contraction occurs before the accessory pathway has regained its excitability. However, the A-V node, with a shorter refractory period than the accessory pathway, is able to conduct the impulse to the ventricles. As the ventricles fire, the accessory pathway, having regained its excitability, is excited and conducts the ventricular impulse retrogradely to excite the atria. A circus movement pathway is set up with orthograde conduction through the A-V node and retrograde conduction through the accessory pathway. AP: accessory pathway. AVN: A-V node. H: His bundles. PAC: premature atrial contraction.

supraventricular tachyarrhythmias, there is evidence obtained from myocardial cells from diseased atria from patients who had arrhythmias showing the presence of automatic impulse activity (29). Automaticity has also been recorded from cells within the mitral valve, the His bundle, and Purkinje fibers (30,31).

Atrial tachyarrhythmias due to enhanced automaticity usually display some degree of A-V nodal block, an observation that is incompatible with a continuous reentrant process in the A-V node. In atrial tachycardias the A-V node is not involved, except to receive rapid stimuli, which, if they exceed the maximal rate of A-V transmission, are partially blocked.

In the case of atrial flutter and atrial fibrillation there is still an unresolved question whether these arrhythmias are due to enhanced ectopic foci or reentry or both. Although the rate in atrial flutter is between 300 and 360 beats per minute, only a portion of the impulses gain access to the ventricular conducting system, because of the inability of the A-V node to conduct at this rapid frequency. Thus, usually a 2:1 block with a regular ventricular rate occurs, because the conducting capacity of the A-V node has been exceeded.

In atrial fibrillation, the ventricular rate becomes irregular because of variable degrees of impulse penetration that concealed conduction in the A-V node.

It should be apparent that in both atrial flutter and atrial fibrillation the ventricular rate is determined by the number of atrial impulses that are capable of traversing the A-V node and entering the His-Purkinje system. Thus, any intervention, whether it be mediated by the autonomic nervous system or by means of a pharmacologic agent acting on the A-V node, will modify the ventricular response, depending on how A-V nodal transmission is affected. The clinical objective in atrial flutter or atrial fibrillation is to adequately control the ventricular rate so that the hemodynamic status of the patient may become stabilized. Aside from converting the

disorder of atrial rhythm and restoring normal sinus rhythm by means of synchronized DC countershock, the therapeutic approach is via the A-V node, which constitutes the weakest link in the conduction path between atria and ventricles. Thus, physiologic or pharmacologic maneuvers that result in a decrease in conduction through the A-V node result in a slowing of the ventricular rate regardless of the effects they have on the frequency of atrial activity.

An entirely different situation, and one that may require a different approach to its management, involves those supraventricular arrhythmias that occur in association with the Wolff-Parkinson-White (WPW) syndrome. Although various hypotheses have been proposed to explain the genesis of WPW beats (23,33), it is generally regarded as being due to the fact that the sinus or atrial impulse is conducted down both the normal and anomalous or accessory pathways to the ventricles (34). Because of the electrophysiologic characteristics of the anomalous pathway, the impulse is transmitted at a faster rate in the accessory path than it is in the normal atrioventricular pathway. The rapid conduction velocity over the anomalous pathway permits the atrial impulse to invade a portion of the ventricular myocardium, resulting in preexcitation of the region (preexcitation syndrome). The delta wave is due to the depolarization of the ventricle around the insertion of the anomalous pathway, from which site further impulse transmission occurs slowly through the ventricular myocardium. The simultaneous slower impulse conduction through the atrioventricular node, on exit from this region, is transmitted rapidly through the remainder of the ventricles via the His-Purkinje system. It is commonly accepted that the paroxysmal atrial tachycardias in patients with WPW are due to a reciprocal mechanism (35–37). The tachyarrhythmia may be initiated by a properly timed premature atrial excitation due to an ectopic atrial beat or a premature ventricular beat that conducts to the atrium in a retrograde manner.

Most frequently, the supraventricular impulse travels in the antegrade direction and utilizes the A-V node and His bundle to reach the ventricular myocardium and returns to the atrium in a retrograde fashion via the anomalous pathway. The ability of the premature atrial impulse to move in the antegrade direction by way of the A-V node is due to the fact that the anomalous pathway possesses a longer refractory period, as opposed to the A-V node. Thus, the two pathways differ with regard to the relative durations of their refractory periods, so that the anomalous pathway is more likely, because of its longer refractory period, to display unidirectional block in response to a premature atrial impulse. On the other hand, the slow conduction through the normal A-V node provides sufficient time for the anomalous pathway to recover from its refractory state, so that antegrade A-V node/His-Purkinje excitation of the ventricular myocardium continues to be propagated in a retrograde manner across the accessory pathway to the atria, thereby setting the stage for a reciprocating tachyarrhythmia in which the wave of excitation enters the ventricles via the A-V node/His-Purkinje system and returns to the atria via the anomalous pathway. The initiating premature impulse can just as easily originate in the ventricles, with retrograde propagation across the anomalous pathway to the atria, whereupon it reenters the A-V nodal system and propagates to the ventricles. In both instances, a premature beat, either atrial or ventricular, initiates the sequence in which retrograde conduction occurs through the anomalous pathway. Thus, a feature common to all cases of WPW associated tachyarrhythmias is the existence of an accessory or anomalous pathway that differs electrophysiologically from the A-V node/His-bundle system.

Therapy for supraventricular tachyarrhythmias depends on the use of physiologic maneuvers or pharmacologic interventions that prevent or alter the electrical events that predispose to initiation of the rhythm disorder (premature atrial or ventricular beats) or that

maintain the reciprocating circuit once a reentry rhythm has occurred. Therefore, the therapeutic objective is to control the abnormal process by diminishing enhanced automaticity or to interrupt a reentry mechanism.

The mechanism by which drugs would be expected to provide beneficial effects would depend on their ability to (a) reduce spontaneous phase-4 diastolic depolarization, which would suppress the development of some atrial and/or ventricular premature beats, (b) depress the rapid upstroke of phase-0 fast sodium current, which would lead to a decrease in conduction velocity of the affected myocardial cells, (c) prolong the refractory period of cardiac cells and make them less likely to serve as a pathway for conduction, and (d) affect the slow calcium current in the A-V node or abnormal cells that have low resting membrane potentials and a slow rate of depolarization.

Paroxysmal Atrial Tachycardia Due to A-V Nodal Reentry

Drugs can act on the A-V nodal or His-Purkinje system by either enhancing or delaying conduction, as reflected by the A-H and H-V intervals. Table 2 lists the effects on the A-V nodal conduction system of several of the more frequently encountered pharmacologic agents, some of which are useful in terminating episodes of A-V nodal reentrant paroxysmal supraventricular tachyarrhythmias.

Digitalis Glycosides

Digitalis glycosides usually prolong the effective refractory period of the fast or slow pathway or both. These effects of the cardiac glycosides result in greater difficulty with induction of tachycardia as well as inability to sustain a reciprocating A-V nodal reentrant mechanism. The most vulnerable point in the system is usually in the antegrade conduction in the slow pathway, and this explains why the tachycardia can be terminated by the digitalis glycosides. Although digitalis slows con-

Table 2. *Effects of drugs on the A-V nodal conduction system*

Drug	A-V conduction system		
	Conduction velocity		Effective refractory period
	A-H	H-V	
Digoxin	D[a]	NC	I
Propranolol	D	NC	I
Procainamide	I[b]	D	D-I[c]
Quinidine	I[b]	D	D-I[c]
Disopyramide	NC	NC	NC
Verapamil	D	NC	I
Ajmaline	NC	D	NC
Amiodarone	D	NC	I
Atropine	I	NC	D

Abbreviations: I = increase; D = decrease; NC = no change.

[a] Due to direct effects of digoxin plus its indirect effect mediated by vagal stimulation.

[b] Due to the vagolytic effects (blocks acetylcholine) that would enhance A-H conduction velocity.

[c] Effective refractory period is decreased initially due to vagolytic action, and it increases later because of direct effect as drug dosage is increased.

duction velocity and lengthens the effective refractory periods of the fast and slow pathways within the A-V node, the important effect is the relative change in these two pathways, which determines whether or not paroxysmal supraventricular tachycardia can occur in a given individual. Thus, a slowing of conduction velocity alone will lengthen the cycle length of the paroxysmal supraventricular tachyarrhythmia, but will not abolish it unless there is a simultaneous increase in the refractory period. The antegrade or slow pathway is highly susceptible to the influence of vagal tone. Thus, interactions such as carotid sinus massage, a Valsalva maneuver, or administration of pharmacologic agents that can enhance vagal actions (digitalis, edrophonium, neostigmine, pressor agents such as phenylephrine) usually can result in abrupt termination of the supraventricular tachyarrhythmia that often ends with a P wave that blocks antegradely because of decreased conduction velocity and an increased refractory period in the slow A-V nodal pathway. Digitalis, by

virtue of its ability to enhance vagal tone, as well as its direct effects on the A-V nodal pathways, is often the agent of choice for prophylaxis against paroxysmal supraventricular tachycardia, although quinidine, procainamide, or propranolol may also be of value prophylactically, because they can suppress premature atrial and/or ventricular beats that often are the precipitating factors in the development of A-V nodal reentrance and supraventricular tachycardia.

β Receptor Blocking Agents

β-Adrenergic receptor blocking agents such as propranolol and alprenolol can be used to interrupt paroxysmal A-V nodal reentrant supraventricular tachyarrhythmias because of their potential to alter the electrophysiologic properties in the A-V node/His-Purkinje pathways. Propranolol delays conduction within the A-V node by increasing the A-H interval, whereas conduction in the H-V region is unaltered. In addition, propranolol increases both the functional and effective refractory periods of the A-V node. Propranolol has no direct effect on either the relative or effective refractory period of the His-Purkinje system.

Therapy with a β-adrenergic receptor blocking agent appears to be of particular value in those instances where paroxysmal atrial tachycardia is precipitated by exercise or emotion. Exercise-induced paroxysmal supraventricular tachycardia frequently is not associated with other evidence of organic heart disease, and it is presumably brought about by the increased sympathetic drive of exercise (38). It usually responds poorly to digitalis or quinidine. The beneficial effects of the β receptor blocking agents in the management of paroxysmal supraventricular tachyarrhythmias are clearly related to inhibition of adrenergic influences on the A-V node. Thus, it is safe to assume that all agents belonging to this class of drugs should result in similar actions in the acute and prophylactic management of patients with paroxysmal supraventricular tachycardia.

Verapamil

Verapamil has been noted to be a most effective treatment for A-V nodal reciprocating tachycardias (39), perhaps because its ability to interfere with the slow calcium current influences the susceptible N region of the atrioventricular node. The electrophysiologic actions of verapamil are markedly different from those of the more commonly used antiarrhythmic agents and can be attributed to the ability of verapamil to slow calcium conductance in the myocardial cell during membrane depolarization without altering the sodium influx. The specific effect on calcium conductance accounts for its negative inotropic effect and is the most likely mechanism by which it exerts its antiarrhythmic actions (40–42). Electrocardiographic studies of the His bundle have shown that verapamil delays A-V conduction proximal to the His bundle without having an effect on intraatrial or intraventricular conduction (43–45), with the effect being independent of autonomic influences (44,45). Verapamil prolongs both antegrade and retrograde conduction within the A-V node (45), an important observation in view of the fact that many cases of paroxysmal supraventricular tachyarrhythmias are known to depend on A-V nodal reentry (46,47).

Amiodarone

Amiodarone has been used extensively in Europe for the control of A-V nodal reciprocating and ectopic atrial arrhythmias. The agent produces an increase in the refractory period and slows conduction in the A-V node, as evidenced by an increase in the A-H interval (48,49). In addition, amiodarone prolongs the refractory period of the atrium as well as that of the ventricles. Supraventricular arrhythmias showed the greatest response to amiodarone, with recurrent paroxysmal atrial flutter and fibrillation being suppressed in 29 of 30

patients (96.6%) and in 57 of 59 patients (96.6%) with paroxysmal supraventricular tachycardia.

Quinidine, Procainamide, and Disopyramide ✗

Supraventricular tachycardias that are caused by a reentrant or reciprocal mechanism within the A-V node may be initiated by atrial extrasystoles, and the tachyarrhythmia frequently can be terminated by vagal maneuvers. Enhancement of vagal tone increases the effective refractory period of the A-V node and delays conduction in the A-H region.

Quinidine, procainamide, and disopyramide are each capable of antagonizing the cholinergic effects of acetylcholine on the A-V node. As indicated in Table 2, procainamide and quinidine produce variable effects on the effective refractory period of the A-V node because of the opposing actions of these agents, in which their anticholinergic effects (atropinelike, Table 2) counteract the direct effects of the drug on the A-V node. Thus, it is only at the higher dose levels that these agents can be expected to prolong the effective refractory period of the A-V node. In a similar manner, atrioventricular conduction velocity is influenced in a variable manner, once again because of opposing effects of cholinergic blockade and direct depressant actions of the pharmacologic agents.

Disopyramide likewise possesses marked anticholinergic actions, but it has less of a direct depressant effect on A-V conduction velocity and effective refractory period (50). The net result of these opposing effects is that the drug produces no significant alteration in the electrophysiologic properties of the A-V conduction system.

Because quinidine, procainamide, and disopyramide have minimal effects on the A-V node, they would not be expected to be as effective as some of the other agents listed in Table 2 with respect to being able to terminate a supraventricular tachyarrhythmia caused by an A-V reciprocating mechanism.

As previously discussed, A-V reciprocating

tachyarrhythmias are frequently precipitated by atrial extrasystoles. Because procainamide, quinidine, and disopyramide can suppress atrial extrasystoles, these agents are of value in the prevention of paroxysms of supraventricular tachycardias.

Each of the three agents will prolong the effective refractory period of atrial muscle. Thus, in those instances where the tachycardia is caused by a reentry mechanism within the atria, procainamide, quinidine, and disopyramide should be effective in terminating the arrhythmia.

We can summarize the foregoing discussion on the pharmacologic basis for treatment of supraventricular tachyarrhythmias by stating that to be effective in the prophylaxis of such rhythm disorders, a drug must (a) prevent the electrical events that predispose to A-V conduction delay required to initiate the reciprocating tachyarrhythmia (atrial premature depolarization) and (b) alter A-V conduction so that reentry is no longer a physiologic possibility.

Supraventricular Tachyarrhythmias Associated with WPW Syndrome

The foregoing discussion on reentrant mechanisms in the WPW syndrome with recurrent tachyarrhythmias provides some basis for a rational approach to therapy in the rhythm disorders. It is important to recognize that there exists in WPW an extranodal accessory A-V pathway with electrophysiologic properties that differ from those of the normal A-V node. Drugs acting on the two pathways may lead to electrophysiologic alterations that may favor or depress impulse transmission, so that the two pathways may become dissimilar, and conduction will be favored by one pathway over the other. An important point to recall is that the A-V nodal fibers have the characteristics of a slow conduction velocity and a short refractory period, both of which are influenced by vagal innervation. Enhanced vagal tone produces a slowing of A-V conduction and a prolongation of the refractory period. Cholinergic blockade produces the opposite effects. The extranodal accessory A-V pathway (bundle of Kent), on the other hand, possesses the properties of fast conduction velocity and a long refractory period. The bypass tract behaves like atrial muscle in response to vagal stimulation in that conduction velocity is enhanced and the refractory period if shortened. Cholinergic blockade would have the opposite effect. Therefore, an intervention that resulted in an increase in vagal tone would interfere with conduction over the normal atrioventricular pathway and enhance impulse transmission over the extranodal accessory A-V pathway. The approach to pharmacologic management of supraventricular tachyarrhythmias associated with the WPW syndrome must consider the direct and indirect effects that any intervention will have on each of the A-V pathways. Table 3 summarizes the electrophysiologic alterations in the A-V node and accessory pathways for several of the more commonly used antiarrhythmic agents.

The paroxysmal tachycardias in WPW are of two basic types. Reciprocating tachycardia is the commonest and constitutes 70 to 80% of all arrhythmias. Atrial flutter/fibrillation

Table 3. *Effects of antiarrhythmic drugs on effective refractory periods of A-V node and accessory pathway in WPW syndrome*

Drug	Effective refractory period	
	A-V node	Accessory pathway
Digoxin	I[a]	D
Propranolol	I	NC
Procainamide	D-I[b]	I
Quinidine	D-I[b]	I
Disopyramide	NC	I
Verapamil	I	NC
Ajmaline	NC	I
Amiodarone	I	I
Atropine	D	I

Abbreviations: I = increase; D = decrease; NC = no change.
[a] Due to direct effects of digoxin plus its indirect effect mediated by vagal stimulation.
[b] Due to vagolytic effect initially, which is then followed by direct effects.

is the second type of arrhythmia specifically associated with the syndrome, and it carries a certain risk for the patient, because it can terminate in ventricular fibrillation. The pharmacologic management of these two types of WPW-associated rhythm disorders requires special attention.

It should be recalled that in the reciprocating tachyarrhythmia of WPW, the refractory periods of the pathways are such that A-V conduction is via the A-V node and His-Purkinje system, whereas the ventriculoatrial impulse is conducted over the accessory pathway back to the atria only to reenter the A-V node. Rarely does the reentry loop operate in the opposite direction. In the latter instance, the QRS complexes are broad, as ventricular preexcitation occurs due to A-V conduction over the accessory pathway. Such QRS complexes may simulate ventricular tachycardia.

The pharmacologic management of paroxysmal supraventricular tachycardia associated with the WPW syndrome is selected to alter one or more links in the reciprocating network. Prophylaxis can be achieved by preventing the atrial and/or ventricular extrasystoles that so frequently precipitate the tachyarrhythmias. Further protection against the paroxysms can be attained by narrowing the interval during which premature beats can dissociate the normal and accessory pathways. Lastly, pharmacologic agents may prolong refractoriness, so that the returning impulse is blocked either in the accessory pathway or in the A-V node. The special electrophysiologic properties of several drugs known to be effective in preventing or terminating WPW-associated tachycardias are discussed in the following section.

The electrophysiologic effects of the cardiac glycosides in the presence of WPW syndrome deserve special consideration because of the drug's potential detrimental effects in the patient with coexisting atrial flutter or atrial fibrillation.

The cardiac glycosides exert their electrophysiologic effects by both direct and indirect mechanisms; the latter occur as a result of

enhancement of vagal tone. Therefore, as shown in Table 3, the cardiac glycosides shorten the refractory period of the accessory pathway—an action that results from an increase in vagal tone that causes atrial muscle (accessory pathway) to repolarize at a fast rate. In addition, conduction velocity in atrial tissue is enhanced. At the same time, digitalis, by enhancing vagal tone, prolongs the refractory period of the A-V node and also delays A-V conduction. The net result of these electrophysiologic changes in the accessory pathway and the A-V node is that antegrade impulse transmission is impeded over the A-V node and facilitated via the accessory pathway.

It is apparent from the foregoing discussion that the digitalis glycosides, by impairing antegrade conduction through the A-V node, will limit the accessibility of an atrial premature impulse to this conduction pathway and therefore prevent the initiation of a reciprocating rhythm. Thus, the primary mechanism by which digitalis exerts a prophylactic action in the patient with reciprocating supraventricular tachyarrhythmias associated with the WPW syndrome is by decreasing the differences in the refractory periods of the two pathways and therefore abolishing the window produced by the discrepant refractory periods in the individual A-V pathways.

It has long been appreciated that patients with the preexcitation syndrome are susceptible to two types of tachyarrhythmias. The first, reciprocating tachycardia, which was mentioned earlier, can be prevented by digitalization, as well as by other agents to be discussed. The second dysrhythmia in WPW is atrial flutter or fibrillation with a rapid ventricular response due to antegrade conduction over the accessory pathway. It is important to recall that the accessory pathway (basically, atrial tissue) possesses a long refractory period and a rapid conduction velocity, as compared with the A-V nodal fibers, which have a slow conduction velocity and short refractory period. In the absence of an A-V bypass tract, the A-V node guards the ventricles against rapid atrial rates by failing to conduct in a 1:1 fashion above a critical rate. Thus, it is not unusual to find a patient with atrial flutter (atrial rate of 300 per minute) with a ventricular rate of 150 as a result of a 2:1 block at the A-V node. In the presence of the preexcitation syndrome, however, the protective effect of the A-V node on the ventricle is bypassed, because the accessory pathway is capable of conducting in a 1:1 manner, so that excessively high ventricular rates can be achieved if atrial flutter or fibrillation develops in the presence of the WPW syndrome. In such an instance, administration of a digitalis glycoside can be hazardous. As digitalis decreases the refractory period of the accessory pathway and enhances conduction velocity in this tissue, more impulses gain access to the ventricle, and a life-threatening ventricular response and ventricular fibrillation may result (51,52). Thus, in patients who have the WPW syndrome and a relatively short refractory period in the accessory pathway, an additional shortening of the refractory pathway can be fatal. Because of the evidence that digitalis can increase the ventricular response during atrial fibrillation in some patients, the use of cardiac glycosides in the preexcitation syndromes should be reserved for those patients in whom elective induction of atrial fibrillation has demonstrated that the patient is not at risk for developing ventricular fibrillation (52). Other pharmacologic agents will be more suitable choices if digitalis is contraindicated because of the reasons discussed earlier. Selection of the appropriate drug will depend on an understanding of its electrophysiologic effects on each of the A-V pathways.

In a patient with the preexcitation syndrome and a rapid ventricular response in the presence of atrial fibrillation, pharmacologic intervention should be directed at depressing conduction and increasing the refractoriness of the accessory pathway. Propranolol decreases conduction via the A-V node and will favor conduction over the accessory pathway (53).

It should be noted that both digitalis and propranolol, by slowing A-V nodal conduction, will allow a greater time for recovery of the accessory pathway and may actually promote a reentry phenomenon (54,55).

On the other hand, a number of agents are known to prolong refractoriness and conduction in the bypass tract. Lidocaine was demonstrated to exert beneficial effects in the clinical setting of WPW and atrial fibrillation, in which the drug immediately abolished antegrade conduction down the bypass tract, thus slowing the ventricular response (56). Because of the ability to administer the drug rapidly by the intravenous route, lidocaine offers a means of controlling these life-threatening arrhythmias. Needless to say, the effect is short-lived and requires continuous intravenous administration. However, it affords an opportunity to stabilize the patient until more permanent measures can be instituted.

The effects of propranolol, as would be expected, contrast with those of lidocaine and resemble the actions of digitalis on A-V nodal impulse transmission. Propranolol does not exert any significant effect on the anomalous pathway. Because of its ability to produce β-adrenergic receptor blockade and remove sympathetic influences on the A-V node, propranolol depresses A-V nodal transmission. The electrophysiologic changes due to propranolol include prolongation of the A-V nodal refractory period and a decrease in conduction velocity. Preexcitation will tend to be accentuated as a result of the electrophysiologic changes in the A-V node (59).

In a patient with a very short refractory period of the accessory bundle, it is possible to initiate episodes of supraventricular tachycardia by an appropriately timed ventricular premature beat. The premature impulse propagates to the atrium over the accessory pathway and returns to the ventricle over the normal A-V node and the His-Purkinje system, thus initiating an episode of supraventricular tachycardia. Propranolol plus procainamide or quinidine will be of value. Propranolol will prevent access of the returning impulse to the A-V node. Procainamide or quinidine will have an effect primarily on the anomalous pathway. Both drugs result in prolongation of the refractory period of the accessory pathway, and they slow both antegrade and retrograde conduction in the bypass tract (58,59). The effect of procainamide or quinidine on the sustaining mechanism of reciprocating tachycardia depends largely on the influence of the drugs on the length of the circulatory wave, that is, the mean conduction velocity times the refractory period. As shown by Sellers et al. (59), to be effective, the drug must increase the length of the refractory period of the different components of the reciprocating circuit more than it decreases the mean conduction velocity of the circulating wave. Thus, some patients may become more symptomatic on therapy, making it impossible to predict the effectiveness of a certain drug on the tachycardia in an individual patient. Another mechanism by which procainamide or quinidine may function is by its influence on the initiating event, premature atrial or ventricular depolarizations. Procainamide is particularly effective in suppressing ventricular premature beats, whereas quinidine is equally effective against both atrial and ventricular premature depolarizations. Procainamide is especially useful when atrial fibrillation supervenes in a patient with a short refractory period of the accessory pathway. Intravenous administration of procainamide results in immediate control of the ventricular rate, as it prolongs the effective refractory period and slows conduction via the anomalous pathway without depressing conduction over the A-V node.

An interesting feature of quinidine and procainamide is that both drugs have a vagolytic effect and thus inhibit the influences of cholinergic innervation to the accessory pathway (atrial muscle) and the A-V node. The influence of vagal stimulation on these structures was discussed previously. It only need be mentioned that inhibition of vagal tone will slow conduction velocity and prolong the refractory period of the accessory pathway and will enhance conduction velocity and decrease

the refractory period of the A-V node. The net result is that procainamide and quinidine favor utilization by the atrial impulse of the normal A-V pathway. This becomes an important consideration when using procainamide or quinidine in WPW with associated atrial flutter and a rapid ventricular response because of 1:1 conduction over the anomalous pathway. Whereas the drugs will suppress impulse transmission over the anomalous pathway, the vagolytic effects of the drugs may promote rapid atrial impulse transmission via the A-V nodal pathway, an event that could be controlled with the addition of propranolol to the therapeutic regimen.

Disopyramide is an antiarrhythmic agent that has been found effective in the management of extrasystoles and tachycardias of both supraventricular and ventricular origin. Disopyramide has minimal effects on the refractory period or conduction velocity of the A-V node. This lack of effect is due to the direct depressant effects of the drug on A-V nodal function being offset by the intense vagolytic actions of disopyramide (60). In patients with the WPW syndrome, disopyramide was shown to prolong the effective refractory period of the anomalous bypass and to prolong antegrade and retrograde conduction times of the accessory pathway. The electrophysiologic effects of disopyramide on the accessory pathway are a result of its direct actions as well as its indirect (vagolytic) actions on the tissue bridging the A-V junction. In many ways, disopyramide resembles quinidine with respect to its cardiac electrophysiologic properties, except that it has minimal effects on conduction in the His-Purkinje system. Because of its depressant effects on the anomalous pathway, disopyramide may have potential therapeutic value for management of the WPW syndrome with atrial flutter or fibrillation (50).

Verapamil is receiving increased attention as an antiarrhythmic agent, particularly in the management of supraventricular tachyarrhythmias. As discussed earlier, verapamil has the ability to inhibit the slow inward calcium current, and this results in a decrease in conduction velocity in the A-V node as well as an increase in the A-V nodal refractory period (61). Antegrade and retrograde conduction times in the anomalous bypass are unaffected in most patients (61). In view of the fact that antegrade conduction of atrial premature beats or of a reciprocating rhythm is by way of the A-V node, verapamil should be effective as a means of terminating tachyarrhythmias associated with the WPW syndrome (62) or in preventing initiation of the event by a premature atrial depolarization.

Whereas studies by Spurrell et al. (61) suggest that verapamil is an effective drug in the treatment of reciprocal tachycardias associated with the WPW syndrome, it may, in some patients, influence the anomalous pathway in an adverse manner and result in ventricular fibrillation.

Ajmaline, a reserpinelike drug, has been used extensively in Europe for management of a variety of cardiac arrhythmias. Ajmaline has been reported to prolong the refractory period and to depress conduction velocity in the accessory pathway and to have minimal effects on A-V nodal transmission, except for a slight prolongation of the H-V interval (63,64). The value of ajmaline in the management of supraventricular tachyarrhythmias is still uncertain, and further clinical studies are needed before its effectiveness relative to other existing agents can be adequately assessed.

A drug of promising potential is the agent amiodarone. Studies by Rosenbaum et al. (48) and Wellens et al. (65) have elucidated the electrophysiologic effects of amiodarone on the anomalous and normal pathways in patients with the preexcitation syndrome. Amiodarone lengthens the refractory period of the accessory pathway. But, as with other drugs, its effects on the accessory pathway are not the same when antegrade and retrograde conductions are compared. Whereas amiodarone uniformly prolongs refractoriness in the anomalous pathway in an A-V direction, prolongation in a V-A direction was observed in only half of the patients studied (65). In all patients in whom tachycardias could still be initiated after treatment with amiodarone, the heart rate during tachycardia was slower than before treatment, a result to be expected, because amiodarone decreases the conduction velocity of the circulatory wave. The electrophysiologic effects of amiodarone suggest that it would be of special value in patients with WPW syndrome and atrial fibrillation. In the latter clinical setting, parenteral administration of amiodarone has proved to be most beneficial in reverting what otherwise would be a life-threatening tachyarrhythmia (66).

From this discussion of the electrophysiologic effects of pharmacologic agents on the anomalous bypass and normal A-V pathways, it is apparent that the drugs used to manage patients with the WPW syndrome can be divided into those that predominantly affect impulse transmission in the A-V node and those that alter impulse transmission in the accessory bundle. Thus, quinidine, procainamide, disopyramide, ajmaline, and amiodarone have major effects in prolonging the refractory period of the anomalous pathway. In contrast, digitalis, β receptor blocking agents, and verapamil prolong refractoriness in the A-V node.

Aside from synchronized cardioversion in emergency situations, drug therapy for reciprocating tachyarrhythmias might best be accomplished with parenteral administration of procainamide or amiodarone, because both can act rapidly on the anomalous bypass and will be considered appropriate treatment for those patients with atrial flutter or fibrillation and rapid conduction over the bypass. Prevention of reciprocating tachyarrhythmias in the WPW syndrome may be accomplished by quinidine or disopyramide, which not only reduce the frequency of premature atrial and ventricular depolarizations but also depress conduction over the accessory pathway. However, because these drugs depress only one of the A-V pathways, it is possible that they could result in a paradoxical increase in the frequency of attacks of reciprocating tachycardia, because a premature beat may dissociate the two pathways. In such cases it might be helpful to combine a second drug, propranolol, along with quinidine to delay conduction in the A-V node.

It is obvious that patients with the WPW syndrome do not compose a homogeneous group. The tachyarrhythmias are the results of different mechanisms, with varied electrophysiologic properties of the two A-V pathways. Each patient with the WPW syndrome and reciprocating tachyarrhythmias should be evaluated with electrophysiologic studies to determine the mechanism of the tachyarrhythmia and the effectiveness of one or more therapeutic interventions.

GENERAL PHARMACOLOGY

Quinidine ✗

For centuries the quinidine alkaloids present in the bark of *Cinchona officinalis* have been used for treatment of malaria. As a result of the use of cinchona for treatment of malaria, it became apparent that cinchona was capable of converting atrial fibrillation to normal sinus rhythm. Clinical investigation showed that of the three major alkaloids present in the bark of the cinchona tree (quinine, quinidine, and cinchonine), quinidine was the most effective antiarrhythmic agent (67). The efficacy and long history of use of quinidine in the treatment of disorders of the cardiac rhythm led to the establishment of quinidine as the prototype antiarrhythmic agent. Despite the introduction of newer antiarrhythmic agents, quinidine still plays a major role in the treatment of chronic cardiac dysrhythmias.

The structure of quinidine (the dextro-rotary isomer of quinine) is shown in Fig. 8. Quinidine shares all the pharmacologic properties of quinine, including antimalarial, antipyretic, oxytocic, and skeletal muscle relaxant actions. However, these actions are also accompanied by all the toxic manifestations observed with the administration of quinine.

Electrophysiologic Actions

The effects of quinidine on atrial myocardium and specialized conduction tissue are a composite of the direct actions of the drug on cardiac tissue electrical properties and the indirect actions of the drug mediated by competitive blockade of muscarinic cholinergic receptors. The net effect of quinidine on the electrical properties of a particular cardiac tissue is dependent on the extent of parasympathetic nervous system innervation, the level of tone exerted by the parasympathetic nervous system, and the dose of quinidine administered. Because of the relatively greater potency of quinidine as a cholinergic muscarinic antagonist versus direct electrophysiologic actions, the anticholinergic actions of quinidine predominate at the lower plasma quinidine concentrations. The anticholinergic actions of quinidine are most apparent during initial oral therapy. Later, when steady-state therapeutic plasma concentrations are achieved, the direct electrophysiologic actions of quinidine tend to predominate. The direct and indirect electrophysiologic actions of quinidine are summarized in Table 4.

Sinoatrial node. Experimental studies have shown quinidine to increase the action-potential duration and to depress the slope of phase-4 depolarization of sinus node pacemaker cells (68). This direct depression of sinus node function is also observed in *in vitro* canine atrial preparations (69).

However, when autonomic innervation is intact in conscious animals and in humans, quinidine manifests either no effect or an increase in sinus heart rate (70,71). Direct depression of sinus node automaticity is counteracted by blockade of vagus-nerve-mediated

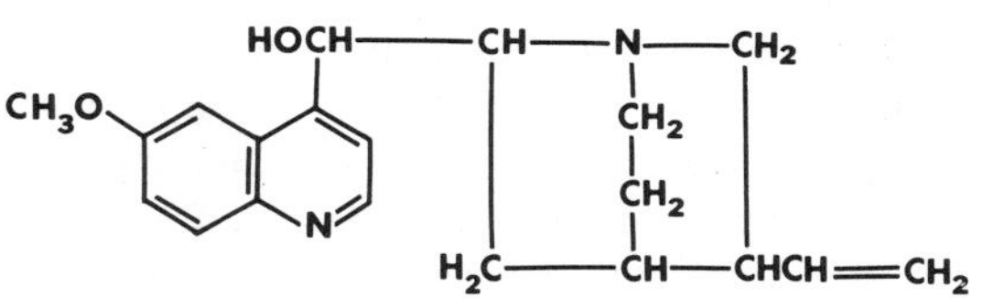

FIG. 8. Quinidine.

Table 4. *Electrophysiologic actions of quinidine, procainamide, and disopyramide at therapeutic plasma concentrations*

Tissue	Direct action	Indirect action	Net effect
Sinus node	Decrease	Increase	No change
Atria			
Automaticity	Decrease		Decrease
Conduction velocity	Decrease	Decrease	Decrease
Refractory periods	Increase	Increase	Increase
A-V node			
Automaticity	Decrease		Decrease
Conduction velocity	Decrease	Increase	No change
Refractory periods	Increase	Decrease	No change or slight increase
His-Purkinje/ventricular muscle			
Automaticity	Decrease		Decrease
Conduction velocity	Decrease		Decrease
Refractory periods	Increase		Increase

depression of sinus node function, sometimes actually resulting in an increased sinus rate. Other factors may also be involved. Deterioration of hemodynamic function as a result of quinidine administration may result in increased sympathetic nervous system tone. This stimulation of sympathetic tone may, in part, be responsible for an increase in sinus heart rate observed after quinidine administration in some patients.

In atrial muscle fibers, quinidine suppresses automaticity by depressing phase-4 depolarization. Atrial pacemakers are more sensitive to depression by quinidine than are ventricular pacemakers (72).

Quinidine administration results in a dose-dependent depression of membrane responsiveness in atrial muscle fibers (73). The maximum rate of phase-0 depolarization and the amplitude of the phase-0 potential are depressed equally at all membrane potentials. Quinidine also decreases atrial muscle excitability, so that a larger current stimulus is needed for initiation of an active response at the normal level of resting membrane potential (71). These actions of quinidine are often termed the "local anesthetic properties" of quinidine. Reduction of membrane responsiveness and reduction of the action-potential

amplitude, as well as the decrease in excitability, are believed to be direct results of a reduction in the rapid influx of sodium into the cell. These changes result in a reduction of conduction velocity in atrial myocardium.

The action-potential duration in atrial myocardium is prolonged only slightly by quinidine administration (73). This action of quinidine results in a small increase in the effective refractory period of atrial myocardium. However, because of the failure of early premature beats to conduct from the site of stimulation as a result of depression of conduction, the effective refractory period is prolonged to a much greater extent than the action-potential duration.

The anticholinergic properties of quinidine also alter the electrophysiologic properties of atrial muscle. Stimulation of the vagus nerve or administration of acetylcholine produces both a slight depolarization of atrial muscle fibers and a shortening of the action-potential duration. These changes in the cellular electrophysiology of atrial muscle fibers result in an increase in conduction velocity and a decrease in the effective refractory periods of atrial myocardium. These actions of acetylcholine are antagonized by administration of quinidine. Atrial muscle fibers are mildly depolarized, and the action-potential duration is prolonged, resulting in a decrease in conduction velocity and an increase in effective refractory periods.

Human electrophysiologic studies have confirmed the results of earlier *in vitro* and *in vivo* electrophysiologic studies. In human electrophysiologic studies, acute quinidine administration slows intraatrial conduction (74) and prolongs the effective refractory period of atrial myocardium (70). The refractory periods of A-V accessory (bypass) pathways are increased after quinidine administration, and conduction velocity is decreased (64). When atrial fibrillation or atrial flutter is induced in patients with A-V accessory pathways, the resultant ventricular rate is slowed by quinidine.

A-V node. Both the direct and indirect actions of quinidine are important in determining the ultimate effect of quinidine on A-V conduction. The indirect (anticholinergic) properties of quinidine prevent vagally mediated prolongation of A-V node refractory periods and depression of A-V node conduction velocity. A-V transmission is thereby facilitated. Quinidine's direct electrophysiologic actions on the A-V node result in a decrease in conduction velocity and an increase in the effective refractory period. These direct actions of quinidine result in depression of A-V conduction. In considering the action of quinidine on A-V transmission, one must be aware of both the direct and indirect actions of quinidine. The direct effects of quinidine are manifested at therapeutic plasma concentrations. It is because of its indirect actions on the A-V node that quinidine must never be the initial drug in the treatment of atrial flutter and possibly atrial fibrillation. In both instances the atria are being stimulated at a rapid rate. The primary objective is to control the ventricular rate, and the second is to restore normal sinus rhythm. Although quinidine is often successful in producing normal sinus rhythm, its administration in the presence of a rapid atrial rate will lead to a further, and dangerous, increase in the ventricular

rate. The effect is a result of the anticholinergic properties of quinidine that result in enhancement of A-V transmission. It is for this reason that digitalis is the drug to be administered before one elects to convert atrial flutter or atrial fibrillation to normal sinus rhythm with quinidine. The direct and indirect effects of digitalis on the A-V node protect against the anticholinergic effects of quinidine. In summary, quinidine has both direct and indirect effects on A-V transmission at therapeutic plasma concentrations. One must be aware of its early anticholinergic or indirect properties that may facilitate A-V transmission and present a hazard when it is given as the initial drug in the presence of atrial flutter.

Human electrophysiologic studies have confirmed earlier electrophysiologic studies in animals that showed dangerous increases in ventricular rate to occur when quinidine was administered in the presence of atrial flutter or atrial fibrillation. Acute quinidine administration has been shown to increase conduction velocity and to decrease the effective refractory period of the A-V node (64,70). The magnitude of the increase in A-V transmission can vary widely between patients, probably because of a wide degree of variation in vagal tone.

His-Purkinje system/ventricular muscle. An important therapeutic action of quinidine is to depress automaticity of ventricular pacemakers by depressing the slope of phase-4 depolarization (75). Depression of pacemakers in the His-Purkinje system is more pronounced than depression of sinus node pacemaker cells. Toxic doses of quinidine may increase the rate of discharge of ventricular pacemakers (76). This increase in ventricular automaticity as a result of quinidine toxicity is due to an increased slope of phase-4 depolarization. A drug-induced decrease in maximum diastolic potential is observed at this time.

Quinidine administration reduces the amplitude of the action potential and produces a parallel shift to the right of the membrane responsiveness curves for Purkinje fibers and ventricular muscle (76). Membrane responsiveness (the maximum rate of phase-0 depolarization) is reduced at all levels of membrane potential without altering the resting membrane potential or intracellular sodium and potassium ion concentrations. Myocardial excitability is also depressed. The depressions of phase-0 depolarization and the action-potential amplitude combined with a decrease in myocardial excitability produce a depression of conduction velocity in the His-Purkinje system and ventricular myocardium. In the surface electrocardiogram, this reduction in conduction velocity is reflected as an increase in the QRS interval.

Quinidine slightly prolongs repolarization in Purkinje fibers and ventricular muscle, resulting in a small increase in the action-potential duration. As in atrial muscle, quinidine administration results in prolongation of the effective refractory period by depression of conduction of premature beats away from the site of origin.

The indirect (anticholinergic) properties of quinidine are not a factor in the actions of quinidine on ventricular muscle and the His-Purkinje system. The effects of the parasympathetic nervous system on the electrical properties of ventricular muscle and His-Purkinje fibers are of minor consequence.

Serum potassium concentrations are a major determinant of the activity of quinidine on cardiac tissue. Low extracellular potassium ion concentrations antagonize the depressant effects of quinidine on membrane responsiveness. High extracellular potassium ion concentrations increase the ability of quinidine to depress membrane responsiveness. The actions of quinidine that are dependent on potassium ion concentration may explain why hypokalemic patients are often unresponsive to the antiarrhythmic effects of quinidine. Caution must be exercised, however, in that excessive extracellular potassium ion concentrations will enhance the depressant actions of quinidine on the A-V node as well as its depressant actions on pacemaker cells. Prolongation of the QRS interval and serious conduction disturbances are more likely to occur at higher plasma quinidine concentrations when hyperkalemia is present.

In human electrophysiologic studies, acute quinidine administration slows conduction in the His-Purkinje system and increases His-Purkinje refractory periods. Ventricular effective refractory periods are increased (64, 70,74).

Electrocardiographic Changes

At normal therapeutic plasma concentrations, quinidine prolongs the PR interval, QRS interval, and QT interval of the surface electrocardiogram. QRS and QT prolongations are more pronounced with quinidine than with other antiarrhythmic agents. The magnitudes of these changes are directly related to the plasma quinidine concentration and are given in Table 5. Toxic concentrations of quinidine produce further slowing of conduction. The QRS and QT intervals are dramatically increased, and secondary repolarization waves may appear.

Hemodynamic Effects

Quinidine is well known to possess a negative inotropic effect on atrial and ventricular myocardium. This effect has been observed in humans (77) and experimental animals (13). At plasma quinidine concentrations in the normal therapeutic range, myocardial depression is not a problem in patients with normal myocardial function. However, depression of myocardial contractility in patients with compromised myocardial function may produce a significant rise in left ventricular end-diastolic pressure, resulting in overt heart failure. In addition, quinidine depresses vascular smooth muscle and results in a decrease in peripheral vascular resistance. This peripheral vasodilation is in part due to blockade of α-adrenergic receptors, with a resultant decrease in adrenergic vasoconstrictor tone (78). The reduction in peripheral vascular resistance, combined with a reduction in cardiac output, can produce dramatic decreases in arterial pressure. The depressant effects of quinidine on the cardiovascular system are more likely

Table 5. *Electrocardiographic changes associated with antiarrhythmic agents*

	PR interval	QRS interval	QT interval corrected for heart rate
Quinidine	No change or increase	Increase	Increase
Procainamide	No change or increase	Increase	Increase
Disopyramide	No change or increase	Increase	Increase
Propranolol	No change or increase	No change	Decrease
Phenytoin	No change or decrease	No change	Decrease
Lidocaine	No change	No change	No change or decrease
Bretylium	No change or increase	No change	No change

to occur with intravenous administration. Intravenous quinidine administration should not be employed routinely for emergency treatment of arrhythmias, because of the potential for producing severe cardiovascular depression. Table 6 lists the important hemodynamic changes associated with quinidine administration.

Toxic Reactions

The cardiac toxicity of quinidine includes atrioventricular and intraventricular block, ventricular tachyarrhythmias, and depression of myocardial contractility. The precipitation of ventricular arrhythmias by toxic doses of quinidine may be related to a marked depression of intraventricular conduction or may be due to an increase in ventricular automaticity. In most patients, toxicity can be controlled by proper adjustment of the dosage or discontinuance of the drug, if necessary.

Quinidine-induced depression of myocardial conduction and contractility can be treated by a number of interventions. Catecholamine administration may improve depressed intraventricular conduction and restore arterial pressure. Cautious administration of molar sodium lactate or sodium bicarbonate may be beneficial (79). Reversal

Table 6. *Hemodynamic actions of antiarrhythmic agents*

	Mean arterial pressure	Peripheral resistance	Cardiac output	Left ventricular end-diastolic pressure
Quinidine	Decrease	Decrease	Decrease	Increase
Procainamide	Decrease	Decrease	Decrease	Increase
Disopyramide	No change	Increase	Decrease	Increase
Propranolol	Decrease	Increase	Decrease	Increase
Phenytoin	Decrease	No change or decrease	No change or decrease	No change or increase
Lidocaine	Decrease	No change	No change or decrease	No change or increase
Bretylium	Decrease	Decrease	No change or increase	No change or decrease

of quinidine cardiotoxicity and hypotension by sodium lactate has been noted even during advanced stages of cardiotoxicity. The empiric use of sodium lactate or sodium bicarbonate to treat quinidine toxicity has some theoretical support, because alkalosis induces potassium shifts from extracellular to intracellular sites and increases binding of quinidine to serum albumin, reducing free quinidine concentrations. On the other hand, alkalosis can result in decreased urinary excretion of the weak base quinidine.

Large doses of quinidine can produce a syndrome known as cinchonism, characterized by ringing in the ears, headache, nausea, visual disturbances or blurred vision, disturbed auditory acuity, and vertigo. Larger doses can produce confusion, delirium, hallucinations, or psychoses. At therapeutic doses, the most commonly observed side effects are related to the gastrointestinal tract: nausea, vomiting, and diarrhea.

In some patients, thrombocytopenia may occur as a result of quinidine administration. Quinidine-induced thrombocytopenia is due to the formation of a plasma protein/quinidine complex that evokes a circulating antibody. The antibody can react with platelets in the presence of quinidine. Platelet counts return to normal on cessation of quinidine therapy. However, administration of quinidine or quinine at a later date can cause reappearance of thrombocytopenia.

Quinidine syncope and/or sudden arrhythmic death, an uncommon but major complication of quinidine therapy, is due to transient or irreversible ventricular tachycardia or ventricular fibrillation. This action of quinidine is not necessarily due to quinidine overdosage; it can occur at therapeutic or subtherapeutic plasma concentrations. The mechanism for these arrhythmias is poorly understood, but they may be a result of slowed myocardial conduction.

Pharmacokinetics

Absorption. Quinidine is almost completely absorbed from the gastrointestinal tract after oral administration. Quinidine sulfate is well absorbed from solution, tablet, and capsule formulations. Peak plasma concentrations are achieved between 2 and 4 hr after oral administration. The bioavailability of oral quinidine gluconate is similarly higher (72–87%), the balance being explained by first-class hepatic metabolism. Intramuscular injection of quinidine gluconate is painful and may cause significant tissue necrosis, as well as incomplete and inconsistent absorption. Peak plasma levels observed after intramuscular injection are greater than those observed after oral administration and are obtained earlier after administration.

Metabolism and excretion. Quinidine is extensively metabolized in the body, primarily by the liver. Major metabolites include 3-hydroxyquinidine and quinidine-N-oxide. Minor metabolites include 2'-oxyquinidinone and O-desmethylquinidine. The 3-hydroxy metabolite of quinidine possesses antiarrhythmic activity that may contribute to the therapeutic action of quinidine with plasma concentrations roughly one-third those of unchanged quinidine. Urinary excretion of conjugated or free metabolites of quinidine accounts for 75 to 90% of administered quinidine. Renal excretion of unaltered quinidine accounts for the remainder. Changes in urinary pH may markedly alter renal clearance of quinidine, a weak base with a pK_a of 8.57. Excretion of the drug increases as the urine is acidified. Dihydroquinidine, a contaminant of quinidine tablet preparations, may be detected in human serum and is an active antiarrhythmic agent.

Kinetics. After intravenous injection, quinidine disposition may be adequately described by a two-compartment model (biphasic exponential excretion). Values for the volume of the central compartment (V_C) and steady-state volume of distribution (V_DSS) are given in Table 7. The initial rapid redistribution phase (alpha-phase) half-life is approximately 6 min. The second, slower elimination phase (beta-phase) half-life is approximately 5 to 8 hr. Renal disease may require a reduction in quinidine dosage or an increase in the dosage

Table 7. *Quinidine pharmacokinetics*

Percentage absorbed after oral administration	70–80%
Clearance	1.5–7.0 ml/min/kg
Volume of distribution	
V_C	0.91 liter/kg
V_DSS	3.03 liters/kg
Plasma $T_{1/2}$	4–8 hr
Percentage excreted unchanged in urine	10–20%
Percentage free (unbound) in plasma	10–20%
Therapeutic plasma concentrations	3–6 µg/ml

interval. Liver disease also requires reduction of quinidine dosage. Renal function decreases with age, and lower doses may be necessary in elderly patients. Simultaneous administration of anticonvulsant drugs can stimulate the metabolism of quinidine and may require an increase in quinidine dosage.

In excess of 80% of plasma quinidine is bound to plasma proteins. Albumin serves as the primary source of binding protein in plasma. Neither heart failure nor renal disease alters the extent of plasma protein binding, although liver disease or hypoalbuminemia decreases plasma protein binding. The nonionized quinidine molecule is preferentially bound to albumin. Quinidine enters red blood cells and is bound to hemoglobin. At equilibrium, red blood cell concentrations are similar to plasma concentrations. In individual patients, there are wide variations in the plasma concentrations of quinidine with a given dosage regimen of the drug, with toxic manifestations correlating with serum or plasma concentration of the drug rather than with the administered dose. It must be appreciated, however, that the serum level may not properly reflect the myocardial concentration of the drug, especially after rapid administration. After rapid administration, the serum-to-cardiac-tissue ratio may be temporarily higher than that present at steady state. Therapeutic plasma concentrations are also dependent on the analytic method used for quantitation. The earliest assays measured the quantity of quini-

dine plus metabolites in serum. The more recently developed assays are specific for quinidine and do not mistakenly measure metabolites as quinidine. Therapeutic plasma concentrations of quinidine as measured by most assay procedures currently in use range from 3 to 6 µg/ml. Toxic manifestations are commonly observed at plasma concentrations in excess of 8 µg/ml. Therapeutic plasma concentrations of quinidine as measured by recently developed specific assays are 2 to 4 µg/ml.

Oral Dosage for Arrhythmia Conversion

One commonly used mode of administration for conversion of atrial flutter or atrial fibrillation is to give an oral dose every 2 hr for a total of five doses. The initial dose usually is 200 mg. If conversion is not attained, the oral dose is increased by 200 mg the next day, and five doses are given. On this regimen, plasma quinidine concentrations of approximately 4.0, 5.0, and 5.8 µg/ml are attained with doses of 200, 400, and 600 mg. A plasma concentration plateau is reached after the sixth dose, so that additional doses do not produce any further increase in the plasma level.

Oral maintenance doses of quinidine are 300 to 600 mg every 6 hr. For intravenous dosing, 6 to 10 mg/kg quinidine gluconate may be given slowly over a period in excess of 30 min. During intravenous dosing, the patient's blood pressure, electrocardiogram, and clinical status must be closely monitored. Intravenous dosing with quinidine is a potentially dangerous procedure, especially in the setting of acute myocardial infarction or hemodynamic compromise.

Contraindications

One of the few absolute contraindications for quinidine is that of complete A-V block with an A-V pacemaker or idioventricular pacemaker that may be suppressed by quinidine. Because of the negative inotropic action of quinidine, congestive heart failure and hypotension are contraindications for quinidine therapy. Digitalis intoxication and hyperkalemia can accentuate the depression of conduction caused by quinidine, and quinidine should be used with extreme care in these conditions. Myasthenia gravis can be aggravated severely by quinidine's actions at myoneural junctions, and quinidine should not be administered.

Indications

Quinidine has withstood the test of time and continues to play an important role in therapy. Primary indications for the use of quinidine include (a) abolishing premature beats of atrial, A-V junctional, and ventricular origin, (b) restoration of normal sinus rhythm in atrial flutter and atrial fibrillation after control of heart rate with digitalis, (c) maintenance of normal sinus rhythm after electrical conversion of atrial arrhythmias, (d) prophylaxis for arrhythmias associated with electrical countershock, and (e) termination of ventricular tachycardia and suppression of repetitive ventricular tachycardia associated with WPW syndrome. By depressing conduction through the A-V accessory pathway, quinidine favors orthograde A-V transmission and prevents the reentry mechanism, which requires the presence of an accessory pathway.

Quinidine is not primarily indicated for either prophylaxis or active treatment of ventricular flutter or ventricular fibrillation. Management of these arrhythmias often requires intravenous drug administration, and quinidine carries significant risk of toxic effects when given by this route.

Patients with atrial flutter or atrial fibrillation are often given a digitalis glycoside, such as digoxin, for the purpose of controlling the ventricular rate and subsequently are given oral quinidine in an effort to restore normal sinus rhythm. In recent years it has been appreciated that the high incidence of digitalis-induced toxicity in such patients is related to the fact that concomitant administration of the two drugs leads to an excessively high plasma concentration of the digitalis glyco-side. The initial increase in plasma digoxin concentration is probably caused by displacement of the cardiac glycoside from tissue stores by quinidine (80). The prolonged rise in plasma digoxin concentrations after the administration of quinidine is most likely related to a reduction in renal clearance of the cardiac glycoside (81). Thus, through the combined effects of reducing the volume of distribution and the renal clearance of digoxin, quinidine can increase the incidence of cardiac-glyco-side-induced toxicity. Therefore, a reduction in digoxin dosage is suggested when the drugs are given concurrently. In addition, frequent assessment of the plasma concentration of digoxin and careful attention to clinical symptoms of toxicity will help to prevent glycoside-induced toxicity.

Procainamide ✗

It has been appreciated for approximately 30 years that the local anesthetic agent procaine hydrochloride was effective against cardiac arrhythmias when the drug was administered intravenously (83). But the use of procaine for treatment of cardiac arrhythmias had several drawbacks: (a) The drug was rapidly hydrolyzed in plasma by butyrocholinesterase and thus had a very short duration of action, making it difficult to achieve and maintain therapeutic plasma concentrations. (b) The potential to produce stimulation of the central nervous system militated against its use. (c) Oral administration did not prove to be effective. A systematic investigation of congeners of procaine was undertaken to identify compounds that had the therapeutic actions of procaine but did not have its drawbacks. Modification of the procaine molecule to produce procainamide yielded a compound with local anesthetic and antiarrhythmic actions that overcame the difficulties observed with the use of procaine (Fig. 9).

Procainamide was reported to be an effective antiarrhythmic drug, and subsequent investigation (83,84) led to its widespread clinical use. The amide group of procainamide

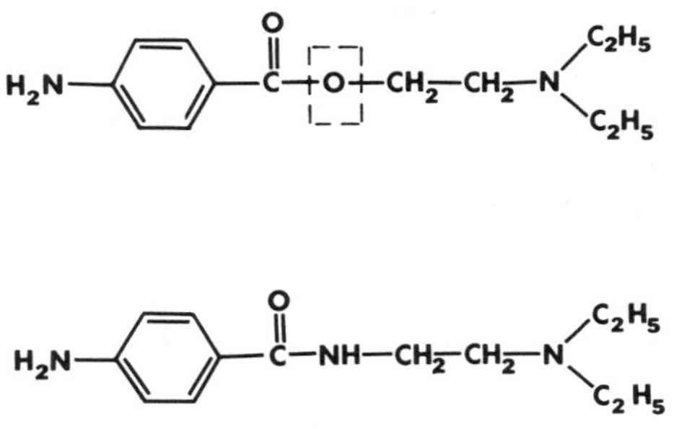

FIG. 9. Chemical structures of procaine (*top*) and procainamide (*bottom*). The ester linkage of procaine is indicated by the broken lines. Esterases in plasma are capable of hydrolyzing the ester linkage. Procainamide is resistant to the action of plasma esterases.

prevents the drug from undergoing hydrolysis by plasma butyrocholinesterase, as occurs with procaine. Thus, procainamide is effective by oral, intramuscular, and intravenous routes, and it lacks the central nervous system effects of procaine.

Electrophysiologic Actions

The direct effects of procainamide on cardiac muscle and specialized conduction fibers are essentially the same as those of quinidine.

Sinoatrial node. Procainamide has a direct effect on the sinoatrial node that leads to a decrease in the rate of spontaneous diastolic depolarization of specialized cells of the node. The direct actions of the drug lead to a decrease in heart rate. The direct negative chronotropic action of procainamide may be counteracted by the anticholinergic properties of procainamide. At therapeutic plasma concentrations, usually no change or only a small increase in heart rate is observed. The direct and indirect actions of procainamide are summarized in Table 6. The vagolytic properties of procainamide are less pronounced than those of quinidine or disopyramide.

Atrial muscle. Procainamide depresses automaticity in specialized atrial muscle fibers by depressing the rate of phase-4 depolarization. Atrial pacemakers are more sensitive to depression than ventricular pacemakers.

Administration of procainamide results in a dose-dependent parallel shift in atrial muscle membrane responsiveness and reduces the amplitude of the phase-0 upstroke potential. The maximum rate of phase-0 depolarization is de-pressed equally at all membrane potentials. Excitability of atrial muscle is also depressed, resulting in a decrease in conduction velocity in atrial muscle.

The action-potential duration of atrial muscle fibers is slightly prolonged by procainamide. This action of procainamide results in only a small increase in the atrial effective refractory period. Most of the increase in the effective refractory period can be attributed to a decrease in membrane responsiveness and failure of early premature beats to conduct from the site of stimulation. The anticholinergic properties of procainamide contribute to the depression of conduction velocity and increase in refractoriness observed with procainamide, although the anticholinergic actions of procainamide are less marked than those of quinidine.

In human electrophysiologic studies, acute procainamide administration results in an increase in atrial muscle refractory periods and a decrease in intraatrial conduction velocity (59,86). Conduction velocity in A-V accessory pathways is depressed, and the effective refractory period is increased (59). In the presence of atrial flutter or atrial fibrillation, in patients with WPW syndrome, procainamide reduces the ventricular rate by decreasing transmission over the accessory pathway, which behaves electrophysiologically like atrial muscle (86).

A-V node. Procainamide has both direct and indirect (anticholinergic) effects on A-V transmission. Direct effects include a decrease in A-V conduction velocity and an increase in A-V node refractoriness. Indirect or anticholinergic effects include a decrease in A-V node refractoriness and an increase in A-V nodal conduction velocity. The special considerations necessary for quinidine administration in the presence of atrial flutter and atrial fibrillation are equally applicable to procainamide administration. Procainamide administration may result in acceleration of ventricular rate due to increased transmission of atrial impulses through the A-V node because of the anticholinergic properties of the drug.

A number of investigators have studied the effects of acute procainamide on A-V conduction in humans. These studies have shown that procainamide's actions on A-V conduction velocity and A-V refractoriness are unpredictable. The effective refractory period of the A-V node can be increased, decreased, or unchanged (85,86). The same variability is seen in the action of procainamide on A-V conduction velocity. Although, in most cases, a decrease or no change in A-V transmission has been seen, in some cases there has been a dramatic increase in A-V transmission. The increase in A-V conduction observed in some patients could be potentially dangerous if atrial fibrillation or atrial flutter is also present.

In toxic doses, procainamide can produce marked depression of A-V conduction. The effects of procainamide on A-V conduction are additive to those of digitalis, and extreme caution must be exercised when using the drugs in combination (87).

His-Purkinje system/ventricular muscle. Procainamide administration results in a decrease in membrane responsiveness and a decrease in the action-potential amplitude of Purkinje fibers and ventricular muscle (76). The phase-0 maximum rate of depolarization is depressed equally at all membrane potentials. Coupled with a decrease in excitability, these changes result in depression of conduction velocity in the His-Purkinje system and in ventricular muscle. The prolongation of ventricular activation due to a decrease in conduction velocity results in prolongation of the QRS interval.

Procainamide administration also results in a slight prolongation of the action-potential duration (76). The effective refractory period is prolonged to a greater degree than the action-potential duration, a result of depression of membrane responsiveness. This action is observed in both ventricular muscle and the His-Purkinje system.

In human electrophysiologic studies, the effects of acute procainamide on conduction and refractoriness in the His-Purkinje system and ventricular muscle are more consistent than the effects on the A-V node. Consistent slowing of conduction and increases in refractoriness are observed in His-Purkinje tissue (86). Higher plasma concentrations result in a greater depression of conduction and a greater increase in refractoriness (86). Ventricular muscle effective refractory periods are increased by procainamide administration (88). Depression of conduction occurs at lower plasma concentrations than that necessary to produce increases in ventricular muscle refractory periods.

Although procainamide has been in clinical use for more than 25 years, its mechanism of action against ventricular arrhythmias is not completely understood. One reason for this is that often the mechanism for the arrhythmia is not entirely clear. Recent observations suggest that procainamide progressively increases the coupling interval before termination of extrasystoles. The reentry of excitation within the ventricle or ventricular conducting system has been postulated as a mechanism for the production of ventricular premature depolarizations. Because procainamide depresses the maximum rate of rise and amplitude of the action potential and increases the effective refractory period, it is postulated that these actions will cause slowing of the reentrant impulse, particularly in abnormal tissue exhibiting slow conduction and unidirectional block. The reduction in responsiveness caused by procainamide could interrupt a reentrant rhythm by converting unidirectional block to bidirectional block. The proposed hypothesis is that procainamide prolongs conduction in the depressed portion of the reentrant pathway such that conduction is further delayed and conduction block finally occurs, thereby terminating the arrhythmia (89).

Procainamide decreases the spontaneous rate of firing in Purkinje fibers by depressing the slope of phase-4 depolarization. This action may account for the effectiveness of procainamide in the treatment of ventricular arrhythmias occurring as a result of enhanced automaticity.

In a manner similar to that of quinidine, changes in extracellular potassium ion concentrations can alter the electrophysiologic properties of procainamide. Increased extracellular potassium concentrations potentiate depression of conduction velocity. Patients with hypokalemia may fail to respond to procainamide, and hyperkalemia will accentuate its depressant actions on myocardial conduction.

Electrocardiographic Changes

Electrocardiographic changes observed with procainamide administration are similar to those observed with quinidine. At normal therapeutic plasma concentrations, procainamide prolongs the PR interval, the QRS interval, and the QT interval of the surface electrocardiogram. The magnitudes of these changes are proportional to the plasma procainamide concentration. The changes in the electrocardiogram observed after procainamide administration are summarized in Table 5. Toxic procainamide plasma concentrations may produce marked QT and QRS prolongation. Enhanced ventricular automaticity and ventricular arrhythmias are often present with excessive procainamide dosage.

Hemodynamic Effects

The hemodynamic alterations produced by procainamide are the same as those of quinidine. However, the hemodynamic alterations produced by procainamide are not as severe as those produced by quinidine. The route of administration, dosage, and rate of administration will determine the magnitude of the hemodynamic responses observed after procainamide administration. Alterations in circulatory dynamics will also vary according to the cardiovascular state of the individual.

Early hemodynamic studies with procainamide suggested that the drug produced both marked depression of myocardial contractility and vasodilation (90). More recent studies have suggested that depression of myocardial contractility and vasodilation are primarily a result of excessive dosage and/or too rapid administration (91). The dose-dependent relationship of these events was demonstrated by investigators studying the hemodynamic effects of procainamide administration on patients undergoing open-heart surgery (92). After a 2-mg/kg injection, systolic blood pressure and right ventricular force decreased by 10% and 12% respectively. At a dose of 4 mg/kg, further decreases in systolic blood pressure and right ventricular force were observed (15% and 21%, respectively). The hypotensive effects are less pronounced after intramuscular administration and seldom occur after oral administration. Blood pressure can be restored by catecholamine administration, which produces vasoconstriction and augments cardiac contractility.

Toxic Reactions

Acute cardiovascular reactions to procainamide administration include hypotension, present to some degree in almost all patients receiving the drug intravenously. After oral administration, hypotensive episodes are infrequent and minor.

Procainamide, unlike procaine, has little potential to produce central nervous system toxicity (90). However, central nervous system stimulation has been observed after rapid intravenous administration of procainamide. An occasional patient may experience mental confusion or hallucinations.

Other toxic reactions to procainamide can include A-V block, intraventricular block, ventricular tachyarrhythmias, and complete heart block. The drug dosage must be reduced or even stopped if severe depression of conduction (severe prolongation of the QRS interval) or repolarization (severe prolongation of the QT interval) occurs in ventricular myocardium. Ventricular tachyarrhythmias leading to syncope or sudden unexpected ventricular fibrillation can occur with procainamide as well as quinidine administration. This toxic manifestation, however, is less common with procainamide administration. In toxic doses, procainamide may increase the slope of phase-4 depolarization in ventricular pacemakers and may produce an increase in ventricular premature beats.

Procainamide administration may also produce nausea, vomiting, and diarrhea, which are dose-related and generally occur with doses in excess of 4 g/day. If these gastrointestinal symptoms remain relatively minor, it is not necessary to discontinue the drug.

An important consideration with chronic use of procainamide concerns the development of a syndrome resembling systemic lupus erythematosus, but without renal or cerebral involvement (93,94). Procainamide has a greater capacity to induce this syndrome than any other chemical. The development of the syndrome depends on both the duration of administration and the total daily dose. The most prevalent symptom is arthralgia. Other signs include skin rash, pleuropneumonic involvement, fever, and hepatomegaly. Symptomatic patients display positive tests for antinuclear factors and for lupus erythematosus cells. Other laboratory tests may differ from clinically observed systemic lupus erythematosus in that no anti-DNA antibodies are formed. The syndrome usually develops after a minimum of 1 month of therapy. Long-term use leads to increased antinuclear antibody titers in over 80% of patients, and more than 30% of patients on long-term procainamide therapy develop a clinical lupus-erythematosus-like syndrome.

The symptoms of lupuslike syndrome disappear within a few days of cessation of procainamide therapy, although the tests for antinuclear factor and lupus erythematosus cells may remain positive for several months.

Pharmacokinetics

Absorption. Oral doses of procainamide are well absorbed from the gastrointestinal tract, with bioavailability of approximately 75%. The remaining fraction can be accounted for by first-pass liver metabolism. Peak plasma concentrations are achieved 60 to 90 min after oral administration. Absorption of intramuscularly administered procainamide is more rapid, with peak plasma levels observed 12 to 45 min after injection (95).

Metabolism and excretion. Procainamide is metabolized extensively in the liver by the enzyme N-acetyltransferase to N-acetylprocainamide. The rate of metabolism of procainamide varies widely between patients and assumes a bimodal distribution of rapid and slow acetylators. The rate of drug acetylation is under genetic control and parallels that of isoniazid, hydralazine, and sulfonamide drugs. Rapid acetylators have higher plasma concentrations of N-acetylprocainamide and excrete larger amounts of N-acetylprocainamide in urine than slow acetylators. Acetylation of procainamide may occur predominantly as a first-pass effect after oral administration, as very little N-acetylprocainamide is formed after intravenous administration. N-acetylprocainamide possesses electrophysiologic actions similar to those of procainamide, although N-acetylprocainamide is less potent. Despite differences observed in the rate of procainamide metabolism by N-acetyltransferase in rapid and slow acetylators, the plasma clearances and therapeutic responses to procainamide are not markedly different in rapid and slow acetylators.

The renal clearance of procainamide is proportional to the creatinine clearance. However, the high rate of renal clearance suggests that both active secretion and filtration are involved in renal excretion of procainamide and N-acetylprocainamide. Although pro-

Table 8. *Procainamide pharmacokinetics*

Percentage absorbed after oral administration	75–90%
Clearance	11.8 ml/min/kg
Volume of distribution	
V_C	0.1 liter/kg
V_CSS	2.2 liters/kg
Plasma $T_{1/2}$	2.0–5.0 hr
Percentage excreted unchanged in urine	50–60%
Percentage free in plasma	85%
Therapeutic plasma concentrations	4–10 μg/ml

cainamide is a weak base, and renal excretion should be increased by urine acidification, conflicting results have been reported on the effect of urinary pH on procainamide excretion, and it is uncertain what effect alterations in urine pH have on procainamide excretion.

Kinetics. After intravenous injection, procainamide plasma concentrations can be adequately described by a two-compartment model. The alpha-phase half-life is approximately 5 min, with a beta-phase half-life of 2 to 5 hr. Further pharmacokinetic data are summarized in Table 8.

Congestive heart failure alters many of the pharmacokinetic parameters that describe procainamide disposition. The steady-state volume of distribution is reduced by 20 to 25%. Renal clearance of the drug is reduced, increasing the plasma half-life. The extent and rate of oral and intramuscular absorption of the drug are reduced. Renal disease also increases the plasma half-life of procainamide. Hemodialysis can effectively increase procainamide clearance and decrease the plasma half-life. Procainamide dosage should, therefore, be altered in the presence of congestive heart failure and decreased renal function. Liver disease does not appear to significantly alter procainamide clearance.

Procainamide is poorly bound to plasma proteins. About 85% of the drug in plasma exists in the unbound state. Myocardial tissue concentrations of procainamide are 2 to 2.5 times those in plasma.

Renal failure shifts procainamide elimination from a renal-dependent to a hepatic-dependent function. Renal disease causes N-acetylprocainamide plasma concentrations to increase dramatically, even after therapy is adjusted to maintain normal therapeutic plasma procainamide concentrations.

The effective plasma procainamide concentration for suppression of ectopic ventricular activity in patients with acute myocardial infarction has been reported to be between 4 and 6 μg/ml. Plasma procainamide concentrations of 2 to 4 μg/ml provide partial protection against ectopic impulse formation. However, recent evidence suggests that recurrent sustained ventricular tachycardia or ventricular fibrillation may be prevented only by procainamide plasma concentrations in excess of 10 μg/ml (96).

The short half-life of procainamide requires that doses be taken every 3 to 4 hr in order to maintain adequate plasma concentrations. Administration at longer intervals increases the incidence of therapeutic failures.

Oral Dosage

Maintenance doses of procainamide for treatment of atrial and ventricular arrhythmias are between 500 and 1,000 mg administered every 4 to 6 hr. Shorter dosage intervals obtain better control of arrhythmias, but poor patient compliance can negate this gain.

Intravenous Dosage

To reduce the occurrence of hypotensive episodes, 100-mg doses may be administered every 5 min by direct slow intravenous injection, at a rate not exceeding 50 mg in any 1 min, until arrhythmia control is achieved or until a cumulative dose of 1 g has been given. To maintain therapeutic levels, an infusion may then be started at a rate of 2 to 6 mg procainamide per minute, depending on the person's renal status and body mass.

The following equation can be used to approximate the plasma procainamide concentration achieved by the foregoing method of administration (91):

$$Y = 0.84 + 0.73(x)$$

where Y is plasma procainamide concentration (μg/ml) and x is cumulative dose of procainamide (mg/kg). For example, if a patient weighing 70 kg were given seven 100-mg intravenous doses at 5-min intervals, the cumulative dose would be 10 mg/kg. The estimated plasma procainamide concentration would be $Y = 0.84 + 0.73(10) = 8.1$ μg/ml.

Procainamide can also be administered as an intravenous infusion, beginning with 500 to 600 mg given over a period of 25 to 30 min. This loading infusion should be followed by a maintenance infusion of 2 to 6 mg/min, based on body weight and renal function.

Intramuscular Dosage

A dose of 0.5 to 1.0 g may be administered intramuscularly every 4 to 8 hr as needed.

Contraindications

The contraindications for procainamide are similar to those for quinidine. Because of its effects on A-V nodal and His-Purkinje conduction, procainamide should be administered with caution to patients with second-degree A-V block and bundle branch block. Parenteral administration may be hazardous in patients with compromised hemodynamic function, as further depression may occur as a result of procainamide's negative inotropic action. Procainamide should not be administered to patients with previous procaine or procainamide sensitivity and should be used with caution in patients with bronchial asthma. Prolonged administration should be accompanied by repeated hematologic studies, as agranulocytosis may occur.

Indications

Although the spectra of action and electrophysiologic effects of quinidine and procain-

amide are similar, the drugs are not interchangeable, as therapeutic response or intolerance may occur to one drug but not the other. The longer duration of action of quinidine limits procainamide use to patients who are intolerant or unresponsive to quinidine.

Clinical studies indicate that procainamide is an extremely effective antiarrhythmic agent when given in sufficient dosage at relatively short (3–4 hr) dosage intervals. It is effective for treatment of premature atrial contractions, paroxysmal atrial tachycardia, and atrial fibrillation of recent onset. Procainamide is only moderately effective in converting atrial flutter or chronic atrial fibrillation to sinus rhythm, although it is of value in preventing reoccurrences of these arrhythmias once they have been terminated by DC cardioversion.

Studies by several investigators indicate that procainamide can decrease occurrences of all types of active ventricular dysrhythmias in patients with acute myocardial infarction who are free from A-V dissociation, serious ventricular failure, and shock. It has been found that 90% of patients with ventricular premature contractions and 80% of patients with ventricular tachycardia respond to procainamide administration (97). The selection of procainamide over quinidine is in many instances a matter of personal preference. For oral administration, the longer duration of action of quinidine is advantageous. For short-term parenteral medication, intravenous or intramuscular procainamide is to be preferred because it is less likely to cause adverse hemodynamic alterations.

Disopyramide ✗

The recent introduction of disopyramide, an orally effective agent capable of suppressing atrial and ventricular arrhythmias, and possessing a longer duration of action than other currently available agents, has been of considerable value for treatment of disorders of cardiac rhythm. The structure of disopyramide is shown in Fig. 10.

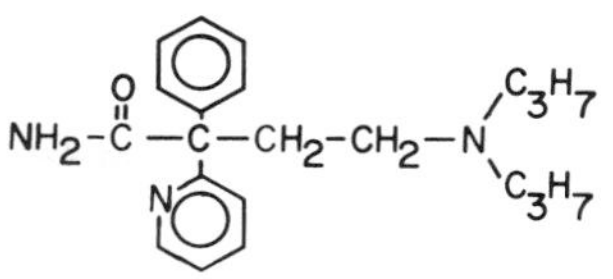

FIG. 10. Disopyramide.

Electrophysiologic Actions

The effects of disopyramide on the myocardium and specialized conduction tissue are a composite of the direct actions of the drug on myocardial electrical properties and indirect actions of the drug mediated by competitive blockade of cardiac cholinergic receptors. The direct actions of disopyramide are those possessed in common with other members of the group I antiarrhythmic agents, and the indirect actions of disopyramide are virtually identical with the actions of atropine and other anticholinergic agents. These direct and indirect properties are shared with other members of the class I antiarrhythmic agents, quinidine and procainamide. Table 4 summarizes the electrophysiologic properties of disopyramide on atrial and ventricular myocardium and specialized conduction tissue.

Sinoatrial node. By virtue of its direct depressant effects, disopyramide reduces the frequency of beating of isolated right atrial tissue preparations that are devoid of intact autonomic nervous system innervation (98). In conscious animals and in humans, the direct depressant actions are counteracted by the anticholinergic properties, so that at therapeutic plasma concentrations of disopyramide, usually no change or a slight increase in sinus heart rate is observed (99,100). Disopyramide should be used cautiously in patients with sinus node dysfunction, as a deterioration in sinus node activity may become manifest (101).

Atrium. Disopyramide reduces membrane responsiveness in atrial muscle and thereby reduces the velocity of atrial conduction (98), a manifestation of its membrane action that places disopyramide into the category of class I antiarrhythmic agents. The action-potential duration in atrial muscle fibers is prolonged

by disopyramide administration, resulting in an increase in the atrial muscle effective refractory period (98). Electrophysiologic studies performed in humans have demonstrated depression of intraatrial conduction and increased atrial muscle refractoriness at therapeutic plasma concentrations (99,100,102). These actions result from direct effects of disopyramide on cardiac membranes and are not a result of the anticholinergic properties of disopyramide, as they occur in patients pretreated with atropine (102).

A-V node. Disopyramide depresses conduction velocity and increases the effective refractory period of the A-V node via a direct action. Additionally, disopyramide increases conduction velocity and decreases the effective refractory period of the A-V node by virtue of its anticholinergic properties (99,100,102). The net effect on A-V transmission will be a result of the interplay of these two opposing actions, a direct depression and an indirect facilitation of A-V nodal transmission. At lower plasma concentrations, the anticholinergic actions predominate, whereas direct depression predominates at toxic concentrations. The same precautions necessary for administration of quinidine or procainamide in the presense of atrial flutter or atrial fibrillation must be exercised with disopyramide to prevent a possible acceleration of ventricular rhythm via facilitation of A-V conduction.

A number of electrophysiologic studies have been performed to examine the effects of disopyramide on A-V conduction in humans (99–102). In these studies, mean plasma disopyramide concentrations ranging from 1.3 to 5.6 μg/ml produced very little change in A-V nodal conduction. No change in conduction velocity and either no change or a small decrease in the effective refractory period were observed. Large doses of disopyramide will depress A-V nodal conduction in animals (103), and this potential may exist clinically.

His-Purkinje system/ventricular muscle. Disopyramide reduces membrane responsiveness in canine Purkinje fibers and ventricular muscle (104,105). This action results in depression of conduction velocity in the His-Purkinje system and ventricular muscle (103,106). Disopyramide also increases the action-potential duration in canine Purkinje fibers and ventricular muscle fibers (104,105), thereby increasing the effective refractory period of ventricular myocardium (106,107). The electrophysiologic actions of disopyramide on ventricular muscle are generally analogous to those of quinidine or procainamide.

The magnitude of the depressant action of disopyramide on membrane responsiveness is dependent on the extracellular potassium concentration (104,105). Greater depression of conduction is seen at higher extracellular potassium ion concentrations. This may, in part, explain the poor response of patients with hypokalemia to class I antiarrhythmic agents. Likewise, hyperkalemia may accentuate the depression of conduction produced by disopyramide.

In electrophysiologic studies performed in humans (99–102), disopyramide has been shown to depress conduction in the His-Purkinje system and to increase the ventricular effective refractory period. These changes are associated with prolongation of the QRS and QT intervals.

Electrocardiographic Changes

The electrocardiographic changes observed after disopyramide administration are similar to those commonly observed with quinidine or procainamide. There is dose-dependent prolongation of the PR, QRS, and QT intervals.

Hemodynamic Effects

At plasma concentrations that produce an antiarrhythmic response, disopyramide produces a significant depression of myocardial contractility (103,108). This action results in an increase in left ventricular end-diastolic pressure and a decrease in cardiac output (103). Administration of disopyramide to patients with compensated heart failure may produce serious depression of cardiac function and lead to overt heart failure. Current data suggest that depression of cardiac function may be greater with disopyramide than that observed at equivalent antiarrhythmic doses of procainamide or quinidine (108).

Disopyramide administration produces vasoconstriction and an increase in peripheral vascular resistance (108) via a direct action on the peripheral vasculature. The exact mechanism responsible for this vasoconstriction is not known. As a result of this increase in peripheral vascular resistance, blood pressure is well maintained despite a fall in cardiac outut.

Although disopyramide is presently available in the United States only for oral administration, clinical trials are in progress using parenteral formulations. The myocardial depressant actions of disopyramide are more marked with parenteral administration, and care must be taken to avoid cardiovascular depression, especially in the setting of acute myocardial infarction. Catecholamine administration can reverse the myocardial depressant effects.

Toxic Reactions

Major toxic reactions to disopyramide include hypotension and cardiac depression. These reactions result from a dose-dependent decrease in myocardial contractility and are primarily observed in patients with poorly compensated heart failure and preexisting cardiac damage. Mild ventricular dysfunction is not an absolute contraindication. Many of the remaining side effects can be attributed to the anticholinergic action of the drug. Dry mouth and urinary hesitancy have been reported in 10 to 40% of patients. Blurred vision, nausea, constipation, and urinary retention have been reported. Central nervous system stimulation and hallucinations can occur, but they are rare. The incidence of severe adverse effects of long-term disopyramide therapy may be less than those observed with quinidine.

Disopyramide can produce depression of A-V nodal and ventricular conduction in some patients. Primary, secondary, and complete heart block have been observed. Ventricular tachycardia or fibrillation associated with prolongation of the electrocardiographic QT interval (109) has been observed with disopyramide administration. This condition closely resembles "quinidine syncope" associated with quinidine administration. The incidence of idiosyncratic ventricular tachyarrhythmias associated with long-term disopyramide therapy is not known. Fortunately, simultaneous use of disopyramide and digoxin does not result in abnormally high plasma concentrations of the cardiac glycoside, as is known to occur with quinidine. Because of the similarity in the antiarrhythmic spectra of disopyramide and quinidine, the former agent may prove clinically advantageous in patients who are receiving digoxin and who require antiarrhythmic therapy with a class I drug.

Pharmacokinetics

Disopyramide is rapidly and almost completely absorbed from the gastrointestinal tract (83%) after oral administration. First-pass liver metabolism occurs, but is not a significant factor in oral use of the drug. Peak plasma disopyramide concentrations are attained within 2 hr after an oral dose.

The clearance of disopyramide from plasma is almost equally divided between renal and hepatic clearances. The metabolism of disopyramide is not well understood; however, the major metabolite, the mono-*N*-dealkylated product, is active as an antiarrhythmic agent. The metabolite accumulates slowly over a period of time, and 25 to 50% of the administered drug can be found in urine in the mono-*N*-dealkylated form. Clearance of disopyramide and its major metabolite from plasma is

dependent on renal excretion, with the remainder appearing in the feces. Plasma clearance exceeds the rate of creatinine clearance, and this implies that active tubular secretion of disopyramide may be involved in renal excretion. Renal clearance of the drug is not altered significantly by changes in urinary pH.

The clearance of disopyramide from plasma is reduced by renal insufficiency and requires a reduction in the dosage of disopyramide to prevent systemic toxicity. Although the rate of renal clearance of disopyramide is not a linear first-order function of the plasma concentration (clearance of disopyramide is more rapid at higher doses and higher plasma concentrations because of the greater fraction of the drug in plasma being in the free, unbound form), clearance values calculated as a function of creatinine clearance can aid in adjustment of the dosage for patients with lowered renal function. Hemodialysis is effective for removal of disopyramide from plasma and can be used in cases involving renal failure or overdose.

The clearance of disopyramide from plasma can be adequately described by a two-compartment (biexponential) model providing for a rapid initial distribution phase (alpha phase) and a slower elimination phase occurring after the drug has been distributed to body tissues (beta phase). The initial distribution-phase (alpha-phase) half-life is approximately 2 min, with a beta-phase half-life of between 5 and 7 hr for patients with normal renal function. Pharmacokinetic values for disopyramide are given in Table 9.

The free plasma concentration, or the fraction of the drug in plasma that is not bound to plasma proteins and is therefore free to exert its pharmacologic effect, is not constant at plasma disopyramide concentrations within the normal therapeutic range. The free plasma concentration increases from 5 to 65% of the total plasma concentration as total plasma disopyramide concentrations are increased from 0.1 to 8 μg/ml. Therefore, an increase in the administered dose may produce a disproportionately large increase in the unbound plasma

Table 9. *Disopyramide pharmacokinetics*

Percentage absorbed after oral administration	83%
Clearance	3.4 ml/min/kg
Volume of distribution	
V_C	0.13 liter/kg
V_DSS	1.29 liters/kg
Plasma $T_{1/2}$	5–7 hr
Percentage excreted unchanged in urine	52%
Percentage free in plasma	15–65% over therapeutic range
Therapeutic plasma concentrations	2–5 µg/ml

drug concentration and a more pronounced pharmacologic effect. As a result of this response and the ability of disopyramide to produce cardiovascular depression, the dosage of the drug must be increased slowly to avoid unwanted side effects.

The effective therapeutic plasma concentration of disopyramide as defined by early clinical trials was between 2 and 4 µg/ml (110, 111). Whereas maintenance of disopyramide plasma concentrations within the range of 2 to 4 µg/ml is effective for suppression of ventricular premature beats and maintenance of normal sinus rhythm after electrical conversion of atrial fibrillation, significantly higher concentrations (4–8 µg/ml) are needed to suppress malignant ventricular arrhythmias (107,112,113).

Quinidine administration alters the plasma kinetics of digoxin, producing an increase in serum digoxin concentrations by unbinding quinidine from tissue stores such as skeletal muscle (80) or by altering the renal clearance of digoxin (81), leading to digoxin toxicity. An increase in serum digoxin concentrations is *not* observed with disopyramide administration.

Oral Dosage

Patients weighing 110 pounds or more, with normal renal and hepatic function, should be given 150 mg every 6 hr. Patients weighing less than 110 pounds should receive 100 mg every 6 hr. More rapid control of arrhythmias

can be obtained with an initial loading dose of 300 mg (200 mg for patients weighing less than 110 pounds), followed by the normal maintenance dose 6 hr later.

Dosage reduction is necessary for patients with hypotension, possible cardiac decompensation, reduced left ventricular function, or cardiomyopathy. The suggested initial dosage in these patients is 100 mg every 6 hr. Renal impairment requires reduction in dosage according to the following schedule (C_{cr} = creatinine clearance):

$C_{cr} > 40$ ml/min	100 mg every 6 hr
$C_{cr} = 15$–40 ml/min	100 mg every 10 hr
$C_{cr} = 5$–15 ml/min	100 mg every 20 hr
$C_{cr} = 1$–5 ml/min	100 mg every 30 hr

Severe refractory ventricular tachycardias may require larger disopyramide dosages for suppression. The dosage should be increased gradually, with electrocardiographic and blood pressure monitoring. In some cases, dosages of 250 to 400 mg every 6 hr may be necessary to effect suppression of more malignant arrhythmias.

Contraindications

Disopyramide should not be administered in the presence of cardiogenic shock, preexisting second- or third-degree A-V block, or known hypersensitivity to the drug. Disopyramide should not be administered in the presence of poorly compensated or uncompensated heart failure, or in the presence of severe hypotension.

As a result of its anticholinergic properties, disopyramide should not be used in patients with glaucoma. Urinary retention and benign prostatic hypertrophy also present relative contraindications to disopyramide therapy. Patients with myasthenia gravis may present with myasthenic crisis after disopyramide administration because of the local anesthetic action of disopyramide at the neuromuscular junction.

If first-degree heart block develops during disopyramide administration, the drug dosage should be reduced. The appearance of second-degree or third-degree heart block (in the absence of an implanted pacemaker) requires withdrawal of the drug. Prolongation of the QRS or QT intervals in excess of 25% also requires lowering of the dosage or discontinuance of the drug.

Patients with congenital prolongation of the QT interval (Jervell-Lang-Nielsen syndrome) should not receive quinidine, procainamide, or disopyramide, because further prolongation of ventricular repolarization and a resultant increase in the QT interval may increase the incidence of ventricular fibrillation.

Indications

The indications for disopyramide are similar to those for quinidine and procainamide, except that disopyramide is not currently approved for use in the prophylaxis of atrial flutter or atrial fibrillation after DC cardioversion. The indications are as follows: (a) unifocal premature (ectopic) ventricular contractions; (b) premature (ectopic) ventricular contractions of multifocal origin; (c) paired premature ventricular contractions (couplets); (d) episodes of ventricular tachycardia (persistent ventricular tachycardia is usually treated by DC cardioversion).

As a result of the additive depression of cardiac conduction produced by disopyramide in the presence of the already depressed conduction produced by cardiac glycosides, disopyramide is not indicated for the treatment of digitalis-induced ventricular arrhythmias.

Lidocaine ✗

Lidocaine was introduced into therapy in 1943 as a local anesthetic agent, and it is still extensively used for that purpose today. It was first used as an antiarrhythmic agent in the late 1940s and early 1950s for treatment of arrhythmias occurring during cardiac catheterization. Widespread use of lidocaine was delayed until the 1960s, when it gained popularity for the treatment of ventricular arrhythmias associated with cardiac surgery, digitalis intoxication, and acute myocardial infarction. Extensive experience has demonstrated lidocaine to be an effective and safe drug for termination of ventricular arrhythmias. The chemical structure of lidocaine is shown in Fig. 11.

Electrophysiologic Actions

The therapeutic usefulness of lidocaine is in large measure due to several specific electrophysiologic properties that give it distinct advantages over other currently available antiarrhythmic agents. In contrast to quinidine and procainamide, lidocaine acts primarily on disturbances of ventricular origin and has a narrow spectrum of antiarrhythmic action.

Sinoatrial node. In isolated tissue, high concentrations of lidocaine (greater than 10^{-4} M) produce a slowing of sinus nodal pacemaker discharge (69,114). At concentrations approximating normal therapeutic plasma concentrations, no alteration in sinus nodal pacemaker discharge is observed. Severe slowing of sinus node automaticity in isolated tissue preparations is not observed even at plasma concentrations 50 to 100 times those observed in humans. It is apparent that the striking sinoatrial nodal depression observed at moderate procainamide, quinidine, or disopyramide concentrations is not observed with lidocaine. When administered in normal therapeutic doses in humans, 1 to 5 mg/kg lidocaine has no effect on the sinus rate.

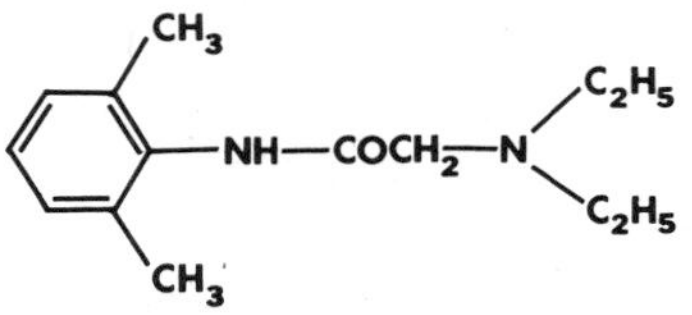

FIG. 11. Lidocaine.

Atria. Early experimental studies suggested that lidocaine produced only small and variable effects on the cardiac action potential in ordinary atrial muscle fibers or specialized conduction fibers of the atria, even when toxic concentrations are used (10^{-4} M) (114). This failure to observe marked electrophysiologic effects of lidocaine may be due to the use of abnormally low extracellular potassium ion concentrations. When the extracellular potassium ion concentrations are increased to levels normally present in the extracellular fluid of humans, the electrophysiologic properties of lidocaine in atrial muscle more closely resemble those of quinidine. Membrane responsiveness is decreased, and the action-potential amplitude is decreased (115). Excitability of atrial muscle is decreased. These changes result in a decrease in atrial muscle conduction velocity. However, the depression of conduction velocity by lidocaine is less marked than that with quinidine or procainamide, even when toxic concentrations of lidocaine are used.

The action-potential duration of atrial muscle fibers is not markedly altered by lidocaine at either normal or subnormal extracellular potassium ion concentrations (114,115). The effective refractory period of atrial myocardium either remains the same or increases slightly after lidocaine administration. Effective refractory periods are not as greatly or consistently increased as with quinidine or procainamide.

The rate of phase-4 depolarization of atrial muscle fiber is depressed by lidocaine. Atrial muscle automaticity is depressed by lidocaine concentrations that do not affect the sinus node (114).

In human electrophysiologic studies, lidocaine failed to alter atrial refractoriness or atrial conduction velocity (116). Conduction in A-V bypass pathways is depressed, and A-V transmission is decreased in the accessory pathway (57).

In summary, lidocaine usually fails to significantly alter atrial refractoriness or conduction velocity. This is the basis for the failure of lidocaine in treatment of supraventricular arrhythmias, except for supraventricular tachycardia using an accessory pathway that may be responsive to lidocaine.

A-V node. Lidocaine minimally alters conduction velocity and the effective refractory period of A-V node (51,116). Lidocaine does not possess anticholinergic properties and will not improve A-V transmission when atrial flutter or atrial fibrillation is present.

In electrophysiologic studies conducted in humans, lidocaine failed to significantly alter atrioventricular nodal refractoriness (57,116). Although lidocaine does not normally alter A-V nodal transmission, it is suggested that lidocaine *not* be administered to patients with atrial flutter or atrial fibrillation, or to patients with second-degree or third-degree A-V block, unless close observation of the hemodynamic and electrophysiologic status is maintained, as both facilitation of A-V transmission and complete A-V block have been reported with the use of lidocaine.

His-Purkinje system. Lidocaine reduces the action-potential amplitude and membrane responsiveness (117). The maximum rate of phase-0 depolarization is most markedly reduced in fibers with reduced resting membrane potentials and in the presence of normal or raised extracellular potassium ion concentrations. The maximum rate of phase-0 depolarization in normal Purkinje fibers with a resting membrane potential of −80 to −90 mV in the presence of extracellular potassium concentrations normally found in humans is depressed less severely by lidocaine than by procainamide or quinidine. Severe depression can be observed in Purkinje fibers, with reduced resting membrane potentials (−70 to −60 mV) occurring as a result of myocardial ischemia. This depression of phase-0 upstroke can be so severe as to produce complete conduction block at lidocaine concentrations in the high therapeutic range (118,119). His-Purkinje excitability is reduced, and combined with the slight depression of phase-0 upstroke velocity, this produces a slight decrease in conduction velocity of the His-Purkinje system.

The action-potential duration in Purkinje

fibers is decreased by lidocaine administration (117). Significant shortening of the action potential and effective refractory period occurs at lower concentrations in Purkinje fibers than in ventricular muscle. As with procainamide and quinidine, lidocaine causes the effective refractory period to lengthen relative to the action-potential duration.

Lidocaine at very low concentrations slows phase-4 depolarization in Purkinje fibers and decreases the spontaneous rate of firing (117–119). At higher concentrations, automaticity in Purkinje fibers may be completely suppressed and phase-4 depolarization completely eliminated. Lidocaine also suppresses automaticity in Purkinje fibers induced by stretch, hypoxia, or catecholamines.

Ventricular muscle. Lidocaine does not alter the resting membrane potential of isolated ventricular muscle fibers. The action-potential duration and effective refractory period are both decreased (117). No changes in the amplitude or the maximum rate of phase-0 depolarization can be observed with lidocaine concentrations in the normal therapeutic range. Myocardial conduction velocity and effective refractory periods are not altered by lidocaine administration.

Electrophysiologic studies in humans have confirmed the foregoing *in vitro* and *in vivo* observations. Lidocaine shortens the effective refractory period of His-Purkinje tissue and does not alter conduction velocity in the His-Purkinje system (116). Ventricular effective refractory periods are not altered by lidocaine. On the basis of lidocaine's action on normal ventricular myocardial tissue and His-Purkinje tissue, it is difficult to suggest a mechanism for antiarrhythmic action. The effects of lidocaine on damaged myocardial tissue may determine its antiarrhythmic action. However, the effect of lidocaine on damaged myocardium is poorly understood. The ability of lidocaine to suppress automaticity in damaged myocardium may be of importance in its antiarrhythmic action, in addition to its effects on conduction velocity and refractory periods (118,119).

Electrocardiographic Changes

The changes in the surface electrocardiogram observed after lidocaine administration are summarized in Table 5. The PR interval, QRS interval, and QT interval usually are unchanged, although the QT interval may be shortened in some patients. This lack of observed electrocardiographic changes with lidocaine is a result of failure of lidocaine to specifically alter conduction velocity in specialized conduction tissues and myocardium.

Hemodynamic Effects

Large doses of lidocaine produce decreases in peak force development and rate of force development in isolated ventricular muscle (120). Studies in the intact canine heart have shown either no change in ventricular performance or a slight positive inotropic effect at normal therapeutic doses (121). At larger doses, dose-dependent decreases in myocardial contractility, cardiac output, and aortic pressure have been noted (122). Studies in the dog after experimental myocardial infarction have shown lidocaine to produce no significant hemodynamic changes at doses up to 200 µg/kg/min (121).

Lidocaine administered as an intravenous bolus at a dose of 1 mg/kg to patients undergoing cardiac surgery produced an increase in myocardial contractility. Doses of 2 mg/kg were not associated with an alteration in myocardial contractility compared with the control state (123). Infusion of either 1.5 mg/kg as an intravenous bolus or 0.3 mg/kg/min intravenous infusion produced no change in the rate of developed pressure, ejection time, time to peak pressure, or right ventricular end-diastolic pressure in a group of 10 patients with heart disease (124). Bolus injection of 100 mg of lidocaine has been shown to produce small and transient decreases in arterial pressure and cardiac output. In the setting of acute myocardial infarction, lidocaine administration fails to significantly alter arterial pressure, right atrial pressure, heart rate, and cardiac output.

Alterations in hemodynamics occurring as a result of administration of lidocaine depend on the status of the patient and on the dose administered. Myocardial contractility and peripheral vascular resistance are depressed only slightly, if at all, by therapeutic doses of lidocaine, but they may be adversely affected by plasma concentrations of lidocaine in excess of normal therapeutic concentrations.

Toxic Reactions

The most common toxic reactions due to lidocaine are primarily results of lidocaine's actions on the central nervous system. Drowsiness is the most commonly observed side effect, and unless it is excessive, it may not be particularly undesirable in patients suffering from acute myocardial infarction (125). Some patients may experience paresthesias, disorientation, and muscle twitching. These undesirable effects may cause the patient to become agitated or frightened, but, of equal importance, they forewarn of more serious deleterious effects. These deleterious effects can include psychosis, respiratory depression, and seizures. Focal seizures often occur just prior to the appearance of generalized tonic-clonic seizures. Convulsions are a dose-related side effect and can be avoided by the simple expedient of controlling the rate of infusion and preventing plasma concentrations from exceeding 5 μg/ml. Diazepam administration will prevent these adverse central nervous effects of lidocaine, and this is the treatment of choice for lidocaine-induced seizures. However, if signs of toxicity are present, lowering the infusion rate or stopping the drug usually will suffice to prevent further toxicity, as lidocaine has a relatively short plasma half-life.

Lidocaine may produce clinically significant hypotension, but this is exceedingly uncommon if the drug is given at moderate dosages. Depression of an already damaged myocardium may result from large doses.

Adverse electrophysiologic effects are uncommon with lidocaine administration. However, lidocaine is contraindicated in the presence of second- or third-degree heart block, because it may increase the degree of heart block and may abolish the idioventricular pacemaker that is maintaining cardiac rhythm. Cardiac pacing should be instituted if lidocaine or other antiarrhythmic drugs must be administered in these instances.

Pharmacokinetics

Absorption. Oral administration of lidocaine has been attempted, but therapeutically efficient blood levels have not been achieved by this route of administration. The failure of oral lidocaine administration is not due to poor intestinal absorption of the drug, but rather is due to extensive first-pass liver metabolism. In excess of 70% of orally administered lidocaine is metabolized by the liver before reaching the systemic circulation. Dizziness, nausea, and vomiting may occur in humans after oral lidocaine administration, and they probably are results of the high circulating plasma concentrations of the mono-N-deethylated and the di-N-deethylated metabolites of lidocaine (monoethylglycine xylidide and glycine xylidide).

Lidocaine is absorbed rapidly after intramuscular injection. Absorption is more rapid after injection into the deltoid muscle (absorption half-life 11.7 min) than into the vastus lateralis and gluteus maximus (absorption half-life 25.7 min).

Metabolism and excretion. Approximately 70% of the lidocaine entering the liver from the systemic circulation is metabolized on a single circulation through the liver. The rate of lidocaine metabolism is therefore critically dependent on hepatic blood flow. Reductions in liver blood flow sharply reduce lidocaine plasma clearance. Lidocaine dosage must be reduced in the presence of decreased liver blood flow or in the presence of deficiencies in liver metabolic function.

Two major metabolites of lidocaine are found in significant concentrations in the blood of patients receiving the drug. The first metabolite, monoethylglycine xylidide, is formed by *N*-deethylation of lidocaine. Monoethylglycine xylidide is as potent an antiarrhythmic agent as lidocaine and has similar convulsant activity. Monoethylglycine xylidide has a plasma half-life of 120 min and is eliminated from plasma primarily by a second *N*-deethylation to form glycine xylidide, the second major metabolite of lidocaine. Glycine xylidide possesses both antiarrhythmic and convulsant activity, although it is only 10 to 26% as potent as lidocaine. Glycine xylidide is both metabolized and excreted by the kidney. It has a plasma half-life of 10 hr.

Accumulation of metabolites during prolonged intravenous administration may help explain why toxicity develops despite plasma lidocaine concentrations that remain in the therapeutic range. About 90% of an administered lidocaine dose appears in the urine as metabolites.

Excretion of unchanged lidocaine by the kidney is a minor route of elimination (10% of dose). Lidocaine is a weak base (pK_a 7.9), and renal clearance is increased by a decrease in urine pH.

Lidocaine crosses the placenta readily from mother to fetus. The drug is then broken down in the fetus or neonate at a rate comparable to that in the mother. The safety of lidocaine for use in pregnancy has not been established.

Kinetics. Lidocaine plasma concentrations after an intravenous dose can be adequately explained by a two-compartment model. The initial distribution-phase (alpha-phase) half-life is 8 min, and the beta-phase half-life is 100 min. Other pharmacokinetic parameters are given in Table 10. A rapid equilibrium is established between tissue and plasma in organs of the body with high blood flows, such as heart, brain, lung, liver, and kidney. The prompt action of lidocaine after intravenous administration is a result of rapid delivery to and uptake in myocardial tissue. Lidocaine then slowly redistributes to other organ systems with lower blood flows. This action accounts for the initial redistribution or alpha phase. The alpha phase (redistribution phase)

Table 10. *Lidocaine pharmacokinetics*

Percentage absorbed after oral administration	<30%
Clearance	10 ml/min/kg
Volume of distribution	
V_C	0.5 liter/kg
V_DSS	1.1 liters/kg
Plasma $T_{1/2}$	100 min
Percentage excreted unchanged in urine	<10%
Percentage free in plasma	60–70%
Therapeutic plasma concentrations	2–5 µg/ml

of lidocaine is extensive and is an important factor in determining dosage regimens for lidocaine.

A number of pathologic conditions alter the disposition and clearance of lidocaine. Heart failure results in significant reductions in both the volume of distribution and plasma clearance of lidocaine. The clinical implication is that patients with congestive heart failure should receive smaller lidocaine dosages. Chronic alcoholic liver disease reduces plasma clearance of lidocaine by as much as 50%. Renal failure and age produce only small and insignificant decreases in lidocaine clearance. However, in elderly and renally compromised patients, lidocaine metabolites can accumulate and produce central nervous system toxicity. The rate of indocyanine green clearance from plasma can be used as a guide for the rate of liver lidocaine clearance.

At usual plasma concentrations, 70% of the total lidocaine is plasma-protein-bound. Alterations of the fraction bound to plasma proteins are minor between different plasma concentrations and are not a factor in dosing schedules.

Therapeutic plasma concentrations range from 2 to 5 µg/ml. Plasma lidocaine concentrations in excess of 6 µg/ml are frequently toxic. Plasma concentrations from 1 to 2.5 µg/ml may suppress ventricular ectopic beats, but plasma lidocaine concentrations of 2.5 µg/ml or greater may be necessary for prevention of ventricular fibrillation.

Dosage

Lidocaine is usually administered intravenously. After a single intravenous bolus injection, the drug disappears rapidly from the plasma because of redistribution of the drug to other tissues. This rapid phase of distribution correlates with the clinically apparent duration of action. The true steady-state plasma half-life of lidocaine is 100 min. Because of these pharmacokinetic properties, lidocaine is administered as an intravenous bolus followed by a constant intravenous infusion.

A. Loading dose (objective is to administer 200 mg in 10–20 min):
   1. 100 mg given over a 2-min period at 10-min intervals, or
   2. 50 mg in 1 min, given four times, 5 min apart, or
   3. 20 mg/min infused for 10 min.
B. Continuous infusion (an infusion-regulating device should be used): 2 to 4 mg/min for 24 to 30 min.
C. To raise plasma concentration acutely if arrhythmia control is lost: 50-mg bolus over 1 min, and simultaneously increase infusion rate to no more than 5 mg/min.
D. In shock, heart failure, and hepatocellular disease: reduce doses by one-half for loading and infusion rates.

Intramuscular administration of lidocaine may also be effective in prevention of ventricular fibrillation. Absorption of lidocaine may be decreased by hemodynamic changes associated with myocardial infarction, and intravenous lidocaine is the preferred mode of administration. Injection of 300 to 400 mg/kg gives persistent therapeutic levels lasting for 2 hr.

Contraindications

Contraindications to the use of lidocaine include the following: (a) hypersensitivity to local anesthetics of the amide type (a very rare occurrence); (b) the presence of complete heart block, because lidocaine suppresses ventricular pacemakers and would result in ventricular standstill; (c) the presence of severe hepatic dysfunction; (d) a previous history of grand mal seizures due to lidocaine; (e) patients 70 years old or older. These conditions are only relative contraindications for the drug if dosage is properly altered.

Indications

In contrast to quinidine and procainamide, lidocaine is much less effective in the treatment of supraventricular arrhythmias (84).

Lidocaine has been shown to be effective for terminating ventricular arrhythmias. Initially it was used primarily in postoperative patients who developed ventricular premature beats or ventricular tachycardia, but it soon gained acceptance in the coronary care unit as a valuable agent for control of ventricular arrhythmias in patients with acute myocardial infarction. Lidocaine administration carries relatively little risk for the patient with acute myocardial infarction, because of its lack of marked depressant effects on the cardiovascular system and the reversibility and short duration of toxic side effects. Routine lidocaine administration may be indicated for all patients with acute myocardial infarction as a result of its ability to prevent ventricular arrhythmias and, most important, ventricular fibrillation, while being easily administered and relatively free of toxic effects. The clinical efficacy of lidocaine in prevention of ventricular fibrillation during acute myocardial infarction is unquestioned.

Lidocaine is the drug of choice for treatment of the electrical manifestations of digitalis intoxication. It may also be used to prevent arrhythmias during countershock in patients who have received digitalis.

Phenytoin

Phenytoin (diphenylhydantoin) is structurally related to the barbiturates and was introduced in 1938 for control of convulsive disorders (126). It was not until 1950 that phenytoin was used for the treatment of cardiac arrhythmias (127). The chemical structure of phenytoin is shown in Fig. 12.

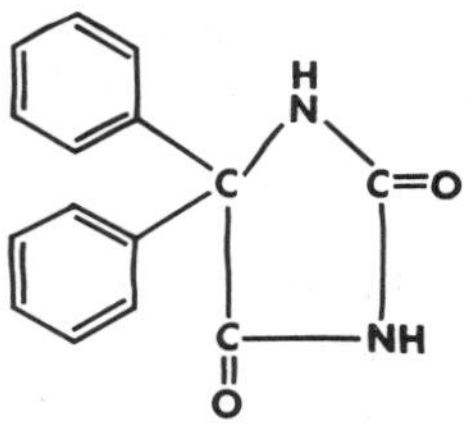

FIG. 12. Phenytoin.

Electrophysiologic Actions

Phenytoin's electrophysiologic actions differ from those of quinidine and procainamide and more closely resemble the electrophysiologic actions of lidocaine.

Sinoatrial node. Supratherapeutic concentrations of phenytoin decrease the slope of phase-4 depolarization in sinus nodal pacemaker cells and depress the spontaneous rate of the sinus node (128). However, concentrations of phenytoin normally observed in humans do not significantly alter sinus rate. When the function of the sinoatrial node or perinodal fibers is altered by disease, sinoatrial pacemaker activity may be impeded by phenytoin and other antiarrhythmic drugs. However, of antiarrhythmic agents currently in use, phenytoin (and possibly lidocaine) produces the least alterations in sinus nodal function, even when sinus nodal function is altered by disease. In humans, phenytoin administration usually fails to alter sinus rate. Hypotension produced after intravenous administration may produce an increase in sympathetic tone and result in an increased sinus heart rate.

Atria. The electrophysiologic effects of phenytoin are disguised by the electrophysiologic properties of the diluent present in commercial preparations of phenytoin. Because of this action of the diluent, one must be careful in examining many of the earliest studies of the electrophysiologic properties of phenytoin using phenytoin preparations that contained the commercial diluent.

The electrophysiologic actions of phenytoin on atrial muscle fibers resemble the actions of lidocaine. Except at very high concentrations, phenytoin usually fails to appreciably alter the action-potential duration or effective refractory period of atrial myocardium (129, 130).

The effect of phenytoin on membrane responsiveness of atrial muscle is dependent on the frequency of stimulation and the extracellular potassium ion concentration (129). When extracellular potassium ion concentrations are less than 3 mM and atrial muscle is paced at a rate below normal sinus rhythm, phenytoin may increase the rate of phase-0 depolarization of atrial muscle. When extracellular potassium ion concentrations are in the range normally observed in humans (3–5 mM) and the atrial muscle is paced at a normal sinus rate, phenytoin depresses the rate of phase-0 depolarization of atrial muscle fibers. Excitability of atrial muscle fibers is not altered by phenytoin. Atrial conduction velocity is either unchanged or slightly depressed after phenytoin administration.

Phenytoin depresses the rate of spontaneous phase-4 depolarization of atrial muscle fibers and decreases the rate of discharge of atrial pacemakers. Atrial pacemakers are more sensitive to depression by phenytoin than are sinus nodal pacemakers (130).

In human electrophysiologic studies, phenytoin failed to significantly alter atrial refractoriness and intraatrial conduction velocity (131). The effects of phenytoin on A-V accessory pathways are unclear, although increases in the effective refractory period have been reported.

A-V node. Phenytoin lacks the anticholinergic properties of quinidine, disopyramide, and procainamide. However, the direct actions of phenytoin on the A-V node facilitate A-V transmission.

In human electrophysiologic studies, phenytoin has been shown to decrease A-V nodal effective refractory periods and to increase A-V nodal conduction velocity (131,132). Depression of A-V conduction has not been observed. Phenytoin reverses digitalis-induced lengthening of the A-V effective refractory period and decreases in A-V conduction velocity. Phenytoin can return A-V transmission toward normal in the digitalis-intoxicated patient (132). In addition, phenytoin can reduce digitalis-induced ventricular automaticity. However, caution should be used when administering phenytoin in the presence of digitalis-induced third-degree heart block. Ventricular automaticity may be depressed before A-V conduction is restored, and the ventricular rate may fall precipitously before being restored to normal.

Because of the increase in A-V transmission observed after phenytoin administration, phenytoin should not be administered to patients with atrial flutter or atrial fibrillation. Phenytoin probably will not be effective in restoring normal sinus rhythm and may produce a dangerous acceleration of the ventricular rate.

His-Purkinje system. The electrophysiologic effects of phenytoin on the His-Purkinje system resemble those of lidocaine. The action-potential duration and effective refractory period to the action-potential duration are increased (133).

Phenytoin's effects on membrane responsiveness have been confusing. Phenytoin can increase the maximum rate of phase-0 depolarization in Purkinje fibers after phase-0 depolarization has been depressed by digitalis overdoses or hypoxia. Restoration of depressed conduction has been observed in the His-Purkinje system after digitalis overdoses. However, normal Purkinje fibers or Purkinje fibers damaged by myocardial ischemia do not respond to phenytoin in the same manner. At normal extracellular potassium ion concentrations, phenytoin produces either no change or a slight decrease in phase-0 maximum rate of depolarization. In a manner similar to that of lidocaine, phenytoin decreases the maximum rate of phase-0 depolarization in diseased, depolarized Purkinje fibers with resting membrane potentials of less than -70 mV. Experiments performed in anesthetized dogs suggest that depression of conduction velocity and increases in ventricular refractoriness are the primary actions of phenytoin in myocardium damaged by myocardial ischemia (134). Im-

provement in cardiac conduction velocity by phenytoin may be limited to that observed in digitalis toxicity.

Phenytoin decreases the rate of phase-4 depolarization in Purkinje tissue and reduces the rate of discharge of ventricular pacemakers. This depression of automaticity is observed with procainamide, quinidine, disopyramide, and lidocaine, as well as with phenytoin (133).

In human electrophysiologic studies, phenytoin has been shown to decrease the effective refractory period of the His-Purkinje system, while leaving conduction velocity unaltered or slightly decreased (131). The effects of phenytoin on ventricular refractoriness are presently unknown. Phenytoin can abolish premature ventricular beats resulting from digitalis intoxication without altering His-Purkinje conduction or refractoriness.

Electrocardiographic Changes

The electrocardiographic changes observed with phenytoin administration are given in Table 5. Because phenytoin improves A-V conduction and shortens the action-potential duration of ventricular myocardium, phenytoin may decrease the PR interval and QT interval of the surface electrocardiogram. The electrophysiologic properties of phenytoin are summarized in Table 11.

Hemodynamic Effects

The effects of phenytoin on the cardiovascular system vary with the dose, mode and rate of administration, and the presence of cardiovascular abnormalities. Rapid administration of phenytoin can produce transient hypotension, a result of peripheral vasodilation and depression of myocardial contractility (135). These effects are due to direct actions of phenytoin on the vascular bed and ventricular myocardium. If large phenytoin doses are given slowly, dose-related decreases in left ventricular force, rate of force development, and cardiac output can be observed, along

Table 11. *Electrophysiologic properties of lidocaine and phenytoin*

Tissue	Effect of lidocaine	Effect of phenytoin
Sinus node	No change	No change
Atria		
Automaticity	Decrease	Decrease
Conduction velocity	No change	No change
Effective refractory period	No change	No change
A-V node		
Automaticity	Decrease	Decrease
Conduction velocity	No change	No change or increase
Effective refractory period	No change	No change or decrease
His-Purkinje/ventricular muscle		
Automaticity	Decrease	Decrease
Conduction velocity	No change	No change
Effective refractory period	Decrease	Decrease

with an increase in left ventricular end-diastolic pressure.

In human subjects, phenytoin doses of 2.5 to 5.4 mg/kg over a 3- to 5-min period failed to produce significant changes in cardiac output, systemic or pulmonary arterial pressures, or peripheral resistance (136). Administration of phenytoin at a rate of 50 mg/min to patients with heart disease resulted in an increase in left ventricular end-diastolic pressure, in addition to a decrease in stroke work and stroke power. There was no significant change in either cardiac index or arterial pressure (137). Phenytoin appears to be superior to quinidine, procainamide, and disopyramide when one considers their hemodynamic effects.

Toxic Reactions

The major toxic effects of phenytoin manifest themselves on the circulatory, central nervous, and hematopoietic systems.

Intravenous phenytoin administration can present a hazard, and initial enthusiasm for its use as an antiarrhythmic agent was tempered by reports of serious cardiovascular toxicity. Respiratory arrest, arrhythmias, and hypotension have been reported with the use of intravenous phenytoin. In most cases, toxicity was due to rapid administration of phenytoin (in excess of 50 mg/min) (138,139).

Even though A-V block and bradycardia are occasionally associated with phenytoin administration (140), much of the rationale for using phenytoin in preference to other antiarrhythmic agents in the treatment of digitalis toxicity lies in the fact that phenytoin usually enhances rather than depresses A-V conduction (132). Depression of conduction is rare, but it is an important factor to be aware of when administering the drug.

It is important to recognize that the diluent supplied with phenytoin is not pharmacologically inert (141), and many of the adverse hemodynamic effects attributed to phenytoin may actually be due to the diluent, which has a pH of 11 and contains 40% propyleneglycol, 10% ethyl alcohol, and water. Because of the high pH of the solution, intravenous administration of phenytoin may cause local irritation of the vein at the site of injection. To prevent pain and irritation at the site of injection, each dose of phenytoin should be followed with an injection of sterile saline to "flush" the vein.

The central nervous system manifestations of phenytoin toxicity can include giddiness, ataxia, tremors, nystagmus on far lateral gaze, diplopia, blurring of vision, slurring of speech, sedation, and ptosis. These symptoms can generally be related to plasma phenytoin levels in patients receiving long-term phenytoin therapy. These central nervous system side effects occur at plasma concentrations of 20 μg/ml or greater, generally at levels that are above the therapeutic range.

Hematologic manifestations of phenytoin toxicity include anemia, pancytopenia, and reticuloendothelial disorders that regress when the drug is discontinued. The drug may also produce a megaloblastic anemia, which responds to folate therapy.

Pharmacokinetics

Absorption. Phenytoin is almost completely absorbed after an oral dose. First-pass liver metabolism does not limit oral bioavailability to an appreciable extent. Phenytoin is poorly and erratically absorbed after intramuscular injection and is not recommended for administration by this route. Peak plasma concentrations after a single oral dose occur approximately 12 hr after ingestion.

Metabolism and excretion. Phenytoin is metabolized to 5-phenyl-t-parahydroxy-phenylhydantoin by hepatic microsomal enzymes. This compound is conjugated in the liver with glucuronic acid and excreted in the urine. About 50 to 75% of a single phenytoin dose is excreted in the urine as the parahydroxy glucuronide metabolite. Several other metabolites have been recovered from urine. Less than 5% of a single dose appears unchanged in the urine.

Kinetics. The kinetics of phenytoin disappearance from plasma are nonlinear and follow Michaelis-Menten kinetics. The nonlinearity and Michaelis-Menten kinetics of phenytoin disposition may be explained by saturation of microsomal enzymes responsible for its metabolism. Most patients can metabolize 10 mg/kg/day by an essentially zero-order kinetic process. The pharmacokinetic parameters of phenytoin are summarized in Table 12.

Table 12. *Phenytoin pharmacokinetics*

Percentage absorbed after oral administration	98%
Clearance	0.02 liter/kg/hr (linear kinetics)
Volume of distribution V_D	0.5–0.8 liter/kg
Plasma $T_{1/2}$	8–60 hr (dose-dependent)
Percentage excreted unchanged in urine	<5%
Percentage free (unbound) in plasma	4–12%
Therapeutic plasma concentrations	10–18 μg/ml

About 93% of plasma phenytoin concentrations are plasma-protein-bound. Small decreases in plasma protein binding may enhance the clinical effect or toxicity of phenytoin by increasing the free plasma concentration of phenytoin without altering its total plasma concentration. Salicylates, sulfonamides, phenylbutazone, and bilirubin all displace phenytoin from plasma proteins and increase free phenytoin concentrations. In uremic patients, twofold to threefold increases in free (unbound) phenytoin concentrations can be observed even though total phenytoin plasma concentrations remain in the "therapeutic" range. Plasma protein binding is also reduced with some hepatocellular diseases. These conditions require reductions in phenytoin doses to maintain free plasma concentrations in the therapeutic range.

Considerable variation in phenytoin plasma levels can occur in patients receiving identical phenytoin doses. Part of this variation may be a result of marked differences in the rate of hepatic metabolism. Some patients have a genetic deficiency in the activity of microsomal enzymes responsible for phenytoin metabolism, whereas others metabolize phenytoin at rates much faster than the normal population. Hepatocellular disease decreases phenytoin clearance.

Therapy with other drugs may alter phenytoin elimination from plasma. Isoniazid interferes with microsomal metabolism of phenytoin, whereas drugs that stimulate microsomal metabolism (barbiturates, etc.) may increase phenytoin clearance. Phenytoin itself may stimulate its own metabolism, so that hepatic phenytoin clearance may increase with the duration of therapy. These factors make individualized therapy and monitoring of plasma phenytoin concentrations mandatory.

Three-fourths of responsive cardiac arrhythmias are abolished at phenytoin plasma concentrations of 10 to 18 μg/ml. Because of a nonlinear relationship between dose and steady-state plasma concentrations, maintenance of consistent levels is difficult.

Oral Dose

To achieve plasma concentrations of 10 to 18 μg/ml within 24 hr, an initial loading dose of 1,000 mg must be given. The dose on the second day is 500 to 600 mg, with maintenance doses of 300 to 400 mg/day thereafter. On the average, a daily dose of 300 mg gives a plasma concentration of 10 μg/ml, and a dose of 500 mg doubles that to 20 μg/ml.

Intravenous Dose

Intravenous doses of 100 mg can be given every 5 min until the arrhythmia is abolished or until 1,000 mg have been given. Oral maintenance therapy should then be started. The plasma half-life is sufficiently long to obviate the need for continuous maintenance infusions.

Contraindications

The contraindications to the use of phenytoin are similar to those for other antiarrhythmic drugs. Thus, the drug should not be used or should be used cautiously in patients with hypotension, severe bradycardia, high-grade A-V block, severe heart failure, and hypersensitivity to the drug. Caution should be exercised when using phenytoin in conjunction with other drugs that alter the metabolism of phenytoin.

Indications

Phenytoin, like lidocaine, has been found to be more effective for treatment of ventricular arrhythmias than supraventricular arrhythmias, and it has been most effective in treating ventricular arrhythmias associated with digitalis toxicity, acute myocardial infarction, open-heart surgery, anesthesia, cardiac catheterization, cardioversion, and angiographic studies.

Phenytoin finds its most effective use in the treatment of ventricular arrhythmias associated with digitalis intoxication. It is extremely effective for the treatment of both supraventricular and ventricular arrhythmias occurring as a result of digitalis. Phenytoin's ability to improve digitalis-depressed A-V conduction is a special feature and is in contrast to other antiarrhythmic agents.

The experience of most investigators has indicated that phenytoin is not effective in the conversion of atrial flutter or atrial fibrillation to normal sinus rhythm, nor is it effective in the treatment of other supraventricular arrhythmias not associated with digitalis toxicity. It should be appreciated that phenytoin, by virtue of its ability to enhance A-V conduction, may increase the ventricular rate in the presence of atrial flutter or atrial fibrillation.

An important application of phenytoin has been as a prophylactic agent to prevent postconversion arrhythmias, particularly in the digitalized patient. Phenytoin administered to the digitalis-sensitized animal has a tendency to increase the threshold for producing ventricular tachycardia.

Phenytoin has been shown to be ineffective in preventing sudden coronary death (ventricular fibrillation) in patients during prolonged therapy in the healing phase of myocardial infarction. For this reason, phenytoin is not a drug of choice for treatment of patients with complicated ventricular arrhythmias due to coronary artery disease.

Propranolol

Propranolol is unique among the antiarrhythmic drugs, for in addition to its ability to abolish certain disorders of cardiac rhythm, it will prevent the effects of the adrenergic nervous system or adrenergic drugs (norepinephrine, epinephrine, isoproterenol, dopamine) on the heart. It is therefore a β-adrenergic receptor blocking agent, and, as such, it will produce a wide variety of effects, both hemodynamic and metabolic, by virtue of the antagonism of adrenergically mediated responses.

Several of the more important physiologic responses mediated by activation of β-adrenergic receptors include (a) increases in heart rate and cardiac contractile force in response to exercise, stress, excitation, etc., (b) an increase in A-V conduction velocity, (c) relaxation of bronchial smooth muscle and a decrease in airway resistance, and (d) release of insulin from β cells in the islets of Langerhans in response to adrenergic stimulation. After propranolol administration, the adrenergic system can no longer initiate the responses indicated.

The clinical use of propranolol, or other β receptor blocking agents, must take into consideration the effects of β-adrenergic receptor blockade and the consequences of such to the overall regulation of the cardiovascular system. Patients with normally functioning cardiovascular systems may be able to tolerate

a blockade of adrenergic transmission to the heart; however, those with compensated heart failure will be dependent on adrenergic tone to maintain adequate cardiac output. Removal of background adrenergic tone by administration of a β-adrenergic receptor blocking agent may precipitate acute congestive heart failure or pulmonary edema.

The chemical structure of propranolol is shown in Fig. 13. Also shown in Fig. 13 are the structures of nadolol and metoprolol, two β-adrenergic agents recently approved for clinical use. Each of these three β-adrenergic receptor blocking agents contains a chiral center. This asymmetric center in the side chain of these compounds gives rise to dextro- and levo-rotary compounds, which can differ greatly in their pharmacologic actions. Only one of the two isomers possesses β-adrenergic receptor blocking activity. However, because the drug is administered as a racemate (containing both *d* and *l* forms), the actions of the non-β-adrenergic blocking components may also be important. With propranolol, the *d* isomer (only the *l* isomer possesses β-adrenergic blocking activity) has direct electrophysiologic actions that resemble those of quinidine and are termed "membrane-stabilizing" properties (12,13). The direct electrophysiologic actions of propranolol are of lesser importance than the β-adrenergic blockade in clinical management of cardiac arrhythmias. The direct membrane-stabilizing action is lacking in nadolol and is present with

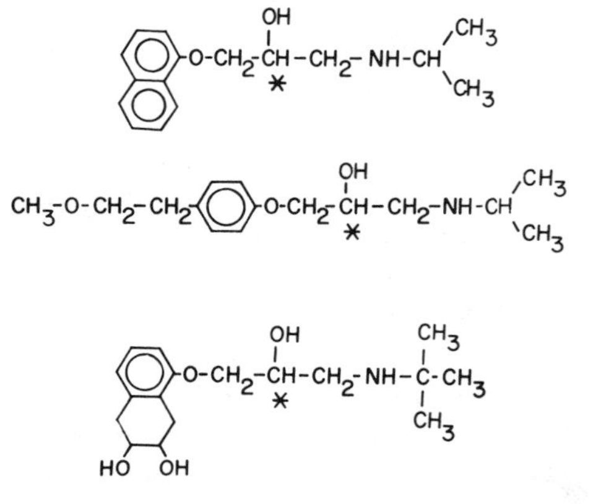

FIG. 13. Chemical structures of propranolol (*top*); metoprolol (*middle*); and nadolol (bottom).

Table 13.

	β blocking activity	Membrane stabilization
Propranolol	β_1, β_2 receptor	+
Metoprolol	β_1 receptor	±
Nadolol	β_1, β_2 receptor	−

metoprolol only at very high doses (Table 13). At present, only propranolol is approved for treatment of cardiac arrhythmias, although both nadolol and metoprolol probably are effective in the treatment of supraventricular arrhythmias.

Electrophysiologic Actions

Unlike the other antiarrhythmic agents previously discussed, propranolol has two separate and distinct actions. The first action involves the consequences of competitive β-adrenergic receptor blockade and the removal of adrenergic influences on the heart (Fig. 14). The second action of propranolol involves the direct myocardial effects (membrane stabilization) that can account for its antiarrhythmic effect against arrhythmias in which enhanced β receptor stimulation does not play a significant role in the genesis of the rhythm disturbance.

Sinoatrial node. Propranolol administration produces a decrease in the spontaneous rate of isolated rabbit atrial preparations (142). This action of propranolol is far more significant in the intact heart, which is under the influence of the sympathetic nervous system as well as circulating catecholamines. The ability of propranolol to block β-adrenergic receptors in the sinoatrial node and prevent the effects of adrenergic influences on this structure is the primary mechanism by which propranolol produces a bradycardia. In addition, doses in excess of those required to produce β receptor blockade can exert a direct negative inotropic action on sinoatrial nodal pacemaker cells (142).

Atria. Propranolol has local anesthetic properties and has actions on the membrane action potential of atrial muscle similar to those of quinidine (143). Membrane responsiveness and action-potential amplitude are reduced, and excitability is decreased. Conduction velocity is reduced. Because the concentrations required to produce these effects have significant β receptor blocking actions, it is impossible to determine if the drug acts by specific receptor blockade or through an action that some have referred to as a "quinidinelike" or "membrane-stabilizing" effect. However, the *d* isomer of propranolol, as well as the *l* isomer, produces these membrane depressant actions.

Propranolol prolongs slightly the action-potential duration and the effective refractory period of atrial tissue. However, at small doses, propranolol has little effect on atrial refractoriness or conduction velocity in humans. Atrial bypass tract conduction and refractoriness are also not altered (57). The effects of supra-β-adrenergic blocking doses have not been studied.

A-V node. Propranolol's effects on A-V node conduction velocity and effective refractory period can be attributed to both β-adrenergic receptor blockade and direct membrane depressant properties (144,145). The effects of propranolol on the A-V node are additive to those produced with digitalis administration. Thus, both drugs are of value, either alone or in combination, in slowing the ventricular rate during atrial flutter or atrial fibrillation. In the presence of digitalis toxicity, propranolol may be contraindicated because of the possibility that it could produce complete A-V block and ventricular asystole. The depressant effects of propranolol on the A-V node are more pronounced than the direct depressant effects of quinidine, because of propranolol's dual mechanism: β-adrenergic receptor blockade and direct depressant actions. Propranolol also does not have the anticholinergic actions of quinidine and other antiarrhythmic agents.

In humans, propranolol administration results in a decrease in A-V conduction velocity and an increase in A-V nodal refractory peri-

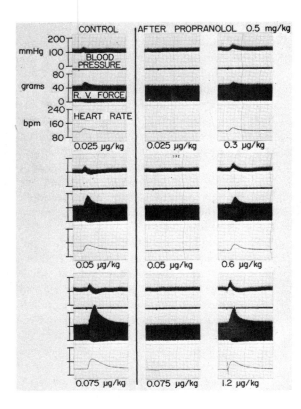

FIG. 14. Effects of β-adrenergic receptor blockade with propranolol on the blood pressure, cardiac force, and heart rate responses to geometrically increasing doses of isoproterenol. Control responses are illustrated on the left. The center column shows the responses to the same doses of isoproterenol after administration of propranolol. The column on the right shows the responses to larger doses than those used previously and illustrates the surmountable nature of the antagonism.

ods. This effect is seen at doses of 0.1 mg/kg administered intravenously (144). When the drug is administered in the absence of atrial pacing, the simultaneous decrease in sinus rate indirectly enhances A-V conduction, because conduction is enhanced at the slower rate. The PR interval, therefore, may not be prolonged after propranolol administration.

His-Purkinje system. Propranolol decreases Purkinje fiber membrane responsiveness and reduces the action-potential amplitude (14). The maximum rate of phase-0 depolarization is depressed at all resting membrane potentials. His-Purkinje tissue excitability is also reduced. These changes result in a decrease in His-Purkinje conduction velocity. However, these electrophysiologic alterations are observed at propranolol concentrations that are in excess of those normally observed in humans.

Propranolol administration produces decreases in the action-potential duration and the effective refractory period of Purkinje fibers. However, increases in the effective refractory period are observed only at levels that exceed those normally observed in the clinical use of the drug.

The most striking electrophysiologic property of propranolol at representative therapeutic concentrations is a depression of catecholamine-stimulated automaticity. Epinephrine and isoproterenol dramatically increase phase-4 depolarization of Purkinje fibers and thereby increase the rate of spontaneous firing. This action of catecholamines is mediated by β-adrenergic receptors and is blocked by the β-adrenergic blocking properties of propranolol. The β-adrenergic blocking action of propranolol is probably responsible for the decrease in ventricular premature beats observed with low or moderate propranolol dosages.

Ventricular muscle. In ventricular muscle fibers, propranolol decreases membrane responsiveness and decreases myocardial excitability (14). The action-potential duration is not prolonged until very high propranolol dosages are used. The necessary concentrations are much higher than those normally obtained, and may be in excess of 100 ng/ml.

Summary. The antiarrhythmic action of propranolol is a result of two separate effects: (a) the β-adrenergic receptor blocking action of the drug and (b) the direct membrane depressant (membrane stabilization or quinidinelike) properties of propranolol. At low plasma concentrations, less than 100 ng/ml, the antiarrhythmic action is a result of β-adrenergic blockade. This action is very effective in reducing A-V transmission and will slow the ventricular rate in the presence of atrial flutter or atrial fibrillation. This action may also reduce the incidence of premature ventricular beats in patients with ischemic heart disease by reducing catecholamine-dependent ventricular automaticity. However, plasma concentrations above 100 ng/ml may be needed to reduce the ventricular rate in some patients with atrial flutter or atrial fibrillation. At this plasma concentration, in addition to β-adrenergic blockade, the direct depressant actions of propranolol on A-V transmission are manifested, and a further reduction in ventricular rate will occur. The high plasma concentrations are necessary in order to observe the direct membrane-stabilizing properties of propranolol, and it is only at the higher plasma propranolol concentrations that the antiarrhythmic properties of propranolol in the treatment of ventricular arrhythmias are commonly manifested (146).

Electrocardiographic Changes

The electrocardiographic changes observed after propranolol administration are summarized in Table 5. Either no change or an increase in the PR interval can be observed. No change in the QRS interval is observed unless large doses are given. The QRS interval may then be prolonged slightly. The QT interval is usually shortened with propranolol administration (147).

Hemodynamic Effects

The majority of studies dealing with the hemodynamic effects of β receptor blockade have been conducted with propranolol. Other β receptor blocking agents have properties that may cause them to produce effects significantly different from those of propranolol, both qualitatively and quantitatively (148). The following discussion applies primarily to propranolol.

The blockade of cardiac β-adrenergic receptors prevents or reduces the usual positive inotropic and chronotropic actions due to catecholamine administration or cardiac sympathetic nerve stimulation. In anesthetized dogs with intact cardiac innervation and intrinsic sympathetic tone, propranolol has been reported to decrease the resting heart rate, myocardial contractile force, and blood pressure (149). The effects of β-adrenergic receptor blockade on the racing performance of normal greyhounds and greyhounds with chronic intrinsic cardiac denervation have been reported (150). β-Adrenergic receptor blockade resulted in an increase in racing time in the normal animal, with only a slight reduction in maximal heart rate. In animals with chronically denervated hearts, racing time was prolonged, cardiac acceleration was severely limited, and the animals finished in a state of collapse. Maximal performance, therefore, is dependent on the cardiac stimulatory action of both sympathetic nerves and circulating catecholamines. Analogous studies in humans (151) were carried out to assess the effects of β-adrenergic receptor blockade on cardiovascular responses to treadmill exercise in normal subjects and subjects with heart disease. In normal subjects, propranolol produced a fall in the endurance time to maximal exercise, which was 40% less on the average than the control. This was associated with decreases in cardiac output (22%), mean arterial pressure (15%), left ventricular minute work (34%), and maximal oxygen uptake (6%). Increases in the arteriovenous oxygen difference (12%) and the central venous pressure (2.8

mm Hg) were noted after β receptor blockade. Similar results were obtained in patients with heart disease who were able to exercise normally. Under conditions of submaximal exercise, propranolol produced similar circulatory responses, with the exception that oxygen uptake was not altered. The decrease in cardiac output was compensated for by an increase in the arteriovenous oxygen difference.

The response of heart size to exercise measured before and after β-adrenergic receptor blockade is an increase in ventricular end-diastolic dimensions, whereas exercise in the normal subject results in a decrease in ventricular dimensions (152,153). Intravenous administration of propranolol produces decreases in the velocity of shortening of myocardial fibers, stroke index, and left ventricular minute work. β-Adrenergic receptor blockade prolongs systolic ejection periods at rest and during exercise and increases ventricular dimensions during exercise. Both alterations tend to increase myocardial oxygen consumption. However, these alterations are offset by factors that tend to reduce oxygen consumption: decreased heart rate and decreased force of contraction. The decrease in oxygen demand produced by a decrease in heart rate and a decrease in force of contraction is usually greater than the increase in oxygen demand produced by an increased heart size and increased ejection time, with a net result that oxygen demand is decreased. The hemodynamic effects of propranolol are summarized in Table 14, illustrating the manner in which propranolol is capable of reducing myocardial oxygen consumption.

Toxic Reactions

The adverse effects associated with propranolol and other β-adrenergic receptor blocking agents are for the most part related to the primary pharmacologic action, that of β receptor blockade.

Cardiac failure has been the most serious adverse effect associated with β receptor blockade. Three possible mechanisms may be

Table 14. *Hemodynamic effects of propranolol*

Decrease in resting heart rate
Decrease in myocardial contractility
   Decrease in stroke volume
   Decrease in ventricular pressure development
   Decrease in rate of ejection
   Increase in ventricular end-diastolic size
Decrease in inotropic and chronotropic responses to exercise

involved: (a) β receptor blockade will decrease the heart rate, which in the normal heart is no serious consequence, but this can lead to a fall in cardiac output in those patients who have a limited stroke volume and who are dependent on an increased heart rate to maintain an adequate output; (b) the increased durations of systole and of diastole that accompany β receptor blockade may decrease cardiac output in patients with valvular regurgitation due to increased regurgitant flow; (c) patients in borderline failure maintain cardiac compensation partly through an increase in cardiac adrenergic tone. The sudden removal of cardiac adrenergic support by β receptor blockade removes the inotropic and chronotropic effects of adrenergic stimulation. In addition to those effects attributable to β receptor blockade, it is important to remember that propranolol possesses direct cardiac depressant effects that become manifest when the drug is administered rapidly by the intravenous route.

Heart failure due to administration of propranolol cannot be managed in the conventional manner with the use of adrenergic inotropic agents because of the presence of β-adrenergic receptor blockade, which will prevent the response of the heart to conventional doses of norepinephrine, isoproterenol, or dopamine. It is true, however, that the effects of β receptor blockade may be overcome by large doses of the adrenergic agents because of the competitive nature of the receptor blockade by propranolol. Such an approach is not convenient or easy to manage and in the case of norepinephrine may prove to be hazardous. The latter drug, when administered in the presence of β receptor blockade, will still be capable of producing peripheral vasoconstriction (an α-mediated effect) at a time when myocardial β receptors are blocked and the heart is unable to respond to the acute increase in outflow impedance (aortic diastolic pressure), leading to the development of acute left ventricular failure. A similar response may be anticipated from dopamine if used under similar circumstances.

The digitalis glycosides are capable of exerting a positive inotropic effect in the presence of β receptor blockade; however, the action of digitalis on the A-V node may be additive to the effect of propranolol, with the result that A-V block will develop. Furthermore, the inotropic effect of digitalis is not manifest immediately, and the delay in onset of action may be a drawback in an emergency situation.

Aminophylline would be a most suitable inotropic agent for the reversal of heart failure induced by propranolol. The drug has an immediate positive inotropic effect, but its action may be accompanied by marked hypotension if given rapidly by the intravenous route. The most suitable agent for treatment of propranolol-induced heart failure would be the polypeptide hormone glucagon. Glucagon will immediately reverse all of the cardiac depressant effects of propranolol, and its use is associated with a minimum of side effects.

Electrical asystole due to depressed pacemaker activity or effects on the A-V node by propranolol may lead to ventricular asystole. It should be remembered that the heart will still respond to mechanical or electrical stimulation in the event that propranolol produces electrical asystole or complete A-V block. Catecholamines will be of little value in restoring cardiac rhythm in the presence of β receptor blockade. Intravenous atropine may be of some value and should be tried in those instances where propranolol produces marked bradycardia. The agent of choice, however, is glucagon.

Hypotension may occur with rapid intravenous administration of propranolol due to direct effects on the vascular smooth muscle

leading to vasodilation. In addition, the cardiac actions due to β receptor blockade and direct myocardial depression further augment the fall in blood pressure.

Hypoglycemia has been reported in diabetic patients on insulin, in children during recovery from anesthesia, and in patients following partial gastrectomy. The mechanism may be related to the fact that β receptor blockade prevents adrenergic stimulation of glycogenolysis in skeletal muscle, which ordinarily would result in an increase in plasma lactate. Lactate is subsequently converted by the liver to glucose, which is added to the plasma pool.

Bronchospasm may occur in asthmatics and in normal subjects. Increased airway resistance has been observed after administration of propranolol as well as other β receptor blocking agents. Aminophylline, intravenously, will counteract the bronchospasm, but isoproterenol will not relax the bronchial smooth muscle in the presence of propranolol. β receptor blocking agents are contraindicated in patients with bronchial asthma or other chronic obstructive lung diseases.

Pregnancy is not interfered with by chronic administration of propranolol, but because the drug does cross the placenta and enters the fetal circulation, fetal cardiac responses to the stresses of labor and delivery will be blocked, as well as those of the mother (154).

It is important to remember that abrupt withdrawal of β-adrenoceptor blocking agents may be potentially dangerous for patients with ischemic heart disease. Increased incidences of angina, coronary spasm, and myocardial infarction can occur in patients who have been abruptly withdrawn from chronic β receptor blockade. The reason for this is unclear. Chronic β-adrenergic blockade may have been masking a deterioration in ischemic heart disease, or long-term β blockade may result in increased endogenous sympathetic activity.

Pharmacokinetics

Absorption. Propranolol is almost completely absorbed from the gastrointestinal tract after a single oral dose. Peak plasma concentrations are observed approximately 2 hr after an oral dose.

Metabolism and excretion. Propranolol is eliminated almost entirely by metabolism. Only 1 to 4% of a dose is recovered as unchanged drug. There are four primary pathways for the metabolism of propranolol: *O*-dealkylation, side-chain oxidation, glucuronic acid conjugation, and ring oxidation.

The major ring-hydroxylated metabolite, 4-hydroxy-propranolol, is observed in plasma only after oral administration. Other ring-hydroxylated metabolites have been identified in human plasma and urine as conjugated sulfates or glucuronides. The ring-hydroxylated metabolites of propranolol are active as β-adrenergic blocking agents, but it is not known to what extent they contribute to β-adrenergic blockade. *O*-dealkylation and side-chain oxidation account for about 20% of single oral doses and 40% of single intravenous doses.

Although propranolol is nearly completely absorbed from the intestinal tract, the systemic availability of propranolol is limited as a result of extensive first-pass extraction by the liver. When small doses of propranolol (5–30 mg) are given orally, only extremely low plasma concentrations of propranolol are detected. Larger doses (40 mg or greater) result in much higher plasma propranolol concentrations. It is uncertain if this hepatic extraction is a result of metabolism or bile excretion or another process. In oral doses above 40 mg, the hepatic extraction is approximately 70% and does not change markedly with propranolol dosage.

Kinetics. A two-compartment (biexponential) model can be used to describe plasma propranolol elimination. Pharmacokinetic parameters of propranolol are given in Table 15.

Propranolol clearance is primarily a function of the liver. In patients with normal hepatic function, clearance is limited by hepatic blood flow. Patients with hepatocellular disease have a decreased rate of propranolol metabolism and a resultant decrease in hepatic

Table 15. *Propranolol pharmacokinetics*

Percentage absorbed after oral administration	40%
Clearance	0.44–0.92 liter/min
Volume of distribution	
V_C	—
V_DSS	3–4 liters/kg
Plasma $T_{1/2}$	2–5 hr
Percentage excreted unchanged in urine	<1%
Percentage free (unbound) in plasma	4–9%
Therapeutic plasma concentrations	>40 ng/ml

clearance. Bioavailability may also be increased as a result of decreased first-pass extraction of propranolol by liver. Hepatocellular disease also decreases the plasma-protein-bound propranolol fraction and increases free propranolol concentrations at a given total plasma propranolol concentration. Hyperthyroidism may increase hepatic propranolol clearance, and hypothyroidism may decrease hepatic propranolol clearance.

Propranolol is highly bound to plasma proteins in humans (85–96%). Plasma protein binding is reduced by uremia and hepatic disease.

Therapeutic plasma propranolol concentrations vary widely and are individualized. β-adrenergic receptor blockade is achieved at plasma concentrations of 5 to 50 ng/ml. Early work suggested that plasma levels of 40 to 85 ng/ml were necessary for suppression of ectopic beats in patients with ischemic heart disease, but later work has suggested that suppression of ventricular arrhythmias may not occur in some patients until plasma concentrations of 100 ng/ml or more are achieved.

The plasma levels resulting from oral administration of propranolol to an individual are remarkably similar on repeated administrations. Between individuals, however, there is wide variation of plasma levels following oral administration, with a sevenfold range in peak plasma levels after the same dose, whereas in the same subject, interindividual plasma concentrations after intravenous administration are remarkably similar. These results were interpreted as suggesting the plasma levels differ after oral administration because of quantitative differences among individuals in the amount or rate of drug passing from the intestinal tract to the systemic circulation.

Oral Dosage

For treatment of supraventricular arrhythmias, 10 to 30 mg three or four times daily usually is sufficient. Treatment of ventricular arrhythmias may require very large doses (320 mg/day or greater) and is highly variable.

Intravenous Dosage

Intravenous administration of propranolol is reserved for life-threatening arrhythmias or those occurring under anesthesia. The usual dose is 1 to 3 mg administered under careful hemodynamic and electrocardiographic monitoring. The rate of administration should not exceed 1 mg (1 ml) per minute, to diminish the possibility of hypotension and cardiac standstill. Sufficient time should be allowed for the drug to reach the heart from the site of injection before administering another dose. No less than 2 min should pass between doses. Additional drug should not be given in less than 4 hr.

Contraindications

The most significant complication of propranolol therapy is depression of cardiac contractility, particularly in patients with congestive heart failure, and, presumably, an increased level of circulating catecholamines. The depression in contractility is thought to result from the β receptor blocking effects of the drug that cause immediate removal of adrenergic support to the myocardium. In addition, when propranolol is used at doses greater than that required to produce β receptor blockade, further cardiac depression may result from the direct effects of the drug on the contractile properties of the heart. Similar depressant effects can occur from rapid intravenous administration of the drug.

The hemodynamic status of the patient is of primary importance when the use of β receptor blocking drugs is under consideration. In the presence of myocardial infarction, extreme caution should be used when propranolol is being administered intravenously. It has been suggested that a β receptor blocking agent with intrinsic sympathomimetic properties would be a suitable alternative drug because it would have less of a myocardial depressant action.

The presence of any degree of A-V block prior to the onset of a tachyarrhythmia is a contraindication to the use of propranolol, because of its ability to further depress A-V transmission. This contraindication will not apply in the presence of a demand ventricular pacing system, in which case one can guard against ventricular standstill.

Propranolol is contraindicated in therapy for patients with frequent ventricular extrasystoles in whom the basic sinus rate is already less than 60 per minute. The β receptor blockade induced by propranolol plus its direct effect on sinoatrial pacemaker cells would further decrease the sinus rate or might induce sinoatrial arrest.

The presence of chronic obstructive airway disease is a contraindication to the use of propranolol. The resulting β receptor blockade would intensify the degree of airway obstruction.

Patients receiving anesthetic agents that tend to depress myocardial contractility (ether, enflurane, halothane) should not receive propranolol. The presence of β receptor blockade would unmask the myocardial depressant effects of the anesthetic agents. The depressant effects of the anesthetic drugs usually are counteracted by a compensatory increase in adrenergic stimulation of the heart.

Indications

Propranolol may be indicated for management of a variety of cardiac rhythm abnormalities that are totally or in part due to enhanced adrenergic stimulation. Thus, β-adrenergic receptor blockade is important with respect to several of the therapeutic actions of propranolol.

In selected cases of sinus tachycardia due to anxiety, pheochromocytoma, or thyrotoxicosis, β receptor blockade will reduce the spontaneous heart rate.

Propranolol alone or in conjunction with digitalis is of value in controlling the ventricular rate in patients with atrial flutter or atrial fibrillation. The mechanism by which propranolol produces its beneficial effect is through blockade of β-adrenergic receptor stimulation at the level of the A-V node. In addition, propranolol can produce a direct depressant effect on A-V transmission if it is administered in large doses or too rapidly by the intravenous route.

By virtue of its ability to delay A-V transmission, propranolol is an important antiarrhythmic agent in the prevention of recurrent supraventricular tachyarrhythmias associated with the WPW syndrome.

Patients with supraventricular extrasystoles and intermittent paroxysms of atrial fibrillation may benefit from the institution of β receptor blockade with propranolol.

The arrhythmias associated with halothane or cyclopropane anesthesia have been attributed to the interaction of the anesthetic with catecholamines and have been suppressed by intravenous administration of 1 to 3 mg of propranolol (155).

An increase in circulating catecholamines has been observed in patients with acute myocardial infarction and has been correlated with the development of arrhythmias (156,157). Orally administered propranolol has neither improved the survival rate nor decreased the incidence of recorded arrhythmias in patients with acute myocardial infarction.

Clinically, tachyarrhythmias associated with digitalis excess, including supraventricular and ventricular extrasystoles and tachycardia, as well as ventricular fibrillation, have been suppressed by intravenously and orally administered propranolol (158–160). In spite of the experimental evidence implicating catecholamines in the genesis of digitalis-related arrhythmias (161,162), there is sufficient experimental and clinical evidence to suggest that the suppression of this group of arrhythmias is not entirely a result of β receptor blockade (146). The dose of dl-propranolol or l-propranolol required to suppress ouabain and acetylstrophanthidin arrhythmias has consistently been greater than that required to prevent epinephrine-induced arrhythmias (12). In addition, d-propranolol suppresses digitalis-induced arrhythmias in experimental animals and in humans, and not all β-adrenergic receptor blocking agents are capable of suppressing digitalis-induced arrhythmias, although they antagonize catecholamine-induced rhythm disturbances, a finding that emphasizes that β-adrenergic blockade alone is unable to antagonize digitalis-induced arrhythmias and that some other property must explain the effectiveness of propranolol against this arrhythmia.

Propranolol has not proved effective in preventing the recurrence of atrial fibrillation after cardioversion, but the combination of propranolol and quinidine is reported to be more effective than quinidine alone. Combined use of propranolol and procainamide has proved effective in patients with persistent ventricular fibrillation.

Propranolol has not been effective in converting chronic atrial fibrillation and flutter. It is likewise ineffective in suppressing ventricular arrhythmias not due to digitalis or to exercise.

Although propranolol has been recommended for treatment of digitalis toxicity, it is not the drug of choice, because of its ability to depress myocardial contractility, depress A-V transmission, and produce bradycardia. Even though propranolol is highly effective in the treatment of digitalis-induced arrhythmias, diphenylhydantoin and lidocaine would be preferred.

Bretylium

Bretylium (Fig. 15) was introduced in 1959 as an agent for treatment of hypertension

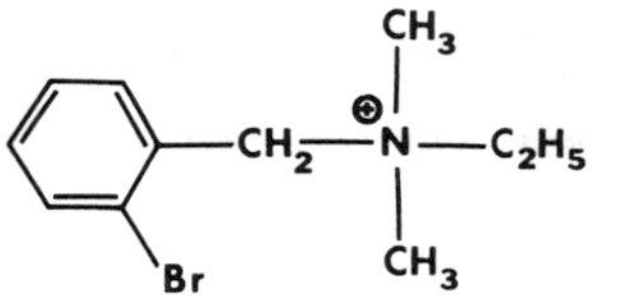

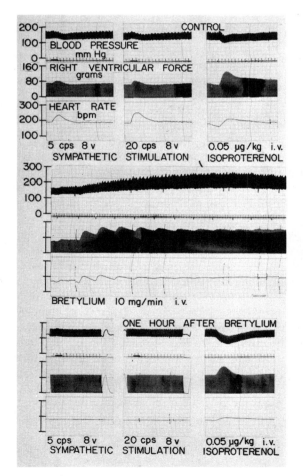

FIG. 15. Bretylium.

(163). It soon proved ineffective for clinical management of hypertension because of rapid tolerance to its antihypertensive effect.

Bretylium's antihypertensive effect is a result of inhibition of norepinephrine release from postganglionic nerve terminals of the sympathetic nervous system (164). Bretylium is highly concentrated in the postganglionic nerve terminals of adrenergic nerves and interferes with norepinephrine release without significantly altering the ultrastructural integrity of adrenergic neuronal vesicles, depressing preganglionic or postganglionic sympathetic nerve conduction, impairing sympathetic ganglionic transmission, depleting neuronal norepinephrine stores, or diminishing the responsiveness of adrenergic receptors to adrenergic agonists. This inhibition of norepinephrine release is preceded by an initial release of catecholamines from adrenergic nerve endings into the general circulation (164) (Fig. 16).

The antiarrhythmic action of bretylium was first suggested by the observation that bretylium prevented atrial fibrillation induced by acetylcholine in dogs made hypokalemic by administration of glucose and insulin (165). Subsequently it was reported that bretylium raised the electrical threshold necessary to induce ventricular fibrillation in the canine heart

FIG. 16. Cardiac effects of direct sympathetic stimulation and isoproterenol before and after administration of bretylium. Bretylium was administered at a rate of 10 mg/min to a dose of 10 mg/kg. The release of endogenous stores of norepinephrine with each administration of bretylium is indicated by the marked rises in arterial pressure, cardiac contractility, and heart rate. One hour after bretylium, stimulation of the sympathetic chain no longer elicits its characteristic effects on cardiac force and heart rate, because of the ability of the drug to block the release of norepinephrine.

(166) and markedly reduced the vulnerability of the human heart to develop ventricular fibrillation under a number of pathologic conditions (167). More important, bretylium suppresses ventricular fibrillation associated with acute myocardial infarction (168–171).

Electrophysiologic Actions

The net effects of bretylium on the electrical and mechanical properties of the heart are a composite of the direct actions of the drug on cardiac tissues and indirect actions mediated via the drug's actions on the sympathetic nervous system. These actions are summarized in Table 16.

Sinoatrial node. Bretylium administration produces an initial brief increase in sinus node automaticity (172–174). This initial increase in heart rate is blocked by cardiac denervation (174) and corresponds temporally with the release of catecholamines from sympathetic nerve terminals. No change (175) or a slight decrease (174,176) in sinus heart rate is generally observed after the initial phase of catecholamine release.

Atria. At therapeutic concentrations, the only significant action of bretylium is to prolong the action-potential duration (177). This action results in prolongation of atrial muscle effective refractory periods (173,174). The action-potential amplitude, excitability, and membrane responsiveness are not altered (177), and there does not appear to be any alteration in intraatrial conduction times (178). Quinidine-like actions (depression of membrane responsiveness and a decrease in conduction velocity in cardiac tissue) that characterize class I antiarrhythmic drugs such as quinidine, procainamide, or disopyramide are not observed with bretylium *in vivo* (173,174) and are observed in *in vitro* tissue preparations only at concentrations that are far in excess of those attained in plasma at therapeutic doses (177). Surgical denervation incompletely reverses the increase in the atrial effective refractory period observed after bretylium administration and suggests that the

Table 16. *Electrophysiologic properties of bretylium*

Tissue	Indirect action[a]	Direct action
Sinus node	Increase	Decrease
Atria		
Conduction velocity	Increase	No change
Refractory period	Decrease	Increase
Automaticity	Increase	No change
A-V node		
Conduction velocity	Increase	Decrease
Refractory period	Decrease	Increase
His-Purkinje/ventricular muscle		
Conduction velocity	Increase	No change
Refractory period	Decrease	Increase
Automaticity	Increase	No change

[a] Results from bretylium-induced release of norepinephrine from adrenergic nerve terminals.

increase in the atrial effective refractory period is a direct action of the drug on atrial muscle (174).

In clinical studies, the only prominent electrophysiologic effect of bretylium in atrial muscle is prolongation of the atrial effective refractory period (173). The effect of bretylium on conduction and refractoriness in A-V accessory pathways is unknown.

A-V node. The direct action of bretylium on the A-V node is to slow A-V nodal conduction velocity and to increase the A-V nodal refractory period (173,174). However, this action is observed primarily with large doses of bretylium. In humans, moderate bretylium doses increase conduction velocity and decrease the A-V nodal refractory period (173). This action may result from the initial catecholamine release, and the net effect of bretylium on A-V transmission with chronic therapy is unknown. However, improvement of A-V transmission as a result of the initial catecholamine release excludes bretylium from clinical use in the presence of atrial fibrillation or atrial flutter, as a dangerous acceleration of ventricular rate may occur. Bretylium should not be administered in the presence of A-V block resulting from digitalis glycoside toxicity. Although the initial phase of catecholamine release will improve A-V transmission, catecholamine release will also potentiate digitalis-induced ventricular automaticity and may lead to ventricular fibrillation (179).

His-Purkinje system/ventricular muscle. Quinidinelike actions (decreased membrane responsiveness and decreased conduction velocity) associated with class I antiarrhythmic agents are not observed with bretylium (18,19,174) and are not responsible for the antifibrillatory actions of the drug. At therapeutic concentrations, the predominant effect of bretylium on the canine Purkinje cell and ventricular muscle is an increase in the action-potential duration (18,19), resulting in an increase in the effective refractory period (174). The increase in the effective refractory period in Purkinje cells and ventricular muscle is greater than that observed with other currently approved antiarrhythmic agents and is the property that distinguishes bretylium as a member of the class III antiarrhythmic agents. Prolongation of the action-potential duration and effective refractory period cannot be explained by the actions of the drug on the sympathetic nervous system, as the action-potential duration and effective refractory periods are prolonged in denervated hearts (174), reserpine-pretreated animals (18), and hearts lacking intact sympathetic nervous system innervation (180).

The initial catecholamine release brings about an increase in Purkinje cell automaticity (18,19) and will increase the rate of a ventricular escape rhythm (174). This increase in the rate of ectopic impulse formation is most prominent in ventricular tissue that has been damaged by myocardial ischemia (181). Reserpine pretreatment prevents the increase in Purkinje cell automaticity (18).

The most prominent electrophysiologic action of bretylium is to raise the intensity of electrical current necessary to induce ventricular fibrillation (166,182–185). This action is dramatic and is more prominent with bretylium than with any other currently available antiarrhythmic agent (disopyramide, lidocaine, phenytoin, procainamide, propranolol, and quinidine) and can be observed in both

normal (166,182,184,185) and ischemic hearts (183,185). Spontaneous conversion of ventricular fibrillation to sinus rhythm in humans has been observed after bretylium administration (186). Chemical defibrillation has not been observed with other antiarrhythmic agents and is a property possessed by bretylium and other experimental quaternary ammonium compounds (186,187). The antifibrillatory actions of bretylium are not believed to result from bretylium's actions on the sympathetic nervous system, as guanethidine, a compound that exerts similar actions on the sympathetic nervous system, fails to exert antifibrillatory effects in canine myocardium (182,188). Bretylium is equally as effective in reserpinized hearts (188) and hearts lacking an intact adrenergic innervation (180) as in normal hearts. UM-360, a structural analogue of bretylium that lacks the catecholamine-releasing action and adrenergic blocking action of bretylium, exerts a similar antifibrillatory action (184).

Currently approved antiarrhythmic agents (quinidine, lidocaine, phenytoin, disopyramide, procainamide, and propranolol) raise the current necessary to defibrillate canine hearts (189). In contrast to this action, bretylium lowers the electrical threshold for successful defibrillation (190). This beneficial action of bretylium was previously reported by Holder et al. (168), who showed an increased rate of successful defibrillations after bretylium administration.

Hemodynamic and Cardiovascular Effects

A unique property of bretylium as an antiarrhythmic agent is its positive inotropic action (191–193). This action is related to the initial release of neuronal stores of norepinephrine associated with bretylium administration.

Bretylium's actions on the sympathetic nervous system include (a) an initial release of neuronal stores of norepinephrine and (b) an inhibition of norepinephrine release resulting from sympathetic nerve stimulation. The initial phase of catecholamine release may be associated with transient hypertension (172, 175), although the most commonly observed side effect of bretylium is hypotension associated with the later development of adrenergic neuronal blockade (166,167,170–172,191). The onset of hypotension is delayed 1 to 2 hr, as the initial catecholamine release maintains arterial pressure prior to this time. Hypotension is most commonly postural, but marked reductions in supine blood pressure have been reported (175,176). Despite decreases in peripheral resistance and arterial pressure, cardiac output is maintained, and pulmonary capillary wedge pressure is not altered (191).

The hazards involved with bretylium administration, especially in the patient with acute myocardial infarction, include its positive inotropic and chronotropic effects, which may aggravate existing myocardial ischemia by further increasing myocardial oxygen requirements. Because bretylium has the potential to interfere with adrenergic tone to the heart and peripheral vasculature, it may cause further deterioration of an already compromised hemodynamic status.

Bretylium has been reported to eliminate heart block and stimulate pacemaker activity (170). The low incidence of heart block of 1.6% in patients treated with bretylium, as compared with 12% in an earlier study, has suggested that bretylium prevents the emergence of heart block.

Toxic Reactions

The most important side effect associated with the use of bretylium is hypotension, a result of peripheral vasodilatation caused by adrenergic neuronal blockade. Hypotension, when it does occur, is reversed readily by intravenous fluid to increase circulating blood volume and by cautious administration of intravenous norepinephrine. Bradycardia resulting from adrenergic neuronal blockade has been observed in some patients receiving bretylium. Nausea, vomiting, and diarrhea have been reported with intravenous administration

and can be minimized by slow infusion. Longer-term problems include swelling and tenderness of the parotid gland, particularly occurring at meal time.

Pharmacokinetics

Bretylium, a quaternary ammonium compound with a fixed positive charge, has poor systemic availability after oral administration. Plasma concentrations after oral administration are erratic, reaching peak concentrations in about 3 hr with only 10 to 30% of an oral dose reaching the general circulation. Bretylium is well absorbed after intramuscular injection, with peak plasma levels being attained within 1 hr.

No metabolites of bretylium have been observed in any animal species, and the drug is excreted almost entirely by renal mechanisms. More than 90% of oral, intramuscular, and intravenous doses are excreted unchanged in the urine over a period of 48 hr. The remaining 10% is excreted over the ensuing 3 days. Renal clearance is rapid and approaches that of total renal blood flow at lower bretylium plasma concentrations. This suggests that active secretion of bretylium takes place in the renal tubules. Clearance of bretylium by the kidney is reduced by renal disease, but it is not known to what extent drug dosage must be altered in such clinical conditions. Renal clearance of bretylium is dependent on the amount in the plasma and is more rapid at lower plasma bretylium concentrations.

Pharmacokinetic values for bretylium are given in Table 17. Bretylium's disappearance from plasma is a multiexponential function and is poorly described by a biexponential function. The concentration of bretylium in plasma has not been correlated with the intensity of its antiarrhythmic response and at the present time cannot be used as a guide for therapy. There is a complex relationship (185) between plasma bretylium concentrations, myocardial bretylium concentrations, and antifibrillatory activity. The electrophysiologic actions (166,182,185) and clinical efficacy

Table 17. *Pharmacokinetics of bretylium*

Percentage absorbed after oral administration	10–30%
Clearance	3–12 ml/kg/min (concentration-dependent)
Volume of distribution	
V_C	5.3 liters/kg
V_DSS	3.4 liters/kg
Plasma $T_{1/2}$	8–13 hr
Percentage excreted unchanged in urine	>90%
Percentage free (unbound) in plasma	100%
Therapeutic plasma concentrations	Not known

(170,171,175) of bretylium are not immediately apparent, and a delay in onset of 3 to 6 hr may occur. Despite the rapid elimination of bretylium from plasma, the antiarrhythmic action of bretylium may persist for 8 to 14 hr or more after intravenous administration (170,171,175).

Dosage and Administration

Bretylium is to be used clinically for treatment of life-threatening ventricular arrhythmias under constant electrocardiographic monitoring. Because there is a delay in onset of its antiarrhythmic action, bretylium is not to be considered or used as a replacement for rapidly acting antiarrhythmic agents currently in use. Patients should either be kept supine during the course of bretylium therapy or be closely observed for postural hypotension. The optimal dose schedule for parenteral administration of bretylium has not been determined. There is comparatively little experience with dosages greater than 30 mg/kg/day, although such doses have been used without apparent adverse effects. The following schedule is suggested.

For immediately life-threatening ventricular arrhythmias, as in ventricular fibrillation. Administer undiluted bretylium at a dosage of 5 mg/kg body weight by rapid intravenous injection. Other usual cardiopulmonary resuscitative procedures, including electrical cardi-

oversion, should be employed prior to and following the injection in accordance with good medical practice. If ventricular fibrillation persists, the dosage may be increased to 10 mg/kg and repeated at 15- to 30-min intervals until a total dose of not more than 30 mg/kg body weight has been given.

For prevention of recurrent ventricular tachycardia and/or fibrillation (intravenous use). Administer a dosage of 5 to 10 mg bretylium per kilogram of body weight by intravenous infusion over a period greater than 8 min. More rapid infusion may cause nausea and vomiting. A second dose may be given in 1 to 2 hr if tachyarrhythmia recurs.

For intramuscular injection. Inject 5 to 10 mg bretylium per kilogram of body weight. Dosage may be repeated in 1 to 2 hr if the arrhythmia persists. Thereafter, maintain with same dosage every 6 to 8 hr.

Intramuscular injection should not be made directly into or near a major nerve, and the sites of injection should be varied on repeated injection.

Maintenance dosage. The diluted bretylium solution may be administered by intermittent intravenous infusion or by constant infusion.

Intermittent infusion. Infuse the diluted solution at a dosage of 5 to 10 mg bretylium per kilogram of body weight over a period greater than 8 min, every 6 hr. More rapid infusion may cause nausea and vomiting.

Constant infusion. Infuse the diluted solution at a dosage of 1 to 2 mg bretylium per minute. Dosage of bretylium should be reduced and discontinued in 3 to 5 days under electrocardiographic monitoring. Other appropriate antiarrhythmic agents should be substituted, if indicated.

Contraindications

The pharmacologic properties of bretylium should dictate in which instances the drug will be contraindicated. The associated release of catecholamines could result in an excessive pressor rise and stimulation of cardiac force and pacemaker activity. The resulting increase in myocardial oxygen consumption in a patient with ischemic heart disease could lead to the development of ischemic pain (angina pectoris).

Patients in a state of circulatory shock should probably not be administered bretylium, because of its delayed sympatholytic action, which would cause further deterioration of the hemodynamic state of the individual.

Indications

Bretylium is not to be considered a first-line antiarrhythmic agent. However, because of its ability to prolong the refractory period of Purkinje fibers and to elevate the electrical threshold to ventricular fibrillation, bretylium has been studied and found useful in the treatment of life-threatening ventricular arrhythmias, principally recurrent ventricular tachycardia and/or ventricular fibrillation, especially when conventional therapeutic agents such as lidocaine or procainamide prove to be ineffective. In addition, bretylium is known to facilitate the ease with which precordial shock reverses ventricular fibrillation (168,190). In the latter instance, because of the emergent nature of the patient's clinical state, the drug is administered intravenously in dosages of 5 to 10 mg/kg as a rapid bolus, followed by external cardiac massage and repeated attempts at electrical defibrillation. It is not unusual for bretylium, when administered in the presence of ventricular fibrillation and accompanied by external cardiac massage, to result in defibrillation and a return to coordinated cardiac rhythm. Bretylium is therefore capable of producing chemical defibrillation when its administration is accompanied by cardiopulmonary resuscitative procedures.

It is important to recognize that the use of bretylium for the prevention of recurrent ventricular tachycardia and/or ventricular fibrillation may lead to apparent disappointing results because of the fact that the onset of its antifibrillatory effect may be delayed for as long as 6 hr. Thus, the drug has a delayed onset of action when given as a slow intravenous infusion. The delay in its onset of action is undoubtedly related to the fact that the drug must achieve a critical concentration in myocardial tissue before it can favorably alter the electrophysiologic properties of the heart. Furthermore, the release of norepinephrine from cardiac nerve endings during the administration of bretylium may actually increase the frequency of ventricular premature complexes, an event that is worsened by rapid intravenous administration of the drug.

It was long assumed that the antifibrillatory effects of bretylium were associated with the ability of bretylium to produce adrenergic neuronal blockade as a result of the drug being accumulated in sympathetic nerve fibers. It is now appreciated that the adrenergic neuronal blocking action is unnecessary for bretylium to produce its protective effects against the recurrence of ventricular tachycardia and/or ventricular fibrillation. Previous administration of a tricyclic antidepressant drug, such as protriptyline or doxepin, which effectively blocks the amine uptake mechanism in adrenergic neurons, will prevent bretylium from gaining access to the adrenergic nerves. Thus, the catecholamine release and subsequent sympatholytic effects of bretylium can be prevented without affecting the electrophysiologic effects of the quaternary amine on the heart, therefore retaining the potential to confer an antifibrillatory effect. This form of pharmacologic antagonism can put to good use when it becomes necessary to avoid excessive hypotension in a patient in need of the protective effects of bretylium.

Present indications for the use of bretylium limit its administration to no longer than 5 days. The drug is available for parenteral use only. However, a limited number of patients known to be at risk of developing recurrent ventricular fibrillation have been managed successfully for long terms by first being administered an intravenous dosing regimen for 24 to 48 hr and then being placed on oral drug (300–600 mg every 6 hr) (171,194,195). Repeated determinations of plasma and urine bretylium concentrations have confirmed the ability of the drug to be absorbed after oral administration (195). More important, bretylium has the potential of becoming an important agent for the management of patients who are at a high risk of sudden coronary death. The low incidences of side effects following chronic administration make bretylium and other quaternary ammonium agents attractive drugs for future study in an attempt to reduce the incidence of sudden coronary death.

Verapamil

Verapamil (Isoptin®, Calan®) (Fig. 17) was intended initially as a synthetic substitute for the smooth-muscle relaxant papaverine. The drug was studied for its peripheral and coronary vasodilator properties in preclinical and clinical settings. Because of its ability to affect coronary vascular smooth muscle, much attention has been focused on the use of verapamil as a therapeutic intervention in the management of patients with variant angina pectoris (Prinzmetal's angina), as well as patients with effort-induced angina pectoris.

Although it was first thought to be a specific inhibitor of β-adrenergic receptors, subsequent experimental studies revealed that verapamil, in addition to possessing antiarrhythmic properties, produced selective inhibition of transmembrane calcium fluxes in myocardial cells by affecting a secondary inward depolarizing current that flows through a slow channel. This current is carried primarily by calcium ions, and voltage changes due to this current are referred to as slow-channel depolarizations or slow responses.

The transmembrane action potentials obtained from cells in the sinoatrial and A-V nodes show potentials with the characteristics of slow-channel calcium currents. Thus, depolarization within the sinoatrial and A-V nodal regions may depend on an inward current through the slow channel and one that is susceptible to the inhibitory effects of verapamil and other slow-channel calcium antagonists, thereby accounting for the use of the agent in supraventricular A-V nodal reentrant arrhythmias (196,197).

Electrophysiologic Actions

When studied in myocardial tissues in clinically relevant concentrations, verapamil fails to elicit effects characteristic of those produced by the class I, II, or III antiarrhythmic drugs. Evidence that excitation-contraction coupling in mammalian heart muscle could be blocked *in vitro* and *in vivo* by pharmacologic means was first presented by Fleckenstein (198). The calcium antagonism by verapamil is considered to be a specific action, as opposed to nonspecific calcium-antagonistic effects obtained with high dosages of barbiturates or certain β-adrenergic receptor blocking agents. Thus, the specific calcium antagonists produce their effects at concentrations at which other pharmacologic actions are negligible. Exposure of guinea pig isolated papillary muscle to increasing concentrations of verapamil (2×10^{-6} M to 1×10^{-5} M) results in a progressive loss of contractility without affecting the membrane resting potential or the action-potential parameters, such as upstroke velocity and height of the overshoot (199). These findings indicate that the transmembrane sodium flux across the fast channel is unchanged by verapamil. The inhibitory effects of verapamil on calcium influx and contractile tension can be overcome by addition of calcium or isoproterenol.

Sinoatrial node. Pacemaker activity in the sinoatrial node has an ionic mechanism completely different from action potentials generated in Purkinje fibers or ordinary atrial muscle cells. Spontaneous phase-4 depolarization,

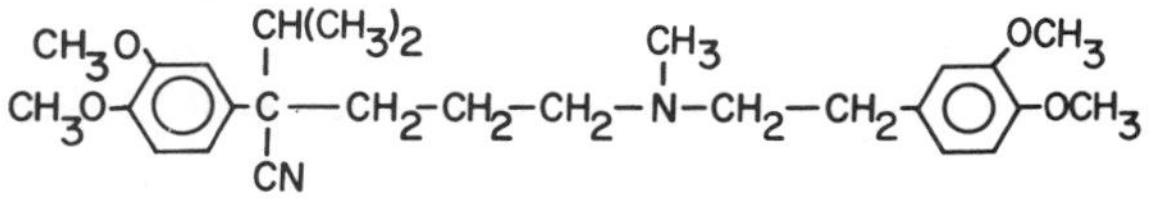

FIG. 17. Verapamil.

a characteristic of normal sinoatrial nodal cells, relies on deactivation of an outward current that is selective for potassium ions and a slow inward current that is carried by sodium and calcium ions. Thus, from the standpoint of verapamil's effect on inward calcium ion fluxes, it is understandable why the drug depresses phase-4 depolarization in the sinoatrial node. Verapamil produces reductions in the rate of rise and the slope of diastolic slow depolarization, the maximal diastolic potential, and the membrane potential at the peak of depolarization in the sinoatrial node (200,201). These findings provide additional support for the belief that the slow-channel calcium current is of primary importance in the genesis of sinoatrial nodal pacemaker activity. *In vivo,* the direct effect of verapamil on sinoatrial nodal function will be manifest as a decrease in heart rate (negative chronotropic effect). However, cardiovascular reflexes in response to the changes in cardiac output and peripheral vascular resistance will result in enhancement of cardiac sympathetic tone, thereby masking the direct negative chronotropic effects of verapamil.

Atrium. Verapamil fails to exert any significant electrophysiologic effects on atrial muscle. Although contractile force is depressed, the only change in the action potential of atrial muscle fibers is a shortening of the early phase of repolarization. This is not unexpected, because the early phase of repolarization or phase 2 is dependent on the slow inward calcium current that is antagonized by verapamil. Electrophysiologic recordings from diseased atrial tissue obtained during surgery have demonstrated that verapamil can inhibit spontaneous diastolic activity, therefore suggesting the participation of the slow-channel calcium current in the genesis of human atrial rhythm disorders (202). These findings are of significance in view of the potential role of verapamil in the clinical management of supraventricular arrhythmias.

A-V node. Action potentials from the nodal region of the A-V junction resemble slow responses, although automaticity is not a property of the true nodal region of the A-V junction. The speed of conduction in the nodal region is quite slow. Conduction block is common, and graded electrical responses are frequent. In addition, refractoriness in A-V nodal tissue outlasts the action-potential duration. These observations suggest that depolarization in A-V nodal cells, like that in sinoatrial nodal tissue, is dependent on an inward current through the slow channel. It is well known that A-V nodal conduction is depressed by pharmacologic agents that block the slow-channel calcium current. Verapamil would therefore be expected to impair conduction across the A-V node and prolong the A-V nodal refractory period at plasma concentrations that show no effect on the His-Purkinje system. A-V nodal reentry, one mechanism for maintaining reciprocating tachycardia, is prevented by verapamil, and this accounts for the effectiveness of verapamil in the treatment of supraventricular tachyarrhythmias (203). This action agrees with the role of the slow-channel calcium current in A-V nodal transmission and the proposed cellular mechanism of action of verapamil.

His-Purkinje system/ventricular muscle. In clinically relevant concentrations, verapamil does not have electrophysiologic effects of the class I antiarrhythmic drugs. When examined in canine Purkinje fiber action potentials, verapamil had no effect on the action-potential amplitude or V_{max} or on resting membrane potential. However, the slope of phase-2 repolarization is increased by verapamil. These changes are consistent with the block of a slow inward current such as that carried by the calcium ion (202). Further evidence for a lack of effect on the His-Purkinje system was obtained from data showing that verapamil failed to produce any change in the QRS and QT_c intervals. The only significant electrocardiographic change was a prolongation of the PR interval, a response consistent with the known effects of the drug on A-V nodal transmission (204).

His-bundle studies have provided further evidence that verapamil is without effect on intraatrial and intraventricular conduction. The predominant electrophysiologic effect is on A-V conduction proximal to the His bundle.

Hemodynamic Effects

Studies on isolated cardiac muscle preparations have shown verapamil to possess a negative inotropic action, a response consistent with its ability to reduce influx of calcium during the rapid phase of depolarization as well as phase 2 of the action-potential plateau. The negative inotropic effect can be counteracted by calcium, catecholamines, glucagon, and digitalis glycosides. When administered to intact animals or to humans, verapamil shows a dose-dependent negative inotropic effect that is modified by reflex sympathetic responses. Verapamil produces peripheral vasodilatation by a direct relaxant effect on vascular smooth muscle. The peripheral vasodilatation results in changes in preload and afterload and changes in cardiac sympathetic tone that exert a complex interplay of factors affecting stroke volume and cardiac output. The negative inotropic action exerted by verapamil and the expected reduction in cardiac output are minimized by the effects of the drug on left ventricular afterload. The usual intravenous dose of verapamil employed for antiarrhythmic effects (10 mg) is not associated with marked alterations in arterial blood pressure, peripheral vascular resistance, heart rate, left ventricular end-diastolic pressure, or contractility. The changes that do occur on intravenous administration are short-lived. It must be recalled that the presence of an intact cardiac sympathetic nervous system markedly attenuates the cardiac depressant effects of the calcium antagonist. On the other hand, profound cardiac depression and disturbances in A-V conduction are more likely to occur when verapamil is administered concomitantly with propranolol or other β-adrenergic receptor blocking agents. The same concerns regarding the negative inotropic effects of verapamil might apply to the patient with severe cardiac decompensation or acute myocardial infarction.

Because of its capacity to modify calcium ion fluxes in vascular smooth muscle and thus interfere with excitation-contracting coupling, verapamil elicits relaxation of peripheral vessels as well as those supplying the myocardium. The coronary vasodilator effects of verapamil plus its ability to decrease myocardial contractility and afterload and thus reduce myocardial oxygen consumption have suggested its use in the management of patients with effort-induced angina pectoris and in variant angina. In the latter instance, where myocardial ischemia is related to coronary vasospasm, the vasodilator effect of verapamil appears to have major importance in preventing the recurrence of ischemic episodes.

The antianginal properties of verapamil have been attributed to its coronary vasodilator effects. However, selective coronary vasodilators have not proved effective in abolishing ischemic symptoms associated with effort-induced angina pectoris. The coronary vasodilator effects of verapamil have been revealed in studies in animals or in isolated perfused hearts. When administered to patients with coronary artery disease, verapamil fails to dilate the diseased coronary vascular segments and does not improve regional coronary blood flow (205,206).

Administration of verapamil to patients with coronary artery disease resulted in a decrease in coronary blood flow at rest and during pacing stress that was of sufficient magnitude to always cause angina pectoris in the period before drug administration (207). Intravenous administration of verapamil results in decreases in mean aortic blood pressure and myocardial oxygen consumption.

Therefore, in patients with exertional or effort-induced angina pectoris, the beneficial effect of verapamil is not primarily due to its coronary vasodilator actions. Instead, verapamil decreases myocardial oxygen consumption, which most likely accounts for its ability to improve exercise tolerance by restoring the balance between myocardial oxygen supply and demand. In the presence of vasospastic or variant angina, the vasodilator effect undoubtedly plays a major role in preventing myocardial ischemia. This effect can be attributed to verapamil's inhibition of the slow-channel calcium flux in coronary vascular smooth muscle and is seen with other slow-channel calcium antagonists as well (208).

Toxic Reactions

The administration of oral verapamil is well tolerated by the majority of patients. Most complaints are with respect to gastrointestinal side effects of constipation and gastric discomfort. Other complaints include vertigo, headache, nervousness, and pruritus.

The intravenous route of administration is associated with transient and mild decreases in blood pressure. However, because the drug has such a prominent effect on cellular fluxes of calcium, rapid intravenous administration or excessive dosage could lead to cardiac depression, both mechanically and electrically, along with peripheral vasodilation and hypotension. Cardiac depression and ventricular asystole are more prone to develop in patients given verapamil while concomitantly receiving propranolol.

Verapamil should not be administered or should be given with great caution to patients with sick-sinus syndrome, disturbances in A-V conduction, or severe congestive heart failure, unless the low output state can be attributed to a persistent rapid atrial tachyarrhythmia, in which case the reversion to sinus rhythm produced by verapamil will lead to improvement in cardiac function.

The combined actions of digitalis and verapamil seem to impose no special deleterious effect unless A-V conduction is already compromised, in which case further impairment of conduction can occur as a result of verapamil's effect on the A-V node, which will add to the effects of digitalis. The negative inotropic effect of verapamil could negate some of the benefits to be derived from the positive inotropic actions of digitalis. Likewise, digitalis glycosides could overcome the negative inotropic effects of verapamil. The potential use of verapamil in patients with acute myocardial infarction from the control of arrhythmias, or as a means of preserving jeopardized ischemic myocardium, has not been established.

Pharmacokinetics

Examination of the hemodynamic effects after a single intravenous dose of verapamil would suggest that the drug possesses a relatively short pharmacologic half-life. The maximum cardiovascular actions are observed within 3 to 5 min, with almost complete return to baseline values within 10 to 20 min. Similar observations with respect to pharmacologic effects have been made in patients with atrial fibrillation, in whom the ventricular rate in response to verapamil was noted to decrease within a few minutes after drug administration, only to resume the initial rate within a short time. On the other hand, measurements of the A-H intervals of His-Purkinje electrocardiograms indicated that a single intravenous dose of verapamil exerted electrophysiologic effects that became apparent within 1 to 2 min, reaching a maximum effect at 10 min, with residual effects being recorded for up to 6 hr.

Studies using oral verapamil have shown that the drug is active by this route of administration, with initial effects being apparent within 2 hr and a maximum effect being obtained within 5 hr, as determined by the ability of the agent to modify the electrophysiologic properties of the A-V node in humans. Thus, in evaluating pharmacokinetic data and the pharmacologic actions of verapamil, one might conclude that the two may not correlate with respect to their temporal relationships. One possibility is that verapamil or an active metabolite accumulates in cardiac tissue and continues to exert electrophysiologic effects independent of the plasma concentration of the drug. On the basis of electrophysiologic studies, there seems to be a preferential uptake by the A-V nodal tissues, because the duration of the depressant effect of verapamil on the A-V node appears to considerably outlast the duration of the hemodynamic actions of the drug.

Although verapamil exhibits almost complete absorption from the gastrointestinal tract, the drug undergoes a substantial degree of metabolism during its first pass through the hepatic portal circulation, so that overall bioavailability is about 10 to 20%. Furthermore, the drug is highly bound by plasma proteins, and only 10% of the drug in the plasma exists in the free form.

Because of the extensive first-pass metabolism of verapamil, only low concentrations of drug can be measured in the plasma, and only negligible amounts are excreted unchanged in the urine and feces. The concentrations of the N-demethylated and N-dealkylated metabolites rise gradually with continued administration of verapamil. Because the pharmacologic activities of the metabolites might contribute to the overall therapeutic response, it is not possible to predict the therapeutic plasma concentration of verapamil. Further study must be conducted to clarify this matter, and renewed approaches to examining the pharmacokinetics of verapamil and its metabolites seem warranted. Table 18 presents a summary of current pharmacokinetic data on verapamil.

Dosage

The studies to date with verapamil have focused primarily on its use in the management of patients with supraventricular tachyarrhythmias, although the drug has potential use in the treatment of patients with effort-induced angina pectoris and variant angina.

In the management of atrial tachyarrhythmias, the most frequently used intravenous dose has been 10 mg or 0.145 mg/kg given as a single injection over 10 to 15 min or longer in order to reduce the potential hazard of inducing left ventricular failure and/or A-V block. A second dose can be repeated in 30 min if the initial response is unsatisfac-

Table 18. *Verapamil pharmacokinetics*

Percentage absorbed after oral administration	90%
Percentage bioavailability due to first-pass metabolism clearance	10–20%
Volume of distribution	6.5 liters/kg
Plasma $T_{1/2}$	3–7 hr
Percentage excreted in:	
Urine (mostly as metabolite)	70%
Feces (mostly as metabolite)	16%
Percentage free in plasma	10%
Therapeutic plasma concentrations	Unknown because of possible contribution of metabolites to therapeutic action

tory. The drug has been given as a continuous infusion at the rate of 0.1 mg/min. Experience in children, although limited, has suggested that an intravenous dose of 3.5 to 5.0 mg has been successful in converting paroxysmal supraventricular tachycardia.

Because of the extensive first-pass hepatic metabolism, the oral dose of verapamil is 8 to 10 times greater than the intravenous dose. Thus, long-term oral dosage for prophylaxis against supraventricular arrhythmias has required doses up to 120 or 160 mg 2 or 3 times daily. The usual starting dosage is 40 to 80 mg every 8 hr. The dosage can be increased over 2 to 3 days if needed, and in the absence of known contraindications a dosage of 720 mg/day is possible. A slow-release form of verapamil is under investigation, and it is likely that a single daily dose of 240 mg may suffice.

Contraindications

Verapamil must be used with extreme caution or not at all in patients who are receiving β-adrenergic receptor blocking agents. Because verapamil has the ability to antagonize the movement of calcium ion via the slow channel, it will exert its primary depressant effects on the sinoatrial and A-V nodes. Thus, the heart rate and A-V conduction velocity will be decreased. In the absence of other therapeutic interventions, the negative chronotropic and dromotropic effects of verapamil will, in part, be overcome by an increase in reflex sympathetic tone. The latter would be prevented by simultaneous administration of a β receptor blocking agent, thus exaggerating the depressant effects of verapamil on heart rate and A-V conduction. Needless to say, the negative inotropic effects of verapamil would be greater in the presence of a β receptor blocking agent, thus adding to the potential of the calcium antagonist to depress ventricular function.

The direct negative chronotropic effects of verapamil preclude its use in patients with sick-sinus syndrome. Because of the dependence of the A-V nodal cells on the slow-channel calcium current, verapamil is contraindicated in those instances where A-V conduction is impaired.

It is noteworthy that the depressant effects of verapamil on sinoatrial and A-V nodal functions, as well as on ventricular muscle contraction, can be overcome by the use of cardiac β-adrenergic receptor agonists such as norepinephrine, dopamine, dobutamine, and isoproterenol. The pancreatic hormone glucagon will likewise reverse the depression of ventricular contraction induced by verapamil, especially if it occurs in the presence of a β receptor blocking agent, in which instance cardiac β receptor agonists are likely to be of minimal value. Whereas digitalis glycosides will reverse the negative inotropic effects of verapamil, they may produce a further decrease in A-V node function.

In patients with congestive heart failure, verapamil must be used with caution, if at all, and further experience is needed in this area.

Because of the dependence on renal function for elimination of verapamil and/or its metabolites, the drug should be used cautiously

and at reduced dosage in patients with impaired renal function.

Indications

Verapamil has been approved by the Food and Drug Administration for use in the United States under the trade names Isoptin® and Calan® after many years of use in Europe and clinical investigation in this country.

Clinical studies indicate that verapamil has a narrow spectrum of antiarrhythmic effectiveness. It appears to be most valuable as an antiarrhythmic drug in the management of patients with atrial tachyarrhythmias, where the negative dromotropic effects on the A-V node lead to control of the ventricular rate or abolish the reentrant mechanism within the A-V node, thus restoring normal sinus rhythm.

Reentrant paroxysmal supraventricular tachycardia involving the sinoatrial or A-V nodes has responded favorably to verapamil, both for the acute attack and for prevention of recurrences of the tachyarrhythmias. There has been some success in reversion of atrial flutter and atrial fibrillation to sinus rhythm, but more often the drug exerts its benefits by virtue of its ability to decrease the ventricular response to the atrial tachyarrhythmia.

A distinct advantage of verapamil in supraventricular tachyarrhythmias is its rapid onset of effect. In paroxysmal supraventricular tachycardia, the drug is 80 to 100% effective in restoring sinus rhythm and offers an advantage over current therapy, which may require the use of digitalis glycosides when vagal maneuvers have failed.

The use of verapamil in tachyarrhythmias associated with the WPW syndrome offers another therapeutic application. Intracardiac recordings have shown that verapamil does not alter the electrophysiologic properties of the atrial bypass tract and thus would be of little value in atrial fibrillation in the presence of an anomalous pathway in which the fibrillatory impulses enter the ventricles via the accessory pathway. However, the ability of ver-

Table 19. *Potential clinical uses of verapamil and other slow-channel calcium antagonists*

Arrhythmias
    Sinoatrial and A-V nodal reentrant tachyarrhythmias (PAT)
    Atrial flutter
    Atrial fibrillation
    Tachyarrhythmias associated with WPW syndrome
Angina pectoris
    Effort-induced angina
    Prinzmetal's angina
Obstructive cardiomyopathy
Essential hypertension
Cardioplegic protection of ischemic heart

apamil to alter A-V nodal conduction may allow the drug to exert a beneficial effect in WPW tachyarrhythmias where the A-V node serves as the pathway for antegrade conduction. Verapamil would prolong the refractoriness of the A-V node and interrupt the reentrant rhythm, even though the electrophysiologic properties of the accessory path are unaffected.

In addition to its use in the management of atrial rhythm disorders, verapamil and other slow-channel antagonists (nifedipine, diltiazem) are known to be effective therapeutic agents in the management of patients with vasospastic angina pectoris (Prinzmetal's angina, variant angina), as well as in effort-induced angina. A wide variety of clinical entities (Table 19) have been reported to be benefited by verapamil and related slow-channel calcium blocking agents. With the recent introduction of verapamil, clinical experience will undoubtedly determine the full extent to which this new class of drugs can be employed.

New Antiarrhythmic Drugs Under Clinical Investigation

Recent years have witnessed an intensified search for new and more effective antidysrhythmic drugs that lack important side effects when administered chronically. Part of the stimulus for new investigative efforts has been the recognition that sudden coronary death constitutes a major problem in the United States, as well as elsewhere in the world, and that the currently available antiarrhythmic agents either are ineffective in the prevention of sudden coronary death or are limited by serious toxicity when administered on a chronic basis. Thus, the development and clinical evaluation of safe, effective, and longlasting antidysrhythmic drugs present an immediate challenge to the cardiovascular pharmacologist. At present, a number of new agents for the management of patients with cardiac rhythm disorders are under clinical trial. This section will present a brief review of those that have been developed to a sufficient extent to permit discussion of their pharmacology and potential therapeutic applications.

Ethmozin

Ethmozin (Fig. 18) is the ethyl ester hydrochloride of 10-(3-morpholinopropronyl)phenothiazine-2-carbonic acid. The agent was developed in the Soviet Union and recently has undergone clinical evaluation in the United States.

Electrophysiologic studies on isolated nonischemic Purkinje fibers from the canine heart have demonstrated that the drug has properties similar to those of lidocaine, so that ethmozin could be categorized as a class I antiarrhythmic agent (209,210). Accordingly, ethmozin produces a dose-dependent decrease in the maximum upstroke velocity of phase-0 depolarization, presumably through inhibition of sodium ion conductance during excitation of the myocardial cell membrane. In addition, ethmozin results in a decrease in the duration of the membrane action potential. Contrary to what is observed with other class I antiarrhythmic agents, however, was the observation that ethmozin did not affect the slope of phase-4 depolarization of spontaneous automatic Purkinje fibers, but did suppress automaticity in Purkinje fibers obtained from canine hearts previously subjected to myocardial ischemia. In the intact dog, ethmozin was

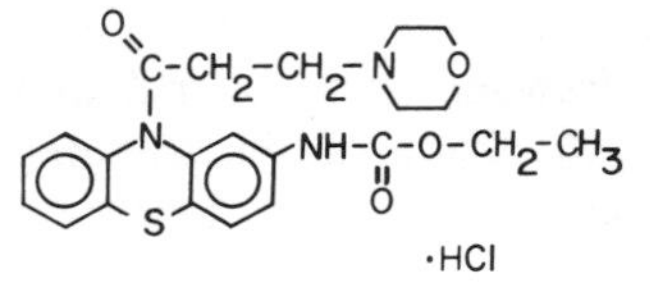

FIG. 18. Ethmozin.

effective in suppressing ventricular arrhythmias that were present after experimentally induced myocardial infarction, and it was reported to be more effective than quinidine (210).

Ethmozin administered at a dose of 500 mg orally to normal volunteers showed a mean elimination half-life of 4 ± 1 hr, with a range of 2.1 to 5.1 hr. Patients with atrial premature contractions and ventricular premature contractions showed significant decreases in ectopic frequency at plasma concentrations that averaged 597 ± 48 ng/ml (range 244–1,300 ng/ml).

The drug was reported to be well absorbed orally and well tolerated, with the only reported symptom being mild nausea. More extensive studies are needed to determine its efficacy and safety. In view of its structural similarity to the phenothiazines, one might expect ethmozin to share some of the side effects of the phenothiazine drugs.

The limited studies to date with ethmozin have used oral maintenance dosages of 75 to 150 mg given every 6 hr. Some clinical trials have been conducted in which the drug was given at an oral dosage of 250 mg every 8 hr. The drug is most likely metabolized via hepatic mechanisms, but only limited information is available on the mechanism of clearance from the body.

Encainide

Encainide, (Fig. 19), 4-methoxy-2'-(1-methyl-2-piperidylethyl)benzanidide hydrochloride, can be categorized as a class I antiarrhythmic agent showing direct membrane depressant properties when studied on canine cardiac Purkinje fibers. At concentrations of 10^{-5} M, encainide reduced the action-potential amplitude and upstroke velocity (maximum

dV/dt). The action-potential duration was reduced, but refractoriness was not affected. Spontaneous diastolic depolarization in Purkinje fibers was depressed by encainide (211).

In closed-chest anesthetized dogs, encainide given at intravenous doses of 0.3 to 2.7 mg/kg was found to prolong conduction in the His-Purkinje system and to prolong intraventricular conduction time. At the same time, the drug was without effect on A-V nodal conduction, nor did it alter ventricular repolarization or refractoriness (212).

Because encainide lacks significant electrophysiologic effects on A-V transmission, it may have particular value in patients in whom alterations in A-V nodal conduction are undesirable. Because the drug depresses H-V and intraventricular conduction, encainide probably should not be used with quinidine or disopyramide. The full potential value of encainide in the treatment of patients with ventricular rhythm disturbances remains to be determined.

Lorcainide

Lorcainide (R15889) is a class I antiarrhythmic agent that has local anesthetic properties (Fig. 20). Experimental animal studies showed the drug to be effective in terminating arrhythmias due to ouabain intoxication and experimentally induced myocardial ischemia. Electrophysiologic studies on Purkinje fiber preparations, as well as on ventricular and atrial muscle, have shown the drug to decrease the rate of rise of the transmembrane action potential and to decrease conduction velocity. The refractory periods of Purkinje fibers and ventricular muscle are prolonged by lorcainide, as is the functional refractory period of

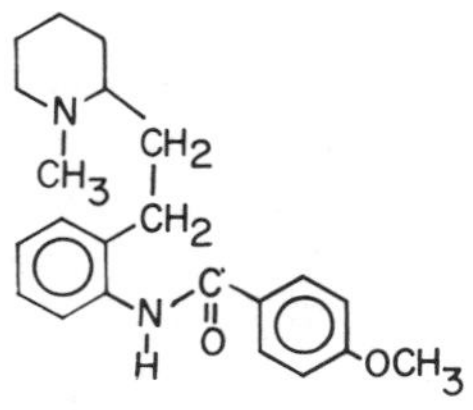

FIG. 19. Encainide.

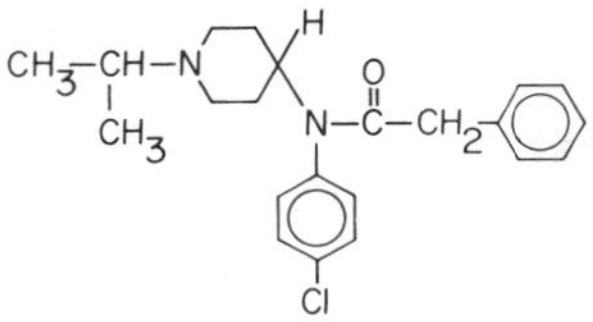

FIG. 20. Lorcainide.

the A-V node. Spontaneous diastolic depolarization of the sinoatrial node, as well as that arising in atrial muscle exposed to toxic concentrations of ouabain or to low extracellular K^+, is depressed by lorcainide (213).

Initial clinical trials with lorcainide have shown encouraging results, in that the drug was found to be effective in 31 of 36 patients with frequent premature contractions and recurrent ventricular tachycardia. In a more sophisticated double-blind crossover study, lorcainide was found to be as effective as mexiletine against ventricular premature contractions. Lorcainide was reported to be effective in preventing recurrent ventricular tachycardias and ventricular fibrillation in patients who were unresponsive to other modes of therapy.

Electrophysiologic studies in humans have shown lorcainide to differ from most other antiarrhythmic drugs and to have a similarity to aprindine in that it produces a decrease in conduction velocity in the atria and A-V node and within the ventricles, the latter being associated with a widening of the QRS complex. Lorcainide depresses sinus node function in humans. Thus, lorcainide produces impairment of impulse generation and conduction by the specialized conduction system of the heart. These effects are more pronounced in patients with previous alterations in cardiac impulse formation and/or conduction.

Whereas lorcainide has little effect on atrial refractory periods in humans, it does increase the refractory period of the A-V node, suggesting that the drug may be effective in controlling the ventricular rate in patients with supraventricular tachyarrhythmias.

As with all new antiarrhythmic agents, the position of lorcainide remains to be established by detailed clinical trials.

N-acetylprocainamide

It has been shown that *N*-acetylprocainamide (Acecainide®) (NAPA) (Fig. 21) is effective in suppressing premature ventricular contractions in placebo-controlled dose-ranging studies; it is currently undergoing intensive clinical evaluation as a class I antiarrhythmic agent. NAPA is a major metabolite of procainamide. Studies in animals and in humans have indicated that NAPA may be as potent as procainamide in the prevention of experimentally induced or clinically occurring arrhythmias. It is of interest that experimental data show that the *N*-acetyl metabolite of procainamide, unlike the parent compound, has a positive inotropic effect. Observations in humans are also suggestive of the drug being able to augment cardiac contractility, because NAPA has been shown to decrease the ratio between preejection period and left ventricular ejection time. In addition, it has also been noted to decrease sinoatrial rate.

The therapeutic range of NAPA plasma concentrations has not been established with certainty. However, in humans, concentrations in plasma as high as 41 μg/ml have been achieved without adverse electrocardiographic and/or hemodynamic signs of toxicity. Maximal antiarrhythmic effects of NAPA have been obtained with a plasma concentration of 30 μg/ml. The antiarrhythmic action of NAPA is reported to persist longer than that of procainamide, an observation that could be consistent with the fact that the elimination half-life of NAPA in patients with normal renal function is approximately twice (6 hr) that of procainamide, thus permitting NAPA to be given every 6 to 8 hr.

Aside from the aforementioned characteristics, NAPA is of clinical interest, because, in

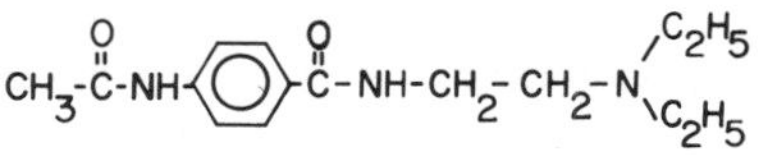

FIG. 21. N-acetylprocainamide.

comparison with procainamide, it shows less tendency to induce the lupuslike syndrome or cause the appearance of antinuclear antibodies when administered chronically. One of the major drawbacks to chronic use of procainamide (more than 3 months) as a prophylactic measure in the management of patients with arrhythmias is its tendency to produce a lupuslike syndrome, with skin rash, fever, arthritis, arthralgia, pleuritic chest pain, and pericarditis, along with a rise in serum antinuclear antibodies (ANA). It is worthy of note that elevated ANA titers developed in only 1 of 5 patients who received NAPA for 1 year, whereas each of 18 patients who received procainamide for 1 year was reported to have an elevated titer. The preliminary data to date would suggest that the major drawback of the lupuslike reaction so common with chronic procainamide may not be as frequent an occurrence with NAPA.

The reason for the difference between procainamide and NAPA with respect to the potential to induce a lupuslike syndrome is not known. It is reasonable to speculate that the toxic effect results from the parent compound or from a metabolite of procainamide that results from metabolism of the aromatic amine moiety of the molecule. The introduction of an acetyl group reduces the formation of the toxic metabolite. It has been demonstrated that procainamide is metabolized by mammalian microsomal oxidative enzymes to a metabolite that can interact with the DNA of *Salmonella typhimurium* to produce mutations. NAPA is inactive in the latter test system, thus supporting the belief that it is less likely to induce the lupuslike syndrome.

Tocainide

Tocainide (W-36095) (Fig. 22) is a new, orally effective analogue of lidocaine that has

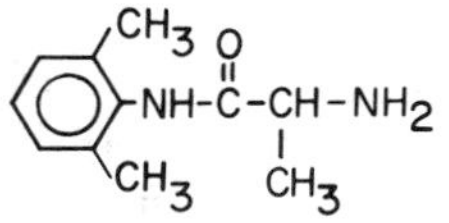

FIG. 22. Tocainide.

proved effective in the management of patients with ventricular premature beats and ventricular tachycardia. The major therapeutic interest in tocainide relates to the fact that it is an orally effective drug with a reported elimination half-life of 13.5 to 14.7 hr, thus allowing an 8- to 12-hr dosing regimen to be used clinically. Because tocainide lacks alkyl substitutions on the terminal nitrogen, it does not undergo first-pass hepatic elimination after oral administration; thus, its hepatic clearance, in contrast to that of lidocaine, is not large. At least 40% of the drug may be excreted unchanged in the urine after oral dosing. The drug is well absorbed from the gastrointestinal tract, with peak serum levels being obtained in 60 to 90 min. Therapeutic plasma concentrations are reported to be 6 to 12 μg/ml and can be achieved with an oral dosing regimen of 400 to 600 mg given every 8 hr (214). About 50% of the drug is bound to plasma protein, a factor that is of significance, because only the free form of the drug is excreted via glomerular filtration.

The spectrum of tocainide's antiarrhythmic action is identical with that of lidocaine, and the drug is classified as a class I antiarrhythmic agent. A number of reports have suggested that tocainide is effective in reducing the frequency of premature ventricular beats, although efficacy was often reported to be associated with side effects. In patients with recurrent ventricular tachycardia, tocainide given at an oral dose of 400 to 800 mg every 8 hr did not appear to reduce the dysrhythmic episodes.

The most commonly observed side effects include anorexia, nausea, vomiting, and abdominal discomfort. More disturbing are the symptoms and signs referable to the central nervous system, which resemble those seen with lidocaine toxicity. Neurologic disturbances include tremor, twitching, headache, disturbances in hearing acuity, paresthesis, dizziness, and lightheadedness. The neurologic side effects are dose-related and appear to subside on reduction in dosage.

The value of tocainide in the prevention

of sudden coronary death due to ventricular fibrillation has been examined experimentally in dogs. Contrary to what one might expect, "therapeutic" plasma concentrations known to be effective in reducing the frequency of premature ventricular beats resulted in a significant increase in the number of dogs developing ventricular fibrillation in response to acute coronary artery occlusion. The electrical threshold for the induction of ventricular fibrillation was not increased by "therapeutic" plasma concentrations, but was increased by dosages (25 mg/kg) that gave a threefold increase in the plasma concentration (18 μg/ml) (215). Such concentrations would not be tolerated clinically. Whether or not the experimental studies can be extrapolated to humans is doubtful, and only further clinical evaluation of tocainide in the prevention of sudden coronary death will provide the necessary answers. Because of its long half-life and systemic availability after oral administration, tocainide deserves to be evaluated clinically.

Mexiletine

Mexiletine (Fig. 23) is classified as a class I antiarrhythmic agent that has pharmacologic properties and antidysrhythmic effects similar to those of lidocaine and tocainide. Like tocainide, it is effective by oral administration, being almost completely absorbed, with peak plasma levels being achieved within 2 to 4 hr. Therapeutic plasma concentrations of 1 to 2 μg/ml can be maintained with doses of 200 to 300 mg every 6 to 8 hr. Daily doses range between 600 and 1,000 mg. The plasma half-life is estimated at 12 hr, although in patients with myocardial infarction, the mean half-life was found to be 16.7 hr, probably because of reduced hepatic blood flow, which would impair drug metabolism.

Mexiletine undergoes extensive hepatic me-

tabolism, and the fraction eliminated via the kidneys is influenced by the urinary pH. Acidification of the urine (pH 5.0) results in a plasma elimination half-life of 2.8 hr, with about 50% of the administered dose appearing in the urine in 48 hr. In the presence of an alkaline (pH 8.0) urine, the half-life is increased to 8.6 hr, with a negligible fraction of the dose appearing in the urine.

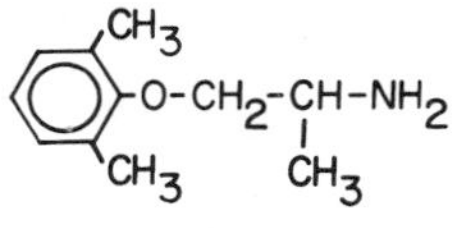

In a number of clinical trials, mexiletine has been reported to be effective in the management of patients with acute and/or chronic ventricular arrhythmias. Initial reports suggest that plasma concentrations between 0.75 and 2.0 μg/ml are effective in the control of dysrhythmias, although mild toxicity has been observed with plasma concentrations of 0.83 to 3.0 μg/ml, and severe toxicity has occurred within the range of 1.0 to 4.4 μg/ml (216).

In a large series of 191 patients with recent myocardial infarction, mexiletine was administered to reduce the frequency of "malignant" ventricular arrhythmias (i.e., ventricular premature beats in excess of 5 per minute; multiform or R-on-T rhythm), ventricular tachycardia, or recurrent ventricular fibrillation. Thirty-two of these patients had persistent ST-segment elevation and were considered to be at risk of developing ventricular fibrillation. Even though mexiletine reduced the frequency of premature ventricular beats, it did not prevent the recurrence of ventricular tachycardia and/or ventricular fibrillation. Whereas mexiletine may prove useful in those patients who appear to be refractory to lidocaine, its potential as an agent for long-term management of patients with electrical instability of the myocardium secondary to ischemia is yet to be determined. The data to date do not permit the conclusion that oral administration of mexiletine will reduce the incidence of sudden coronary death in patients who survive acute myocardial infarction.

Most of the side effects related to the use of mexiletine occur during the initial period of administration. Because the drug has a large volume of distribution in excess of 500 liters, and a long plasma half-life, achieving a steady

FIG. 23. Mexiletine.

state may require several days or relatively large initial intravenous dosages. Thus, the side effects on initiation of therapy often are related to the period when blood and tissue concentrations fluctuate before reaching equilibrium, especially when the intravenous route is used.

The first signs of toxicity are manifest by a fine tremor of the hands, followed by dizziness and blurred vision. Hypotension, sinus bradycardia, and widening of the QRS complex have been noted as the most common unwanted cardiovascular effects. The side effects are less common with long-term oral maintenance. Reducing or delaying the next dose usually reduces the severity of the undesirable side effects. The oral dosing regimen for mexiletine has been with dosages of 200 to 300 mg every 8 hr. It is estimated that 12 mg/kg/day in divided doses will be adequate to maintain therapeutic plasma concentrations.

Amiodarone

The benzofuran derivative amiodarone (Cordarone®) (Fig. 24) was introduced initially as a coronary artery dilator for use in patients with angina pectoris. Subsequent studies in animals and isolated cardiac muscle preparations demonstrated that pretreatment with amiodarone produced marked prolongation of the duration of atrial and ventricular action potentials. Thus, amiodarone may be classified as a class III antiarrhythmic drug (217). In humans, chronic administration of amiodarone is associated with sinus bradycardia and prolongation of the QT_c interval. One aspect of the electrophysiologic effects of amiodarone of extreme clinical utility is the ability of the drug to prolong the refractory period of the accessory pathway associated with WPW syndrome (218). It is this clinical set-

ting in which amiodarone has promise as a therapeutic agent. Although published clinical experience with amiodarone is sparse, there is a suggestion that the drug will be of potential benefit in the wide spectrum of atrial and ventricular rhythm disorders.

Amiodarone has been administered at an intravenous dose of 5 to 10 mg/kg slowly. Although its effects on ventricular contractility are negligible, amiodarone will produce vasodilatation, and higher doses will result in a negative inotropic effect. The oral dosage is reported to be between 200 and 800 mg daily. It is of special interest to note that amiodarone has been reported effective in a small number of patients who exhibited repetitive ventricular tachycardia. Because the electrophysiologic effects of amiodarone on the ventricular myocardium differ from those of the classic antiarrhythmic agents, this drug may constitute a significant addition to the therapy for patients with life-threatening cardiac arrhythmias.

The clinical development of amiodarone will be hampered by the side effects noted with prolonged amiodarone administration. In addition to imparting a slate gray or bluish color to the skin, amiodarone administration is associated with yellowish brown corneal deposits. The corneal microdeposits do not interfere with vision and are reversible after discontinuing the drug. Amiodarone may alter thyroid function, as well as the levels of serum-protein-bound iodine and thyroxine.

There are limited pharmacokinetic data pertaining to amiodarone, but preliminary data would suggest that the elimination half-life may be as long as 30 to 45 days after the cessation of chronic therapy. The long half-life is a reflection of the deposition of the drug in many body tissues. The antiarrhythmic effect may persist for extended periods if myocardial tissue serves as a site of deposition.

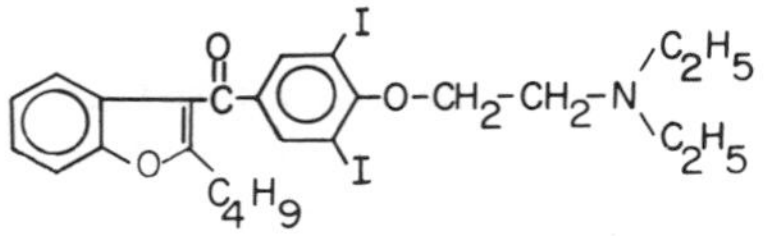

FIG. 24. Amiodarone.

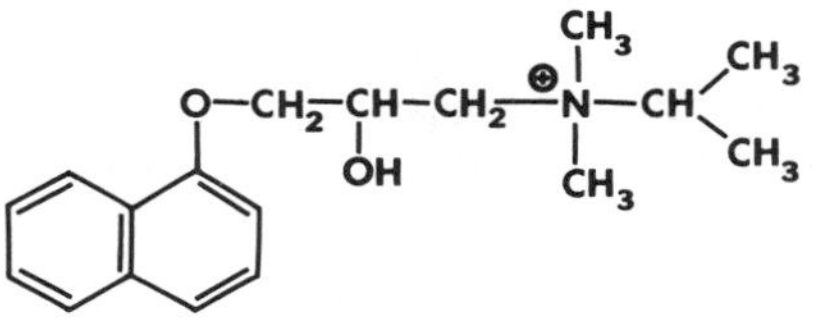

FIG. 25. Pranolium.

Whereas the long $T_{1/2}$ constitutes an advantage over presently available drugs, it also implies that the drug may need to be given days to weeks before its full antiarrhythmic effect becomes manifest.

Quaternary Ammonium Compounds as Potential Antiarrhythmic and/or Antifibrillatory Drugs

Preliminary experimental and clinical results with bretylium and other related drugs would suggest that the quaternary ammonium ion derivatives of antiarrhythmic agents may possess certain characteristics (as yet undefined) that will render them especially useful as antiarrhythmic and antifibrillatory drugs.

The structural modification of propranolol to give N,N-dimethylpropranolol (UM-272, Pranolium®) (Fig. 25) results in an agent that is devoid of β-adrenergic receptor blocking properties, but that retains the direct membrane effects of the parent compound. Pranolium has been effective in reversing experimentally induced cardiac rhythm disorders, including those resulting from acute myocardial infarction. The quaternary derivative of propranolol has been shown to increase the experimentally determined electrical threshold for ventricular fibrillation in nonischemic as well as ischemic canine hearts (219). At a dose of 10 mg/kg, pranolium prevented the induction of ventricular fibrillation by a 60-Hz train of impulses delivered during the vulnerable period of the cardiac cycle.

In a limited clinical trial in which pranolium was administered by the intravenous route, the drug was reported to be effective in restoring sinus rhythm in patients with ventricular tachycardia, some of whom were unresponsive to conventional antiarrhythmic drugs (220).

Contrary to common belief about the absorption of monoquaternary drugs after oral absorption, pranolium has been shown to elicit antidysrhythmic effects when given orally to dogs with experimentally induced arrhythmias. Furthermore, the drug is absorbed well after sublingual administration, leading to a rapid antiarrhythmic response in the experimental animal without producing adverse hemodynamic effects.

Recently, a second quaternary compound, clofilium (4-chloro-N,N-diethyl-N-heptylbenzene butanaminium) (Fig. 26) has been reported to prolong the action-potential duration and effective refractory period of canine Purkinje fibers without changing the rate of rise, amplitude, resting potential, or rate of diastolic depolarization (187). Clofilium increased the canine ventricular fibrillation threshold, and as seen with several quaternary ammonium compounds (bretylium, pranolium), clofilium administration was accompanied by several instances of spontaneous defibrillation without the use of DC countershock.

The introduction of bretylium has provided initial clinical evidence to demonstrate the exciting potential of quaternary ammonium compounds as antifibrillatory drugs. Because the use of bretylium is associated with acute functional alterations in sympathetic nervous system activity, its use in emergent clinical situations is made difficult, and its chronic use is compromised by orthostatic hypoten-

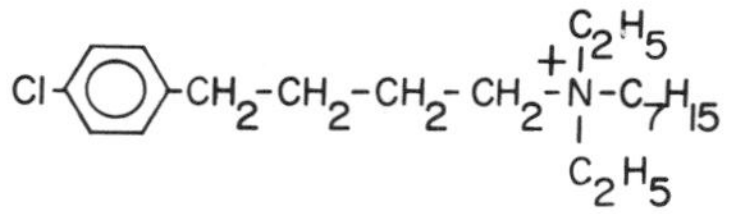

FIG. 26. Clofilium.

sion. Thus, the potential development of pranolium and/or clofilium as antifibrillatory agents is an important consideration in light of the fact that sudden coronary death, which claims over 450,000 lives each year in the United States, is usually due to ventricular fibrillation. The ability to offer a pharmacologic intervention for such a catastrophic event has been a long-sought goal for pharmacologists interested in the area of antidysrhythmic drugs. It is important to recognize, therefore, that the electrical rhythm disturbances leading to ventricular fibrillation, and ventricular fibrillation itself, are preventable and reversible events. Thus, the ischemic heart that is highly vulnerable to developing ventricular fibrillation must be protected if sudden coronary death is to be prevented or its incidence reduced. Conventional antiarrhythmic drugs of the class I and II types are unlikely to be of significant value. Mere reductions in the number and/or severity of ventricular ectopic beats, the usual measure of antiarrhythmic drug efficacy, is unlikely to result in protection against the development of ventricular fibrillation. The quaternary ammonium drugs such as bretylium, pranolium, and clofilium will undoubtedly receive intensive experimental and clinical evaluation to determine their proper roles in the prevention of sudden coronary death, a goal that has not been achieved to date with conventional antiarrhythmic agents.

REFERENCES

1. Elharrar, V., and Zipes, D. P. (1977): Cardiac electrophysiologic alterations during myocardial ischemia. *Am. J. Physiol.,* 233:H329–H345.
2. Wit, A. L., and Bigger, J. T. (1975): Possible electrophysiological mechanisms for lethal arrhythmias accompanying myocardial ischemia and infarction. *Circulation* [*Suppl. III*] 51–52:III-96–III-114.
3. Bigger, J. T., Dresdale, R. J., Heissenbuttel, R. H., Weld, F. M., and Wit, A. L. (1977): Ventricular arrhythmias in ischemic heart disease: Mechanism, prevalence, significance, and management. *Prog. Cardiovasc. Dis.,* 19:255–295.
4. Lazzara, R., El-Sherif, N., Hope, R. R., and Scherlag, B. J. (1978): Ventricular arrhythmias and electrophysiological consequences of myocardial ischemia and infarction. *Circ. Res.,* 42:740–749.

5. Weidmann, S. (1955): The effect of the cardiac membrane potential on the rapid availability to the sodium carrier system. *J. Physiol.,* 127:213–224.
6. Hoffman, B. F., Kao, C. Y., and Suckling, E. E. (1957): Refractoriness in cardiac muscle. *Am. J. Physiol.,* 190:473–482.
7. Noble, D. (1966): Application of Hodgkin-Huxley equations to excitable tissues. *Physiol. Rev.,* 46:1–50.
8. Van Dam, R. T., Moore, E. N., and Hoffman, B. F. (1963): Initiation and conduction of impulses in partially depolarized cardiac fibers. *Am. J. Physiol.,* 204:1133–1144.
9. Katz, R. L., and Epstein, R. A. (1968): The interaction of anesthetic agents and adrenergic drugs to produce cardiac arrhythmias. *Anesthesiology,* 29:763.
10. Besterman, E. M. M., and Friedlander, D. H. (1965): Clinical experiences with propranolol. *Postgrad. Med. J.,* 41:526–535.
11. Johnstone, M. (1966): Propranolol during halothane anesthesia. *Br. J. Anaesth.,* 38:516–529.
12. Lucchesi, B. R., Whitsitt, L. S., and Stickney, J. L. (1967): Antiarrhythmic effects of beta-adrenergic blocking agents. *Ann. N.Y. Acad. Sci.,* 139:940–951.
13. Parmley, W. W., and Braunwald, E. (1967): Comparative myocardial depressant and antiarrhythmic properties of *d*-propranolol, *d,l*-propranolol, and quinidine. *J. Pharmacol. Exp. Ther.,* 158:11–21.
14. Davis, L. D., and Temte, J. V. (1968): Effects of propranolol on the transmembrane potentials of ventricular muscle and Purkinje fibers of the dog. *Circ. Res.,* 22:661–677.
15. Gibson, D., and Sowton, E. (1969): The use of beta-adrenergic receptor blocking drugs in dysrhythmias. *Prog. Cardiovasc. Dis.,* 12:16–39.
16. Schamroth, L. (1966): Immediate effects of intravenous propranolol on various cardiac arrhythmias. *Am. J. Cardiol.,* 18:438–443.
17. Gettes, L. S., and Surawicz, B. (1967): Long-term prevention of paroxysmal arrhythmias with propranolol therapy. *Am. J. Med. Sci.,* 254:257–265.
18. Wit, A. L., Steiner, C., and Damato, A. N. (1970): Electrophysiologic effects of bretylium tosylate on single fibers in canine specialized conducting system and ventricle. *J. Pharmacol. Exp. Ther.,* 173:344–356.
19. Bigger, J. T., and Jaffe, C. C. (1971): Effect of bretylium tosylate on electrophysiologic properties of ventricular muscle and Purkinje fibers. *Am. J. Cardiol.,* 27:82–91.
20. Singh, B. N., and Vaughan-Williams, E. M. (1970): The effect of amiodarone, a new anti-anginal drug, on cardiac muscle. *Br. J. Pharmacol.,* 39:657–667.
21. Singh, B. N., Jewitt, D. E., Downey, J. M., et al. (1976): Effects of amiodarone and L8040, novel antianginal and antiarrhythmic drugs, on cardiac and coronary hemodynamics and on cardiac intracellular potentials. *Clin. Exp. Pharmacol. Physiol.,* 3:427–442.
22. Han, J., Malozzi, A. N., and Moe, G. K. (1968): Sino-atrial reciprocation in the isolated rabbit heart. *Circ. Res.,* 22:355–362.
23. Allessi, M. A., Bonke, F. J. M., and Schopman,

F. J. G. (1974): Circus movement in rabbit heart atrial muscle as a mechanism of tachycardia. *Circulation*, 33:54–62.

24. Mendez, D., and Moe, G. K. (1966): Demonstration of a dual AV nodal conduction system in the isolated rabbit heart. *Circ. Res.*, 19:378–393.

25. Bailey, J. R., Andersen, G. J., and Pippenger, D. (1973): Reentry within the isolated canine bundle of His: Possible mechanism for reciprocating rhythm. *Am. J. Cardiol.*, 32:808–813.

26. Narula, O. S. (1974): Sinus node reentry: A mechanism of supraventricular tachycardia. *Circulation*, 50:1114–1128.

27. Wu, D., Amat-Y-Leon, F., Denes, P., et al. (1973): Demonstration of dual A-V nodal pathways in patients with paroxysmal supraventricular tachycardia. *Circulation*, 48:549–555.

28. Varghese, P. H., Damato, A. H., Curacta, A. T., et al. (1974): Intraventricular conduction delay as a determinant of atrial echo beats. *Circulation*, 49:805–810.

29. Singer, D. H., Ten-Eick, R. E., and DeBoer, A. A. (1973): Electrophysiologic correlates of human atrial tachyarrhythmias. In: *Cardiac Arrhythmias*, edited by L. S. Dreifus and W. Likoff, p. 97–119. Grune & Stratton, New York.

30. Hoffman, B. F., and Cranefield, P. F. (1964): Physiologic basis of cardiac arrhythmias. *Am. J. Med.*, 37:670–684.

31. Wit, A. L., and Cranefield, P. F. (1976): Triggered activity in cardiac muscle fibers of the simian mitral valve. *Circ. Res.*, 38:85–98.

32. Lau, S. H., Stein, E., Rosowsky, D. B., et al. (1967): Atrial pacing and atrioventricular conduction in anomalous atrioventricular excitation (Wolff-Parkinson-White syndrome). *Am. J. Cardiol.*, 19:354–359.

33. Scherf, D., and Bornemann, C. (1967): Two cases of the preexcitation syndrome. *J. Electrocardiol.*, 2:177–184.

34. Hunter, A., Papp, C., and Parkinson, J. (1940): The syndrome of short P-R interval, apparent bundle branch block, and associated paroxysmal tachycardia. *Br. Heart J.*, 2:107–122.

35. Castellanos, A., Chapunoff, E., Castillo, C., et al. (1970): His bundle electrograms in two cases of Wolff-Parkinson-White (pre-excitation) syndrome. *Circulation*, 41:399–411.

36. Boineau, J. P., and Moore, E. N. (1970): Evidence for propagation of activation across an accessory atrioventricular connection in types A and B preexcitation. *Circulation*, 41:375–397.

37. Durrer, D., Schoo, L., Schuilenburg, R. M., et al. (1967): The role of premature beats in the initiation and termination of supraventricular tachycardia in the Wolff-Parkinson-White syndrome. *Circulation*, 36:644–662.

38. Gibson, D., and Sowton, E. (1969): The use of beta-adrenergic receptor blocking drugs in dysrhythmias. In: *Current Status of Drugs in Cardiovascular Disease*, edited by C. K. Friedberg, p. 160–179. Grune & Stratton, New York.

39. Heng, M. K., Singh, B. N., Roche, A. H. G., et al. (1975): Effects of intravenous verapamil on cardiac arrhythmias and on the electrocardiogram. *Am. Heart J.*, 90:487–498.

40. Singh, B. N., and Hauswirth, O. (1974): Comparative mechanisms of action of antiarrhythmic drugs. *Am. Heart J.*, 87:367–382.

41. Singh, B. N., and Vaughan-Williams, E. M. (1972): A fourth class of anti-dysrhythmic action? Effect of verapamil on ouabain toxicity, on atrial and ventricular intracellular potentials and on other features of cardiac function. *Cardiovasc. Res.*, 6:109–119.

42. Cranefield, P. F., Aronson, R. S., and Wit, A. L. (1974): Effect of verapamil on the normal action potential and on a calcium dependent slow response of canine cardiac Purkinje fibers. *Circ. Res.*, 34:204–213.

43. Neuss, H., and Schlepper, M. (1971): Der Einfluss von verapamil auf die atrioventrickulare Uberleitung. Lokalisation des Wirkungsortes mit His bundel Elecktrogrammen. *Verh. Dtsch. Ges. Kreislaufforsch.*, 37:433–441.

44. Husaini, M. H., Kvasnicka, J., Ryden, L., et al. (1973): Action of verapamil in sinus node, atrioventricular and intraventricular conduction. *Br. Heart J.*, 35:734–737.

45. Roy, P. R., Spurrell, R. A. J., and Sowton, G. E. (1974): The effect of verapamil on the cardiac conduction system in man. *Postgrad. Med. J.*, 50:270–275.

46. Goldreyer, B. N., and Bigger, J. T. (1971): The site of reentry in paroxysmal supraventricular tachycardia in man. *Circulation*, 43:15–26.

47. Goldreyer, B. N., and Damato, A. N. (1971): The essential role of atrioventricular conduction delay in the initiation of paroxysmal supraventricular tachycardia. *Circulation*, 43:679–687.

48. Rosenbaum, M. B., Chiale, P. A., Ryba, D., et al. (1974): Control of tachyarrhythmias associated with Wolff-Parkinson-White syndrome by amiodarone hydrochloride. *Am. J. Cardiol.*, 34:215–223.

49. Touboul, P., Porte, J., Huerta, F., et al. (1975): Electrophysiological effects of amiodarone in man. *Am. J. Cardiol.*, 35:173A.

50. Spurrell, R. A. J., Thorburn, C. W., Camm, J., et al. (1975): Effects of disopyramide on electrophysiological properties of specialized conduction system in man and on accessory atrioventricular pathway in Wolff-Parkinson-White syndrome. *Br. Heart J.*, 37:861–867.

51. Wellens, H. J. J., and Durrer, D. (1974): Wolff-Parkinson-White syndrome and atrial fibrillation. Relation between refractory period of the accessory pathway and ventricular rate during atrial fibrillation. *Am. J. Cardiol.*, 34:777–782.

52. Sellers, T. D., Jr., Bashore, T. M., and Gallagher, J. J. (1977): Digitalis in the pre-excitation syndrome. Analysis during atrial fibrillation. *Circulation*, 56:260–267.

53. Rosen, K. M., Barwolf, C., and Ehsani, A. (1972): Effects of Lidocaine and propranolol on the normal and anomalous pathways in patients with pre-excitation. *Am. J. Cardiol.*, 30:801–809.

54. Wu, D., Wyndham, C., Amat-Y-Leon, F., et al. (1975): The effects of ouabain on induction of atrio-

ventricular nodal re-entrant paroxysmal supraventricular tachycardia. *Circulation,* 52:201–207.

55. Wu, D., Denes, P., Dhingra, R., et al. (1974): The effects of propranolol on induction of A-V nodal re-entrant paroxysmal tachycardia. *Circulation,* 50:665–667.

56. Josephson, M. E., Kastor, J. A., and Kitchen, J. G., III (1975): Lidocaine in Wolff-Parkinson-White syndrome with atrial fibrillation. *Ann. Intern. Med.,* 84:44–45.

57. Rosen, K. M., Lau, S. H., Weiss, M. B., D'Amato, A. N. (1970): The effect of lidocaine on atrioventricular and intraventricular conduction in man. *Am. J. Cardiol.,* 25:1–5.

58. Mandel, W., Laks, M., Obayaski, K., et al. (1973): Electrophysiological features of the WPW syndrome: Modification by procainamide. *Circulation* [*Suppl. 4*], 48:195A.

59. Sellers, T. D., Jr., Campbell, W. F., Bashore, T. M., et al. (1977): Effects of procainamide and quinidine sulfate in the Wolff-Parkinson-White syndrome. *Circulation,* 55:15–22.

60. Birkhead, J. S., and Vaughan-Williams, E. N. (1977): Dual effect of disopyramide on atrial and atrioventricular conduction and refractory periods. *Br. Heart J.,* 39:657–660.

61. Spurrell, R. A. J., Krikler, D. M., and Sowton, E. (1974): Effects of verapamil on electrophysiological properties of anomalous atrioventricular connection in Wolff-Parkinson-White syndrome. *Br. Heart J.,* 36:256–264.

62. Schamroth, L., Krikler, D. M., and Garrett, C. (1972): Immediate effects of intravenous verapamil in cardiac arrhythmias. *Br. Med. J.,* 1:660–662.

63. Chiale, P. A., Przybyiski, J., Halpern, M. S., et al. (1977): Comparative effects of ajmaline on intermittent bundle branch block and the Wolff-Parkinson-White syndrome. *Am. J. Cardiol.,* 39:651–657.

64. Wellens, H. J. J., and Durrer, D. (1974): Effect of procaine amide, quinidine and ajmaline in the Wolff-Parkinson-White syndrome. *Circulation,* 50:114–120.

65. Wellens, H. J. J., Lie, K. I., Bar, F. W., et al. (1976): Effect of amiodarone in the Wolff-Parkinson-White syndrome. *Am. J. Cardiol.,* 38:189–194.

66. Daubert, J. C., and Couffault, J. (1977): Etude clinique de *l*-amiodarone injectable. *Coeur Med. Interne,* 16:415–421.

67. Wenckebach, K. F. (1914): *Die unregelmassige Herztatigkeit und ihre klinische Bedeutung.* W. Engelmann, Leipziz.

68. West, T. C., and Amory, D. W. (1960): Single fiber recording of the effect of quinidine at atrial and pacemaker sites of the isolated right atrium of the rabbit. *J. Pharmacol. Exp. Ther.,* 130:183–193.

69. Chiba, S., Kobayashi, M., and Furrekawa, Y. (1979): Effects of disopyramide on SA nodal pacemaker activity and contractility of the isolated blood-perfused atrium of the dog. *Eur. J. Pharmacol.,* 57:13–19.

70. Josephson, M. E., Seides, S. F., Batsford, W. P., Weisfogel, G. M., Akhtar, M., Caracta, A. R., Lau, S. H., and Damato, A. N. (1974): The electrophysiological effects of intramuscular quinidine on the atrioventricular conducting system in man. *Am. Heart J.,* 87:55–64.

71. Wallace, A. G., Cline, R. E., Sealy, W. C., Young, W. G., and Froyer, W. G. (1966): Electrophysiologic effects of quinidine. *Circ. Res.,* 19:960–969.

72. Nye, C. E., and Roberts, J. (1966): The reactivity of atrial and ventricular pacemakers to quinidine. *J. Pharmacol. Exp. Ther.,* 152:67–74.

73. Vaughan-Williams, E. M. (1958): Mode of action of quinidine on isolated rabbit atria interpreted from intracellular records. *Br. J. Pharmacol.,* 13:276–287.

74. Hirschfeld, D. S., Ueda, C. T., Rowland, M., and Scheinman, M. M. (1977): Clinical and electrophysiological effects of intravenous quinidine in man. *Br. Heart J.,* 39:309–316.

75. Weidmann, S. (1955): Effects of calcium ions and local anesthetics on electrical properties of Purkinje fibers. *J. Physiol. (Lond.),* 129:568–582.

76. Hoffman, B. F. (1958): Action of quinidine and procaine amide on single fibers of dog ventricle and specialized conduction system. *An. Acad. Bras. Cien.,* 29: 365–368.

77. Stern, S. (1971): Hemodynamic changes following separate and combined administration of beta blocking drugs and quinidine. *Eur. J. Clin. Invest.,* 1:432–436.

78. Schmid, P. G., Nelson, L. D., Mark, A. L., Herstad, D. D., and Abboud, F. M. (1974): Inhibition of adrenergic vasoconstriction by quinidine. *J. Pharmacol. Exp. Ther.,* 188:124–134.

79. Bellet, S., Hamdan, G., Somlyo, A., and Lara, R. (1959): The reversal of cardiotoxic effects of quinidine by molar sodium lactate. An experimental study. *Am. J. Med. Sci.,* 237:165–189.

80. Doherty, J. E., Straub, K. D., Murphy, M. L., deSoyza, N., Bissett, J. K., and Kane, J. J. (1980): Digoxin-quinidine interaction: Changes in canine tissue concentrations from steady state with quinidine. *Am. J. Cardiol.,* 45:1196–1200.

81. Leaky, E. B., Carson, J. A., Bigger, J. T., and Butler, V. P. (1979): Reduced renal clearance of digoxin during chronic quinidine administration. *Circulation* [*Suppl. II*], 60:II-16 (abstract).

82. Burstein, C. L. (1946): Treatment of acute arrhythmias during anesthesia by intravenous procaine. *Anesthesiology,* 7:113–121.

83. Mark, L. C., Kayden, H. J., Steele, J. M., Cooper, J. R., Berlin, I., Rovenstine, E. A., and Brodie, B. B. (1951): The physiological disposition and cardiac effects of procaine amide. *J. Pharmacol. Exp. Ther.,* 102:5–15.

84. Bigger, J. T., and Heissenbuttal, R. H. (1961): The use of procainamide and lidocaine in the treatment of cardiac arrhythmias. *Prog. Cardiovasc. Dis.,* 11:515–534.

85. Ogunkelu, J. B., Damato, A. N., Akhtar, M., Reddy, C. P., Caracta, A. R., and Lau, S. H. (1976): Electrophysiologic effects of procainamide in subtherapeutic to therapeutic doses on human atrioventricular conducting system. *Am. J. Cardiol.,* 37:724–731.

86. Sellers, T. D., Campbell, R. W. F., Bashore, T. M., and Gallagher, J. J. (1977): Effects of procainamide and quinidine sulfate in the Wolff-Parkinson-White syndrome. *Circulation,* 55:15–27.

87. Helfant, R. H., Scherlag, B. J., and Damato, A. N. (1967): The electrophysiological properties of diphenylhydantoin sodium (Dilantin) as compared to procaine amide in the normal and digitalis intoxicated heart. *Circulation,* 36:108–118.

88. Kastor, J. A., Josephson, M. E., Guss, S. B., and Horowitz, L. N. (1977): Human ventricular refractoriness. II. Effects of procainamide. *Circulation,* 56:462–467.

89. Giardina, E. G. V., and Bigger, J. T. (1973): Procaine amide against re-entrant ventricular arrhythmias. *Circulation,* 48:959–970.

90. Kayden, H. J., Brodie, B. B., and Steele, J. M. (1957): Procaine amide. *Circulation,* 15:118–126.

91. Giardina, E. G., Heissenbuttel, R. H., and Bigger, J. T. (1973): Intermittent intravenous procaine amide to treat ventricular arrhythmias. *Ann. Intern. Med.,* 78:183–193.

92. Harrison, D., Sprouse, H., and Morrow, A. G. (1963): The antiarrhythmic properties of lidocaine and procainamide. *Circulation,* 28:486–491.

93. Ladd, A. T. (1962): Procainamide induced lupus erythematosus. *N. Engl. J. Med.,* 267:1357–1358.

94. Colman, R. W., and Sturgill, B. C. (1965): Lupuslike syndrome induced by procainamide. *Arch. Intern. Med.,* 115:214–216.

95. Karlsson, E. (1978): Clinical pharmacokinetics of procainamide. *Clinical Pharmacokinetics,* 3:97–107.

96. Greenspan, A. M., Horowitz, L. N., Spielman, S. R., and Josephson, M. E. (1980): Large dose procainamide therapy for ventricular tachyarrhythmia. *Am. J. Cardiol.,* 46:453–468.

97. Koch-Weser, J., Klein, S. W., Foo-Canto, L. L., Kastor, J. A., and DeSanctis, R. W. (1969): Arrhythmia prophylaxis with procainamide in acute myocardial infarction. *N. Engl. J. Med.,* 281:1253–1260.

98. Sekiya, A., and Vaughan-Williams, E. M. (1963): A comparison of the antifibrillatory actions and effects on intracellular cardiac potentials of pronethalol, disopyramide, and quinidine. *Br. J. Pharmacol.,* 21:473–481.

99. Josephson, M. E., Caract, A. R., Lau, S. H., Gallagher, J. J., and Damato, A. N. (1973): Electrophysiological evaluation of disopyramide in man. *Am. Heart J.,* 86:771–778.

100. Befeler, B., Castellanos, A., Wells, D. E., Vagueiro, M. C., and Yeh, B. K. (1975): Electrophysiologic effects of the antiarrhythmic agent disopyramide phosphate. *Am. J. Cardiol.,* 35:382–389.

101. LaBarre, A., Strauss, H. C., Scheinman, M. M., Evans, G. T., Bashore, T., Tiedeman, J. S., and Wallace, A. G. (1979): Electrophysiologic effects of disopyramide phosphate on sinus node function in patients with sinus node dysfunction. *Circulation,* 59:226–235.

102. Birkhead, J. S., and Vaughan-Williams, E. M. (1977): Dual effect of disopyramide on atrial and atrioventricular conduction and refractory periods. *Br. Heart J.,* 39:657–660.

103. Yeh, B. K., Sung, P. K., and Scherlag, B. J. (1973): Effects of disopyramide on electrophysiological and mechanical properties of the heart. *J. Pharm. Sci.,* 62:1924–1929.

104. Danilo, P., Hordof, A. J., and Rosen, M. R. (1977): Effects of disopyramide on electrophysiologic properties of canine cardiac Purkinje fibers. *J. Pharmacol. Exp. Ther.,* 201:701–710.

105. Kus, T., and Sasyniuk, B. I. (1978): The electrophysiological effects of disopyramide phosphate on canine ventricular muscle and Purkinje fibers in normal and low potassium. *Can. J. Physiol. Pharmacol.,* 56:139–149.

106. Levites, R., and Anderson, G. J. (1979): Electrophysiological effects of disopyramide phosphate during experimental myocardial ischemia. *Am. Heart J.,* 98:339–344.

107. Patterson, E., Gibson, J. K., and Lucchesi, B. R. (1980): Electrophysiologic effects of disopyramide phosphate on reentrant ventricular arrhythmia in conscious dogs after myocardial infarction. *Am. J. Cardiol.,* 46:792–799.

108. Walsh, R. A., and Horwitz, L. D. (1979): Adverse hemodynamic effects of intravenous disopyramide compared with quinidine in conscious dogs. *Circulation,* 60:1053.

109. Meltzer, R. S., Robert, E. W., McMorrow, M., and Martin, R. P. (1978): Atypical ventricular tachycardia as a manifestation of disopyramide toxicity. *Am. J. Cardiol.,* 42:1049–1053.

110. Deano, D. A., Wu, D., Mautner, R. K., Sherman, R. H., Ehsani, A. E., and Rosen, K. M. (1977): The antiarrhythmic efficacy of intravenous therapy with disopyramide phosphate. *Chest,* 71:597–606.

111. Vismara, L. A., Mason, D. T., and Amsterdam, E. A. (1974): Disopyramide phosphate: Clinical efficacy of a new oral antiarrhythmic drug. *Clin. Pharmacol. Ther.,* 16:330–335.

112. Josephson, M. E., and Horowitz, L. N. (1979): Electrophysiologic approach to therapy of recurrent sustained ventricular tachycardia. *Am. J. Cardiol.,* 43:631–642.

113. Benditt, D. G., Pritchett, E. L. C., Wallace, A. G., and Gallagher, J. J. (1979): Recurrent ventricular tachycardia in man: Evaluation of disopyramide therapy by intracardiac electrical stimulation. *Eur. J. Cardiol.,* 9:255–276.

114. Mandel, W. J., and Bigger, J. T. (1970): Effect of lidocaine on sinoatrial node and atrial fibers. *Am. J. Cardiol.,* 25:113–124.

115. Singh, B. N., and Vaughan-Williams, E. M. (1971): Effects of altering potassium concentrations on the action of lidocaine and diphenylhydantoin on rabbit atrial and ventricular muscle. *Circ. Res.,* 29:286–295.

116. Josephson, M. E., Caracta, A. R., Lau, S. H., Gallagher, J. J., and Damato, A. N. (1972): Effects of lidocaine on refractory periods of man. *Am. Heart J.,* 84:778–786.

117. Davis, L. D., and Temte, J. V. (1969): Electrophysiologic actions of lidocaine on canine ventricular muscle and Purkinje fibers. *Circ. Res.,* 24:639–655.

118. Lazzara, R., Hope, R. R., El-Sherif, N., and Scherlag, B. J. (1978): Effects of lidocaine on hypoxic and ischemic cardiac cells. *Am. J. Cardiol.,* 41:872–879.

119. Allen, J. D., Brennan, F. J., and Wit, A. L. (1978): Actions of lidocaine on transmembrane potentials

of subendocardial Punkinje fibers surviving in infarcted canine hearts. *Circ. Res.,* 43:470–481.

120. Nelson, D. H., and Harrison, D. C. (1965): A comparison of the negative inotropic effects of procaine
amide, lidocaine, and quinidine. *Physiologist,* 8:
241A.

121. Robinson, S. L., Shroll, M., and Harrison, D. C.
(1969): The circulatory response to lidocaine in experimental myocardial infarction. *Am. J. Med. Sci.,*
258:260–269.

122. Austen, W. G., and Moran, J. M. (1965): Cardiac
and peripheral vascular effects of lidocaine and procaine amide. *Am. J. Cardiol.,* 16:701–707.

123. Collinsworth, K. A., Summer, M. K., and Harrison,
D. C. (1974): The clinical pharmacology of lidocaine
as an antiarrhythmic drug *Circulation,* 50:1217–
1230.

124. Grossman, J. J., Cooper, J. A., and Frieden, J.
(1969): Cardiovascular effects of infusion of lidocaine on patients with heart disease. *Am. J. Cardiol.,*
24:191–197.

125. Jewitt, D. E., Kishon, Y., and Thomas, M. (1968):
Lignocaine in the management of arrhythmias after
acute myocardial infarction. *Lancet,* 1:266–270.

126. Merritt, H. H., and Putnam, T. J. (1938): Sodium
diphenylhydantoinate in the treatment of convulsive
disorders. *J.A.M.A.,* 111:1068–1073.

127. Harris, A. S., and Kokernot, R. H. (1950): Effects
of diphenylhydantoin sodium and phenobarbital sodium upon ectopic ventricular tachycardia in acute
myocardial infarction. *Am. J. Physiol.,* 163:505–516.

128. Strauss, H. C., Bigger, J. T., Bassett, A. L., and
Hoffman, B. F. (1968): Actions of diphenylhydantoin on the electrical properties of isolated rabbit
and canine atria. *Circ. Res.,* 23:463–477.

129. Singh, B. N., and Vaughan-Williams, E. M. (1971):
Effect of altering potassium concentration on the
action of lidocaine and diphenylhydantoin on rabbit
atrial and ventricular muscle. *Circ. Res.,* 29:286–
294.

130. Rosati, R. A., Alexander, J. A., Schaal, S. F., and
Wallace, A. G. (1967): Influence of diphenylhydantoin on electrophysiological properties of the canine
heart. *Circ. Res.,* 21:757–765.

131. Caracta, A. R., Damato, A. N., Josephson, M. E.,
Ricciutti, M. A., Gallagher, J. J., and Lau, S. H.
(1973): Electrophysiologic properties of diphenylhydantoin. *Circulation,* 47:1234–1241.

132. Scherlag, B. J., Helfant, R. H., and Damato, A. N.
(1968): The contrasting effects of diphenylhydantoin
and procaine amide on A-V conduction in the digitalis intoxicated and the normal heart. *Am. Heart
J.,* 75:200–205.

133. Bigger, J. T., Bassett, A. L., and Hoffman, B. F.
(1968): Electrophysiologic effects of diphenylhydantoin on canine Purkinje fibers. *Circ. Res.,* 22:221–
236.

134. El-Sherif, N., and Lazzara, R. (1978): Reentrant
ventricular arrhythmias in the late myocardial infarction period. 5. Mechanism of action of diphenylhydantoin. *Circulation,* 57:465–472.

135. Mixter, C. G., Moran, J. M., and Austen, W. G.
(1966): Cardiac and peripheral vascular effects of
diphenylhydantoin. *Am. J. Cardiol.,* 17:332–338.

136. Conn, R. D., Kennedy, J. W., and Blackman, J. R.
(1967): The hemodynamic effects of diphenylhydantoin. *Am. Heart J.,* 73:500–505.

137. Lieberson, A. D., Schumacher, R. R., Childress,
R. H., Boyd, D. L., and Williams, J. F. (1967):
Effects of diphenylhydantoin on left ventricular
function in patients with heart disease. *Circulation,*
36:692–699.

138. Karliner, J. S. (1967): Intravenous diphenylhydantoin sodium in cardiac arrhythmias. *Dis. Chest,*
51:256–269.

139. Russell, M. A., and Bousvaros, G. (1968): Total
results from diphenylhydantoin administered intravenously. *J.A.M.A.,* 206:218–223.

140. Conn, R. D. (1965): Diphenylhydantoin sodium in
cardiac arrhythmias. *N. Engl. J. Med.,* 272:277–282.

141. Louis, S., Kutt, H., and McDowell, F. (1967): The
cardiocirculatory changes caused by intravenous dilantin and its solvent. *Am. Heart J.,* 74:523–529.

142. Pitt, W. A., and Cox, A. R. (1968): The effect of
the beta-adrenergic antagonist propranolol on rabbit
atrial cells with the use of the ultramicroelectrode
technique. *Am. Heart J.,* 76:242–248.

143. Vaughan-Williams, E. M. (1966): Mode of action
of beta-receptor antagonists on cardiac muscle. *Am.
J. Cardiol.,* 18:399–405.

144. Berkowitz, W. D., Wit, A. L., Lau, S. H., Steiner,
C., and Damato, A. N. (1969): The effects of propranolol on cardiac conduction. *Circulation,* 40:
855–862.

145. Whitsitt, L. S., and Lucchesi, B. R. (1969): The
effects of beta-adrenergic receptor blockade and glucagon on the atrioventricular transmission system.
Circ. Res., 23:585–595.

146. Woosley, R. L., Kornhauser, D., Smith, R., Reele,
S., Higgins, S. B., Nies, A. S., Shand, D. G., and
Oates, J. A. (1979): Suppression of chronic ventricular arrhythmias with propranolol. *Circulation,* 60:
819–821.

147. Stern, S., and Eisenberg, S. (1969): The effect of
propranolol (Inderal) on the electrocardiogram of
normal subjects. *Am. Heart J.,* 77:192–195.

148. Gibson, D. G. (1974): Pharmacodynamic properties
of beta-adrenergic receptor blocking drugs in man.
Drugs, 7:8–38.

149. Nakano, J., and Kusakari, T. (1966): Effect of beta-
adrenergic blockade on the cardiovascular dynamics. *Am. J. Physiol.,* 210:833–837.

150. Donald, D. E., Terguson, P. A., and Milburn, S. E.
(1969): Effect of beta-adrenergic receptor blockade
on racing performance of greyhounds with normal
and denervated hearts. *Circ. Res.,* 22:127–137.

151. Epstein, S., Robison, B. F., Kahler, R. L., and
Braunwald, E. (1965): Effects of beta-adrenergic
blockade on cardiac response to maximal and submaximal exercise in man. *J. Clin. Invest.,* 44:1745–
1753.

152. Sonnenblick, E. H., Braunwald, E., Williams
J. F. J., and Glick, G. (1965): Effects of exercise
on myocardial force velocity relations in intact unanesthetized man: Relative roles of changes in heart
rate, sympathetic activity, and ventricular dimensions. *J. Clin. Invest.,* 44:2051–2062.

153. Sowton, E., and Hamer, J. (1966): Hemodynamic

changes after beta-adrenergic blockade. *Am. J. Cardiol.,* 18:317–320.

154. Reed, R. L., Cheney, C. B., Fearon, R. E., Hook, R., and Hehre, F. W. (1974): Propranolol therapy during pregnancy: A case report. *Anesth. Analg.,* 53:214A.

155. Johnstone, M. (1966): Propranolol during halothane anesthesia. *Br. J. Anaesth.,* 38:516–529.

156. Norris, R. M., Coughey, D. E., and Scott, P. J. (1968): Trial of propranolol in acute myocardial infarction. *Br. Med. J.,* 2:398–400.

157. Sowton, E. (1968): Beta-adrenergic blockade in cardiac infarctions. *Prog. Cardiovasc. Dis.,* 10:561–572.

158. Gibson, D., and Sowton, E. (1969): The use of beta-adrenergic receptor blocking drugs in dysrhythmias. *Prog. Cardiovasc. Dis.,* 12:16–39.

159. Naggar, C. Z., and Alexander, S. (1976): Propranolol treatment of VPB's. *N. Engl. J. Med.,* 294:903–904.

160. Nixon, J. V., Pennington, W., Bitter, W., and Shapiro, W. (1978): Efficacy of propranolol in the control of exercise-induced or augmented ventricular ectopic activity. *Circulation,* 57:115–122.

161. Erlij, D., and Mendez, R. (1964): The modification of digitalis intoxication by excluding adrenergic influences on the heart. *J. Pharmacol. Exp. Ther.,* 144:97–103.

162. Roberts, J., Ryuta, I., Reilly, J., and Cairoli, V. J. (1963): Influence of reserpine and BTM-10 on digitalis induced ventricular arrhythmias. *Circ. Res.,* 13:149–158.

163. Boura, A. L. A., Green, A. F., McCoubrey, A., Laurence, D. R., Moulton, R., and Rosenheim, M. L. (1959): Darenthin: Hypotensive agent of a new type. *Lancet,* 2:17–21.

164. Boura, A. L. A., and Green, A. F. (1959): The actions of bretylium: Adrenergic neurone blocking and other effects. *Br. J. Pharmacol.,* 14:536–548.

165. Leveque, P. E. (1965): Antiarrhythmic action of bretylium. *Nature,* 207:203–204.

166. Bacaner, M. (1966): Bretylium tosylate for suppression of induced ventricular fibrillation. *Am. J. Cardiol.,* 17:528–534.

167. Bacaner, M. (1968): Treatment of ventricular fibrillation and other acute arrhythmias with bretylium tosylate. *Am. J. Cardiol.,* 21:530–543.

168. Holder, D. A., Sniderman, A. D., Fraser, G., and Fallen, E. L. (1977): Experience with bretylium tosylate by a hospital cardiac arrest team. *Circulation,* 55:541–544.

169. Terry, G., Vellani, C. W., Higgins, M. R., and Doig, A. (1970): Bretylium tosylate in treatment of refractory ventricular arrhythmias complicating myocardial infarction. *Br. Heart J.,* 32:21–25.

170. Day, H. W., and Bacaner, M. (1974): Use of bretylium tosylate in the management of acute myocardial infarction. *Am. J. Cardiol.,* 27:177–189.

171. Bernstein, J. G., and Koch-Weser, J. (1972): Effectiveness of bretylium tosylate against refractory ventricular arrhythmias. *Circulation,* 45:1024–1034.

172. Anderson, J. L., Patterson, E., Wagner, J. G., Stewart, J. R., Behm, H. L., and Lucchesi, B. R. (1980): Oral and intravenous bretylium disposition. *Clin. Pharmacol. Ther.,* 28:468–478.

173. Touboul, P., Porte, J., Huerta, F., and Belahaye, J. F. (1976): Etude des proprietes electrophysiologiques du tosylate de bretylium chez l'homme. *Arch. Mal. Coeur,* 69:503–511.

174. Waxman, M. B., and Wallace, A. G. (1972): Electrophysiologic effects of bretylium tosylate on the heart. *J. Pharmacol. Exp. Ther.,* 183:264–274.

175. Romhilt, D. W., Bloomfield, S. S., Lipicky, R. J., Welch, R. M., and Fowler, N. O. (1972): Evaluation of bretylium tosylate for the treatment of premature ventricular contractions. *Circulation,* 45:800–807.

176. Cohen, H. C., Gozo, E. G., Langendorf, R., Kaplan, B. M., Chan, A., Pick, A., and Glick, G. (1973): Response of resistant ventricular tachycardia to bretylium. *Circulation,* 47:331–340.

177. Papp, J. G., and Vaughan-Williams, E. M. (1969): The effect of bretylium on intracellular cardiac action potentials in relation to its anti-arrhythmic and local anesthetic activity. *Br. J. Pharmacol.,* 37:380–399.

178. DeAzevedo, I. M., Watanabe, Y., and Dreifus, L. S. (1974): Electrophysiologic antagonism of quinidine and bretylium tosylate. *Am. J. Cardiol.,* 33:633–638.

179. Gillis, R. A., Clancy, M. M., and Anderson, R. J. (1973): Deleterious effects of bretylium in cats with digitalis-induced ventricular tachycardia. *Circulation,* 47:974–983.

180. Namm, D. H., Wang, C. M., El-Sayad, S., Copp, F. C., and Maxwell, R. A. (1975): Effects of bretylium on rat cardiac muscle: The electrophysiological effects and its uptake and binding in normal and immunosympathectomized rat hearts. *J. Pharmacol. Exp. Ther.,* 193:194–207.

181. Cardinal, R., and Sasyniuk, B. I. (1978): Electrophysiological effects of bretylium tosylate on subendocardial Purkinje fibers from infarcted hearts. *J. Pharmacol. Exp. Ther.,* 204:159–174.

182. Bacaner, M. B. (1968): Quantitative comparison of bretylium with other antifibrillatory drugs. *Am. J. Cardiol.,* 21:504–512.

183. Bacaner, M. B., and Schrienemachers, D. (1968): Bretylium tosylate for suppression of ventricular fibrillation after experimental myocardial infarction. *Nature,* 220:494–496.

184. Kniffen, F. J., Lomas, T. E., Counsell, R. E., and Lucchesi, B. R. (1975): The antiarrhythmic and antifibrillatory actions of bretylium and its *o*-iodobenzyltrimethyl ammonium analog, UM-360. *J. Pharmacol. Exp. Ther.,* 192:120–128.

185. Anderson, J. L., Patterson, E., Conlon, M., Pasyk, S., Pitt, B., and Lucchesi, B. R. (1980): Kinetics of antifibrillatory effects of bretylium: Correlation with myocardial drug concentrations. *Am. J. Cardiol.,* 46:583–591.

186. Sanna, G., and Arcidiacono, R. (1973): Chemical ventricular defibrillation of the human heart with bretylium tosylate. *Am. J. Cardiol.,* 32:982–987.

187. Steinberg, M. I., and Malloy, B. B. (1979): Clofilium—a new antifibrillatory agent that selectively increases cellular refractoriness. *Life Sci.,* 25:1397–1406.

188. Cervoni, P., Ellis, C. H., and Maxwell, R. A. (1971): The antiarrhythmic action of bretylium in normal, reserpine-pretreated, and chronically denervated

dog hearts. *Arch. Int. Pharmacodyn. Ther.*, 190:91–102.

189. Babbs, C. F., Yim, G. K. W., Whistler, S. J., Tacker, W. A., and Geddes, L. A. (1979): Elevation of ventricular defibrillation threshold in dogs by antiarrhythmic drugs. *Am. Heart J.*, 98:345–350.

190. Tacker, W. A., Niebauer, M. J., Babbs, C. F., Combs, W. J., Halin, B. M., Barber, M. A., Bourland, J. D., and Geddes, L. A. (1980): *Crit. Care Med.*, 8:177–180.

191. Chatterjee, K., Mandel, W. J., Vyden, J. K., Parmley, W. W., and Forrester, J. S. (1973): Cardiovascular effects of bretylium tosylate in acute myocardial infarction. *J.A.M.A.*, 223:757–760.

192. Markis, J. E., and Koch-Weser, J. (1971): Characteristics and mechanisms of inotropic and chronotropic actions of bretylium tosylate. *J. Pharmacol. Exp. Ther.*, 178:94–102.

193. Graham, J. D., and Chandler, B. M. (1973): The effects of lidocaine, propranolol, procainamide, and bretylium tosylate: A unique property of an antiarrhythmic agent. *Can. J. Physiol. Pharmacol.*, 51:763–773.

194. MacAlpin, R. N., Zalis, E. G., and Kivowitz, C. F. (1970): Prevention of recurrent ventricular tachycardia with oral bretylium tosylate. *Ann. Intern. Med.*, 72:909–912.

195. Anderson, J. L., Patterson, E., Wagner, J. G., Johnson, T., Lucchesi, B. R., and Pitt, B. (1972): Clinical pharmacokinetics of intravenous and oral bretylium tosylate in survivors of ventricular tachycardia or fibrillation. *J. Cardiovasc. Pharm.*, 1:660–662.

196. Schamroth, L., Krikler, D. M., and Garrett, C. (1972): Immediate effects of intravenous verapamil in cardiac arrhythmias. *Br. Med. J.*, 1:660–662.

197. Feigl, D., and Ravid, M. (1979): Electrocardiographic observations on the termination of supraventricular tachycardia by verapamil. *J. Electrocardiogr.*, 12:129–136.

198. Fleckenstein, A. (1964): Die bedentung der energiereidren phosphate fur knotracktilitat und tonus des myokards. *Verh. Dtsch. Ges. Inn. Med.*, 70:81–99.

199. Fleckenstein, A. (1968): Prog. Vth Eur. Congr. Cardiol., Athens, 1968, p. 255–269.

200. Zipes, D. P., and Fischer, J. C. (1974): Effects of agents which inhibit the slow channel on sinus node automaticity and atrioventricular conduction in the dog. *Circ. Res.*, 34:184–192.

201. Okada, T. (1976): Effect of verapamil on electrical activities of SA node, ventricular muscle, and Purkinje fibers in isolated rabbit hearts. *Jpn. Circ. J.*, 40:329.

202. Rosen, M. R., Wit, A. L., and Hoffman, B. F. (1975): Electrophysiology and pharmacology of cardiac arrhythmias. IV. Cardiac effects of verapamil. *Am. Heart J.*, 89:665–673.

203. Rinkenberger, R. L., Prystowsky, E. N., Heger, J. J., Troup, P. J., Jackman, W. M., and Zipes, D. P. (1980): Effects of intravenous and chronic oral verapamil administration in patients with supraventricular tachyarrhythmias. *Circulation,* 62:996–1010.

204. Heng, M. K., Singh, B. N., Roche, A. H. G., Norris, R. M., and Mercer, C. J. (1975): Effects of intravenous verapamil on cardiac arrhythmias and on the electrocardiogram. *Am. Heart J.*, 90:487–498.

205. Luebs, E. D., Cohan, A., Zaleski, E. J., and Bing, R. J. (1966): Effect of nitroglycerin, intensain, isoptin and papaverine on coronary blood flow in man. Measured by coincidence counting technic and rubidium[84]. *Am. J. Cardiol.*, 17:535–541.

206. Singh, B. N., Ellrodt, G., and Peter, C. T. (1978): Verapamil: A review of its pharmacological properties and therapeutic uses. *Drugs,* 15:169–197.

207. Terlinz, J., and Furbow, M. E. (1980): Antianginal and myocardial metabolic properties of verapamil in coronary artery disease. *Am. J. Cardiol.*, 46:1019–1025.

208. Gunther, S., Muller, J. E., Mudge, G. H., and Grossman, W. (1981): Therapy of coronary vasoconstriction in patients with coronary artery disease. *Am. J. Cardiol.*, 47:157–162.

209. Ruffy, R., Rozenshtrauker, L. V., Elharrar, V., and Zipes, D. P. (1977): Cardiac electrophysiologic properties of ethmozin. *Clin. Res.*, 25:557A (abstract).

210. Danilo, P., Langan, W. B., Rosen, M. R., and Hoffman, B. F. (1977): Effects of the phenothiazine analog, EN-313, on ventricular arrhythmias in the dog. *Eur. J. Pharmacol.*, 45:127–139.

211. Gibson, J. K., Somani, P., and Basset, A. L. (1978): Electrophysiologic effects of encainide (MJ9067) on canine Purkinje fibers. *Eur. J. Pharmacol.*, 52:161–169.

212. Harrison, D. C., Winkle, R., Sami, M., and Mason, J. (1980): Encainide: A new and potent antiarrhythmic agent. *Am. Heart J.*, 100:1046–1054.

213. Carmeliet, E., Janssen, P. A. J., Morsboom, R., Van Neuten, J. M., and Zhonneux, R. (1978): Antiarrhythmic, electrophysiological and hemodynamic effects of lorcainide. *Arch. Int. Pharmacodyn. Therm.*, 231:104–130.

214. Winkle, R. A., Meffin, P. J., and Harrison, D. C. (1978): Long-term tocainide therapy for ventricular arrhythmias. *Circulation,* 57:1008–1016.

215. Schnittger, I., Griffin, J. C., Hall, R. J., and Winkle, R. A. (1978): Effects of tocainide on ventricular fibrillation threshold. *Am. J. Cardiol.*, 42:76–81.

216. Zipes, D. P., and Troup, P. J. (1978): New antiarrhythmic agents. *Am. J. Cardiol.*, 41:1005–1024.

217. Singh, B. N., and Vaughan-Williams, E. M. (1970): The effect of amiodarone, a new anti-anginal drug, on cardiac muscle. *Br. J. Pharmacol.*, 39:657–667.

218. Wellens, H. J. J., Lie, K. I., Bar, F. W., Wesdorp, J. C., Dohmen, H. J., Duren, D. R., and Durrer, D. (1976): Effect of amiodarone in the Wolff-Parkinson-White syndrome. *Am. J. Cardiol.*, 38:189–194.

219. Kniffen, F. J., Schuster, D. P., and Lucchesi, B. R. (1973): Antiarrhythmic and electrophysiologic properties of UM-272, dimethyl quaternary propranolol, in the canine heart. *J. Pharmacol. Exp. Ther.*, 187:260–268.

220. Reele, S., Woosley, R. L., Kornhauser, D., Carr, K., and Shand, D. (1978): Antiarrhythmic efficacy of pranolium in man. *Clin. Res.*, 26:264A.

Cardiovascular Pharmacology, Second Edition,
edited by Michael Antonaccio.
Raven Press, New York © 1984.

Calcium Antagonists

Ravinder K. Saini

The Squibb Institute for Medical Research, Princeton, New Jersey 08540

Medical treatment of patients with ischemic heart disease has improved greatly during the past two decades (1). Nitrates continue to play a vital role in therapy, although their mechanism(s) of action are still incompletely delineated after a century of use. The introduction of β blockers (specifically propranolol in this country) provided a second highly effective and extremely safe therapeutic modality for relieving angina, reducing blood pressure, and antagonizing certain cardiac arrhythmias (2,3). Recently, another new group of agents, used extensively in Europe and Japan for over 10 years, has shown promise in American clinical studies. These investigational drugs, which act by directly antagonizing the effect of calcium ions (Ca^{2+}) on both myocardial contractility and coronary arterial tone, are collectively known as Ca^{2+} antagonists. Their effect, according to Fleckenstein (4), is explained by selective blockade of the slow channel of the cell membrane—i.e., by interference with the transmembrane Ca^{2+} influx. However, recently some investigators (5,6) have suggested that other sites of action may be also important. The exact mechanism(s) of action of these agents are gradually being elucidated, and the new understanding is reflected in new terminology. Although many still use the term "Ca^{2+} antagonist," the more exact term "Ca^{2+} slow-channel blockers" was recently proposed.

Historically, the development of slow-channel blockers dates back to the early 1960s, at which time some German scientists (7,8)

observed that prenylamine, a newly developed coronary dilator, and verapamil, another phenylalkylamine with coronary dilating properties, exerted negative inotropic effects on isolated cat and rabbit myocardium and also depressed cardiac performance in the canine heart-lung preparation. This potent cardiodepressant effect of these two new agents appeared to distinguish them from classic vasodilators, because drugs such as nitroglycerin and papaverine with potent smooth-muscle-relaxing properties depress cardiac muscle only at high concentrations. Because the inotropic and chronotropic effects of prenylamine and verapamil were quite opposite to those elicited by catecholamines, the new drugs were first believed to be adrenergic blocking agents (9,10). However, Fleckenstein et al. (11) were among the first to report that the effects of both prenylamine and verapamil differed from β-adrenergic receptor antagonists. They observed that both agents depressed cardiac contractility without altering the height of the contour of the monophasic action potential, and they concluded that the drugs acted as uncouplers of excitation-contraction coupling. The action of these drugs was attributed to inhibition of the influx of Ca^{2+} into the myocardial cells. Consequently, the agents were called Ca^{2+} antagonists (11).

ROLE OF CALCIUM IN THE HEART

Calcium ions are widely recognized as playing important roles in the overall maintenance of homeostasis, in the contractile process of the heart, smooth muscle, and skeletal muscle, in glandular secretion, and in the release of neurotransmitters (4,12–14). In view of this, it is rather surprising that Ca^{2+} antagonists can be used therapeutically, having apparently a rather selective action on the cardiovascular system, without important side effects. It was a century ago that Sidney Ringer (15) established the importance of calcium in cardiac contraction. It is now well recognized that activation of contraction results from elevation of the intracellular concentration of calcium above 10^{-7} M. This, in turn, removes the inhibitory influence of the troponin-tropomyosin protein complex on the interaction between actin and myosin (16); actin filaments are displaced relative to myosin filaments, and contraction ensues (17) (Fig. 1). Thus, the calcium that enters the cell during the plateau of the action potential plays an essential role, coupling myocardial excitation to contraction, although there is some evidence that the transmembrane flux of calcium may merely trigger the release of larger quantities of the ion from intracellular stores and that it is the latter that actually activates the contractile mechanism (Fig. 1). Extracellular calcium is bound to the cell surface coat, and intracellular calcium is sequestered in the sarcoplasmic reticulum. In skeletal muscle, the calcium that triggers contraction comes mainly from internal stores in the plentiful sarcoplasmic reticulum. In cardiac muscle, the sarcoplasmic reticulum is not so plentiful, and the calcium current that flows from the cell surface to the interior during the action-potential plateau plays a more important role than in skeletal muscle. In vascular smooth muscle, membrane calcium may play an even more important role in contraction and maintenance of tone. The lumina of coronary and systemic arteries may be altered by changes in smooth-muscle tone induced by the movement of calcium across the membranes of smooth-muscle cells. If extracellular calcium is prevented from penetrating the cell membrane, muscular contraction will be prevented (18). In addition, vascular

smooth muscle will relax, producing vasodilatation, and cardiac muscle will contract less powerfully. In addition to its role in contraction of heart muscle, calcium is important for the generation and conduction of the cardiac impulse. Reduction of calcium ions results in atrioventricular (A-V) block. In reentrant supraventricular tachyarrhythmias, the A-V node is considered to be the site of the recurrent pathway. Like digitalis, but by a different mechanism, agents that inhibit calcium flux tend to block conduction within the A-V node and depress reentrant circuits, thereby preventing or arresting supraventricular tachycardia. After-depolarizations are also inhibited by these agents. Thus, the genesis of extrasystoles is depressed. Overwhelming evidence has accumulated in the last two decades indicating that calcium ions are required during excitation in order to activate the biochemical processes that utilize adenosine triphosphate (ATP) for contraction. The rapid rise in free intracellular calcium resulting from the increased transmembrane calcium influx and a simultaneous liberation of calcium from endoplasmic stores initiates the splitting of ATP by the calcium-dependent ATPase of the myofibrils, so that phosphate-bond energy is transformed into mechanical work. Therefore, contractility is reversibly lost on calcium withdrawal. Thus, calcium ions not only trigger the contractile process but also control quantitatively the output of mechanical tension by regulating the amount of ATP that is metabolized during activity (20). The splitting of ATP will in turn give rise to intensified glycolytic and oxidative recovery processes that have to refill the high-energy phosphate stores. This explains that the whole chain of metabolic reactions following contraction is "calcium-sensitive."

ELECTROPHYSIOLOGY OF THE HEART

Although the precise mechanism of excitation-contraction coupling in most contractile tissues is still uncertain, information is availa-

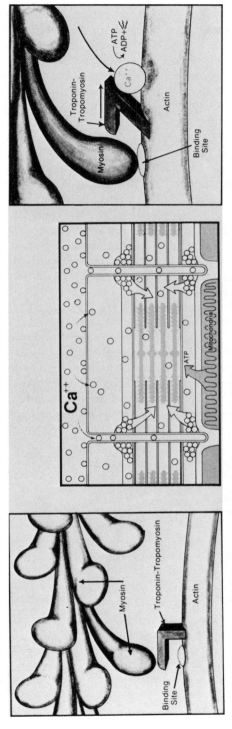

FIG. 1. Calcium's general role in muscle contraction. **Left:** In the resting state, regulatory protein tropomyosin prevents interaction of the contractile proteins actin and myosin, thereby preventing contraction. **Center:** When the cell is stimulated, calcium enters the cell during upstroke and the plateau of the action potential. Transmembrane calcium current associated with the action potential also triggers release of calcium from internal stores in sarcoplasmic reticulum. **Right:** When the cytoplasmic calcium concentration exceeds 10^{-7} M, calcium binds to the regulatory protein troponin, removing the inhibitory action of troponin; actin and myosin then interact to cause contraction. Free myoplasmic calcium is then actively pumped back into the sarcoplasmic reticulum. When the cytoplasmic calcium is again reduced below 10^{-7} M, the muscle relaxes. (From Bigger, ref. 132, with permission.)

ble from voltage clamp studies (20,21) that clarifies the ionic basis of depolarization in excitable membranes. Ions are believed to traverse the membrane through pores and channels. The conducted cardiac impulse can be viewed as a traveling wave of ion permeability and conductance changes that transiently reverse membrane polarity. Different ions (Na^+, K^+, Cl^-, Ca^{2+}) carry charges into and out of the cell; i.e., positive ions moving into the cell and negative ions moving out of the cell tend to depolarize it, and vice versa.

An understanding of the role of calcium fluxes in cellular electrophysiology requires an appreciation of the electrical activity of cardiac cells. The cardiac action potential can be divided into five phases (Fig. 2): phase 0, rapid depolarization; phase 1, early repolarization; phase 2, plateau; phase 3, rapid repolarization; phase 4, diastole. The shape of the cardiac action potential varies among the different types of cardiac cells (22,23). For example, cells in the sinoatrial (SA) and A-V nodes (Fig. 3) depolarize at a much slower rate than do cells in Purkinje fibers and atrial and ventricular contractile fibers. Microelectrode studies have shown the existence of two different currents responsible for the development

of the cardiac action potential: a rapid inward sodium current causing the rapid depolarization (phase 0) and a slow inward current carried mostly, but not exclusively, by calcium responsible for the plateau (24). The reason for slow conduction in the nodal cells is the nonexistence of fast sodium channels. Hence, depolarization is brought about by the slow inward calcium instead of sodium current (Fig. 3). Because of their dependence on calcium, sinus and A-V nodal cells are very sensitive to calcium-blocking agents.

The resting transmembrane potential during phase 4 (diastole) is maintained by a high intracellular K^+ concentration. Also, the cardiac cell actively extrudes Na^+ from its interior (22), so that the extracellular Na^+ concentration greatly exceeds the intracellular Na^+ concentration.

Rapid Inward Current

The rapid upstroke or action-potential spike during phase 0 is caused by a voltage-dependent increase in sodium conductance resulting in the rapid inward sodium current. Voltage-clamp studies have indicated that the fast sodium channel has rapid activation and inacti-

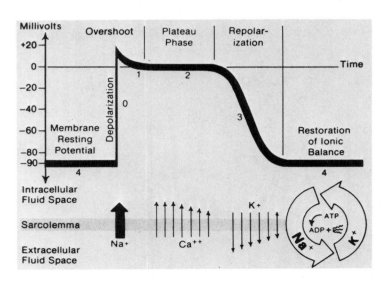

FIG. 2. Schematic of transmembrane cardiac action potential. (From Bigger, ref. 132, with permission.)

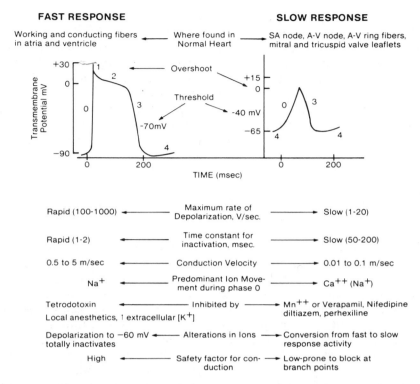

FIG. 3. Diagrammatic characterization of differences between fast and slow inward currents of cardiac action potential.

vation kinetics; its threshold for activation is between −60 and −70 mV, with a correspondingly high resting potential (Fig. 3). It has a large-amplitude action potential with a rapid rate of rise and rapid conduction velocity (0.5–5 m/sec), ensuring a high safety factor for conduction. The atrial and ventricular muscle fibers dependent on the fast channel for activation respond to a stimulus in an all-or-none fashion, and under physiologic conditions the recovery of excitability is prompt with the completion of repolarization. Furthermore, the fast sodium channel is dependent on the extracellular sodium and can be blocked by tetrodotoxin (a toxin produced by the Japanese puffer fish), low-sodium media, or local anesthetics (25). The passage of rapid inward sodium current is controlled by "gates" that open or close in response to voltage changes across the membrane (22,26,27).

Slow Inward Current

The slow and sustained inward calcium current develops when the cell has been depolarized from −90 mV to about −30 mV (Fig. 3). Activation of the slow current determines to a large extent the last part of the action-potential upstroke in most atrial, ventricular, and Purkinje fibers. It is responsible for excitation-contraction coupling and the plateau phase of the action potential (28). The slow channel is particularly significant in the early upstroke of the action potential in the A-V node. The kinetics of activation and inactivation of the slow inward current are several orders of magnitude slower than those of the fast channel (25,29,30), and the threshold voltage for activation is much lower (31,32). It reaches its maximum value when membrane potential is in the range of −20 to 0 mV (30).

Although the slow channel is often called a calcium channel, calcium and sodium are charge carriers for this channel (33). The fact that an action potential continues in calcium-free solutions is accounted for by assuming that sodium ions can take the place of calcium ions during this slow component. The contribution of sodium to the slow inward current under normal conditions is complex and differs among species and cardiac tissues. The resting membrane potential, action-potential amplitude, and overshoot in fibers with slow-channel activity are much smaller, and also the conduction velocity is about one-tenth (0.01–0.1 m/sec) that of fast-channel-dependent fibers (Fig. 3). Although the major ionic species contributing to slow inward current is calcium, Reuter (25,31) has estimated that the so-called slow channels are about 100 times more selective for calcium than for sodium or potassium, justifying the use of the term "calcium channel." However, such channels have not yet been identified as distinct anatomic structures and could be considered as specific protein macromolecular structures that traverse the lipid bilayer at various locations (34,35). Divalent cations with ionic radii similar to that of calcium (Ba^{2+} or Sr^{2+}) can pass through the calcium channel, whereas ions whose radii differ markedly from that of calcium (Mn^{2+}, Co^{2+}, Ni^{2+}, La^{3+}) can block these channels and inhibit passage of calcium (34–36). These latter inorganic metal ions may be considered to selectively inhibit slow-channel activity, but clinical interest in their use is limited in view of their potent general effects. However, an almost identical effect is produced by other compounds such as verapamil, nifedipine, and diltiazem, in concentrations not influencing the fast-channel activity. This effect has provided the basis for categorizing such agents as slow-channel blockers.

Modulation of Slow Inward Current

Sympathetic activity or stimulation by β-adrenergic receptor agonists such as isoproter-

enol, epinephrine, and cyclic AMP increases the magnitude of the slow current (31,37), whereas β receptor antagonists reduce calcium influx (4). Reuter and Scholz (38) investigated the mechanisms involved through which catecholamines exert their effects. Using isolated Purkinje fibers, they showed that enhancement of slow current by catecholamines is due to an increase in calcium conductance through the slow channel, without any marked alterations in the kinetics of the slow inward current or selectivity of the slow channel. Similar results were obtained with methylxanthines, histamine, and angiotensin (37). Addition of cyclic AMP also induces the "slow response" by modifying the ionic currents during the cardiac action potential (39). Cyclic AMP may activate a protein kinase that catalyzes a critical phosphorylation reaction at the inner gate of the slow channel (25,37). That cyclic AMP plays an important role is suggested by the oscillations in cyclic AMP levels during the cardiac cycle, with the peak occurring midway through the rise in tension (40,41). In addition, cyclic GMP, which opposes the effects of cyclic AMP, causes a reduction in the slow inward current (42). Thus, the magnitude of the slow inward current is determined by the number of slow channels opened and by the availability of cyclic AMP required to promote phosphorylation of a protein at the inner surface of the membrane (37). ATP has also been proposed to increase the slow inward current, probably by chelating intracellular calcium adjacent to the sarcolemma, resulting in a large electrochemical driving force for the inward calcium current during the plateau phase of the action potential (37,43).

In addition to the slow calcium channel, calcium ion influx could occur via a sodium-calcium carrier mechanism (44). The magnitude of this Na^+-Ca^{2+} exchange is dependent on the relative intracellular and extracellular concentrations of sodium (45). This carrier mechanism is electrogenic in nature (46) and is susceptible to inhibition by lanthanum (47).

Importance of Slow Current in Myocardial Ischemia

Unlike the situation with fast-channel activity, the threshold for activation of the slow channel is in the range of −30 to −40 mV. Such an action potential is particularly prone to arise in partially depolarized fibers, as in myocardial ischemia. This may contribute to the appearance of so-called unidirectional block and reentrant excitation due to excessively depressed conduction that is of importance in the genesis of ectopic tachyarrhythmias (23). Pacemaker cells of the SA node and cells in the proximal regions of the A-V node have slowly rising action potentials and reduced rates of conduction and are activated largely by the slow inward current. Such slow potentials, by their effect on cell metabolism, can cause depolarization of the cells within the ischemic region, resulting in anomalous automaticity due to the decremental reduction they induce. This anomalous or triggered automaticity can be seen in cells in the coronary sinus and other locations and occasionally has been partly responsible for supraventricular tachyarrhythmias in humans. Triggered automaticity can be abolished by calcium antagonists. This approach may have clinical applicability as well. On the other hand, because slow-response action potentials are seen under normal physiologic conditions in the sinus and A-V nodes, calcium antagonists may exacerbate the sick-sinus syndrome or potentiate A-V block.

DELETERIOUS EFFECTS OF CALCIUM OVERLOADING ON THE HEART

The increased exploration of calcium antagonists as potential therapeutic agents is due to the increasingly recognized importance of calcium as a mediator of myocardial injury induced by myocardial ischemia (48,49).

Cardiac muscle depends almost exclusively on aerobic metabolism for the genesis of ATP required for maintenance of cell viability and contractile function. This aerobic generation of ATP occurs in the mitochondria—organelles that oxidize substrate and conserve the energy liberated in the form of ATP. Mitochondria also utilize energy obtained from substrate oxidation to extrude calcium from the organelles themselves and transport it into the cytosol. Under normal physiologic conditions, intracellular free calcium is maintained within the range of 10^{-7} to 10^{-8} M. Thus, a massive concentration gradient (of the order of 10,000 : 1) exists from extracellular calcium to intracellular calcium. During myocardial cell damage by ischemia, or when mitochondria are exposed to elevated levels of calcium, as in reperfusion arrhythmias, calcium moves down the concentration gradient and enters the cytosol (Fig. 4). The massive calcium influx eventually impinges on mitochondria, resulting in the shunting of mitochondrial energy from production of ATP to increased mitochondrial calcium efflux. Excessive "bombardment" of mitochondria by pathologically augmented intracellular calcium concentration results in intramitochondrial deposition of granular deposits of calcium phosphate (50–52). This is reflected by ultrastructural changes, indicative of irreversible cell injury, as well as macroscopic evidence of excessive free calcium within the tissue, as reflected by augmented avidity for radiolabeled tracers, like [99m]TC-pyrophosphate (53). In experimental animals, the extent to which intracellular calcium accumulation occurs following ischemia correlates well with the calcium content of isolated mitochondria and with the impaired mechanical performance of the left ventricle. In such experimental situations, reperfusion with calcium-free blood tends to minimize the reperfusion injury (54), or exposure to calcium-blocking agents leads to preservation of the structures and function of the left ventricle and precludes the accumulation of calcium by the mitochondria (48,51).

The energy required for myocardial contractility under physiologic conditions is derived from hydrolysis of ATP. The enzymatic

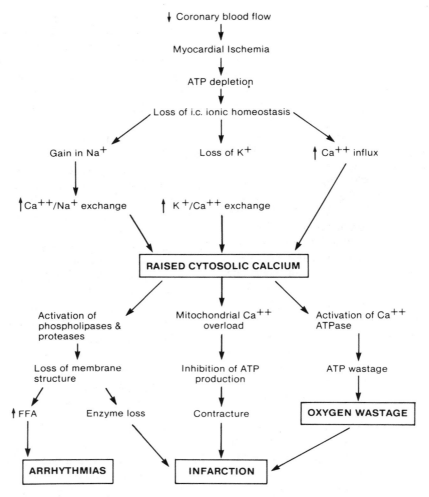

FIG. 4. Possible metabolic mechanisms whereby a decrease in the coronary flow results in massive calcium overloading, resulting in myocardial infarction and the development of arrhythmias.

processes involved for production of this energy are dependent on the intracellular calcium concentration and are modulated by calcium activated ATPase (Fig. 4). The excessively high intramitochondrial calcium "overloading" during ischemia results in potentiation of ATP hydrolysis, with consequent depletion of the intracellular high-energy phosphate stores required for maintenance of cell viability (Fig. 4).

Excessive influx of calcium during ischemia could also lead to increased degradation of membrane phospholipids (Fig. 4), impairing membrane structure and ultimately giving rise to detergentlike molecules potentially capable of inducing malignant arrhythmias (55,56). Examples of potentially detergentlike molecules are long-chain fatty acids esterified with Coenzyme A, acyl carnitine, and lysophosphoglycerides that accumulate in large quantities in the ischemic myocardium (55,57). Thus, the use of calcium antagonists to inhibit massive calcium influx induced by ischemia not only would preserve the jeopardized myocardium but also would tend to reduce the accumulation of noxious metabolites (48).

MECHANISMS OF ACTION OF CALCIUM ANTAGONISTS

The basic mechanism of action of calcium antagonists, (more precisely, the exact site of their action) is not yet clarified. This is reasonable, for it is clear that there are numerous sites, both intracellular and extracellular, at which calcium antagonists might be expected to modify excitation-contraction coupling. These drugs do not act according to the traditional concepts of an agonist–antagonist relationship. Rather, several distinct mechanisms could be operating, owing to their structural diversity and pharmacologic properties.

A number of agents that inhibit the slow inward current (Fig. 6) are now available and indeed are of great potential value in the treatment of numerous cardiovascular disorders. Most experimental and clinical experience has been obtained with four drugs: verapamil, nifedipine, perhexiline, and diltiazem. The calcium antagonists have now been further subdivided into those altering the kinetics of calcium flux (verapamil) and those altering total calcium conductance (diltiazem, nifedipine), presumably by their differential effects on the two different gates in the calcium channel of cardiac tissue (58). For example, nifedipine reduces the number of slow channels available for transporting calcium, without changing the rate at which calcium transport occurs through any intact remaining channel. For this reason, the effects of nifedipine are not dependent on heart rate. In contrast, verapamil not only alters the number of channels available for transport but also markedly affects the kinetics of transport. In particular, it appears to delay recovery from inactivation after an electrical stimulus resulting in calcium transport, and accordingly its effects are markedly dependent on heart rate.

Recently, the concept (59) has emerged that there are at least two calcium-activation systems in mammalian smooth muscle. The first can be blocked by the typical calcium antagonists and is preferentially involved in producing phasic mechanical activity. The other mechanism, resistant to calcium blockers, is preferentially involved in producing tonic mechanical activity and is suppressed by sodium nitroprusside.

In isolated cardiac muscle, depression of contractility was demonstrated without any alteration in the upstroke velocity of the action potential, only with slight abbreviation of the plateau phase (4,60). From these experiments and others demonstrating an effect on the action potential after Na^+ flux was inhibited, Fleckenstein concluded that calcium antagonists act by selective inhibition of the calcium influx through the cell membrane. If this mechanism were the only explanation for their action, calcium antagonists should inhibit ^{45}Ca uptake by the cells when measured with the lanthanum methods. However, none of the available calcium antagonists at concentrations that depress cardiac contractility *in vitro* cause any diminution in uptake of lanthanum-resistant ^{45}Ca (5,61). Thus, it is probably incorrect to consider these agents as specific competitive calcium-channel blockers (25). As summarized by Henry (62), the calcium antagonists vary markedly in chemical structure, and their inhibitory effects on the slow inward current are not always completely corrected by increases in external calcium concentration or mimicked by reduction in external calcium concentration.

Although all electrophysiologic evidence indicates that calcium antagonists produce reduction in the maximum slow-channel conductance, recent studies have shown that fast sodium channels could also be affected at concentrations somewhat greater than required to block slow inward current. This has been shown for D600 (methoxyverapamil) and diltiazem, but not for nifedipine (63,64). In contrast, verapamil, but not nifedipine, is capable of blocking an outward K^+ current that occurs during repolarization (62,65). Furthermore, the negative inotropic effects and calcium-antagonist properties of verapamil and D600 are associated with the (−)-isomers, whereas the (+)-isomer is a sodium-channel blocker (66). Many of the experimental and clinical studies have used racemic mixtures. It is unclear at the present time whether or not any of the other drugs shown in Fig. 6 have these differential effects in their optical isomers. The impairment of inward current by verapamil and D600 is frequency- and voltage-dependent, consistent with their ability to retard or voltage-shift the recovery from channel inactivation or to reduce the availability of calcium to the channel (67). The frequency-dependent inhibition by these agents resembles the inhibitory action of local anesthetics on the sodium channel (68); however, nifedipine exhibits a less marked frequency-dependent inhibition of response (69). Additionally, both verapamil and D600 have been shown in binding studies to inhibit cardiac muscarinic (70) and liver α-adrenergic receptors (71), but they do not affect the Na^+-Ca^{2+} exchange mechanism discussed earlier (72).

In view of the heterogeneity of structure and varying electrophysiologic and vascular actions of these agents, it is premature to ascribe all of their effects to "calcium-channel blockade." Thus, it has been proposed (6, 73,96) that there may be either a qualitative or quantitative difference in the response of the slow channels in vascular smooth-muscle cells and A-V nodal cells to calcium antagonists. All calcium antagonists, in addition to inhibiting the slow calcium influx in the cardiac tissue, reduce intracellular calcium in vascular smooth muscle as well. This is demonstrated by their rather remarkable effectiveness in preventing coronary vasospasms, the cause of variant angina; i.e., these agents inhibit the contraction of vascular smooth muscle. The mechanisms involved in reducing calcium influx, however, may have little to do with their effect on the slow current that is readily shown in the cardiac tissue. It has been suggested recently (74,75) that calcium antagonists may bind to the calcium-dependent regulatory protein or calmodulin. Because this protein may serve as the calcium-binding protein of the smooth-muscle contractile machinery (75), this may represent their site of action as calcium antag-

onists in vascular smooth muscle. Zelis and Flaim (6) have recently reviewed the mechanisms involved in vascular smooth-muscle contraction (Fig. 5). Accordingly, the contraction could be initiated either by activation of potential-dependent calcium channels (PDC) or by activation of receptor-operated channels (ROC) by norepinephrine (NE) in this case. The passage of calcium ion through ROC can trigger release of calcium from storage sites in the sarcolemmal membrane (site 3 in Fig. 5) or sarcoplasmic reticulum (site 4). When the intracellular calcium concentration increases, the combination of calcium and calmodulin activates myosin light-chain kinase (site 5), resulting in phosphorylation of the light chains of myosin (MLC-P) and thus allowing actin and myosin to interact to induce contraction (site 6). Relaxation occurs when a phosphatase-mediated (P-TASE) dephosphorylation of MLC-P predominates (site 7) over the MLC-mediated phosphorylation reaction. MLC kinase activity decreases when the MLC-kinase-calmodulin-calcium complex is dissociated because of uptake of calcium into intracellular storage sites in the sarcolemma (site 8), mitochondria (site 9), and sarcoplasmic reticulum (site 10) or when calcium is extruded from the cell through a calcium-activated pump (site 11) or passively via sodium-calcium exchange (site 14).

The preliminary data (76) indicate that verapamil inhibits calcium influx in the smooth muscle through the ROC (site 2) by blocking the trigger release of sarcolemmal calcium (site 3). Diltiazem, on the other hand, stimulates the sodium-potassium pump (site 14), and the reduced intracellular sodium drives passive sodium-calcium exchange (sites 12 and 13). It may also stimulate energy-dependent calcium extrusion (site 11). Furthermore, these data indicate that inhibition of NE-induced intracellular calcium accumulation by verapamil peaks early and then declines, whereas diltiazem produced a steady, slow, progressive inhibition of intracellular calcium accumulation. They also explain the findings that verapamil inhibits vascular smooth-mus-

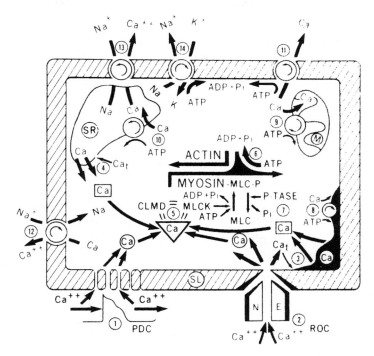

FIG. 5. Schematic representation of the mechanisms involved in vascular smooth-muscle contraction and relaxation. CLMD, calmodulin; MLCK, myosin light-chain kinase; SL, sarcolemma; SR, sarcoplasmic reticulum; M, mitochondria; PDC, potential-dependent calcium channels; Ca_t, trigger calcium; [Ca], calcium from intracellular sites (SL and SR); (Ca), calcium from extracellular sources. The reaction ATP → ADP + Pi is sometimes abbreviated as ATP →. (From Zelis and Flaim, ref. 6, with permission.)

cle oxygen consumption, whereas diltiazem stimulates it (77). Based on the foregoing discussion, it would be premature to suggest any definitive conclusions regarding the dominant mechanisms of action of drugs with calcium-antagonistic effects.

PHARMACOLOGY OF CALCIUM ANTAGONISTS

Figure 6 lists the drugs grouped together as calcium antagonists by Fleckenstein (4). Besides these heterogeneous compounds, several other drugs are known to interfere with the availability of calcium for contraction of smooth muscle. The relaxant effects of diazoxide, nitroglycerin, papaverine, and hydralazine depend to a great extent on their interference with the mobilization of intracellular calcium (78). This is unlike calcium antagonists, which block the influx of extracellular

calcium (4). Another difference between the smooth-muscle relaxants and calcium antagonists is that depression of cardiac contractility is characteristic only for the latter group of drugs (4,79).

The question in the minds of many physicians and researchers is this: When will the calcium antagonists be available for use in the United States? In December 1980, the cardiorenal advisory committee of the FDA recommended approval of intravenous verapamil (in use in Germany since 1962) as an antiarrhythmic agent, more precisely for treating paroxysmal supraventricular tachycardia. It is contraindicated in patients with known sinoatrial or wide QRS-segment tachycardia. In 1981, verapamil in its oral form was approved for all forms of angina pectoris. Nifedipine (in use in the United Kingdom since 1977), in oral form, was also recommended by the FDA in early 1981 for vasospastic and

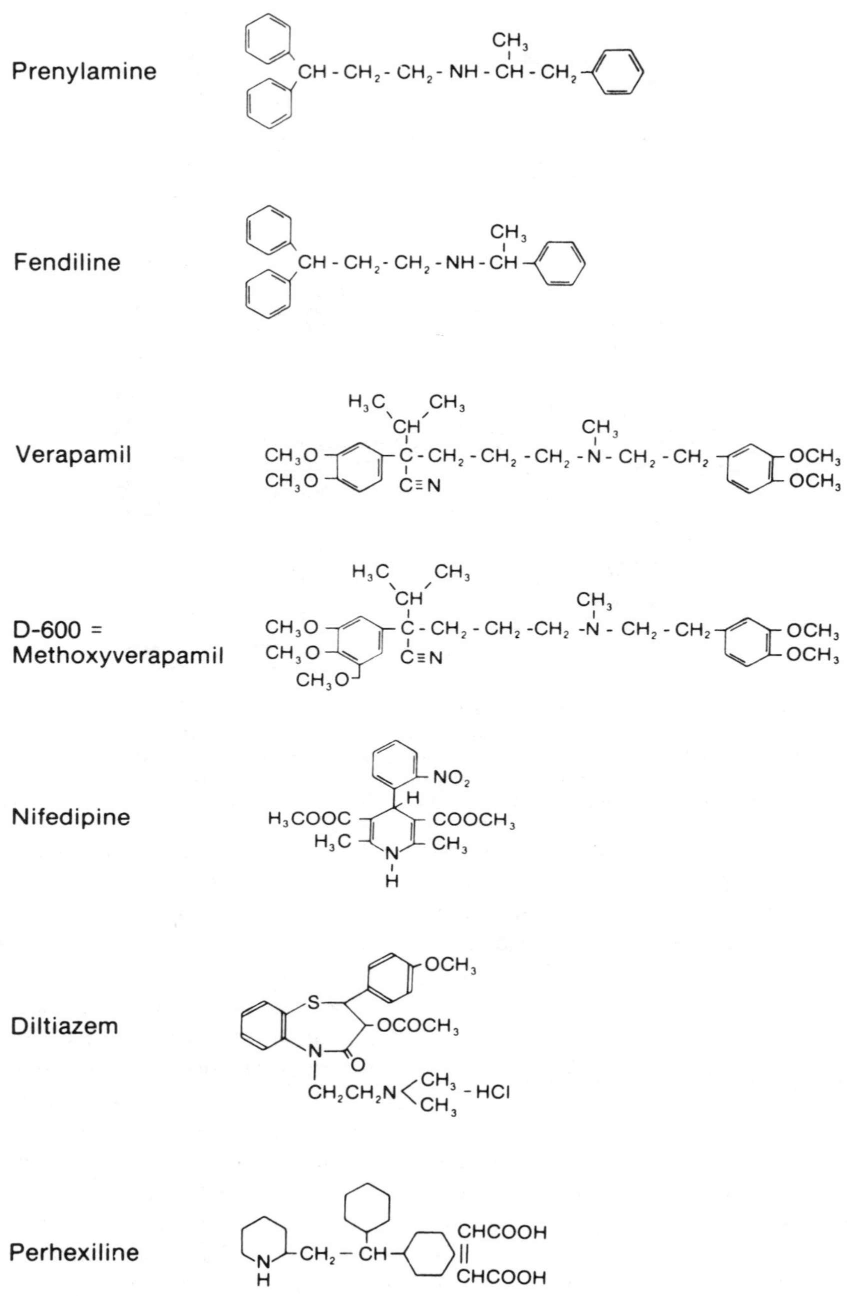

FIG. 6. Chemical structures of several calcium antagonists.

chronic stable angina. Diltiazem (in use in Japan since 1974) has undergone extensive clinical studies in the United States, and in 1981 it was approved (in oral form) for angina pectoris. Yet another calcium antagonist, lidofla- zine (in use in Belgium since 1969), was approved for angina pectoris unresponsive to conventional β blocker and nitrate therapy, but additional trials were recommended by the FDA in patients with ischemic heart disease, sinus rhythm, and angina pectoris to determine whether or not the drug causes ventricular arrhythmias. Other calcium antagonists that have been used in Europe and are under consideration or are undergoing clinical testing in the United States are perhexiline (in use in Germany since 1975) and flunarizine (in use in Germany since 1977).

The subsequent discussion, however, will be focused on (±)-verapamil, nifedipine, and diltiazem, the agents receiving the most clinical attention in the United States.

Verapamil

Verapamil (Isoptin®, Calan®), the prototype calcium antagonist, is a synthetic papaverine derivative (Fig. 6) and was first introduced as a smooth-muscle relaxant with potent peripheral and coronary vasodilator properties. However, recently it has been reported (80) that the smooth-muscle-relaxing effects are weaker than those exerted by nitroglycerin and nifedipine.

Electrophysiologic Effects

The electrophysiologic effects of verapamil are most pronounced in SA and A-V nodal cells. Cellular depolarization in these areas is determined primarily by the slow (calcium) inward current, as discussed earlier, which leads to a slow action potential. The direct electrophysiologic actions of verapamil on the heart are particularly evident in partially depolarized or ischemic myocardium (81–83). Verapamil, for example, has been shown to reduce the conduction delay in ischemic myocardium (82–84,260), in contrast to agents possessing a fast-channel-blocking property (lidocaine), which increase the ischemia-induced conduction delay (85). Theoretically, impairment of slow inward current by verapamil should further retard conduction through the ischemic myocardium and thus facilitate the production of reentry arrhythmias. This latter outcome could be due to an increase in extracellular K^+ (86) and release of catecholamines (87) in the ischemic zone

after coronary occlusion resulting in a decrease in the membrane potential. The aforementioned paradoxical effect of verapamil could be explained by the hemodynamic effects of reduction in afterload and reduction in the size of ischemic injury (82), rather than its electrophysiologic actions (88). If this happens, blockade of the slow response that prolongs conduction delay might be offset by its hemodynamic effects, resulting in improved conduction. In other studies (89) in open-chest dogs, low doses of verapamil (plasma level less than 150 ng/ml) prolonged the P-P interval from 397 to 442 msec and the A-H interval (His-bundle electrogram) from 65 to 94 msec. However, at higher drug levels (less than 400 ng/ml), the P-R and A-H intervals increased to 554 and 136 msec, respectively, and 50% of the animals had second- or third-degree A-V block due to excessive prolongation of A-V conduction. The QRS duration, Q-T interval, and H-V intervals were not affected even at the highest plasma drug levels (400–2,000 ng/ml). Similar dose-dependent prolongation of the P-R interval in dogs has been reported by other investigators (90,91). The depressant effect on the rate of SA node discharge (negative chronotropic) and the inhibition of conduction velocity through the A-V node (negative dromotropic) induced by verapamil do not appear to be mediated via the autonomic nervous system, because they occur in the presence of autonomic blockade with atropine and propranolol (92,93). Thus, prolongation of A-V nodal refractoriness and slowing of conduction by verapamil provides the theoretical basis for its clinical effectiveness in controlling reentrant paroxysmal supraventricular arrhythmias (90).

The results from various clinical studies are in substantial agreement with the experimental data. For example, in patients in sinus rhythm, verapamil, intravenously, had no effect on R-R, QRS, and Q-Tc intervals of the electrocardiogram (94). The P-R interval, reflecting A-V conduction, increased after therapeutic doses (10 mg i.v., 120 mg orally) of verapamil (94,95) (Table 1). Furthermore, verapamil at 0.15 mg/kg intravenously prolonged

TABLE 1. *Effects of intravenous verapamil on electrocardiograms in patients with sinus rhythm*

Interval (msec)	Before verapamil	After verapamil	No. of patients	Significance
R-R	743.0 ± 38	738.0 ± 27	15	N.S.[a]
P-R	186.1 ± 6.2	205.4 ± 8.1	13	$p < 0.001$
QRS	65.5 ± 4.1	66.1 ± 4.6	13	N.S.
Q-T$_c$	457.8 ± 9.9	451.0 ± 6.6	12	N.S.

[a] N.S.: not significant.
From Heng et al. (94), with permission.

the A-H interval without altering the H-V interval (96).

Effects on Coronary Circulation

By inhibiting excitation-contraction coupling in vascular smooth muscle, verapamil has been shown to cause marked vasodilatation in most peripheral vascular beds, including mesenteric and canine hindlimb preparations (4,97). It is also an extremely potent coronary vasodilator (98), and it increases coronary blood flow to a much greater extent than papaverine and reduces myocardial oxygen uptake (8). Nayler and Szeto (99) have demonstrated that, like propranolol, verapamil decreases myocardial oxygen demand, but whereas propranolol consistently increases coronary vascular resistance, verapamil has the opposite effect, even during the hypotensive phase of the drug's action.

Verapamil was initially believed to be a competitive β-adrenergic receptor antagonist because it appeared to antagonize cardiac adrenergic effects (100). However, subsequent studies (97) showed that verapamil decreased the vascular responsiveness to α and β receptor stimulants and to angiotensin receptors in the dog. Coronary vasoconstriction induced by cardiac glycosides was also blocked by verapamil (101), as well as vasoconstriction induced by tetraethylammonium in large and small coronary arteries (102). Thus, the relaxant effect of verapamil on smooth muscle is due to inhibition of calcium influx, a critical step in the excitation-contraction process that

is not dependent on the receptor type responsible for stimulation. The vasodilating effect of verapamil can be blocked or totally abolished by increasing the extracellular calcium concentration (103) and is unaffected by β-adrenergic receptor antagonists, catecholamine depletion, or vagotomy (104).

Experimental studies have shown that verapamil given soon after coronary artery ligation increases flow distal to the ligature, as indicated by direct measurement of retrograde coronary flow (105), by the tracer microsphere technique (162), or by plastic casts made of the coronary vasculature. This enhanced collateral flow to the ischemic area may be due to a reduction in coronary arteriolar resistance in collateral vessels supplying the ischemic zone or in vessels in the ischemic zone distal to the ligature (105).

Vasodilator Effects

Verapamil is a potent peripheral vasodilator, although its smooth-muscle-relaxing effects are weaker than those exerted by nitroglycerin and nifedipine (4,80). In open-chest dogs, administration of verapamil yielding plasma levels less than 150 ng/ml (fluorometric assay) produced little hemodynamic change. However, larger doses (14–22 mg, plasma level as high as 2,000 ng/ml) induced marked decreases in arterial pressure, heart rate, left ventricular *dP/dt*, peripheral resistance, and cardiac output (89,162). In a separate study, Angus et al. (93) reported a dose-dependent peripheral vasodilatation, with reflex increases in myocardial contractility and heart rate. In conscious animals, verapamil produced dose-related reductions in stroke volume, mean aortic pressure, maximum *dP/ dt,* and total peripheral resistance, as well as an increase in heart rate (106,107,166). Propranolol pretreatment blocked the reflex cardiac stimulation, but the vasodilatation was unaffected, consistent with the fact that the vascular effects of verapamil were mediated through a mechanism independent of peripheral β receptor stimulation (93,106). Verapamil, in contrast to nifedipine, has a greater propensity to exert direct myocardial depressant effects. Nevertheless, in antiarrhythmic doses, precipitation of cardiac failure is unusual (108,109).

In healthy subjects, verapamil at 7.5 to 12.5 mg i.v. increased heart rate and cardiac index and decreased peripheral resistance, mean aortic pressure, and mean pulmonary pressure (110). One patient had second-degree A-V block, and three others exhibited prolongation of the P-R interval (110,111). In other studies (108) involving patients with coronary artery disease, verapamil (0.1-mg/kg bolus followed by 0.005 mg/kg/min infusion) markedly lowered mean aortic pressure and systemic vascular resistance. Simultaneously, all indices of left ventricular performance markedly improved. The cardiac index and ejection fraction significantly increased. No significant changes were noted in the heart rate after verapamil administration. The peripheral vasodilating effect of verapamil probably leads to a reflex tachycardia, offsetting the direct bradycardia caused by SA node depression (112) and helping to maintain the cardiac output. Even with atrial pacing, verapamil at 0.1 mg/ kg had only a mild negative inotropic effect in patients with normal left ventricular function (113). In summary, verapamil depresses the rate of spontaneous SA nodal discharge (negative chronotropic effect), prolongs A-V nodal conduction (negative dromotropic effect), and depresses myocardial contractility (negative inotropic effect). However, its potentially negative inotropic effect is compensated

for by its vasodilatory effect (108,114). These effects are rapid in onset, are dose-dependent, and are rapidly dissipated within 10 min after acute intravenous administration.

Side Effects and Contraindications

Adverse effects of oral and intravenous verapamil occur in approximately 10% of patients, but only 1% of such patients require discontinuation of the drug (114,115). Orally administered verapamil is extremely well tolerated, with a very low incidence of gastric intolerance, constipation, vertigo, facial flushing, headache, nervousness, and pruritus. However, the side effects encountered during intravenous administration are in part due to its pharmacologic properties. The most common is a transient and mild decrease in arterial blood pressure and occasional A-V conduction disturbances (94,116). Serious side effects of intravenous verapamil, such as hypotension, bradycardia, and even ventricular asystole, have been reported in patients receiving concomitant β receptor antagonists (117–119) and in patients with severe hypertrophic cardiomyopathy (120). In patients with impaired function of SA node or impaired A-V conduction, intravenous verapamil may cause sinus bradycardia, sinus arrest, shock, and heart block (121).

The main contraindications (Table 2) to the use of verapamil are the presence of advanced heart failure, sick-sinus syndrome, second- or third-degree A-V block, digitalis toxicity, and hypotension (115,122). Also, coadministration of verapamil and β blockers should be avoided; β blockade abolishes the compensatory reflex tachycardia induced by verapamil, and the cardiodepressant effects of these agents are additive (112). Hepatotoxicity due to verapamil has been documented (123); hence, this complication should be considered if a patient receiving verapamil has an abnormal liver function test.

Therapy for Toxic Effects

In most cases, intravenous atropine sulfate (1 mg) can shorten prolonged A-V conduction

TABLE 2. *Comparative contraindications of β blocking agents, verapamil, and nifedipine*

Contraindications	β blockade	Verapamil	Nifedipine
Absolute			
Sinus bradycardia	++	0/+	0
Sick-sinus syndrome	++	+	0
A-V conduction defects	+	++	0
Digitalis toxicity			
with A-V block[a]	+	++	0
Bronchospasm	++	0	0
Heart failure	++	+	0
Hypotension	+	+	+
Relative			
Digitalis without toxicity	Care	Care	0
β blockade	0	Care	Hypotension
Verapamil therapy	Care	0	Hypotension

[a] Contraindication to rapid intravenous administration.
From Opie (121), with permission.

(124). Calcium gluconate, 1 to 2 g infused over 5 min (10–20 ml) and later maintained at 5 mM/hr, helps in heart failure. Norepinephrine also will rapidly reverse excessive bradycardia or hypotension. Should pharmacologic measures fail, external massage and cardiac pacing should be initiated and maintained to provide necessary support until verapamil's short-lived effects attenuate. Verapamil is not effectively removed by dialysis (125).

Absorption, Fate, and Excretion

Verapamil is almost completely absorbed (> 90%) after oral administration. However, because of extensive first-pass hepatic metabolism, only about 20% of the drug is bioavailable (Table 3). Measurable electrophysiologic effects (prolongation of P-R interval) have appeared at 2 hr and peaked at 5 hr after a single dose (68,115). A slow-release form of verapamil has an onset of action of 6 hr and a duration of about 14 hr (126). Absorption following oral administration varies from 88 to 92%. After intravenous administration, the hypotensive effect is short-lived, but the negative dromotropic effect is more sustained. The peak hypotensive effect occurs at 5 min, and by 10 to 20 min the effect is dissipated

(121,127). However, the onset of the negative dromotropic effect is within 1 to 2 min; it peaks at 10 to 15 min and is still detectable after 6 hr. This indicates preferential uptake and binding of verapamil by the A-V nodal tissues (115).

The drug exhibits a biexponential decline after both oral and intravenous administrations, with an initial distribution phase lasting from 18 to 35 min (Table 3) and a much slower elimination phase with a half-life varying from 3 to 7 hr (127,128). Seventy percent of an oral or intravenous dose is excreted by the kidney, and 15% is eliminated via the gastrointestinal route. Only 3 to 4% is excreted unchanged in the urine. The first-pass metabolism in the liver by the oral route accounts for the marked differences between the oral and intravenous doses required to obtain similar physiologic effects (128). Thus, oral doses must be 8 to 10 times larger than intravenous doses to achieve comparable plasma verapamil levels. Ninety percent of verapamil in the serum is bound to protein (128). Therapeutic plasma verapamil concentrations lie in the range of 100 to 300 ng/ml.

A large number of metabolites are produced by hepatic metabolism by *N*-alkyl cleavage of the homoveratryl and methyl groups and by *O*-demethylation (129). However, it is un-

TABLE 3. *Pharmacokinetics of calcium antagonists*

	(±)-Verapamil	Nifedipine	Diltiazem
Dosage			
Oral (mg/8 hr)	80–160	10–20	60–90
Intravenous (μg/kg)	150	5–15	75–150
Absorption			
Oral (%)	>90	>90	>90
Bioavailability (%)	10–22	65–70	<20
Onset of action			
Sublingual (min)	—	3	—
Oral (min)	<30	<20	<30
Peak effect	10–15 min i.v.	1–2 hr orally	30 min orally
	5 hr orally		
Therapeutic plasma con-	15–100	25–100	30–130
centration (ng/ml)	(3.2×10^{-8}—2×10^{-7} M)	(7×10^{-8}—2×10^{-7} M)	(7×10^{-8}—3×10^{-7} M)
Protein binding (%)	90	90	80
Plasma half-time			
Initial fast (α) (min)	15–30	150–180	20
Slow (β) (hr)	3–7	5	4
Metabolism	Extensive first-pass he-	Extensively metabo-	Extensively deacety-
	patic extraction (70%	lized to an inert free	lated
	of oral dose)	acid and lactone	
Excretion			
Renal (%)	50 first day (70 total)	70 first day (80 total)	35 (total)
Fecal (%)	15	<15	65

Adapted from Henry (68).

clear to what extent these metabolites contribute to the drug's therapeutic effects (130). One of the major metabolites (norverapamil) correlates well with the concentration of the parent drug (131,186). Norverapamil is about 20% as potent as verapamil in terms of systemic hemodynamic effects and coronary vasodilation (132). No accumulation of either compound has been documented. Further studies will be required to fully assess the pharmacologic properties of such metabolites, because they may contribute to the overall therapeutic actions of verapamil.

Analogues of Verapamil

Methoxyverapamil or D600 (Fig. 6) is a slow-channel antagonist (4), but it has greater myocardial depressant effect and offers no advantage over verapamil. It has been used for over 12 years by biologists as a standard tool to study the effects of calcium ions.

Dimeditiapramine (Ro 11–1781, Tiapamil®, Larocord®) is an achiral analogue of verapamil, with replacement of cyano and iso-

propyl groups with 1,3-tetraoxadithiane substitutions (133) (Fig. 7). Tiapamil is 2 to 10 times less potent than verapamil but is less cardiodepressant (134,135,288). Like verapamil, however, it slows A-V conduction and causes coronary vasodilation (135,288). Tiapamil has been reported to have antifibrillatory activity as well as the ability to reduce infarct size in experimental animals (136).

Nifedipine

Nifedipine (Bay a 1040, Procardia®, Adalat®) is a dihydropyridine derivative (137) that bears no structural similarity to other already known vasoactive or cardioactive drugs (Fig. 6). Nifedipine is not a nitrate, and its ortho NO_2 group is not essential for its pharmacologic activity (138). In recent years, multiple dihydropyridine derivatives have been synthesized (niludipine, nimodipine, etc.) and are receiving investigative attention (Table 4).

Electrophysiologic Effects

Nifedipine appears to facilitate rather than suppress A-V conduction. Any direct suppres-

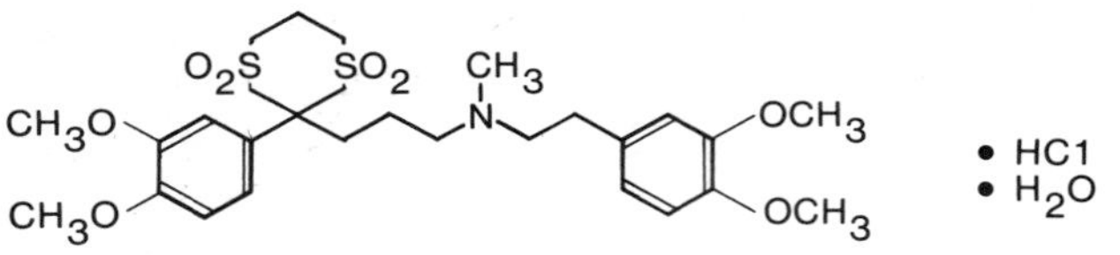

● HC1
● H$_2$O

FIG. 7. Chemical structure of Ro 11–1781.

sive effects of nifedipine on A-V nodal conduction seem weak because of the low dose used (one-tenth that of verapamil and diltiazem) and are overcome by a reflex increase in the sympathetic tone due to a fall in blood pressure (140).

In chronically instrumented dogs, nifedipine at 0.01 to 0.04 mg/kg had no discernible effect on A-V conduction, unlike verapamil (91). However, in equipotent hypotensive doses, nifedipine shortened the P-R interval, in contrast to verapamil, which results in prolongation of the P-R interval (89,91,95). Recently it was demonstrated that nifedipine at 0.1 mg/kg slightly decreased the magnitude of conduction delay in the ischemic myocardium at 15 min of ischemia, which corresponded with the peak plasma levels of nifedipine (141). However, conduction delay in the remainder of the study was essentially unaltered by nifedipine (141).

High concentrations of nifedipine (10^{-6} M), in sharp contrast to verapamil, failed to reduce the atrial excitability of isolated guinea pig atria (91) and had minimal effects on the resting potential and on maximal rate of rise of the action potential (64). However, it did depress the plateau phase of the action potential. At such high concentrations (10^{-6} M), nifedipine also caused dose-dependent prolongations of the atrial refractory period of the iso-

lated guinea pig atria and of the A-V node in the rabbits (90), but the dose–response curve was much less steep than for verapamil.

In clinical settings, nifedipine at 7.5 μg/kg intravenously did not affect the A-H and H-V intervals of His-bundle electrograms (96), unlike verapamil. The lack of any significant electrophysiologic properties, particularly in the conduction system, explains in part the lack of antiarrhythmic activity of the drug (141–143). Hence, in combination with β receptor antagonists and digoxin, it should theoretically be less hazardous than verapamil (121,163).

Effects on Coronary Circulation

The virtual absence of a detrimental effect of nifedipine on the A-V node could be due to its greater preference for vascular smooth muscle (144,145), resulting in, primarily, coronary and peripheral vasodilation. For example, in the blood-perfused A-V nodal preparation, verapamil increased both blood flow through the A-V nodal artery and A-V conduction time, in the same dose range. In contrast, blood flow was about 10 times more sensitive to nifedipine than was conduction (91). Dose selection is critical for studies with nifedipine, because excessive blood pressure reduction may be deleterious to the ischemic

TABLE 4. *Chemical structure of closely related dihydropyridine analogues of nifedipine*

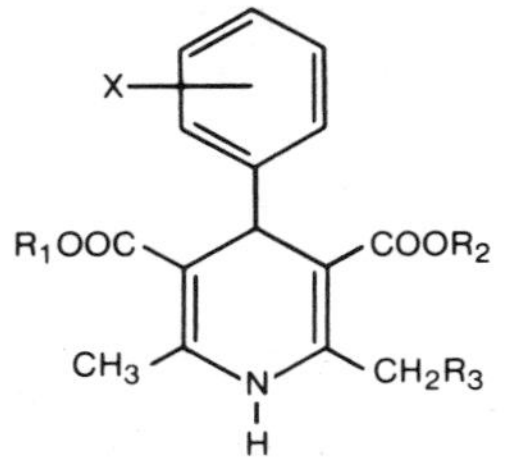

X	R$_1$	R$_2$	R$_3$	Compound
2–NO$_2$	Me	Me	H	Nifedipine
2–NO$_2$	(CH$_3$)$_2$CH$_2$CH$_2$	Me	H	Nisoldipine
2–CF$_3$	Et	Me	H	SKF – 24,260
3–NO$_2$	Me	Et	H	Nitrendipine
3–NO$_2$	nPrOCH$_2$CH$_2$	nPrOCH$_2$CH$_2$	H	Niludipine
3–NO$_2$	iPr	MeOCH$_2$CH$_2$	H	Nimodipine
3–NO$_2$	Et	Et	OH	FR – 7534
3–NO$_2$	Me	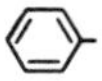 ⬡–CH$_2$N(CH$_3$)CH$_2$CH$_2$	H	Nicardipine

myocardium (155). Nifedipine at 5 µg/kg had minimal effects on the electrophysiology of the A-V node, but this dose caused pronounced increases in coronary sinus flow and a decrease in coronary resistance in the dog *in situ* (146). The degree of coronary vasodilation has been measured by evaluating the reactivity of isolated coronary artery strips in reducing K+-induced contracture. In equimolar doses, nifedipine was the most potent coronary vasodilator, being several thousand times more potent than papaverine (147).

Nifedipine at 0.43 mg/kg sublingually in conscious dogs caused a 65% increase in coronary flow and a 38% reduction in coronary resistance (148). These effects were sustained for periods of about 45 to 60 min. However, in anesthetized closed-chest dogs, nifedipine given intravenously at 10 µg/kg increased coronary blood flow by 142% at 2 min, and the duration of the effect was more than 30 min (149). Similar effects on coronary circulation were obtained in anesthetized open-chest dogs (150,151) and anesthetized pigs (152), resulting in a decrease in myocardial oxygen consumption (150,153) and a reduction in the size of the ischemic area in canine hearts (154,155). These beneficial effects exerted by nifedipine in the ischemic myocardium have been attributed to its ability to increase collateral flow (150,154,156) by stimulation of the latent preexistent interarterial coronary anastomoses (157) and by increasing phosphorylase *a* activity in the endocardial layers (158). However, it is unclear whether or not the latter metabolic effect of nifedipine has any relationship to its ability to redistribute myocardial blood flow in the ischemic myocardium (158). More recently, it has been demonstrated that, like adenosine (159), nifedipine also redistributes blood flow from endocardium to epicardium, depending on the extent of coronary occlusion in anesthetized open-chest dogs (160). The nifedipine-induced increase in coronary flow was associated with increases in inferior caval flow (venous return) and pulmonary arterial flow (cardiac output). In contrast, nitroglycerin tended to reduce venous return and car-

diac output (148). In the isolated blood-perfused canine heart, nifedipine as a coronary dilator was equipotent compared with nitroglycerin but more potent than dipyridamole, carbochromen, verapamil, papaverine, and khellin (148).

Vasodilator Effects

Nifedipine is one of the most potent vasodilators; it promptly relaxes isolated arteries contracted by KCl, norepinephrine, serotonin, and cardioactive glycosides (4). It is as potent as nitroglycerin, but in contrast to the situation with nitrates, the induced relaxations are sustained. The lack of a direct depressant action on the SA node and the absence of antisympathetic effect result in reflex increases in heart rate and contractility in response to peripheral vasodilatation induced by nifedipine. Thus, in this respect, the overall hemodynamic effects of nifedipine closely resemble those of conventional vasodilators. The direct depressant effect of nifedipine caused by inhibition of the slow channel in the heart is largely nullified by the drug's peripheral vasodilator properties (161). Thus, on a relative basis, nifedipine has less negative inotropic and chronotropic properties than verapamil and diltiazem. Administration to conscious dogs at 0.43 mg/kg sublingually decreased total peripheral resistance by 42% but did not produce any significant reduction in aortic mean blood pressure (148). In addition, heart rate and cardiac output increased by 62% and the contractile force (LV *dP/dt*) was augmented by 16% (148). In anesthetized dogs, similar results were obtained with nifedipine given as a bolus followed by slow intravenous infusion (150,156). In anesthetized pigs, Verdouw et al. (152) found that nifedipine decreased arterial pressure but had minor effects on cardiac output, coronary blood flow, left ventricular *dP/dt*, and systolic wall thickening. These authors concluded that nifedipine had no direct effects on the myocardium, but acted primarily by reducing afterload. It has been suggested that in conscious dogs nifedipine may not induce major changes in mean aortic blood pressure, because of a reflex increase in cardiac output (148,154,164). Thus, any direct negative inotropic action of nifedipine may be masked by a positive inotropic influence due to reflex sympathetic activation. By means of ultrasonic length gauges in the ischemic zone in anesthetized dogs it was found that nifedipine at 1 μg/kg/min, unlike nitroglycerin and nitroprusside, markedly improved (31%) shortening of ischemic segments, resulting in improved performance in ischemic zones (165). Nifedipine produced greater increases in coronary flow than in aortic flow, indicating selectivity of the drug for the coronary vascular bed (153,154). Recently, nifedipine has been demonstrated to antagonize ergonovine and K^+-induced coronary spasms in anesthetized dogs (167,168). Similar results have been documented in patients with variant angina, where nifedipine abolished symptomatic coronary artery spasms (169,170). The antispasmodic actions of nifedipine may account for its role in vasospastic angina. Nifedipine used in combination with hypothermic, potassium-based cardioplegia provided significant additional myocardial protection over cardioplegia alone (171–173). Recently, nifedipine has been demonstrated to have a potent anti-platelet-aggregating effect against ADP, epinephrine, and collagen-induced platelet aggregation in human platelet-rich plasma (174). Its effectiveness against digitalis-induced arrhythmias has also been documented (194).

The hemodynamic effects of nifedipine in humans resemble those observed in dogs. In patients undergoing cardiac catheterization for coronary artery disease, nifedipine at 20 mg sublingually produced increases in heart rate (+21%), cardiac output (+25%), and maximal dP/dt (+13%). Total peripheral resistance declined (−17%). Other hemodynamic variables, including mean aortic pressure, ejection fraction, and mean circumferential shortening velocity, did not change significantly (175). In addition, myocardial perfusion of underperfused segments was increased after intracoronary injection of 100

μg of nifedipine (175). After 20 mg of nifedipine sublingually, improved perfusion of normal zones and zones supplied by stenotic coronary arteries was also documented by thallium scintigraphy (175). These clinical observations indicate that nifedipine augments coronary flow in humans.

Side Effect and Contraindications

The mild side effects exerted by nifedipine are mainly from its vasodilatory effects. Headache occurs in about 5% of patients on chronic therapy, but hypotension, digital dysesthesias, flushing, dizziness, nausea and vomiting, tiredness, sedation, and leg edema occur less frequently (176). Sodium retention after nifedipine has recently been reported, but this is largely resolved by giving it in combination with diuretics (177). Only 4.7% of patients on chronic therapy with nifedipine have developed intolerable side effects that have led to discontinuation.

A small fraction of patients develop exacerbation of ischemic symptoms after 30 min of nifedipine administration (178–180). This possible detrimental effect could be induced by imbalancing myocardial oxygen supply and demand, resulting in severe hypotension in the presence of severe fixed obstruction, or by producing a coronary steal (155). No tolerance has been reported for nifedipine. The pulmonary, hepatic, and renal functions are unaltered, and so is the hematopoietic system (176).

The only absolute contraindication to nifedipine therapy is hypotension (Table 2). The use of nifedipine in combination with β receptor antagonists significantly increases exercise tolerance in patients with effort angina (163,181,182), but care must be taken about the possibility of heart failure (183). Similar beneficial effects of combination therapy have been reported in hypertensive patients (184, 185).

Absorption, Fate, and Excretion

After oral or sublingual administration of nifedipine, more than 90% of the administered drug is absorbed (Table 3). Only 20 to 30% of nifedipine is removed from portal blood by the liver, yielding a systemic bioavailability of more than 65% (187). The drug is detectable in the serum 3 min after sublingual administration and 20 min after oral administration. The peak blood concentration occurs 1 to 2 hr after oral use (Table 3). The total duration of action is 8 to 12 hr. Nifedipine at 15 μg/kg intravenously produced approximately the same concentration–time curve as 150 μg/kg orally or sublingually (187). The main metabolic pathway consists of oxidation to a "free acid," a small fraction of which is converted to a lactone (188). These metabolites are pharmacologically inert and do not tend to accumulate in the body during long-term administration (188). Intact nifedipine is 90% bound to plasma proteins, whereas the "free acid" is only 54% bound. Approximately 70 to 80% of the metabolized drug is eliminated via the kidney, and 90% of the urinary excretion occurs during the first 24 hr. Only trace amounts of intact nifedipine appear in the urine. There is some reabsorption through enterohepatic circulation. Only 15% of the metabolized drug is eliminated through the gastrointestinal tract.

Biexponential analysis of the disappearance of nifedipine in plasma yields an initial fast half-life of 2.5 to 3 hr and a terminal slow half-life of 5 hr (Table 3). Nifedipine does not appear to interact with other drugs and can be safely administered together with nitrates, β blockers, digoxin, furosemide, anticoagulants, and antihypertensive and antidiabetic agents (176).

A slow-release formulation (Adalat® retard) of nifedipine is now available and can be given twice daily, instead of the four times daily administration. Nifedipine cannot be given intravenously because of light sensitivity.

Analogues of Nifedipine

Only recently, a number of dihydropyridine analogs of nifedipine have been developed which have relatively less undesirable actions of nifedipine and are "selective" in increasing blood flow in various organs (Table 4).

Niludipine (Bay a 7168) is 1,4-dihydropyridine that is closely related to nifedipine in chemical structure and in cardiac actions. However, niludipine has more depressant effect on A-V conduction than nifedipine, producing dose-related decreases in heart rate, systemic blood pressure, and coronary resistance in open-chest pentobarbital-anesthetized dogs (189). It was found that coronary blood flow increased even when heart rate and blood pressure decreased. This effect may be due to increased venous return (189). Also, prolonged hypotension was observed that outlasted the increase in coronary blood flow. Other investigators (190), using chloralose-anesthetized dogs, found increases in heart rate and renal blood flow accompanied by a reduction in mean aortic pressure. Niludipine was 3 to 10 times more potent than nifedipine in dilating the coronary artery in canine heart-lung and isolated fibrillating heart preparations (190). In closed-chest anesthetized dogs, niludipine increased the coronary blood flow by 200% at 2 min after injection of 25 μg/kg. The duration of the effect was more than 60 min, in contrast to 30 min observed with nifedipine (149). Recently, niludipine has been shown to have a potent antihypertensive effect in conscious renal-hypertensive dogs (191), antiarrhythmic activity in a canine model of acute myocardial ischemia (192), and an antianginal effect in patients (193).

Nisoldipine (Bay k 5552) has nonidentical ester groups on the dihydropyridine molecule and has been reported to have relative specificity for dilation of the coronary vascular bed. It is the most potent known calcium antagonist, having minimal effects on heart rate or cardiac contractility (162,195). Nisoldipine has been shown to reduce myocardial oxygen consumption, to decrease peripheral resistance, and to increase coronary flow in both normal and ischemic myocardium by increasing total coronary collateral perfusion in conscious as well as anesthetized dogs (162,195) and in humans (196). Antiarrhythmic efficacy of nisoldipine in a canine model of myocardial ischemia has also been described (192).

Nimodipine (Bay e 9736) was synthesized on the basis of earlier reports that cerebral vascular smooth muscle may be more sensitive to the effects of calcium antagonists than is peripheral vascular smooth muscle (197,198). Nimodipine is a compound having selective actions on cerebral vessels and having little effect on arterial pressure (199). It may provide rational therapy for cerebrovascular disorders that involve reduced perfusion or vasospasms. Nimodipine has cerebral vasodilator actions at doses that do not decrease systemic blood pressure, unlike papaverine, nitrates, or adenosine (199). In addition, it has been found to have protective actions in several *in vitro* and *in vivo* models of cerebral ischemia (200–204) and hypoxia (200).

Nicardipine (YC-93) is a potent, water-soluble vasodilator with selectivity for cerebral and coronary vascular beds in animal and human studies (205). Chronic administration of nicardipine to dogs caused typical calcium-antagonistic actions on the myocardium, resulting in bradycardia and heart block at high doses. However, this agent is also a potent inhibitor of cyclic AMP phosphodiesterase, which may in part contribute to its vasodilating actions (206).

FR 7534 is an agent that possesses the advantage over nifedipine of being light-stable in solution. It has been found to produce a sustained increase in ischemic myocardial blood flow in a model of complete coronary occlusion (150,208,209) and during a partial coronary artery constriction, provided aortic blood pressure is maintained constant (210).

Nitrendipine (Bay e 5009) is a dihydropyridine with nonidentical ester functions that has been synthesized as an antihypertensive drug (211).

Diltiazem

Diltiazem (CRD-401, Cardiem®) (Fig. 6) is a 1,5-benzothiazepine derivative that is claimed to be a potent calcium antagonist and coronary vasodilator (212). It lacks significant negative inotropic actions (213,252), as does niludipine, the newly reported analogue of nifedipine. At present, some aspects of the mechanism of action of diltiazem are not completely clear. It has been suggested that, unlike other calcium antagonists, diltiazem causes inhibition of stimulated calcium influx by interacting with the calcium pathway involved in excitation, rather than competing with calcium for the entry (214). Accordingly, the term "calcium antagonist" may be inappropriate for diltiazem and perhaps should be replaced by a more descriptive term, such as "calcium-influx inhibitor" (214).

Electrophysiologic Effects

The electrophysiologic effects exerted by diltiazem are more akin to those of verapamil than those of nifedipine (90). Voltage clamp studies on bullfrog atrium revealed that diltiazem decreased slow inward current (215, 216). Low concentrations of diltiazem (1 μg/ml) reduced the plateau of the action potential and shortened the duration in both ventricular and Purkinje fibers without any change in the maximum rate of rise (V_{max}) or resting potential (215). Contractile tension of ventricular muscle was markedly decreased. At high concentrations (5 μg/ml), V_{max} in both ventricular muscle and Purkinje fiber decreased by about 20%, without any change in the resting potential. Diltiazem also blocked the spontaneous firing that appeared in depolarized Purkinje fibers and abolished the automaticity elicited in electrically depolarized ventricular muscle (215). In other studies (92,139) diltiazem, like verapamil, suppressed A-V nodal conduction and prolonged refractory periods in humans and in the excised rabbit A-V nodal preparation. In an animal model of myocardial ischemia, diltiazem at 0.4 mg/kg i.v. significantly reduced the ischemia-induced conduction delay in anesthetized dogs (82). This is in contrast to lidocaine, which increased conduction delay.

In human subjects, with and without sinus or A-V node dysfunction, diltiazem did not depress sinus activity in healthy subjects, but marked inhibition was observed in patients with sick-sinus syndrome (217). Ventricular automaticity was little affected. However, as occurs after verapamil, A-V conduction was significantly depressed (217,218), and no difference was observed between healthy and A-V block patients. Diltiazem had no apparent effects on atrial refractoriness, atrial echo zone, or the accessory pathway system. Thus, diltiazem mainly affects the sinus and A-V conduction systems. Its effect on the sinus node may present a hazardous problem in patients with the sick-sinus syndrome, whereas its effect on the A-V node will have therapeutic value in patients with A-V nodal reentrant arrhythmias.

Effects on Coronary Circulation

Diltiazem is a potent dilator of the large-conductance coronary arteries and of coronary collaterals (219). This is because of selective and specific inhibition of calcium influx into the smooth-muscle cells of the coronary arteries. In anesthetized dogs, diltiazem at 0.003 to 1 mg/kg increased coronary blood flow by about 50% when the blood pressure was allowed to fall and by 100% when the blood pressure was maintained constant (220,221). However, coronary flow did not increase beyond the fixed stenosis in the circumflex artery, but increased in the border zone, probably because of opening of the collaterals and redistribution of blood flow (222). A similar increase in coronary flow was observed in conscious dogs (223), in conscious rats (224), and in anesthetized pigs (225).

Vasodilator Effects

In addition to the potent coronary vasodilator effect, diltiazem reduces systemic blood pressure and heart rate and increases right atrial pressure and aortic blood flow in a dose-dependent manner (162,221). Diltiazem at 0.1 mg/kg increased coronary flow by 100% in anesthetized dogs and resulted in 25, 37, and 10% increases in femoral, carotid, and renal blood flows, respectively (220,221,226). At 0.3 and 1 mg/kg, myocardial contractility (LV dP/dt) increased, preceded by an initial decrease (221). However, others have reported a consistent decrease (162) or no change in contractile force (252). Despite a definite decrease in mean systemic blood pressure, appreciable changes were not observed in pulse pressure, suggesting that diltiazem decreased both systolic and diastolic blood pressures (221). Diltiazem has been reported to have a direct effect on the myocardium, exerting a noncompetitive β blocking action; i.e., a weak negative chronotropic and inotropic action (227,228). Reduction in ST-segment elevation following brief coronary occlusion, with a subsequent decrease in myocardial oxygen consumption, could be due to the previously mentioned hemodynamic profile (223,229,234). Both Bourassa et al. (220) and Millard (225) reported that in anesthetized animals diltiazem decreased systemic vascular resistance and heart rate. This resulted in increased tissue blood flow to border areas around an ischemic zone and improved endo/epi ratios. Blood flow in the central ischemic zone, however, remained unchanged, but the coronary collateral flow was redistributed within the ischemic region, favoring primarily subendocardium (162,229).

Similar improvements in myocardial function and blood flow distribution by diltiazem have been reported by several investigators using animal models of brief coronary occlusion (230), global ischemia in isolated perfused guinea pig heart (231), complete occlusion gradually achieved by ameroid constrictors (232), and pacing-induced ischemia in conscious dogs with partial coronary stenosis (233). In all of these animal models, the probable mechanism(s) of protection could be metabolic: i.e., preservation of mitochondrial function by diminishing the breakdown of ATP and lowering the tissue levels of lactic acid and free fatty acids, which reduces the tissue acidosis, with a resultant increase in the enzymatic activity necessary for tissue metabolism (234); the hemodynamic action of the agent; i.e., increased collateral blood flow and a decrease in myocardial work load (222,239), by improving shortening in the ischemic segments (165,233) and by inhibition of neurogenically mediated coronary vasospasms (246). In a model of chronic myocardial infarction in conscious dogs, the increased myocardial flow after diltiazem at 100 μg/kg i.v. was greater in the subepicardial layer of the ischemic area than in the subendocardial layer (235). There was no significant reduction in infarct size after diltiazem, either determined by CPK analysis or estimated by flow measurements (229,235). This is in contrast to the findings in studies conducted by Bush et al. (236). Preliminary studies have indicated that diltiazem may increase survival time after acute ligation in anesthetized pigs because of improvement in myocardial blood flow and suppression of ventricular premature contractions (237). Diltiazem at 500 μM inhibited platelet aggregation of human and rabbit platelets induced by ADP, by collagen, and by arachidonic acid (174,238).

In patients, diltiazem has been shown to produce coronary artery vasodilation and decreases in cardiac output, venous return, and heart rate (64). The reductions in cardiac work and stroke work after diltiazem were attributed to decreased venous return and prolongation of systemic circulation time (239). The diuretic and vasodilating actions of diltiazem did not further aggravate the symptoms of congestive heart failure (240,245). In patients undergoing cardiac catheterization for coronary disease or hypertension, diltiazem at 60 mg orally produced small decreases in heart rate (-6.2%), systolic aortic pressure (-9.1%), cardiac index (-5.2%), and peripheral resistance (-4.1%) (241). In several clinical studies, diltiazem has shown marked efficacy in variant angina (242,243) and angina of effort (244,245).

Side Effects and Contraindications

Diltiazem has been reported to have a low incidence of side effects (243) and thus should provide significant advantages over current prophylactic therapy for Prinzmetal's angina. A-V nodal conduction disturbances may accompany intravenous administration (247). Drug rash, dizziness, headaches, flushing, and gastrointestinal discomfort have been reported in some patients (248). Diltiazem may exert a direct inhibitory action on renal tubular resorption of sodium (240,249). The contraindications to diltiazem therapy are the same as reported for verapamil.

Absorption, Fate, and Excretion

Diltiazem is rapidly and completely absorbed after oral administration, appearing in the plasma within 15 to 30 min after administration (250,251). The peak concentration occurs after 30 min, and the plasma half-life is about 4 hr (Table 3). Approximately 80% of the drug is protein-bound, and 65% of the drug is metabolized by the liver, with the remainder being excreted by the kidneys. The main metabolic pathway is deacetylation, N-demethylation, and O-demethylation (251).

COMPARATIVE HEMODYNAMIC EFFECTS OF CALCIUM ANTAGONISTS

The similarities and differences in the cardiovascular responses to verapamil, nifedipine, and diltiazem are listed in Table 5. Nifedipine, on a weight basis, is the most potent agent in all of its pharmacologic actions (235), whereas verapamil and diltiazem are intermediate. The significance of these differences is apparent when examining the net effects of these agents. Because nifedipine is a potent vasodilator (Table 5), it elicits a strong β-adrenergic response. This, in turn, counterbalances its negative inotropic, chronotropic, and dromotropic effects (96,153). The net effect of nifedipine is therefore relatively pure vasodilatation, with little resultant electrophysiologic or inotropic effect. In contrast, doses of verapamil that exert the same degree of vasodilatation as does nifedipine produce greater negative dromotropic effects (96), and reflexly induced β-adrenergic activity may not completely offset these direct electrophysiologic effects. Equipotent doses (that doubled

TABLE 5. *Pharmacologic effects of some slow-channel inhibitors[a]*

Effect	Verapamil (Isoptin)	Nifedipine (Adalat)	Diltiazem (Herbesser)
Nonspecific sympathetic antagonism	+	−	++
Local anesthetic effect on nerve	1.6 × procaine	0	Equal to procaine
Depression of fast response in heart muscle	±	0	↓
Heart rate (in conscious state)	↑↓	↑	+++
Atrioventricular conduction (depression)	++++	±	+++
Slow-channel inhibition in heart	+++	+++	+++
Inhibition of EC[b] coupling in vascular smooth muscle (with coronary and peripheral vasodilatation)	+++	++++	+++

[a] The effect of each drug is indicated by 0, ++, +++, or ++++, with 0 meaning no effect and ++++ being the most potent effect.
[b] EC: excitation-contraction.
From Ellrodt et al. (253), with permission.

coronary flow in anesthetized dogs) of verapamil (100 μg/kg) and diltiazem (100 μg/kg) caused prolongation of A-V conduction time and functional refractory period as well. In contrast, nifedipine (3 μg/kg) had no significant effect on these variables (144). Thus, administration of verapamil and diltiazem to increase coronary blood flow may be accompanied by A-V nodal conduction disturbances. However, low doses of verapamil can be used for its antiarrhythmic effects, with minimal hemodynamic consequence (115). In equimolar clinical doses (0.04–0.17 mg/kg i.v.), verapamil, unlike diltiazem, decreased left ventricular function, despite equal changes in heart rate and aortic pressure (252). No negative inotropic effect was produced by diltiazem even after full β blockade (252), in contrast to the situation with verapamil, where the negative inotropic effects were potentiated by concurrent administration of β-adrenergic receptor antagonists (106).

COMPARISON OF THE HEMODYNAMIC EFFECTS OF CALCIUM ANTAGONISTS, β BLOCKERS, AND NITRATES

Calcium antagonists have definite advantages over β blockers and nitrate therapy. For example, all calcium antagonists are potent coronary vasodilators, in contrast to β blockers, which constrict coronary vessels. This unquestionable property of coronary vasodilatation with reduction in the afterload could be of therapeutic potential in patients who are intolerant to β blockers or in whom β blockers are contraindicated because of bronchospasms or peripheral vascular disease.

Nitrates improve ventricular function by decreasing the preload produced by extracardiac vasodilatation, in combination with a reduced afterload. Such agents decrease mean aortic pressure and regional myocardial flow to both normally perfused and underperfused poststenotic areas. In contrast, calcium antagonists increased blood flow to both normal and poststenotic underperfused areas, in spite of a decrease in mean aortic pressure, reflecting primary coronary vasodilation (175). Calcium antagonists, unlike nitrates, have no action on the venous capacitance beds (153,254), indicating minimal or no effect on the preload.

THERAPEUTIC APPLICATIONS OF CALCIUM ANTAGONISTS

The clinical indications for the various calcium antagonists are not identical, as might be expected from their variable electrophysio-

logic and pharmacologic properties. Therefore, their net therapeutic effects must be anticipated and interpreted individually, because
these agents produce a complex interplay of
simultaneous alterations in preload, afterload,
contractility, heart rate, A-V conduction, and
coronary blood flow (252,253). The value of
calcium antagonists as therapeutic agents is
no longer in doubt. Nifedipine and diltiazem
are efficacious in relieving angiospastic angina,
and verapamil is the drug of choice for termination of supraventricular reentrant tachycardias. In addition, these drugs may be of value
for the treatment of other disease states (e.g.,
angina pectoris, hypertension, cardiomyopathy, cerebral vasospasm, cardiac preservation). The clinical applications will be briefly
summarized, in view of the ever increasing
number of clinical studies concerning indications for calcium antagonists.

Angiospastic Angina

Recently, coronary vasospasms have been
implicated as the pathogenetic mechanism of
variant angina, the syndrome in which patients develop spontaneous episodes of chest
pain associated with reversible ST-segment elevation (255). Hemodynamic monitoring has
demonstrated that pain and evidence of ischemia precede any increase in the major determinants of myocardial oxygen demand (256).
Because the calcium blockers are extremely
potent coronary vasodilators, there has been
great interest in treating variant angina with
these agents. The probable mechanism(s) of
action could work at two levels: (a) by antagonizing the vasospastic components of the arterial occlusion; (b) by decreasing the calcium
content of the red blood cells (257). This combination of effects decreases the resistance to
flow through the larger vessels and allows an
improved supply of blood to the tissues. In
addition, the available red blood cells can ful-
fill their function at the microcirculatory level
because they regain their normal flexibility
(257).

Verapamil (258,261), nifedipine (169,170),
and diltiazem (242,243) have all been shown
to be strikingly effective in controlling frequent attacks of variant angina resistant to
β blockers with or without nitrates. Repeated
attacks of ventricular fibrillation complicating
attacks of variant angina have also been shown
to respond to calcium antagonists (259). Also,
such agents have been shown to consistently
block the coronary spasms and ST elevation
provoked by ergonovine in patients with variant angina (262). However, nifedipine was
most efficacious in preventing coronary spasm.
The combination of a long-acting nitrate and
a calcium antagonist may be more effective
than either agent alone in preventing attacks
of variant angina (263). This is in contrast
to combining a calcium antagonist with β
blockers, where the recurrent episodes of variant angina were aggravated (264).

Classic Angina Pectoris

Prophylactic use of calcium antagonists in
angina pectoris was suggested by their potent
coronary vasodilator property. In addition, by
decreasing peripheral vascular resistance or
afterload and reducing myocardial contractility, these agents may decrease myocardial oxygen consumption and thereby improve the relation between myocardial oxygen supply and
demand. However, reflex β-adrenergic stimulation may oppose these direct effects (Fig.
8).

The efficacy of verapamil as primary therapy for classic angina has been well documented with (265) and without (266,285,286)
propranolol. Significant reductions in the frequency of anginal episodes and nitroglycerin
consumption and improvements in exercise
tolerance have recently been demonstrated.
Nifedipine has been extensively studied in the
treatment of classic angina, although it appears to be less effective for treatment of anginal syndromes not attributable to coronary
spasms (176). Double-blind trials with nifedipine showed reductions in exercise-induced
ischemic ST-segment depression in patients
treated for periods ranging from 2 weeks to

3 years (176,267). Tachyphylaxis to the hemo-dynamic effects of nifedipine has not been re-ported in experimental animals (146) or in humans (267). Current evidence indicates that therapy with nifedipine plus β receptor block-ade yields better results than either agent alone (121,163,176). A composite analysis from eight double-blind placebo studies has indi-cated that nifedipine may increase anginal symptoms in up to 11% of patients (179). This could be due to imbalance between oxygen supply and demand, resulting from a reflex increase in myocardial contractility or heart rate. Alternatively, coronary collateral flow may be redistributed in such a way that a coronary steal occurs (155).

The results of the few double-blind studies with diltiazem have shown less prominent beneficial effects than observed with other cal-cium antagonists (244,245).

Different pharmacologic approaches to therapy for angina may be more effective than others in a given patient, depending on the pathophysiologic mechanism responsible for myocardial ischemia. For example, when fixed obstructive coronary disease is the only mech-anism producing ischemia, then propranolol, nitrates, or the calcium antagonists, either singly or in combination, may be equally effec-tive. However, if coronary spasms play a ma-jor role in the genesis of myocardial ischemia, the calcium blockers may be more effective because of their coronary vasodilator action. In clinical situations in which β antagonists and calcium antagonists are equally effective, calcium antagonists may have advantages over β blockers in patients who also have broncho-spastic disorders (268).

Cardiac Arrhythmias

The antiarrhythmic effects of calcium an-tagonists are due to their direct electrophysio-logic actions (114,115). The experimental data thus far indicate that the depression of the slow response by calcium antagonists in pathologic tissues may abolish arrhythmias due to reentry as well as automaticity. Nifedi-pine appears to have no direct antiarrhythmic effects in patients (141–143), but has been shown to possess antiarrhythmic properties in experimental animals (269,270). This differ-ence in response could be due to the fact that nifedipine has verapamil-like effects on the conduction system in animals (73) but not hu-mans (96). Diltiazem has not been studied much for its antiarrhythmic properties, al-though its known electrophysiologic effects on A-V conduction (218) are suggestive of antiar-rhythmic efficacy similar to that of verapamil.

Verapamil is the drug of choice for treat-ment of reentrant supraventricular tachycar-dia, irrespective of whether reentry is in-tranodal or occurs in association with an accessory pathway (96,271,272). Verapamil probably acts by lengthening the effective and functional refractory period of the A-V node and prolonging the A-V nodal conduction time. At the cellular level, it may be counter-acting the increase in intracellular calcium concentration induced by decreased mito-chondrial calcium-binding activity (273). Ver-apamil does not appear to be a very effective drug for treatment of ventricular arrhythmias (94,114), except in instances in which such arrhythmias arise because of coronary vaso-spasm with transmural myocardial ischemia. The role of the slow response in the genesis of ischemic ventricular arrhythmias is contro-versial (274). Because ischemia impairs local conduction, the inhibitory effects of a calcium antagonist should further accentuate impaired conduction. However, in dogs with experi-mental ischemia it was shown that verapamil improved conduction in the ischemic zones (82–84,260). The reason for this paradoxical effect is not clear. It may be due to verapamil-induced hemodynamic and coronary effects, resulting in marked improvement in the elec-trophysiologic performance of the ischemic heart (82,88). However, recently (275) it has been reported that the salutary effects of cal-cium antagonists on the conduction delay may not be attributable to their vasodilating ac-tions, because only at high doses (30 μg/kg) was nifedipine able to reduce conduction delay in the ischemic zone. Thus, a direct salutary effect on the ischemic cells may be responsible for their favorable effect on the ischemia-induced conduction delay (275).

Arterial Hypertension

All calcium antagonists are arterial vasodilators. Therefore, they are potentially useful in treating systemic arterial hypertension. Nifedipine in this respect exerts the most potent vasodilatory effect, with the least adverse electrophysiologic effects. Nifedipine administered orally or sublingually promptly reduced systolic and diastolic pressures in patients with severe hypertension (276). Therefore, in hypertensive emergencies, oral nifedipine may be a valuable alternative to intravenous diazoxide or nitroprusside (277). Verapamil (116,278) and diltiazem (279) have been found to produce only small decreases in blood pressure, without affecting the plasma renin concentration. However, both nifedipine, and verapamil were found to be effective in patients with chronic hypertension (289). Thus, calcium antagonists may be useful for the treatment of mild hypertension complicated by coronary disease or impaired ventricular performance or both. The mechanism of antihypertensive effect is not clear, but it may involve diminution of vascular tone maintained by postsynaptic α_2-adrenergic receptors (280).

Preservation of Myocardium

Numerous studies in experimental animals have indicated the beneficial potential of calcium antagonists in salvaging ischemic myocardium. However, it is unknown whether or not such salutary effects result in lower morbidity and mortality from acute myocardial infarction if the intervention is applied in the early phases of coronary occlusion in humans. There are several ways in which calcium antagonists could protect the ischemic myocardium (Fig. 8). By inhibiting slow-channel transport, such agents produce negative inotropic effects. Under these conditions, myocar-

dial ATP consumption is reduced, leaving ATP available for maintaining intracellular homeostasis, particularly with respect to calcium and sodium. This, in turn, prevents mitochondrial calcium overloading, thereby possibly ensuring their functional survival (49,51). The hemodynamic properties of reducing myocardial contractility and reducing afterload would tend to reduce myocardial oxygen requirements. Their potent coronary vasodilator action could enhance collateral blood flow, even in the presence of a fixed coronary occlusion, thereby ensuring tissue viability (154). The massive influx of calcium during reperfusion, responsible for structural damage, could also be minimized by calcium antagonists (48,52). Finally, by preventing the development of coronary spasm, these agents may prevent the occurrence of or may relieve myocardial ischemia. Nifedipine (146,155,172), verapamil (50,105,162,281–283), and diltiazem (230,234,235) have been shown convincingly to alter regional myocardial blood flow after coronary occlusion in the dog and to exert variable effects on the size and manifestation of myocardial infarction. Recently, verapamil has been shown to have beneficial hemodynamic and metabolic effects in animals with hemorrhagic shock (284).

Hypertrophic Cardiomyopathy

In patients with hypertrophic cardiomyopathy, the degree of dynamic obstruction to ejection of blood from the left ventricle is directly related to the inotropic state of the myocardium. Adrenergic β receptor antagonists, which decrease the inotropic state of the myocardium, have been effective for this disorder, but there remain many patients in whom control of symptoms is inadequate. Thus, neither medical nor surgical therapy has been uniformly successful in this condition. In addition, arrhythmias arising on the basis of slow-channel activity may cause sudden death in hypertrophic cardiomyopathy. Of the various calcium antagonists, verapamil is the most suitable for treatment of this condition, be-

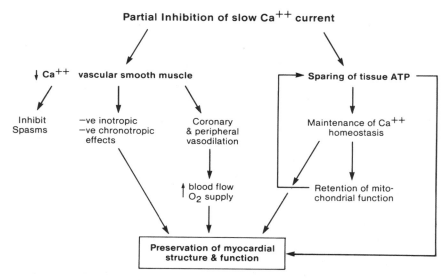

FIG. 8. Proposed scheme of the possible pathways involved in the protective effects of drugs inhibiting slow-channel calcium transport (calcium antagonists).

cause it exerts a potent negative inotropic effect without any marked reflex β-adrenergic stimulatory response. Its net inotropic effect, therefore, may be negative if the dose used does not cause significant peripheral arterial vasodilatation (120). It has been reported that short- or long-term therapy with verapamil reduces the basal left ventricular outflow gradient, with minor changes in the cardiac index, resulting in sustained improvement in exercise tolerance during chronic therapy (111,120, 287).

REFERENCES

1. Singh, B. N. (1980): Drug lag: Therapeutic implications in antiarrhythmic and antianginal therapy in the U.S.A. *Primary Cardiol.,* 5:37–41.
2. Connolly, M. E., Kersting, E., and Dollery, C. T. (1976): The clinical pharmacology of beta-adrenoceptor blocking drugs. *Prog. Cardiovasc. Dis.,* 19:203–234.
3. Singh, B. N., and Jewitt, D. E. (1974): Beta-adrenergic receptor blocking drugs in cardiac arrhythmias. *Drugs,* 7:426–461.
4. Fleckenstein, A. (1977): Specific pharmacology of calcium in myocardium, cardiac pacemakers and vascular smooth muscle. *Annu. Rev. Pharmacol. Toxicol.,* 17:149–166.
5. Church, J., and Zsoter, T. T. (1980): Calcium antagonistic drugs. Mechanism of action. *Can. J. Physiol. Pharmacol.,* 58:254–263.
6. Zelis, R., and Flaim, S. F. (1981): Calcium influx blockers and vascular smooth muscle. Do we really understand mechanisms? *Ann. Intern. Med.,* 94:124–126.
7. Lindner, E. (1960): Phenyl-propyl-diphenyl-propylamin, eine neue Substanz mit coronargefaber-weiternder Wirkung. *Arzneim. Forsch.,* 10:569–573.
8. Haas, H., and Hartfelder, G. (1962): α-isopropyl-α-(*n*-methylhomoveratryl)-γ-aminopropyl)-3,4-dimethoxy-phenylacetonilril, eine Substanz mit coronargefaberweiternden Eigenschaften. *Arzneim. Forsch.,* 12:549–558.
9. Melville, K. I., and Benfey, B. C. (1965): Coronary vasodilatory and cardiac adrenergic blocking effects of iproveratril. *Can. J. Physiol. Pharmacol.,* 43:339–342.
10. Haas, H., and Busch, E. (1967): Vergleichende Untersuchungen der wirkung von α-isopropyl-α(*n*-methyl-*N*-homoveratryl)-γ-aminopropyl)-3,4-dimethoxy-phenylacetonitril, seiner Derivate sowie einiger anderer Coronardilatatoren und β-receptor-affiner Substanzen. *Arzneim. Forsch.,* 17:257–271.
11. Fleckenstein, A., Kammermeier, H., Doring, H., and Freund, H. J. (1967): Zum Wirkungs-mechanismus neuartiger Koronardilatatoren mit gleichzeitig Sauerstoff-einsparenden Myokard-Effekten, Prenylamin und Iproveratril. *Z. Kreislaufforsch.,* 56:716–744, 839–853.
12. Driefuss, J. J., Grau, J. D., and Nordmann, J. J. (1975): Calcium movements related to neurohypophysical hormone secretion. In: *International Symposium on Calcium Transport in Contraction and Secretion,* edited by E. Carafoli and F. Clementi, pp. 271–290. North Holland, Amsterdam.
13. Devis, G., Somers, G., Van Obberghen, E. N., and Malaisse, W. J. (1975): Calcium antagonists and islet

function: Inhibition of insulin by verapamil. *Diabetes,* 24:547–551.

14. Luccioni, R., Vague, P. H., Luccioni, F., and Gerard, R. (1978): Abnormalities of insulin secretion in coronary patients: Effects of perhexiline maleate. In: *Perhexiline Maleate: Proceedings of a Symposium,* pp. 71–88. Excerpta Medica, Amsterdam.

15. Ringer, S. (1882): A further contribution regarding the influence of the different constituents of the blood on the contraction of the heart. *J. Physiol.,* 4:29–42.

16. Huxley, A. F. (1971): The activation of striated muscle and its mechanical response. *Proc. R. Soc.,* 178:1–27.

17. Ebashi, S., and Endo, M. (1968): Calcium ion and muscle contraction. *Prog. Biophys. Mol. Biol.,* 18:123–183.

18. Andersson, K. E. (1979): Effects of calcium and calcium antagonists on excitation-contraction coupling in striated and smooth muscle. *Acta Pharmacol. Toxicol.,* 43:5–14.

19. Fleckenstein, A. (1968): Experimental heart failure due to disturbances in high-energy phosphate metabolism. In: *Proceedings of the Fifth European Congress of Cardiology,* Athens, pp. 255–269.

20. Fozzard, H. A., and Beeler, G. W. (1976): The voltage clamp and cardiac electrophysiology. *Circ. Res.,* 37:403–413.

21. Hauswirth, O., and Singh, B. N. (1978): Toxic mechanisms in heart muscle in relation to the genesis and the pharmacological control of cardiac arrhythmias. *Pharmacol. Rev.,* 30:5.

22. Coraboeuf, E. (1976): Ionic basis of electrical activity in cardiac tissues. *Am. J. Physiol.,* 234:101–116.

23. Cranefield, P. F. (1975): *Conduction of the Cardiac Impulse.* Futura, New York.

24. Coraboeuf, E., Deroubaix, E., and Hoerter, J. (1976): Control of ionic permeabilities in normal and ischemic heart. *Circ. Res.,* 38:I-92–97.

25. Reuter, H. (1979): Properties of two inward membrane currents in the heart. *Annu. Rev. Physiol.,* 41:413–424.

26. Noble, D. (1975): *The Initiation of Heart Beat.* Clarendon Press, Oxford.

27. Hodgkin, A. L., and Huxley, A. F. (1952): A quantitative description of membrane current and its application to conduction and excitation in nerve. *J. Physiol. (Lond.),* 117:500–544.

28. Weidmann, S. (1974): Heart: Electrophysiology. *Annu. Rev. Physiol.,* 36:155–169.

29. Reuter, H. (1973): Divalent cations as charge carriers in excitable membranes. *Prog. Biophys. Mol. Biol.,* 26:1–43.

30. Beeler, G. W., and Reuter, H. (1977): Reconstruction of the action potential of ventricular myocardial fibers. *J. Physiol. (Lond.),* 268:177–210.

31. Reuter, H., and Scholz, H. (1977): A study of the ion selectivity and the kinetic properties of the calcium dependent slow inward current in mammalian cardiac muscle. *J. Physiol. (Lond.),* 264:17–47.

32. McDonald, T. F., and Trautwein, W. (1978): Membrane currents in cat myocardium: Separation of inward and outward components. *J. Physiol. (Lond.),* 274:193–216.

33. Goldman, Y., and Morad, M. (1977): Ionic membrane conductance during the time course of the cardiac action potential. *J. Physiol. (Lond.),* 268:655–695.

34. Diamond, J. M., and Wright, E. M. (1969): Biological membranes: The physical basis of ion and nonelectrolyte selectivity. *Annu. Rev. Physiol.,* 31:581–646.

35. Williams, R. J. P. (1970): The biochemistry of sodium, potassium, magnesium and calcium. *Q. Rev. Chem. Soc.,* 24:331.

36. Rosenberger, L., and Triggle, D. J. (1978): Calcium, calcium translocation and specific calcium antagonists. In: *Calcium in Drug Action,* edited by G. B. Weiss, pp. 3–31. Plenum Press, New York.

37. Sperelakis, N., and Schneider, J. A. (1976): A metabolic control mechanism for calcium ion flux that may protect the ventricular myocardial cell. *Am. J. Cardiol.,* 37:1079–1085.

38. Reuter, H., and Scholz, H. (1977): The regulation of the calcium conductance of cardiac muscle by adrenaline. *J. Physiol. (Lond.),* 264:49–62.

39. Tsein, R. W., Gilies, W. R., and Greengard, P. (1972): Cyclic AMP mediates the effects of adrenaline on cardiac Purkinje fibers. *Nature (New Biol.),* 260:101–108.

40. Brooker, G. (1973): Oscillation of cyclic adenosine monophosphate concentration during the myocardial contraction cycle. *Science,* 182:933–934.

41. Wollenberger, A., Babskii, E. B., and Bogdanova, E. A. (1973): Cyclic changes in levels of cAMP and cGMP in frog myocardium during the cardiac cycle. *Biochem. Biophys. Res. Commun.,* 55:446–452.

42. Ten Eick, R., Nawrath, H., and Trautwein, W. (1976): On the mechanism of the negative inotropic effects of acetylcholine. *Pfluegers Arch.,* 301:207–213.

43. Cheneval, J. P., Hyde, A., and Blondel, B. (1972): Heart cells in culture: Metabolism, action potential and transmembrane ionic movements. *J. Physiol. (Paris),* 64:413–430.

44. Reuter, H. (1974): Exchange of calcium ions in the mammalian myocardium. *Circ. Res.,* 34:599–605.

45. Glitsch, H. G., Reuter, H., and Scholz, H. (1970): The effect of internal sodium concentration on calcium fluxes in isolated guinea-pig auricles. *J. Physiol. (Lond.),* 209:25–43.

46. Pitts, B. J. R. (1979): Stoichiometry of sodium-calcium exchange in cardiac sarcolemmal vesicles: Coupling to the sodium pump. *J. Biol. Chem.,* 254:6232–6235.

47. Reeves, J. P., and Sutko, J. L. (1979): Sodium-calcium ion exchange in cardiac membrane vesicles. *Proc. Natl. Acad. Sci. U.S.A.,* 76:590–594.

48. Henry, P. D., Schuchleib, R., Davis, J., Weiss, E. S., and Sobel, B. E. (1977): Myocardial contracture and accumulation of mitochondrial calcium in ischemic rabbit heart. *Am. J. Physiol.,* 233:H677–684.

49. Nayler, W. G., and Grinwald, P. (1981): Calcium entry blockers and myocardial function. *Fed. Proc.* 40:2855–2861.

50. Reimer, K. A., Lowe, J. E., and Jennings, R. E. (1977): Effect of calcium antagonist verapamil on

necrosis following temporary coronary artery occlusion in dogs. *Circulation,* 55:581–587.

51. Nayler, W. G., Ferrari, R., and Williams, A. (1980): Protective effect of pretreatment with verapamil, nifedipine and propranolol on mitochondrial function in the ischemic and reperfused myocardium. *Am. J. Cardiol.,* 46:242–248.
52. Tanabe, M., Fujiwara, S., Ohta, N., Shimamoto, N., and Hirata, M. (1980): Pathophysiological significance of coronary collaterals for preservation of the myocardium during coronary occlusion and reperfusion in anesthetized dogs. *Cardiovasc. Res.,* 14:288–294.
53. Coleman, R. E., Klein, M. S., Ahmed, S. A., Weiss, E. S., and Sobel, B. E. (1977): Mechanisms contributing to myocardial accumulation of technetium-99m stannous pyrophosphate after coronary arterial occlusion. *Am. J. Cardiol.,* 39:55–59.
54. Ashraf, M., White, F., and Bloor, C. M. (1978): Ultra-structural influences of reperfusing dog myocardium with calcium-free blood after coronary artery occlusion. *Am. J. Pathol.,* 90:423–428.
55. Sobel, B. E., Corr, P. B., Robinson, A. K., Goldstein, R. A., Witkowski, F. X., and Klein, M. S. (1978): Accumulation of lysophosphoglycerides with arrhythmogenic properties in ischemic myocardium. *J. Clin. Invest.,* 62:546–553.
56. Corr, P. B., and Sobel, B. E. (1980): The role of biochemical factors in ventricular dysrhythmia accompanying ischemia. *Adv. Cardiol.,* 27:346–360.
57. Opie, L. H. (1979): Role of carnitine in fatty acid metabolism of normal and ischemic myocardium. *Am. Heart J.,* 97:375–388.
58. Antman, E. M., Stone, P. H., Muller, J. E., and Braunwald, E. (1980): Calcium channel blocking agents in the treatment of cardiovascular disorders. *Ann. Intern. Med.,* 93:875–885.
59. Golenhofen, K., and Weston, A. H. (1976): Differentiation of calcium activation systems in vascular smooth muscle. In: *Ionic Actions on Vascular Smooth Muscle,* edited by E. Betz, pp. 21–25. Springer-Verlag, Berlin.
60. Nakajima, N., Hoshiyama, M., Yamashita, U., and Kiyomoto, A. (1975): Effect of diltiazem on electrical and mechanical activity of isolated ventricular muscle of guinea pig. *Jpn. J. Pharmacol.,* 25:383–392.
61. Van Breemen, C., Farinas, B. R., Casteels, R., Gerba, P., Wuytack, F., and Deth, R. (1973): Factors controlling cytoplasmic calcium concentration. *Philos. Trans. R. Soc. Lond.,* 265:57–71.
62. Henry, P. D. (1979): Calcium ion antagonists: Mechanism of action and clinical applications. *Prac. Cardiol.,* 5:145–156.
63. Galper, J. B., and Catterall, W. A. (1979): Inhibition of sodium channels by D600. *Mol. Pharmacol.,* 15:174–178.
64. Nabata, H. (1977): Effects of calcium-antagonistic coronary vasodilators on myocardial contractility and membrane potentials. *Jpn. J. Pharmacol.,* 27:239–249.
65. Chen, C. M., and Gettes, L. S. (1977): Effects of verapamil in premature and non-premature sodium

dependent action potentials at various potassium levels. *Circulation,* 56:III-127 (abstract).
66. Satoh, K., Yangisawa, T., and Taira, N. (1979): Effects on AV conduction and blood flow of enantiomers of verapamil and of tetrodotoxin injected into the posterior and anterior spetal artery of the AV node preparation of the dog. *Naunyn Schmiedebergs Arch. Pharmacol.,* 308:89–98.
67. Ehara, T., and Kaufman, R. (1978): The voltage and time-dependent effects of (−) verapamil on the slow inward current in isolated cat ventricular myocardium. *J. Pharmacol. Exp. Ther.,* 207:49–55.
68. Henry, P. D. (1980): Comparative pharmacology of calcium antagonists: Nifedipine, verapamil and diltiazem. *Am. J. Cardiol.,* 46:1047–1058.
69. Bayer, R., Kaufman, R., Lee, J. H., and Henekes, R. (1977): Effects of nifedipine on contraction and monophasic action potential of isolated cat myocardium. *Naunyn Schmiedebergs Arch. Pharmacol.,* 302:217–226.
70. Cavey, D., Vincent, J. P., and Lazdunski, M. (1977): Muscarinic receptor of heart cell membranes. Association with agonists, antagonists and antiarrhythmic agents. *F.E.B.S. Lett.,* 84:110–114.
71. Blackmore, P. F., El-Refai, M., and Exton, J. H. (1979): Alpha-adrenergic blockade and inhibition of A23187 mediated Ca^{++} uptake by verapamil in rat liver cells. *Mol. Pharmacol.,* 15:598–606.
72. Fossett, M., DeBarry, J., Lenoir, M. C., and Lazdunski, M. (1977): Analysis of molecular aspects of Na$^+$ Ca^{++} uptakes by embryonic cardiac cells in culture. *J. Biol. Chem.,* 252:6112–6117.
73. Endo, M., Yanagisawa, T., and Taira, N. (1978): Effect of verapamil and nifedipine on the ventricular automaticity of dog. *Naunyn Schmiedbergs Arch. Pharmacol.,* 302:235–238.
74. Hidaka, H., Yamaki, T., and Asano, M. (1979): Selective inhibitors of Ca^{++} binding modulator of PDE produce vascular relaxation and inhibit actin-myosin interaction. *Mol. Pharmacol.,* 15:49–59.
75. Hartshorne, D. J. (1980): Biochemical basis of contraction of vascular smooth muscle. *Chest,* 78:140–149.
76. Irwin, J. M., and Flaim, S. F. (1980): Effects of diltiazem on cellular ^{45}Ca and ^{22}Na in vascular smooth muscle. *Fed. Proc.,* 39:1071 (abstract).
77. Irwin, J. M., Ratz, P. H., and Flaim, S. F. (1980): Diltiazem: A calcium antagonist which stimulates oxygen consumption rate by increasing Na$^+$- K$^+$ pump activation in vascular smooth muscle. *Circulation,* 62:III-10 (abstract).
78. Rahwan, R. G., Piascik, M. F., and Witiak, D. T. (1979): Role of calcium antagonism in the therapeutic action of drugs. *Can. J. Physiol. Pharmacol.,* 57:443–460.
79. Nayler, W. C., and Szeto, F. (1972): Effect of verapamil on contractility, oxygen utilization and calcium exchangeability in mammalian heart muscle. *Cardiovasc. Res.,* 6:120–128.
80. Mikkelsen, E., Anderson, K. E., and Lederballe, P. O. (1979): Verapamil and nifedipine inhibition of contractions induced by potassium and noradrenaline in human mesenteric arteries and veins. *Acta Pharmacol. Toxicol.,* 44:110–190.

81. Hordof, A. J., Edie, R., Malm, J. R., Hoffman, B. F., and Rosen, M. R. (1976): Electrophysiologic properties and response to pharmacologic agents of fibers from diseased human atria. *Circulation,* 54:774–790.

82. Nakaya, H., Hattori, Y., and Kanno, M. (1980): Effects of calcium antagonists and lidocaine on conduction delay induced by acute myocardial ischemia in dogs. *Jpn. J. Pharmacol.,* 30:587–597.

83. Dersham, G. H., and Han, J. (1981): Actions of verapamil on Purkinje fibers from normal and infarcted tissue. *J. Pharmacol. Exp. Ther.,* 216:261–264.

84. Elharrar, V., Graum, W. E., and Zipes, D. P. (1977): Effect of drugs on conduction delays and incidence of ventricular arrhythmias induced by acute coronary occlusion. *Am. J. Cardiol.,* 39:544–549.

85. Kupersmith, J., Antman, E. M., and Hoffman, B. F. (1975): In vitro electrophysiological effects of lidocaine in canine acute myocardial infarction. *Circ. Res.,* 36:84–91.

86. Opie, L. H., Nathan, D., and Lubbe, W. F. (1979): Biochemical aspects of arrhythmogenesis and ventricular fibrillation. *Am. J. Cardiol.,* 43:131–148.

87. Corr, P. B., and Gillis, R. A. (1978): Autonomic neural influences on the dysrhythmias resulting from myocardial infarction. *Circ. Res.,* 43:1–9.

88. Brooks, W. W., Verrier, R. L., and Lown, B. (1980): Protective effect of verapamil on vulnerability to ventricular fibrillation during myocardial ischemia and reperfusion. *Cardiovasc. Res.,* 14:295–302.

89. Mangiardi, L. M., Hariman, R. J., McAllister, R. G., Bhargara, V., Surawicz, B., and Shebatai, R. (1978): Electrophysiologic and hemodynamic effects of verapamil: Correlation with plasma drug concentrations. *Circulation,* 57:366–372.

90. Wit, A. L., and Cranefield, P. F. (1974): Effect of verapamil on SA and AV nodes of rabbits and the mechanism by which it arrests reentrant AV nodal tachycardia. *Circ. Res.,* 35:413–425.

91. Raschack, M. (1976): Differences in the cardiac actions of the calcium antagonists verapamil and nifedipine. *Arzneim. Forsch.,* 26:1330–1333.

92. Zipes, D. P., and Fischer, J. C. (1974): Effects of agents which inhibit the slow channel on SA node automaticity and AV conduction in the dog. *Circ. Res.,* 34:184–192.

93. Angus, J. A., Dhumma-Upahorn, P., Cobbin, L. B., and Goodman, A. H. (1976): Cardiovascular action of verapamil in the dog with particular reference to myocardial contractility and AV conduction. *Cardiovasc. Res.,* 10:623–632.

94. Heng, M. K., Singh, B. N., Roche, A. H. G., Norris, R. M., and Mercer, C. J. (1975): Effects of intravenous verapamil on cardiac arrhythmias and on the EKG. *Am. Heart J.,* 90:487–498.

95. Koike, Y., Shimamura, K., Shudo, I., and Saito, H. (1979): Pharmacokinetics of verapamil in man. *Res. Commun. Chem. Pathol. Pharmacol.,* 24:37–47.

96. Rowland, E., Evans, T., and Kriker, D. (1979): Effect of nifedipine on AV conduction as compared with verapamil: Intracardiac electrophysiological study. *Br. Heart J.,* 42:124–127.

97. Greenberg, S., and Wilson, W. R. (1974): Iproveratril: A non-specific antagonist of peripheal vascular reactivity. *Can. J. Physiol. Pharmacol.,* 52:266–271.

98. Winbury, M. M., Howe, B. B., and Hefner, M. A. (1969): Effect of nitrates and other coronary dilators on large and small coronary vessels: An hypothesis for the mechanism of action of nitrates. *J. Pharmacol. Exp. Ther.,* 168:70–95.

99. Nayler, W. G., and Szeto, J. (1972): Effect of verapamil on contractility, oxygen utilization and calcium exchangeability in mammalian heart muscle. *Cardiovasc. Res.,* 6:120–128.

100. Melville, K. I., and Benfey, B. G. (1965): Coronary vasodilator and cardiac adrenergic blocking effects of iproveratril. *Can. J. Physiol. Pharmacol.,* 43:339–342.

101. Fleckenstein, A., and Fleckenstein-Grun, G. (1975): Further studies on the neutralization of glycoside-induced contractures of coronary smooth muscle by Ca^{++} antagonistic compounds. *Naunyn Schmiedebergs Arch. Pharmacol.,* 287:R38 (abstract).

102. Harder, D. R., Belardinelli, L., Sperelakis, N., Rubio, R., and Berne, R. M. (1979): Differential effects of adenosine and nitroglycerin on the action potentials of large and small coronary arteries. *Circ. Res.,* 44:176–182.

103. Fleckenstein, A. (1976): On the basic pharmacologic mechanism of nifedipine in relation to therapeutic efficacy. In: *The Third International Adalat Symposium,* edited by A. D. Jatene and P. R. Lichtlen, pp. 1–18. Excerpta Medica, Amsterdam.

104. Rowe, G. G., Stenlund, R. R., Thomsen, J. R., Corliss, R. J., and Sialer, S. (1971): The systemic and coronary hemodynamic effects of iproveratril. *Arch. Int. Pharmacodyn. Ther.,* 193:381–390.

105. DaLuz, P. L., DeBarros, L. F. M., Leite, J. J., Pileggi, F., and Decourt, L. V. (1980): Effect of verapamil on regional coronary and myocardial perfusion during acute coronary occlusion. *Am. J. Cardiol.,* 45:269–275.

106. Newman, R. R., Bishop, V. S., Peterson, D. F., Leroux, E. J., and Horowitz, L. D. (1977): Effect of verapamil on left ventricular performance in conscious dogs. *J. Pharmacol. Exp. Ther.,* 201:723–730.

107. Satoh, K., Yanagisawa, T., and Taira, N. (1980): Coronary vasodilator and cardiac effects of optical isomers of verapamil in the dog. *J. Cardiovasc. Pharmacol.,* 2:309–318.

108. Ferlinz, J., Easthope, J. L., and Aranow, W. S. (1979): Effects of verapamil on myocardial performance in coronary disease. *Circulation,* 59:313–319.

109. Hamer, A., Peter, T., Platt, M., and Mandel, W. J. (1981): Effect of verapamil on supraventricular tachycardia in patients with overt and concealed Wolff-Parkinson-White syndrome. *Am. Heart J.,* 101:600–612.

110. Vincenzi, M., Allegri, P., Gabaldo, S., Maiolino, P., and Ometto, R. (1976): Hemodynamic effects caused by i.v. administration of verapamil in healthy subjects. *Arzneim. Forsch.,* 26:1221–1223.

111. Rosing, D. R., Kent, K. M., Maron, B. J., and Epstein, S. E. (1979): Verapamil therapy: A new approach to the pharmacologic treatment of hy-

pertrophic cardiomyopathy. *Circulation,* 60:1208–1213.

112. Singh, B. N., and Roche, A. H. G. (1977): Effects of intravenous verapamil on hemodynamics in patients with heart disease. *Am. Heart J.,* 94:593–599.

113. Seabra-Gomes, R., Rickards, A., and Sutton, R. (1976): Hemodynamic effects of verapamil and practolol in man. *Eur. J. Cardiol.,* 4:79–85.

114. Singh, B. N., Ellrodt, G., and Peter, C. T. (1978): Verapamil: A review of its pharmacological properties and therapeutic use. *Drugs,* 15:169–197.

115. Singh, B. N., Collett, J. T., and Chew, C. Y. C. (1980): New perspectives in the pharmacologic therapy of cardiac arrhythmias. *Prog. Cardiovasc. Dis.,* 22:243–301.

116. Lederballe-Pederson, O. (1978): Does verapamil have a clinically significant antihypertensive effect. *Eur. J. Clin. Pharmacol.,* 13:21–24.

117. Benaim, M. E. (1972): Asystole after verapamil. *Br. Med. J.,* 2:169–170 (letter).

118. Boothby, C. B., Garrard, C. S., and Pickering, D. (1972): Verapamil in cardiac arrhythmias. *Br. Med. J.,* 2:349.

119. Hagemeijer, F. (1978): Verapamil in the management of supraventricular tachycardia occurring after a recent myocardial infarction. *Circulation,* 57:751–755.

120. Epstein, S. H., and Rosing, D. R. (1981): Verapamil: Its potential for causing serious complications in patients with hypertrophic cardiomyopathy. *Circulation,* 64:437–441.

121. Opie, L. H. (1980): Calcium antagonists. *Lancet,* 1:806–810.

122. Carrasco, H. A., Fuenmayor, A., Barboza, J. S., and Gonzalez, G. (1978): Effect of verapamil on normal SA node function and sick sinus syndrome. *Am. Heart J.,* 96:760–771.

123. Brodsky, S. J., Cutler, S. S., Weiner, D. A., and Klein, M. D. (1981): Hepatotoxicity due to treatment with verapamil. *Ann. Intern. Med.,* 94:490–491.

124. Husaini, M. H., Kvasnicka, J., Ryden, I., and Holmberg, S. (1973): Action of verapamil on SA node, AV and intraventricular conduction. *Br. Heart J.,* 35:734–737.

125. Spiegelhalder, B., and Eichelbaum, M. (1977): Determination of verapamil in human plasma by mass fragmentography using stable labelled verapamil as internal standard. *Arzneim. Forsch.,* 27:94–97.

126. Schlepper, M., Thormann, J., and Schwarz, F. (1975): The pharmacodynamics of oral verapamil and verapamil retard as judged by their negative dromotropic effects. *Arzneim. Forsch.,* 25:1452–1455.

127. Dominic, J. A., Bourne, D. W. A., Tan, T. G., Kirsten, E. B., and McAllister, R. G. (1981): Pharmacology of verapamil. III. Pharmacokinetics in normal subjects after i.v. drug administration. *J. Cardiovasc. Pharmacol.,* 3:25–38.

128. Schomerus, M., Spiegelhalder, B., Stieren, B., and Eichelbaum, M. (1976): Physiological disposition of verapamil in man. *Cardiovasc. Res.,* 10:605–612.

129. Eichelbaum, M., Ende, G., Remberg, M., Schomerus, M., and Dengler, H. J. (1979): The metabolism of DL-[¹⁴C]verapamil in man. *Drug Metab. Dispos.,* 7:145–148.

130. Nuegebauer, G. (1978): Comparison of cardiovascular actions of verapamil and its major metabolites in the anesthetized dogs. *Cardiovasc. Res.,* 12:247–254.

131. Woodcock, B. G., Hopf, R., and Kaltenbach, M. (1980): Verapamil and norverapamil plasma concentrations during long-term therapy in patients with hypertrophic obstructive cardiomyopathy. *J. Cardiovasc. Res.,* 2:17–23.

132. Bigger, J. T., Jr. (1980): A Primer on Calcium Ion Antagonists, pp. 1–11. Knoll Pharmaceutical Co.

133. Ramuz, H. (1978): A new calcium antagonist, Ro 11–1781 and its metabolites. *Arzneim. Forsch.,* 28:2048–2051.

134. Eigenmann, R., Gerold, M., and Haeusler, G. (1978): Cardiovascular effects of calcium antagonists in chronically instrumented conscious dogs. *Experientia,* 34:923.

135. Cocco, G., Chu, D., and Strozzi, C. (1979): Dimeditiapramine, a new calcium antagonist in the management of supraventricular tachycardia in patients with acute myocardial infarction. *Clin. Cardiol.,* 2:131–134.

136. Saini, R. K., and Antonaccio, M. J. (1982): Antiarrhythmic, antifibrillatory activities and reduction of infarct size following the calcium antagonist Ro 11–1781 (Tiapamil) in anesthetized dogs. *J. Pharmacol. Exp. Ther.,* 221:29–36.

137. Vater, W., Kroneber, G., Hoffmeister, F., et al. (1972): Zur Pharmakologie von Nifedipine (Bay a 1040). *Arzneim. Forsch.,* 22:1–14.

138. Rodenkirchen, R., Bayer, R., Steiner, R., et al. (1979): Structure activity studies on nifedipine in isolated cardiac muscle. *Naunyn Schmiedebergs Arch. Pharmacol.,* 310:69–78.

139. Kawai, C., Konishi, T., Matsuyama, E., and Okazaki, H. (1981): Comparative effects of three calcium antagonists, diltiazem, verapamil and nifedipine on the SA and AV nodes. *Circulation,* 63:1035–1042.

140. Narimatsu, A., and Taira, N. (1976): Effects on AV conduction of calcium antagonistic coronary vasodilators, local anesthetics and quinidine injected into the posterior and anterior septal artery of AV node preparation in the dog. *Naunyn Schmiedebergs Arch. Pharmacol.,* 294:169–177.

141. Fujimoto, T., Peter, T., Hamamoto, H., et al. (1981): Effects of nifedipine on conduction delay during ventricular myocardial ischemia and reperfusion. *Am. Heart J.,* 102:45–52.

142. Gutovitz, A. L., Cole, B., Henry, P. D., Sobel, B. E., and Roberts, R. (1977): Resistance of ventricular dysrhythmia to nifedipine, a calcium antagonist. *Circulation,* 56:III-179 (abstract).

143. Padeletti, L., Brat, A., Franchi, F., et al. (1980): The cardiac electrophysiological effects of nifedipine. *Br. J. Clin. Pract.,* 8:27–31.

144. Taira, N., Motomura, S., Narimatsu, A., and Iijima, T. (1975): Experimental pharmacological investigations of effects of nifedipine on AV conduction in comparison with other coronary vasodilators. In: *Second International Adalat Symposium,* edited by

W. Lochner, W. Braasch, and G. Kroneberg, pp. 40–48. Springer-Verlag, Berlin.

145. Ono, H., Himori, N., and Taira, N. (1977): Chrontropic effects of coronary vasodilators as assessed in the isolated blood perfused SA node preparation of the dog. *Tohoku J. Exp. Med.*, 121:383–390.

146. Schmier, J., Bruckner, U. B., Mittman, U., and Wirth, R. H. (1976): Intracoronary collaterals and intramyocardial blood flow distribution in dogs following nifedipine administration compared with controls. In: *Third International Adalat Symposium,* edited by A. D. Jatene and P. R. Lichtlen, pp. 42–49. Excerpta Medica, Amsterdam.

147. Fleckenstein-Grun, G., Freckenstein, A., Byon, Y. K., and Kim, K. W. (1976): Mechanism of action of calcium antagonists in the treatment of coronary disease with special reference to perhexiline maleate. In: *Proceedings of a Symposium on Perhexiline Maleate,* pp. 140–150. Excerpta Medica, Amsterdam.

148. Gross, R., Kirchheim, H., and von Olshausen, K. (1979): Effects of nifedipine on coronary and systemic hemodynamics in the conscious dogs. *Arzneim. Forsch.*, 29:1361–1368.

149. Ogawa, K., Wakamasu, Y., Ito, T., et al. (1981): Comparative coronary vasodilatory effects of nifedipine and niludipine. *Arzneim. Forsch.*, 31:770–773.

150. Jolly, S. R., Hardman, H. F., and Gross, G. J. (1981): Comparison of two dihydropyridine calcium antagonists on coronary collateral blood flow in acute myocardial ischemia. *J. Pharmacol. Exp. Ther.*, 217:20–25.

151. Saini, R. K., Fulmor, I. E., and Antonaccio, M. J. (1982): Effect of tiapamil and nifedipine during critical coronary stenosis and in the presence of adrenergic beta-receptor blockade in anesthetized dogs. *J. Cardiovasc. Pharmacol.*, 4:770–776.

152. Verdouw, P. D., Ten Cate, F. J., and Hugenholtz, P. G. (1980): Effect of nifedipine on segmental myocardial function in the anesthetized pig. *Eur. J. Pharmacol.*, 63:209–212.

153. Vater, W., and Schlossmann, K. (1976): Effects of nifedipine on the hemodynamics and the oxygen consumption of the heart in animal experiments. In: *Proceedings of the Third International Adalat Symposium,* edited by A. D. Jatene and P. R. Lichtlen, p. 33. Excerpta Medica, Amsterdam.

154. Henry, P. D., Shuchleib, L. J., Borda, R., et al. (1978): Effects of nifedipine on myocardial perfusion and ischemic injury in dogs. *Circ. Res.*, 43:372–380.

155. Selwyn, A. P., Welman, E., Fox, P., et al. (1979): The effects of nifedipine on acute myocardial ischemia and infarction in dogs. *Circ. Res.*, 44:16–23.

156. Henry, P. D., Schuchleib, R., Clark, R. E., and Perez, J. E. (1979): Effect of nifedipine on myocardial ischemia: Analysis of collateral flow, pulsatile heat and regional muscle shortening. *Am. J. Cardiol.*, 44:817–824.

157. Kanazawa, T., Suzuki, N., Ino-oka, E., et al. (1974): Effect of nifedipine on intercoronary collateral circulation. *Arzneim. Forsch.*, 24:1267–1274.

158. Ichihara, K., Ichihara, M., and Abiko, Y. (1979): Effect of verapamil and nifedipine on ischemic myocardial metabolism in dogs. *Arzneim. Forsch.*, 29:1509–1514.

159. Gallagher, K. P., Folts, J. D., Shebuski, R. J., et al. (1980): Subepicardial vasodilator reserve in the presence of critical stenosis in dogs. *Am. J. Cardiol.*, 46:67–73.

160. Weintraub, W. S., Hattori, S., Agarwal, J., et al. (1981): Variable effect of nifedipine on myocardial blood flow at three grades of coronary occlusion in the dog. *Circ. Res.*, 48:937–942.

161. Polese, A., Fiorentini, C., Olivari, M. T., and Guazzi, M. D. (1979): Clinical use of a calcium antagonistic agent, nifedipine in acute pulmonary edema. *Am. J. Med.*, 66:825–831.

162. Warltier, D. C., Meils, C. M., Gross, G. J., and Brooks, H. L. (1981): Blood flow in normal and acutely ischemic myocardium after verapamil, diltiazem, nisoldipine—a new dihydropyridine calcium antagonist. *J. Pharmacol. Exp. Ther.*, 218:296–302.

163. Tweddel, A. C., Beattie, J. M., Murray, R. G., and Hutton, I. (1981): Combination of nifedipine and propranolol in the management of patients with angina pectoris. *Br. J. Clin. Pharmacol.*, 12:229–233.

164. White, S. W., Porges, W. L., and McRitchie, R. J. (1974): Coronary hemodynamic effects of nifedipine (Bay a 1040) and glyceryl trinitrate in unanesthetized dogs. *Clin. Exp. Pharmacol. Physiol.*, 1:77–86.

165. Perez, J. E., Sobel, B. E., and Henry, P. D. (1980): Improved performance of ischemic canine myocardium in response to nifedipine and diltiazem. *Am. J. Physiol.*, 239:658–663.

166. Smith, J. H., Goldstein, J. M., Griffith, K. M., et al. (1976): Regional contractility: Selective depression of ischemic myocardium by verapamil. *Circulation*, 54:629–635.

167. Margolis, B., Verrier, R. L., and Lown, B. (1980): Influence of ergonovine-induced coronary artery spasm on vulnerability to ventricular fibrillation. *Am. J. Cardiol.*, 45:455 (abstract).

168. Perez, J. E., Lucas, C., and Henry, P. D. (1980): Experimental coronary artery spasms in dogs: Relief by nifedipine and nitroglycerin. *Circulation*, 62:III-253 (abstract).

169. Goldberg, S., Reichek, N., Wilson, J., et al. (1979): Nifedipine in the treatment of Prinzmetal's (variant) angina. *Am. J. Cardiol.*, 44:804–810.

170. Antman, E., Muller, J., Goldberg, S., et al. (1980): Nifedipine therapy for coronary artery spasms. *N. Engl. J. Med.*, 302:1269–1273.

171. Magee, P. G., Flaherty, J. T., Bixler, T. J., et al. (1979): Comparison of myocardial protection with nifedipine and potassium. *Circulation*, 60:I151–157.

172. Clark, R. E., Christlieb, I. Y., Henry, P. D., et al (1979): Nifedipine: A myocardial protective agent. *Am. J. Cardiol.*, 44:825–831.

173. Magovern, G. J., Dixon, C. M., and Burkholder, J. A. (1981): Improved myocardial protection with nifedipine and potassium-based cardioplegia. *J. Thorac. Cardiovasc. Surg.*, 82:239–244.

174. Ono, H., and Kimura, M. (1981): Effect of calcium antagonistic vasodilators, diltiazem, nifedipine, perhexilline, and verapamil on platelet aggregation in vitro. *Arzneim. Forsch.*, 31:1131–1134.

175. Lichtlen, H., Engel, J., Wolf, R., and Amende, I. (1980): The effect of the calcium antagonistic drug

nifedipine on coronary and left ventricular dynamics in patients with coronary artery disease. In: *Calcium Antagonismus,* edited by A. Fleckenstein and H. Roskamm, pp. 270–281. Springer-Verlag, Heidelberg.

176. Ebner, F., and Dunschede, H. B. (1976): Hemodynamics, therapeutic mechanism of action and clinical findings of Adalat use based on world-wide clinical trials. In: *Third Adalat Symposium,* edited by A. D. Jatene and P. R. Lichtlen, pp. 283–300. Excerpta Medica, Amsterdam.

177. Lewis, G. R. J. (1981): Slow channel-inhibiting drugs in treatment of hypertension. In: Calcium inhibiting drugs in cardiovascular therapy: Mechanism of action and application, edited by B. Surawicz and A. Maseri (*in press*).

178. Rodger, C., and Stewart, A. (1978): Side-effects of nifedipine. *Br. Med. J.,* 1:1619–1620 (letter).

179. Jariwalla, A. G., and Anderson, E. G. (1978): Side effects of drugs, production of ischemic cardiac pain by nifedipine. *Br. Med. J.,* 1:1181–1182.

180. Keidar, S., Marmor, A., Grenadier, E., and Palant, A. (1979): Nifedipine and Prinzmetal's angina. *Circulation,* 59:195 (letter).

181. Ekelund, L. G., and Oro, L. (1979): Antianginal efficacy of nifedipine with and without a beta blocker, studied with exercise test. A double-blind randomized subacute study. *Clin. Cardiol.,* 2:203–211.

182. Lynch, P., Dargie, H., Krikler, S., and Krikler, D. (1980): Objective assessment of antianginal treatment: A double-blind comparison of propranolol, nifedipine and their combination. *Br. Med. J.,* 281:184–187.

183. Anastassiades, C. J. (1980): Nifedipine and beta blocker drugs. *Br. Med. J.,* 281:1251–1252.

184. Opie, L. H., and White, D. A. (1980): Adverse interaction between nifedipine and beta blockade. *Br. Med. J.,* 281:1462.

185. Dean, S., and Kendall, M. J. (1981): Adverse interaction between nifedipine and beta blockade. *Br. Med. J.,* 282:1322 (letter).

186. Johnston, A., Burgess, C. D., and Hamer, J. (1981): Systemic availability of oral verapamil and effect on PR interval in man. *Br. J. Clin. Pharmacol.,* 12:397–400.

187. Jakobsen, P., Lederballe-Pedersen, O., and Mikkelsen, E. (1979): Gas chromatographic determination of nifedipine and one of its metabolites using electron capture detector. *J. Chromatogr.,* 162:81–87.

188. Schlossmann, K., Medenwald, H., and Rosenkranz, H. (1975): Investigation on the metabolism and protein binding of nifedipine. In: *Second International Symposium on Adalat,* edited by W. Lochner, W. Braasch, and G. Kroneberg, pp. 33–39. Excerpta Medica, Amsterdam.

189. Taira, N., Narimatsu, A., Satoh, K., et al. (1979): Cardiovascular actions of niludipine (Bay a 7168), a new dihydropyridine vasodilator in the dog. *Arzneim. Forsch.,* 29:246–255.

190. Hashimoto, K., Takeda, K., Katano, Y., et al. (1979): Effect of niludipine on the cardiovascular system. *Arzneim. Forsch.,* 29:1368–1373.

191. Hiwatari, M., and Taira, N. (1979): Antihypertensive effect of niludipine in conscious renal-hypertensive dogs. *Arzneim. Forsch.,* 29:1373–1376.

192. Fagbemi, O., and Parratt, J. R. (1981): Suppression by orally administered nifedipine, nisoldipine and niludipine of early life-threatening arrhythmias resulting from acute myocardial ischemia. *Br. J. Pharmacol.,* 74:12–14.

193. Maeda, K., Tanaka, C., Yagi, Y., et al. (1981): Treatment of angina pectoris patients with niludipine—a new calcium antagonistic drug. *Arzneim. Forsch.,* 31:830–834.

194. Spracklen, F. H. N., and Lazarus, L. H. (1980): Nifedipine for digitalis induced arrhythmias. *S. Afr. Med. J.,* 57:1046.

195. Kazda, S., Garthoff, B., Meyer, H., et al. (1980): Pharmacology of a new calcium antagonist—nisoldipine (Bay k 5552). *Arzneim. Forsch.,* 30:2144–2162.

196. Vogt, A., Newhaus, K. L., and Kreuzer, H. (1980): Hemodynamic effects of the new vasodilator drug, Bay k 5552, in man. *Arzneim. Forsch.,* 30:2162–2164.

197. Allen, G. S., and Banghart, S. B. (1979): Cerebral arterial spasm (part 9): In vitro effects of nifedipine on serotonin, phenylephrine and potassium induced contractions of canine basilar and femoral arteries. *Neurosurgery,* 4:37–41.

198. Shimizu, K., Ohta, T., and Toda, N. (1980): Evidence for greater susceptibility of isolated dog cerebral arteries to calcium antagonists than peripheral arteries. *Stroke,* 11:261–266.

199. Kazda, S., Hoffmeister, F., Garthoff, B., et al. (1979): Prevention of the post-ischemic impaired reperfusion of the brain by nimodipine. *Acta Neurol. Scand.,* 60:358–359.

200. Hoffmeister, F., Kazda, S., and Krause, H. P. (1979): Influence of nimodipine on the post-ischemic changes of brain function. *Acta Neurol. Scand.,* 60:302–303.

201. Towart, R., and Perzborn, E. (1981): Nimodipine inhibits carbocyclic thromboxane-induced contractions of cerebral arteries. *Eur. J. Pharmacol.,* 69:213–215.

202. Towart, R. (1981): Selective inhibition of serotonin induced contractions of rabbit vascular smooth muscle by calcium antagonistic dihydropyridines (nimodipine). *Circ. Res.,* 48:650–657.

203. Towart, R. (1981): Predilective relaxation by the calcium antagonist, nimodipine of isolated cerebral blood vessels contracted with autologus blood. *Br. J. Pharmacol.,* 74:268P–269P.

204. Towart, R., and Kazda, S. (1980): Selective inhibition of serotonin-induced contractions of rabbit basilar artery by nimodipine. *I.R.C.S. Med. Sci.,* 8:206.

205. Takenaka, T., Usuda, S., Nomura, T., et al. (1976): Vasodilator profile of a new 1,4-dihydropyridine derivative—YC-93. *Arzneim. Forsch.,* 26:2172–2178.

206. Sakamoto, N., Terai, M., Takenaka, T., et al. (1978): Inhibition of cAMP phosphodiesterase by YC-93, a potent vasodilator. *Biochem. Pharmacol.,* 27:1269–1274.

207. Narimatsu, A., Satoh, K., and Taira, N. (1978): Assessment of the coronary vasodilator action of

SK&F 24260 in the dog. *Clin. Exp. Pharmacol. Physiol.*, 5:107–115.

208. Jolly, S. R., and Gross, G. J. (1979): Effect of FR 7534, a new calcium antagonist, on myocardial oxygen demand. *Eur. J. Pharmacol.*, 54:289–293.

209. Jolly, S. R., and Gross, G. J. (1980): Improvement in ischemic myocardial blood flow following a new calcium antagonist. *Am. J. Physiol.*, 239:163–171.

210. Gross, G. J., Waltier, D. C., Jolly S. R., and Hardman, H. F. (1980): Comparative effects of FR 7534, nitroglycerin and dipyridamole on regional myocardial blood flow and contractility during partial coronary artery occlusion in the dog. *J. Cardiovasc. Pharmacol.*, 2:797–813.

211. Meyer, V. H., Bossert, F., Wehinger, E., et al. (1981): Synthesis and comparative pharmacological studies with non-identical ester function compounds. *Arzneim. Forsch.*, 31:407–409.

212. Nagao, T., Ikeo, T., and Sato, M. (1977): Influence of calcium ions on responses to diltiazem in coronary arteries. *Jpn. J. Pharmacol.*, 27:330–332.

213. Nagao, T., Millard, R. W., Schwartz, A., and Franklin, D. (1979): Augmented ischemic myocardial function by recruitment of collateral flow reserve with diltiazem. *Circulation*, 59,60:II-260 (abstract).

214. Van Breemen, C., Hwang, O. K., and Meisheri, K. D. (1979): Mechanism of inhibitory action of diltiazem on vascular smooth muscle contractility. *J. Pharmacol. Exp. Ther.*, 218:459–463.

215. Saikawa, T., Nagamoto, Y., and Arita, M. (1977): Electrophysiological effects of diltiazem, a new slow channel inhibitor, on canine cardiac fibers. *Jpn. Heart J.*, 18:235–245.

216. Yatani, A. (1976): Effect of CRD-401 (diltiazem) on membrane currents and contractile tension of bullfrog atrium. *Jpn. J. Clin. Exp. Med.*, 53:562.

217. Sugimoto, T., Ishikawa, T., Kaseno, K., et al. (1980): Electrophysiological effects of diltiazem in patients with impaired sinus or AV node function. *Angiology*, 31:700–709.

218. Oyama, Y., Imai, Y., Nakaya, H., et al. (1978): Effects of diltiazem HCl on the cardiac conduction: A clinical study of His bundle electrogram. *Jpn. Circ. J.*, 42:1257–1264.

219. Sato, M., Nagao, T., Yamaguchi, I., et al. (1971): Pharmacological studies on a new 1,5-benzothiazepine derivative—CRD-401. *Arzneim. Forsch.*, 21:1338–1343.

220. Bourassa, M. G., Cote, P., Theroux, P., et al. (1980): Hemodynamics and coronary flow, following diltiazem administration in anesthetized dogs and in humans. *Chest*, 78:224–230.

221. Sakai, K., Shiraki, Y., and Nabata, H. (1981): Cardiovascular effects of a new coronary vasodilator, SG-75. Comparison with nitroglycerin and diltiazem. *J. Cardiovasc. Pharmacol.*, 3:139–150.

222. Nagao, T., Murata, S., and Sato, M. (1975): Effect of diltiazem on developed coronary collaterals in the dog. *Jpn. J. Pharmacol.*, 25:281–288.

223. Yabe, Y., Abe, H., Yoshimura, S., et al. (1979): Effect of diltiazem on coronary hemodynamics and its clinical significance. *Jpn. Heart J.*, 20:83–93.

224. Flaim, S. F., and Zelis, R. F. (1980): Regional distribution of cardiac output in conscious rats at rest and during exercise. Effects of diltiazem. *Chest* [*Suppl.*], 78:187–192.

225. Millard, R. W. (1980): Changes in cardiac mechanics and coronary blood flow of regionally ischemic porcine myocardium induced by diltiazem. *Chest* [*Suppl.*], 78:193–199.

226. Ishikawa, H., Matsushima, M., Matsui, H., et al. (1978): Effect of diltiazem HC1 on renal hemodynamics of dogs. *Arzneim. Forsch.*, 28:402–406.

227. Yamada, K., Shimamura, T., and Nakajima, H. (1973): Studies on diltiazem. (V): Antiarrhythmic actions. *Jpn. J. Pharmacol.*, 23:321–328.

228. Briley, M., Cavero, I., Langer, S. Z., and Roach, A. G. (1980): Evidence against beta-adrenoceptor blocking activity of diltiazem, a drug with calcium antagonist properties. *Br. J. Pharmacol.*, 69:669–673.

229. Nakamura, M., Kikuchi, Y., Senda, Y., et al. (1980): Myocardial blood flow following experimental coronary occlusion. Effects of diltiazem. *Chest* [*Suppl.*], 78:205–209.

230. Nagao, T., Matlib, M. A., Franklin, D., et al. (1980): Effects of diltiazem on regional myocardial function and mitochondria after brief coronary occlusion. *J. Mol. Cell. Cardiol.*, 12:20–43.

231. Jolly, S. R., Menahan, L. A., and Gross, G. J. (1981): Diltiazem in myocardial recovery from global ischemia and reperfusion. *J. Mol. Cell. Cardiol.*, 13:359–372.

232. Franklin, D., Millard, R. W., and Nagao, T. (1980): Responses of coronary collateral flow and dependent myocardial mechanical function to the calcium antagonist, diltiazem. *Chest*, 78:200–204.

233. Sasayma, S., Takahashi, M., Nakamura, M., et al. (1981): Effect of diltiazem on pacing-induced ischemia in conscious dogs with coronary stenosis: Improvement of post-pacing deterioration of ischemic myocardial function. *Am. J. Cardiol.*, 48:460–466.

234. Weishaar, R., Ashikawa, K., and Bing, R. J. (1979): Effect of diltiazem, a calcium antagonist, on myocardial ischemia. *Am. J. Cardiol.*, 43:1137–1143.

235. Nakamura, M., Koiwaya, Y., Yamada, A., et al. (1979): Effects of diltiazem, a new antianginal drug, on myocardial blood flow following experimental coronary occlusion. In: *Ischemic Myocardium and Antianginal Drugs*, edited by M. M. Winbury and Y. Abiko, pp. 129–142. Raven Press, New York.

236. Bush, L., Romson, J., Ash, J., and Lucchesi, B. R. (1981): Reduction of ischemic injury by diltiazem in a model of regional ischemia and reperfusion. *Fed. Proc.*, 40:691 (abstract).

237. Krusling, L., Rice, B. J., and Millard, R. W. (1981): Diltiazem, a calcium antagonist, increases survival time after acute coronary artery ligation in anesthetized pigs. *Fed. Proc.*, 40:673 (abstract).

238. Shinjo, A., Sasaki, Y., Inamsu, M., et al. (1978): In vitro effect of the coronary vasodilator diltiazem on human and rabbit platelets. *Thromb. Res.*, 13:941–955.

239. Kusukawa, R., Kinoshita, M., Shimono, Y., et al. (1977): Hemodynamic effects of a new anti-anginal drug, diltiazem HCl. *Arzneim. Forsch.*, 27:878–883.

240. Kinoshita, M., Kusukawa, R., Shimono, Y., et al. (1979): Effect of diltiazem HC1 upon sodium diure-

sis and renal function in chronic congestive heart failure. *Arzneim. Forsch.,* 29:676–681.

241. Kinoshita, M., Motomura, M., Kusukawa, R., et al. (1979): Comparison of hemodynamic effects between beta blocking agents and a new anti-anginal drug, diltiazem HCl. *Jpn. Circ. J.,* 43:587–598.

242. Pepine, C., Feldman, R. L., Whittle, J., et al. (1981): Effect of diltiazem in patients with variant angina: A randomized double blind trial. *Am. Heart J.,* 101:719–725.

243. Schroeder, J. S., Rosenthal, S., Ginsburg, R., et al. (1980): Medical therapy of Prinzmetal's variant angina. *Chest,* 78:231–233.

244. Koiwaya, Y., Nakamura, M., and Mitsutake, A. (1981): Increased exercise tolerance after oral diltiazem, a calcium antagonist, in angina pectoris. *Am. Heart J.,* 101:143–149.

245. Low, R. I., Takeda, P., Lee, G., et al. (1981): Effects of diltiazem-induced calcium blockade upon exercise capacity in effort angina due to chronic coronary artery disease. *Am. Heart J.,* 101:713–718.

246. Mudge, G. H., Grossman, W., Mills, R. M., et al. (1976): Reflex increase in coronary vascular resistance in patients with ischemic heart disease. *N. Engl. J. Med.,* 295:1333–1337.

247. Tubau, J. F., Cote, P., and Bourassa, M. G. (1980): Systemic and coronary hemodynamic effects of intravenous diltiazem in patients with coronary artery disease. *Am. J. Cardiol.,* 45:439 (abstract).

248. Tanaka, E. (1978): Long term administration of diltiazem in ischemic heart disease. *Med. Consult. New Remed.,* 15:587.

249. Kinoshita, M., Kusukawa, R., Shimono, Y., et al. (1978): Effect of diltiazem HCl on renal hemodynamics and urinary electrolyte excretion. *Jpn. Circ. J.,* 42:553–560.

250. Kohno, K., Takeuchi, Y., Etoh, A., et al. (1977): Pharmacokinetics and bioavailability of diltiazem (CRD-401) in dog. *Arzneim. Forsch.,* 27:1424–1428.

251. Meshi, T., Sugihara, J., and Sato, Y. (1971): Metabolic fate of CRD-401. *Chem. Pharm. Bull. (Tokyo),* 19:1546–1556.

252. Walsh, R., Badke, F., and O'Rourke, R. (1981): Differential effects of systemic and intracoronary calcium channel blocking agents on global and regional left ventricular function in conscious dogs. *Am. Heart J.,* 102:341–350.

253. Ellrodt, G., Chew, C. Y. C., and Singh, B. N. (1980): Therapeutic implications of slow channel blockade in cardio-circulatory disorders. *Circulation,* 62:669–679.

254. Hagemann, K., Lochner, W., and Niehues, B. (1975): Studies on the extracardial effects of nifedipine in anesthetized dogs. In: *Second Adalat Symposium,* edited by W. Lochner, W. Braasch, and W. Kroneberg, pp. 49–54. Springer-Verlag, New York.

255. Maseri, A., L'Abbate, A., Pesola, A., et al. (1977): Coronary vasospasms in angina pectoris. *Lancet,* 1:713–717.

256. Maseri, A., L'Abbate, A., Chierchia, S., et al. (1979): Significance of spasms in the pathogenesis of ischemic heart disease. *Am. J. Cardiol.,* 44:788–792.

257. Van Nueten, J. M., and Vanhoutte, P. M. (1980): Improvement of tissue perfusion with inhibitors of

calcium ion flux. *Biochem. Pharmacol.,* 29:479–481.

258. Johnson, S. M., Mauritson, D. R., Willerson, J. T., and Hillis, L. D. (1981): A controlled study of verapamil for Prinzmetal's variant angina. *N. Engl. J. Med.,* 304:862–866.

259. Lown, B. (1979): Symposium on nifedipine and calcium flux inhibition in the treatment of coronary artery spasms and myocardial ischemia. *Am. J. Cardiol.,* 44:780–782.

260. Hamamoto, H., Peter, T., Fujimoto, T., and Mandel, W. J. (1981): Effect of verapamil on conduction delay produced by myocardial ischemia and reperfusion. *Am. Heart J.,* 102:350–358.

261. Freeman, W. R., Peter, T., and Mandel, W. J. (1981): Verapamil therapy in variant angina pectoris refractory to nitrates. *Am. Heart J.,* 102:358–362.

262. Waters, D. D., Theroux, P., Szlachcic, J., et al. (1981): Provocative testing with ergonovine to assess the efficacy of treatment with nifedipine, diltiazem and verapamil in variant angina. *Am. J. Cardiol.,* 48:123–130.

263. Raizner, A. E., Gaston, W., Chahine, R. A., et al. (1981): The effectiveness of combined verapamil and nitrate therapy in Prinzmetal's variant angina. *Am. J. Cardiol.,* 45:439 (abstract).

264. Yasue, H., Omote, S., Takizawa, A., et al. (1978): Pathogenesis and treatment of angina pectoris at rest as seen from its response to various drugs. *Jpn. Circ.,* 42:1–10.

265. Leon, M. B., Rosing, D. R., Bonow, R. D., et al. (1981): Clinical efficacy of verapamil alone and combined with propranolol in treating patients with chronic stable angina. *Am. J. Cardiol.,* 48:131–139.

266. Carlens, P. (1981): Effect of intravenous verapamil on exercise tolerance and left ventricular function in patients with severe exertional angina pectoris. *J. Cardiovasc. Pharmacol.,* 3:1–10.

267. Moskowitz, R. M., Piccini, P. A., Nacarelli, G., and Zelis, R. (1979): Nifedipine therapy for stable angina pectoris. *Am. J. Cardiol.,* 44:811–816.

268. Hills, E. A. (1970): Iproveratril and bronchial asthma. *Br. J. Clin. Prac.,* 24:116.

269. Ribeiro, L. G. T., Brandon, T. A., Debauche, T. L., Moroko, P. R., and Miller, R. R. (1981): Antiarrhythmic and hemodynamic effects of calcium channel blocking agents during coronary artery reperfusion. *Am. J. Cardiol.,* 48:69–74.

270. Bergey, J. L., McCallum, J. D., and Nocella, K. (1981): Antiarrhythmic evaluation of verapamil, nifedipine, perhexiline and SKF 525-A in four canine models of cardiac arrhythmias. *Eur. J. Pharmacol.,* 70:331–343.

271. Matsuyama, E., Konishi, T., Okazaki, H., et al. (1981): Effects of verapamil on accessory pathway properties and induction of circus movement tachycardia in patients with the Wolff-Parkinson-White syndrome. *J. Cardiovasc. Pharmacol.,* 3:11–24.

272. Hamer, A., Peter, T., Platt, M., et al. (1981): Effects of verapamil on supraventricular tachycardia in patients with overt and concealed WPW syndrome. *Am. Heart J.,* 101:600–612.

273. Sugiyama, S., Kitazawa, M., Kotaka, K., et al. (1981): Mechanism of the antiarrhythmic action of verapamil. *J. Cardiovasc. Pharmacol.,* 3:801–806.

274. Lazzara, R., El-Sherif, N., Hope, R. R., and Scherlag, B. J. (1978): Ventricular arrhythmias and electrophysiological consequences of myocardial ischemia and infarction. *Circ. Res.,* 42:740–749.

275. Nakaya, H., Haltori, Y., Sakuma, I., and Kanno, M. (1981): Effects of calcium antagonists on coronary circulation and conduction delay induced by myocardial ischemia in dogs: A comparative study with other coronary vasodilators. *Eur. J. Pharmacol.,* 73:273–281.

276. Guazzi, M., Olivari, M. R., Polese, A., et al. (1977): Nifedipine, a new antihypertensive with rapid action. *Clin. Pharmacol. Ther.,* 22:528–532.

277. Kuwajima, I., Ueda, K., Kamata, C., et al. (1978): A study on the effects of nifedipine in hypertensive crises and severe hypertension. *Jpn. Heart J.,* 19:455–467.

278. Anavekar, S. N., Christophidis, N., Louis, W. J., et al. (1981): Verapamil in the treatment of hypertension. *J. Cardiovasc. Pharmacol.,* 3:287–292.

279. Sakuri, T., Kurita, T., Nagano, S., et al. (1972): Antihypertensive, vasodilating and sodium diuretic actions of CRD-401. *Acta Urol. Jpn.,* 18:695–707.

280. Van Meel, J., Dejonge, A., Kalkman, H. O., et al. (1981): Vascular smooth muscle contraction initiated by postsynaptic alpha₂ receptor activation is induced by an influx of extracellular calcium. *Eur. J. Pharmacol.,* 69:205–208.

281. Smith, H. J., Singh, B. N., Nisbet, H. D., et al. (1975): Effects of verapamil on infarct size following experimental coronary occlusion. *Cardiovasc. Res.,* 9:569–578.

282. Sherman, L. G., Liang, C. S., Boden, W. E., and Hood, W. B. (1981): Effect of verapamil on mechanical performance of acutely ischemic and reperfused myocardium in the conscious dog. *Circ. Res.,* 48:224–232.

283. Osakada, G., Kumada, T., Gallagher, K. P., et al. (1981): Reduction of exercise-induced ischemic regional myocardial dysfunction by verapamil in conscious dogs. *Am. Heart J.,* 101:707–712.

284. Hackel, D. B., Mikat, E. M., Reimer, K., and Whalen, G. (1981): Effects of verapamil on heart and circulation in hemorrhagic shock in dogs. *Am. J. Physiol.,* 241:12–17.

285. Hecht, H. S., Chew, C. Y. C., Burnam, M. H., et al. (1981): Verapamil in chronic stable angina: Amelioration of pacing-induced abnormalities of left ventricular ejection fraction, regional wall motion, lactate metabolism and hemodynamics. *Am. J. Cardiol.,* 48:536–543.

286. Subramanian, B., Bowles, M., Lahiri, A., et al. (1981): Long term antianginal action of verapamil assessed with quantitated serial treadmill stress testing. *Am. J. Cardiol.,* 48:529–535.

287. Rosing, D. R., Condit, J. R., Maron, B. J., et al. (1981): Verapamil therapy: A new approach to the pharmacologic treatment of hypertrophic cardiomyopathy: III. Effects of long term administration. *Am. J. Cardiol.,* 48:545–553.

288. Eigenmann, L., Blaber, L., Nakamura, K., Thorens, S., and Haeusler, G. (1981): Tiapamil, a new calcium antagonist. *Arzneim. Forsch.,* 31:1393–1410.

Cardiovascular Pharmacology, Second Edition,
edited by Michael Antonaccio.
Raven Press, New York © 1984.

Cardiovascular Actions of the Prostaglandins

Philip J. Kadowitz, Howard L. Lippton, Dennis B. McNamara,
Michael S. Wolin, and *Albert L. Hyman

*Departments of Pharmacology and *Surgery, Tulane University School of Medicine,
New Orleans, Louisiana 70112*

"Prostaglandin" is a term coined by von Euler to describe the active principle derived from acidic lipid extracts of seminal fluid that possess potent smooth-muscle-stimulating and vasodepressor activities (1,2). Structural assignment of these oxidized fatty acids has been an active area of investigation since the early 1960s. This chapter emphasizes the actions of the prostaglandins and related metabolites on the peripheral and pulmonary circulations. Comprehensive reviews on various aspects of prostaglandin biosynthesis, physiology, and pharmacology can be found in *Advances in Prostaglandin and Thromboxane Research,* a series edited by Bengt Samuelsson and Radolfo Paoletti (3–5).

20-Carbon polyunsaturated fatty acids derived from dietary sources or by desaturation and chain elongation of the essential fatty acid linoleic acid are biosynthetically transformed into prostaglandins and related tissue hormones (6). These fatty acids, or more specifically arachidonic acid (5,8,11,14-eicosatetraenoic acid), are transported in a protein-bound state and stored in the phospholipids in cell membranes of all tissues in the body (7). Metabolic activities such as respiration and oxidative phosphorylation appear to be dependent on these essential fatty acids. A variety of stimuli are believed to activate the release of arachidonic acid, in a Ca^{2+}-dependent manner, from storage in the 2 position of phospholipid membranes. Release of the fatty acid is

considered the rate-limiting step that determines in large measure the amount of substrate available for synthesis of prostaglandins and related metabolites (8). Two enzymes compete for the released fatty acid in a manner that is specific to the physiological or pharmacological state of the tissue under study. The cyclooxygenase enzyme complex, present in virtually every tissue in the body, converts arachidonic acid to prostaglandins, and this system is inhibited by the nonsteroidal antiinflammatory drugs (NSAID), such as aspirin and indomethacin (9). The lipoxygenase system also competes for released arachidonic acid, in a manner that appears to be tissue-specific and currently is not well understood, to give rise to hydroperoxy fatty acids (HPETE), which can be converted to the recently identified leukotrienes or reduced to hydroxy fatty acids (HETE) (10). Inactivation of the prostaglandins is catalyzed by chemical hydrolysis or 15-hydroxy prostaglandin dehydrogenase (PGDH), an enzyme that generates 15-keto prostaglandins (11). The relative metabolic activity of this enzyme (PGDH) determines the extent to which prostaglandin regulation is limited to the organ that produces them. Pulmonary PGDH activity is high, and thus after uptake of prostaglandins, the lung functions as an important metabolic organ to clear venous blood of the active prostaglandins (E and F series prostaglandins, but not PGI_2). Also, the lung can be viewed as an endocrine organ because it has great capacity to produce prostaglandins (predominantly PGI_2) that can be released into the arterial circulation (3,12). Prostaglandins and the thromboxanes are not stored in tissues, but these potent substances, when formed in various organs, are involved in the modulation of cardiovascular function and platelet aggregation.

The prostaglandins are a group of closely related molecules that possess a cyclopentane ring, derived from the 20-carbon fatty acid, with two adjacent hydrocarbon side chains. Prostaglandins derived from arachidonic acid possess a double bond adjacent to the cyclopentane ring on each side chain, and thus have the subscript 2. The substrates 8,11,14- and 5,8,11,14,17-eicosapentaenoic acids can also be converted to the 1 and 3 prostaglandin series, but they may be of minor importance, because they are present in low concentrations in most organ systems. The membrane-bound cyclooxygenase enzyme is responsible for synthesis of the prostaglandin ring structure by the addition of two molecules of molecular oxygen to the 20-carbon polyunsaturated fatty acid. Heme or heme-proteins are required for the cyclooxygenase reaction, which first generates the endoperoxide prostaglandin G (PGG), containing a hydroperoxy group in the 15 position (13). Cyclooxygenase also possesses peroxidase activity to reduce the 15-hydroperoxy group to the hydroxyl that is the eventual site of inactivation by the PGDH enzyme (14). The endoperoxide prostaglandin H (PGH) is believed to be the species released from the cyclooxygenase enzyme, and the conversion of PGG to PGH requires an electron-donating species that may be uric acid (15). Nonsteroidal antiinflammatory drugs such as aspirin block the cyclooxygenase reaction. PGH_2 is unstable in aqueous medium and decomposes with a half-life of about 5 min, primarily to prostaglandins E_2 and D_2 (16). Sulfhydryl groups and metals enhance the formation of $PGF_{2\alpha}$, which may be a major mechanism for increasing its production (17). Enzymes specific to the tissue or cell type com-

pete for PGH_2 to synthesize a variety of prostaglandins, including PGI_2 or thromboxane A_2. Thromboxanes possess a six-member oxane ring formed by an enzymatic rearrangement of the endoperoxy-cyclopentane ring of PGH_2. PGH_2 possesses smooth-muscle-stimulating activity and induces platelet aggregation, but because of the conversion to more potent metabolites, its physiological role is not considered to be clearly defined.

Prostaglandin I_2 (PGI_2) and thromboxane A_2 (TxA_2) currently appear to be the most active and major metabolites of PGH_2 associated with the cardiovascular system. Prostacyclin synthetase, a membrane-bound enzyme in vascular tissue, synthesizes PGI_2 (18). PGI_2 possesses potent vasodilator and platelet-aggregation inhibitory activity that is associated with increased intracellular levels of cyclic AMP (18). The inactivation of PGI_2 occurs with a half-life of 5 min and involves a hydrolysis reaction to 6-keto-$PGF_{1\alpha}$, a relatively inactive metabolite (19). TxA_2 is synthesized in platelets by the membrane-bound thromboxane synthetase, an enzyme with a secondary catalytic activity that results in the decomposition of PGH_2 into malondialdehyde (MDA) and 17-carbon hydroxy fatty acids (HHT) (20). The decomposition reaction is also catalyzed by Fe^{2+} (21). Contraction of smooth muscle along with platelet aggregation and the release reaction are induced by TxA_2 at a 10-fold lower concentration than PGH_2 (22). TxA_2 is inactivated by a hydrolysis reaction, with a half-life of about 30 sec, to the relatively inactive metabolite TxB_2 (22).

Additional conversions of PGH_2 to PGD_2, PGE_2, and $PGF_{2\alpha}$ may be physiologically significant. The enzymes PGE and PGD isomerase have differential distributions in tissues. PGE synthetase appears to be a particulate enzyme that possesses a glutathione (GSH) dependence that is not associated with stoichiometric oxidation of GSH (21). PGD synthetase appears to be a soluble enzyme without a GSH dependence. Heme proteins in the presence of thiol groups catalyze the formation of $PGF_{2\alpha}$, but native and boiled enzyme preparations have been found to possess comparable PGF isomerase activity (23). The formation of $PGF_{2\alpha}$ may also occur through NADPH-dependent reduction of the 9- and 11-keto groups of PGE_2 and PGD_2, respectively, by the hydroxy prostaglandin reductase enzymes (25). PGE_2 and PGD_2 increase cyclic AMP levels in some tissues (24). Generalizations with reference to the physiological functions of prostaglandins D, E, and F cannot be made.

Lipoxygenase is a second enzyme that may compete with cyclooxygenase for the arachidonic acid that is released from the phospholipid stores. This enzyme is not distributed in all tissues and has been found in platelets, leukocytes, and the lung (26–28). The lipoxygenase enzymes are classified based on the fatty acid hydroperoxide (HPETE) generated when arachidonic acid is examined as a substrate. Platelets synthesize 12-HPETE, whereas leukocytes generate 5-HPETE and 15-HPETE. The various HPETEs can be converted to the recently characterized leukotrienes that appear to be potent mediators of immediate and subacute hypersensitivity reactions (10). It is believed that 5-HPETE and 15-HPETE are enzymatically converted into leukotriene A (5-LTA_4 or 15-LTA_4), which contains a very reactive 5,6- or 14,15-epoxide group (29). An adduct formed with glutathione gives rise to the leukotriene C (LTC_4) series, and the removal of glutamate results in leukotriene D (LTD_4) (10). 5-LTC_4 and 5-LTD_4 have been identified as the major constituents of the slow-reacting substance of anaphylaxis (SRS-A) (10). The cysteine adduct of LTA_4 is leukotriene E_4. These agents possess potent contractile activity on smooth muscle (30). Dihydroxy fatty acids, termed leukotriene B (LTB), are formed by the enzymatic and nonenzymatic decomposition of LTA_4 (27). Several of the hydroxy (HETE) and dihydroxy fatty acids (LTB_4) are potent chemotactic factors for the migration of the various leukocytes (31). HPETEs also inhibit the formation of PGI_2 (32). Complex interactions appear to exist between the lipoxygenase and cyclooxygenase pathways that may serve in important regulatory processes, but these interactions are currently too poorly understood to be discussed in a concise manner.

SYSTEMIC VASCULAR ACTIONS OF PROSTAGLANDINS

Data illustrating the effects of PGI_2 on systemic arterial pressure, cardiac output, and systemic vascular resistance in the anesthetized cat are summarized in Table 1. Cardiac output was determined by the thermodilution technique after injecting a preset volume of 0.9% saline solution at room temperature into the left atrium and computing cardiac output by detecting blood temperature changes with a thermistor-tipped catheter placed in the ascending aorta. Systemic vascular resistance was calculated by dividing mean aortic pressure (mm Hg) by cardiac output (ml/min) and was expressed as mm Hg/ml/min. Rapid bolus injections of PGI_2, the major metabolite of PGH_2 in vascular tissue, into the right atrium produced significant dose-related decreases in mean aortic pressure. Cardiac output, as measured at the peak of the aortic depressor response by the thermodilution technique, was increased significantly, and systemic vascular resistance was decreased at each dose of PGI_2 studied (Table 1). The influence of lung transit on systemic vascular responses to PGI_2 was compared in this same group of cats. PGI_2 was injected into the left atrium by way of a transseptally placed catheter and into the right atrium by way of a catheter in that chamber. Both of these catheters were positioned under fluoroscopic guidance. PGI_2 decreased systemic vascular resistance when injected into the left or the right atrium. The reductions in mean aortic pressure and systemic vascular resistance in response to PGI_2 were not significantly different when PGI_2 was injected into the left or into the right side of the circulation. These experiments indicate that PGI_2 is not inactivated in passage through the feline pulmonary vascular bed, and they are in agreement with

TABLE 1. *Influence of right atrial injections of PGI$_2$ on hemodynamics in anesthetized cats (N = 8)*

	Aortic pressure (mm Hg ± SEM)	Cardiac output (ml/min ± SEM)	Systemic vascular resistance (mm Hg/ml/min ± SEM)
Control	173 ± 8	463 ± 32	0.388 ± 0.034
PGI$_2$, 0.3 μg	160 ± 8[a]	504 ± 36[a]	0.332 ± 0.034[a]
Control	167 ± 7	485 ± 32	0.352 ± 0.024
PGI$_2$, 1 μg	144 ± 6[a]	566 ± 34[a]	0.259 ± 0.015[a]
Control	154 ± 8	467 ± 38	0.335 ± 0.024
PGI$_2$, 3 μg	117 ± 9[a]	549 ± 40[a]	0.217 ± 0.034[a]

[a] $p < 0.05$ when compared with corresponding control; paired comparison.

studies showing that PGI$_2$ is not inactivated in the lungs of other species, including the dog, rat, and rabbit (33–35).

The influence of lung transit on responses to PGE$_1$ was also investigated in the cat. Whereas reductions in systemic arterial pressure and systemic vascular resistance were similar when PGI$_2$ was injected into the right or the left side of the circulation, this was not what was observed with PGE$_1$ (36). This monoenoic prostaglandin caused greater decreases in systemic arterial pressure and systemic vascular resistance when injected into the left side of the circulation and lung transit was avoided on the first pass. The observation that "PGI$_2$-like" substances are released spontaneously into the circulation and that PGI$_2$ is not inactivated in the lung suggests that PGI$_2$ may serve as a circulating hormone that could act to maintain the peripheral vascular bed in a dilated state (37). Thus, there is an important difference between PGI$_2$ and other prostaglandins formed from arachidonic acid and PGH$_2$. PGI$_2$ is not inactivated by the pulmonary circulation and is equipotent as a vasodilator when given intraarterially or intravenously, whereas other prostaglandins such as PGE$_1$ and PGE$_2$ do not escape pulmonary metabolism and are much less active when given intravenously (34–36). Thus, PGI$_2$ could serve to maintain the peripheral vascular bed in a dilated state because of the fact that it escapes pulmonary inactivation and because it is a potent peripheral vasodilator substance (34,36,41). The actions of PGI$_2$ on vas-

cular smooth muscle from a number of organ systems have been reported (38). PGI$_2$ relaxes strips from mesenteric, celiac, and coronary arteries (30,40) and increases blood flow in the canine coronary, renal, and mesenteric vascular beds (34,41,42). The systemic vascular effects of PGI$_2$ and PGE$_1$ have been compared in the regional circulation in cats, and these data are shown in Fig. 1. In these experiments, blood flow to the small intestine, kidney, and hindquarters is maintained constant with a pump, so that changes in perfusion pressure directly reflect changes in resistance to the flow of blood in the regional vascular bed. In these experiments, intraarterial injections of graded doses of PGI$_2$ and PGE$_1$ into the intestinal, renal, and hindquarter vascular beds produced dose-related decreases in perfusion pressure. In terms of relative vasodilator activity, the effects of PGI$_2$ were greater in the feline intestine than in the kidney or hindquarters. This observation suggests that an increase in circulating levels of PGI$_2$ in the cat would be expected to increase blood flow (cardiac fraction) to the intestine to a greater extent than to the kidney or skeletal muscle (36). Because the prostacyclin-generating capacity of the gastrointestinal tract is greater than that of other organs, enhanced local synthesis of PGI$_2$ would also be expected to have a marked effect on blood flow to the intestine and the fraction of cardiac output going to the gastrointestinal tract (39,43). Differential sensitivity to vasodilator responses to PGI$_2$ was also found in the regional circulation in the

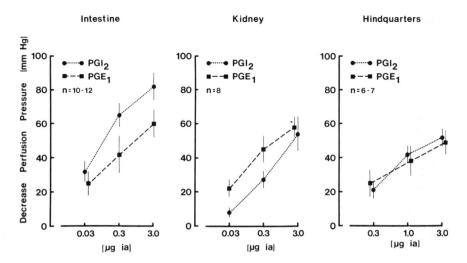

FIG. 1. Dose–response curves comparing the effects of intraarterially injected PGI_2 and PGE_1 in the feline intestinal (mesenteric), renal (kidney), and hindquarter vascular beds (*n* indicates number of animals). Because flow was maintained constant in these experiments, decreases in perfusion pressure directly reflect decreases in regional vascular resistance in cats.

dog (34,52). In these experiments, PGI_2 was 10-fold more active in increasing blood flow to the mesenteric vascular bed than to the renal vascular bed. In the regional circulation in the dog, PGE_1 and PGI_2 had similar vasodilator activities (34,42). In terms of the regional circulation, PGI_2 also had marked vasodilator activity in the coronary vascular bed in intact-chest dogs (41).

PGI_2 is rapidly degraded to 6-keto-$PGF_{1\alpha}$, a breakdown product that has little, if any, biologic activity (34). However, 6-keto-$PGF_{1\alpha}$ and its parent compound, PGI_2, may be converted to 6-keto-PGE_1, a biologically active metabolite, by the 9-hydroxy prostaglandin dehydrogenase pathway that is present in the liver and platelets (44,45). The actions of 6-keto-PGE_1 on systemic arterial pressure, cardiac output, and systemic vascular resistance in the cat are summarized in Table 2. 6-Keto-PGE_1 decreased systemic arterial pressure and increased cardiac output, indicating that this recently discovered metabolite of PGI_2 decreases systemic vascular resistance (46). In addition, the influence of lung transit on systemic vascular responses to 6-keto-PGE_1 was studied in the cat. Reductions in systemic arte-

rial pressure and systemic vascular resistance were similar when 6-keto-PGE_1 was injected into the right or the left atrium (46,47). These results demonstrate that 6-keto-PGE_1 is not converted to less active metabolites in passage through the feline pulmonary vascular bed, and they are in agreement with studies in several species, including the rat, dog, and newborn lamb (47–49). The ability of 6-keto-PGE_1 to dilate the peripheral vascular bed was first shown in the rat kidney (49). This substance has since been reported to dilate the canine renal and feline hindquarter and mesenteric vascular beds (50–52). The comparative effects of infusions of PGI_2, 6-keto-$PGF_{1\alpha}$, and 6-keto-PGE_1 on the feline intestinal vascular bed were also studied. Infusion of PGI_2 or 6-keto-PGE_1 into the intestinal bed at a rate of 1 μg/min caused a marked reduction in mesenteric perfusion pressure. The fall in perfusion pressure or intestinal vascular resistance was rapid in onset and was well maintained during the period of infusion of PGI_2 or 6-keto-PGE_1. In contrast, infusion of 6-keto-$PGF_{1\alpha}$, the stable breakdown product of PGI_2, into the superior mesenteric artery produced no change in mesenteric perfusion pressure. In addition,

TABLE 2. *Effects of injections of 6-keto-PGE$_1$ into the superior vena cava on systemic arterial pressure, cardiac output, and systemic vascular resistance (N = 7)*

	Aortic pressure (mm Hg)	Cardiac output (liters/min)	Systemic vascular resistance (mm Hg/liter/min)
Control	151 ± 12	0.44 ± 0.04	375 ± 59
6-keto-PGE$_1$ (1 μg)	134 ± 11^a	0.56 ± 0.07^a	294 ± 61^a
Control	161 ± 4	0.43 ± 0.04	402 ± 48
6-keto-PGE$_1$ (3 μg)	128 ± 3^a	0.52 ± 0.05^a	266 ± 31^a
Control	163 ± 5	0.43 ± 0.04	401 ± 41
6-keto-PGE$_1$ (10 μg)	115 ± 7^a	0.58 ± 0.04^a	211 ± 29^a
Control	159 ± 7	0.44 ± 0.04	373 ± 30
6-keto-PGE$_1$ (30 μg)	98 ± 4^a	0.58 ± 0.06^a	188 ± 29^a

$^a p < 0.05$ when compared with corresponding control; paired comparison.

aortic pressure was not altered during infusion of PGI$_2$, 6-keto-PGF$_{1\alpha}$, and 6-keto-PGE$_1$ into the superior mesenteric artery. Thus, 6-keto-PGE$_1$, like PGI$_2$, is not inactivated in the lung and is equipotent to PGI$_2$ in its ability to decrease mesenteric and systemic vascular resistance. PGI$_2$ is inactivated in transit through the peripheral vascular bed (38).

In addition to their actions on vascular smooth muscle, PGI$_2$ and 6-keto-PGE$_1$ inhibit the platelet aggregation that is involved in physiological and pathophysiological processes such as coagulation and thromboembolus formation (24,38,53–58). Although other prostaglandins, including PGE$_1$, PGE$_2$, and PGD$_2$, have been reported to affect platelet aggregation, PGI$_2$ and 6-keto-PGE$_1$ appear to be the most potent inhibitors of aggregation (53–56). PGI$_2$ and 6-keto-PGE$_1$ inhibit platelet aggregation induced by a number of aggregating substances, including collagen, arachidonic acid, epinephrine, and thrombin (55–58). The influence of 6-keto-PGE$_1$ on human platelet aggregation stimulated by arachidonic acid and adenosine diphosphate (ADP) is illustrated in Fig. 2: Platelet-rich plasma (PRP) is prepared from whole blood by centrifugation. The degree of platelet aggregation is measured with a platelet aggregometer, a photometric device that monitors aggregation by continuous recording of light transmittance. PRP is turbid, and when an aggregating agent is added, the formation of platelet aggregates is accompanied by a clearing in the PRP, and thus light transmittance through the sample is increased. These experiments show that when incubated in human PRP, 6-keto-PGE$_1$ produces a dose-related inhibition of aggregation induced by arachidonic acid and ADP. Although 6-keto-PGE$_1$ has been shown to inhibit platelet aggregation in doses similar to those of PGI$_2$, evidence to the contrary has been reported; however, both agents appear to produce their platelet effects by the same mechanism (55–58). PGI$_2$ and 6-keto-PGE$_1$ inhibit aggregation through the stimulation of cyclic AMP accumulation in platelets (55–58). Because there is a direct correlation between the extent to which a "PGI$_2$-like" molecule elevates platelet cyclic AMP levels and inhibits aggregation, the abilities of PGI$_2$ and 6-keto-PGE$_1$ to stimulate adenylate cyclase may determine their relative biologic activities (55–58). Because the production of 6-keto-PGE$_1$ may occur enzymatically on conversion of PGI$_2$ or its hydrolysis product, 6-keto-PGF$_{1\alpha}$, by the 9-hydroxy prostaglandin pathway, a part of the vasoactive and antiaggregatory properties of PGI$_2$ may be due to conversion to 6-keto-PGE$_1$ (55,59). The presence of this

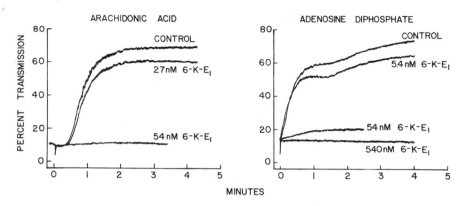

FIG. 2. Left: Tracings from typical experiments illustrating the inhibition of arachidonic-acid-induced (0.41 mM) aggregation by prostaglandin 6-keto-E_1 (27 and 54 nM) in human platelet-rich plasma. **Right:** Tracings from typical experiments illustrating the inhibition of ADP-induced (2 μM) aggregation by prostaglandin 6-keto-E_1 (5.4, 54, and 540 nM).

enzyme system has been reported in both liver and platelet; however, its presence and activity in other organ systems are uncertain (44, 45,59).

$PGF_{2\alpha}$, PGE_2, and PGD_2 are additional products of arachidonic acid metabolism that possess diverse activities in the peripheral vascular bed (42,60,61). $PGF_{2\alpha}$ is a vasoconstrictor that can increase vascular resistance in the mesenteric and hindquarter vascular beds, whereas PGE_2 and PGD_2 dilate vascular smooth muscle in peripheral organ systems, including the kidney and skeletal muscle (60,61). Although PGD_2 is an isomer of PGE_2, vascular responses to these two prostaglandins may be qualitatively different (60–62). Responses to PGD_2 in the feline intestinal vascu-

lar bed shown in Fig. 3 are biphasic. At low doses, the predominant response to bolus injections is vasoconstriction, whereas at higher doses the predominant response is vasodilation. Infusions of PGD_2 at 1.0, 0.3, and 0.1 μg/min produce a biphasic response, with an initial vasoconstrictor component that is early in onset. However, in the mesenteric vascular bed, responses to intraarterial injections and infusion of PGE_2 are also dilator, even at high doses and concentrations. These data may support the hypothesis that the gastrointestinal tract, like blood platelets, contains separate and specific receptors for PGE_2 and PGD_2 (60–63). In addition, the relative vasodilator effects of PGE_2 are organ-dependent, and the effects of PGD_2 depend on both organ and

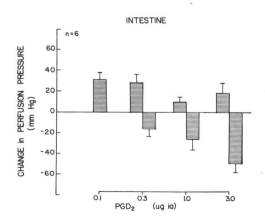

FIG. 3. Influence of intraarterial (bolus) injections of PGD_2 on perfusion pressure in the feline intestinal (mesenteric) vascular bed. Because blood flow was maintained constant, changes in perfusion pressure directly reflect changes in mesenteric vascular resistance (*n* indicates number of cats).

dose in the cat and in the dog (42,52,60–62,64).

INFLUENCE OF PROSTAGLANDINS ON VASCULAR RESPONSES

In addition to their abilities to directly affect isolated vascular smooth muscle and alter vascular resistance in the peripheral vascular bed, prostaglandins have been shown to inhibit vasoconstrictor responses to pressor hormones and sympathetic nerve stimulation (52,64–68). Data illustrating the effects of infusion of PGI$_2$ (1 μg/min) on responses to norepinephrine, sympathetic nerve stimulation, and angiotensin II in the feline mesenteric vascular bed are shown in Fig. 4. In these studies, the blood flow to the superior mesenteric artery was held constant, so that changes in perfusion pressure directly reflected changes in intestinal vascular resistance. The nerve plexus surrounding the

superior mesenteric artery was carefully placed on an electrode, permitting stimulation of sympathetic postganglionic fibers at various frequencies. Pressor hormones were injected into the perfusion circuit close to the superior mesenteric artery. Control responses to nerve stimulation, norepinephrine, and angiotensin were frequency- and dose-dependent and were reproducible with respect to time. During infusion of PGI$_2$ at 1 μg/min, vasoconstrictor responses to norepinephrine and angiotensin were decreased significantly at all doses of the pressor hormones studied, whereas responses to nerve stimulation were decreased significantly at stimulus frequencies of 1 and 3 Hz. Responses to nerve stimulation and pressor hormones returned to control values or higher values 30 min after the PGI$_2$ infusion was ended. Because responses to nerve stimulation and norepinephrine were decreased to similar extents, the present data suggest that the ef-

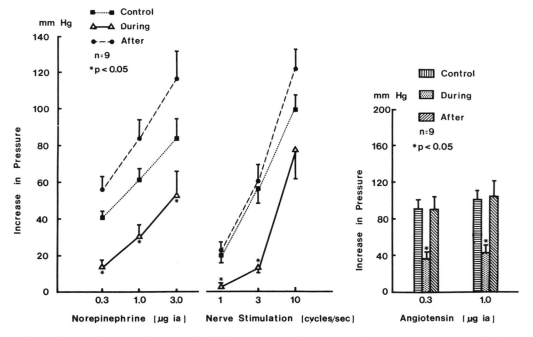

FIG. 4. Effects of infusion of prostacyclin, PGI$_2$, on mesenteric vasoconstrictor responses to nerve stimulaton and to intraarterial injections of norepinephrine and angiotensin in cats. Responses to nerve stimulation and the pressor hormones were obtained before (control), during infusion of PGI$_2$ (1 μg/min), and 30 min after the end of the prostaglandin infusion (n indicates number of cats). Responses were compared using Dunnett's test for multiple-range analysis.

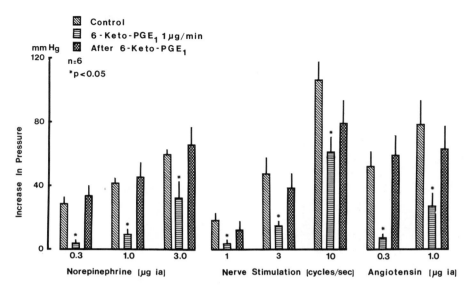

FIG. 5. Influences of infusion of 6-keto-PGE$_1$ on mesenteric vasoconstrictor responses to sympathetic nerve stimulation and intraarterial injections of norepinephrine and angiotensin II. Responses to nerve stimulation and the vasoconstrictor hormones were obtained before (control), during infusion of 6-keto-PGE$_1$ (1 μg/min), and 30 min after the termination of the prostaglandin infusion. Responses were compared using Dunnett's test for multiple-range analysis (n indicates number of animals).

fects of PGI$_2$ were mainly postjunctional in nature. In addition, responses to norepinephrine and angiotensin II were also decreased to similar extents, suggesting that the postjunctional effects of PGI$_2$ were nonspecific (65). 6-Keto-PGE$_1$ and PGE$_1$, which possess biologic activity similar to that of PGI$_2$, inhibit vasoconstrictor responses to pressor hormones and nerve stimulation in the feline mesenteric vascular bed, and these data are presented in Fig. 5. Because intraarterial infusion of 6-keto-PGE$_1$ and PGE$_1$ at 1 μg/min significantly decreases responses to norepinephrine, angiotensin II, and nerve stimulation, these prostaglandins, like PGI$_2$, influence the response to vasoconstrictor stimuli postjunctionally and in a nonspecific manner (65,69,70). In contrast, experiments in the feline hindquarters vascular bed under similar conditions suggest that the effects of prostaglandins on vasoconstrictor responses may depend on the organ system under study (52,69,70). The influences of 6-keto-PGE$_1$ on responses to norepinephrine, angiotensin II, and stimulation of the lumbar sympathetic nerves are presented in

Table 3. In the control period, responses to pressor hormones and nerve stimulation were dose- and frequency-related and reproducible with respect to time. Infusion of 6-keto-PGE$_1$ at 3 μg/min significantly decreased the hindquarter pressor response to nerve stimulation, whereas responses to norepinephrine and angiotensin II were unchanged during continuous infusion of 6-keto-PGE$_1$. Responses to nerve stimulation returned to control values 30 min after the 6-keto-PGE$_1$ infusion was terminated. Infusion of PGE$_1$ or PGE$_2$ at 3 μg/min into the abdominal aorta significantly decreased responses to nerve stimulation (0.1, 0.3, 1.0, and 3.0 Hz) and angiotensin II, whereas the hindquarter responses to norepinephrine and tyramine were unchanged by continuous infusion of PGE$_1$ and PGE$_2$. Because 6-keto-PGE$_1$, PGE$_1$, and PGE$_2$ did not alter constrictor responses to intraarterial injections of norepinephrine, these data suggest that the predominant effects of E-series prostaglandins in the hindquarters vascular bed were prejunctional in nature.

The lack of effect of PGE$_1$ and PGE$_2$ on

TABLE 3. *Effects of infusion of 6-keto-PGE$_1$ on hindquarter vasoconstrictor responses to norepinephrine, sympathetic nerve stimulation, and angiotensin II in six cats*[a]

	Change in perfusion pressure (mm Hg $\pm$ SE)		
	Control	During 6-keto-PGE$_1$ infusion (3 μg/min)	30 min after end of infusion
Norepinephrine (μg i.a.)			
0.3	34 ± 4	27 ± 5	40 ± 5
1.0	62 ± 6	63 ± 11	71 ± 8
3.0	84 ± 6	89 ± 14	108 ± 9
Nerve stimulation (cycles/sec)			
0.3	19 ± 3	5 ± 2[b]	20 ± 5
1.0	53 ± 9	21 ± 6[b]	58 ± 9
3.0	106 ± 12	64 ± 8[b]	103 ± 10
10.0	151 ± 13	116 ± 10[b]	150 ± 12
Angiotensin II (μg i.a.)			
0.3	81 ± 8	53 ± 6[b]	83 ± 9
1.0	144 ± 16	135 ± 14	152 ± 15

[a] Responses were obtained before (control), during 6-keto-PGE$_1$ infusion, and 30 min after 6-keto-PGE$_1$ infusion was ended. Responses were compared using Student's t test for paired analysis.
[b] $p < 0.05$.

vasoconstrictor responses to tyramine suggests that the pool of norepinephrine released by tyramine is not the same as that released by nerve stimulation. Because release of norepinephrine by nerve stimulation has a necessary requirement for calcium, whereas norepinephrine release by tyramine is a calcium-independent process, the present data provide indirect support that PGEs alter adrenergic responses by interfering with the availability of calcium for the release mechanism (71).

Infusion of PGE$_1$ and PGE$_2$ reduced hindquarter responses to angiotensin II, suggesting that inhibition of an adrenergic component by PGEs in the angiotensin response may be possible (52). Support for this interpretation has been obtained in a number of vascular beds where angiotensin II augments the vasoconstrictor response to adrenergic nerve stimulation by both facilitating release and inhibiting neuronal uptake of transmitter by sympathetic nerve endings (72–76). The influence of prostaglandins on vasoconstrictor responses to pressor hormones and sympathetic nerve stimulation may also depend on the species studied. Data illustrating the effects of infusion of PGE$_1$ (1 μg/min) on responses to norepinephrine, angiotensin II, and sympa-

thetic nerve stimulation in the rabbit hindquarter vascular bed are shown in Fig. 6; the effects of PGE$_2$ and PGI$_2$ were similar to those of PGE$_1$. The responses to all vasoconstrictor stimuli were decreased significantly and to similar extents during continuous infusion of PGE$_1$, PGE$_2$, and PGI$_2$. In contrast to studies in the cat, these data suggest that the actions of PGE$_1$, PGE$_2$, and PGI$_2$ in the hindquarter vascular bed were postjunctional and nonspecific in nature (52,70). Thus, the ability of prostaglandins to alter vasoconstrictor responses to pressor hormones and sympathetic nerve stimulation depends on both organ and species. Sympathetic stimulation and vasoactive hormones increase the synthesis and release of prostaglandins in a number of adrenergically innervated organs (66). Prostaglandins have been shown to attenuate release of the adrenergic transmitter and inhibit responses to norepinephrine, angiotensin, and nerve stimulation in a number of regional vascular beds, including the hindpaw, hindquarters, intestine, kidney, and spleen (62–71, 77,78). Thus, it has been suggested that prostaglandins may act as modulators of adrenergic neurotransmission to vascular smooth muscle and play an important role

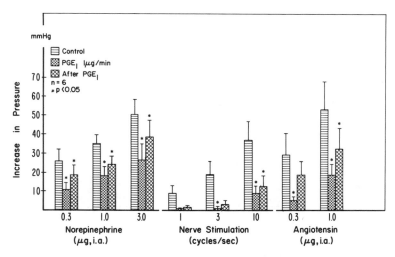

FIG. 6. Effects of infusion of PGE_1 (1 μg/min) on responses to vasoconstrictor hormones and nerve stimulation in the rabbit hindquarter vascular bed. Dose–response curves for norepinephrine and angiotensin and the frequency–response curve for nerve stimulation were determined before, during, and 30 min after the PGE_1 infusion (n indicates number of animals). Data were compared by Student's t test for paired analysis.

in the regulation of vasomotor tone in the systemic vascular bed. The actions of prostaglandins on peripheral vascular resistance may be dependent on their ability to alter vasoconstrictor responses to pressor hormones and nerve stimulation and influence the release of norepinephrine from adrenergic nerves.

INFLUENCE OF PROSTAGLANDINS IN THE LUNG

The lung is a major organ for the synthesis of prostaglandins, thromboxane A_2, and prostacyclin. The effects of bolus injections of arachidonic acid and of primary prostaglandins on the pulmonary vascular bed in intact-chest dogs and cats are shown in Figs. 7 and 8. All of the bisenoic prostaglandins, the PGH_2 analogue, and arachidonic acid increased lobar arterial pressure in dogs and cats in a dose-dependent manner. In dogs, under conditions of controlled pulmonary lobar blood flow, $PGF_{2\alpha}$ was about 10-fold more active than PGE_2, which in turn was about 10 to 20 times more active than arachidonic acid. In dogs, the stable endoperoxide analogue is about 10-fold more active than

$PGF_{2\alpha}$. Although not shown in Fig. 7, the pressor activities of PGF_2 and PGD_2 were quite similar in dogs. Arachidonic acid, $PGF_{2\alpha}$, PGD_2, and the PGH_2 analogue all increased transpulmonary pressure and small intrapulmonary vein pressures in dogs. This analogue is thought to mimic the effects of TxA_2. The increases in lobar arterial and small-vein pressures in response to the stable analogue, the prostaglandins, and arachidonic acid were similar when the lobe was ventilated or when ventilation was arrested at end-expiration. In addition to increasing lobar vascular pressures, arachidonic acid increased airway resistance and decreased dynamic lung compliance, and in this respect it is similar to, but much less potent than, $PGF_{2\alpha}$, PGD_2, and the PGH_2 analogue. The effects of arachidonic acid on canine and feline pulmonary vascular beds and airways were blocked after administration of indomethacin or meclofenamate (2.5–5 mg/kg i.v.).

In intact-chest cats, $PGF_{2\alpha}$ was a very potent vasoconstrictor agent in that pulmonary vascular resistance was nearly doubled at a dose of 10 ng (Fig. 8). In cats, $PGF_{2\alpha}$ was approximately 10 to 30 times more active than

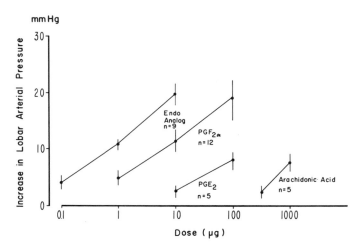

FIG. 7. Dose–response curves comparing increases in lobar arterial pressure in response to graded doses of an endoperoxide (PGH_2) analogue, $PGF_{2\alpha}$, PGE_2, and arachidonic acid in intact-chest dogs (n indicates number of animals). Blood flow to the left lower lobe was maintained constant with a pump. All substances were injected rapidly as a bolus into the perfused lobar artery, and all responses were dose-related.

PGD_2, whereas $PGF_{2\alpha}$ was 100 to 300 times more potent than PGE_2. Arachidonic acid, when administered as a rapid bolus injection, was less active than PGE_2 (Fig. 8). Although the data are not shown in Fig. 8, the stable PGH_2 analogue was similar to $PGF_{2\alpha}$ in intact-chest cats. The effects of the endoperoxide, PGH_2 (not an analogue), on the canine pulmonary vascular bed were also studied, and the endoperoxide itself, when injected as a 2-μg bolus into the perfused lobar artery, produced a small increase in lobar arterial and small-vein pressures and decreased aortic pressure in dogs. The endoperoxide, PGH_2, was far less active than its stable analogue in increasing pulmonary lobar vascular resistance in dogs. The endoperoxide, PGH_2, also had modest pressor activity in the feline pulmonary vascular bed, where it was approximately 100-fold less active than its stable analogues. Under resting conditions, PGH_2 did not dilate the pulmonary vascular bed.

In contrast to the effects of primary prostaglandins, PGH_2, and stable PGH_2 analogues, PGI_2 had vasodilator activity in the pulmonary vascular bed. PGI_2 produced small but significant reductions in lobar arterial and small-vein pressures without affecting left atrial pressure. Although the effects of PGI_2 were quite modest under resting conditions in dogs when existing vasomotor tone was low, they were greatly enhanced when pulmonary vascular resistance was increased by infusion of a stable PGH_2 analogue. In the cat pulmonary vascular bed, PGI_2 caused small dose-related decreases in lobar arterial pressure without affecting left atrial pressure (Fig. 9). The pulmonary vasodilator effects of PGI_2 were also greatly enhanced in cats when pulmonary vascular resistance was increased by infusion of a PGH_2 analogue (Fig. 9). The foregoing experiments show that PGI_2 is the only known product of the arachidonic acid cascade that has vasodilator activity in the pulmonary vascular bed of the mature animal. The newly discovered metabolite of PGI_2, 6-keto-PGE_1, also dilated the pulmonary vascular bed. Thus, PGI_2 and 6-keto-PGE_1 have unique activity in the pulmonary vascular bed.

It has been reported that PGI_2 is the major product of arachidonic acid and PGH_2 metabolism in isolated vascular tissue. However, when administered as a rapid bolus, arachidonic acid had pressor activity. It has also

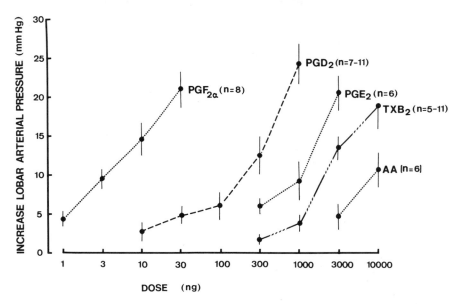

FIG. 8. Dose–response relationships comparing increases in lobar arterial pressure in response to bolus intralobar injections of graded doses of $PGF_{2\alpha}$, PGD_2, PGE_2, TxB_2, and arachidonic acid in intact-chest cats (*n* indicates number of animals). Blood flow to the left lower lobe was held constant with a pump. All responses were dose-related.

been reported that arachidonic acid decreases pulmonary vascular resistance in cats and dogs when administered by infusion. In both species, arachidonic acid had no significant dilator activity when pulmonary vascular resistance was at resting levels. However, when pulmonary vascular resistance was increased by infusion of a PGH_2 analogue or 15-methyl-$PGF_{2\alpha}$, arachidonic acid infusions decreased lobar arterial pressure in dogs and cats. A possible explanation for the divergent responses to arachidonic acid is provided by the biochemical studies to be discussed next.

A typical radiochromatographic scan obtained following thin-layer chromatography of the products of incubation of [1-^{14}C]PGH_2 with cat lung microsomes is shown in Fig. 10. The endoperoxide metabolites were identified by co-migration with authentic prostaglandin standards. A characteristic pattern of three major peaks can be seen (Fig. 10). The two more polar peaks co-chromatographed with standard TxB_2 and 6-keto-$PGF_{1\alpha}$, the stable breakdown products of TxA_2 and PGI_2, respectively. The fastest-running peak, which

moved slightly behind the compound DL-12-hydroxystearic acid, was 12-L-hydroxyl-5,-8,10-heptadecatrienoic acid (HHT), formed by chemical decomposition of PGH_2 and the action of thromboxane synthetase. TxB_2 and 6-keto-$PGF_{1\alpha}$ were not found in the incubation mixture of PGH_2 with heat-inactivated microsomes (Fig. 10). Instead, PGH_2 appeared to undergo decomposition to PGD_2, PGE_2, and $PGF_{2\alpha}$. The TxB_2 peak was abolished and HHT formation was lowered in the presence of 20-mM imidazole (Fig. 10), an inhibitor of thromboxane synthetase. Addition of 10-mM tranylcypromine, an inhibitor of prostacyclin synthetase, to an incubation mixture resulted in the disappearance of 6-keto-$PGF_{1\alpha}$ as well as a decrease in the production of both TxB_2 and HHT (Fig. 10). The effects of changing enzyme concentrations on product formation at fixed PGH_2 substrate concentration were also investigated. At 10 μM PGH_2 concentrations, increasing the microsomal protein concentration resulted in an increase in TxB_2 formation. Above 1.5 μg protein per microliter of incubation medium, no further

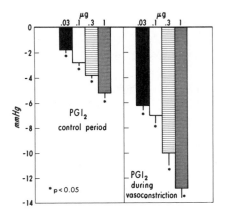

FIG. 9. Dose–response relationships for PGI$_2$ in the feline pulmonary (lobar) vascular bed under conditions of controlled pulmonary blood flow. Bars on the left side show that PGI$_2$ caused small dose-related decreases in lobar arterial pressure when vasomotor tone was at control levels. However, responses to PGI$_2$ were greatly enhanced when vasomotor tone was increased by infusion of a stable prostaglandin endoperoxide analogue. Left atrial pressure was unchanged in these experiments.

increase in product formation was observed. In contrast, the formation of 6-keto-PGF$_{1\alpha}$ continued to rise gradually until 3 μg protein per microliter of incubation medium; hence, at this concentration, both TxB$_2$ formation and 6-keto-PGF$_{1\alpha}$ formation had reached a maximum. It was observed that in buffer alone, approximately 15% of PGH$_2$ was converted to HHT because of nonenzymatic breakdown and that in response to variations in the microsomal protein concentration, the formation of HHT paralleled the formation of TxB$_2$, with HHT formation about 15% greater than that of TxB$_2$. The effects of vary-

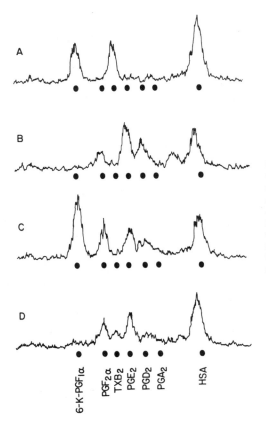

FIG. 10. Radiochromatogram of the products isolated from incubation of 5-μM PGH$_2$ with 300 μg of microsomal protein from cat lung in 100 μliter of 0.1-M potassium phosphate buffer, pH 7.4, for 2 min at 37°C. **A:** Cat lung microsomes; TxB$_2$ and 6-keto-PGF$_{1\alpha}$ conversions 23.4 and 17.2%, respectively. **B:** Microsomes boiled for 10 min. **C:** Microsomes + 20-mM imidazole. **D:** Microsomes + 10-mM tranylcypromine. Migration of authentic prostaglandin standards is indicated. HSA denotes DL-12-hydroxystearic acid.

ing PGH_2 concentration on the formation of TxB_2 and 6-keto-$PGF_{1\alpha}$ were investigated. A hyperbolic curve was observed for the production of 6-keto-$PGF_{1\alpha}$, and prostacyclin synthetase became saturated with PGH_2 at a substrate concentration of about 60 μM. TxB_2 production increased linearly with increasing PGH_2 concentration, reaching saturation only after a substrate concentration of 100 μM. More TxB_2 was formed than 6-keto-$PGF_{1\alpha}$ except at concentrations of PGH_2 below 10 μM. The maximum formation of TxB_2 was about seven times more than that of 6-keto-$PGF_{1\alpha}$ after saturation of both enzymes with substrate.

In most organ systems that have been studied, the unsaturated fatty acid precursor, arachidonic acid, which can be derived from the breakdown of cell membrane phospholipids, is converted into the endoperoxide intermediates by the membrane-bound cyclooxygenase (79). The endoperoxide intermediate (PGH_2) is then converted by terminal enzymes into primary prostaglandins, thromboxane A_2 (TxA_2), or prostacyclin (PGI_2) (16,18,22, 23,26). The distribution and activity of terminal enzymes determine the patterns and relative amounts of vasoactive products formed from PGH_2 metabolism in an organ system (38,80). PGI_2 has been reported to be the major product formed from arachidonate and endoperoxide metabolism in vascular tissue (18,32,39,40). This substance inhibits platelet aggregation and relaxes isolated vascular smooth muscle from a variety of organs (18,32,39,40). PGI_2 increases blood flow in the coronary, renal, and mesenteric vascular beds in dogs (34,41,42). The data presented in this chapter show that PGI_2 decreased systemic arterial pressure in a dose-related manner in anesthetized cats. Because cardiac output measured at the nadir of the decrease in systemic arterial pressure was increased, the decrease in systemic arterial pressure reflects a decrease in systemic vascular resistance. The reductions in systemic arterial pressure and systemic vascular resistance in response to left or right atrial injections of PGI_2 were similar,

indicating that prostacyclin is not inactivated in transit across the pulmonary vascular bed. The observation that this locally formed substance that inhibits platelet aggregation and relaxes vascular smooth muscle is not inactivated in the lung suggests that this substance can function as a circulating hormone (33–35). The systemic vascular effects of PGI_2 were further investigated in the hindquarter, renal, and mesenteric vascular beds in the cat. PGI_2 decreased perfusion pressure in a dose-dependent manner in the three regional vascular beds. Inasmuch as blood flow was maintained constant with a pump, the reductions in perfusion pressure reflect a decrease in vascular resistance in the regional vascular beds in the cat. These data suggest that reductions in vascular resistance in the mesenteric, renal, and hindquarter vascular beds contribute to the reductions in sytemic arterial pressure and systemic vascular resistance in response to PGI_2 in the cat. In terms of relative vasodilator activity, the effects of PGI_2 were greater in the feline intestine than in the renal or hindquarter vascular bed. This suggests that an increase in circulating levels of PGI_2 would serve to increase blood flow to the intestine to a greater extent than to the kidney or skeletal muscle (36). The vasodilator activity of PGI_2 was also greater in the intestine in the dog, as compared with the kidney (34). Therefore, because the prostacyclin-generating capacity of the gastrointestinal tract is greater than that of other organs, enhanced local synthesis of PGI_2 would also have a marked effect on blood flow to the intestine and the fraction of cardiac output going to the gastrointestinal tract.

Results of studies in anesthetized dogs show that the prostaglandin precursor, arachidonic acid, is converted into substances that decrease systemic arterial pressure and that have vasodilator activity in the renal, mesenteric, and coronary vascular beds (41,42,68,81,82). Responses to the essential fatty acid precursor were blocked by cyclooxygenase inhibitors such as indomethacin and meclofenamic acid, indicating that the responses were due to formation of vasodilator metabolites in the cyclo-oxygenase pathway (41,42,68,81,82). The endoperoxide, PGH_2, also has good vasodilator activity in the peripheral vascular bed in the dog (41,83). However, it is uncertain whether this is due to the activity of PGH_2 itself or to the subsequent formation of PGI_2 or dilator prostaglandins. PGI_2 is the major product formed from PGH_2 metabolism in vascular tissue and in the peripheral vascular bed in the dog and cat, prostacyclin had potent vasodilator activity (34,36,41,42). PGE_2 also had good vasodilator activity, whereas PGD_2 had moderate vasodilator activity in the coronary and renal vascular beds (41,82). $PGF_{2\alpha}$ had little activity in the coronary or renal vascular bed, whereas PGD_2 and $PGF_{2\alpha}$ had pressor activity in the mesenteric vascular bed (41, 42,82). The effects of thromboxane A_2 on regional vascular resistance are uncertain because this substance is so unstable at physiological conditions. However, several PGH_2 analogues that are reported to mimic the actions of thromboxane A_2 have potent vasoconstrictor activity in the peripheral vascular bed (82).

Prostacyclin and 6-keto-$PGF_{1\alpha}$ can be converted into a biologically active metabolite, 6-keto-PGE_1, by the 9-hydroxy prostaglandin dehydrogenase pathway that has been described in the liver and platelets (44,45). This biologically active metabolite inhibits platelet aggregation by a cyclic-AMP-dependent mechanism and has marked vasodilator activity equivalent to or greater than that of PGI_2 in the regional circulation in the cat and the dog (49–51).

In addition to their ability to directly alter the tone of vascular smooth muscle in the peripheral vascular bed, prostaglandins have the capacity to modify responses to sympathetic nerve stimulation and vasoconstrictor hormones (52,62,64–71). In general, PGE_1 and PGE_2 have inhibitory effects on vasoconstrictor responses, and in some organ systems the effects of these agents are greater on sympathetic nerve stimulation than to exogenous norepinephrine. These data suggest that E-se-

ries prostaglandins may serve to modulate the effects of the sympathetic nervous system in the peripheral vascular bed. PGD_2 and $PGF_{2\alpha}$ also have the ability to influence responses to vasoconstrictor stimuli in the peripheral vascular bed (52,62). PGI_2 possesses the ability to inhibit vasoconstrictor responses to sympathetic nerve stimulation and pressor hormones (62,67). The effects of PGI_2 on vasoconstrictor responses are dose-related and reversible, and the effects of PGI_2 are not due to subsequent formation of 6-keto-$PGF_{1\alpha}$, because that breakdown product had no activity. Responses to nerve stimulation and pressor hormones were decreased to approximately the same extent, indicating that the actions of PGI_2 were for the most part postjunctional in nature. In addition, responses to norepinephrine and to angiotensin were reduced to a similar extent, suggesting that the inhibitory effects of PGI_2 are nonspecific in nature. The effects of PGI_2 and of 6-keto-PGE_1 on responses to nerve stimulation and pressor hormones were very similar in the feline intestinal vascular bed. The effects of both substances were postjunctional and nonspecific in nature, and these agents have nearly identical capacities to inhibit in a reversible manner responses to nerve stimulation and pressor hormones. Neither PGI_2 nor 6-keto-PGE_1 is inactivated in the lung, and they could serve as circulating hormones by acting to modulate the vasoconstrictor effects of sympathetic nerve stimulation and pressor hormones. Moreover, PGI_2 or 6-keto-PGE_1 would modulate vasoconstrictor responses in a nonspecific manner, whereas PGE_2 would act mainly at the level of the adrenergic terminal to inhibit release of norepinephrine in some systems (66).

In regard to the lungs, these studies show that when injected as a rapid bolus, the prostaglandin precursor, arachidonic acid, increases pulmonary lobar arterial pressure in intact-chest dogs and cats (81,84,85). Inasmuch as pulmonary blood flow was held constant and left atrial pressure was unchanged, the rise in lobar arterial pressure reflects an increase in pulmonary lobar vascular resistance in both species. The primary prostaglandins (PGE_2, PGD_2, and $PGF_{2\alpha}$), as well as PGH_2 and a stable PGH_2 analogue and thromboxane B_2, all increase pulmonary vascular resistance in dogs and cats (81,84–88). In the dog, in addition to increasing lobar arterial pressure, arachidonic acid, the bisenoic prostaglandins, and the PGH_2 analogue all increase small intrapulmonary vein pressure (89). The increases in lobar arterial and small-vein pressures suggest that these substances increase pulmonary vascular resistance by constricting intrapulmonary veins and upstream segments believed to be small arteries (89). This could increase the amount of fluid leaving the pulmonary capillary bed, which could interfere with gas exchange and ultimately lead to the formation of pulmonary edema.

Arachidonic acid has also been shown to increase transpulmonary airway pressure when the lung is ventilated at constant volume with a positive pressure (84). In experiments in which the effects of arachidonic acid on lung function were further investigated, the increase in transpulmonary pressure was associated with a transient rise in lung resistance and a sustained decrease in dynamic compliance (90). The endoperoxide analogue, $PGF_{2\alpha}$, and PGD_2 all increased lung resistance and decreased dynamic compliance, and in this regard they were similar to, but much more potent than, arachidonic acid (90–92). In contrast, PGI_2 had modest bronchodilator activity in the cat when bronchomotor tone was elevated, whereas 6-keto-PGE_1 had greater bronchodilator activity than PGI_2 (93,94). The effects of PGE_2 on the pulmonary vascular bed and on the airways were modest when this substance was injected in the same doses as PGD_2 or $PGF_{2\alpha}$ (84–86). Pulmonary vasoconstrictor, bronchoconstrictor, and systemic vasodepressor responses to arachidonic acid were blocked after administration of indomethacin, a cyclooxygenase inhibitor (81,84–86,90). These data suggest that the effects of arachidonic acid on the airways and pulmonary and peripheral vascular beds are due to conversion of the substrate into vasoac-

tive and bronchoactive metabolites in the cyclooxygenase pathway. The pulmonary vasoconstrictor response to arachidonic acid is associated with increased synthesis of E- and F-like prostaglandins; however, it is not known if PGD_2 or TxB_2 is produced by the lung in the intact dog (84). The effects of arachidonic acid or the endoperoxide analogue on the pulmonary vascular bed were not dependent on the presence of platelets or other formed elements in that the response to these substances was not diminished when the lung was perfused with a dextran solution (84, 86,87). These findings suggest that the substrate is converted to vasoactive substances by the lung itself and that platelet aggregation or release of vasoactive products from the platelets plays little or no role in this response.

In contrast to the pressor effects of $PGF_{2\alpha}$, PGD_2, and PGE_2 or the PGH_2 analogue, which may mimic the effects of TxA_2 on the pulmonary vascular bed, the newly discovered bicyclic prostaglandin, PGI_2, had vasodilator activity in the canine and feline pulmonary vascular beds (34,84,95). Stable PGI_2 analogues were also found to have vasodilator activity in the lung (96). 6-Keto-PGE_1, a newly discovered PGI_2 metabolite, also had vasodilator activity in the pulmonary vascular bed (46,47). The pulmonary vasodilator effects of PGI_2 and 6-keto-PGE_1 were modest under resting conditions but were greatly enhanced when pulmonary vascular resistance was increased actively by infusion of a vasoconstrictor substance (46,47,95). Although PGI_2 had vasodilator activity, arachidonic acid, when administered as a bolus, consistently increased pulmonary vascular resistance in intact dogs and cats and in isolated dog lung (81,84, 85,90,97). These results suggest that under physiological conditions in the intact state the predominant products formed in the lung when arachidonate is injected as a bolus are vasoconstrictor in nature (TxA_2 or prostaglandin E, F, or D). Alternatively, it is possible that both vasoconstrictor and vasodilator metabolites are formed but that the activity of the vasoconstrictor overshadows the action of any simultaneously formed PGI_2-like substances. It has been reported that PGI_2 is the predominant metabolite formed from arachidonic acid and endoperoxide intermediates in vascular tissue (38). Indeed, we have observed that slow infusions of arachidonic acid decrease lobar vascular resistance in intact dogs and cats and decrease bronchomotor tone in cats (98–100). However, these vasodilator and bronchodilator effects are observed only when pulmonary vascular or airway tone is enhanced (98–100). The explanation for the divergent responses to rapidly injected arachidonic acid and slowly infused arachidonic acid is uncertain at the present time. It is, however, possible that when excessive amounts of substrate are converted to PGH_2, the endothelial prostacyclin synthetase may be overwhelmed and the endoperoxide may isomerize to PGD_2 and PGE_2 or be reduced to $PGF_{2\alpha}$.

We have reported that administration of cyclooxygenase inhibitors such as indomethacin and meclofenamate results in a slow, gradual increase in pulmonary vascular resistance in intact dogs (101). It has been shown that a PGI_2-like substance is continually released by the lung (37). We have therefore suggested that under resting conditions, the pulmonary vascular bed is maintained in a dilated state by production of a vasodilator product in the cyclooxygenase pathway (101). Recent evidence suggests that this vasodilator product in the cyclooxygenase pathway is a PGI_2-like substance (98,99,102).

Recent results of biochemical studies demonstrate that cat lung microsomes generate predominately 6-keto-$PGF_{1\alpha}$ and TxB_2, the stable metabolites of the vasoactive substances of PGI_2 and TxA_2, respectively (102). The formation of 6-keto-$PGF_{1\alpha}$, TxB_2, and HHT from PGH_2 by the lung microsomes is inhibited by heat denaturation, indicating that these were enzymatic reactions. Small amounts of PGD_2, PGE_2, and $PGF_{2\alpha}$ were formed in the incubation with microsomes and became more apparent at high PGH_2 concentrations (102). However, in the present assay we did not quantitatively distinguish between enzymic

conversion and chemical decomposition of PGH_2 to these products in aqueous medium. Thromboxane synthetase, which catalyzes the conversions of PGH_2 to TxA_2 and to HHT, was selectively inhibited by imidazole in our study (102). Tranylcypromine markedly inhibited prostacyclin synthetase, but partially inhibited thromboxane synthetase as well. Our experiments indicate that the formation of HHT parallels the formation of TxB_2 in relation to changing microsomal protein concentrations. Furthermore, the formation of HHT is approximately equal to that of TxB_2 when correction is made for the nonenzymatic breakdown of PGH_2 to HHT, which is approximately 15%. These observations suggest that equal productions to TxB_2 and HHT are catalyzed by one enzyme. The present biochemical studies show that metabolism of PGH_2 varies, depending on substrate availability. Prostacyclin synthetase became saturated at a lower substrate concentration than thromboxane synthetase, and thromboxane biosynthesis dominated the metabolism of the endoperoxide except at low PGH_2 concentration (10 μM), where prostacyclin formation occurred to a similar extent. Our studies show that arachidonic acid, when delivered at high concentrations, increases pulmonary arterial pressure and pulmonary vascular resistance in intact-chest cats, whereas vasodilation can occur at lower doses and with low infusion rates of the precursor acid (98,99). Our results offer a possible explanation for these divergent responses (98,99,102). Administration of high concentrations of arachidonic acid may result in production of large amounts of PGH_2, leading to the predominant formation of TxA_2 relative to PGI_2, with subsequent pulmonary vasoconstriction (102). However, at low concentrations of PGH_2, which would occur at lower doses or infusion rates of arachidonic acid, PGI_2 production may be equivalent to or slightly less than that of TxA_2. Consequently, because of the longer half-life of PGI_2 (3 min versus 30 seconds for TxA_2), pulmonary vasodilation could result.

ACKNOWLEDGMENTS

We wish to thank Ms. Jan Ignarro for help in preparing the manuscript. The research in this chapter was supported in part by NIH grants HL-11802, HL-15580, and HL-18070. Mr. Lippton is currently a second year medical student at the College of Medicine, University of Florida, Gainesville, Florida. Dr. Wolin is a postdoctoral fellow supported by a National Research Service Award (grant number HL-06225).

REFERENCES

1. von Euler, U. S. (1935): Ueber die spezlfische blutdrucksenkende Substanz des menschlichen Prostataund Samen-blasensekretes. *Klin. Wochenschr.*, 14:1182–1183.
2. von Euler, U. S. (1936): On the specific vasodilating and plain muscle stimulating substances from accessory genital glands in man and certain animals. *J. Physiol. (Lond.)*, 88:213–234.
3. Samuelsson, B., Ramwell, P. W., and Paoletti, R. (editors) (1980): *Advances in Prostaglandin and Thromboxane Research, Vol. 6.* Raven Press, New York.
4. Samuelsson, B., Ramwell, P. W., and Paoletti, R. (editors) (1980): *Advances in Prostaglandin and Thromboxane Research, Vol. 7.* Raven Press, New York.
5. Samuelsson, B., Ramwell, P. W., and Paoletti, R. (editors) (1980): *Advances in Prostaglandin and Thromboxane Research, Vol. 8.* Raven Press, New York.
6. Marcus, A. J. (1978): The role of lipids in platelet function: With particular reference to the arachidonic acid pathway. *J. Lipid Res.*, 19:793–825.
7. Ramwell, P. W., Leovey, E. M., and Sintentos, A. L. (1977): Regulation of the arachidonic acid cascade. *Biol. Reprod.*, 16:70–87.
8. Lapetina, E. G., Schmitges, C. J., Chandrabrose, K., and Cuatrecas, P. (1978): Regulation of phospholipase activity in platelets. In: *Advances in Prostaglandin and Thromboxane Research*, edited by C. Galli, G. Galli, and G. Porcellati, Vol. 3, pp. 127–135. Raven Press, New York.
9. Ferreira, S. H., Moncada, S., and Vane, J. R. (1971): Indomethacin and aspirin abolish prostaglandin release from the spleen. *Nature [New Biol.]*, 231:237–239.
10. Samuelsson, B., Hammarstrom, S., Murphy, R. C., and Borgeat, P. (1980): Leukotrienes and slow reacting substances of anaphylaxias (SRS-A). *Allergy*, 35:375–381.
11. Anggard, E. (1971): Studies on the analysis and metabolism of the prostaglandins. *Ann. N.Y. Acad. Sci.*, 180:200–215.
12. Vane, J. R. (1972): The role of the lungs in the metabolism of vasoactive substances. In: *Pharmacology and Pharmacokinetics*, edited by T. Teorell, R. L. Dedrich, and P. G. Condliffe, pp. 195–207. Plenum Press, New York.
13. Ogino, N., Ohki, S., Yamamoto, S., and Hayaishi, O. (1978): Prostaglandin endoperoxide synthetase from bovine vesicular glands—inactivation and activation by heme and other metaloporphyrins. *J. Biol. Chem.*, 253:5061–5068.
14. Ohki, S., Ogino, N., Yamamoto, S., and Hayaishi, O. (1979): Prostaglandin hydroperoxidase, an integral part of prostaglandin endoperoxide synthetase from bovine gland microsomes. *J. Biol. Chem.*, 254:829–836.
15. Ogino, N., Ohki, S., Yamamoto, S., and Hayaishi, O. (1979): Isolation of an activator for prostaglandin hydroperoxidase from bovine vesicular gland cytosol and its identification as uric acid. *Biochem. Biophys. Res. Commun.*, 87:184–191.
16. Nugteren, D., and Christ-Hazelhof, E. (1980): Chemical and enzymatic conversions of the prostaglandin endoperoxide PGH_2. In: *Advances in Prostaglandin and Thromboxane Research*, edited by B. Samuelsson, P. W. Ramwell, and R. Paoletti, Vol. 6, pp. 129–137. Raven Press, New York.
17. Chan, J., Nsgasawa, M., Takeguchi, C., and Sih, C. (1975): On agents favoring prostaglandin F formation during biosynthesis: *Biochemistry*, 14:2987–2991.
18. Moncada, S., Gryglewski, R., Bunting, S., and Vane, J. (1976): An enzyme isolated from arteries that transforms prostaglandin endoperoxides to an unstable substance that inhibits platelet aggregation. *Nature*, 263:663–665.
19. Isakson, P., Raz, A., Denny, S., Pure, E., and Needleman, P. (1977): A novel prostaglandin is the major product of arachidonic acid metabolism in rabbit heart. *Proc. Natl. Acad. Sci. U.S.A.*, 71:101–105.
20. Sun, F. (1977): Biosynthesis of thromboxanes in human platelets. I. Characterization and assay of thromboxane synthetase. *Biochem. Biophys. Res. Commun.*, 74:1432–1440.
21. Yamamoto, S., Ohki, S., Ogino, N., Shimizu, T., Yoshimoto, T., Watanabe, K., and Hayaishi, O. (1980): Enzymes involved in the formation and further transformation of the prostaglandin endoperoxides. In: *Advances in Prostaglandin and Thromboxane Research*, edited by B. Samuelsson, P. W. Ramwell, and R. Paoletti, Vol. 6, pp. 27–34. Raven Press, New York.
22. Hamberg, M., Sevensson, J., and Samuelsson, B. (1975): Thromboxanes: A new group of biologically active compounds derived from prostaglandin endoperoxides. *Proc. Natl. Acad. Sci. U.S.A.*, 72:2994–2998.
23. Nugteren, D., and Hazelhof, E. (1973): Isolation and properties of intermediates in prostaglandin biosynthesis. *Biochim. Biophys. Acta*, 326:448–461.
24. Tateson, J., Moncada, S., and Vane, J. (1977): Effects of prostacyclin (PGX) on cyclic AMP concentrations in human platelets. *Prostaglandins*, 13:389–399.
25. Yuan, B., Tai, C., and Tai, H.-H. (1980): 9-Hydroxy-

prostaglandin dehydrogenase from rat kidney—purification to homogeneity and partial characterization. *J. Biol. Chem.*, 255:7439–7443.

26. Hamberg, M., and Samuelsson, B. (1974): Prostaglandin endoperoxides. Novel transformations of arachidonic acid in human platelets. *Proc. Natl. Acad. Sci. U.S.A.*, 71:3400–3404.

27. Borgeat, P., and Samuelsson, B. (1979): Arachidonic acid metabolism in polymorphonuclear leukocytes: Effects of ionophore A23187. *Proc. Natl. Acad. Sci. U.S.A.*, 76:2143–2152.

28. Walker, J. L. (1980): Interrelationships of SRSA production and arachidonic acid metabolism in human lung tissue. In: *Advances in Prostaglandin and Thromboxane Research*, edited by B. Samuelsson, P. W. Ramwell, and R. Paoletti, Vol. 6, pp. 115–119. Raven Press, New York.

29. Lundberg, U., Radmark, O., Malmsten, C., and Samuelsson, B. (1981): Transformation of the 15-hydroperoxy-5,9,11,13-eicosatetraenoic acid into novel leukotrienes. *F.E.B.S. Lett.*, 126:127–132.

30. Hedqvist, P., Dahlen, S.-E., Gustafsson, L., Hammarstrom, S., and Samuelsson, B. (1980): Biological profile of leukotriene C_4 and D_4. *Acta Physiol. Scand.*, 110:331–333.

31. Goetzl, E. J., and Pickett, W. C. (1980): The human PMN leukocyte chemotactic activity of complex hydroxy-eicosatetraenoic acids (HETES). *J. Immun.*, 125:1789–1791.

32. Moncada, S., Gryglewski, R., Bunting, S., and Vane, J. (1976): A lipid peroxide inhibits the enzyme in blood vessel microsomes that generates from prostaglandin endoperoxides the substance (prostaglandin X) which prevents platelet aggregation. *Prostaglandins*, 12:715–733.

33. Armstrong, J. M., Lattimer, N., Moncada, S., and Vane, J. R. (1978): Comparison of the vasodepressor effects of prostacyclin and 6-oxo-prostaglandin $F_{1\alpha}$ with those of prostaglandin E_2 in rats and rabbits. *Br. J. Pharmacol.*, 63:125–130.

34. Kadowitz, P. J., Chapnick, B. M., Feigen, L. P., Hyman, A. L., Nelson, P. K., and Spannhake, E. W. (1978): Pulmonary and systemic vasodilator effects of the newly discovered prostaglandin, PGI_2. *J. Appl. Physiol.*, 45:408–413.

35. Waldman, H. M., Alter, I., Kot, P. A., Rose, J. C., and Ramwell, P. W. (1978): Effect of lung transit on systemic depressor responses to arachidonic acid and prostacyclin in dogs. *J. Pharmacol. Exp. Ther.*, 204:289–293.

36. Lippton, H. L., Paustian, P. W., Mellion, B. T., Nelson, P. K., Feigen, L. P., Chapnick, B. M., Hyman, A. L., and Kadowitz, P. J. (1979): Cardiovascular actions of prostacyclin (PGI_2) in the cat. *Arch. Int. Pharmacodyn. Ther.*, 241:121–130.

37. Gryglewski, R. J., Korbut, R., Ogetkiewicz, A., Splawinski, J., Wojtaszek, B., and Swies, J. (1978): Lungs as a generator of prostacyclin: Hypothesis on physiological significance. *Naunyn Schmiedebergs Arch. Pharmacol.*, 304:45–50.

38. Moncada, S., and Vane, J. R. (1979): Pharmacology and endogenous roles of prostaglandin endoperoxides, thromboxane A_2 and prostacyclin. *Pharmacol. Rev.*, 30:293–331.

39. Bunting, S., Gryglewski, R., Moncada, S., and Vane, J. R. (1976): Arterial walls generate from prostaglandin endoperoxides a substance (prostaglandin X) which relaxes strips of mesenteric and coelias arteries and inhibits platelet aggregation. *Prostaglandins*, 12:897–913.

40. Dusting, G. J., Moncada, S., and Vane, J. R. (1977): Prostacyclin (PGX) is the endogenous metabolite responsible for relaxation of coronary arteries induced by arachidonic acid. *Prostaglandins*, 13:3–16.

41. Hyman, A. L., Kadowitz, P. J., Lands, W. E. M., Crawford, C. G., Fried, J., and Barton, J. (1978): Coronary vasodilator activity of 13,14-dehydroprostacyclin methyl ester: Comparison with PGI_2 and other prostanoids. *Proc. Natl. Acad. Sci. U.S.A.*, 75:3522–3526.

42. Chapnick, B. M., Feigen, L. P., Hyman, A. L., and Kadowitz, P. J. (1978): Differential effects of prostaglandins in the mesenteric vascular bed. *Am. J. Physiol.*, 4:H326–332.

43. Pade-Asciak, C. (1976): A new prostaglandin metabolite of arachidonic acid. Formation of 6-keto-$PGF_{1\alpha}$ by the rat stomach. *Experientia*, 32:291–294.

44. Wong, P.Y.-K., Malik, K. U., Desiderio, D. M., McGiff, J. C., and Sun, F. F. (1980): Hepatic metabolism of prostacyclin (PGI_2) in the rabbit: Formation of a potent novel inhibitor of platelet aggregation. *Biochem. Biophys. Res. Commun.*, 93:486–494.

45. Wong, P.Y.-K., Lee, W. H., Chao, P.H.-W., Reiss, R. F., and McGiff, J. C. (1980): Metabolism of prostacyclin by 9-hydroxyprostaglandin dehydrogenase in human platelets. *J. Biol. Chem.*, 255:9021–9024.

46. Hyman, A. L., and Kadowitz, P. J. (1980): Vasodilator actions of prostaglandin 6-keto-E_1 in the pulmonary vascular bed. *J. Pharmacol. Exp. Ther.*, 213:468–472.

47. Nandiwads, P., Hyman, A. L., Feigen, L. P., and Kadowitz, P. J. (1980): Cardiopulmonary actions of prostaglandin 6-keto-E_1 in the anesthetized dog. *Arch. Int. Pharmacodyn. Ther.*, 245:118–128.

48. Lock, J. E., Olley, P. M., Coceani, F., Hamilton, F., and Doubilet, G. (1979): Pulmonary and systemic vascular responses to 6-keto-PGE_1 in the conscious lamb. *Prostaglandins*, 18:303–309.

49. Quilley, C. P., Wong, P.Y.-K., and McGiff, J. C. (1979): Hypotensive and renovascular actions of 6-keto-prostaglandin E_1, a metabolite of prostacyclin. *Eur. J. Pharmacol.*, 57:273–276.

50. Feigen, L. P., Chapnick, B. M., Hyman, A. L., King, L., Marascalo, B., and Kadowitz, P. J. (1980): Peripheral vasodilator effects of prostaglandins: Comparison of 6-keto-prostaglandin E_1 with prostacyclin and escape from prostaglandin E_2 in the mesenteric vascular bed. *J. Pharmacol. Exp. Ther.*, 214:528–534.

51. Lippton, H. L., Chapnick, B. M., Hyman, A. L., and Kadowitz, P. J. (1980): Inhibition of vasoconstrictor responses by 6-keto-PGE_1 in the feline mesenteric vascular bed. *Prostaglandins*, 19:299–310.

52. Lippton, H. L., Chapnick, B. M., and Kadowitz, P. J. (1981): Influence of prostaglandins on vasoconstrictor responses in the hindquarters vascular bed of the cat. *Prostaglandins and Medicine*, 6:183–202.

53. de Gaetana, G., and Garattini, S. (editors) (1978):

Platelets: A Multidisciplinary Approach. Mario Negri Institute for Pharmacological Research, Milan.

54. de Gaetano, G., and Garattini, S. (1978): *Platelets: A Multidisciplinary Approach.* Raven Press, New York.

55. Wong, P.Y.-K., McGiff, J. C., Sun, F. F., and Lee, W. H. (1979): 6-Keto-prostaglandin E_1 inhibits the aggregation of human platelets. *Eur. J. Pharmacol.,* 60:245–248.

56. Miller, O. V., Aiken, J. W., Shebuski, R. J., and Gorman, R. R. (1980): 6-Keto-prostaglandin E_1 is not equipotent to prostacyclin (PGI_2) as an antiaggregatory agent. *Prostaglandins,* 20:391–400.

57. Pontecorvo, E. G., Meyers, C. B., Lippton, H. L., and Kadowitz, P. J. (1981): Inhibition of platelet aggregation by 6-keto-PGE_1: Lack of an effect on cyclic GMP levels. *Prostaglandins and Medicine,* 6:473–483.

58. Gorman, R. R., Bunting, S., and Miller, O. V. (1977): Modulation of human platelet adenylate cyclase by prostacyclin (PGX). *Prostaglandins,* 13:377–388.

59. Quilley, C. P., McGiff, J. C., Lee, W. H., Sun, F. F., and Wong, P.Y.-K. (1980): 6-Keto-PGE_1: A possible metabolite of prostacyclin having platelet antiaggretory effects. *Hypertension,* 2:524–531.

60. Feigen, L. P., and Chapnick, B. M. (1979): Evidence for separate PGD_2 and $PGF_{2\alpha}$ receptors in the canine mesenteric vascular bed. *Prostaglandins,* 18:221–233.

61. Lippton, H. L., Paustian, P. W., Sporl, L., and Kadowitz, P. J. (1980): Comparative effects of PGD_2 and PGE_2 in the regional circulation of the cat. *Prostaglandins and Medicine,* 5:365–373.

62. Lippton, H. L., Cassin, S., and Kadowitz, P. J. (1980): Comparative effects of PGD_2 and PGE_2 on vasoconstrictor responses in the feline intestinal vascular bed. *Prostaglandins and Medicine,* 5:297–305.

63. Simon, B., Kather, H., and Kommerell, B. (1979): Regional differences of prostaglandin D_2-sensitive adenylate cyclase activity in the human alimentary tract. *Biochem. Pharmacol.,* 28:3465–3466.

64. Chapnick, B. M., Paustian, P. W., Klainer, E., Joiner, P. D., Hyman, A. L., and Kadowitz, P. J. (1976): Influence of prostaglandins E, A and F on vasoconstrictor responses to norepinephrine, renal nerve stimulation and angiotensin in the feline kidney. *J. Pharmacol. Exp. Ther.,* 196:44–52.

65. Lippton, H. L., Chapnick, B. M., Hyman, A. L., and Kadowitz, P. J. (1979): Inhibition of vasoconstrictor responses by prostacyclin (PGI_2) in the feline mesenteric vascular bed. *Arch. Int. Pharmacodyn. Ther.,* 241:214–233.

66. Hedqvist, P. (1977): Basic methods of prostaglandin action on autonomic neurotransmission. *Annu. Rev. Pharmacol. Toxicol.,* 17:259–279.

67. Kadowitz, P. J., Sweet, C. S., and Brody, M. J. (1971): Differential effects of prostaglandins E_1, E_2, F_1 and F_2 on adrenergic vasoconstriction in the dog hindpaw. *J. Pharmacol. Exp. Ther.,* 177:641–649.

68. Fink, G. D., Chapnick, B. M., Goldberg, M. R., Paustian, P. W., and Kadowitz, P. J. (1977): Influence of prostaglandin E_2, indomethacin and reserpine on renal vascular responses to nerve stimula-

tion, pressor and depressor hormones. *Circ. Res.,* 41:172–178.

69. Brody, M. J., and Kadowitz, P. J. (1974): Prostaglandins as modulators of the autonomic nervous system. *Fed. Proc.,* 33:48–60.

70. Gottlieb, A. L., Lippton, H. L., Parey, S. E., Paustian, P. W., and Kadowitz, P. J. (1980): Blockade of vasoconstrictor responses by prostacyclin (PGI_2), PGE_2 and PGE_1 in the rabbit hindquarters vascular bed. *Prostaglandins and Medicine,* 4:1–11.

71. Hedqvist, P. (1972): Prostaglandin-induced inhibition of vascular tone and reactivity of the cat's hindleg *in vivo. Eur. J. Pharmacol.,* 17:157–162.

72. Zimmerman, B. G., and Gomez, J. (1965): Increased response to sympathetic stimulation in the cutaneous vasculature in the presence of angiotensin. *Int. J. Neuropharmacol.,* 4:185–193.

73. Palaic, D., and Khairallah, P. A. (1967): Inhibition of noradrenaline uptake by angiotensin. *J. Pharm. Pharmacol.,* 19:396–397.

74. Panisset, J., and Bourdois, P. (1968): Effect of angiotensin on the response to noradrenaline and sympathetic nerve stimualtion and on ^{3}H-noradrenaline uptake in cat mesenteric blood vessels. *Can. J. Physiol. Pharmacol.,* 46:125–131.

75. Kadowitz, P. J., Sweet, C. S., and Brody, M. J. (1972): Influence of angiotensin I, angiotensin II and cocaine on adrenergic vasoconstrictor responses in the dog hindpaw. *J. Pharmacol. Exp. Ther.,* 183:275–283.

76. Hughes, J., and Roth, R. H. (1971): Evidence that angiotensin enhances transmitter release during sympathetic nerve stimulation. *Br. J. Pharmacol.,* 41:239–255.

77. Hedqvist, P., and Brundin, J. (1969): Inhibition by prostaglandin E_1 of noradrenaline release and of effector response to nerve stimulation in the cat spleen. *Life Sci.,* 8:389–395.

78. Hedqvist, P. (1970): Control by prostaglandin E_2 of sympathetic neurotransmission in the spleen. *Life Sci.,* 9:269–278.

79. Anggard, E., and Samuelsson, B. (1966): Prosynthesis of prostaglandins from arachidonic acid in guinea pig lung. *J. Biol. Chem.,* 240:3518–3521.

80. Pace-Asciak, C. R. (1977): Oxidative biotransformations of arachidonic acid. *Prostaglandins,* 13:811–817.

81. Kadowitz, P. J., Spannhake, E. W., Greenberg, S., Feigen, L. P., and Hyman, A. L. (1977): Comparative effects of arachidonic acid, bisenoic prostaglandins and an endoperoxide analog on the canine pulmonary vascular bed. *Can. J. Physiol. Pharmacol.,* 55:1369–1377.

82. Feigen, L. P., Chapnick, B. M., Flemming, J. E., Flemming, J. M., and Kadowitz, P. J. (1977): Renal vascular effects of endoperoxide analogs, prostaglandins and arachidonic acid. *Am. J. Physiol.,* 233:H573–579.

83. Feigen, L. P., Chapnick, B. M., Gorman, R. R., Hyman, A. L., and Kadowitz, P. J. (1978): The effect of PGH_2 on blood flow in the canine renal and superior mesenteric vascular beds. *Prostaglandins,* 16:803–813.

84. Hyman, A. L., Mathe, A. A., Matthews, C. C., Ben-

nett, J. T., Spannhake, E. W., and Kadowitz, P. J. (1978): Modification of pulmonary vascular responses to arachidonic acid by alterations in physiologic state. *J. Pharmacol. Exp. Ther.,* 207:388–401.

85. Kadowitz, P. J., and Hyman, A. L. (1980): Comparative effects of thromboxane B_2 on the canine and feline pulmonary vascular bed. *J. Pharmacol. Exp. Ther.,* 213:300–305.

86. Kadowitz, P. J., and Hyman, A. L. (1977): Influences of a prostaglandin endoperoxide analog on the canine pulmonary vascular bed. *Circ. Res.,* 40:282–287.

87. Kadowitz, P. J., Gruetter, C. A., McNamara, D. B., Gorman, R. R., Spannhake, E. W., and Hyman, A. L. (1977): Comparative effects of the endoperoxide PGH_2 and an analog on the pulmonary vascular bed. *J. Appl. Physiol.,* 42:953–958.

88. Kadowitz, P. J., Joiner, P. D., and Hyman, A. L. (1975): Effects of prostaglandins E_2 on pulmonary vascular resistance in intact dog, swine and lamb. *Eur. J. Pharmacol.,* 31:72–80.

89. Hyman, A. L., Spannhake, E. W., and Kadowitz, P. J. (1978): Prostaglandins and the lung. A state of the art review. *Am. Rev. Respir. Dis.,* 117:111–136.

90. Spannhake, E. W., Lemen, P. J., Wegmann, M. J., Hyman, A. L., and Kadowitz, P. J. (1978): Effects of arachidonic acid and prostaglandins on lung function in the intact dog. *J. Appl. Physiol.,* 44:397–495.

91. Spannhake, E. W., Lemen, R. J., Wegmann, M. J., Hyman, A. L., and Kadowitz, P. J. (1978): Analysis of the airway effects of a PGH_2 analog in the anesthetized dog. *J. Appl. Physiol.,* 44:406–415.

92. Wasserman, M. A., DuCharme, E. W., Griffin, R. L., DeGraaf, G. L., and Robinson, F. G. (1977): Bronchopulmonary and cardiovascular effects of prostaglandins D_2 in the dog. *Prostaglandins,* 13:255–269.

93. Spannhake, E. W., Levin, J. L., Mellion, B. T., Gruetter, C. A., Hyman, A. L., and Kadowitz, P. J. (1980): Reversal of 5-HT-induced bronchoconstriction by PGI_2: Distribution of central and peripheral actions. *J. Appl. Physiol.,* 49:521–527.

94. Spannhake, E. W., Levin, J. L., Hyman, A. L., and Kadowitz, P. J. (1981): 6-Keto-PGE_1 exhibits more potent bronchodilatory activity in the cat than its precursor, PGI_2. *Prostaglandins,* 21:267–275.

95. Hyman, A. L., and Kadowitz, P. J. (1979): Pulmonary vasodilator activity of prostacyclin (PGI_2) in the intact cat. *Circ. Res.,* 45:404–409.

96. Hyman, A. L., Chapnick, B. M., Kadowitz, P. J., Lands, W. E. M., Crawford, C. G., Fried, J., and Barton, J. (1977): Unusual pulmonary vasodilator activity of a novel prostacyclin analog: Comparison with endoperoxides and other prostanoids. *Proc. Natl. Acad. Sci. U.S.A.,* 12:5711–5715.

97. Wicks, T. C., Rose, J. C., Johnson, M., Ramwell, P. W., and Kot, P. A. (1976): Vascular response to arachidonic acid in the perfused canine lung. *Circ. Res.,* 38:167–171.

98. Spannhake, E. W., Hyman, A. L., and Kadowitz, P. J. (1980): Dependence of the airway and pulmonary vascular effects of arachidonic acid upon route and rate of administration. *J. Pharmacol. Exp. Ther.,* 212:584–590.

99. Hyman, A. L., Spannhake, E. W., and Kadowitz, P. J. (1980): Divergent actions of arachidonic acid on the feline pulmonary vascular bed. *Am. J. Physiol.,* 239:H40–46.

100. Levin, J. R., Spannhake, E. W., Hyman, A. L., and Kadowitz, P. J. (1982): Analysis of airway responses to dihomo-γ-linolenic acid in the cat. *J. Pharmacol. Exptl. Ther.,* 223:169–176.

101. Kadowitz, P. J., Chapnick, B. M., Joiner, P. D., and Hyman, A. L. (1975): Influences of inhibitors of prostaglandin synthesis on the canine pulmonary vascular bed. *Am. J. Physiol.,* 299:941–946.

102. She, H. S., McNamara, D. B., Spannhake, E. W., Hyman, A. L., and Kadowitz, P. J. (1981): Metabolism of prostaglandin endoperoxide by microsomes from cat lung. *Prostaglandins,* 21:531–541.

Cardiovascular Pharmacology, Second Edition,
edited by Michael Antonaccio.
Raven Press, New York © 1984.

Platelets and Platelet Aggregation Inhibitors

*Friedel Seuter and **Alexander Scriabine

*Institute of Pharmacology, Bayer AG, Wuppertal, West Germany; and **Miles Institute for Preclinical Pharmacology, New Haven, Connecticut 06509

Platelets are oval disks 2 to 3 μm in diameter found in the blood of mammals. They are involved in blood coagulation; they can adhere to the blood vessel walls, release many bioactive compounds, and aggregate to each other. Because of these properties, platelets are important in initiating hemostasis, thromboembolism, and perhaps atherogenesis.

Hemostasis can be defined as the spontaneous arrest of bleeding from damaged blood vessels. It comprises a chain of events that includes vascular contraction, platelet adhesion to the injured vessel wall, release of platelet contents, aggregation of platelets, formation of platelet plug, and subsequent consolidation of the platelet plug with fibrin.

Thrombosis or formation of thrombus is a pathological exaggeration of hemostasis; it is often initiated by damage to the blood vessel wall, e.g., atherosclerotic lesions. The aggregation of platelets represents an initial and possibly even triggering event, especially in arterial thrombosis. Subsequent fibrin formation stabilizes the thrombus. In venous thrombosis, the role of platelets is not fully understood, but it seems to be less important than in the arterial system; fibrin formation may well be the primary event.

Blood coagulation is the interaction of clotting factors leading to fibrin formation. It is not dependent on the presence of the blood vessel wall; it can occur *in vitro* and also *in vivo* during normal hemostasis.

This chapter deals with the physiological role of platelets and with drugs known to inhibit their aggregation. These drugs are potentially useful in therapy for thrombosis. There is a need for new antithrombotic drugs, because thromboembolism is the major cause of morbidity and mortality in the senior segment of our population, and the presently available therapy is unsatisfactory.

PLATELET MORPHOLOGY

Recent advances in our knowledge of platelet morphology and function were made possible by development of the electron microscope. The electron microscopic studies performed during the last two decades revealed the morphological complexity of platelets (1). Granules, dense bodies, mitochondria, and glycogen particles were identified as platelet components. Platelets were found to possess three different systems of channels: open canalicular system, dense tubular system, and circumferential microtubules (Fig. 1). Three morphologically and functionally distinct zones were identified in platelets. The peripheral zone of the platelet consists of the exterior coat, unit membrane, and the submembrane area. This trilaminar membrane is similar to the plasma membrane of other blood and tissue cells. Its major role is to maintain the homeostasis of platelets; it is involved in adhesion and aggregation. The submembrane area contains filaments that are closely associated with the cell surface; they help to maintain

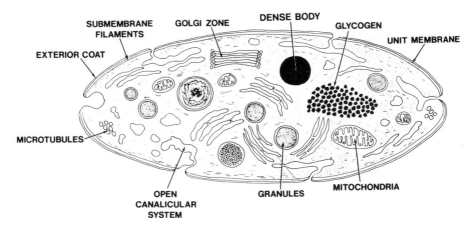

FIG. 1. A platelet and its contents.

the discoid shape of platelets and participate in the formation and stabilization of pseudopods. The sol-gel zone consists of microtubules and microfilaments; it is involved in support of platelet form. The microtubules are believed to represent the storage form of the actin component of thrombosthenin.

One of the functions of the microtubules is to orient the wave of contraction leading to expulsion of the platelet contents. After platelet activation, a centralization can be observed simultaneously with pseudopod formation at the periphery (Fig. 2). The organelle zone contains granules, dense bodies, and mitochondria; it is involved in secretory function. Granules are numerous, and each is 0.2 to 0.3 μm in diameter; they are rich in phospholipids and in lysosomal enzymes. They contain mucopolysaccharides, glycoproteins, fibrinogen, serotonin, norepinephrine, adenosine triphosphate (ATP), and adenosine diphosphate (ADP). Granules that are opaque to the electron beam are referred to as dense bodies. The dense bodies contain ATP, ADP, serotonin, calcium, and catecholamines. They are storage organelles for products secreted by platelets during the release reaction. With the increase in uptake of serotonin, the electron density of dense bodies also increases. The opacity of the dense body is, however, not dependent on the serotonin per se. Serotonin is transported across the platelet membrane as a calcium chelate, and calcium is responsible for the opacity of the dense bodies. The α granules contain platelet factor 4 (PF$_4$, heparin-neutralizing factor), fibrinogen, a mitogenic factor inducing intimal proliferation (3), and β-thromboglobulin, with a not-yet-identified function. Mitochondria support energy requirements of platelets and contain ATP and typical mitochondrial enzymes, including monoamine oxidase. An electron micrograph of normal platelets is shown in Fig. 2.

BIOCHEMICAL COMPOSITION OF PLATELETS AND VESSEL WALL

Platelets contain sodium, potassium, magnesium, calcium, and phosphorus. Potassium is readily exchangeable, whereas calcium is tightly bound to platelet lipids and proteins. Platelet phosphorus is either lipid- or protein-bound. Protein-bound phosphorus is more easily exchangeable than lipid-bound phosphorus. The following phosphatides are known to be present in human platelets: serine phosphoglycerides, choline phosphoglycerides, ethanolamine phosphoglycerides, inositol phosphatides, and sphingomyelin (4).

Platelets contain proteins as well as free amino acids. Taurine, glutamic acid, glycine, alanine, and aspartic acid are found in relatively higher concentrations. Platelets also

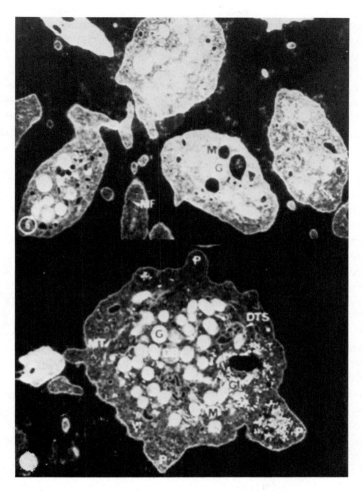

FIG. 2. Normal human platelets immediately after addition of collagen in an aggregometer (2). DB = dense bodies; DTS = dense tubular system; G = granules; Gly = glycogen particles; M = mitochondria; MF = microfibrils; MT = microtubules; P = pseudopods.

contain threonine, serine, proline, valine, leucine, lysine, phosphoethanolamine, and phosphoserine. Among platelet proteins, thrombosthenin occupies a unique position. Like muscle actomyosin, thrombosthenin is involved in contractile activity that leads to changes in platelet shape and in the release reaction. It constitutes about 50% of platelet proteins. Platelets contain more ATP than most other tissues. ATP is consumed during clotting and clot retraction; it is also involved in contraction of thrombosthenin.

Platelets contain oxidases, peroxidases, de-

hydrogenases, phosphatases, esterases, aminopeptidases, glucuronidases, and phosphorylases. The presence of glucose-6-phosphate dehydrogenase and 6-phosphogluconic dehydrogenase suggests platelet capacity to oxidize carbohydrates by the hexose monophosphate pathway.

Platelets contain a variety of monosaccharides, including glucose, galactose, mannose, fructose, ribose, glucosamine, galactosamine, and glucuronic and sialic acids. The total carbohydrate content of human platelets is 8.5% of dry weight. Platelet sialic acid consists primarily of N-acetylneuraminic acid. The sulfated and nonsulfated mucopolysaccharide fractions have been isolated from platelets.

Most of the blood serotonin is present in platelets. Platelets cannot synthesize serotonin, but they concentrate it by passive and active transport mechanisms. Serotonin is taken up from plasma as a complex containing Ca^{2+}. Platelets also can take up epinephrine and norepinephrine. The uptake mechanism for these amines is active and is not identical with that of serotonin. Platelets cannot concentrate these catecholamines to the same extent as they can concentrate serotonin. Histamine can be formed in platelets by histidine decarboxylase. It is present in high concentrations only in platelets of rabbits. Only traces of ribonucleic acid (RNA) are present in platelets; deoxyribonucleic acid (DNA) is essentially absent.

Cytochemical methods have contributed substantially to elucidation of platelet components. However, not every substance can be identified by a specific reaction, and substances soluble in fixatives are difficult to identify (5). The limitations of cytochemical techniques also involve precise determination of whether the substance is normally present in platelets or is being absorbed from plasma.

Since the discovery of thromboxane A_2 (TXA_2) in platelets and prostacyclin (PGI_2) in the vessel wall, their importance with regard to thromboregulation has been discussed intensively. TXA_2 and PGI_2 are two highly active metabolites of the arachidonate pathway (6–10) (Fig. 3). Arachidonic acid is liberated from phospholipids in the cell membrane by membrane-bound phospholipases following activation by platelet-aggregating agents (e.g., thrombin, collagen, ADP). Arachidonic acid is then metabolized by the fatty acid cyclooxygenase to the labile prostaglandin endoperoxides (PGG_2, PGH_2). Thromboxane synthetase rapidly tranforms the endoperoxides to TXA_2, a strong vasoconstrictor and aggregation-inducing agent; its half-life in an aqueous solution is 30 sec at $37°C$ (11). Further transformation occurs to the stable breakdown product thromboxane B_2. The arachidonic acid serves also as a substrate for lipoxygenase and generates 12-L-hydroxy-5,8,10,14-eicosatetraenoic acid (HETE) (Fig. 3). In addition to forming TXA_2, the endoperoxides are broken down to the prostaglandins PGD_2, (a relatively strong inhibitor of platelet aggregation), PGE_2, $PGF_{2\alpha}$, and 12-L-hydroxy-5,8,10-heptadecatrienoic acid (HHT), plus malondialdehyde (Fig. 3).

Prostacyclin (PGI_2), a vasodilator and the most active inhibitor of platelet aggregation known, is not synthesized in platelets but in the vessel wall, mainly by the microsomal fraction of its own precursor arachidonic acid, and is broken down to the stable 6-keto-$PGF_{1\alpha}$ within 2 min in an aqueous solution at $37°C$ (11).

Another enzyme in the platelet membrane is adenylate cyclase (Fig. 3), which regulates platelet function via cyclic adenosine monophosphate (cAMP), cytoplasmic calcium, and release of platelet components.

ROLE OF PLATELETS IN BLOOD COAGULATION AND HEMOSTASIS

The platelet factor responsible for acceleration of coagulation is platelet factor 3, a phospholipoprotein present primarily in the platelet membrane (Fig. 3). Platelet factor 3 catalyzes the interaction of factor Xa, factor V, and Ca^{2+} to activate prothrombin (factor II). Its chemical structure and localization are not yet exactly known (9).

Recent experimental evidence suggests that the role of platelets in coagulation is considerably more complex and involves many more factors. According to Walsh (12,13), platelets possess procoagulant activity that is not dependent on platelet factor 3. At least two additional mechanisms may be involved in the effect of platelets on coagulation. The first mechanism involves the alteration of platelet surface and activation of factor XII by exposure of platelets to ADP. The second mechanism involves initiation of coagulation by collagen-stimulated platelets in the presence of

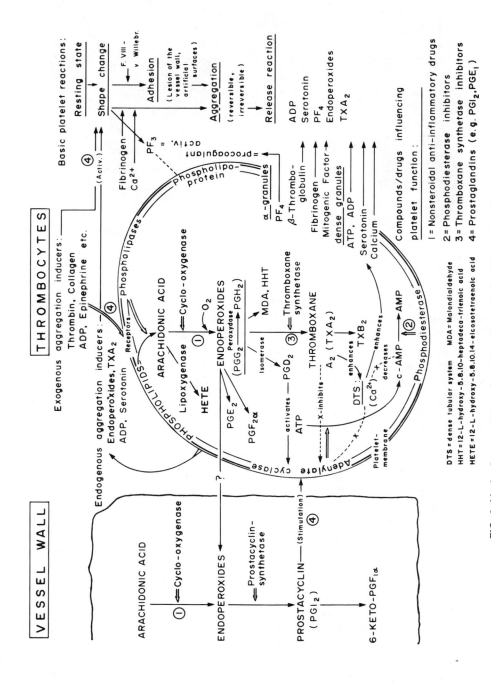

FIG. 3. Mechanisms regulating platelet function and platelet/vessel wall interactions.

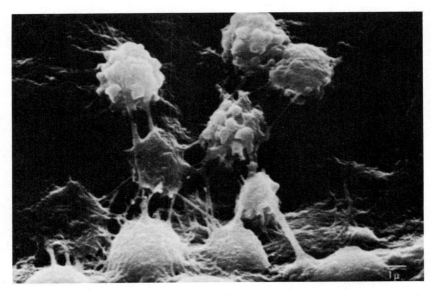

FIG. 4. Adhesion of platelets to endothelial surface of rabbit aorta. Note that platelets adhere to each other as well as to vascular wall. ×6,072. (Courtesy of Dr. H. W. Carter, Merck Institute, Rahway, N.J.)

factor XI, but in the absence of factor XII. This leads eventually to formation of factor Xa. Platelet factor 4 (PF$_4$, heparin-neutralizing activity, HNA) is a platelet protein present in the α granule fraction (10). PF$_4$ is liberated during the release reaction. Its role in hemostasis is poorly understood. However, increased plasma levels of PF$_4$ have occasionally been reported in thromboembolic diseases.

Hemostasis involves a variety of physiological mechanisms, the interplay of which leads to cessation of bleeding. Hemostasis depends on the contraction of the injured blood vessels, adhesion of platelets to the injured vessel wall, aggregation of platelets to each other, and coagulation of blood plasma around the formed platelet plug. The platelets do not adhere to normal endothelial cells but do adhere to vascular basement membrane in gaps between the endothelial cells. The adhesiveness of platelets to the vessel wall and the aggregation to each other (Fig. 4) are dependent on platelet activation. These processes are associated with the reduction in platelet levels of cAMP and inhibition of adenylate cyclase in the platelet membrane.

Activated platelets differ from normal platelets in the following ways (14): (a) They lose their normal disc shape to become spiny spheres. (b) They promote coagulation by stimulating the formation of thrombin. Thrombin, in addition to its coagulant activity, also aggregates platelets. (c) Their electrophoretic mobility is diminished. (d) They can clump together. This clumping or aggregation is reversible, and platelets can return to the inactivated state.

The adhesiveness of platelets to the vessel wall is markedly increased by several substances that are present in normal vessel walls. These include collagen, epinephrine, and ADP, which are known as aggregating agents. ADP and epinephrine cause biphasic aggregation of platelets, as measured by an aggregometer in citrated platelet-rich plasma (PRP) under constant stirring. The first phase is caused by the added compounds, and the second phase is due to the release of ADP, TXA$_2$, and other aggregating substances from platelets. The first phase of ADP- or epinephrine-induced platelet aggregation involves a change in platelet shape leading to formation of pseudopods and of a relatively loose aggregate of

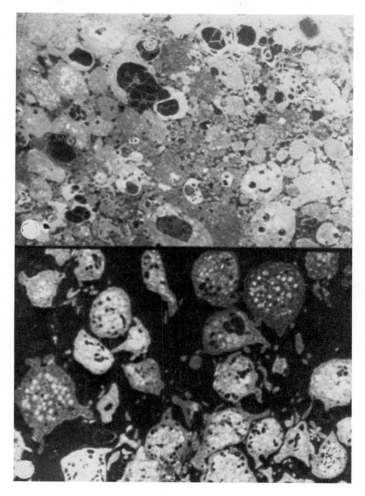

FIG. 5. ADP-induced aggregation (threshold concentration causing a biphasic response in the control) of human platelets without **(top)** and with **(bottom)** ASA (10 μg/ml, 10-min preincubation) (2).

platelets with some fibrin fibers. During the second phase of aggregation, platelets are much more tightly packed together to form a dense aggregate (Fig. 5). If the second phase is blocked by acetylsalicylic acid (ASA), a loose, reversible first-phase aggregate results (Fig. 5). Collagen-induced aggregation is monophasic and is due to the release reaction only (Fig. 6).

Both the adhesiveness and the aggregation of platelets, as well as the ability of platelets to promote coagulation, are involved in a delicate interplay that leads to formation of he-

mostatic plugs, with the aim to maintain the vascular integrity.

ROLE OF PLATELETS IN THROMBOSIS

Arterial Thrombosis

The role of platelets in arterial thrombosis is similar to their role in hemostasis. This is not surprising, because arterial thrombosis can be viewed as an exaggeration of the hemostatic process. As in the hemostatic reaction, plate-

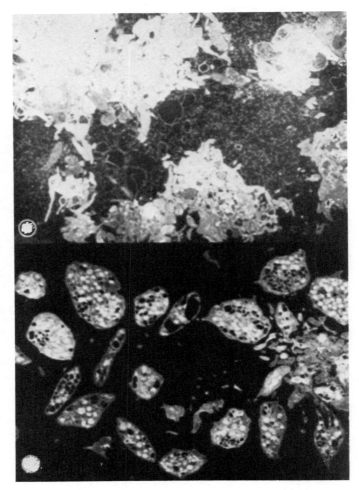

FIG. 6. Collagen-induced aggregation of human platelets without **(top)** and with **(bottom)** ASA (10 μg/ml, 10-min preincubation) (2).

lets adhere to the damaged vessel wall and aggregate to each other, releasing ADP, TXA₂, etc., and initiating the chain of events leading to the formation of a white thrombus that is composed primarily of platelets. Substantial endothelial damage and contact of platelets with collagen fibers, basement membrane, and microfibrils of the vessel wall are required to initiate arterial thrombosis. Collagen is probably the most effective component of the vascular wall in causing adhesion and aggregation of platelets. Activation of Hageman factor by collagen initiates blood coagula-

tion and accumulation of fibrin and therefore further stabilization of thrombi. Thrombogenesis, particularly propagation of thrombi, is dependent on the availability of fibrin. With the activation of the fibrinolytic state, thrombosis is less likely to progress. Thrombogenesis and thrombolysis are both highly dynamic processes; they should be viewed as being in continuous progress in a living organism. It is a pathological exaggeration of one or a deficiency of the other that leads to the formation of thrombi. Adhesion and aggregation of platelets are not the sole factors determining arterial thrombogenesis. The rheological conditions in the arteries (e.g., turbulence of blood flow created by atherosclerotic plaques or other types of vascular damage) promote deposition of platelets at the site of vascular injury. Platelet thrombi that develop at the site of atherosclerotic plaques may precipitate a terminal event by the occlusion of coronary and cerebral arteries.

Venous Thrombosis

Platelets are less clearly involved in the development of venous thrombosis than in arterial thrombosis. The factors contributing to venous thrombosis are circulatory stasis, excessive generation of thrombin, formation of fibrin, and platelet aggregation. There is no clear intimal lesion in the venous wall that is associated with thrombogenesis. In venous thrombosis, platelets, blood cells, and fibrin are intermixed.

The relatively greater importance of excessive fibrin formation, as compared with platelet aggregation, in venous thrombogenesis has its therapeutic implication. Anticoagulants, which inhibit fibrin formation, are the therapy of choice in venous thrombosis, and classic inhibitors of platelet aggregation such as aspirin do not consistently benefit patients with venous thromboembolic diseases.

THROMBOGENIC THEORY OF ATHEROSCLEROSIS

Thrombosis is often the final event in occlusive atherosclerotic vascular disease. According to the thrombogenic theory of atherosclerosis, thrombosis also precedes the development of atherosclerotic plaques. Damage to vascular endothelium leads to formation of microthrombi, which become organized, eventually infiltrated with cholesterol, and become atherosclerotic plaques. This theory was first proposed by Rokitansky in 1852, but it was not widely accepted (15). In recent years the thrombogenic theory of atherosclerosis has received renewed attention (16). The following observations favor the involvement

of thrombosis in the pathogenesis of atherosclerosis:

1. The major components of thrombi, platelets and fibrin, are found in atherosclerotic plaques.
2. Components of plaques, foam cells and cholesterol clefts, are present in organized thrombi.
3. Multiluminal channels are present in the atherosclerotic artery. Formation of such channels is typical for organization of thromboemboli.
4. Fibrous tissue and collagen, not lipids, are the major components of complicated atherosclerotic plaques.
5. In animals, experimentally induced thrombi can be transformed into atherosclerotic plaques.

If the thrombogenic theory of atherosclerosis is correct, platelet adhesion and aggregation play roles in the pathogenesis of atherosclerosis. In spite of the foregoing observations, the majority of investigators in this field are not willing to accept the thrombogenic theory. A recent hypothesis on the pathogenesis of atherosclerosis involves endothelial injury, platelet thrombosis, proliferations of medial smooth-muscle cells, and intimal thickening as the initial events in plaque formation (17). But even in this theory there is a role for platelets: The factor or factors causing proliferation of cells may have been released from platelets (3).

We have recently shown (18) that damage to arterial vessels in rats and rabbits by a thrombogenic stimulus produces marked intimal proliferation in relatively short time intervals (Fig. 7). Similar proliferation is found using a standard laboratory diet, indicating that high levels of lipids are not necessary to produce the initial stages of atherosclerotic plaques. These plaques resemble those found in humans.

PLATELET RELEASE REACTION

In hemostasis, as well as in thrombosis, adhesion and aggregation of platelets lead to re-

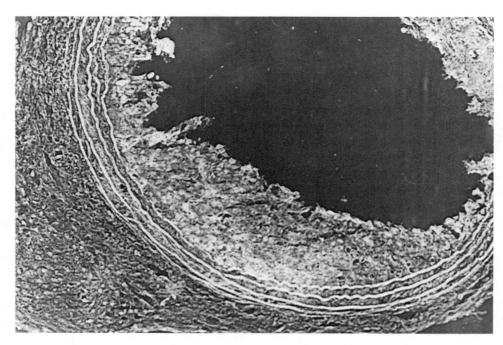

FIG. 7. Cross section of a chilled (−15°C) carotid artery of a rat fed a lipid-rich diet for 4 weeks.

lease of platelet contents, including endoperoxides, TXA_2, serotonin, and ADP, which in turn cause further adhesion and aggregation (6,11,19–24). This process is viewed as a self-activating chain reaction. There are two types of release reactions: (a) selective release of some platelet constituents, a release from which platelets usually recover; (b) generalized release of all constituents associated with lysis of platelets. The selective platelet release reaction represents a specific secretory mechanism similar to that involved in the release of epinephrine from the adrenal medulla. The substances released during the selective platelet release reaction by exogenous or endogenous inducers like thrombin, collagen, or ADP are located in the platelet granules (Fig. 3); the substances located in cytoplasm, mitochondria, or membranes are retained. The process of selective release is energy-dependent. The energy is derived from glycolysis, as well as from oxidative phosphorylation. The release reaction proceeds in three steps: initiation, transmission, and expulsion. Initiation

sensitizes the platelet to stimuli; unlike the next two steps, it does not require energy. Transmission involves the activation of intracellular transmitters including Ca^{2+} and cAMP. The expulsion step involves the movement of granules to the sites of expulsion and actual expulsion of contents of granules. In addition to endoperoxides and TXA_2, serotonin, ADP, the platelet mitogenic factor and β-thromboglobulin, calcium, K^+, and Mg^{2+} ions are released from the dense bodies and α granules (10). The time course of release of calcium parallels that of ADP. This is suggestive of a common site of granular storage for calcium and ADP, namely the α granule fraction.

Numerous substances induce the platelet release reaction. Some substances (e.g., collagen and immunocomplexes) induce a selective release at low concentrations and a generalized release at high concentrations. Serotonin, epinephrine, and ADP cause a selective platelet release reaction. The second phase of *in vitro* platelet aggregation in response to addition of ADP represents the release reaction. Drugs that inhibit the release reaction (e.g., ASA or other nonsteroidal antiinflammatory agents) inhibit the second phase but not the first phase of ADP-induced platelet aggregation. Thrombin and high concentrations of collagen that are able to stimulate adenylate cyclase directly cause release from all three types of granules: dense, α, and lysosomal granules (25).

ROLES OF cAMP AND CYTOPLASMIC Ca^{2+} IN PLATELET AGGREGATION

According to the current hypothesis, the aggregation of platelets is correlated with a decrease in platelet cAMP. The intracellular cAMP levels are determined by at least two enzymes (Fig. 3): adenylate cyclase, which catalyzes the formation of cAMP from ATP, and phosphodiesterase, which catalyzes the formation of 5-AMP from cAMP. Compounds that enhance the accumulation of cAMP, such as prostacyclin (PGI$_2$), prostaglandin D$_2$ (PGD$_2$), and prostaglandin E$_1$ (PGE$_1$), stimulate adenylate cyclase. Others, such as theophylline, papaverine, and dipyridamole, inhibit phosphodiesterase. Adenylate cyclase stimulants, as well as phosphodiesterase inhibitors, inhibit platelet aggregation (7,8,26).

Platelet cyclic guanosine monophosphate (cGMP) concentrations are also correlated with changes in platelet function. ADP, serotonin, epinephrine, norepinephrine, and Ca^{2+} increase cGMP levels and aggregate platelets. The roles of cyclic nucleotides in the regulation of platelet function are described in more detail elsewhere (27–29).

The role of cytoplasmic calcium as either trigger or second messenger in regulation of the platelet aggregation response via cAMP, with participation of TXA$_2$ and PGI$_2$, is not fully understood (7,8). It has been hypothesized (8) that TXA$_2$ might cause mobilization of Ca^{2+} from storage sites, which could inhibit the adenylate cyclase and enhance the release reaction (Fig. 3). On the other hand, cAMP might be inhibitory for the mobilization of Ca^{2+}.

METHODS OF PRODUCING AGGREGATION OF PLATELETS

The classic method for studying aggregation of platelets *in vitro* is the turbidimetric or optical-density technique of Born (30). The technique involves preparation of PRP from citrated blood by centrifugation (usually at 100–200 × g for 5–20 min). A small sample of PRP is stirred (usually at 1,000–1,200 rpm) at 37°C in a cuvette in a special apparatus called an aggregometer. A light beam of a photometer is directed through the plasma sample. Changes in optical density (light transmittance) caused by formed platelet aggregates are continuously recorded. The pen deflection indicates platelet aggregation; progression of aggregation parallels an increase in light transmittance. ADP, collagen, epinephrine, serotonin, thrombin, arachidonic acid, etc., are used as aggregating agents. Typical aggregation curves illustrating the effects of standard inhibitors on the aggregation of human and rat platelets are shown in Figs. 8 and 9.

This technique is useful for evaluating drug effects (relative potency, onset, and duration of action) *in vitro* or *ex vivo* (animals, humans), as well as for detecting hyperaggregable states in patients. Blood samples are taken before and at various intervals after drug treatment, and the sensitivities of platelets to various aggregating agents are determined.

Changes in platelet morphology are accompanied by changes in the light-scattering properties of platelet suspensions. Michal and Born (32) modified the cuvette chamber of the aggregometer to measure light scattering. Measurement of the initial phase of a change in light scattering indicates the rate of the morphological change in platelets. In the presence of ethylenediaminetetraacetic acid (EDTA), aggregating agents cause only morphological changes without aggregation. Inhibitors of platelet aggregation, such as adenosine, also

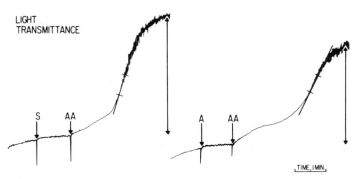

FIG. 8. Effect of aspirin (A; 8 μg/ml) on arachidonic acid (AA; 166 μg/ml)-induced aggregation of platelets. S = saline (10 μl). Note: aspirin produced lag in onset and decrease in the height of the aggregation curve.

inhibit the initial morphological change of platelets.

Breddin (33) proposed a platelet aggregation test (PAT I) that does not involve addition of exogenous aggregating agents. The aggregation of platelets by this test represents the platelet release reaction in the presence of a hypothetical plasma factor. This factor is present during vascular and infectious diseases and is activated by contact with glass, ADP, and polysaccharides. The disadvantages of Breddin's test include its subjectivity and difficulties in quantitation of the results. The method is inadequate to measure a decrease in the aggregability of platelets. Born's method is more sensitive to environmental changes than Breddin's PAT I. Results obtained with the two methods probably express different functional properties of platelets. In the presence of platelet damage, the two procedures give different results.

Recently, Breddin's test was improved by the introduction of continuous photometric recording of spontaneous platelet aggregation, the so-called PAT II (34). A further improvement was obtained with the PAT III (35,36), which allows measurements of spontaneous aggregation and induced aggregation by aggregating agents (Born technique). For evaluation of spontaneous platelet aggregation, PRP is rotated in a disc-shaped cuvette at 20 rpm and 37°C. The aggregation response is recorded according to the Born method. The test was developed in order to detect individu-

als with hyperaggregable platelets; these individuals are considered high-risk patients.

Within the wide variety of platelet aggregation tests, especially *ex vivo*, the method of Wu and Hoak (37) should be mentioned. With this technique the platelet–aggregate ratio is determined. Blood is drawn in an EDTA/formalin solution and in an EDTA solution only. This method is based on the idea that aggregates present in the blood are centrifuged down after fixation and, depending on their concentration, are expected to change the platelet count ratio. To what extent this ratio represents the actual circulating platelet aggregates, or the aggregates formed during blood withdrawal, is still an open question.

Tests for platelet adhesiveness must be sharply distinguished from tests for aggregation of platelets. The possible significance of the adhesiveness of platelets to glass in disease was suggested by Hellem (38) and Salzman (39). Platelet adhesiveness, or, as it should be called, platelet retention, is measured with glass-bead columns. The phenomenon of platelet retention in the glass-bead column involves adhesion of platelets to glass, the sticking of platelets to other platelets, and the trapping of larger aggregates in the spaces between glass beads. The common principle for various methods of measuring platelet retention is that platelet counts are performed before and after blood has been exposed to glass beads for variable periods of time. Platelet retention is expressed as the number of adhered platelets

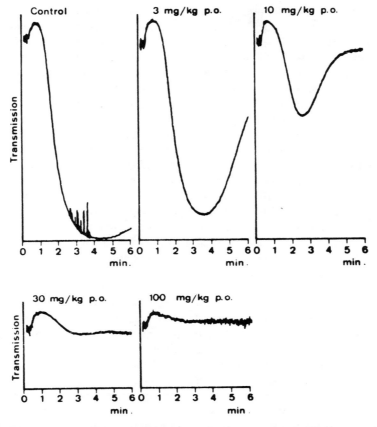

Fig. 9. Dose–response relationships for ASA after administration of a single dose to rats; evaluation of collagen-induced aggregation in citrated PRP (according to reference 31).

or as the percentage of platelets that adhere to the beads. The clinical diagnostic results with platelet adhesiveness in thromboembolic diseases or "prethrombotic" states have been conflicting and inconsistent. However, increased platelet retention was reported in patients with atherosclerosis, hypertension, hyperlipemia, and diabetes mellitus and in postoperative states. More detailed information on platelet function tests can be found elsewhere (40).

EXPERIMENTAL THROMBOSIS *IN VIVO*

The evaluation of platelet aggregation inhibitors for *in vivo* antithrombotic activity usually begins with pretreatment of animals with the test drugs and determination of the sensitivity of their platelets to various aggregating agents. The relative potency, the onset, and the duration of action of platelet aggregation inhibitors are determined with this technique. The major disadvantage of this approach is that it measures inhibition of platelet aggregation, not the actual antithrombotic activity.

Various modifications of the *in vivo/in vitro* technique have been published. The microaggregates of platelets are measured in venous blood by hemocytometry (41). Platelet aggregation is also estimated with platelet counts, which are reduced with the increased tendency of platelets to aggregate.

Another *in vivo* technique to measure platelet aggregation is screen filtration (42,43). This involves measurement of arterial pressure before and after an extracorporeal filter, with a pore size of approximately 20 μm. Platelet aggregates partially occlude the filter; this increases the arterial pressure in circulation proximal to the filter and lowers it distal to the filter. ADP or other aggregating agents are used to produce aggregation. A potential advantage of the screen filtration technique or filter loop technique is that platelet aggregation is produced *in vivo*.

Potential antithrombotic drugs have been tested for their effects on bleeding time in mice, rats, and rabbits (44,45). Standard incisions are made in the skin of the animal, and the time to cessation of bleeding is measured with a stopwatch. In mice and rats, the tips of the tails can be cut, and micropuncture of the venules in the mouse mesentery has been used for bleeding-time determinations. Under these conditions, aspirin prolongs bleeding time. The bleeding-time technique represents an unspecific but efficient screening procedure for potential antithrombotic drugs in small animals. The main disadvantage of the technique is that it measures hemostatic reaction rather than thrombogenesis. The drugs interfering with hemostasis can be expected to have antithrombotic activity. The reverse is not necessarily true. Many potential antithrombotic drugs do not prolong the bleeding time, at least when used at therapeutic doses. There is also some doubt that the antithrombotic effects of ASA are related to the prolongation of the bleeding time. There is no correlation between other platelet function tests and bleeding time.

Techniques to produce thrombi in animals involve surgical intervention and/or damage to the vascular wall. Local thrombi can be produced by electrical stimulation of larger arteries, by their partial occlusion, or by inverting their branches into the lumen of the main vessels (46). Localized thrombi can be produced by electrical stimulation of the mesenteric and brain vessels in various species of animals. Imipramine, aspirin, and papaverine increase the threshold for the current necessary to cause thrombus formation (47). In hamster cheek-pouch preparations, microthrombi can be produced by electrical stimulation of venules, and antithrombotic drugs partially prevent the obstruction of venules by thrombi (48). Advances in biolaser methods have permitted precise quantitation of the damage to blood vessels, which leads to reproducible production of thrombi (49). The rabbit ear-chamber biolaser system has been adapted to evaluation of antithrombotic drugs. The laser beam produces a microburn that leads to the formation of a small thrombus. The advantages of this technique lie in its reproducibility and the fact that it can be performed in conscious animals.

To examine thrombus formation quantitatively and to test drug effects, endothelial trauma was induced in the jugular vein in rats with a high-energy-output ruby laser (50). ASA, administered prophylactically, showed a significant protective effect against laser-induced thrombosis.

Of the many methods used to produce experimental thrombosis (51), few meet the following requirements: (a) the experimental conditions (animal species, age, body weight, anesthesia, equipment, training of technicians) are standardized; (b) the results are reproducible (i.e., they are predictable within a defined range); (c) reference standards are effective; (d) animal models verify *in vitro* results (e.g., platelet aggregation inhibition).

We have attempted to develop models for the evaluation of potential antithrombotic drugs (52–56). In 1975, Meng was able to consistently produce thrombi in the jugular vein in rats by chilling ($-12°C$) a small-vessel segment (52,53). This model was further standardized by Schmidt (54). The thrombi were removed 4 hr after their production, and their weight or hemoglobin content was determined. This method was adapted to the arterial system (e.g., the carotid artery in rats) using a silver clip in addition to the freezing at $-15°C$ (55,56). Arterial thrombi were also produced consistently in 4 hr. Under our experimental conditions, Virchow's triad appears to be fulfilled: vessel damage by endothelial lesion; altered rheology; possibly stimulation of blood clotting. Reference standards (e.g., ASA and heparin) were highly active, showing significant and reproducible results in many experiments (57). The same methods (52–56) are also useful for assessment of fibrinolytic activity of test compounds. The fibrinolytic enzymes streptokinase and urokinase reduced by more than 80% the weights of thrombi already formed (56,57). Many potential antithrombotic compounds (drugs affecting platelet function, anticoagulants, fibrinolytics, etc.) have been compared in these

models under identical experimental conditions with the known reference standards (Tables 1 and 2) (57). Only some of the compounds showed satisfactory activity (57).

Extracorporeal arteriovenous (A-V) shunts utilize production of thrombi that develop in plastic Y or T tubes of the shunts (45). Platelet aggregation inhibitors, including aspirin, are known to reduce the weight of thrombi in A-V shunts. The major disadvantages of the A-V shunt technique include the presence of artificial surfaces, nonphysiological turbulence, and the use of anesthesia.

Experimental thrombosis has also been pro-

TABLE 1. *Antithrombotic activity (prophylaxis) of potential antithrombotic drugs (platelet aggregation inhibitors, anticoagulants, fibrinolytics, etc.) on experimental thrombosis (rat)*

Compound	Dose (mg/kg)	Route	Efficacy (inhibition of thrombus formation)	A = arterial V = venous
Platelet-function-influencing compounds:				
Acetysalicylic acid (ASA)	3	p.o.	≥ 50%	A, V
Bay g 6575	0.3	p.o.	≥ 50%	A, V
	0.03	i.v.	> 50%	A
Bay i 7351	0.3	p.o.	> 50%	A, V
BL 3459	3	p.o.	< 30%	A
			< 50%	V
Bencyclane	30	p.o.	NE	A, V
	10	i.v.	NE	A, V
Carbocromen	10	i.v.	NE	A, V
Dipyridamole	30/100	p.o.	NE	A
			< 30%	V
Flurbiprofen	10	p.o.	NE	V
Imidazole	100	p.o.	NE	A, V
Indomethacin	10	p.o.	< 50%	V
			NE	A
Phenylbutazone	3–10	p.o.	≥ 50%	A, V
Phthalazinol	100	p.o.	NE	A, V
Prostacyclin	100 µg	i.v.	NE	A, V
Sulfinpyrazone	30/100	p.o.	NE	V
			< 50% NS	A
Suloctidil	30	p.o.	< 30%	A, V
	3	i.v.	< 30%	A, V
Anticoagulants:				
Heparin	1–3	s.c.	≥ 50%	A, V
	0.3	i.v.	> 50%	V
Phenprocoumon	5 × 0.25	p.o.	< 50%	A, V
Fibrinolytics:				
Streptokinase	2 × 10,000 units	i.v.	> 50%	V
Urokinase	1,000 units	i.v.	> 50%	A, V

NE = no effect. NS = not significant

TABLE 2. *Antithrombotic activity* (thrombolysis) *of potential antithrombotic drugs* (*platelet aggregation inhibitors, anticoagulants, fibrinolytics, etc.*) *on experimental thrombosis* (*rat*)

Compound	Dose (mg/kg)	Route	Efficacy (reduction in thrombus weight)	A = arterial V = venous
Platelet-function-influencing compounds:				
Acetylsalicylic acid (ASA)	2 × 100	p.o.	NE	A, V
Bay g 6575	2 × 1	p.o.	>50%	V
	2 × 0.3	p.o.	>50%	A
Bay i 7351	2 × 3	p.o.	>50%	V
	2 × 1	p.o.	>50%	A
Dipyridamole	2 × 30/100	p.o.	NE	A
Indomethacin	2 × 3	p.o.	NE	A
Phenylbutazone	2 × 30/100	p.o.	NE	A
Anticoagulants:				
Heparin	3	s.c.	NE	A, V
	1	i.v.	NE	A, V
Fibrinolytics:				
Steptokinase	2 × 10,000–15,000 units	i.v.	>50%	A, V
Urokinase	2 × 2,500 units	i.v.	>50%	A, V

NE = no effect

duced by injection of the proteolytic enzyme pronase, which removes the intimal and muscularis layers of the vessel wall (58). Dipyridamole and aspirin were found to reduce the incidence of thrombotic occlusions caused by pronase.

Decompression sickness is another model for evaluation of antithrombotic drugs (59). Decompression at a too-rapid rate results in the formation of small air bubbles in the circulation. The adherence of platelets to air bubbles leads to the release reaction and further aggregation. There is a remarkable similarity to thrombogenesis. The total platelet count in divers subjected to decompression is reduced after diving, even without any symptoms of decompression sickness. Inhibitors of platelet aggregation prevent the drop in platelet count in divers and in experimental animals subjected to decompression. Experimental decompression sickness has been produced in rabbits, rats, and minipigs. The severity of experimental decompression sickness was correlated with platelet aggregates, and thrombi were found by autopsy of the animals.

During the last few years, experimental evidence has accumulated that patients with thromboembolic diseases have reduced platelet survival times. To determine platelet survival, the ^{51}Cr method of Aster and Jandl (60) is usually used. Autologous platelets are labeled with ^{51}Cr. Radioactivity is measured in platelet concentrate from blood samples obtained at regular intervals after reinfusion of labeled platelets. The normal platelet survival time in humans is 6.7 ± 0.21 days.

Harker et al. (61) attempted to establish an experimental animal model with reduced platelet survival time by infusions of homocysteine to baboons. Homocysteine produces extensive general endothelial damage and reduces platelet survival time. This effect is antagonized by dipyridamole and sudoxicam.

Arachidonic-acid-induced mortality in animals is also used as a model of experimental thrombosis (62,63). Sodium arachidonate is injected into a marginal ear vein in rabbits, causing death of the animals in minutes. Silver et al. (62) found platelet thrombi in the pulmonary capillaries. Other authors found, after arachidonic acid injection, a marked increase in TXA_2 production, measured as TXB_2 (63). These findings suggest that in addition to the formation of platelet aggregates, vasoconstriction can be observed. Cyclooxygenase inhibitors (ASA, indomethacin, phenylbutazone, sulfinpyrazone), and to a lesser degree thromboxane synthetase inhibitors (e.g., imidazole derivatives), are active. Whole heparin and some antiaggregating agents are inactive (63). We suggested that this model detects compounds that interfere with the metabolism of arachidonic acid, but not the antithrombotic drugs in general (63).

THROMBOREGULATION BY TXA$_2$ AND PGI$_2$

The findings of Hamberg et al. (22) in 1975 that TXA_2 is generated by platelets, and those of Moncada et al. (64) and Gryglewski et al. (65) in 1976 that PGI_2 is generated by the vessel wall, led to the hypothesis of a homeostatic function for these two unstable metabolites of arachidonic acid. To what extent intravascular thrombus formation is controlled by TXA_2 and PGI_2 alone or in combination with other substances (e.g., adenine nucleotides, thrombin) warrants further investigation (20,21). Also, it is not clear how various pharmacological agents interfere with the balance of TXA_2 and PGI_2, and it remains to be determined if thromboxane synthetase inhibition will offer a more promising approach than cyclooxygenase inhibition for treatment of thromboembolic diseases. Cyclooxygenase inhibitors influence both thromboxane formation in platelets and prostacyclin generation in the vessel wall (Fig. 3). The inhibition of the vessel wall cyclooxygenase is the likely cause for the suggested anti-thrombogenic effect of nonsteroidal antiinflammatory drugs (e.g., ASA). According to the initial hypothesis of Vane et al., endoperoxides (PGG$_2$ and PGH$_2$) formed in platelets are the substrates for the vessel wall cyclooxygenase. It is now known that the vessel wall can form PGI_2 from its own endogenous precursors. In addi-

tion, release of endoperoxides from platelets seems to occur only under certain conditions, such as inhibition of thromboxane synthetase by imidazole (66,67). Prostacyclin is metabolized to many breakdown products, a process that takes place more rapidly than the nonenzymatic transformation to 6-keto-PGF$_{1\alpha}$ (68). The fact that PGI_2, unlike the classic prostaglandins (PGE$_2$, PGF$_{2\alpha}$), is not inactivated during the first pulmonary passage has supported the assumption that prostacyclin might be a circulating hormone (68–70). However, at physiologically occurring plasma levels, PGI_2 neither inhibits platelet aggregation nor modulates platelet sensitivity (71).

It has now been shown that vessel wall cyclooxygenase is less sensitive to nonsteroidal antiinflammatory agents than is platelet cyclooxygenase and that the nucleus-free platelets are not able to synthesize this protein *de novo* after irreversible acetylation by aspirin (67,72–75).

It has been concluded that only at high doses does ASA block both the platelet cyclooxygenase and the vessel wall cyclooxygenase, whereas at low doses of ASA only the platelet cyclooxygenase is blocked. The so-called paradoxical effect on bleeding time after low and high aspirin doses found by O'Grady et al. (76) was not confirmed by others (77–79) and was not observed in our own animal experiments.

PHARMACOLOGY OF PLATELET AGGREGATION INHIBITORS

Inhibitors of platelet aggregation were classified in accordance with their sites of action in various phases of aggregation or their assumed mechanisms of action (14). Drugs that interfere with the induction of aggregation at the membrane site include adenosine, its 2-chloro derivative, ATP, and AMP, which are specific inhibitors of ADP-induced aggregation and probably act independent of the arachidonate pathway (7). α-Adrenergic blocking agents specifically inhibit epinephrine-induced platelet aggregation, presumably at the induction phase. At low concentrations, heparin selectively blocks thrombin-induced platelet aggregation. The serotonin antagonists methysergide and cyproheptadine inhibit serotonin-induced aggregation of platelets. This effect is highly specific. The known specific inhibitors of the induction reaction include fibrinogen degradation products and sulfhydryl-group inhibitors such as *p*-chloromercury benzene sulfonate.

Transmission is inhibited by substances that increase cAMP levels by virtue of either stimulation of adenyl cyclase (e.g., PGE_1, PGI_2, PGD_2) or inhibition of phosphodiesterase (e.g., theophylline, papaverine, dipyridamole). The transmission and expulsion phases of the platelet release reaction are energy-dependent. Therefore, inhibitors of energy production block transmission and the aggregation of platelets.

Blockade of the expulsion phase of the selective platelet release reaction is effectively achieved by nonsteroidal antiinflammatory agents such as aspirin and indomethacin. Some antihistamines (diphenhydramine) and antidepressants (desmethylimipramine) have multiple sites of action but affect the release reaction at lower concentrations than other phases of aggregation.

Specific inhibition of thromboxane synthetase is considered as a new approach in antithrombotic therapy.

The pharmacologic effects of inhibitors of platelet aggregation are discussed next. The chemical structures of less well known compounds are shown in Table 3.

Of the many compounds that influence platelet function (aggregation, retention, etc.) *in vitro* at relatively high concentrations, only a few may be considered antiplatelet drugs. Apart from side effects, many of the substances cannot be administered at high enough doses to produce sufficiently high blood concentrations (165). Therefore, inhibitors active *in vitro* should be tested *ex vivo* and *in vivo* (intravascular platelet aggregation, experimental thrombosis) in animal experiments prior to their clinical evaluation. Presently,

only three platelet aggregation inhibitors are used clinically as antiplatelet drugs: ASA, dipyridamole, and sulfinpyrazone.

ASA

Many investigators have described the inhibitory effects of ASA on platelet aggregation (7,11,31,77,166–171). ASA acetylates plasma proteins and donates the acetate group for incorporation in platelet components (172). However, there is no conclusive evidence that acetylation is the only mechanism for the platelet aggregation inhibitory activity of ASA. Recent studies have suggested the possible importance of the arachidonate pathway in the mechanism of the platelet aggregation inhibitory action of ASA. As discussed earlier, formation of PG endoperoxides increases the tendency of platelets to aggregate. ASA, as well as indomethacin, inhibits cyclooxygenase, the enzyme controlling the formation of endoperoxides from arachidonic acid. It was therefore suggested that the platelet aggregation inhibitory activity of aspirin is due to irreversible inhibition of the platelet cyclooxygenase (11,173,174). Inhibition of cyclooxygenase in washed platelets by nonsteroidal and antiinflammatory agents leads to decreases in the formation of endoperoxides, TXA_2, and HHT and an increase in the formation of HETE (Fig. 3) from ^3H-arachidonic acid as a substrate (175).

Under certain experimental conditions, ASA can be shown to inhibit platelet adhesion to foreign surfaces or to altered elements of the vessel wall (77,176,177). ASA is the classic inhibitor of the platelet release reaction, including the procoagulatory activity (PF_3, PF_4). It antagonizes the second phase of ADP- or epinephrine-induced aggregation, as well as collagen-, thrombin-, and serotonin-induced platelet aggregation. These effects are observable *in vitro* as well as *ex vivo;* they are dose- and time-related. Various investigators disagree on the absolute and relative potency of ASA. Most differences are attributable to the *in vitro* experimental conditions, especially the preincubation time (31,178). If

TABLE 3. *Chemical structures of some platelet aggregation inhibitors*

Generic name or experimental drug code number	Structure	Chemical Abstracts name	References
Adenosine-derivatives		a. $R_1 = H$; $R_2 = OH$; $R_3 = H$ b. $R_1 = H$; $R_2 = OH$; $R_3 = NH_2$ a = 6-hydroxyaminopurine riboside b = 2-amino-6-hydroxy-aminopurine riboside	80
AN 162		N–(2–Diethylaminoethyl)–N–(2–hydroxy–2–phenyl–ethyl) 2,5–dichloroaniline	81
AY-16804		5–oxo–1–cyclopentene–1–heptanoic acid	82
BAY g 6575 = Nafazatrom		3-methyl–1–[2–(2–naphthyl–oxy) ethyl]–2–pyrazolin–5–one	56
BAY i 7351		4,4'–dichloro–N,N'–bis [(1–methyl–4–piperidinyl)–methyl]–2,2'–dithiobis–benzamide	83, 84
Bencyclane		N–[3–(1–Benzyl–cycloheptyloxy)–propyl]–N,N–dimethylamine	85–89
Benorylate		p–Acetamido–phenylacetyl–salicylate	90
BL-3459		6–methyl–1, 2, 3, 5,–tetra–hydroimidazo [2, 1–b] quinazolin–2–one	91–94
BL-4162 A = Anagrelide		6,7–dichloro–1,5–dihydro–imidazo [2, 1–b] quinazolin–2 (3 H)–one monohydro–chloride	95

Continued

TABLE 3. Continued

Generic name or experimental drug code number	Structure	Chemical Abstracts name	References
Carbocromene		3–(2–Diethylaminoethyl) 4–methyl–7–(carbethoxy–meth–oxy)–2–oxo–1,2–chromene–hydrochloride	96–97
Cyproheptadine		4–(5 H–Dibenzo [a, d] cyclohep–ten–5– ylidene)–1–methylpi–peridine	98–102, 169, 234
Dipyridamole and derivatives: Dipyridamole = RA 8		2,6–bis(diethanolamino)–4,8–dipiperidinopyrimido–[5,4–d] pyrimidine	57, 103–108, 168, 175, 182, 200–207, 191–194, 196–199, 211–222
RA 233		2,6–bis–(diethanolamino)–4–piperidino–pyrimido–[5,4–d] pyrimidine	26, 106, 108–110, 168, 196, 202, 203, 223
RA 433		2, 4, 6, Trimorpholinopyrimido–[5,4–d]–pyrimidine	111, 168, 196, 202, 223
Ditazol = S 222		4,5–diphenyl–2–bis–(2–hy–droxyethyl) aminoxazol	112–116
EMD 26644		2–[4,5–Bis (p–chlorophenyl) –oxazolyl–(2)–thio]–propionic acid	117
Flurbiprofen		2–(2–Fluoro–4–biphenylyl) propionic acid	118–119
Gliclazide = S 1702		1–(4–methylbenzene–sulfonyl–3,3–[azabicyclo (3.3.0) octyl]–urea	120–121
GP 44296			122

Continued

TABLE 3. Continued

Generic name or experimental drug code number	Structure	Chemical Abstracts name	References
GP 45840		N–(2,6–dichlorophenyl)–o– aminophenylacetic acid	122
Hydroxychloro– quine		7–chloro–4–[4–[ethyl–(2– hydroxyethyl) amino]–1–me– thylbutylamino]quinoline	45, 123
Inolamine		3–phenyl–4–diethyl–amino– ethyl–5–imino–1, 2, 4–oxo– diazoline	124
K 3920 = Indobufen		2–[p–(1–oxo–2–isoindolinyl) phenyl] butyric acid	125
KC-6141		1–methyl–2–mercapto–5– (3–pyridyl)–imidazole	126–127
Methergoline			128
Methysergide		9, 10–Didehydro–N– [1–(hydroxymethyl) propyl]–1,6–dimethyl– ergoline–8–carboxamide	98
Nictindol = L 8027		3–(2–isopropylindolyl)–3– pyridylketone	129–131, 181
Nitrofurantoin		1–[[(5–Nitro–2–furanyl) methylene] amino]–2,4– imidazolidine dione	132
ONO-747		17–Ethyl–11, 15–dihydroxy–9– oxoprosta–2, 13–dien– oic acid	232

Continued

TABLE 3. Continued

Generic name or experimental drug code number	Structure	Chemical Abstracts name	References
OPC-3689 = Cilostamide		N–cyclohexyl–N–methyl–4–(1,2–dihydro–2–oxo–6–quinolyloxy) butyramide	133
Phenidone		1–Phenyl–3–pyrazolidone	134
Phthalazinol = EG 626		7–ethoxycarbonyl–6,8–di–methyl–4–hydroxymethyl–1 (2 N)–phthalazinone	135–137
Proquazone		1–isopropyl–7–methyl–4–phenyl–2 (1 H)–quinazolinone	138
Pyridinol carbamate		2,6–pyridinedimethanol–bis [N–methylcarbamate]	137, 139
RMI 6792		N–(2–diethylaminoethyl)–N–(2–hydroxy–2–phenylethyl)–2,5–dichloroaniline	140–141
RMI 10393		α–[p–(fluoren–9–ylidenemethyl) phenyl]–2–piperidine–ethanol	140–141
SH 869			107, 114 203, 209
Sudoxicam			142
Sulindac = MK 231		cis–5–fluoro–2–methyl–1–[p–(methylsulfinyl)–benzylidenyl]–indene–3–acetic acid	143–144

Continued

TABLE 3. Continued

Generic name or experimental drug code number	Structure	Chemical Abstracts name	References
Suloctidil = CP 556 S		1-(4-isopropyl-thiophenyl)-2-n-octylaminopropanol	145–148
Suprofen = R 25061		α-Methyl-4-(2-thienylcarbonyl) benzeneacetic acid	149
Ticlopidine		5-(2-chlorobenzyl)-4, 5, 6, 7-tetrahydrothieno [3, 2-c] pyridine hydrochloride	150–155
Verapamil		α-Isopropyl-α-[(N-methyl-N-homoveratryl)-γ-aminopropyl]-3,4-dimethoxyphenyl-acetonitril	156
Viquidil			157
VK 744		2-[(2-aminoethyl) amino]-4-morpholinothieno-(3,2-D)-pyrimidine dihydrochloride	108, 114, 158–161, 168, 196, 210, 223
VK 774		4-morpholino-2-piperazino-thieno-(3,2-D) pyrimidine dihydrochloride	107, 108 159, 162 168, 209
WY 23049		2-(p-chlorophenyl)-4-thia-zoleacrylic acid	163
Y-3642			164

a 10-min preincubation time is used, ASA inhibits the collagen-induced aggregation in citrated PRP in concentrations ranging from 1 to 3 μg/ml, and most of the other clinically used drugs are less potent (31). *Ex vivo* in rats, ASA was effective in oral doses as low as 3 mg/kg; at 30 mg/kg orally, these effects persisted for up to 2 days (31). If extremely high concentrations of collagen are used, ASA may have no inhibitory effect; this suggests that collagen may aggregate platelets by more than one mechanism. ASA is usually active in models of experimentally induced thrombosis, although sometimes contradictory results are obtained (55). Using a new quantitative and well-standardized technique, we found that ASA has a moderate activity on both venous and arterial thrombus formation in different animal species (52–55,179).

Rabbits pretreated with ASA are protected against arachidonic-acid-induced thromboembolic death (62); the effect is dose-dependent, and the protection is complete at 100 mg/kg orally (63). This effect can be observed with other nonsteroidal antiinflammatory agents and may be due, at least in part, to inhibition of pulmonary TXA$_2$ generation (63). The bleeding time is prolonged after administration of ASA. This may be due to interference with the function of platelets that causes the initial arrest of bleeding. There is a discrepancy between the doses of ASA required to inhibit platelet aggregation and those used in clinical trials to prevent thrombosis. The known facts do not, however, justify a conclusion that ASA has an anti-thrombogenic effect.

The major side effect of ASA is its ability to produce gastrointestinal bleeding in some patients. Benorylate, a lipid-soluble ester of aspirin and *p*-aminophenol, was described to be similar to ASA as an inhibitor of collagen-induced platelet aggregation, and it causes little or no gastrointestinal bleeding (90). We were not able to demonstrate any *ex vivo* effect of benorylate on collagen-induced aggregation after administration to rats at doses up to 100 mg/kg orally (179).

Other Nonsteroidal Antiinflammatory Agents

In the series of nonsteroidal antiinflammatory agents (NSAIA) (e.g., ASA, amidopyrine, flufenamic acid, indomethacin, ibufenac, ibuprofen, mefenamic acid, paracetamol, phenylbutazone, sodium salicylate, suprofen) there is good correlation between antiinflammatory activity and inhibition of collagen-induced platelet aggregation (149,180). Drugs such as phenylbutazone and indomethacin inhibit primarily the release reaction (180). Indomethacin inhibits collagen-, sodium-arachidonate-, and the second phase of epinephrine- or ADP-induced aggregation of human platelets *in vitro* at concentrations in the range of 1 μg/ml (7,31).

Other NSAIA with platelet aggregation inhibitory activity include ditazol, EMD 26644, flurbiprofen, GP 45840, K 3920 (indobufen), nictindol (L 8027), proquazone, sudoxicam, sulindac, and Y-3642 (Table 3).

It was found that ditazol inhibited the release reaction *in vitro,* but primary ADP-induced aggregation was not significantly affected. It did not prolong the bleeding time in rats. The oxazole derivative ditazol also inhibited the formation of electrically induced thrombosis in rabbits in a similar manner as ASA. Coupling of the compound to a synthetic polymer markedly reduced its thrombogenicity (112–116).

EMD 26644 was active in normal volunteers after a single oral dose of 250 mg in inhibiting spontaneous platelet aggregation, according to Breddin's PAT I, but rather weak effects were obtained on ADP-induced aggregation (Born's technique). Further development was discontinued because of side effects (117).

Flurbiprofen is active *in vitro* as an inhibitor of the release reaction at concentrations below 1 μg/ml and is at least as potent as indomethacin (118,119).

A potent inhibitor of the release reaction is *N*-(2,6-dichlorophenyl)-*o*-aminophenylacetic acid (GP 45840). It antagonized the second phase of ADP-induced aggregation of human platelets at concentrations 500 to 1,000 times lower than those of sulfinpyrazone (122).

K 3920 (indobufen) is another NSAIA that inhibits the release reaction *in vitro* (125).

Nictindol (L 8027) is a strong inhibitor of collagen-induced aggregation, but not ADP-induced aggregation, *in vitro* (129–131). In addition to its thromboxane synthetase inhibitory properties, it also inhibits cyclooxygenase. In this respect nictindol differs from imidazole, which is a selective TXA_2 antagonist (181).

Proquazone, a quinazolinone derivative, is a potent inhibitor of collagen-induced platelet aggregation and of the release reaction *in vitro* ($IC_{50} = 0.15$–0.35 μM) as well as *ex vivo* (ID_{50} in rabbits 3.4 mg/kg p.o.). In this respect, proquazone is more potent than ASA. The primary ADP-induced aggregation is influenced by proquazone only at very high concentrations (138).

Two other quinazolinone derivatives, BL 3459 (91–94) and BL 4162 A (95), are very active compounds in inhibiting both the primary and secondary aggregation phases produced by ADP, collagen, or other release-inducing agents. The effective *in vitro* concentrations (IC_{50}) of BL 3459 range from 0.1 to 0.5 μg/ml in the rabbit PRP regardless of the aggregating agent; the *ex vivo* ID_{50} is 0.1 to 0.4 mg/kg i.p. By oral administration to rats or dogs, BL 3459 at 2 to 3 mg/kg produces a 50% inhibition. In addition, BL 3459 has significant oral activity in some experimental models of thrombosis (screen filtration pressure, endotoxemic death in rats, thrombosis induced by electric current in the carotid artery in dogs or by laser beam in the microvasculature in rabbit ear). The bleeding time in guinea pigs is slightly prolonged by the drug.

A close analogue to BL 3459 is BL 4162 A, which has broad-spectrum efficacy similar to that of BL 3459, including inhibition of the primary phase of ADP-induced aggregation. This last property is considered advantageous in comparison to the inhibitors of the release reaction.

Sudoxicam inhibits the release reaction at concentrations below 1 μg/ml; it inhibits experimentally induced thrombus formation in dogs. Prolongation of the bleeding time with sudoxicam has been observed in mice and rats (142).

Sulindac is a weak inhibitor of collagen-induced aggregation. The compound is of interest because of its more active sulfide metabolite (143,144).

Suprofen has been shown to have an effect on collagen-induced platelet aggregation equally as strong as that of indomethacin. The primary wave of ADP-induced aggregation is not inhibited. It is believed to inhibit cyclooxygenase and the release reaction (149).

Y-3642, a tetrahydrothienopyridine derivative, is another inhibitor of the release reaction with a favorable therapeutic index (164).

The typical NSAIAs are inhibitors of the release reaction only, and they differ from each other primarily in potency, with the exception of ASA, which has a unique long-lasting effect. The safety margin for most of them is low, and widespread use as antithrombotic agents is therefore doubtful.

Sulfinpyrazone

Sulfinpyrazone (SULF), a uricosuric agent with little antiinflammatory activity, is a pyrazole compound structurally related to phenylbutazone. At high concentrations *in vitro*, it was found, like ASA, to inhibit cyclooxygenase (175), collagen-induced aggregation, and the platelet release reaction (7,31). *Ex vivo* these effects were demonstrable only at irrelevantly high doses (31); they were not found at therapeutic doses in patients (169). However, *in vivo* it inhibited collagen-induced platelet aggregation in a dose-related manner; this was correlated with the plasma levels of sulfinpyrazone (195). The *in vivo* effects were attributed to an active metabolite. Sulfinpyrazone was shown to be a competitive inhibitor of prostaglandin synthesis in platelets (183). Its ability to protect rabbits from arachidonate-induced death (63) may be due to its interference with arachidonic acid metabolism. Sulfinpyrazone prolongs a reduced platelet survival time and restores platelet survival to normal in patients (184–186).

At 40 mg/kg p.o., sulfinpyrazone had no effect on bleeding time in mice (187). However, sulfinpyrazone inhibited the adherence of pig platelets to fibrinogen-coated surfaces (188) and diminished the adherence of rabbit platelets to the vessel wall (189). It is conceivable that the antithrombotic activity of sulfinpyrazone in humans (it lowers the incidence of thrombosis in patients with A-V shunts) (190) and in rats (at higher i.v. doses it antagonizes electrically induced thrombosis in rat carotid arteries) (210) is not determined by its ability to prevent aggregation of platelets to each other but rather by prevention of their adherence to the vascular wall.

In experimental thrombosis produced in rats by freezing of a small-vessel segment, sulfinpyrazone has only weak, if any, antithrombotic activity (57). Further elucidation of possible mechanisms of the antithrombotic action of sulfinpyrazone is likely to contribute to further understanding of the role of platelets in thrombosis.

Dipyridamole and Derivatives

Dipyridamole (RA 8), other pyrimidopyrimidines (RA 233, RA 433), and thienopyrimidines (VK 744, VK 774), or a close analogue, SH 869, inhibit the first phase of ADP-induced platelet aggregation, which may be advantageous from a theoretical point of view.

Dipyridamole

Dipyridamole (DIP) was developed as a coronary vasodilator. At high concentrations it inhibits *in vitro* ADP-induced aggregation and the release reaction *in vitro* (7,31,103, 105,106,191,196,200). However, in contrast to its weak effects in PRP, which are possibly caused by a DIP-α_1-acid-glycoprotein complex, DIP is very active in suspensions of washed human platelets (203). The antiaggregatory effects of DIP may be due to inhibition of the platelet phosphodiesterase (135, 192,193,201) and might be of importance in reinforcing the adenylate-cyclase-stimulating activity of compounds such as prostaglandins (194). Besides the platelet phosphodiesterase, DIP also inhibits adenosine deaminase in erythrocytes and blocks the uptake of adenosine by platelets and red blood cells (108,197–199). Both effects may lead to an increase in the availability of adenosine that inhibits platelet aggregation. *Ex vivo*, in clinical doses, DIP does not inhibit platelet aggregation (31,169,170). The transient fall in platelet count following intravenous ADP injection into experimental animals, which is attributed to intravascular aggregation, was inhibited by DIP (107). Reduced *in vitro* and *ex vivo* platelet adhesion/retention to glass beads was found by some authors, but not by others (106,168,169,171,196). DIP normalizes decreased platelet survival (204) and also prevents platelet consumption in homocysteinemic baboons (61). Bleeding time was prolonged when measured at the tip of the mouse tail (196). However, when administered in therapeutic doses to humans, DIP did not prolong the bleeding time (179,207), but it prolonged the effects of PGI$_2$ on the bleeding time (211). Antithrombotic effects of DIP were observed in some experimental models of thrombosis (104,168,169,196,202) but not in others (57,182,206). Recent findings regarding potentiation of the antiaggregatory effect of PGI$_2$ by DIP and its ability to stimulate endogenous PGI$_2$ production are uncertain (194,212–217). Likewise contradictory is the suggested inhibition of TXA$_2$ formation (216–221). A direct interaction with thromboxane synthetase may exist only at irrelevantly high concentrations (175,220,222).

DIP Derivatives

Of the series of compounds related to DIP, most (RA 233, RA 433, SH 869, VK 744, VK 774) are more potent *in vitro* inhibitors of ADP-, collagen-, and thrombin-induced aggregation than DIP (106,108,111,114,158, 159,162,168,196,203). However, they are less potent than DIP in inhibiting adenosine uptake (106,108). RA 233 and SH 869 were active at 10^{-6} to 10^{-7} M as inhibitors of ADP-, thrombin-, and collagen-induced aggregation in washed human platelets, as well as in PRP (203). In contrast to DIP, these compounds showed little capacity to form complexes with acid glycoproteins (203). Also, other platelet functions (e.g., retention of platelets to glass beads or adherence to foreign surfaces) were affected by these compounds (106,158, 168,196). The drugs differed in relative potency. The decrease in circulating platelets after ADP injection in experimental animals was inhibited by SH 869 and VK 774. VK 744 prevented electrically induced thrombosis in carotid arteries of rats (210); RA 233, RA 433, and VK 744 prevented thrombosis in mesenteric vessels (196); RA 233 and RA 433 had antithrombotic activity in A-V shunts (202). Like DIP, these compounds appeared to exert their antithrombotic activity by inhibiting phosphodiesterase (26,109). RA 233, RA 433, and VK 744 prevented the adherence of intravenously injected Walker-256 carcinosarcoma cells to the vascular endothelium in the rat mesentery. They also prevented lethal pulmonary embolism (223). RA 233 was also effective in reducing metastases of ascites tumor cells in mice (110).

The first clinical trials with the DIP derivatives were less encouraging. At low doses the drugs had no *ex vivo* pharmacological effects. Concurrently with the effect on platelet function, serious side effects (anorexia, nausea, etc.) were observed, leading to discontinuation of the trial (160,162). In addition, in animal experiments an occasional long-lasting hypotension was observed (107,196) that may have interfered with assessment of the antithrombotic activities of these drugs (168).

Ticlopidine, a thienopyridine derivative, by repeated administration, was shown to inhibit both the first and second phases of ADP-induced aggregations, but not collagen-induced aggregation (150,151,155). Ticlopidine, when given orally to rats, inhibited ADP-, collagen-, thrombin-, arachidonic-acid-, and prostaglandin-endoperoxide/TXA_2-induced thrombosis (153). These effects were long-lasting, with a half-life of about 48 hr. With a single oral dose of 100 mg/kg p.o. we were not able to demonstrate any effect on collagen-induced aggregation in rats (179).

With repeated daily administration, ticlopidine was active in preventing experimentally induced thrombosis (lactic-acid-induced pulmonary thrombosis in rats; ADP- and collagen-induced transient thrombocytopenia and thromboembolic death in rats and mice) (152). The mode of action of ticlopidine as an inhibitor of platelet aggregation is believed to be activation of basal- and PGE_1-stimulated adenylate cyclase activity (154). Ticlopidine prolongs bleeding time (155).

Adenosine and Its Derivatives

Adenosine-induced inhibition of ADP-induced platelet aggregation was discovered by Born and Cross (224). The active concentrations of adenosine ranged from 0.03 to 0.1 μg/ml (31). The mechanism of inhibitory action of adenosine involves competitive inhibition of ADP. Other hypotheses have proposed that transport of adenosine through the cell membrane consumes energy required for aggregation and that adenosine forms an inhibitory adenosine carrier complex in the cell membrane. Adenosine exerts its inhibitory effect without being taken up by the platelet. In plasma, adenosine is rapidly destroyed by adenosine deaminase. Among adenosine derivatives, the most potent is 2-chloroadenosine (225); its duration of action is considerably longer than that of adenosine. This is due to the fact that, unlike adenosine, 2-chloroadenosine is not deaminated in plasma. Therapeutic use of 2-chloroadenosine is precluded by its high toxicity. Several other naturally occurring adenosine derivatives, including ATP and AMP, inhibit ADP-induced platelet aggregation (7), but none is as potent as either adenosine or 2-chloroadenosine. 2-Amino-6-hydrox-yaminopurine riboside has been shown to be 5 to 10 times as potent as adenosine, whereas 2-chloroadenosine is only 1 to 3 times as potent (80).

Prostaglandins

PGE$_1$ inhibits the aggregation of platelets (226). This effect is attributed to PGE$_1$-induced stimulation of adenylate cyclase and subsequent accumulation of cAMP. PGE$_1$ is one of the most potent inhibitors of the primary phase of ADP-induced platelet aggregation known; it is active at 5×10^{-8} M. Recent studies with prostaglandin precursors and prostaglandin synthetase inhibitors suggest that prostaglandin formation is involved in the platelet release reaction and subsequent aggregation. During arachidonic-acid-, collagen-, or epinephrine-induced platelet aggregation, prostaglandin intermediates (the endoperoxides designated PGH$_2$ and PGG$_2$) are formed (227,228). They are metabolized to the highly potent platelet aggregating substance TXA$_2$ and to PGI$_2$, the most potent inhibitor of platelet aggregation known so far.

Besides TXA$_2$ and PGI$_2$ formation, the endoperoxides are found in the enzymatic conversion of arachidonic acid to PGE$_2$, PGF$_{2\alpha}$, and PGD$_2$ and cause aggregation of human platelets at low (10–330 ng/ml) concentrations. PGD$_2$ inhibits aggregation of platelets; its potency is similar to that of PGE$_1$ (229, 230). Some of the synthetic prostaglandin derivatives also inhibit aggregation of platelets. 5-Oxo-1-cyclopentene-1-heptanoic acid (AY-16,804) inhibits ADP-induced aggregation of rat platelets in vitro and in vivo. Ay-16,804 is comparable in potency to sulfinpyrazone (82).

A very potent inhibitor of platelet aggregation is the PGE$_1$ derivative ONO-747; it is 16 times as potent as PGE$_1$ as an inhibitor of ADP-induced aggregation in human PRP. It is also active ex vivo in rats and rabbits (232).

Most prostaglandins are rapidly eliminated from the circulation. Their use in antithrombotic therapy is therefore severely limited.

Hydroxychloroquine

Hydroxychloroquine reduces the incidences of postoperative deep-vein thrombosis and pulmonary embolism in humans (123). It inhibits thrombus formation and reduces platelet consumption in the extracorporeal shunt in rabbits without increasing bleeding time (45). The maximal antithrombotic effect, as judged by the decrease in thrombus weight, is obtained at 1 hr after oral administration of hydroxychloroquine at 25 mg/kg. The effect is still present 72 hr after a single oral dose of the drug. ASA also inhibits thrombus formation in extracorporeal shunts, but, unlike hydroxychloroquine, it prolongs bleeding time in humans. There is presently no sufficient evidence for direct association of the antithrombotic activity and the effects of hydroxychloroquine on platelet functions.

Antiserotonin and Antihistaminic Drugs

Substances that inhibit serotonin-induced platelet aggregation include the tricyclic compound cyproheptadine and drugs such as methergoline and methysergide. Cyproheptadine as an antihistaminic and antiserotonin agent (99) inhibits aggregation of platelets induced by serotonin, collagen, ADP, thrombin, and antigen-antibody complexes at relatively high concentrations in vitro (98,234). It is effective against serotonin at considerably lower concentrations that those required against other aggregating agents. Unlike nonsteroidal antiinflammatory agents, cyproheptadine also antagonizes the first phase of ADP-induced platelet aggregation. Cyproheptadine is bound firmly by the platelet membrane; this leads to a stabilizing effect at the membrane level that could explain its aggregation inhibitory activity (100). The platelet aggregation inhibitory activity of cyproheptadine was correlated by Gaut (233) with its ability to inhibit uptake of deoxyglucose. Nonsteroidal antiinflammatory drugs and tricyclic antidepressants do not antagonize deoxyglucose uptake by platelets. In hamster cheek-pouch preparations, cyproheptadine antagonizes thrombus formation caused by electrical stimulation of venules. Cyproheptadine enhances the inhibitory effects of dipyridamole or aspirin on collagen-induced aggregation of guinea pig platelets (98). Combinations of antithrombotic drugs may represent a useful approach to therapy for thrombosis, and cyproheptadine may have a place in such combinations. Cyproheptadine has been reported to increase the survival time of rats with renal transplants and to inhibit rejection in humans (102). In extracorporeal bypass studies in dogs, cyproheptadine was shown to inhibit traumatized dog platelets from aggregation on the oxygenator membranes and subsequent deposition in the lungs (102). However, an *ex vivo* effect of cyproheptadine on platelet aggregation in humans has not been shown (169). Like cyproheptadine, another antiserotonin drug, methergoline, antagonizes not only serotonin- but also ADP- and collagen-induced aggregation of rabbit platelets. It is particularly effective against aggregation caused by combined administration of serotonin and epinephrine (128). Methysergide inhibits serotonin-induced aggregation of human platelets at concentrations similar to those of cyproheptadine, but its dose–response curve is steeper (98). Many commonly used antihistamines (e.g., promethazine) interfere with platelet functions *in vitro*, particularly platelet aggregation, but only at concentrations considerably greater than those obtainable *in vivo* with therapeutic doses of these drugs (146,235,239).

Cardiovascular/Cerebrovascular Drugs

Among these drugs, the α-adrenergic blocking agents (e.g. phentolamine and dihydroergotamine) and the β blocking agent propranolol should be mentioned. Depending on the aggregating agent (epinephrine, norepinephrine, ADP, collagen, thrombin, etc.), different

results have been obtained, both qualitative and quantitative (7,168,169,236). Their effects are mediated through different receptor sites; this is discussed is more detail elsewhere (169). Propranolol is active at concentrations that may be achieved with clinical doses (208). A direct action on the platelet membrane (stabilizing effect like that of tricyclic compounds, e.g., imipramine; interference with calcium availability) has been suggested (237,238).

Many other vasoactive drugs, particularly vasodilators, have been shown to inhibit platelet functions. The standard vasodilator, papaverine, is active *in vitro* and *in vivo* (31,240, 241). It also inhibits platelet phosphodiesterase, and this is a probable mechanism of its platelet aggregation inhibitory activity (135).

Bencyclane, a cerebral/peripheral vasodilator and antispasmodic compound, has been shown to inhibit ADP-, collagen-, and epinephrine-induced platelet aggregation *in vitro* (31,85–87), as well as spontaneously enhanced aggregation (36) in 10^{-5} M concentration (86). However, no significant *ex vivo* activity has been revealed (31,86,89); thrombus formation induced by topical ADP was inhibited (85). Intravenously administered bencyclane in monkeys prevented an increase in the screen-filtration pressure induced by ADP and serotonin (88).

Carbochromen, a coronary vasodilator, inhibits dose-dependent platelet aggregation *in vitro*, as studied by the techniques of Born (30) and Breddin (33). It is active only at high concentrations (96) that may not be obtainable *in vivo* at therapeutically used doses. After repeated intravenous administration to dogs, the drug was weakly effective *ex vivo* as an inhibitor of ADP-induced aggregation (97).

Imolamine, an antianginal drug, at concentrations ranging from 50 to 100 μg/ml *in vitro*, inhibited collagen-induced platelet aggregation and the second phases of ADP- and epinephrine-induced aggregation (124).

Sodium nitroprusside, an antihypertensive drug, inhibits platelet aggregation (ADP-, epinephrine-, and thrombin-induced) and the release reaction *in vitro* (ED_{50} ca. 10^{-5} M). It is also active *ex vivo* during infusion to rabbits (209). Use of this drug by infusion in the initial phase of myocardial infarction is believed to be beneficial (170).

Suloctidil, a drug developed for treatment of cerebral and peripheral vascular insufficiencies, inhibited platelet aggregation in human PRP *in vitro* when the aggregation was induced by thrombofax or collagen (147). It was also active with repeated oral administration to volunteers (147). In the rat, we were not able to show any *ex vivo* efficacy (179). The bleeding time and platelet retention to glass were not modified after ingestion of suloctidil (147). Antithrombotic properties of the compound in experimental thrombosis have been described (145,146,148).

Verapamil, a Ca^{2+} antagonist and an antianginal agent, is less potent than papaverine against ADP-induced aggregation of rat and dog platelets *in vitro*. At 1 to 5 mg/kg p.o., verapamil inhibits ADP-, and lauric-acid-induced thrombocytopenia in rats and rabbits (156).

Viquidil is a cerebral vasodilator that antagonizes ADP- or epinephrine-induced aggregation of human platelets *in vitro* at 10^{-5} M and is comparable to papaverine in potency (157).

Xantinol nicotinate, used in the treatment of arterial peripheral and cerebrovascular insufficiencies, inhibited spontaneous platelet aggregation, according to Breddin (33), by intravenous but not oral administration of single doses (242). With long-term administration, xantinol nicotinate inhibited collagen-induced, but not ADP-induced, aggregation (243).

Another vasoactive drug used in peripheral vascular insufficiencies is pentoxifylline. It showed activity in ADP- and serotonin-induced platelet aggregation *in vivo* in monkeys after intravenous administration (244). Inhibition of phosphodiesterase may represent the mechanism of platelet aggregation inhibitory activity of pentoxifylline (245).

TXA$_2$ Inhibitors and Antagonists

Imidazole and methylimidazole, at relatively high concentrations, are inhibitors of platelet aggregation. They are also selective inhibitors of thromboxane synthetase (231). From a theoretical point of view, inhibition of thromboxane synthesis may represent an ideal approach to the treatment of thrombo-embolic diseases (7).

KC 6141, a mercaptoimidazole derivative, inhibited arachidonic-acid- and collagen-induced aggregation of platelets in rabbit PRP ($EC_{50} = 10^{-4}$–10^{-5} M) and had little, if any, effect on ADP-induced aggregation (126). Platelet retention was also inhibited after oral administration to rats (126), as was thrombus formation in an extracorporeal shunt (127).

Pyridinolcarbamate and phthalazinol (EG 626) are considered as TXA$_2$ antagonists (7,137). Their potency in influencing platelet function is very weak *in vitro,* particularly that of pyridinolcarbamate (7,31,139). EG 626 is a phosphodiesterase inhibitor (135). Recently, the TXA$_2$ antagonistic action of EG 626 was questioned, and a PGI$_2$ potentiating effect was proposed (136).

Miscellaneous Drugs

Among drugs that inhibit the aggregation of platelets are anesthetics, diuretics, antibiotics, tranquilizers, hypolipemics, hypoglycemics, and other classes of drugs. The antipsychotic drug chlorpromazine inhibits aggregation of platelets *in vitro* and inhibits adhesion of human platelets to glass beads. At clinically used doses, however, chlorpromazine has no clearly demonstrable effect on platelets (246).

Because thromboembolic disorders are common in diabetics, it is of particular interest that gliclazide, a sulfonylurea derivative with hypoglycemic activity, also inhibits platelet aggregation, presumably by interfering with the ability of platelets to synthesize glycogen (120,121). Other sulfonylurea derivatives have also been reported to inhibit platelet aggregation (247–250).

Nitrofurantoin inhibits the first phase of ADP-induced aggregation of human platelets *in vitro* at 10 μM (132). Even higher plasma concentrations of the drug can be obtained following oral administration of nitrofurantoin at 200 mg. At this dose, nitrofurantoin prolongs bleeding time in humans. The drawbacks of nitrofurantoin therapy include a short duration of action; its activity disappears as rapidly as the drug is eliminated from the circulation. Also, the reported neurotoxicity of nitrofurantoin presents a problem for its chronic use. Another compound that inhibits the first phase of ADP-induced aggregation is a dibenzazepine derivative, GP 44,296. It is more potent than phenylbutazone, oxyphenbutazone, or sulfinpyrazone in inhibiting collagen-induced platelet aggregation *in vitro* (122).

Among a series of compounds investigated by MacKenzie (140,141), α-[*p*-(fluoren-9-ylidenemethyl)phenyl]-2-piperidineethanol (RMI 10,393) and *N*-(2-diethylaminoethyl)-*N*-(2-hydroxy-2-phenylethyl)-2,5-dichloroaniline (RMI 6792) inhibited ADP-induced platelet aggregation *in vitro* and *in vivo*. In guinea pigs, RMI 10,393 was effective against ADP *in vivo* at lower concentrations than *in vitro*.

The first phase of ADP-induced aggregation of human platelets is inhibited by 2-(*p*-chlorophenyl)-4-thiazoleacrylic acid (WY 23,049) (163). As an *in vitro* inhibitor of collagen-induced platelet aggregation, WY 23,049 is less potent than ASA; however, it is more potent than ASA in protecting rats from ADP-induced platelet loss.

Derivatives of benzamidine, phenylguanidine, and benzylamine inhibited collagen-, thrombin-, and ADP-induced aggregation of platelets, possibly by preventing interaction between ADP and platelet membrane (251).

A hypolipemic drug, clofibrate, antagonized aggregation of human platelets induced by latex particles (252) and reduced platelet adhesiveness (253). *In vitro* incubation of human platelets with clofibrate at 100 to 200 μg/ml

decreased the sensitivity of platelets to ADP and epinephrine. The platelets of patients with familial hyperbetalipoproteinemia are hypersensitive to the aggregating agents ADP, collagen, and epinephrine. Clofibrate at 2 g/day antagonizes this hypersensitivity without any significant effect on plasma lipids and lipoproteins (254). The mechanism of action of clofibrate on platelets remains to be determined.

Polyphloretin phosphate, a known prostaglandin inhibitor, inhibits platelet aggregation induced by thrombin and protamine (255). This inhibitory effect is mediated by larger molecular components of polyphloretin phosphate. The small molecular components have no inhibitory activity. It is possible that the platelet aggregation inhibitory activity of polyphloretin phosphate is associated with its antiprostaglandin effects.

The only phospholipid with a consistent inhibitory activity on the platelet release reaction is lysolecithin (256). It is effective *in vitro* at 0.1 mM.

AN 162, a dichloroaniline derivative, inhibits aggregation of platelets induced by ADP, collagen, and thrombin in human PRP (81). Inhibition of platelet aggregation by AN 162 was also observed after oral administration of the drug to guinea pigs (81).

A very potent inhibitor of platelet function is OPC-3689 (cilostamide), which inhibits collagen- and first-phase ADP-induced aggregation at micromolar concentrations (133). This compound is also active after administration to rats, inhibiting collagen- and ADP-induced aggregation (179). OPC-3689 may exert its activity by inhibiting phosphodiesterase, which increases cAMP levels in platelets (133).

Phenidone, a pyrazolidone derivative, appears to be interesting because of its simultaneous inhibition of cyclooxygenase and lipoxygenase (134).

In addition to the compounds mentioned earlier, which are used primarily for indications other than thrombosis, a great deal of effort has been made in our laboratories to find new specific antithrombotic drugs. Bay i 7351, at micromolar concentrations, is a very potent inhibitor of platelet aggregation *in vitro* as well as *ex vivo* in experimental animals at 10 mg/kg orally (83,84). It is active against a wide variety of aggregating agents and inhibits the first phase of ADP-induced aggregation. Also, the TXA_2 formation in washed platelet suspensions is inhibited dose-dependently by Bay i 7351 (84). Experimentally induced thrombosis (52–55) is prevented after both prophylactic and therapeutic administration of the drug at low doses (57,83).

Another compound, Bay g 6575, has exhibited excellent efficacy in experimental thrombosis (52–57). The drug itself is not a platelet aggregation inhibitor; its antithrombotic activity may be due to stimulation of prostacyclin formation in the vessel wall (257).

The foregoing discussion illustrates that many compounds with different chemical structures influence platelet function. The recent developments and tendencies observed in this field are discussed elsewhere (258).

CLINICAL STUDIES WITH PLATELET AGGREGATION INHIBITORS

The presently available experimental and clinical data suggest that inhibitors of platelet aggregation are potentially useful in the prevention and treatment of thrombosis, particularly arterial thromboembolic disorders. Among those, coronary artery diseases, e.g., myocardial infarction (MI), and cerebrovascular diseases are most important. The use of antiplatelet drugs seems also to be indicated in other thromboembolic conditions (e.g., peripheral vascular diseases, renal diseases, valvular heart diseases or prosthetic devices, shunts, dialyzer membranes, and catheters) that are often associated with hyperaggregability of platelets.

Eventually, appropriate antithrombotic drugs will be tested in long-term studies for prophylactic effects in the treatment of myocardial infarction or cerebrovascular disorders (transient ischemic attacks or TIAs, stroke). An observation that a drug inhibits ADP- or collagen-induced platelet aggregation, even in humans, is hardly sufficient to justify large expenditures of either private or public funds required for long-term prophylactic studies. The clinical investigators in the field of thrombosis have made numerous attempts to provide additional evidence of effectiveness in preliminary short-term trials. Some of these attempts have been successful.

In many studies performed during the last two decades with ASA, DIP, and SULF, positive and negative results have been obtained (168,169). To prove clinical efficacy of potential antithrombotic drugs, a precise diagnosis of the thrombotic event is required. In venous thrombosis, ^{125}I-fibrinogen leg scanning is often complemented with phlebography and Doppler ultrasound. The incidence of pulmonary embolism is used as an endpoint. Some trials were weakened by the fact that the endpoints were based mainly on clinical observations. In arterial thrombosis (e.g., induced by prosthetic devices), platelet survival is used as an indicator. This parameter appears to correlate well with the incidence of thromboembolic processes. In the large-scale clinical trials, particularly in MI, primary endpoints have been death or definite MI documented by EKG and enzyme changes or autopsy; secondary endpoints have been angina pectoris, arrhythmia, stroke, TIAs, etc.

SULF has proved to be effective in normalizing the shortened platelet survival in patients with prosthetic heart valves (259,260). In cerebrovascular disorders the value of anticoagulant therapy remains controversial (261). On the other hand, platelet aggregation inhibitors look more and more attractive for therapy of thromboembolic strokes, including TIAs (262). Approximately one-third of untreated TIA patients can be expected to develop strokes within 5 years after the initial diagnosis. The effects of antithrombotic drugs can be studied in patients with amaurosis fugax by observing the passage of platelet aggregates through the retinal arteries. SULF has been effective in preventing attacks of amaurosis fugax (263).

In the Canadian cooperative study with ASA and SULF in threatened stroke, SULF alone was completely ineffective, and it did not diminish the incidences of stroke and death when administered in combination with ASA (264). More encouraging were the findings with SULF in coronary artery disease. In the Anturane Reinfarction Trial, a double-blind, multicenter clinical trial, a significant reduction in cardiac death by 48.5% (4.9 vs. 9.5% of annual death rate) was achieved during the first year after MI (265). The sudden death rate was reduced by 57.2% (2.7 vs. 6.3%), a statistically significant difference. It is still a matter of debate whether or not inhibition of platelet aggregation is the mechanism of SULF in reducing the sudden death rate. It has been suggested that prevention of arrhythmias or lowering of blood uric acid might represent the mechanism of action of SULF in prevention of sudden death. In venous thrombosis, platelets are not likely to play the major role, but SULF has been claimed to be effective in the treatment of recurrent venous thrombosis (269).

DIP, similar to SULF, causes a prolongation of platelet survival time in patients with prosthetic heart valves (204,205,268). In most of the other successful studies, DIP has been used in combination with another drug (anticoagulant, platelet aggregation inhibitor). This includes its use in cardiac valve replacement (266,267) or in MI in the Persantin-Aspirin Re-Infarction Study (PARIS). There is, at present, no evidence that DIP alone is effective in cerebral ischemic diseases (amaurosis fugax, TIAs, stroke) (168,169,171,270,271) or in MI (171). Positive trends have been found with DIP in renal allografts (272). The role of platelet aggregation inhibitor in renal diseases is not clear. In long-term dialysis, ASA may be beneficial (282). Promising results have been reported with SULF, DIP, and ASA in peripheral vascular diseases (171). DIP is ineffective in venous thromboembolism (273).

ASA does not prolong a shortened platelet survival in prosthetic heart valves (205). However, combination of this drug with anticoagu-

lants may be beneficial (274). The prophylactic activity of ASA in postoperative venous embolism is difficult to assess presently. The available results are contradictory, possibly because of differences in types of surgery involved. In two prospective randomized trials, deep-vein thrombosis (DVT) and pulmonary embolism were diagnosed clinically (275,276) and DVT by leg scanning (277). Both studies showed positive trends in favor of ASA. In a third trial by the British Medical Research Council (BMRC study), no benefits were observed in the ASA group, using ^{125}I-fibrinogen uptake to determine the incidence of DVT (278). However, 600 mg of ASA per day may not represent a sufficient dosage for therapy for venous thromboembolism. At higher doses, ASA may interfere with arachidonate metabolism in the lungs, preventing formation of the vasoconstrictory endoperoxides and thromboxane. In orthopedic surgery, particularly in hip replacement, ASA appears to be effective, if diagnosis is made clinically (273–279), but negative results have also been reported (77).

The anticoagulants, on the contrary, are clearly useful in the treatment of venous thrombosis, although their usefulness in arterial thrombosis remains highly controversial.

Considerable interest in the use of platelet aggregation inhibitors to prevent cerebral ischemia was aroused by the findings with ASA in two well-designed trials. Fields et al. (280,281) found in their AITIA studies (Aspirin in Transient Ischemic Attacks) with non-surgical and surgical patients statistically significant differences in favor of ASA when death, infarction, and continuation of TIA activity were considered together. ASA therapy seemed particularly successful in patients with a history of multiple episodes of TIAs. In individuals with stenotic lesions in the region of the carotid artery, the ASA patients had markedly fewer TIAs. But ASA had no distinct effect on incidence of stroke, on mortality, or on cerebral infarction when considered separately. In the Canadian collaborative double-blind trial (264) with ASA and SULF in threatened stroke, ASA was effective ($p < 0.05$) in reducing the incidence of death or stroke. But only male (not female) patients benefited (48% reduction in the risk of stroke and death). It was suggested that ASA can inhibit PGI_2 formation in the vessel wall in women only at lower doses than those used in men, because of higher PGI_2 (283).

The frequency of amaurosis fugax attacks is also reduced by ASA (270).

If thromboembolic processes are involved in the pathogensis of MI, platelet aggregation inhibitors should be effective in the treatment of myocardial ischemia and infarction. Their effectiveness was suggested by experiments in dogs in which myocardial necrosis was prevented by ASA (284). In an epidemiological retrospective study, the Boston Collaborative Drug Surveillance Group found a reduced frequency of acute MI in heavy aspirin users (285). Some prospective randomized double-blind trials on the prevention of secondary MI by ASA have been performed: Elwood et al. (286) found no significant effect with 300 mg ASA daily, although positive trends were indicated by life-table analysis. In the trial of the Coronary Drug Research Group (287), total mortality was reduced from 8.3% in the placebo group to 5.8% in the ASA group. Nonfatal MI occurred in 3.7% of the

patients in the ASA group, compared with 4.2% of those in the control group. The beneficial trend in favor of ASA was not statistically significant. Breddin et al. (288) found in the German-Austrian 2-year prospective study reductions by ASA of the total mortality and coronary death rate by 42.3% and 46.3%, respectively. This effect reached statistical significance in some subgroups (e.g. reduction of coronary death rate in male patients). An excellent comprehensive survey of experimental and clinical studies with ASA in thromboembolic disorders, citing more than 300 references, was published by Jobin (77).

Two further recently finished prospective trials with ASA in MI are the AMIS (Aspirin Myocardial Infarction Study) (289) and PARIS (Persantin-Aspirin Re-Infarction Study) (290) studies. The daily dose of ASA in AMIS was 1 g, and in PARIS 324 mg ASA, plus 75 mg DIP. The results of these randomized, double-blind, placebo-controlled trials are shown in Table 4.

In comparison to placebo groups, mortality was increased by 11% in the AMIS study and decreased by 18% in the PARIS study. The PARIS results are more consistent with those of previous studies than are the results of AMIS, but no conclusion can be drawn regarding overall mortality as a primary end-

TABLE 4. *Two trials of ASA in MI*

	Incidence (%)				
	AMIS		PARIS		
	ASA	Placebo	ASA	ASA/DIP	Placebo
Overall mortality[a]	10.8	9.7	10.5	10.7	12.8
Three-year mortality	9.6	8.8	9.0	9.4	11.4
Coronary mortality	8.7	8.0	8.0	7.7	10.1
Sudden coronary death	2.7	2.0	5.6	3.7	4.4
Coronary incidence[b]	14.1	14.8	14.0	13.8	18.5
Nonfatal definite MI	6.3	8.1	6.9	7.9	9.9
Incidence of definite stroke	1.2	2.0	1.1	1.2	2.0
Death: all causes or definite MI	—	—	16.0	16.8	20.9

[a] All causes of death with follow-up periods of 41 months in the PARIS study and 39 months in the AMIS study.

[b] Coronary death or definite nonfatal MI.

point. The increased mortality in the ASA group (AMIS) is explained by the higher incidence of risk factors before treatment. The greatest differences between the results of the two trials (PARIS and AMIS) were obtained in nonfatal MI. The incidence of nonfatal MI was reduced by 30% in the PARIS trial and 22% in the AMIS trial. However, these differences were not statistically significant. Consistent with previous findings was the reduction of stroke incidence by ASA.

Although the effects obtained with presently used drugs (ASA, SULF, DIP) are not very dramatic, new and more powerful inhibitors of platelet aggregation may prove to be useful in therapy for thromboembolic diseases.

REFERENCES

1. White, J. G. (1974): Current concepts of platelet structural physiology and pathology. *Hum. Pathol.,* 5:1–6.
2. Voigt, W. H., and Seuter, F.: Unpublished results.
3. Ross, R., Glomset, J., Kariya, B., and Harker, L. A. (1974): A platelet-dependent serum factor that stimulates the proliferation of arterial smooth muscle cells in vitro. *Proc. Natl. Acad. Sci. U.S.A.,* 71:1207–1210.
4. Marcus, H. J., and Zucker, M. B. (1965): *The Physiology of Blood Platelets.* Grune & Stratton, New York.
5. Maupin, B., and Gineste, J. (1968): Cytochemistry of blood platelets. In: *Advances in Experimental Biology and Medicine. Vol. 3: Platelets in Haemostasis,* edited by C. Haanen and J. Jurgens, pp. 49–61. S. Karger, Basel.
6. Moncada, S., and Vane, J. R. (1977): The discovery of prostacyclin—a fresh insight into arachidonic acid metabolism. In: *Biochemical Aspects of Prostaglandins and Thromboxanes,* edited by N. Kharasch and J. Fried, pp. 155–177. Academic Press, New York.
7. Busse, W.-D., and Seuter, F. (1979): Influence on thromboxane and malondialdehyde synthesis in human thrombocytes by various inhibitors of platelet function. In: *Arachidonic Acid Metabolism in Inflammation and Thrombosis,* edited by K. Brune and M. Baggiolini, pp. 127–137. Birkhäuser, Basel.
8. Gorman, R. R. (1979): Modulation of human platelet function by prostacyclin and thromboxane A₂. *Fed. Proc.,* 38:83–88.
9. Schafer, A. I., and Handin, R. I. (1979): The role of platelets in thrombotic and vascular disease. *Prog. Cardiovasc. Dis.,* 22:31–52.
10. Kaplan, K. L., Broekman, M. J., Chernoff, A., Lesznik, G. R., and Drillings, M. (1979): Platelet α-granule proteins: Studies on release and subcellular localization. *Blood,* 53:604–618.

11. Moncada, S., and Vane, J. R. (1979): Mode of action of aspirin-like drugs. *Adv. Intern. Med.,* 24:1–22.
12. Walsh, P. N. (1974): Platelets, blood coagulation and hemostasis. In: *Platelets and Thrombosis,* edited by S. Sherry and A. Scriabine, pp. 23–43. University Park Press, Baltimore.
13. Walsh, P. N. (1978): The significance of platelet coagulant activities in hemostasis and thrombosis. In: *Platelet Function Testing,* edited by H. J. Day, H. Holmsen, and M. B. Zucker, p. 436. DHEW publication no. (NIH) 78–1087.
14. Vermylen, J., de Gaetano, G., and Verstraete, M. (1973): Platelets and thrombosis. In: *Recent Advances in Thrombosis,* edited by L. Poller, pp. 113–150. Churchill Livingstone, London.
15. Rokitansky, C. (1852): *A Manual of Pathological Anatomy. Vol. 4,* translated by G. E. Day. Sydenham Society, London.
16. Spaet, T. H., Gaynor, E., and Stermerman, M. B. (1974): Thrombosis, atherosclerosis, and endothelium. *Am. Heart J.,* 87:661–668.
17. Ross, R., and Glomset, J. A. (1973): Atherosclerosis and the arterial smooth muscle cell. *Science,* 180:1332–1339.
18. Seuter, F., Sitt, R., and Busse, W.-D. (1980): Experimentally induced thromboatherosclerosis in rats and rabbits. *Folia Angiologica,* 28:85–87.
19. Mürer, E. H., and Day, H. J. (1974): Observations on the platelet release reaction. In: *Platelets and Thrombosis,* edited by S. Sherry and A. Scriabine, pp. 1–22. University Park Press, Baltimore.
20. Cooper, D. R., Lewis, G. P., Lieberman, G. E., Webb, H., and Westwick, J. (1979): ADP metabolism in vascular tissue, a possible thrombo-regulatory mechanism. *Thromb. Res.,* 14:901–914.
21. Born, G. V. R. (1980): Haemodynamic and biochemical interactions in intravascular platelet aggregation. In: *Blood Cells and Vessel Walls: Functional Interactions,* pp. 61–77. Ciba Foundation Symposium Excerpta Medica, Amsterdam.
22. Hamberg, M., Svensson, J., and Samuelsson, B. (1975): Thromboxanes: A new group of biologically active compounds derived from prostaglandin endoperoxides. *Proc. Natl. Acad. Sci. U.S.A.,* 72:2994–2998.
23. Hamberg, M., Svensson, J., and Samuelsson, B. (1974): Prostaglandin endoperoxides: A new concept, concerning the mode of action and release of prostaglandins. *Proc. Natl. Acad. Sci. U.S.A.,* 71:3824–3828.
24. Holmsen, H. (1978): Platelet secretion. Current concepts and methodological aspects. In: *Platelet Function Testing,* edited by H. J. Day, H. Holmsen, and M. B. Zucker, p. 112. DHEW publication no. (NIH) 78–1087.
25. Harker, L. A. (1977): Platelets. In: *Recent Advances in Haematology,* edited by A. V. Hoffbrand, M. C. Brain, and J. Hirsh, pp. 349–373. Churchill Livingstone, London.
26. Mills, D. C. B. (1974): Factors influencing the adenylate cyclase system in human blood platelets. In: *Platelets and Thrombosis,* edited by S. Sherry and A. Scriabine, pp. 45–67. University Park Press, Baltimore.

27. Gerrard, J. M., Peller, J. D., and White, J. G. (1978): The role of cyclic AMP in platelet physiology. In: *Platelet Function Testing,* edited by H. J. Day, H. Holmsen, and M. B. Zucker, p. 552. DHEW publication no. (NIH) 78–1087.

28. Haslam, R. J. (1978): Cyclic nucleotides in platelet function. In: *Platelet Function Testing,* edited by H. J. Day, H. Holmsen, and M. B. Zucker, p. 487. DHEW publication no. (NIH) 78–1087.

29. Salzman, E. W. (1978): Interrelations of prostaglandins and cyclic AMP. In: *Platelet Function Testing,* edited by H. J. Day, H. Holmsen, and M. B. Zucker, p. 513. DHEW publication no. (NIH) 78–1087.

30. Born, G. V. R. (1962): Aggregation of blood platelets by adenosine diphosphate and its reversal. *Nature,* 194:927–929.

31. Seuter, F. (1976): Inhibition of platelet aggregation by acetylsalicylic acid and other inhibitors. *Haemostasis,* 5:85–95.

32. Michal, F., and Born, G. V. R. (1971): Effect of rapid shape change of platelets on the transmission and scattering of light through plasma. *Nature [New Biol.],* 231:220–222.

33. Breddin, K. (1968): *Die Thrombozytenfunktion bei haemorrhagischen Diathesen, Thrombosen, und Gefässkrankheiten.* Schattauer Verlag, Stuttgart.

34. Jäger, W., Kutschera, J., Wendeberg, H., Kauschmann, R., Riese, W., Pietsch, U., Berger, E., and Bennert, C. (1974): Die fortlaufende Messung der Plättchenaggregation ohne Zugabe von Aggregationsauslösern. *Blut,* 29:184–194.

35. Breddin, K., Grun, H., Krzywanek, H. J., and Schremmer, W. P. (1975): Zur Messung der "spontanen" Thrombozytenaggregation. Plättchenaggregationstest III. Methodik. *Klin. Wochenschr.,* 53: 81–89.

36. Breddin, K., Grun, H., Krzywanek, H. J., and Schremmer, W. P. (1976): On the measurement of spontaneous platelet aggregation. The platelet aggregation test. III. Methods and first clinical results. *Thrombos. Haemostas.,* 35:669–691.

37. Wu, K. K., and Hoak, J. C. (1974): A new method for the quantitative detection of platelet aggregates in patients with arterial insufficiency. *Lancet,* 2:924–926.

38. Hellem, A. J. (1960): The adhesiveness of human blood platelets in vitro. *Scand. J. Clin. Lab. Invest.* [*Suppl. 51*], 12:1–117.

39. Salzman, E. W. (1963): Measurement of platelet adhesiveness. A simple in vitro technique demonstrating an abnormality in von Willebrand's disease. *J. Lab. Clin. Med.,* 62:724–735.

40. Day, H. J., Holmsen, H., and Zucker, M. B. (1972): (editors) (1973): *Platelet Function Testing.* DHEW publication no. (NIH) 78–1087.

41. Solis, R. T., Wright, C. B., and Gibbs, M. B. (1972): A model for quantitating in vivo platelet aggregation. *Bibl. Anat.,* 12:223–228.

42. Hornstra, G. (1970): A method for the determination of thrombocyte aggregation in circulating rat blood. *Experientia,* 26:111–112.

43. Broersma, R. J., Dickerson, G. D., and Sullivan, M. S. (1973): The determination of platelet aggregation by filtration pressure in circulating dog blood. *Thromb. Diath. Haemorrh.,* 29:201–210.

44. Jaques, L. B., and Millar, G. J. (1964): Determination of bleeding time in experimental animals. In: *Blood Coagulation, Hemorrhage and Thrombosis,* edited by L. M. Tocantins and L. A. Kazal. Grune & Stratton, New York.

45. Rosenberg, F. J., Phillips, P. G., and Druzba, P. R. (1974): Use of a rabbit extracorporeal shunt in the assay of antithrombotic and thrombotic drugs. In: *Platelets and Thrombosis,* edited by S. Sherry and A. Scriabine, pp. 223–234. University Park Press, Baltimore.

46. Constantine, J. W., Coleman, G. L., and Purcell, I. M. (1972): Inversion of an arterial branch: A technique for inducing thrombosis. *Atherosclerosis,* 16: 31–36.

47. Spilker, B. A., and Van Balken, H. (1973): Formation and embolization of thrombi after electrical stimulation. On the method and evaluation of drugs. *Thromb. Diath. Haemorrh.,* 30:352–362.

48. Callahan, A. B., Lutz, B. R., Fulton, G. P., and Degelman, J. (1960): Smooth muscle and thrombus thresholds to unipolar stimulation of small blood vessels. *Angiology,* 11:35–39.

49. Fleming, J. S., Buchanan, J. O., King, S. P., Cornish, B. T., and Bierwagen, M. E. (1974): Use of the biolaser in the evaluation of antithrombotic agents. In: *Platelets and Thrombosis,* edited by S. Sherry and A. Scriabine, pp. 247–262. University Park Press, Baltimore.

50. Meng, K., and O'Dea, K. (1974): The protective effect of acetylsalicylic acid on laser-induced venous thrombosis in the rat. *Naunyn Schmiedebergs Arch. Pharmacol.,* 283:379–388.

51. Henry, R. L. (1962): Methods for inducing experimental thrombosis. *Angiology,* 13:554–577.

52. Meng, K. (1975): Tierexperimentelle Untersuchungen zur antithrombotischen Wirkung von Acetylsalicylsäure. *Ther. Ber.,* 47:69–79.

53. Meng, K. (1976): Tierexperimentelle Thrombose und Behandlung mit Acetylsalicylsäure. *Med. Welt,* 27:1359–1362.

54. Schmidt, R. (1975): Eine neue Methode zur Erzeugung von Thromben durch Unterkühlung der Gefässwand und ihre Anwendung zur Prüfung von Acetylsalicylsäure und Heparin. Inaugural dissertation, Giessen.

55. Meng, K., and Seuter, F. (1977): Effect of acetylsalicylic acid on experimentally induced arterial thrombosis in rats. *Naunyn Schmiedebergs Arch. Pharmacol.,* 301:115–119.

56. Seuter, F., Busse, W.-D., Meng, K., Hoffmeister, F., Möller, E., and Horstmann, H. (1979): The antithrombotic activity of BAY g 6575. *Arzneim. Forsch.,* 29:54–59.

57. Seuter, F., Meng, K., and Busse, W.-D. (1979): Effect of antithrombotic drugs on experimental thrombosis. *Thrombos. Haemostas.,* 42:211 (abstract).

58. Mayer, J. E., and Hammond, G. L. (1973): Dipyridamole and aspirin tested against an experimental model of thrombosis. *Ann. Surg.* 178:108–112.

59. Philip, R. B., Schacham, P., and Gowdey, C. W. (1971): Involvement of platelets and microthrombi

in experimental decompression sickness: Similarities with disseminated intravascular coagulation. *Aerosp. Med.*, 42:494–502.

60. Aster, R. H., and Jandl, J. H. (1964): Platelet sequestration in man. I. Methods. *J. Clin. Invest.*, 43:843–855.

61. Harker, L. A., Slichter, S. J., Scott, C. R., and Ross, R. (1974): Homocysteinemia: Vascular injury and arterial thrombosis. *N. Engl. J. Med.*, 291:537–543.

62. Silver, M. J., Hoch, W., Kocsis, J. J., Ingerman, C. M., and Smith, J. B. (1974): Arachidonic acid causes sudden death in rabbits. *Science*, 183:1085–1087.

63. Seuter, F., and Busse, W.-D. (1979): Arachidonic acid induced mortality in animals—an appropriate model for the evaluation of antithrombotic drugs? In: *Arachidonic Acid Metabolism in Inflammation and Thrombosis*, edited by K. Brune and M. Baggiolini, pp. 175–183. Birkhäuser, Basel.

64. Moncada, S., Gryglewski, R. J., Bunting, S., and Vane, J. R. (1976): An enzyme isolated from arteries transforms prostaglandin endoperoxides to an unstable substance that inhibits platelet aggregation. *Nature*, 263:663–665.

65. Gryglewski, R. J., Bunting, S., Moncada, S., Flower, R. J., and Vane, J. R. (1976): Arterial walls are protected against deposition of platelet thrombi by a substance (prostaglandin X) which they make from prostaglandin endoperoxides. *Prostaglandins*, 12:685–713.

66. Needleman, P. (1979): Prostacyclin in blood vessel-platelet interactions: Perspectives and questions. *Nature*, 279–14–15.

67. Baenziger, N. L., Becherer, P. R., and Majerus, P. W. (1979): Characterization on prostacyclin synthesis in cultured human arterial smooth muscle cells, venous endothelial cells and skin fibroblasts. *Cell*, 16:967–974.

68. Salmon, J. A., Mullane, K. M., Dusting, G. J., Moncada, S., and Vane, J. R. (1979): Elimination of prostacyclin (PGI$_2$) and 6-oxo-PGF$_{1\alpha}$ in anaesthetized dogs. *J. Pharm. Pharmacol.*, 31:529–532.

69. Gryglewski, R. J. (1978): A new circulatory hormone: Prostacyclin. *Bull. Acad. R. Med. Belg.*, 133:470–477.

70. Vane, J. R., and Moncada, S. (1980): Prostacyclin. In: *Blood Cells and Vessel Walls: Functional Interactions*, pp. 79–97. Ciba Foundation Symposium Excerpta Medica, Amsterdam.

71. Steer, M. L., MacIntyre, D. E., Levine, L., and Salzman, E. W. (1980): Is prostacyclin a physiologically important circulating anti-platelet agent? *Nature*, 283:194–195.

72. Baenziger, N. L., Dillender, M. J., and Majerus, P. W. (1977): Cultured human skin fibroblasts and arterial cells produce a labile platelet-inhibitory prostaglandin. *Biochem. Biophys. Res. Commun.*, 78:294–301.

73. Livio, M., Villa, S., and de Gaetano, G. (1978): Aspirin, thromboxane and prostacyclin in rats: A dilemma resolved? *Lancet*, 1:1307.

74. Jaffe, E. A., and Weksler, B. B. (1979): Recovery of endothelial cell. Prostacyclin production after in-

hibition by low doses of aspirin. *J. Clin. Invest.*, 63:532–535.

75. Burch, J. W., Baenziger, N. L., Stanford, N., and Majerus, P. W. (1978): Sensitivity of fatty acid cyclooxygenase from human aorta to acetylation by aspirin. *Proc. Natl. Acad. Sci. U.S.A.*, 75:5181–5184.

76. O'Grady, J., and Moncada, S. (1978): Aspirin: A paradoxical effect on bleeding-time. *Lancet*, 2:780.

77. Jobin, F. (1978): Acetylsalicylic acid, hemostasis and human thromboembolism. *Seminars in Thrombosis and Hemostasis*, 4:199–240.

78. Rajah, S. M., Penny, A., and Kester, R. (1978): Aspirin and bleeding-time. *Lancet*, 2:1104.

79. Godal, H. C., Eika, C., Dybdahl, J. H., Daae, L., and Larsen, S. (1979): Aspirin and bleeding-time. *Lancet*, 1:1236.

80. Kikugawa, K., Iizuka, K., Higuchi, Y., Hirayama, H., and Ichino, M. (1972): Platelet aggregation inhibitors. 2. Inhibition of platelet aggregation by 5'-, 2-, 6-, and 8-substituted adenosines. *J. Med. Chem.*, 15:387–390.

81. MacKenzie, R. D., and Blohm, T. R. (1971): Effects of *N*-(2-diethylaminoethyl)-*N*-(2-hydroxy-2-phenylethyl)-2,5-dichloroaniline (AN 162) on platelet function and blood coagulation. *Thromb. Diath. Haemorrh.*, 26:577–587.

82. Muirhead, C. R. (1973): The filter loop technique as a method of measuring platelet aggregation in the flowing blood of the rat; the inhibitory activity of 5-oxo-1-cyclopentene-1-heptanoic acid (AY 16,804) on platelet aggregation. *Thromb. Diath. Haemorrh.*, 30:138–147.

83. Seuter, F., Busse, W.-D., Hörlein, U., Böshagen, H., Hoffmeister, F., and Philipp, E. (1979): BAY i 7351, a new platelet inhibitor, and antithrombotic compound. *Thrombos. Haemostas.*, 42:368 (abstract).

84. Busse, W.-D., and Seuter, F., Hörlein, U., Böshagen, H., Hoffmeister, F., and Philipp, E. (1979): Inhibition of thromboxane synthesis and other platelet functions by BAY i 7351, a new antithrombotic compound. *Thrombos. Haemostas.*, 42:213 (abstract).

85. Kovacs, I. B., Csalay, L., and Csakvary, G. (1971): Antithrombotic and fibrinolytic effect of bencyclane. *Arzneim. Forsch.*, 21:1553–1556.

86. Jäger, W., Scharrer, I., Satkowski, U., and Breddin, K. (1975): Thrombozytenaggregationshemmende Wirkung von Bencyclan in vitro und in vivo. *Arzneim. Forsch.*, 25:1938–1944.

87. Ponari, O., Civardi, E., Dettori, A. G., Megha, A., Poti, R., and Bulletti, G. (1976): In vitro effects of bencyclan on coagulation, fibrinolysis and platelet function. *Arzneim. Forsch.*, 26:1532–1538.

88. Ambrus, J. L., Ambrus, C. M., Gastpar, H., Sapvento, P. J., Weber, F. J., and Thurber, L. E. (1976): Study of platelet aggregation in vivo. I. Effect of bencyclan. *J. Med. (Basel)*, 7:439–447.

89. Rieger, H., Klose, H. J., Schmid-Schönbein, H., and Wurzinger, L. (1978): The effect of orally administered bencyclane on spontaneous platelet aggregation (PA) as a function of bencyclane concentration in coded samples. *Thromb. Res.*, 12:353–356.

90. Kang, A. H., Beachey, F. H., and Katzman, R. L. (1974): The effect of benorylate on collagen-induced

platelet aggregation. *Scand. J. Rheum.*, 3:126–128.

91. Fleming, J. S., Buyniski, J. P., and Bierwagen, M. E. (1974): Use of in vivo animal models in the evaluation of antithrombotic agents. *Circulation* [*Suppl. III*], 50:300.

92. Beverung, W. N., and Partyka, R. A. (1975): 6-Methyl-1,2,3,5-tetrahydroimidazo[2,1-*b*]quinazolin-2-one, a potent inhibitor of ADP-induced platelet aggregation. *J. Med. Chem.*, 18:224–225.

93. Fleming, J. S., Buchanan, J. O., and Buyniski, J. P. (1976): The effect of a potent inhibitor of platelet aggregation, BL-3459, on adrenaline-induced myocardial necrosis in beagle dogs. *Eur. J. Pharmacol.*, 40:57–62.

94. Fleming, J. S., Buyniski, J. P., Cavanagh, R. L., and Bierwagen, M. E. (1975): Pharmacology of a potent, new antithrombotic agent, 6-methyl-1,2,3,5-tetrahydroimidazo[2,1*b*]quinazolin-2-one hydrochloride monohydrate (BL-3459). *J. Pharmacol. Exp. Ther.*, 194:435.

95. Fleming, J. S., and Buyniski, J. P. (1979): A potent new inhibitor of platelet aggregation and experimental thrombosis, Anagrelide (BL-4162 A). *Thromb. Res.*, 15:373–388.

96. Resag, K., Melzer, G., and Nitz, R. E. (1976): Untersuchungen zur Hemmung der Thrombozytenaggregation durch Carbochromen. *Arzneim. Forsch.*, 26:209–213.

97. Woyke, M., Cwajda, H., and Wojcicki, J. (1978): Platelet aggregation and adhesiveness as well as blood lipids level in dogs treated with di-(1-isoquinolinyl)-di-(pyridyl-2)-butane and carbocromen. *Pol. J. Pharmacol. Pharm.*, 30:77–81.

98. Minsker, D. H., Jordan, P. T., and MacMillan, A. (1974): Inhibition of platelet aggregation by cyproheptadine. In: *Platelets and Thrombosis*, edited by S. Sherry and A. Scriabine, pp. 161–176. University Park Press, Baltimore.

99. Stone, C. A., Wenger, H. C., Ludden, C. T., Stavorski, J. M., and Ross, C. A. (1961): Antiserotonin-antihistamine properties of cyproheptadine. *J. Pharmacol. Exp. Ther.*, 131:73–84.

100. Gaut, Z. N. (1973): Binding of cyproheptadine (*N*-methyl-^{14}C) by human blood platelets: Inhibition by phenothiazines and tricyclic antidepressants. *J. Pharmacol. Exp. Ther.*, 185:171–176.

101. Aledort, L. M., Taub, R., Burrows, E., Leiter, E., Glabman, S., Haimov, M., Nirmul, G., and Berger, S. (1974): Use of inhibitors of platelet function in renal rejection phenomena. In: *Platelets and Thrombosis*, edited by S. Sherry and A. Scriabine, pp. 263–271. University Park Press, Baltimore.

102. Ross, J. N., Brown, C. H., Harness, M. K., Greenberg, D., Tacker, M. M., and Kennedy, J. H. (1974): Role of platelet aggregation in prolonged extracorporeal respiratory support. *Circulation* [*Suppl. II*], 49–50:219–235.

103. Emmons, P. R., Harrison, M. J. G., Honour, A. J., and Mitchell, J. R. A. (1965): Effect of dipyridamole on human platelet behavior. *Lancet*, 2:603–606.

104. Didisheim, P. (1968): Inhibition by dipyridamole of arterial thrombosis in rats. *Thromb. Diath. Haemorrh.*, 20:257–266.

105. Griguer, P., Brochier, M., and Raynaud, R. (1975): Etude de l'effet inhibiteur du dipyridamole sur l'adhésivite et l'agregation plaquettaires "in vitro" et "in vivo." *Ann. Cardiol. Angeiol.* (*Paris*) [*Suppl.*], 24:2–36.

106. Rifkin, P. L., and Zucker, M. B. (1973): The effect of dipyridamole and RA 233 on human platelet function in vitro. *Thromb. Diath. Haemorrh.*, 29:694–700.

107. Holmes, I. B., Smith, G. M., and Freuler, F. (1977): The effect of intravenous adenosine diphosphate on the number of circulating platelets in experimental animals: Inhibition by prostaglandin E₁, dipyridamole, SH-869 and VK-774. *Thrombos. Haemostas.*, 37:36–46.

108. Philp, R. B., Francey, I., and McElroy, F. (1973): Effects of dipyridamole and five related agents on human platelet aggregation and adenosine uptake. *Thromb. Res.*, 3:35–50.

109. Smith, J. B., and Mills, D. C. B. (1970): Inhibition of adenosine 3′5′ cyclic monophosphate phosphodiesterase. *Biochem. J.*, 120:20.

110. Ambrus, J. L., Ambrus, C. M., and Gastpar, H. (1978): Studies on platelet aggregation in vivo. VI. Effect of a pyrimido-pyrimidine derivative (RA 233) on tumor cell metastasis. *J. Med.* (*Basel*), 9:183–186.

111. Elkeles, R. S., Hampton, J. R., Honour, A. J., Mitchell, J. R. A., and Prichard, J. S. (1968): Effect of a pyrimido-pyrimidine compound on platelet behavior in vitro and in vivo. *Lancet*, 2:751–754.

112. Caprino, L., Borrelli, F., and Falchetti, R. (1973): Effect of 4,5-diphenyl-2-*bis*-(2-hydroxyethyl)aminoxazol (ditazol) on platelet aggregation, adhesiveness and bleeding time. *Arzneim. Forsch.*, 23:1277–1283.

113. Caprino, L., Borrelli, F., Falchetti, R., Cafiero, C., and Gandolfo, G. M. (1977): Ditazole activity and its interaction with urokinase on experimental thrombosis. *Haemostasis*, 6:310–317.

114. de Gaetano, G., Tonolli, M. C., Bertoni, M. P., and Roncaglioni, M. C. (1977): Ditazole and platelets. I. Effect of ditazole on human platelet function in vitro. *Haemostasis*, 6:127–136.

115. de Gaetano, G., Cavenaghi, A. E., and Stella, L. (1977): Ditazole and platelets. II. Effect of ditazole on in vivo platelet aggregation and bleeding time in rats. *Haemostasis*, 6:190–196.

116. Mari, D., Cattaneo, M., Gattinoni, A., and Dioguardi, N. (1977): Thrombogenicity of an artificial surface is decreased by the antiplatelet agent ditazol. *Thromb. Res.*, 12:59–66.

117. Jacobi, E., Leopold, G., Lissner, R., and Maisenbacher, J. (1978): Human-pharmacological investigations on the platelet adhesiveness- and aggregation-inhibiting effect of EMD 26644, and oxazolyl-thio-propionic acid derivative. *Int. J. Clin. Pharmacol.*, 16:136–141.

118. Nishizawa, F. E., Wynalda, D. J., Suydam, D. E., and Molony, B. A. (1973): Flurbiprofen, a new potent inhibitor of platelet aggregation. *Thromb. Res.*, 3:577–588.

119. Cremoncini, C., Vignati, E., Valente, C., and Dossena, M. G. (1977): Platelet adhesiveness, thromboelastogram, prothrombin activity and partial

thromboplastin time during treatment with flurbiprofen. *Curr. Med. Res. Opin.,* 5:135–140.

120. Desnoyers, P., Labaume, J., Anstett, M., Herrera, M., Pesquet, J., and Sebastien, J. (1972): The pharmacology of S-1702, a new highly effective oral antidiabetic drug with unusual properties. Part III. Antistickiness activity, fibrinolytic properties and hemostatic parameters study. *Arzneim. Forsch.,* 22:1691–1695.

121. Vainer, H., and Verry, M. (1974): Effets "in vitro" du gliclazide, nouvel agent hypoglycemiant, sur les plaquettes humanines normales. *Thromb. Res.* 4:523–538.

122. Jobin, F., and Gagnon, F. T. (1971): Inhibition of human platelet aggregation by a dibenzazepine compound (GP 44296) and by *N*-(2,6-dichlorophenyl)-*o*-aminophenylacetic acid (GP 45840). *Can. J. Physiol. Pharmacol.,* 49:479–481.

123. Carter, A. E., Eban, R., and Perzett, R. D. (1971): Prevention of post-operative deep venous thrombosis and pulmonary embolism. *Br. Med. J.,* 1:312–314.

124. Tremoli, E., Maderna, P., Cocuzza, E., and Mantero, O. (1979): Platelet antiaggregating activity of imolamine: *In vitro* studies. *Pharmacol. Res. Commun.,* 11:31.

125. Di Perri, T., Vittoria, A., and Laghi Pasini, F. (1979): Inhibition of platelet aggregation by a new synthetic compound: 2-(*p*-oxo-2-isoindolinyl)phenyl]butyric acid (K 3920). *Arzneim. Forsch.,* 29:104–106.

126. Umetsu, T., and Kato, T. (1978): Effect of KC-6141 on rabbit platelet aggregation in vitro and rat platelet retention. *Thrombos. Haemostas.,* 39:167.

127. Umetsu, T., and Sanai, K. (1978): Effect of KC-6141, an anti-aggregating compound on experimental thrombosis in rats. *Thrombos. Haemostas.,* 39:74–83.

128. Fregnan, G. B. (1972): The inhibitory effect of metergoline (an anti-5-hydroxytryptaminic agent) on rabbit platelet aggregation. *Pharmacology,* 7:115–125.

129. Damas, J., and Deby, C. (1976): Correlation between inhibition by anti-inflammatory substances of arachidonic acid-induced hypotension and of prostaglandin biosynthesis in vitro. *Biochem. Pharmacol.,* 25:981–985.

130. Gryglewski, R. J. (1978): Screening for inhibitors of prostaglandin and thromboxane biosynthesis. In: *Advances in Lipid Research, Vol. 16,* edited by R. Paoletti and D. Kritchevsky. Academic Press, New York.

131. Gryglewski, R. J., Korbut, R., Ocetkiewicz, A., and Stachura, J. (1978): In vivo method for quantitation of anti-platelet potency of drugs. *Naunyn Schmiedebergs Arch. Pharmacol.,* 302:25–30.

132. Rossi, E. C., and Levin, N. W. (1973): Inhibition of primary ADP-induced platelet aggregation in normal subjects after administration of nitrofurantoin (Furadantin). *J. Clin. Invest.,* 52:2457–2467.

133. Hidaka, H., Hayashi, H., Kohri, H., Kimura, Y., Hosokawa, T., Igawa, T., and Saitoh, Y. (1979): Selective inhibitor of platelet cyclic adenosine monophosphate phosphodiesterase, cilostamide, inhibits platelet aggregation. *J. Pharmacol. Exp. Ther.,* 211:26–30.

134. Blackwell, G. J., and Flower, F. J. (1978): 1-Phenyl-3-pyrazolidone: An inhibitor of cyclo-oxygenase and lipoxygenase pathways in lung and platelets. *Prostaglandins,* 16:417–425.

135. Asano, T., Ochiai, Y., and Hidaka, H. (1977): Selective inhibition of separated forms of human platelet cyclic nucleotide phosphodiesterase by platelet aggregation inhibitors. *Mol. Pharmacol.,* 13:400–406.

136. Tanaka, K., Harada, Y., and Katori, M. (1979): EG-626: Not a thromboxane A₂ antagonist, but a PGI₂ potentiator in platelet aggregation. *Prostaglandins,* 17:235–237.

137. Shimamoto, T., Takashima, Y., Kobayashi, M., Moriya, K., and Takabashi, T. (1976): A thromboxane A₂-antagonistic effect of pyridinolcarbamate and phthalazinol. *Proc. Jpn. Academy,* 52:591.

138. Holmes, I. B. (1977): A comparison of the effect of proquazone, a new non-steroidal antiinflammatory compound, and acetylsalicylic acid on blood platelet function, in vitro and in vivo. *Arch. Int. Pharmacodyn. Thor.,* 228:136–152.

139. N. N. (1972): Pyridimolcarbamat. *Wiener Klin. Wochenschr.,* 84:200–201.

140. MacKenzie, R. D. (1974): New pharmacological approaches to inhibition of platelet aggregation. In: *Platelets and Thrombosis,* edited by S. Sherry and A. Scriabine, pp. 235–246. University Park Press, Baltimore.

141. MacKenzie, R. D., Blohm, T. R., and Steinbach, J. M. (1972): Effects in vivo of α-[*p*-(fluoren-9-ylidenemethyl)phenyl]-2-piperidineethanol (RMI 10, 393) on platelet aggregation and blood coagulation. *Biochem. Pharmacol.,* 21:707–717.

142. Constantine, J. W., and Purcell, I. M. (1973): Inhibition of platelet aggregation and of experimental thrombosis by sudoxicam. *J. Pharmacol. Exp. Ther.,* 187:653–665.

143. Green, D., Given, K. M., Ts'ao, C., Whippie, J. P., and Rossi, E. C. (1977): The effect of a new nonsteroidal anti-inflammatory agent, sulindac, on platelet function. *Thromb. Res.,* 1:283–289.

144. Minsker, D. H., Jordan, P., Ling, P., and Welch, T. (1977): The effect of sulindac and sulindac metabolites on arachinonate-induced lethality in rabbits; effect on human, guinea pig, dog, and rat platelet activity. *Thromb. Res.,* 11:217–226.

145. Roba, J., Claeys, M., and Lambelin. G. (1976): Antiplatelet and antithrombogenic effect of suloctidil. *Eur. J. Pharmacol.,* 37:265–274.

146. Gurewich, W., and Lipinski, B. (1976): Evaluation of antithrombotic properties of suloctidil in comparison with aspirin and dipyridamole. *Thromb. Res.,* 9:101–108.

147. de Gaetano, G., Miragliotta, G., Roncuccu, R., Lansen, J., and Lambelin, G. (1976): Suloctidil: A novel inhibitor of platelet aggregation in human beings. (1). *Thromb. Res.,* 8:361–371.

148. Roba, J., Bourgain, R. Andries. R., Claeys, M., van Opstal, W., and Lambelin, G. (1976): Antagonism by suloctidil of arterial thrombus formation in rats. *Thromb. Res.,* 9:585–594.

149. de Clerck, F., Vermylen, J., and Reneman, R.

(1975): Effects of suprofen, an inhibitor of prostaglandin biosynthesis, on platelet function, plasma
coagulation and fibrinolysis. I. In vitro experiments.
Arch. Int. Pharmacodyn. Ther., 216:263–279.

150. Thebault, J. J., Blatrix, C. E., Blanchard, J. F., and
Panak, E. A. (1975): Effects of ticlopidine, a new
platelet aggregation inhibitor in man. *Clin. Pharmacol. Ther.*, 18:485–490.

151. Thebault, J. J., Blatrix, C. E., Blanchard, J. F., and
Panak, E. A. (1977): The interactions of ticlopidine
and aspirin in normal subjects. *J. Int. Med. Res.*,
5:405–411.

152. Tomikawa, M., Ashida, S., Kakihats, K., and Abiko,
Y. (1978): Anti-thrombotic action of ticlopidine, a
new platelet aggregation inhibitor. *Thromb. Res.*,
12:1157–1164.

153. Ashida, S., and Abiko, Y. (1978): Inhibition of platelet aggregation by a new agent, ticlopidine. *Thrombos. Haemostas.*, 40:542–550.

154. Ashida, S. I., and Abiko, Y. (1979): Mode of action
of ticlopidine in inhibition of platelet aggregation
in the rat. *Thrombos. Haemostas.*, 41:436–449.

155. David, J. L., Monfort, F., Herion, F., and Raskinet,
R. (1979): Compared effects of three dose-levels of
ticlopidine on platelet function in normal subjects.
Thromb. Res., 14:35–49.

156. Kreiskott, H., and Hofmann, H. P. (1973): Tierexperimentelle Untersuchungen zur Hemmung der
Thrombozytenaggregation durch Verapamil in vitro
und in vivo. *Arzneim. Forsch.*, 23:1555–1560.

157. Lecrubier, C., Uzan, A., and Samama, M. (1972):
Action in vitro d'un nouveau vasodilatateur céré-
bral, viquidil, sur l'agrégation des plaquettes san-
guines. *Arzneim. Forsch.*, 22:1334–1336.

158. Sixma, J. J., and Trieschnigg, A. M. (1971): The
inhibition of the function of human blood platelets
in vitro by VK 744. *Acta Med. Scand. [Suppl. 525]*,
237.

159. Slater, S. D., Turpie, A. G. G., Douglas, A. S.,
and McNicol, G. P. (1972): Effect in vitro on platelet
function of two compounds developed from the py-
rimido-pyrimidines. *J. Clin. Pathol.*, 25:427–432.

160. Sixma, J. J., Trieschnigg, A. M. C., de Graaf, S.,
and Bouma, B. N. (1972): In vivo inhibition of human platelet function by VK 744. *Scand. J. Haematol.*, 9:226–230.

161. Philp, R. B., Francey, I., and Warren, B. A. (1978):
Comparison of antithrombotic activity of heparin,
ASA, sulfinpyrazone and VK 744 in a rat model
of arterial thrombosis. *Haemostasis*, 7:282–293.

162. Ten Cate, J. W., Gerritsen, J., and Van Geet-Wei-
jers, J. (1972): In vitro and in vivo experiences with
VK 774. A new platelet function inhibitor. *Pathol.
Biol. (Paris) [Suppl.]*, 20:76–81.

163. Fenichel, R. L., Dougherty, J.-A., and Alburn,
H. E. (1974): Inhibition of platelet aggregation by
2-(p-chlorophenyl)-4-thiazoleacrylic acid (WY-
23,049)-comparison with acetylsalicylic acid. *Biochem. Pharmacol.*, 23:3273–3282.

164. Nakanishi, M., Imamura, H., and Goto, K. (1971):
Potentiation of the ADP-induced platelet aggregation by collagen and its inhibition by a tetrahydrothienopyridine derivative (Y-3642). *Biochem. Pharmacol.*, 20:2116–2118.

165. de Gaetano, G., Donati, M. B., and Garattini, S.
(1975): Drugs affecting platelet function tests. Their
effects on haemostasis and surgical bleeding.
Thromb. Diath. Haemorrh., 34:285–297.

166. Weiss, H. J., Aledort, L. M., and Kochwa, S. (1968):
The effect of salicylates on the hemostatic properties
of platelets in man. *J. Clin. Invest.*, 47:2169–2180.

167. Rosenberg, F. J., Gimber-Phillips, P. E., Groblew-
ski, G. E., Davison, C., Phillips, D. K., Goralnick,
S. J., and Canhill, E. D. (1971): Acetylsalicylic acid:
Inhibition of platelet aggregation in the rabbit. *J.
Pharmacol. Exp. Ther.*, 179:410–418.

168. Mustard, J. F., and Packham, M. A. (1975): Platelets, thrombosis and drugs. *Drugs*, 9:19–76.

169. Weiss, H. J. (1976): Antiplatelet drugs—a new pharmacologic approach to the prevention of thrombosis.
Am. Heart J., 92:86–102.

170. Baumgartner, H. R. (1977): Wirkungsmechanismen
von Plättcheninhibitoren. *Ther. Umsch.*, 34:341–
346.

171. Tsu, E. C. (1978): Antiplatelet drugs in arterial
thrombosis: A review. *Am. J. Hosp. Pharm.*, 35:
1507–1515.

172. Al-Mondhiry, H., Marcus, A. J., and Spaet, T. H.
(1970): On the mechanism of platelet function inhibition by acetylsalicylic acid. *Proc. Soc. Exp. Biol.
Med.*, 133:632–636.

173. Willis, A. L. (1974): An enzymatic mechanism for
the antithrombotic and antihemostatic actions of aspirin. *Science*, 183:325–327.

174. Hamberg, M., Svensson, J., and Samuelsson, B.
(1974): Mechanism of antiaggregating effect of aspirin on human platelets. *Lancet*, 2:223–224.

175. Bailey, J. M., Bryant, R. W., Feinmark, S. J., Mak-
heja, A. N. (1977): Differential separation of thromboxanes from prostaglandins by one and two-dimen-
sional thin layer chromatography. *Prostaglandins*,
13:479–392.

176. Baumgartner, H. R., and Muggli, R. (1974): Effect
of acetylsalicylic acid on platelet adhesion to suben-
dothelium and the formation of mural thrombi.
Thromb. Diath. Haemorrh. [Suppl.], 60:345.

177. Cazenave, J. P., Kinlough-Rathbone, L., Packham,
M. A., and Mustard, J. F. (1978): The effect of
acetylsalicylic acid and indomethacin on rabbit
platelet adherence to collagen and the subendothe-
lium in the presence of a low or high hematocrit.
Thromb. Res., 13:971–981.

178. Rosenberg, F. J., Gimber-Phillips, P. E., Groblew-
ski, G. E., Davison, C., and Phillips, D. K. (1971):
Acetylsalicylic acid: Inhibition of platelet aggregation in the rabbit. *J. Pharmacol. Exp. Ther.*, 179:
410–418.

179. Seuter, F.: Unpublished results.

180. O'Brien, J. R. (1968): Effect of antiinflammatory
agents on platelets. *Lancet*, 1:894–895.

181. Prancan, A. V., Lefort, J., Chignard, M., Gerozissis,
K., Dray, F., and Vargaftig, B. B. (1979): L 8027
and 1-nonylimidazole as non selective inhibitors of
thromboxane synthesis. *Eur. J. Pharmacol.*, 60:287–
297.

182. Danese, C. A., Voleti, C. D., and Weiss, H. J. (1971):
Protection by aspirin against experimentally induced

thrombosis in dogs. *Thromb. Diath. Haemorrh.*, 25:288–296.

183. Ali, M., and McDonald, J. W. D. (1977): Effects of sulfinpyrazone on platelet prostaglandin synthesis and platelet release of serotonin. *J. Lab. Clin. Med.*, 89:868–875.

184. Sacle, P., Battock, D., and Genton, E. (1975): Effects of clofibrate and sulfinpyrazone on platelet survival time in coronary artery disease. *Circulation*, 52:473–476.

185. Mustard, J. F., Murphy, E. A., Robinson, G. A., Rowsell, H. C., Ozge, A., and Crookston, J. H. (1964): Blood platelet survival. *Thromb. Diath. Haemorrh.* [*Suppl.*], 13:245–275.

186. Weily, H. S., and Genton, E. (1970): Altered platelet function in patients with prosthetic mitral valves: Effects of sulfinpyrazone therapy. *Circulation*, 42:967–972.

187. Herrmann, R. G., and Lacefield, W. B. (1974): Effect of antithrombotic drugs on in vivo experimental thrombosis. In: *Platelets and Thrombosis*, edited by S. Sherry, and A. Scriabine, pp. 203–221. University Park Press, Baltimore.

188. Packham, M. A., Jenkins, C. S. P., Kinlough-Rathbone, R. L., and Mustard, J. F. (1971): Agents influencing platelet adhesion to surfaces and the release reaction. *Circulation* [*Suppl. 2*], 44:67 (abstract).

189. Davies, J. A., and Menys, V. C. (1979): Effect of sulphinpyrazone (SP) aspirin (ASA) and dipyridamole (DP) on platelet-vessel wall interaction after oral administration to rabbits. *Thrombos. Haemostas.*, 42:197.

190. Kaegi, A., Pineo, G. F., Shimizu, A., Trivedi, H., Hirsch, J., and Gent, M. (1974): Arteriovenous shunt thrombosis. Prevention by sulfinpyrazone. *N. Engl. J. Med.*, 290:304–306.

191. Didisheim, P. T., and Fuster, V. (1978): Actions and clinical status of platelet-suppressive agents. *Semin. Hematol.*, 15:55–72.

192. Mills, D. C. B., and Smith, J. B. (1971): The influence on platelet aggregation of drugs that affect the accumulation of adenosine $3',5'$-cyclic monophosphate in platelets. *Biochem. J.*, 121:185–196.

193. Rozenberg, M. C., and Walker, C. M. (1973): The effect of pyrimidine compounds on the potentiation of adenosine inhibition of aggregation, on adenosine phosphorylation and phosphodiesterase activity of blood platelets. *Br. J. Haematol.*, 24:409–418.

194. Moncada, S., and Korbut, R. (1978): Dipyridamole and other phosphodiesterase inhibitors act as antithrombotic agents by potentiating endogenous prostacyclin. *Lancet*, 1:1286–1289.

195. Buchanan, M. R., Rosenfeld,, J., and Hirsch, J. (1978): The prolonged effect of sulfinpyrazone on collagen-induced platelet aggregation in vivo. *Thromb. Res.*, 13:883–892.

196. Horch, U., et al. (1970): Pharmacology of dipyridamole and its derivatives. *Thromb. Diath. Haemorrh.* [*Suppl.*], 42:253–266.

197. Bunag, R. D., Douglas, C. R., Imai, S., and Berne, R. M. (1963): In vitro inhibition of adenosine deaminase by persantin. *Fed. Proc.*, 22:642.

198. Born, G. V. R., and Mills, D. C. (1969): Potentiation of the inhibitory effect of adenosine on platelet aggregation by drugs that prevent its uptake. *J. Physiol.* (*Lond.*), 202:41.

199. Subbarao, L., Ricinsky, B., Rausch, M. A., et al. (1977): Binding of dipyridamole to human platelets and to alpha 1 acid glycoprotein and its significance for the inhibition of adenosine uptake. *J. Clin. Invest.*, 60:936–943.

200. Cucuianu, M. P., Nishizawa, E. E., and Mustard, J. F. (1971): Effect of pyrimidopyrimidine compounds on platelet function. *J. Lab. Clin. Med.*, 77:958–974.

201. McElroy, F. A., and Philp, R. B. (1975): Relative potencies of dipyridamole and related agents as inhibitors of cyclic nucleotide phosphodiesterases: Possible explanation of mechanism of inhibition of platelet function. *Life Sci.*, 17:1479–1494.

202. Didisheim, P., and Owen, C. A. (1970): Effect of dipyridamole (Persantin®) and its derivatives on thrombosis and platelet function. *Thromb. Diath. Haemorrh.* [*Suppl.*], 42:267–275.

203. Niewiarowski, S., Lukasiewicz, H., Nath, N., and Sha, A. T. (1975): Inhibition of human platelet aggregation by dipyridamole and two related compounds and its modification by acid glycoproteins of human plasma. *J. Lab. Clin. Med.*, 86:64–76.

204. Harker, L. A., and Slichter, S. J. (1974): Arterial and venous thromboembolism: Kinetic characterization and evaluation of therapy. *Thromb. Diath. Haemorrh.*, 31:188–203.

205. Harker, L. A., and Slichter, S. J. (1970): Studies of platelet and fibrinogen kinetics in patients with prosthetic heart valves. *N. Engl. J. Med.*, 283:1302–1305.

206. Philp, R. B., and Lemieux, V. (1968): Comparison of some effects of dipyridamole and adenosine on thrombus formation, platelet adhesiveness and blood pressure in rabbits and rats. *Nature*, 218:1072–1074.

207. Harker, L. A., and Slichter, S. J. (1972): Platelet and fibrinogen consumption in man. *N. Engl. J. Med.*, 287:1000–1005.

208. Frishman, W. H., Weksler, B., Christodoulou, J. P., Smithen, C., and Killip, T. (1974): Reversal of abnormal platelet aggregability and change in exercise tolerance in patients with angina pectoris following oral propranolol. *Circulation*, 50:887–896.

209. Glusa, E., Markwardt, F., and Stürzebecher, J. (1974): Effects of sodium nitroprusside and other pentacyanonitrosyl complexes on platelet aggregation. *Haemostasis*, 3:249–256.

210. Philp, R. B., Francey, I., and Warren, B. A. (1978): Comparison of antithrombotic activity of heparin, ASA, sulfinpyrazone and VK 744 in a rat model of arterial thrombosis. *Haemostasis*, 7:282–293.

211. Villa, S., and de Gaetano, G. (1979): Aspirin, dipyridamole, prostacyclin (PGI_2) and bleeding time in rats. *Thrombos. Haemostas.*, 42:242.

212. Masotti, G., Poggesi, L., Galanti, G., and Neri Serneri, G. G. (1979): Stimulation of prostacyclin by dipyridamole. *Lancet*, 1:1412.

213. Di Minno, G., Silver, M. J., and de Gaetano, G. (1979): Ingestion of dipyridamole reduces inhibitory effect of prostacyclin on human platelets. *Lancet*, 2:701–702.

214. Di Minno, G., de Gaetano, G., and Silver, M. J.

(1979): Dipyridamole (D) reduces the effectiveness of prostaglandin (PG)I$_2$, PGD$_2$ and PGE$_1$ as inhibitors of platelet aggregation in human platelet-rich plasma (PRP). *Thrombos. Haemostas.*, 42:198.

215. Pedersen, A. K. (1978): Dipyridamole and platelet aggregation. *Lancet*, 2:270.

216. Horrobin, D. F., Ally, A. I., and Manku, M. S. (1978): Dipyridamole and platelet aggregation. *Lancet*, 2:270.

217. Best, L. C., Martin, T. J., McGuire, M. B., Preston, F. E., Russell, R. G. G., and Segal, D. S. (1978): Dipyridamole and platelet function. *Lancet*, 2: 846.

218. Ally, A. I., Manku, M. S., Horrobin, D. F., et al. (1977): Dipyridamole: A possible potent inhibitor of thromboxane A$_2$ synthetase in vascular smooth muscle. *Prostaglandins*, 14:607–609.

219. Best, L. C., McGuire, M. B., Jones, P. B. B., Holland, T. K., Martin, T. J., Preston, F. E., Segal, D. S., and Russel, R. G. B. (1979): Mode of action of dipyridamole of human platelets. *Thromb. Res.*, 16:367–379.

220. Moncada, S., Flower, R. F., and Russell-Smith, N. R. (1978): Dipyridamole and platelet function. *Lancet*, 2:1257–1258.

221. Neri Serneri, G. G., Gensini, G. F., Abbate, R., Favilla, S., and Laureano, R. (1979): Modulation by diypridamole of the arachidonic acid metabolic pathway in platelets. An in vivo and in vitro study. *Thrombos. Haemostas.*, 42:197.

222. Busse, W.-D. (1980): Personal communication.

223. Gastpar, H. (1970): Stickiness of platelets and tumor cells influenced by drugs. *Thromb. Diath. Haemorrh.* [*Suppl.*], 42:291–303.

224. Born, G. V. R., and Cross, M. J. (1963): The aggregation of blood platelets. *J. Physiol.* (*Lond.*), 168: 178–195.

225. Born, G. V. R. (1964): Strong inhibition by 2-chloroadenosine of the aggregation of blood platelets by adenosine diphosphate. *Nature*, 202:95–96.

226. Kloeze, J. (1969): Relationship between chemical structure and platelet-aggregation activity of prostaglandins. *Biochim. Biophys. Acta*, 187:285–292.

227. Hamberg, M., Svensson, J., Wakabayashi, T., and Samuelsson, B. (1974): Isolation and structure of two prostaglandin endoperoxides that cause platelet aggregation. *Proc. Natl. Acad. Sci. U.S.A.*, 71:345–349.

228. Hamberg, M., and Samuelsson, B. (1974): Prostaglandin endoperoxides. Novel transformations of arachidonic acid in human platelets. *Proc. Natl. Acad. Sci. U.S.A.*, 71:3400–3404.

229. Smith, J. B., Silver, M. J., Ingerman, C., and Kocsis, J. J. (1974): Prostaglandin D$_2$ inhibits the aggregation of human platelets. *Thromb. Res.*, 5:291–299.

230. Smith, J. B., Ingerman, C. M., and Silver, M. J. (1976): Formation of prostaglandin D$_2$ during endoperoxide-induced platelet aggregation. *Thromb. Res.*, 9:413–418.

231. Puig-Parellada, and Planas, J. M. (1977): Action of selective inhibitor of thromboxane synthetase on experimental thrombosis induced by arachidonic acid in rabbit. *Lancet*, 40.

232. Castaner, J., and Hillier, K. (1977): ONO-747. *Drugs of the Future*, 2:320–322.

233. Gaut, Z. N. (1974): Influence of various substances which induce and inhibit aggregation on the uptake of deoxyglucose by human blood platelets. *J. Pharmacol. Exp. Ther.*, 190:180–186.

234. Aledort, L. M., Berger, S., Goldman, B., and Puszkin, E. (1974): Antiserotonin and antihistamine drugs as inhibitors of platelet function. In: *Platelets and Thrombosis*, edited by S. Sherry and A. Scriabine, p. 149. University Park Press, Baltimore.

235. Thomson, C., Forbes, C. D., and Prentice, C. R. M. (1973): A comparison of the effects of antihistamines on platelet function. *Thromb. Diath. Haemorrh.*, 30:547–556.

236. Sacchetti, G., Bellani, D., Montanari, C., and Gibelli, A. (1973): Effects "in vitro" of some cardiovascular drugs and other agents on human platelet aggregation. *Thromb. Diath. Haemorrh.*, 29:190–195.

237. Rubegni, M., Provvedi, D., Bellini, P. G., Bandinelli, C., and De Mauro, G. (1975): Propranolol and platelet aggregation. *Circulation*, 52:964–965.

238. Weksler, B. B., Gillick, M., and Pink, J. (1977): Effect of propranolol on platelet function. *Blood*, 49:185–196.

239. Ungaro, P. C., Beck, T. M., McCaa, W. M., and Hershgold, E. J. (1973): The in vivo and in vitro effect of antihistamines on platelet aggregation. *Thromb. Diath. Haemorrh.*, 30:597–601.

240. Markwardt, F., Barthel, W., Glusa, E., and Hoffmann, A. (1967): Untersuchungen über den Einfluss von Papaverin auf Reaktionen der Blutplättchen. *Naunyn Schmiedebergs Arch. Pharmacol.*, 257:420–431.

241. Markwardt, F., Barthel, W., Glusa, E., and Hoffmann, A. (1966) Der Einfluss von Papaverin auf Funktionen der Blutplättchen. *Experientia*, 22:578–579.

242. Steger, W. (1973): Die Beeinflussung des Plättchenagglutinationstestes durch Xantinol-nicotinat. *Med. Welt*, 24:301–302.

243. Seidel, G., and Endell, W. (1977): Effect of Xanthinol nicotinate treatment on platelet aggregation. *Int. J. Clin. Pharmacol.*, 15:139–143.

244. Gastpar, H., Ambrus, J. L., Ambrus, C. M., Spavento, P., Weber, F. J., and Thurber, L. E. (1977): Study of platelet aggregation in vivo. III. Effect of pentoxifylline. *J. Med.* (*Basel*): 8:191–197.

245. Stefanovich, F. (1974): Concerning specificity of the influence of pentoxifylline on various cyclic phosphodiesterases. *Res. Commun. Chem. Pathol. Pharmacol.*, 8:673.

246. Warlow, C., Ogston, D., and Douglas, A. S. (1973): The effect of chlorpromazine and antihistamines on human blood platelets in vitro and in vivo. *Bibl. Anat.*, 12:249–253.

247. Voss, D., Fuchs, G., Schneider, D., and Schneider, J. (1972): Der Einfluss des oralen Antidiabetikums Glibornurid auf Blutgerinnung, Thrombozyten und Fibrinolyse. *Arzneim. Forsch.*, 22:2219–2221.

248. Scholz, C., Losert, W., and Hoder, A. (1975): Experimentelle Untersuchungen zum Mechanismus der durch Sulfonylharnstoffe verursachten Hemmung der Thrombozytenaggregation. 1. Mitteilung: Prob-

lemstellung und Methoden. *Arzneim. Forsch.*, 25: 38–46.

249. Losert, W., Hoder, A., and Scholz, C. (1975): Experimentelle Untersuchungen zum Mechanismus der durch Sulfonylharnstoffe verursachten Hemmung der Thrombozytenaggregation. 2. Mitteilung: Beeinflussung der Blutglukose und der Thrombozytenaggregation durch orale Antidiabetika. *Arzneim. Forsch.*, 25:170–179.

250. Scholz, C., Hoder, A., and Losert, W. (1975): Experimentelle Untersuchungen zum Mechanismus der durch Sulfonylharnstoffe verursachten Hemmung der Thrombozytenaggregation. 3. Mitteilung: Bedeutung von Prostaglandinen und cAMP für den aggregationshemmenden Effekt und andere Wirkungen von Sulfonylharnstoffen. *Arzneim. Forsch.*, 25:347–361.

251. Glusa, E., Barthel, W., and Markwardt, F. (1974): The influence of benzamidine derivatives on human platelet function. *Thromb. Diath. Haemorrh.*, 31: 172–178.

252. Glynn, M. F., Murphy, E. A., and Mustard, J. F. (1967): Effect of clofibrate on platelet economy in man. *Lancet*, 2:447–488.

253. Carson, P., McDonald, L., Pickard, S., Pilkington, T., Davies, B., and Love, F. (1963): Effect of atromid on platelet stickiness. *Atherosclerosis*, 3:619–622.

254. Carvalho, A. C. A., Colman, R. W., and Lees, R. S. (1974): Clofibrate reversal of platelet hypersensitivity in hyperbetalipoproteinemia. *Circulation*, 50:570–574.

255. Swedenborg, J. (1974): Inhibitory effect of polyphloretin phosphate upon platelet aggregation and hemodynamic and respiratory changes caused by thrombin and protamine. *J. Pharmacol. Exp. Ther.*, 188:214–221.

256. Besterman, E. M. M., and Gillett, M. P. T. (1971): Inhibition of platelet aggregation by lysolecithin. *Atherosclerosis*, 14:323–330.

257. Vermylen, J., Chamone, D. A. F., and Verstraete, M. (1979): Stimulation of prostacyclin release from vessel wall by BAY g 6575, an antithrombotic compound. *Lancet*, 1:518–520.

258. Rehse, K. (1978): Entwicklungstendenzen in der Chemie der Antithrombotika. *Dtsch. Apoth. Ztg.*, 118:1853–1858.

259. Weily, H. S., and Genton, E. (1970): Altered platelet function in patients with prosthetic mitral valves: Effects of sulfinpyrazone therapy. *Circulation*, 12:967–972.

260. Weily, H. S., Steele, P. P., Davies, H., et al. (1974): Platelet survival in patients with substitute heart valves. *N. Engl. J. Med.*, 290:534–539.

261. Genton, E., Barnett, H. J. M., Fields, W. S., et al. (1977): Cerebral ischemia: the role of thrombosis and of antithrombotic therapy. *Stroke*, 8:150–175.

262. Yatsu, F. M. (1977): Stroke therapy: Status of antiplatelet aggregation drugs (editorial). *Neurology (Minneap.)*, 27:503–504.

263. Evans, G. (1972): Effect of drugs that suppress platelet surface interaction on incidence of amaurosis fugax and transient cerebral ischemia. *Surg. Forum*, 23:239–241.

264. Barnett, H. J., and Canadian Cooperative Study Group (1978): A randomized trial of aspirin and sulfinpyrazone in threatened stroke. *N. Engl. J. Med.*, 299:53–59.

265. Anturane Reinfarction Trial Research Group (1978): Sulfinpyrazone in the prevention of cardiac death after myocardial infarction. *N. Engl. J. Med.*, 298:289–295.

266. Sullivan, J. M., Harken, D. E., and Gorlin, R. (1968): Pharmacologic control of thromboembolic complications of cardiac-valve replacement. A preliminary report. *N. Engl. J. Med.*, 279:576–580.

267. Sullivan, J. M., Harken, D. E., and Gorlin, R. (1971): Pharmacologic control of thromboembolic complication of cardiac-valve replacement. *N. Engl. J. Med.*, 284:1391.

268. Weily, H. S., Steele, P. P., Davies, H., Pappas, G., and Genton, E. (1974): Platelet survival in patients in substitute heart valves. *N. Engl. J. Med.*, 290:534–536.

269. Steele, P., Weily, H. S., and Genton, E. (1973): Platelet survival and adhesiveness in recurrent venous thrombosis. *N. Engl. J. Med.*, 288:1148.

270. Harrison, M. J. G., Marshall, J., Meadows, J. C., and Ross Russel, R. W. (1971): Effect of aspirin in amaurosis fugax. *Lancet*, 2:743.

271. Acheson, J., Danta, G., and Hutchinson, E. C. (1969): Controlled trial of dipyridamole in cerebral vascular disease. *Br. Med. J.*, 1:614.

272. Mathew, T. H., Clyne, D. H., Nanra, R. S., Kincaid-Smith, P., Saker, B. M., Morris, P. J., and Marshall, V. C. (1974): A controlled trial of oral anticoagulants and dipyridamole in cadaveric renal allografts. *Lancet*, 1:1307.

273. Salzman, E. W., Harris, W. H., and De Sanctis, R. W. (1971): Reduction in venous thromboembolism by agents affecting platelet function. *N. Engl. J. Med.*, 284:1287–1292.

274. Dale, J., Myhre, E., Storstein, O., et al. (1977): Prevention of arterial thromboembolism with acetylsalicylic acid. *Am. Heart J.*, 94:101–111.

275. Loew, D., Wellmer, H. K., Baer, U., Merguet, H., Rumpf, P., Petersen, H., Bromig, G., Persch, W. F., Marx, F. J., and von Bary, S. M. (1974): Postoperative Thromboembolieprophylaxe mit Acetylsalicylsäure. *Dtsch. Med. Wochenschr.*, 99:565–572.

276. Loew, D. (1976): Die deutsche multizentrische Doppelblindstudie zur Prüfung der Thromboseprophylaxe mit ASS. *Med. Welt*, 27:1374–1376.

277. Clagett, G. P., Schneider, P., Rosoff, C. B., and Salzman, E. W. (1975): The influence of aspirin on postoperative platelet kinetics and venous thrombosis. *Surgery*, 77:61–74.

278. British Medical Research Council (1972): Effect of aspirin on postoperative venous thrombosis. *Lancet*, 2:441–445.

279. Zekert, F., Kohn, P., and Vormittag, E. (1976): Eine randomisierte Studie über die postoperative Thromboseprophylaxe mit Acetylsalicylsäure. *Med. Welt*, 27:1372–1373.

280. Fields, W. S., Lemak, N. A., Frankowski, R. F., and Hardy, R. J. (1977): Controlled trial of aspirin in cerebral ischemia, Part I. *Stroke*, 8:301–316.

281. Fields, W. S., Lemak, N. A., Frankowski, R. F.,

and Hardy, R. J. (1978): Controlled trial of aspirin in cerebral ischemia, Part II: Surgical group. *Stroke,* 9:309–319.

282. Harter, H. R., Burch, J. W., and Majerus, P. W. (1979): Prevention of thrombosis in patients on hemodialysis by low-dose aspirin. *N. Engl. J. Med.,* 301:577–579.

383. Vaisrub, S. (1978): On teaching an old dog new tricks. *J.A.M.A.,* 240:2288.

284. Haft, H., Gershengorn, K., Kranz, P. D., et al. (1972): Protection against epinephrine-induced myocardial necrosis by drugs that inhibit platelet aggregation. *Am. J. Cardiol.,* 30:838–843.

285. Boston Collaborative Drug Surveillance Group (1974): Regular aspirin intake and acute myocardial infarction. *Br. Med. J.,* 1:440–443.

286. Elwood, P. C., Cochrane, A. L., and Burr, M. L. (1974): A randomized controlled trial of acetylsalicylic acid in the secondary prevention of mortality from myocardial infarction. *Br. Med. J.,* 1:436–440.

287. Coronary Drug Project Research Group (1976): Aspirin in coronary heart disease. *J. Chronic Dis.,* 29:625–642.

288. Breddin, K., Uberla, K., and Walter, E. (1977): German-Austrian multicenter two years prospective study on the prevention of secondary myocardial infarction by ASA in comparison to phenprocoumon and placebo. *Thrombos. Haemostas.,* 38:168 (abstract).

289. Aspirin Myocardial Infarction Study Research Group (1980): A randomized, controlled trial of aspirin in persons recovered from secondary myocardial infarction. *J.A.M.A.,* 243:661–669.

290. Krol, W. F. (1980): *The Aspirin Myocardial Infarction Study and the Persantine Aspirin Re-infarction Study—Design and Results.* Symposium of the Aspirin Foundation, London.

Cardiovascular Pharmacology, Second Edition,
edited by Michael Antonaccio.
Raven Press, New York © 1984.

Prostacyclin–Thromboxane Interactions in Hemostasis

B. J. R. Whittle and S. Moncada

Department of Prostaglandin Research, Wellcome Research Laboratories, Beckenham, Kent BR3 3BS, United Kingdom

Prostaglandins are synthesized from 20-carbon polyunsaturated fatty acids containing three, four, or five double bonds. These fatty acids are present in the phospholipids of the cell membranes of all mammalian tissues (4). The main precursor of prostaglandins in humans is eicosatetraenoic acid, more commonly called arachidonic acid, which gives rise to the prostaglandins (PGs) containing two double bonds, such as PGE_2, $PGF_{2\alpha}$, PGD_2, and prostacyclin, as well as thromboxane A_2 (Fig. 1). The arachidonic acid in the cell membrane is derived either from elongation and desaturation of the essential fatty acid linoleic acid, found in vegetables in the diet, or from the arachidonic acid content of meats from farm animals. Dihomo-γ-linolenic acid gives rise to prostaglandins that contain only one double bond, such as PGE_1. However, PGE_1 occurs only at very low levels in mammals, and the physiological importance of other prostaglandins derived from this fatty acid is largely unknown.

Arachidonic acid is released from membrane phospholipids by the enzyme phospholipase A_2, which can be activated by many different stimuli (4,10). Perturbation of the cell membrane, including only very slight chemical or mechanical stimulation, suffices to activate the enzyme. Once released, arachidonic acid is rapidly metabolized into oxygenated products by two distinct pathways.

One pathway involves lipoxygenase enzymes, which can give rise to a recently characterized family of products, the leukotrienes (19) (Fig. 1). These products have proinflammatory actions, and the bronchoconstrictor mediator SRS-A is now known to be a leukotriene. The second pathway for arachidonic acid metabolism involves the enzyme cyclooxygenase (earlier known as prostaglandin synthetase), which forms an unstable cyclic endoperoxide, PGG_2 (Fig. 1). Aspirinlike drugs inhibit subsequent prostaglandin formation by inhibiting this enzyme (23). The endoperoxide PGG_2 is in turn converted to another unstable endoperoxide, PGH_2 (the half-lives of both are about 5 min at 37°C in aqueous solution). PGH_2 is broken down either enzymatically or nonenzymatically to the stable prostaglandins PGE_2, $PGF_{2\alpha}$, and PGD_2 (Fig. 1) and to the 17-carbon hydroxy acid 12-hydroxy-5,8,10-heptadecatrienoic acid and malondialdehyde (7,29). The prostaglandin endoperoxides are also transformed by two distinct enzymes into prostacyclin and into thromboxane A_2 (TXA_2). Both of these products are chemically unstable, rapidly breaking down to 6-oxo-$PGF_{1\alpha}$ and thromboxane B_2, respectively, under physiological conditions (Fig. 1).

Isolation and identification of unstable intermediates in the metabolic pathway of arachidonic acid (namely, prostaglandin endoperoxides PGG_2 and PGH_2, TXA_2 and

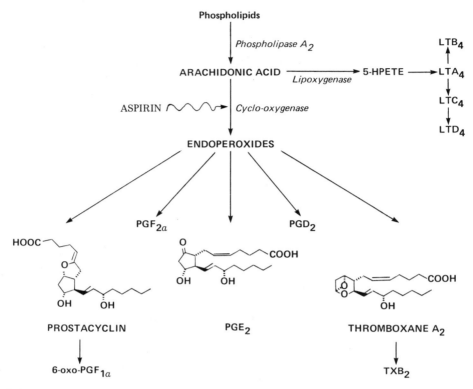

FIG. 1. Pathways of metabolism of arachidonic acid to cyclooxygenase and lipoxygenase products.

prostacyclin) have greatly increased our understanding of the physiology of platelets and their interactions with the vessel wall. These findings have also led to speculation that prostacyclin and TXA$_2$, rather than PGE$_2$ or PGF$_{2\alpha}$, are the most physiologically important products of arachidonic acid metabolism (12,15).

The discovery of these unstable intermediates has prompted a hypothesis that explains some facets of cardiovascular disease on the basis of disturbances in the balance of these compounds in the interactions between platelets and the vessel wall, whether these disturbances are drug-induced or are caused by pathological changes (12,15).

PROSTACYCLIN

Biosynthesis

Prostacyclin has been shown to be the main cyclooxygenase produce of arachidonic acid

in all arteries and veins so far tested (13). The ability of large-vessel wall to synthesize prostacyclin is greatest at the intimal surface and progressively decreases toward the adventitia. Production of prostacyclin by cultured cells from vessel walls also shows that endothelial cells are the most active producers of prostacyclin. Not much is known about prostacyclin formation in the microcirculation, although microvessels, mainly capillaries, isolated from rat cerebrum can generate predominantly prostacyclin. The gastric mucosa, which contains a dense matrix of microvessels, is also a potent source of prostacyclin formation (27).

Initially it was demonstrated that a microsomal preparation of vessel wall, even in the absence of cofactors, could utilize prostaglandin endoperoxides, but not arachidonic acid, to synthesize prostacyclin (13). Later it was shown that fresh vascular tissue could utilize both precursors, although the endoperoxides are much better substrates. Moreover, vessel microsomes, fresh vascular rings, or endothelial cells treated with the cyclooxygenase inhibitor indomethacin could, when incubated with platelets, generate a prostacyclin-like antiaggregating activity. The release of this substance was inhibited by 15-hydroperoxy arachidonic acid (15-HPAA) and other fatty acid hydroperoxides known to be inhibitors of prostacyclin formation. From all these data it was suggested that the vessel wall can synthesize prostacyclin not only from its own endogenous precursors but also from prostaglandin endoperoxides released by the platelets (Fig. 2). This latter proposal, that biochemical cooperation between platelet and vessel wall exists at least *in vitro,* has proved somewhat controversial. Others have suggested that some degree of vascular damage may be necessary for the endoperoxide to be utilized by prostacyclin synthetase or that endoperoxides from platelets cannot be utilized by some other cells under certain experimental conditions. More recent experiments have shown that feeding of endoperoxides to endothelial cells suspended in platelet-rich plasma takes place *in vitro,* but only when the platelet number approaches the normal blood levels (25). It should be stressed, however, that the concept of endoperoxides released from platelets being

utilized by endothelial cells has not yet been fully evaluated *in vivo.*

It is possible that adherence of the platelet to the vessel wall, known to be one of the first responses to injury, could well provide the close proximity that would be needed for such cooperation between platelets and endothelial cells. It is also possible that other formed elements of blood, such as white cells, which produce endoperoxides and TXA$_2$, could interact with the vessel wall to promote formation of prostacyclin. Moreover, leukocytes themselves may generate prostacyclin in whole blood, especially in the presence of thromboxane synthetase inhibitors. Thus, prostacyclin might modulate white cell behavior and help control white cell activity during the inflammatory response.

Effects on Platelets

Prostacyclin is the most potent endogenous inhibitor of platelet aggregation yet discovered. It is 30 times more potent than PGE$_1$ and more than 1,000 times more active than adenosine. Prostacyclin applied locally in low concentrations inhibits thrombus formation due to ADP in the microcirculation of the hamster cheek pouch. When infused intravenously in the rabbit, it prevents electrically

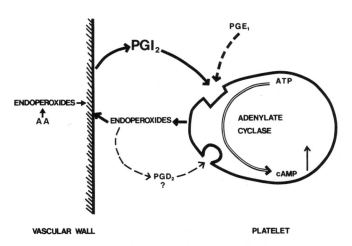

FIG. 2. Interactions of prostacyclin (PGI$_2$), PGE$_1$, and PGD$_2$ with the platelet cAMP system.

induced thrombus formation in the carotid artery, increases bleeding time, and inhibits platelet aggregation, tested *ex vivo*. The duration of these antiaggregating effects *in vivo* is short, and they disappear within 15 to 30 min of administration. Prostacyclin disaggregates platelets *in vitro* in aggregometer cuvettes and in experimental extracorporeal circuits where platelet clumps have formed on collagen strips. Moreover, it inhibits thrombus formation in a coronary artery model in the dog when given locally or systemically and protects against sudden death (thought to be due to platelet clumping) induced by intravenous arachidonic acid in rabbits.

Prostacyclin is unstable, and its activity disappears within 10 min at 22°C at neutral pH or within 15 sec on boiling. In acidic solutions, prostacyclin is rapidly hydrolyzed to 6-oxo-PGF$_{1\alpha}$, the half-life at pH 3 being less than 30 sec. Prostacyclin has an extended stability in plasma and in blood *in vitro* that appears to be associated with binding to albumin. It is stabilized as a pharmaceutical preparation

by freeze-drying and can be reconstituted for clinical use in an alkaline glycine buffer.

Mechanism of Action on Platelets

Prostacyclin inhibits platelet aggregation by stimulating adenylate cyclase, leading to an increase in cAMP levels in the platelets (Fig. 2). The breakdown product 6-oxo-PGF$_{1\alpha}$ has only very weak antiaggregating activity and is almost devoid of activity on platelet cAMP. As with the antiaggregatory activity, prostacyclin is more potent than PGE$_1$ and PGD$_2$ in elevating cAMP levels in platelets. The antiaggregating actions of prostacyclin are augmented by phosphodiesterase inhibitors such as theophylline (Fig. 3) and dipyridamole, which allow accumulation of cAMP. Prostacyclin is also a strong direct stimulator of adenylate cyclase in isolated membrane preparations.

Prostacyclin, PGE$_1$, and PGD$_2$ increase adenylate cyclase activity by acting on two distinct receptors on the platelet membrane.

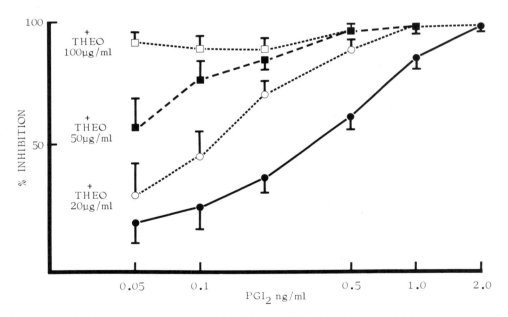

FIG. 3. Potentiation of prostacyclin-induced inhibition of ADP-induced human platelet aggregation by the phosphodiesterase inhibitor theophylline. Theophylline was preincubated 1 min with platelet-rich plasma prior to subsequent 1-min incubation with prostacyclin.

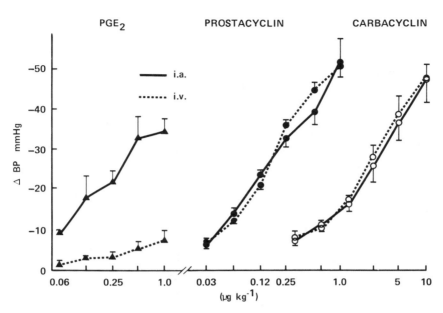

FIG. 4. Vasodepressor actions of prostacyclin, a stable analogue, carbacyclin, and PGE_2 on systemic arterial blood pressure in the anesthetised rat following intravenous or intraarterial bolus injection.

PGE_1 and prostacyclin appear to act at similar sites, whereas PGD_2 acts on another. It is thus likely that the previously recognized PGE_1 receptor in platelets is in fact the prostacyclin receptor (Fig. 2).

Vasodilator Actions

Prostacyclin relaxes most vascular strips *in vitro,* including rabbit celiac and mesenteric arteries, bovine coronary arteries, lamb ductus arteriosus, and human and baboon cerebral and vertebral arteries. Furthermore, prostacyclin antagonizes the contraction induced by spasmogens contained in cerebrospinal fluid obtained from patients with cerebral arterial vasospasm following subarachnoid hemorrhage. Likewise, prostacyclin in low concentrations causes a small relaxation of isolated segments of canine basilar arteries, and prostacyclin can antagonize the constrictor effects of 5-hydroxytryptamine and $PGF_{2\alpha}$. Local application of prostacyclin to the exposed cerebral microvasculature in the cat and dog causes pronounced vasodilation of both large and small arterioles. Prostacyclin is a potent

hypotensive agent following intravenous or intraarterial administration, lowering systemic arterial blood pressure (Fig. 4) and increasing local blood flow through many organs. Prostacyclin is a potent vasodilator in the gastric microcirculation in dog and rat, where it also inhibits gastric acid secretion and mucosal ulceration. It is possible that prostacyclin is involved in modulating blood flow and functional hyperemia in the gastric mucosa (27). Prostacyclin is a potent hypotensive agent when infused in anesthetized dogs, and in primates, prostacyclin at doses as low as 10 to 20 ng/kg/min can lower systemic arterial blood pressure. In anesthetized rabbit or rat, prostacyclin causes a fall in blood pressure and is some 10-fold more potent than PGE_2 following intravenous administration. Prostacyclin is at least 100 times more active as a vasodepressor than its degradation product, $6-oxo-PGF_{1\alpha}$. In the renal circulation in the dog, prostacyclin infused intravenously reduces renal vascular resistance and increases blood flow and urinary excretion of sodium, potassium, and chloride ions at doses below those needed for a systemic effect. There is increasing evidence that prostacyclin mediates the release of renin from the renal cortex.

Although the chemical half-life for prostacyclin at physiological temperatures and pH is short, the biological activity of prostacyclin *in vivo* is often more short-lived. This suggests that the effects *in vivo* are limited by biological inactivation rather than solely by chemical breakdown. Unlike the more classic prostaglandins of the E and F series, prostacyclin had comparable vasodepressor actions when injected by the intraaortic and intravenous routes in rats, rabbits, and dogs (Fig. 4), suggesting that pulmonary degradation is not of primary importance in prostacyclin inactivation. The failure of prostacyclin to be metabolized during passage through the lung indicates that it is not a substrate for the pulmonary uptake system required for metabolism by the enzyme 15-hydroxyprostaglandin dehydrogenase (15-PGDH) in the intact lung, because prostacyclin is a substrate for the enzyme itself *in vitro*. In contrast, the breakdown product 6-oxo-PGF$_{1\alpha}$ is not a good substrate for this enzyme. Prostacyclin is metabolized during passage through the peripheral circulation, liver, and kidney, although the rate and nature of the metabolic processes are complex. Studies on the composition of the urinary metabolites of prostacyclin following its infusion in rats indicate that it can undergo the metabolic transformations described for the more classic prostaglandins. Thus, products resulting from 15-dehydrogenation, Δ^{13} reductase, β-oxidation, 19- and 20-hydroxylation, and oxidation have been identified. Likewise, 6-oxo-PGF$_{1\alpha}$ resulting from chemical breakdown of prostacyclin *in vivo* may be further metabolized, and studies in dogs have indicated rapid elimination of both prostacyclin and 6-oxo-PGF$_{1\alpha}$ from the plasma following intravenous infusion (16).

One of the more recently described metabolites of hepatic metabolism of prostacyclin *in vitro* is 6-oxo-PGE$_1$. This chemically stable product may arise from transformation of either prostacyclin itself or 6-oxo-PGF$_{1\alpha}$ via a 9-hydroxyprostaglandin dehydrogenase pathway present in the liver and may account for up to 7% of the total products (30). Like prostacyclin, this compound is a vasodilator and inhibitor of platelet aggregation. The presence of this dehydrogenase in platelets raises the possibility that under certain conditions platelets may actually produce 6-oxo-PGE$_1$ from prostacyclin. Although this putative platelet metabolite is less active than prostacyclin as an antiaggregating agent (Table 1), this biotransformation may play an interesting intermediate role in the regulation of prostacyclin interactions in hemostasis.

THROMBOXANE A$_2$

Biosynthesis

Arachidonic acid, as well as the prostaglandin endoperoxides PGG$_2$ and PGH$_2$, induces platelet aggregation that is accompanied by the formation of an unstable vasoconstrictor substance identified as thromboxane A$_2$ (8). Thromboxane A$_2$ (TXA$_2$), which breaks down to thromboxane B$_2$, has a chemical half-life at body pH and temperature of 30 sec, although the presence of albumin appears to stabilize the molecule. The activity of the "rabbit aorta-contracting substance" or RCS described first by Piper and Vane can be accounted for by these endoperoxides and TXA$_2$. The enzyme that synthesizes TXA$_2$ from PG endoperoxides was localized in the high-speed particulate fraction of human and horse blood platelets (14). The enzyme has been solubilized and separated from the cyclooxygenase, and detailed studies of human and bovine platelet thromboxane synthetase have been carried out.

Other cells capable of synthesizing TXA$_2$ include rabbit and human polymorphonuclear leukocytes, macrophages from mouse, rat, and guinea pig, and human lung fibroblasts. Tissues shown to have TXA$_2$-generating capacity include rabbit and cat spleen, rabbit iris and conjunctiva, guinea pig lung, human umbilical artery, rabbit pulmonary artery, and rabbit and rat kidney, although the exact location or cellular type possessing TXA$_2$ synthetase in these tissues is not known. However, it may also be in some instances that the production of TXA$_2$ by tissues is due to the presence of platelets or migratory cells.

Actions on Platelets

Addition of the cyclic endoperoxides PGG$_2$ and PGH$_2$ to platelet suspensions induces aggregation and release of the platelet constituents (29). However, Hamberg, Samuelsson, and colleagues showed that during platelet aggregation induced by arachidonic acid or the endoperoxides, a further product, TXA$_2$, is also generated. TXA$_2$ is a more potent inducer of aggregation than the endoperoxides themselves, and it was proposed that TXA$_2$ is the arachidonic acid metabolite that mediates platelet aggregation and the release reaction stimulated under pathophysiological circumstances by such agents as collagen (8). The question whether the endoperoxides have proaggregatory activity in their own right or only after conversion to TXA$_2$ has yet to be fully answered. When their further metabolism to thromboxane is blocked by thromboxane synthetase inhibitors, PGG$_2$ and PGH$_2$ may exert a direct activity on platelets as pharmacological agents, perhaps on the TXA$_2$ receptors. Interestingly, stable 9-11-epoxy endoperoxide analogues that possess proaggregatory and vascular actions are thought to act as thromboxane mimics. However, it is possible that under normal conditions when platelets are activated and the endogenous arachidonic acid cascade is triggered, the prostaglandin endoperoxides thus generated will exert their "physiological role" through conversion to the more potent TXA$_2$. The interaction of products of arachidonic acid metabolism with the so-called third pathway of platelet aggregation (believed to be cyclooxygenase- and ADP-independent) is unknown (11,24). Phospholipase A$_2$ activation may be involved, an idea strengthened by the isolation and identification of a platelet-activating factor (PAF) released from platelets during aggregation. PAF seems to be released by the action of a phospholipase A$_2$, and it aggregates platelets independently of arachidonate and ADP. The biological significance of PAF during human platelet aggregation remains to be elucidated. It thus seems likely that normal "physiological" platelet aggregation is a multifactorial phenomenon in which there is participation by several proaggregating substances. The relative importance of each could depend on the situation in which platelet aggregation occurs (for example, in hemostatic plug, thrombus on an ulcerated atherosclerotic plaque).

Many stimuli that aggregate platelets, including ADP, thrombin, collagen, epinephrine, arachidonic acid, and physical stimuli, cause a decrease in cAMP levels in the platelets. Indeed, the decrease in cAMP induced by PGH$_2$ can be inhibited by thromboxane synthetase inhibitors, suggesting that TXA$_2$ formation itself can decrease platelet cAMP and thus lead to aggregation.

Vascular Actions

TXA$_2$ is, in general, more potent in contracting vascular and airway smooth muscle when studied *in vitro* than are the endoperoxides. However, the biological responses to the endoperoxides PGG$_2$ and PGH$_2$ may be complicated by the ability of most tissues to convert these intermediates into further biologically active products. For example, application of PGH$_2$ contracts strips of human and baboon basilar, middle cerebral, and vertebral arteries suspended in an isolated-organ bath or in superfusion cascade. Thus, despite the partial conversion to prostacyclin, which relaxes these tissues, the direct vasoconstrictor action of the endoperoxide is observed under these conditions. The actions of TXA$_2$ can be determined following its generation *in vitro*, usually by rapidly incubating PGH$_2$ with platelet microsomes. This TXA$_2$ generated exogenously can potently contract isolated segments of rabbit aorta, human umbilical artery, guinea pig trachea, bovine and pig coronary artery, and lamb ductus arteriosus. In studies on helically cut strips prepared from large cerebral conductance arteries, TXA_2, like $PGF_{2\alpha}$, caused contraction of this vascular tissue. Likewise, TXA_2 (generated from arachidonic acid in aliquots of human platelet-rich plasma) contracted isolated segments of human basilar artery. Contraction of rabbit basilar arteries *in vitro* has also been demonstrated with a stable carbocyclic thromboxane analogue. TXA_2 is also a powerful vasoconstrictor in vascular beds *in vivo* in the dog and cat. In the guinea pig, TXA_2 can elevate tracheal inflation pressure, and more recent studies indicate that in this species the potent bronchoconstrictor actions of the leukotrienes may be an indirect action brought about by endogenous release of TXA_2 from the lung. TXA_2 generated directly in blood from arachidonic acid is also a potent vasoconstrictor in the gastric vasculature in the dog, and it can bring about extensive mucosal damage.

INTERACTIONS BETWEEN PROSTACYCLIN AND THROMBOXANE A_2

Prostaglandin endoperoxides, being precursors of substances with opposing biological properties (Fig. 1), have an important pivotal role in the regulation of hemostasis. On the one hand, TXA_2 produced predominantly by the platelets is a strong vasoconstrictor and induces platelet aggregation. On the other hand, prostacyclin produced by the vessel wall is a potent vasodilator and the most potent naturally occurring inhibitor of platelet aggregation known (Table 1). Each substance likewise has opposing effects on cAMP concentrations in platelets and gives a balanced control mechanism that will therefore affect thrombus and hemostatic plug formation (Table 2).

A number of diseases may be related to an imbalance in the prostacyclin-TXA_2 system (12,15,21). Platelets from patients with arterial thrombosis, deep venous thrombosis, or recurrent venous thrombosis produce higher levels of PG endoperoxides and TXA_2, and these platelets have a shortened survival time *in vivo*. Platelets from rabbits made atherosclerotic by dietary manipulation and platelets from patients who have survived myocardial infarction appear abnormally sensitive to aggregating agents and also produce higher levels of TXA_2 than do those of controls. Elevated TXB_2 levels have been demonstrated in the blood of patients with Prinzmetal's angina. Furthermore, studies on thromboxane levels in coronary sinus blood of patients with unstable angina suggest that local TXA_2 release is associated with recent episodes of angina, but it is difficult to distinguish whether the release was cause or effect. Although platelet aggregation results in TXA_2 generation, platelets may form and release TXA_2 under other pathological conditions. Arrhythmias resulting from coronary ligation in the dog may also be related to TXA_2 production.

Platelets from diabetic rats display in-

TABLE 1. *Inhibition of ADP-induced platelet aggregation by prostanoids following 1-min incubation in human platelet-rich plasma*

	ID_{50} (ng-ml^{-1})	Relative potency
PGI_2	0.4 ± 0.1	1
PGI_3	0.7 ± 0.2	0.57
6-oxo-$PGF_{1\alpha}$	282 ± 37	0.0014
6-oxo-PGE_1	6 ± 0.7	0.07
PGE_1	21 ± 3	0.02
PGD_2	11 ± 2	0.04
6β-PGI_1	116 ± 20	0.0034
6α-PGI_1	350 ± 30	0.001
Carbacyclin	11 ± 3	0.04

TABLE 2. *Opposing biological properties of prostacyclin and thromboxane A_2*

PGI_2	TXA_2
Antiaggregatory	Proaggregatory
Vasodilator	Vasoconstrictor
Bronchodilator	Bronchoconstrictor
Cytoprotective	Ulcerogenic

creased release of TXA_2, whereas their blood vessels show reduced production of prostacyclin; these effects are reversed by chronic insulin treatment. Prostacyclin production by blood vessels from patients with diabetes is depressed and circulating levels of 6-oxo-$PGF_{1\alpha}$ are reduced in diabetic patients with proliferative retinopathy, although the direct association between reduced prostacyclin production and diabetic retinopathy is not fully explored.

Thrombocytopenic purpura (TTP), like diabetes, is associated with formation of microvascular thromboemboli, and a deficiency in prostacyclin production may be responsible for the increased platelet consumption that occurs in TTP. This deficiency is postulated to be secondary to lack of a "plasma factor" that is thought to normally stimulate endogenous prostacyclin production. Prostacyclin production is significantly lower in umbilical and placental vessels from preeclamptic patients than in those from normally pregnant women.

Increased prostacyclin production, resulting from accumulation of the as-yet-undefined "plasma factor" that stimulates prostacyclin synthesis, has been suggested to explain the hemostatic defect in uremic patients (18). Patients with Bartter's syndrome excrete in the urine approximately four times as much 6-oxo-$PGF_{1\alpha}$ as do control patients, which has led to the suggestion that overproduction of prostacyclin mediates both the hyperreninemia and the hyporesponsiveness to pressor agents observed in these patients. Enhanced prostacyclin production by blood vessels of spontaneously hypertensive rats has been demonstrated, although in clinical studies there may be diminished excretion of 6-oxo-$PGF_{1\alpha}$ in the urine of patients with essential hypertension.

In general, it seems that in diseases where there is a tendency for thrombosis to develop, TXA_2 production is elevated or prostacyclin production reduced or that both situations occur, whereas the opposite is found in some diseases associated with an increased bleeding tendency.

The detection of prostacyclin formation in the choroid plexus points to a potential physiological role in preventing platelet aggregation and thrombus formation in the cerebroventricular system. Alterations in prostacyclin-mediated processes may be one of the mechanisms underlying the hemodynamic changes observed in certain pathological situations. Cerebral arterial spasm, following subarachnoid hemorrhage, involves damage to the arterioles and the deposition of platelet aggregates and thrombi. Under these conditions there is likely to be a major imbalance between the formation and actions of prostacyclin and of TXA_2 (26). Other vasoactive and thrombus-promoting substances may further interact to aggravate the situation.

Prostacyclin and thromboxane may interact in other physiological and pathological situations, such as in the pulmonary system and in the inflammatory process. The breakdown product 6-oxo-$PGF_{1\alpha}$ has been identified in the inflammatory exudate of chronic granulomas. Moreover, prostacyclin induces erythema when injected into rabbit skin, although it is less active than PGE_2. Prostacyclin also potentiates carrageenin-induced edema in the rat paw, increases vascular permeability, and enhances vascular permeability induced by other inflammatory mediators, probably by its potent vasodilator actions. It is also more potent than PGE_2 in enhancing carrageenin-induced hyperalgesia in rats, although its activity is short-lived. Because of these effects, prostacyclin could be involved, along with other prostaglandins, as well TXA_2, in the genesis and maintenance of some of the signs of the acute inflammatory reaction (9). On the other hand, 6-oxo-PGF$_{1\alpha}$ is produced by macrophages, and it may be produced by other formed elements of blood, such as white cells. The fact that prostacyclin inhibits chemotaxis of human PMNs, without inhibiting phagocytosis, and inhibits white cell margination in the hamster cheek-pouch model suggests that prostacyclin might also play a role in modulating white cell movement during inflammation. At this stage, however, the precise role of prostacyclin in the inflammatory process, in relation to other products of arachidonic acid metabolism, including the lipoxygenase products and the leukotrienes, has not been evaluated.

The release of PGE$_2$, PGF$_{2\alpha}$, and RCS (TXA$_2$ and the endoperoxides) was first identified by Piper and Vane in the effluent from normal or sensitized lungs *in vitro* after different stimuli. The main metabolites of arachidonic acid via the pulmonary cyclooxygenase pathway lung are now recognized as TXA$_2$ and prostacyclin. TXA$_2$ is a bronchoconstrictor and vasoconstrictor, whereas prostacyclin, although not a very potent bronchodilator in humans, is effective in antagonizing bronchoconstriction induced by other agents and is also a vasodilator. The release of these compounds appears to be compartmentalized, the parenchyma being the tissue source of TXA$_2$, and tracheal and vascular tissue being the source of prostaglandinlike material and probably prostacyclin. There could therefore be a balance between these compounds in the modulation of pulmonary function. It is also possible that pathological conditions divert the pathway of synthesis away from prostacyclin and toward TXA$_2$, or lead to increased concentration of prostaglandin endoperoxides. These products are bronchoconstrictors and probably stimulants of vagal lung "irritant" receptors.

INFLUENCE OF DIET ON THROMBOXANE AND PROSTACYCLIN PRODUCTION

Before the discovery of prostacyclin, it was suggested that the use of dietary dihomo-γ-linolenic acid could offer a positive approach for prevention of thrombosis. This acid is the precursor of PGE$_1$, PGG$_1$, and thromboxane A$_1$, and these substances are not proaggregatory for platelets; indeed, PGE$_1$ is a relatively potent antiaggregatory agent. However, use of dihomo-γ-linolenic acid in an attempt to redirect the synthetic machinery of platelets is not the most rational approach to prevention of thrombosis, because the endoperoxides PGG$_1$ and PGH$_1$ are not substrates for a comparable prostacyclin synthesis. Therefore, an accumulation of these substances or their precursor could adversely affect the prostacyclin protective mechanism.

Eicosapentaenoic acid, the precursor of the prostaglandins with three double bonds (17), may, however, lead to the formation of an antiaggregating agent, probably PGI$_3$, whereas thromboxane A$_3$ has a weaker proaggregating activity than TXA$_2$. Thus, the use of this fatty acid could potentially afford dietary protection against intravascular thrombosis, for it would swing the balance toward the antithrombotic nature of the system. Indeed, the low incidence of myocardial infarction in Eskimos and their increased tendency to bleed could probably be due to the high content of eicosapentaenoic acid and low contents of linoleic and arachidonic acids in their diet, and therefore in their tissues (2). It has been proposed for many years that a reduction in the incidence of myocardial infarction can be associated with a reduction in blood cholesterol levels. The additional finding that the prostacyclin-thromboxane system is also involved in hemostasis gives great importance to future research into the effects of dietary polyunsaturated fats (22). It is possible, for example, that the polyunsaturated fats as a group have less relevance to the prevention of cardiovascular disease than a single substance of that group, such as eicosapentaenoic acid. The Eskimos obtain their tissue eicosapentaenoic acid from a diet of marine animals. Interestingly enough, the fat content of most common fish is 8 to 12% eicosapentaenoic acid. This acid represents more than 20% of the more exotic sea foods, such as scallops, oysters, and red caviar.

Linoleic acid is an essential fatty acid needed for construction of membrane phospholipids. It is generally agreed that animals, including humans, have the enzymatic machinery to elongate and desaturate this acid to arachidonic acid. Linolenic acid is the vegetable oil that, if elongated and desaturated, would lead to eicosapentaenoic acid. Clearly, therefore, it is important to know whether or not humans can convert linolenic acid to eicosapentaenoic acid, not least because the latter is found as a constituent of brain cell lipids.

EFFECTS OF INHIBITORS OF ARACHIDONIC ACID METABOLISM

Inhibitors of Cyclooxygenase

As a consequence of the discovery of prostacyclin there has been the need to carefully reexamine the rationale and use of aspirin as an antithrombotic compound. Because aspirin inhibits cyclooxygenase, it can prevent production of TXA_2 in platelets, but also production of prostacyclin in vascular tissue (Fig. 1). Aspirin binds covalently to the active site of cyclooxygenase and therefore inhibits the enzyme in platelets for their entire life-span, platelets being unable to synthesize new protein. Furthermore, aspirin also has an effect on the platelet precursors in the bone marrow. Inhibition of the vascular cyclooxygenase, however, may persist for a much shorter period because of the capability of the tissue to generate new cyclooxygenase enzyme. In addition, the cyclooxygenase of human skin fibroblasts and of arterial smooth-muscle cells appears less sensitive to inhibition by aspirin than that of human platelets. Although some studies carried out in humans following aspirin ingestion suggest some separation between the tissue sensitivities to inhibition, the doses that can be employed to clearly demonstrate such an action are under debate, and detailed findings are reviewed elsewhere (12).

In rabbits, aspirin has a biphasic effect on cutaneous bleeding time and on the formation of platelet clumps in an extracorporeal system. Low doses increase the bleeding time and are antithrombotic, but with higher doses neither effect occurs. This striking dose-related change has been attributed to the low dose affecting only platelet cyclooxygenase and allowing prostacyclin production to continue unabated, whereas with high doses of aspirin both vascular and platelet cyclooxygenases are inhibited. Whether or not this selectivity of action of low-dose aspirin regimens will produce beneficial actions in thromboembolic disorders is currently under intense clinical investigation and discussion.

Thromboxane Synthetase Inhibitors

Several groups of compounds have been reported to inhibit TXA_2 formation. Nictindole (L8027) was found to reduce TXA_2 production and concurrent platelet aggregation, but it did not appear to inhibit cyclooxygenase in the concentrations used. Another experimental compound, N-0164 (a prostaglandin antagonist on smooth muscle and platelets), and several prostaglandin analogues have also been shown to inhibit TXA_2 formation (5). The finding that imidazole also inhibits TXA_2 production (14) has led to the synthesis of many substituted derivatives of greater potency and selectivity than the parent molecule. Such derivatives include 1-benzylimidazole and 1-butylimidazole, as well as an ethoxy benzoic acid derivative (UK-37248) that recently has been administered to humans.

Theoretically, a selective inhibitor of thromboxane synthetase should prove to be a superior antithrombotic agent to aspirin by allowing prostacyclin to be formed by vessel walls or other cells either from their own endoperoxides or from those released from platelets. From *in vitro* studies it can be demonstrated that when platelets are treated with a thromboxane synthetase inhibitor, the endoperoxides are available for utilization by the vessel wall. Interestingly, in the presence of a thromboxane synthetase inhibitor, arachidonic acid or collagen added to blood *in vitro* leads to the formation of 6-oxo-PGF$_{1\alpha}$ rather than TXB$_2$. Because platelets cannot synthesize prostacyclin, this must reflect formation in another cell type. Such a redivision of metabolic pathways away from a proaggregating agent toward a potent antiaggregating agent, if it were to occur in the clinical setting, would be extremely beneficial in the control of thrombotic episodes. This would be especially important in those diseases where TXA$_2$ is not the primary mediator of platelet activation and aggregation. Indeed, recent evidence points to the superiority of thromboxane synthetase inhibitors over aspirin in experimental thrombotic models. Because cyclooxygenase inhibitors reduce the efficacy of the thromboxane synthetase inhibitors, this supports the involvement of the prostacyclin-generating systems in their mechanisms of action. On this basis, a thromboxane antagonist acting at the receptor level, which could not redirect endoperoxide metabolism, may be of less value than a thromboxane synthetase inhibitor, though this awaits direct study.

Lipid Peroxides

15-Hydroperoxy arachidonic acid (15-HPAA), a lipid peroxide, is a potent inhibitor of prostacyclin generation by vessel wall microsomes or by fresh vascular tissue. Other fatty acid peroxides and their methyl esters behave similarly. Interestingly, high concentrations of lipid peroxides have been demonstrated in advanced atherosclerotic lesions. Lipid peroxidation induced by free-radical formation is known to occur in vitamin E deficiency, the ageing process, and perhaps also in the hyperlipidemia that accompanies atherosclerosis. Thus, accumulation of lipid peroxides in, for example, atheromatous plaques could predispose to thrombus formation by inhibiting generation of prostacyclin by the vessel wall. It has been demonstrated that human atheromatous plaques from some patients are incapable of prostacyclin production. Furthermore, prostacyclin generation by athero-

sclerotic arterial tissue has also been shown to be significantly lower than that from normal artery tissue, but no difference was found between early and advanced atherosclerotic lesions. This suggests that the early "fatty streak" may be a biochemically critical stage of the atherosclerotic process. In the rat, application of 15-HPAA to the outside of mesenteric vessels increased the rate of thrombus formation in response to superfusion with ADP. Prostacyclin may also play a role in the regulation of cell growth in the vascular wall, and therefore the smooth-muscle proliferation observed in atherosclerotic plaques might be a consequence of inhibition of prostacyclin generation by lipid peroxides. It could therefore be valuable to explore whether or not a reduction in lipid peroxide formation, perhaps by inhibiting peroxidation, could influence the development of atherosclerosis and arterial thrombosis. Vitamin E acts as an antioxidant, and perhaps the enthusiasm for its use in arterial disease in the past had in fact a biochemical rationale.

A raised concentration of low-density lipoprotein (LDL) is regarded as one of the risk factors associated with ischemic heart disease, whereas high-density lipoprotein (HDL) is thought to protect against the disease. Nordoy and associates showed that LDL reduces the release of a prostacyclinlike substance by human endothelial cells, and others later showed that LDL inhibited and HDL stimulated prostacyclin synthesis. A mixture of low LDL and high HDL also stimulated prostacyclin synthesis. Gryglewski and Szczeklik (6) have confirmed that LDL inhibits prostacyclin synthesis, and, additionally, they observed that the LDL fraction (but not the HDL) of lipoproteins taken from a group of hyperlipidemics contained lipid peroxides at concentrations several times higher than those in the total serum. Thus, it is possible that the lipid peroxide associated with LDL inhibits prostacyclin synthesis and that this inhibition explains the correlation between LDL and ischemic heart disease.

CLINICAL POTENTIAL OF PROSTACYCLIN AND ITS ANALOGUES

Prostacyclin and its stable analogues have many potential clinical applications for management of thromboembolic disorders and prevention of platelet aggregation during interaction with the artificial surfaces of extracorporeal circulatory systems (1). Prostacyclin may also be valuable in the treatment of peripheral vascular disease, its local intraarterial administration leading to alleviation of pain, regression of necrosis, and healing of ulcers in cases of advanced arteriosclerosis obliterans in humans (20). It is likely that prostacyclin or its analogues will find use in conditions where excessive platelet aggregation is involved, such as thrombotic thrombocytopenic purpura (3) or myocardial infarction. Some of the complications of preeclampsia and the platelet component of the rejection process during transplantation surgery may also respond to prostacyclin therapy. These latter applications, however, are at the moment more speculative, and further work is needed before a definite therapeutic role for prostacyclin can be assigned for such uses.

Prostacyclin or its analogues may also prove valuable in the clinical control of cerebrovascular ischemic conditions, cerebral vasospasm, and thrombotic stroke (26). The increased risk of postoperative cerebral complications resulting from obstruction of the microcirculation by microaggregates that follows cardiopulmonary bypass is likely to be reduced by the use of prostacyclin in the extracorporeal circuit.

The circulation of blood through extracorporeal systems brings blood into contact with artificial surfaces, which obviously cannot generate prostacyclin. In the course of such procedures, the formation of microaggregates, thrombocytopenia, and loss of platelet hemostatic function occur, contributing to the bleeding problems following charcoal hemoperfusion and prolonged cardiopulmonary bypass in humans. Prostacyclin administration improves hemocompatibility during charcoal hemoperfusion in dogs and humans, and studies in dogs and humans suggest that prostacyclin can be used as an alternative to heparin for hemodialysis. In cardiopulmonary bypass experiments in dogs, using a bubble oxygenator, prostacyclin in combination with heparin preserved both platelet number and function, with minimal fibrinogen consumption and deposition on the arterial filters. Preservation of platelet number and function by prostacyclin during extracorporeal oxygenation with a membrane has likewise been demonstrated.

Prostacyclin can potentiate the affects of heparin and itself has a small indirect anticoagulant effect. Platelets stimulated by low doses of aggregating agents accelerate clotting by providing a surface on which coagulation factors can combine and react more efficiently. Prostacyclin, by preventing platelet activation, can inhibit the shortening of clotting time produced when either kaolin or collagen is incubated with platelet-rich plasma. In addition, it is known that platelets can release antiheparin activity, which thereby can reduce the anticoagulant effect of heparin *in vitro*. Prostacyclin, by inhibiting this release and by preventing the development of procoagulant activity, can enhance the action of heparin. Because heparin therapy in some patients is complicated by thrombocytopenia and thromboembolic episodes and *in vitro* can cause platelet aggregation and potentiate aggregation to other aggregating agents, prostacyclin therapy will allow a substantial reduction or even elimination of heparin during hemodialysis, especially if anticoagulation is contraindicated.

The instability of prostacyclin is considered useful in limiting its biological activity when used for extracorporeal circulations. However, the possibility of developing a short-acting chemically stable analogue with a biological profile similar to that of prostacyclin for such uses has been considered.

One of the first chemically stable analogues to be described was a 5,6-dihydro analogue, 6β-PGI$_1$, whose structure is shown in Fig.

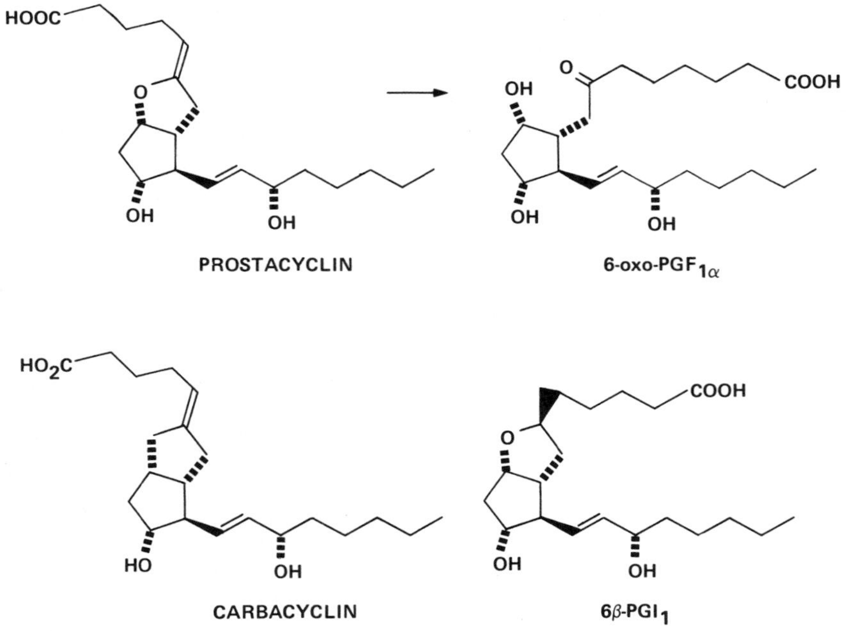

FIG. 5. Chemical structures of prostacyclin, its breakdown product 6-oxo-PGF$_{1\alpha}$, and two stable analogues.

5. This analogue inhibits human platelet aggregation *in vitro* (Table 1), being some 250 times less active than prostacyclin. The epimer, 6α-PGI$_1$, is less active on the cardiovascular parameters and platelet aggregation. In a study of isolated guinea pig heart and bovine coronary artery strips, a divergent profile of activity of both epimers of PGI$_1$ with prostacyclin has been observed. Thus, although these compounds have many of the properties of the parent compound, these 5,6-dihydro analogues cannot be considered as very close mimics of prostacyclin.

The synthesis of carbocyclic analogues of prostacyclin has recently been described. The chemically stable prostacyclin analogue (5E) 6a-carbaprostaglandin I$_2$ (carbacyclin, Fig. 5) has proved to be a potent inhibitor of platelet aggregation in human plasma (Table 1). Carbacyclin is active against human platelet aggregation induced by ADP, archidonic acid, and collagen, and it also inhibits platelet aggregation in plasma from a variety of species, including dog and rabbit (28). As with prostacyclin, the antiaggregating action of carbacyclin is enhanced by the phosphodiesterase inhibitor theophylline. The antiaggregating activities of other carbocyclic prostacyclin analogues have also been reported.

Carbacyclin is a potent inhibitor of *ex vivo* platelet aggregation when infused intravenously in the rabbit and dog, being one-tenth as active as prostacyclin. Consideration of its concurrent effects on BP indicates that carbacyclin is a close mimic of prostacyclin. This analogue is also effective *in vivo* in reducing thrombus formation in dog coronary arteries. Studies with carbacyclin in anesthetized baboons have also shown inhibition of platelet aggregation *ex vivo* following intravenous or intragastric administration.

The antiaggregating action of carbacyclin is short-lived once the infusion is terminated. As with prostacyclin, its inhibitory action on platelet aggregation *ex vivo* in the dog and rabbit is no longer significant 10 min after infusion. Thus, although carbacyclin is chemically stable at physiological temperatures and pH (no loss in biological activity could be detected in aqueous samples stored for 30 days at pH 7 at room temperature), its similar duration of activity to prostacyclin suggests that in the rabbit and dog, both prostacyclin and carbacyclin are rapidly metabolized. Studies in the rat indicate that carbacyclin is not inactivated during passage through the pulmonary circulation, because the analogue had comparable vasodepressor activities when administered by intravenous or intraarterial injection (Fig. 4). Although, like prostacyclin, carbacyclin may not be a substrate for the pulmonary transport system required for metabolism by 15-PGDH enzyme in intact lung, it may be metabolized readily in other organs such as the kidney or in vascular tissue.

Carbacyclin is thus a close mimic of prostacyclin, with respect to its hemodynamic and platelet actions, and it is chemically stable but metabolically unstable. Such analogues should be of clinical value for the same uses proposed for prostacyclin. The development of potent stable prostacyclin analogues with biological profiles very close to that of the parent compound thus represents the first stage in drug design. The next step is the development of analogues with selective biological actions. However, the desirable degree of selectivity between such parameters as platelet inhibition and cardiovascular activity is as yet unknown, because both activities are clearly of importance in many of the proposed clinical uses. Rational design of newer analogues will therefore depend on the clinical experience gained with the parent, prostacyclin. The development of orally active prostacyclin analogues with long-lasting duration of action in humans will provide drugs for the control of platelet aggregation and thromboembolic disorders superior to those known at present and may well form the basis of future antithrombotic therapy.

REFERENCES

1. Bunting, S., Moncada, S., Vane, J. R., Woods, H. F., and Weston, M. J. (1979): Prostacyclin improves hemocompatibility during charcoal hemoperfusion. In: *Prostacyclin*, edited by J. R. Vane and S. Bergström, pp. 361–369. Raven Press, New York.

2. Dyerberg, J., Bang, H. O., Stoffersen, E., Moncada, S., and Vane, J. R. (1978): Eicosapentaenoic acid and prevention of thrombosis and atherosclerosis? *Lancet*, 2:117–119.

3. FitzGerald, G. A., Roberts, L. J., II, Maas, D., Brash, A. R., and Oates, J. A. (1981): Intravenous prostacyclin in thrombotic thrombocytopenic purpura. In: *Clinical Pharmacology of Prostacyclin*, edited by P. J. Lewis and J. O'Grady, p. 81. Raven Press, New York.

4. Flower, R. J. (1978): Prostaglandins and related compounds. In: *Inflammation*, edited by J. R. Vane and S. H. Ferreira, pp. 374–422. Springer-Verlag, New York.

5. Gorman, R. R., Shebuski, R. J., Aiken, J. W., and Bundy, G. L. (1981): Analysis of the biological activity of azoprostanoids in human platelets. *Fed. Proc.*, 40:1997–2000.

6. Gryglewski, R. J., and Szczeklik, A. (1981): Prostacyclin and atherosclerosis. In: *Clinical Pharmacology of Prostacyclin*, edited by P. J. Lewis and J. O'Grady, pp. 89–95. Raven Press, New York.

7. Hamberg, M., Svensson, J., and Samuelsson, B. (1974): Prostaglandin endoperoxides. A new concept concerning the mode of action and release of prostaglandins. *Proc. Natl. Acad. Sci. U.S.A.*, 71:3824–3828.

8. Hamberg, M., Svensson, J., and Samuelsson, B. (1975): Thromboxanes: A new group of biologically active compounds derived from prostaglandin endoperoxides. *Proc. Natl. Acad. Sci. U.S.A.*, 72:2994–2998.

9. Higgs, G. A., Moncada, S., and Vane, J. R. (1980). The mode of action of antiinflammatory drugs which prevent the peroxidation of arachidonic acid. In: *Clinics in Rheumatic Diseases*, edited by E. C. Huskisson, pp. 675–693. W. B. Saunders, London.

10. Lapetina, E. G. (1982): Regulation of arachidonic acid production: Role of phospholipase C and A_2. In: *Trends in Pharmacological Science*, pp. 115–118. Elsevier, Amsterdam.

11. Marcus, A. J. (1978): The role of lipids in platelet function with particular reference to the arachidonic acid pathway. *J. Lipid Res.*, 19:793–826.

12. Moncada, S. (1982): Biological importance of prostacyclin. *Br. J. Pharmacol.*, 76:3–31.

13. Moncada, S., Gryglewski, R. J., Bunting, S., and Vane, J. R. (1976): An enzyme isolated from arteries transforms prostaglandin endoperoxides to an unstable substance that inhibits platelet aggregation. *Nature*, 263:663–665.

14. Moncada, S., Needleman, P., Bunting, S., and Vane J. R. (1976): Prostaglandin endoperoxide and thromboxane generating systems and their selective inhibition. *Prostaglandins*, 12:323–325.

15. Moncada, S., and Vane J. R. (1979): Pharmacology and endogenous roles of prostaglandin endoperoxides, thromboxane A_2 and prostacyclin. *Pharmacol. Rev.*, 30:292–331.

16. Mullane, K. M., Moncada, S., and Vane, J. R. (1979): Formation and disappearance of prostacyclin in the circulation. In: *Prostacyclin*, edited by J. R. Vane and S. Bergstrom, pp. 221–244. Raven Press, New York.

17. Needleman, P., Raz, A., Minkes, M. S., Ferrendelli

J. A., and Sprecher, H. (1979): Triene prostaglandins: Prostacyclin and thromboxane biosynthesis and unique biological properties. *Proc. Natl. Acad. Sci. U.S.A.*, 76:944–948.

18. Remuzzi, G., Marchesi, D., Livio, M., Schieppati, A., Mecca, G., Donati, M. B., and de Gaetano, G. (1980): Prostaglandins, plasma factors and hemostasis in uremia. In: *Hemostasis, Prostaglandins and Renal Disease,* edited by G. Remuzzi, G. Mecca, and G. de Gaetano, pp. 273–281. Raven Press, New York.

19. Samuelsson, B., Hammarström, S., Murphy, R. C., and Borgeat, P. (1980): Leukotrienes and slow reacting substance of anaphylaxis (SRS-A). *Allergy,* 35:375–381.

20. Szczeklik, A., and Gryglewski, R. J. (1981): Treatment of vascular disease with prostacyclin. In: *Clinical Pharmacology of Prostacyclin,* edited by P. J. Lewis and J. O'Grady, pp. 159–167. Raven Press, New York.

21. Silver, M. J., Smith, J. B., McLean, M. I., and Bills, T. K. (1980): Prostaglandins and thromboxanes: Current concepts. In: *Hemostasis, Prostaglandins and Renal Disease,* edited by G. Remuzzi, G. Mecca, and G. de Gaetano, pp. 154–173. Raven Press, New York.

22. Ten Hoor, F., De Dekere, E. A. M., Haddeman, E., Hornstra, G., and Quadt, J. F. A. (1980): Dietary manipulation of prostaglandin and thromboxane synthesis in heart, aorta and blood platelets of the rat. In: *Advances in Prostaglandin and Thromboxane Research, Vol. 8,* edited by B. Samuelsson, P. W. Ramwell, and R. Paoletti, pp. 1771–1781. Raven Press, New York.

23. Vane, J. R. (1971): Inhibition of prostaglandin synthesis as a mechanism of action for aspirin-like drugs. *Nature [New Biol].,* 231:232–235.

24. Vargaftig, B. B. (1980): Arachidonic acid, platelets and blood pressure. In: *Hemostasis, Prostaglandins and Renal Disease,* edited by G. Remuzzi, G. Mecca, and G. de Gaetano, pp. 207–215. Raven Press, New York.

25. Weksler, B. B., Reinus, J., and Eldor, A. (1981): Interactions between platelets and prostaglandins: Modulation of prostacyclin production and action on platelets. In: *Prostaglandins and Cardiovascular Disease,* edited by R. Johnson Hegyeli pp. 125–138. Raven Press, New York.

26. Whittle, B. J. R., and Moncada, S. (1981): Therapeutic potential of prostacyclin and its stable analogues in cerebrovascular and thrombotic diseases. In: *Cerebrovascular Diseases: New Trends in Surgical and Medical Aspects,* edited by H. Barnett, P. Paoletti, E. Flamm, and G. Brambilla, pp. 151–165. Elsevier/North Holland, Amsterdam.

27. Whittle, B. J. R. (1980): Actions of prostaglandins on gastric mucosal blood flow. In: *Gastrointestinal Mucosal Blood Flow,* edited by L. P. Fielding, pp. 180–191. Churchill Livingstone, London.

28. Whittle, B. J. R., Moncada, S., and Vane, J. R. (1981): Biological activities of some metabolites and analogues of prostacyclin. In: *Medical Chemistry Advances,* edited by F. G. De Las Heras and S. Vega, pp. 141–158. Pergamon Press, London.

29. Willis, A. L. (1978): Platelet aggregation mechanisms and their implications in haemostasis and inflammatory disease. In: *Inflammation,* edited by J. R. Vane and S. H. Ferreira, pp. 138–205. Springer-Verlag, Berlin.

30. Wong, P. Y. K., Lee, W. H., Quilley, C. P., and McGiff, J. C. (1981): Metabolism of prostacyclin: Formation of an active metabolite in the liver. *Fed. Proc.,* 40:2001–2004.

Cardiovascular Pharmacology, Second Edition,
edited by Michael Antonaccio.
Raven Press, New York © 1984.

Pharmacologic Basis of the Treatment of Circulatory Shock

Allan M. Lefer and James A. Spath, Jr.

*Department of Physiology, Jefferson Medical College, Thomas Jefferson University,
Philadelphia, Pennsylvania 19107*

INTRODUCTION

The treatment of circulatory shock has been as varied as its causes. Thus, in hemorrhagic shock, the addition of volume in the form of whole blood, plasma, or crystalloid solutions has been recommended, and in endotoxin shock, administration of antibiotics coupled with fluid therapy has been used routinely. Treatment of cardiogenic shock has involved minimizing the work of the injured myocardium. Moreover, the reduced mean arterial blood pressures occurring in virtually all types of circulatory shock have prompted the use of a variety of vasopressor agents in the treatment of shock. Despite the variety of approaches to the treatment of circulatory shock based on correcting recognized abnormalities associated with shock states, treatment of circulatory shock from whatever cause remains a difficult problem. A consideration of both the hemodynamic and the subcellular alterations that occur in shock is necessary in order to understand fully the basis of the therapeutics of the shock state.

DEFINITION OF CIRCULATORY SHOCK, AN ANALYSIS OF ITS CAUSE

Wiggers and Ingraham (1) defined hemorrhagic shock as a progression of three physiological conditions: simple hypotension, impending shock, and irreversible shock. The first of these states requires no treatment other than removal of the immediate cause. Thus, in the case of hemorrhage, cessation of blood loss would be sufficient for return of cardiovascular function to normal. The second phase requires treatment to correct and, if left uncorrected, proceeds to the third stage, irreversible shock. Thus, impending shock involves cellular derangements that become irreversible and lead to death despite generally accepted therapeutic modalities. It is generally held that hypoperfusion of peripheral vascular beds occurs after some degree of hypotension and precedes the development of circulatory shock. Thus, knowledgeable treatment of states of circulatory shock must define both the cause of hypotension and the consequences of hypoperfusion.

Hemodynamic causes of any hypotensive low-flow state, *per se,* are easily defined. Thus, reduced blood pressure is the result of decreased flow (i.e., cardiac output) or reduced peripheral vascular tone or resistance. A decreased blood volume or a decreased activation of cardiac β-receptors results in a decreased filling pressure, a decreased heart rate, or a decreased level of myocardial contractility, all of which decrease cardiac output and promote hypotension. A decreased intramural tension in the resistance vessels of the peripheral vasculature would also promote hypotension. A decrease in vessel tension would arise from a decreased blood volume in the vessel as a result of an absolute loss of total blood volume, altered segmental resistances (i.e., large and small arteries and veins), loss of capillary integrity, and osmotic and ionic shifts within the vasculature. The segmental vascular resistances would be altered by the neurohumoral outflow to them and by osmotic and ionic shifts affecting the contractility of the vascular smooth muscle.

Thus, shock states involve altered function of the heart and the peripheral vasculature. The relative contribution of cardiac failure and peripheral vascular failure to circulatory shock has been the subject of debate among investigators for several years. Obviously, either a progressive decline in the ability of the myocardium to develop sufficient systolic tension or the continuing loss of peripheral vascular tone or integrity would result in death. In considering the various hemodynamic patterns which develop in hemorrhagic, endotoxic, cardiogenic, splanchnic artery occlusion and burn shock, we will review the hemodynamic evidence for cardiac failure or peripheral vasculature collapse in each of these types of circulatory shock.

Hemorrhagic Shock

Hemorrhagic shock is a frequent consequence of a severe, prolonged decrease in the circulating blood volume and is characterized by a marked decrease in blood pressure and cardiac output. Other clinical signs of this type of shock reflect the response of the cardiovascular and respiratory systems to decreased cardiac output and reduced peripheral blood flow. Increased sympathoadrenal discharge, resultant increased levels of circulating norepinephrine and epinephrine, as well as release of angiotension and vasopressin act to increase peripheral resistance and stimulate the myocardium following hemorrhage. The degree of increased total peripheral resistance with hemorrhage varies greatly with the species and within individuals of a given species. Although total peripheral resistance may increase only

moderately with hemorrhage, recent studies indicate that peripheral vascular beds undergo selective vasoconstriction during acute blood loss. Studies of hemorrhaged dog, cat, monkey, and man reveal that one or more of the splanchnic organs undergo profound vasoconstriction with a concomitant severe decrease in blood flow, out of proportion to the decrease in blood pressure. Significant reductions in cutaneous and renal blood flow, and a moderate to severe decrease in muscle blood flow, also appear to be common findings in studies of hemorrhagic shock.

A great number of studies of hemorrhagic shock have employed the Lamson modification of the Wiggers technique for inducing shock. The response of the anesthetized dog to the Wiggers-Lamson protocol is shown in Fig. 1. Experimental hemorrhagic shock is routinely induced by bleeding the animal into a constant-pressure reservoir to a preselected pressure. This model obviates the effectiveness of the compensatory responses of the animal, since a vasopressor response promotes additional loss of blood to the reservoir. The hemorrhaged animal will progressively lose blood into the reservoir up to a certain point known as the "maximal bleedout." Within 1 hr, the animal begins to take blood back into the circulatory system from the reservoir. This process is known as "uptake." The lower the preset reservoir pressure, the sooner the animal will begin to take up blood from the reservoir. The uptake of blood indicates the beginning of circulatory decompensation. Thus, it is customary to permit the animal to take up a fixed percentage of the maximum bled volume after which the remainder of the reservoir blood is reinfused within a few minutes. Following reinfusion, the animal is monitored until recovery or death.

Thus, in hemorrhagic shock the initial traumatic event is hypovolemia with resultant decreased cardiac output and hypotension. The duration of oligemia and hypotension is determined by the investigator and by the reflex compensatory response of the animal. Uptake of blood from the reservoir signals decompen-

Experimental Hemorrhagic Shock

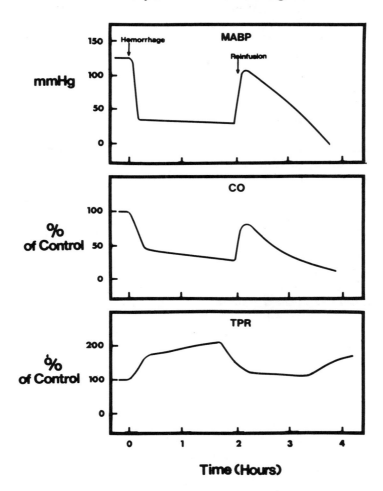

FIG. 1. Hemodynamics of experimental hemorrhagic shock using the Lamson reservoir technique. MABP = mean arterial blood pressure in mm Hg; CO = cardiac output in percent of the zero time control value; TPR = total peripheral resistance in percent of the zero time control value. A 4-hr time course for the shock protocol has been selected for simplicity of presentation.

sation which portends cardiovascular collapse following reinfusion.

Because of variable bleedout volumes of animals subjected to the constant-pressure protocol, the constant-volume technique has also been used to study the hemodynamic response of hemorrhaged animals. This technique requires determining the blood volume of the animals and removing a designated portion of that volume. Forsyth et al. (2), employing radioactive microspheres in studying the re-

sponse of conscious monkeys to hemorrhagic shock, removed 10 to 50% of the circulating blood volume in three stages over a 2-hr period. Loss of 30% of the blood volume provoked decreases in mean arterial blood pressure (MABP), central venous pressure (CVP), cardiac output (CO), and arterial blood pH. Cardiopulmonary stimulation was indicated by increased heart and respiratory rates. A 50% loss of blood volume produced even greater decreases in MABP and cardiac output, but the CVP and arterial pH were comparable to control animals. This return to normal levels of arterial pH reflects the compensatory effects of hyperventilation induced in response to hemorrhage. Following loss of 50% of the blood volume, blood flows to the kidney, skin, and skeletal muscle were reduced to 10 to 20% of the prehemorrhage level, respectively, whereas blood flow to the pancreas and spleen were 8% of the normovolemic level. The percentage of the cardiac output perfusing the heart, brain, small intestine, and hepatic artery increased following hemorrhage.

Rutherford and Trow (3) confirmed the results of Forsyth et al. (2) also in the conscious monkey. However, these authors bled the animals to 40 mm Hg until 15% of the shed volume was taken up after about 2 to 3 hr of oligemia. The remainder of the shed blood was reinfused at that time. Following reinfusion, it was necessary to infuse a volume of Ringer's solution in order to return MABP to prehemorrhage levels. Moreover, a continuous infusion of crystalloid solution failed to maintain MABP at normotensive levels, and the animals died of cardiorespiratory arrest 5 to 15 hr after reinfusion. Death supervened at a time when cardiac output, regional blood flows, and arterial pH were normal and the arterial blood pressure only moderately reduced. These results indicate that: (a) commonly measured hemodynamic parameters may not predict survival and (b) cellular dysfunction originating during the oligemic period may prevent survival despite efforts to normalize circulatory function. Rutherford and Trow (3) suggested the absence of cardiac failure in their preparation, since the cardiac output, cardiac work, and CVP were normal just prior to death. However, following reinfusion, an increased diastolic filling pressure was necessary to return cardiac output and cardiac work to normal levels. Thus, volume support may forestall impending cardiac failure during hemorrhage.

Cardiac decompensation during hemorrhage has been demonstrated by Gomez and Hamilton (4) and by Crowell and Guyton (5)

and is generally believed to contribute to the lethal outcome of circulatory shock. Selective vasoconstriction has also been implicated in collapse of the circulatory system in hemorrhagic shock, either through the direct metabolic deterioration of hypoperfused tissues (6) or through extravasation of fluid in the peripheral beds (7). Thus, early in hemorrhage, fluid enters the vascular space as hematocrit and plasma protein progressively decline. However, with the development of decompensation (i.e., uptake from the reservoir), fluid again begins to leave the vascular system, probably because of increased postcapillary resistance. Further loss of volume, perfusion pressure, and blood flow would then promote additional metabolic alterations which are of negative survival value.

Endotoxin Shock

The general pattern of hemodynamic changes following the experimental administration of bacterial endotoxin appears in Fig. 2. The initial blood pressure response to endotoxin and hemorrhage are similar. However, the combined decrease in MABP and cardiac output following hemorrhage provokes little change or an increase in total peripheral resistance (TPR). Usually, endotoxin elicits little change or a modest decrease in cardiac output coupled with a fall in MABP and a decreased TPR. However, in many clinical cases of septic shock, cardiac output may actually be increased. This does not necessarily indicate enhanced perfusion of peripheral tissues, however, since a great degree of shunting may occur. The quantitative variability in the hemodynamic response to endotoxin is as great as that following hemorrhage. Thus, in addition to reflex alterations in sympathetic activity, endotoxin induces local effects on the microcirculaton in a variety of tissues.

As in the case of hemorrhage, a redistribution of the cardiac output is among the reflex circulatory changes in response to endotoxin. Wyler et al. (8) reported an increase in coronary flow following endotoxin administration

Experimental Endotoxic Shock

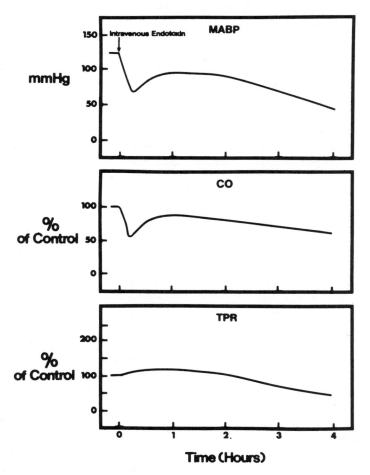

FIG. 2. Hemodynamics of experimental endotoxin shock after intravenous injection of *E. coli* endotoxin. See Fig. 1 for details.

in monkeys. This, coupled with the decreased TPR, could account for the initial increase in cardiac output following endotoxin. In contrast to hemorrhage, neither the absolute flow measured with radioactive microspheres nor the percentage of the cardiac output perfusing the kidneys, skin, or muscle is reduced 40 min after endotoxin. The hypoperfusion of the gastrointestinal tract is consistent with hemorrhaged monkeys. Moreover, the selective vasoconstriction following endotoxin was indicated by a reduced percentage of the cardiac output reaching the pancreas and spleen at

a time when the percentage of the cardiac output perfusing the gastrointestinal tract increased 67%. The occurrence of altered metabolic activity was indicated by a decrease in arterial pH 24 hr after administration of endotoxin at a time when the arterial blood gases and hematocrit levels were not changed significantly. In this regard, Winslow et al. (9) reported significantly greater blood lactate in patients who failed to survive bacteremic shock despite a variety of therapeutic measures. Furthermore, altered cardiac output or stroke work in the face of increased left ventricular filling pressures suggested impaired cardiac function in patients in septic shock.

The possibility of a direct effect of endotoxin on the myocardium has been the subject of considerable debate. Solis and Downing (10) advocated a direct cardiotoxic effect on the myocardium. However, endotoxin failed to alter the contractile response of isolated cardiac tissue (11). Late in endotoxin shock, cardiac failure commonly occurs (11,12). Elkins et al. (13) attributed this endotoxin-induced myocardial failure to prolonged coronary hypoperfusion. However, coronary hypoperfusion may be a canine response to endotoxin, since Wyler et al. (8) failed to demonstrate coronary hypoperfusion in the monkey.

Cardiogenic Shock

Cardiac hypofunction is the principal criterion in the definition of cardiogenic shock (i.e., shock in which a portion of the ventricular myocardium fails to develop significant degrees of tension during systole). Decreased systolic tension produces a decrease in stroke volume and a fall in mean arterial blood pressure (Fig. 3). A fall in blood pressure should activate a sympathetic discharge to the heart and blood vessels. However, the response of the vessels is variable following coronary embolization.

In open-chest dogs (14), a moderate increase in total peripheral resistance occurred associated with a moderate decrease in MABP, heart rate, and contractility 1 hr following coronary embolism. In this study, cardiac output and coronary blood flow were halved but mesenteric and femoral blood flows were reduced out of proportion to the decrease in cardiac output.

A different pattern of flow distribution occurred in conscious monkeys following coronary artery ligation. At the time when total flow to the gastrointestinal tract was unaltered, the percentage of the CO perfusing the pancreas and spleen was reduced to about 50% of the control values. Thus, cardiogenic shock may involve hypoperfusion of cardiac origin, but the consequences of reduced blood flow to the periphery should be considered when defining the cause of the ensuing circulatory collapse. Moreover, the hemodynamic response to myocardial infarction should not be equated with the syndrome of cardiogenic shock. Following myocardial infarction, the blood pressure and cardiac index may be elevated or normal in the presence of normal or elevated filling pressure. Uncomplicated cardiogenic shock presents a decreased cardiac index, decreased aortic pressure, and increased diastolic filling pressure.

Burn Shock

Burns over 35% of the body surface initially do not produce shock. However, secondary to the burn injury, circulatory shock may develop with hypovolemic, endotoxic, or cardiac components (see Fig. 4). Thus, Deets and Glaviano (15) reported normal values of CVP, MABP, and heart rate 4 hr after burn-induced trauma in dogs. At the same time, cardiac output was significantly decreased whereas the TPR and hematocrit were increased. Since the central venous pressures remained in normal range, the authors suggested that the decreased cardiac output was of myocardial origin. However, the authors caution that study of a larger population of burned dogs might reveal a significant decrease in CVP which could account for the cardiac output in thermal injury. In this regard, Shoemaker et al. (16) also reported a decreased CO and increased TPR in patients soon after severe burns. Cardiac performance curves on these patients indicated decreased left ventricular stroke work secondary to decreased CVP following fluid loss from the area of injury. Administration of fluid produced increased cardiac index, stroke work, and central blood volume and decreased TPR for several days after thermal injury. However, in the preterminal period, all hemodynamic parameters except heart rate decreased. Moreover, assessment of cardiac performance in the preterminal period indicated myocardial depression.

Experimental Cardiogenic Shock

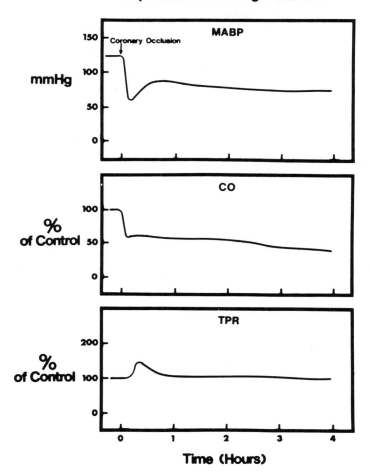

FIG. 3. Hemodynamics of experimental cardiogenic shock after occlusion of a significant portion of coronary flow to the left ventricle. See Fig. 1 for details.

The myocardial depression at this time may be due to toxic factors released from the burn site or elsewhere, coupled with continued loss of volume despite fluid therapy. Thus, it appears that burn shock has an etiology involving both cardiac and peripheral vascular components.

Splanchnic Artery Occlusion Shock

Splanchnic arterial occlusion shock (SAO) occurs following a marked decrease in blood flow to the gastrointestinal tract. Clinically,

mesenteric infarction with shock is found chiefly in elderly patients and is associated with long-standing hypoperfusion of the gastrointestinal tract attributed to primary cardiac or peripheral vascular disease (i.e., abdominal aortic and splanchnic vascular atherosclerosis). The experimental model of SAO shock constitutes occlusion of one or more of the splanchnic vessels (i.e., the celiac axis, the superior and inferior mesenteric arteries) for a fixed duration. Following a period of splanchnic ischemia, the occluding clamps are released and the hemodynamic response

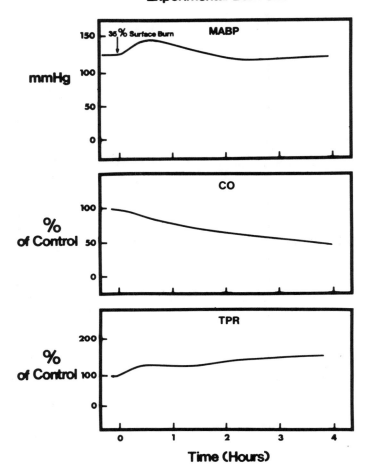

FIG. 4. Hemodynamics of experimental burn shock after a 35% surface burn. See Fig. 1 for details.

of the animal monitored. Figure 5 depicts the typical hemodynamic response to 2 hr of splanchnic arterial occlusion in the cat (17). Following control measurements, the major arteries serving the splanchnic viscera were clamped for 2 hr. SAO produced a transient rise in blood pressure and cardiac output, probably due to a redistribution of flow and to reflex vascular adjustments. The blood pressure, cardiac output, and peripheral resistance remain normal during the period of splanchnic ischemia. Following release of the occlusive clamps, a transient fall in MABP occurs. The fall in MABP initiates reflex vaso-

constriction to restore MABP. Although some recovery does occur, MABP and cardiac output undergo progressive severe decline to shock levels. SAO shock results in the release of toxic substances from the occluded splanchnic region into the circulation. The action of these toxic substances on the heart and lungs has been strongly implicated in the pathophysiology of circulatory shock (18,19).

Conclusion

In describing the hemodynamic patterns found in various types of circulatory shock,

Experimental SAO Shock

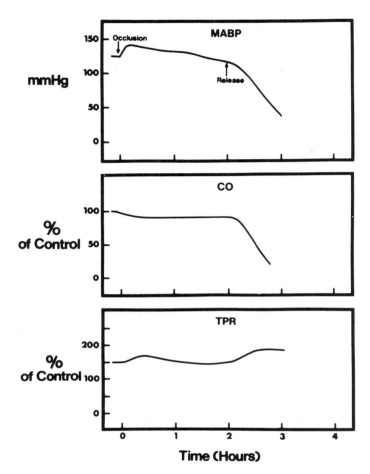

FIG. 5. Hemodynamics of experimental splanchnic artery occlusion (SAO) shock after ligation of the celiac and mesenteric arteries for 2 hr and release of the occlusive clamps. See Fig. 1 for details.

the initial traumatic event is seen to evoke various primary and secondary effects. Thus, a decrease in blood volume or injury to the myocardium primarily produces a decrease in cardiac output. Additionally, septicemia produces decreased peripheral resistance, whereas severely reduced splanchnic flow results in both peripheral vascular and cardiac dysfunction. The primary effects of the shock-inducing event produces variable degrees of sympathoadrenal activation or inhibition which vary with (a) the type of initial traumatic event, (b) the condition of the animal, (c) the species studied, and (d) the duration of the shock state. However, despite the variety of causes of circulatory shock, it has become apparent that all forms of shock involve a redistribution of blood flow to the peripheral tissues of the body. These alterations in vascular perfusion and redistribution of blood flow may result from direct sympathetic activation, inhibition or alterations in the level of circulating vasoactive agents, and the metabolic activity of the vascular smooth muscle within an organ. As a consequence, flow in certain organs declines to a level which does not fully support aerobic metabolism. Indeed, the flow may be so reduced that those metabolic processes required for cellular integrity (e.g., ionic pumps) are no longer maintained. These relationships among hypoperfusion, altered metabolism, and cellular dysfunction are common in all types of circulatory shock regardless of the cause of the initial traumatic event or the specific pattern of the hemodynamic response to the shock state. Thus, pharmacologic management of all forms of circulatory shock requires critical examination of the cellular consequences of the low-flow shock state.

CELLULAR CONSEQUENCES OF SHOCK

Cellular aspects of shock are now well appreciated as a crucial aspect of the shock process. In order to understand fully the basic pathophysiologic mechanism of shock, we must search for abnormal cellular processes as a consequence of the shock state. In general, investigations have called attention to certain aspects of cellular biology during circulatory shock. These are (a) general ultrastructural alterations of the cell, (b) specific perturbations and abnormal processes in key subcellular organelles, and (c) modifications in cellular metabolism with particular emphasis on energy transformation. These findings provide insight into the pathophysiology of the shock state and identify potential target areas for the treatment of circulatory shock.

One of the basic sequelae of shock, which is often used as a definition of shock, is "inadequate perfusion of tissue cells." Hypoperfusion can lead to ischemia as shock progresses and as the circulatory system deteriorates. Along with ischemia, hypoxia and acidosis also occur. Although specific events occur in certain tissues and cell types, there appears to be a generalized cellular response to most types of circulatory shock.

One of the basic cellular responses to a variety of types of shock is cell swelling. In general, most cells swell in response to ischemia, presumably due to inhibition of cell metabolism and the subsequent accumulation of cellular water, although the evidence for this is largely indirect (e.g., isotopic tracer studies, serum/tissue electrolyte ratios, osmolality of plasma, and extracellular compartment size). Hemorrhage has been shown to induce nuclear swelling in certain cells of the cerebral cortex (e.g., nucleus ceruleus), although not in the cerebellar cortex. Although swelling may be an early response to ischemia, several other types of ultrastructural alterations occur. Mitochondria have been shown to swell and to undergo degenerative changes such as invagination and breakup of internal cristae (20–22) in response to hemorrhage, endotoxin, or hypoxia. These changes occur in such diverse organs as liver, posterior pituitary, mesenteric arteries, kidney, and skeletal muscle (20–23).

In addition to these mitochondrial changes, important alterations occur in other subcellular organelles (see Fig. 6). Thus, the usually ordered endoplasmic reticulum is frequently splayed and scattered about the cytoplasm, gaps in the cell membrane can be more readily observed, large channel invaginations in the sarcoplasmic reticulum can be seen, nuclear envelope damage occasionally results, zymogen granules and other secretory granules are often broken or lysed (i.e., sometimes only remnants of their membrane are present), and there is a more prominent appearance of the lysosomal vacuole apparatus (24,25). Lysosomes may be increased or decreased in number depending on the metabolic and functional status of the cell. However, lysosomes usually appear as distended structures with large prominent vacuoles. These vacuoles may be filled with cell debris or with a relatively clear substance containing perhaps a lipid-like material.

In addition to the ultrastructural evidence, physiological and biochemical studies also show mitochondrial damage in shock. In general, there appears to be a significant degree of uncoupling of oxidative phosphorylation as reflected in a decreased mitochondrial P/O ratio (i.e., ratio of high-energy phosphate

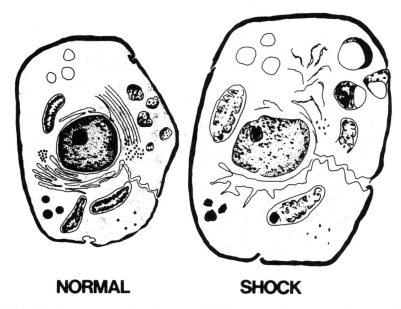

NORMAL　　**SHOCK**

FIG. 6. Cellular alterations in circulatory shock in an idealized normal somatic cell **(left)** and in a similar cell after severe shock **(right)**. Note the cell swelling, damage to cell and endoplasmic reticulum membranes, mitochondrial disruption, lysosomal swelling and vacuole formation, nuclear damage, and the presence of residual bodies in the cell. These changes have been reported in a variety of cell types in different types of circulatory shock.

bonds generated per mole of oxygen consumed) (26–28), although DePalma et al. (29) were unable to find significant changes in liver mitochondrial P/O ratios in hemorrhagic shock. Perhaps even more significant is the well-documented decrease in state 3 respiratory activity (i.e., that O_2 consumption occurring during phosphorylation in the presence of ADP and P_i) and in respiratory control ratios (RCR) indicative of uncoupling of oxidative phosphorylation (28,30,31). These changes are much more prominent in liver than in heart mitochondria (31), perhaps related to the degree of cellular acidosis present. In this regard, hepatocyte pH drops from about 7.1 to 5.9 in hemorrhagic shock, whereas myocardial cell pH appears to increase from 6.6 to 7.2 under the same conditions. Recently, efforts have been made to determine the subcellular basis for the impairment of mitochondrial function. One factor that is known to be crucial to mitochondrial function is the permeability and transport characteristics of the mitochondrial mem-

brane. Thus, as mitochondrial function deteriorates, enhanced Na^+ entry and greater K^+ loss from cells occur. Whether these ionic changes induce mitochondrial failure or whether they are a consequence of mitochondrial damage is not clear at this time. Moreover, Ca^{2+} transport across rat liver mitochondrial membranes is seriously impaired early in endotoxemia (32). This may be a critical step in mitochondrial damage, although more direct data are needed to interpret these findings.

Another possibility that has received attention of late is that lysosomes release large amounts of acid hydrolases early in shock, and these hydrolytic enzymes effectively attack and destroy the mitochondria during shock. This attractive hypothesis has been verified *in vitro* by Mellors et al. (33), who added lysosomal extracts to mitochondrial fractions *in vitro* and found significant damage of the mitrochondria by the lysosomal enzymes. The major lysosomal factor apparently responsible for mitochondrial swelling and uncoupling was a phospholipase (33). Recently, Nicholas et al. (34) extended these findings by showing that lysosomal enzymes also inhibited mitochondrial calcium transport. Other investigators have attempted to relate the increased activity of the cation-activated ATPases of mitochondrial membranes (35) to the defect in mitochondrial function. At present, not enough information is available, but this type of study may provide insight into the basic cellular mechanisms upset by the shock state.

Cell membrane function is another area of cell integrity that appears to be altered during shock. Although ultrastructural damage can occasionally be observed in the cell membrane, no quantitative morphometric analysis of cell membrane integrity during shock is presently available. These studies would be extremely difficult to perform, and interpretation would be subject to a variety of criticisms (i.e., sampling population size, fixation artefacts, etc.). Nevertheless, physiological investigations indicate that significant alterations in cell membrane function occur during circulatory shock. As an example, transport of Na^+ and K^+ across liver cell membranes is impaired in hemorrhagic shock (36). This membrane defect can be corrected by early treatment with fluid therapy. Another approach has been to measure the resting transmembrane potential (E_m) of muscle cells as an index of both active transport mechanisms of the cell membrane and the excitability of muscle cells. These studies indicate that a decrease in E_m on the order of 20 mV occurs in skeletal muscle cells during hemorrhagic shock (37–40). This change in membrane potential is associated with a decrease in extracellular water and an increase in intracellular Na^+. Presumably, these fluid and ionic changes are related to changes in the ratio of the $[K^+]_i / [K^+]_o$, a primary determinant of the resting membrane potential. Once E_m decreases, the rate of rise and amplitude of the muscle action potential also decreases, which can result in impaired excitation of muscle. Although these changes per se are probably not responsible for cell death, they contribute to conditions which re-

sult in cell damage during shock. Comparable findings in cardiac and vascular smooth muscle, although technically more difficult, would lend support to the work of Shires and co-workers in establishing the role of impaired cell excitation in the shock process.

Lysosomes are subcellular organelles which play a key role in the economy and life cycle of most mammalian cells. Lysosomes take many forms, shapes, and sizes, and may contain differing amounts of a variety of acid hydrolases. Despite this heterogeneity of form and function, lysosomes appear to play a relatively similar role in many organs during a variety of types of circulatory shock. In general, during hemorrhagic, endotoxic, bowel ischemic, cardiogenic, and pancreatitis shock, lysosomes undergo marked degenerative changes. These changes occur principally in the organs which become ischemic or hypoxic during the shock state. Usually these tissues are the splanchnic structures (i.e., liver, pancreas, spleen, intestine), and sometimes other areas are involved such as kidney and skeletal muscle. In cardiogenic shock induced by myocardial infarction, there is a direct myocardial lysosomal involvement as well. Janoff, Weissmann, and co-workers were the first investigators (41,42) to recognize the importance of lysosomal changes in the pathophysiology of circulatory shock. These workers showed substantial increases in plasma activities of several lysosomal enzymes during endotoxin, traumatic (e.g., Noble-Collip drum shock), and bowel ischemia shock. Since then, many groups have substantiated and extended these findings in hemorrhagic (43–46), endotoxic (11,31,47), cardiogenic (48,49), bowel ischemia (50,51), traumatic (52,53), and acute pancreatitis (54) shock. Thus, lysosomal involvement is well documented in circulatory shock.

The major source of lysosomal enzymes appears to be the splanchnic organs, particularly the liver and pancreas (46,55). These changes in lysosomes appear to be related to the permeability of the lysosomal membrane, the configuration of the vacuolar apparatus of lysosomes, and the amount and type of acid hydrolase within the lysosome. Since lysosomes contain proteases, lipases, phospholipases, sulfatases, glucuronidases, glucosidases, and other acid hydrolases, their disruption and subsequent release of enzymes into the surrounding cytoplasm can be quite devastating to the structural integrity and metabolic functions of the cell. The role of lysosomes in autolysis and cell death appears to be highly significant, but the exact mechanisms of these changes are not completely understood at present.

LYSOSOMAL HYDROLASE—MYOCARDIAL DEPRESSANT FACTOR SYSTEM IN SHOCK

Toxic humoral factors have been postulated to be mediators of circulatory shock. One of the more prominent of these factors is a myocardial depressant factor (MDF) discovered by Brand and Lefer in 1966 (56). MDF, obtained from the blood of shock animals, has been partially characterized. It has a molecular weight of about 500 and appears to be a peptide or related substance (e.g., a glycopeptide). MDF appears to contain about 3 to 5 amino acid residues, but may be bound to a carrier molecule such as a plasma protein during some stage in its formation or transport to the circulatory system. MDF activity has been shown to be unrelated to salt or to the presence of anesthetic (i.e., pentobarbital) and to be independent of freezing and thawing of plasma (57).

During the development of the shock state, MDF gradually accumulates in the plasma, approximately in proportion to the severity of the splanchnic ischemia present. MDF is quite potent, since it exerts a marked cardiodepressant effect at a plasma concentration of a few nanograms per milliliter. Moreover, MDF has been found in the plasma of several mammalian species including the cat, rabbit, guinea pig, dog, baboon, and man (58). It also appears that a common pathophysiological mechanism exists in a variety of types of

shock, since MDF is formed in hemorrhagic, endotoxic, cardiogenic, splanchnic ischemic, burn, and acute pancreatitis shock (58). Since MDF has now been confirmed by laboratories in Great Britain, Sweden, Japan, Mexico, Germany, and by several in the United States, it appears to be a reasonably well-established finding in shock states (19,49,59–64).

MDF formation is intimately related to splanchnic ischemia and the disruption of certain subcellular organelles (i.e., lysosomes and zymogen granules). Ischemia of the pancreas is more severe than that of other splanchnic organs during shock. Forsyth et al. (2) recently found that hemorrhage decreased blood flow to the liver by 36% and to the intestine by 69%, but a 93% decrease was observed in pancreatic blood flow in monkeys. Although this splanchnic hypoperfusion allows for emergency shunting of blood flow to the coronary and cerebral circulations, a prolonged deficit of flow to the splanchnic region can lead to deleterious consequences which ultimately compromise the survival of the animal.

The formation of MDF results from the integration of several diverse physiological phenomena on both the organ system level (i.e., peripheral circulatory compensation by neural and humoral mechanisms) and the subcellular level (i.e., alteration of subcellular particles and the subsequent interaction of enzymes in a combination not usually operative under normal conditions). Figure 7 summarizes some of these relationships which appear to be a common pathway in a variety of forms of circulatory shock, regardless of the traumatic event which initiates the shock state.

As a result of development of shock (e.g., by hemorrhage, myocardial infarction, etc.), systemic hypotension usually occurs. Although hypotension is not an absolute requirement for the subsequent events, it usually occurs after the initial shock-producing event. Hypotension invariably leads to pancreatic ischemia by a variety of pathophysiologic processes. Passively, the resistance vessels supplying the pancreas narrow as the hydrostatic

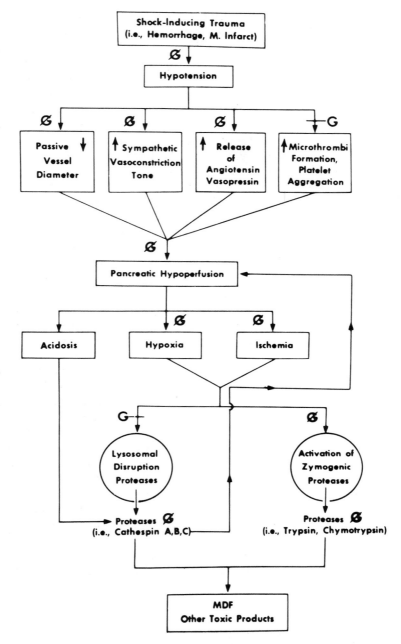

FIG. 7. Schematic diagram of the present working hypothesis of the mechanisms involved in the formation of MDF during shock. (From *Steroids and Shock,* edited by T. M. Glenn, University Park Press, Baltimore, 1974, p. 237.)

pressure within them falls. Additionally, neurohumoral constrictor mechanisms are activated by the shock-inducing trauma and the hypotension. In this regard, sustained sympathetic activity releases increasing amounts of norepinephrine at the neuroeffector junctions, and, humorally, there is an enhanced release of angiotension II and vasopressin into the circulating blood. All of these events contribute to an active vasoconstriction and lead to a further reduction in pancreatic blood flow. Finally, hypotension promotes alterations in the physical properties of the blood cells and platelets which can lead to platelet aggregation and microthrombi formation, two factors which can obstruct these blood vessels, resulting in further curtailment of splanchnic blood flow.

As a consequence of the state of hypoperfusion locally, the splanchnic area becomes hypoxic, ischemic, and acidotic. The severe decrease in PO_2 of the lymph draining these areas, as well as the autolytic changes in hepatic and pancreatic cells during shock (46), are findings which strongly implicate splanchnic ischemia as an important factor in these processes. The exocrine pancreas appears to be particularly susceptible to the consequences of the resultant hypoxia and ischemia.

These factors are the major stimuli for the disruption of lysosomes and the activation of zymogenic proteases in pancreatic acinar cells. As a result of the widespread lysosomal disruption, many acid hydrolases, including a variety of proteases (i.e., cathepsins, B, C), are released into the cytoplasm of the pancreatic cells. Moreover, additional zymogenic proteases are also activated by hypoxia (e.g., trypsinogen is activated to form trypsin). Although acidosis *per se* may not directly release lysosomal proteases, the lowered pH increases their activity, thus promoting their hydrolytic actions.

The activated and released proteases hydrolyze many cellular proteins, cleaving off a variety of biologically active peptides, somewhat analogous to the formation of tissue kinins. One of the small peptides released by this "au-tolytic proteolysis" in the pancreas is MDF.

MDF is usually formed within the pancreas during shock, but can also be produced in the isolated perfused pancreas under conditions of hypoxia or ischemia. The fact that unincubated pancreatic hemogenates do not form appreciable amounts of MDF indicates that MDF is not a normal endogenous storage product of the pancreas, but rather is produced by some catalytic process occurring during autolysis of pancreatic tissue (46). Moreover, although pancreatectomy can prevent MDF formation during shock, survival is only slightly improved by this procedure, largely because of severe disturbances in carbohydrate metabolism which result from removal of the endocrine portion of the pancreas (i.e., islets of Langerhans). A more effective means of preventing pancreatic autolysis and MDF formation is the ligation of the pancreatic ducts several weeks prior to the induction of shock. This procedure prevents MDF production and significantly improves survival. At present, the pancreas appears to be the major source of MDF, but may not be the only source of this toxic factor (65).

Once MDF is formed, it is released through damaged cell membranes into the pancreatic extracellular fluid space. From there, it is transported by the systemic capillaries and also by the lymphatic vessels into the venous circulation where it is carried to the heart. The dynamics of these processes are not fully understood at present, but a portion of the MDF may be bound to a carrier molecule (e.g., in the lymph) as depicted in Fig. 8.

One of the criteria of a shock factor is that it functionally impairs a critical organ system, thus contributing to the lethality of shock. MDF fulfills this criterion by virtue of its cardiodepressant action. This negative inotropic effect appears to be a direct action on the myocardium, since it occurs in isolated papillary muscles, in isolated perfused hearts, as well as in intact animals. Whole plasma (or ultrafiltrates of plasma), containing concentrations of MDF present in shock animals, depresses contractility by about 50% in isolated cardiac

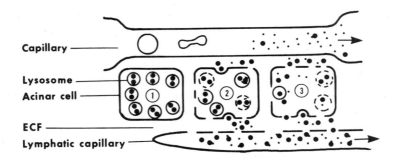

FIG. 8. Diagram of potential mechanisms of transport of MDF from the pancreatic acinar cell and pancreatic extracellar fluid (ECF) space to the systemic circulation. Large dots represent lysosomal enzymes and carrier proteins. Small dots represent peptides and other low-molecular-weight substances such as MDF. MDF thus appears to be transported both in systemic and lymphatic capillaries as the free molecule. It appears also to be transported in the bound form almost exclusively by the lymphatic vessels. Acinar cells 1, 2, and 3 represent progressively more severe stages of autolysis in response to the ischemia and hypoxia of the shock state. (From *Klin. Wochenschr.,* 52:358–370, 1974.)

muscle strips, that is, developed tension declines at a fixed muscle length.

MDF depresses developed tension by about 80% within 2 min in isolated hearts perfused under conditions of constant perfusion pressure. This depression occurs in hearts electrically driven at a constant rate, and in the absence of a significant change in coronary flow. These findings suggest that MDF exerts a direct effect on the contractile apparatus of the heart or on excitation-contraction coupling (64). This conclusion is further supported by the observation that MDF exerts no detectable effect on the electrophysiological properties of the myocardial cell membrane. Moreover, increasing the extracellular calcium concentration threefold can completely reverse the cardiodepressant action of MDF. Perhaps the most compelling finding of the cardiodepressant action of MDF is in normal animals (i.e., in amounts which elevate the plasma activity to that present in shock animals) where MDF decreases cardiac contractility by about 50% within 1 hr (46). Thus, MDF can significantly depress the heart in an otherwise normal animal.

In addition to its negative inotropic effect, MDF also exerts two potentially important actions which contribute to its positive feedback action in shock. These actions are (a) constriction of the splanchnic vasculature, and

(b) depression of the fixed macrophages of the reticuloendothelial system (RES). The splanchnic vasoconstrictor effect enhances the appearance of lysosomal enzymes in the circulation. These hydrolytic enzymes damage the endothelium of the vascular system, sensitize the heart to the actions of MDF, and promote the formation of additional MDF (66). Thus, MDF compromises an already reduced splanchnic flow, leading to the formation of additional MDF in typical positive feedback fashion.

The other positive feedback action of MDF is the impairment of RES function. MDF appears to impair phagocytosis of the fixed macrophages (e.g., Kupffer cells of the liver). This action effectively depresses the system which normally removes toxic factors from the blood. The RES appears to be necessary for the clearance of MDF and lysosomal enzymes (67). Therefore, by inhibiting the RES, MDF promotes conditions which favor elevated plasma MDF activities.

MDF fulfills the basic criteria necessary for validation of a shock factor (68). It is either absent entirely or present in very low concentrations in nonshocked animals. It is produced by many different mammalian species in a variety of shock states. It has been parially isolated and purified from the blood of animals in shock. MDF exerts severe pathophysiologic disturbances on vital organ systems, which lead to impaired homeostasis and increased mortality. Finally, MDF is present in man during shock states and thus appears to be a clinically significant factor in the pathogenesis of human circulatory shock.

OTHER TOXIC FACTORS

A summary of the general characteristics, chemical properties, and biological actions of the known toxic factors in shock is presented in Table 1. This has been reviewed by Lefer (68), and the following is a synopsis of this review. The factors have diversity in their chemical properties. They range from small molecules with molecular weights less than 1,000 to quite complex molecules having molecular weights greater than 1,000,000. Some of the factors have been partially characterized chemically [e.g., hemochromogen, some of the lysosomal hydrolases, myocardial depressant factor (MDF), and reticuloendothelial depressant substance (RDS)], whereas very little is known about the identity of the others. None of the toxic factors has been completely characterized in specific molecular terms. Knowledge of the chemical structure could lead to information about the metabolism and the clearance of a toxic factor and ultimately to the synthesis of molecular analogues which could be useful in the antagonism of that factor which may be of value in the treatment of circulatory shock. Despite the lack of the chemical identity of the toxic factors, we can evaluate each factor in terms of its fulfillment of the basic criteria of a shock factor, and, thus, determine its significance in the pathophysiology of shock.

The first criterion for a shock factor, namely, that the factor not be present in high amounts in control animals, is essentially satisfied by all of the factors in Table 1. Any factor that failed to satisfy this elementary requirement could not be seriously considered as a true shock factor.

The second criterion is that the factor be present in a variety of types of shock. The

finding that certain factors occur in types of shock having diverse etiologies is striking. Moreover, of all the investigators who have studied the formation of a specific toxic factor in shock, none has found a type of shock in which that factor was not present.

A third criterion is that the factor be isolated in a relatively pure state. At present, the factors reported by Fukuda (69), Thal and co-workers (19,70), and Clowes and colleagues (71), as well as by others, have not been isolated in sufficient purity to warrant further consideration of their chemical nature. However, those factors which have been partially purified (i.e., lysosomal hydrolases, RDS, and MDF) and those about which chemical properties are known (i.e., hemochromogen and endotoxin) can be said to have partially satisfied the third criterion.

A fourth criterion is that the shock factor be capable of exerting an effect which compromises the survival of the organism. All of the factors listed induce shock or at least exert severe disturbances in the normal function of the cardiorespiratory or the reticuloendothelial system when injected into normal animals. Thal and co-workers (19,70) have not injected their factor into intact normal animals, but they have perfused the lungs of the shock animal, thus partially fulfilling this requirement. Although all the factors described in Table 1 are capable of exerting a biological effect that can be considered detrimental to survival, the factors have variable toxicity. Some toxic factors appear to exert part or all of their detrimental effects indirectly by releasing other agents, which in turn act as toxic factors, and thus the original factors, in a sense, are "secondary" toxic factors. These "secondary" factors usually have high molecular weights. In contrast, the primary factors, usually of low molecular weight, either depress the heart directly, induce hypotension, which may be a cardiac or a peripheral vascular effect, or impair phagocytosis. Some shock factors also exert effects on other organs or loci in addition to the ones cited above (i.e., MDF also constricts the splanchnic vasculature, Thal's fac-

TABLE 1. *General characteristics, chemical properties, and biological actions of known toxic factors in shock*

Names of factor	Species	Forms of shock	Chemical properties	Type of molecule
Lysosomal hydro-lases	Dog	SAO	MW 25,000–200,000	Proteins
	Cat	Hemorrhagic Endotoxic Cardiogenic	Water soluble Heat labile Nondialyzable	
Hemochromogen	Dog	SAO	MW 68,000	Hemoglobin deriva-tive
		Acute pancreati-tis Hemorrhagic	Nondialyzable	
Endotoxin	Rabbit	Endotoxic	MW 200,000–2,-000,000	Lipopolysaccharide
	Dog	Hemorrhagic SAO Catecholamine	Nondialyzable	
Reticuloendothelial depressant sub-stance (RDS)	Dog Cat	Hemorrhagic SAO	MW 10,000 Dialyzable Can be frozen Soluble in methylene chloride	Unknown
Myocardial depres-sant factor (MDF)	Cat Dog Rabbit Baboon Man	Hemorrhagic Endotoxic SAO Cardiogenic Pancreatitis Burn	MW 500–1,000 Dialyzable Can be frozen H_2O soluble Not soluble in methylene chloride	Peptide glycopeptide
Fukuda's factor	Dog	Hemorrhagic Endotoxic	H_2O soluble Heat labile Precipitated by ammonium sulfate Probably large MW	Appears to be pro-tein
Thal's factor	Dog	SAO	Unknown	Unknown
Clowe's factor	Dog	Septic	MW 1,000–3,000	Possibly peptide

(From *Circ. Res.*, 32:129–139, 1973.)

tor stimulates vascular smooth muscle, etc.). However, these actions probably are not of primary importance in the toxic actions of the factors, although they may play some role in the overall effectiveness.

Regarding the final criterion, namely, the presence of the factors in plasma from human subjects in shock, only MDF and endotoxin have been identified in the plasma of patients having a variety of forms of shock, although Thal's factor and hemochromogen have each been found in one shock patient.

TABLE 1. *Continued*

Origin in body	Biological actions	Prevention of formation of factor	Comments
Ischemic splanchnic region Liver Pancreas Spleen Intestine Kidney	Sensitive heart to other toxic factors Cause hypotension Constrict pancreatic vessels Participate in the formation of MDF	Pharmacological doses of glucocorticoids	Found in lymph in shock Slight hemodynamic effect in presence of intact RE system Action not blocked by glucocorticoids
Blood absorbed by damaged intestinal mucosa	Unclear whether there are direct effects Hypotension	Unknown	Occurs in patients Does not depress myocardium
Ischemic intestine Absorbed through damaged intestinal mucosa	Unclear, may release vasoactive agents	Nonabsorbable antibiotics	Does not depress myocardium Found in lymph Germ-free animals not protected in shock
Ischemic splanchnic region (possibly intestine)	Depresses phagocytosis by fixed macrophages May depress heart Impairs survival	Unknown	Passively transferred to another animal Formed despite absence of intestinal flora
Ischemic splanchnic region Pancreas is major source	Negative inotropic effect Constricts splanchnic resistance vessels May depress RE system	Pharmacological doses of glucocorticoids Trasylol Lymph diversion	Found in lymph and in pancreatic autolysates in shock Occurs in plasma of patients in shock
Ischemic splanchnic region (particularly liver)	Hypotension	Pharmacological doses of corticoids	Passively transferred to another animal Not blocked by glucocorticoids
Ischemic splanchnic region	Induces lesion in lung Stimulates vascular smooth muscle	Phenoxybenzamine	May not be one factor
Probably splanchnic region	Increases pulmonary vascular resistance Induces focal alveolar collapse and right heart failure	Glucocorticoids Trasylol (partially effective)	Activity is free of endotoxin

There are many interesting similarities among the various shock factors. All of the shock factors listed appear to originate in the splanchnic region: endotoxin, hemochromogen, and RDS from the intestine; MDF from the pancreas; Fukuda's factor from the liver; lysosomal enzymes from throughout the splanchnic region but primarily from the liver and the pancreas; and Clowe's and Thal's factors from an unidentified site somewhere in the splanchnic region.

Several of the shock factors are transported from their site of origin by the lymphatic system, particularly the high-molecular-weight factors (i.e., endotoxin and lysosomal enzymes). MDF also appears to be in part transported via the lymphatics, which may indicate that at some stage in formation it is bound to a larger molecule. The other low-molecular-weight factors (i.e., RDS and Clowe's factor) appear to be taken up by the microcirculation in the region in which they are formed. In the cases of hemochromogen and Fukuda's factor, the routes of transport are not clear, although some of the hemochromogen is absorbed via the damaged intestinal mucosa or via mucosal capillaries into the systemic circulation.

Once transported to the systemic circulation, either directly or via the lymphatic system, the factors are then distributed to virtually all the peripheral tissues. However, it is not known to what extent any of these factors can penetrate the blood-brain barrier. Despite the similar origin of the shock factors, there is a diversity in the target organs on which the shock factors exert deleterious effects. Thus, MDF and, to a lesser degree, lysosomal enzymes have a cardiodepressant action, Thal'a and Clowe's factors primarily exert a damaging effect on the lungs, RDS acts on the fixed macrophages of the reticuloendothelial system (i.e., in the liver and perhaps in the spleen), and lysosomal hydrolases (and perhaps endotoxin) appear to exert a damaging effect on the splanchnic vasculature. However, the precise target organs of Fukuda's factor and endotoxin are not clearly established at the present time.

The target organs which are known to be adversely affected by shock factors are clearly among the more vital organs (i.e., heart, lungs, peripheral vasculature, and reticuloendothelial system) and are obviously necessary for the continuing functioning of the organism. Perhaps the brain may be spared because of its unique situation (i.e., the blood-brain barrier), although there is no evidence that the brain is, in fact, free of humorally induced effects.

Clearly, any consideration of the therapeutics of circulatory shock must consider the presence of these toxic factors. Perhaps a systemic effort at counteracting these factors would be more useful than classical pharmacologic approaches to shock, which have been largely disappointing.

THERAPEUTICS OF CIRCULATORY SHOCK

The use of pharmacologic agents to normalize hemodynamic parameters in shock has been largely directed toward modifying the autonomic response of the cardiovascular system to the shock state. Thus, vasoconstrictor and cardiotonic agents have been given to augment the response of the sympathetic system, whereas α- and β-adrenergic blocking agents have been administered to inhibit sympathetic activity in various types of circulatory shock. The rationale for the use of sympathomimetic drugs in shock is to support adequate blood flow to the brain and heart by increasing MABP and cardiac output. However, application of pressor agents with strong vasoconstrictor activity (e.g., norepinephrine) increases vascular resistance while MABP increases. This pharmacologic increase in TPR is deleterious to local organ function since it exacerbates the already reduced tissue perfusion and increased TPR that occurs in many types of shock. These findings (i.e., increased sympathetic activity, increased TPR, reduced tissue perfuson in shock) suggested the use of α-adrenergic blocking agents to improve tissue perfusion in low-flow states. In addition, the use of adrenergic agents has been advocated in those situations where MABP and TPR decrease late in shock. In contrast, inhibition of B-adrenergic activity would act to increase TPR and, therefore, increase systemic arterial blood pressure.

The variability of the hemodynamic response to the several types of circulatory shock has already been discussed. This phenomenon, combined with the variability of pharmacologic manipulation of such a dynamic state, presage the difficulties of the pharmacologic management of circulatory shock. Thus, rational therapeutics require evaluation of the physiologic state prior to treatment and knowledge of the pharmacologic response to sympathomimetic agents and sympathetic blockers used in the treatment of shock.

SYMPATHOMIMETIC AGENTS

Hemorrhagic Shock

The use of sympathomimetic agents and, in particular norepineprine, has long been advocated in cases of hypovolemic shock in which restoration of volume fails to return the MABP to an acceptable level. Although norepinephrine increases myocardial contractility, its effect on cardiac output is variable. Furthermore, total peripheral resistance is significantly elevated at commonly administered therapeutic dose levels. Moreover, even if the cardiac output is increased, the magnitude of the increase may not be sufficient for a beneficial action in shock. Although norepinephrine may transiently improve coronary or cerebral blood flow, it does not improve survival (72). In fact, administration of norepinephrine to hemorrhaged dogs has been associated with increased hemorrhagic lesions in the gastrointestinal tract, splanchnic viscera, and kidneys (73). These lesions arise as a result of prolonged severe tissue hypoxia secondary to hypoperfusion. The hypoperfusion of hemorrhagic shock is exaggerated by the peripheral α-adrenergic vasoconstrictor action of norepinephrine. Norepinephrine has been known to decrease survival in a variety of types of shock (74).

In contrast to norepinephrine, isoproterenol has little, if any, α-adrenergic vasoconstriction activity, but considerable β-adrenergic activity. Isoproterenol has been used to stimulate the heart and to reduce peripheral vascular resistance during hemorrhagic shock. These actions should increase tissue flood flow and ameliorate hypoxic tissue damage in hemorrhagic shock. However, the beneficial effects of isoproterenol require prolonged administration. Thus, Grega et al. (75) infused either isoproterenol or another β-agonist, nylidrin, into hemorrhaged dogs for 2 hr. They found decreased intestinal damage in treated dogs; survival was improved only slightly. Myers et al. (76) infused a similar dose of isoproterenol several times after the induction of hemorrhage and found that the ability of isoproterenol to dilate the splanchnic vasculature was severely blunted 2 to 3 hr after hemorrhage. Apparently, the effects of prolonged hypoperfusion minimize the vasodilating action of isoproterenol. In addition, the excessive stimula-

tion of the heart can produce arrhythmias, excessive demand on oxygen delivery, and even myocardial necrosis (77).

The search for a suitable vasodilator in the treatment of hemorrhagic shock has centered more recently on the norepinephrine precursor, dopamine (78). Dopamine has a cardiotonic effect and has been shown to increase cardiac output in hemorraghed dogs (79). Dopamine also can selectively dilate the renal and splanchnic vascular beds in hemorrhaged dogs. However, despite these actions, dopamine appears only slightly effective in promoting survival in experimental hemorrhagic shock (80).

Endotoxin Shock

Lansing and Hinshaw (81) found dopamine to increase survival in dogs subjected to endotoxic shock. Furthermore, dopamine has been shown to increase myocardial contractility, but not aortic pressure in endotoxic shock (14). This inotropic effect of dopamine was accompanied by decreases in coronary and mesenteric resistance. At lower doses, dopamine induced renal vasodilation. Thus, the positive inotropic and selective vasodilating properties of dopamine suggest a mechanism of the possible beneficial effect of this drug in endotoxin shock (82).

Norepinephrine, isoproterenol, and nylidrin have also been studied in endotoxin shock, the results being similar to those obtained in hemorrhagic shock. Norepinephrine infusion increased MABP and aortic flow in dogs given endotoxin, but MABP was elevated out of proportion to the increase in aortic flow, indicating an increased TPR. Although endotoxin alone, or endotoxin plus norepinephrine, increased mesenteric and renal vascular resistance, the combined effect of endotoxin plus norepinephrine produced a greater increase in resistance than either alone (14). Similar effects have been reported clinically in septic shock (83) and argue against the use of norepinephrine in the treatment of endotoxin shock.

Just as in studies of hemorrhagic shock, the

logic persisted that increased survival in endotoxin shock would be found in animals given
β-adrenergic agents to stimulate the heart and
increase peripheral blood flow. However, the
experimental evidence is unclear. Starzecki
and Spink (84) reported increased survival in
dogs given isoproterenol, but Tadepalli and
Buckley (85) did not find improvement in dogs
given nylidrin and subjected to endotoxin
shock. This difference in the protective effect
of the two β-adrenergic agents may have been
related to the dose of *E. coli* endotoxin administered. The nylidrin-treated dogs were given
a dose of endotoxin that was nearly threefold
greater than isoproterenol-treated dogs. Moreover, each agent has its own characteristic profile of side effects, some of which may be beneficial or detrimental during shock.

Cardiogenic Shock

Vasopressors and positive inotropic agents
have been used routinely in the treatment of
cardiogenic shock. Positive inotropic agents
are usually employed to increase cardiac output by directly stimulating the undamaged
portion of the myocardium. In turn, vasopressors are often administered to increase cardiac
contractility by augmenting coronary flow as
perfusion pressure increases. Such therapeutic
approaches produced variable results with regard to hemodynamic response and survival
(86,87). Norepinephrine infusion to maintain
systolic pressure between 90 and 100 mm Hg
generally increased cardiac output, but elevated MABP out of proportion to the increased output (i.e., peripheral resistance increased markedly) (88). Excessive elevation
of MABP with vasopressor agents adversely
increased the work of the heart in myocardial
infarction (89).

Several studies have considered the modification of infarct size by pharmacological
agents. Following coronary artery ligation, an
ischemic area develops which progressively increases in size. Factors which limit infarct size
would either prevent or delay the occurrences
of cardiogenic shock. Puri (90) studied the

effect of norepinephrine or isoproterenol on
infarct size by measuring velocity of shortening in ischemic and nonischemic areas of myocardial tissue and reasoned that norepinephrine exerts an infarct-reducing effect, whereas
isoproterenol does not. However, norepinephrine has been shown to increase infarct size
in animals following coronary artery ligation
and to induce myocardial damage in otherwise
normal animals (91).

An infarct-enhancing effect was also attributed to isoproterenol by Maroko et al. (92)
and by Shell and Sobel (93). These investigators assessed infarct size by elevation of the
S-T segment of epicardial leads and by serum
creatine phosphokinase (CPK) activity and
postmortem histology. Increased infarct size
associated with isoproterenol administration
or with electrically induced tachycardia could
be produced as late as 3 days after experimental coronary artery ligation (92).

Dopamine infusion (10 to 20 μg/kg/min)
increased heart rate and aortic, coronary, renal, and mesenteric blood flows following coronary embolization in dogs. The greater infusion rate tended to increase resistance to blood
flow, whereas the lesser infusion rate decreased total, renal, and mesenteric vascular
resistances (14). It is this ability of dopamine
to dilate mesenteric and renal resistance vessels while stimulating the myocardium that
suggests its potential usefulness in the treatment of cardiogenic shock.

ALPHA- AND BETA-ADRENERGIC BLOCKADE

Hemorrhagic Shock

The use of α-adrenergic blocking drugs in
the treatment of hemorrhagic shock has produced equivocal results, especially with regard
to survival, since the classical study of Nickerson (74) showing an improved survival in patients in severe shock. Some of the divergent
results of α-adrenergic blockade can be attributed to the variety of experimental designs
employed, which ranged from animals sub-

jected to a moderate oligemia (94) to animals subjected to severe oligemic stress (95). Another important consideration is the time of administration of the blocking agent [i.e., whether it is prior to (95,96) or following (97–100) hemorrhage]. Administration of the α-blocker prior to hemorrhage would tend to reduce absolute blood loss if animals were bled to a constant hypotensive level and, thus, influence the severity of the shock model itself. This can lead to erroneous conclusions.

The most commonly used α-adrenergic blocking agents are phenoxybenzamine and dibenamine. Increased survival of hemorrhaged dogs has been reported using these agents. Schumer (98) reported 86% survival of dogs given phenoxybenzamine (1 mg/kg) after 45 and 65% loss of blood volume over 2 hr. Increased survival was associated with preservation of omental flow and normalization of blood metabolites. Lotz et al. (97) reported increased survival of hemorrhaged dogs given dibenamine 30 min after hemorrhage, although survival was not improved if the drug was administered 85 min after hemorrhage. The beneficial effect of early blockade may have been related to an increase in circulating blood volume early in the course of oligemia.

Alpha-adrenergic blockade has been combined with volume support following the oligemic period of hemorrhagic shock. This is to ensure that the dilated vasculature has an adequate fluid volume to maintain a blood pressure that is compatible with life. Improved survival has been found with α-blockade plus fluid therapy (100,101), but the beneficial effect of combined blockade and volume may have been solely the result of normalization of circulating blood volume.

Bond et al. (95) recently demonstrated that α-adrenergic blockade with droperidol prior to hemorrhage maintained myocardial blood flow throughout the oligemic and postoligemic period in dogs. Moreover, substrate utilization and myocardial performance at equal preload and afterload were unaffected, yet all dogs subsequently died following reinfusion. These re-

sults suggest that α-adrenergic blockade may preserve myocardial function in hemorrhagic shock, but that such preservation, *per se,* does not necessarily indicate improved survival. Thus, many other factors contribute to the lethality of the shock state.

Investigators who advocate the use of α-adrenergic blockade in hemorrhagic shock seek to obviate the deleterious effects of prolonged vasoconstriction, leading to ischemic damage of vital organs. Conversely, other investigators recommend the use of β-adrenergic blockade based on the supposition that failure of peripheral vasoconstriction after prolonged hemorrhagic hypotension leads to death. Experimental support for the latter hypothesis is scant. Berk et al. (102), who favor propranolol therapy in shock, show equal mortality (78%) in untreated or β-blocked dogs subjected to hemorrhagic shock. An increase in survival was observed only if propranolol was coupled with administration of atropine, ouabain, hypertonic glucose, sodium bicarbonate, and calcium chloride. Zierott et al. (100) also showed that pretreatment with propranolol actually shortened the oligemic period and aggravated the metabolic alterations concomitant with hemorrhagic hypotension. Administration of propranolol to induce an effective β-blockade appears to have little, if any, efficacy in the treatment of hemorrhagic shock.

Endotoxin Shock

Halmagyi et al. (103) studied the effects of combined α- and β-adrenergic blockade of dogs subjected to endotoxin shock. Premedication of dogs with phenoxybenzamine or propranolol or combination of the two agents failed to improve survival above that found in nontreated controls. In fact, administration of propranolol in dogs given a lethal dose of endotoxin accelerated the decline of the animals. These investigators suggested different mechanisms in the pathogenesis of endotoxic and hemorrhagic shock, since combined adrenergic receptor blockade (97,100) was effective in hemorrhagic but not in endotoxic shock. However, some of these investigators subsequently demonstrated that survival following α-blockade was improved only if large volumes of low-molecular-weight dextran were administered. Perhaps if dextran had been given to animals given endotoxin, survival would have been improved. Such a result would indicate a common mechanism, though not necessarily a directly adrenergic mechanism, involved in the lethality of both endotoxic and hemorrhagic shock. In this regard, others have shown an improvement in survival time following endotoxin administration in dogs given sufficient dextran to maintain central venous pressure until death, under conditions in which propranolol alone accelerated circulatory collapse.

The clinical effectiveness of adrenergic blockade in the treatment of septic shock is not easily evaluated because of the difficulty in obtaining control data under comparable conditions. Such difficulties are illustrated by the studies of Berk et al. (104), which advocate the use of propranolol in the treatment of septic shock. However, in order to significantly improve survival, the negative inotropic and hypoglycemic effects of propranolol must be eliminated.

Just as the effectiveness of β-blockade in shock is not clear, the efficacy of α-blockade in septic shock is also questionable. The beneficial effect of α-blockade is not easily is not easily dissociated from supportive volume therapy with serum or low-molecular-weight dextran.

Cardiogenic Shock

Use of adrenergic blockade in the treatment of cardiogenic shock has been somewhat limited, perhaps because large increases in total peripheral resistance do not occur frequently in cardiogenic shock, and because of hesitancy to alter stimulation of the already impaired myocardium. However, α-adrenergic blockade has been shown to increase cardiac output subsequent to a decrease in afterload in car-

diogenic shock. Hirsch and Glick (105) demonstrated an improved cardiac output and a significantly greater mesenteric blood flow in dogs subjected to coronary embolization and treated with phenoxybenzamine compared to untreated controls. Despite the effective α-adrenergic blockade, all dogs died within 24 to 26 hr of embolization.

Administration of propranolol has been shown to limit the severity and extent of the myocardial infarction process following coronary artery occlusion in dogs (92). Apparently the β-adrenergic blocking agent decreased myocardial oxygen consumption and cardiac work in the ischemic myocardium. Such an effect could be useful, but caution is advised because of the marked negative inotropic effect of propranolol. However, the β-adrenergic blocker, practolol, has the advantage of increasing myocardial efficiency and limiting infarct size in the absence of any negative inotropic action (106). Further studies of practolol in cardiogenic shock may be of considerable interest.

GLUCAGON

Clinical assessment of the efficacy of glucagon in cardiogenic shock in difficult for the same reasons that apply to evaluation of adrenergic blocking drugs in the treatment of septic shock. Glucagon has a moderate positive inotropic effect independent of β-blockade and some potential antiarrhythmic properties. However, as with most positive inotropic agents, glucagon has recently been demonstrated to increase infarct size (92). Glucagon, therefore, appears of questionable value in the treatment of cardiogenic shock.

Acute injection of glucagon decreased aortic pressure, increased heart rate, and increased cardiac output in dogs when administered 1 to 4 hr after injection of endotoxin. Compared to the preendotoxic response, the stimulating action of glucagon on cardiac output was reduced after endotoxin (107). Despite these apparently favorable hemodynamic effects, the ability of glucagon to promote survival in septic shock has not been established.

More studies have been directed at assessing the possible beneficial effect of glucagon in hemorrhagic shock than in other forms of circulatory shock (108–112). Glucagon has several potentially beneficial effects when administered in animals subjected to hemorrhagic shock. Among these effects are its ability to increase cardiac output, reduce total peripheral resistance, and possibly dilate the mesenteric and renal vascular beds. Tibblen et al, (112) showed that bolus injections of glucagon normalized aortic, coronary, renal, and mesenteric blood flows of dogs when administered 5 to 10 min after hemorrhage. Unfortunately, observations were not carried out to observe the sequential effects of glucagon in hemorrhaged animals. In other studies, infusion of glucagon for 30 min (110) or until death (108) following the reinfusion of shed blood did not increase survival, nor did prolonged infusion of glucagon effect any favorable hemodynamic alterations (54).

The effect of glucagon infusion in hypovolemic monkeys differs somewhat from that of hemorrhaged dogs. Schumer et al. (111) reported decreased lactate production, decreased acid production, and increased omental blood flow 6 hr after loss of 50% of the blood volume in monkeys. The authors suggested that such results indicate a beneficial effect of glucagon in primates. However, Bowman et al. (109) found that, although glucagon infusion increased cardiac output, mean blood pressure, and renal blood flow during oligemia, its hemodynamic effects were largely attenuated following reinfusion of shed blood. In addition to the blunted hemodynamic response of glucagon, it was ineffective in preserving renal tubular integrity in hemorrhaged monkeys. For these reasons, the authors concluded that the therapeutic value of glucagon in the treatment of hemorrhagic shock is questionable.

Glucagon was shown not to increase survival in dogs during hemorrhagic shock, partially because the splanchnic vasadilator action of glucagon could not offset the marked splanchnic vasoconstrictor action of the sympathetic nervous system during hemorrhagic shock. Moreover, glucagon has been shown to labilize lysosomal membranes in shock (54) and thus contribute to proteolysis and toxic factor formation during shock. These are additional reasons for questioning the use of glucagon in the treatment of shock.

CARDIAC GLYCOSIDES

Cardiac glycosides have been used in the treatment of cardiogenic shock in an effort to increase the contractility of normal and ischemic myocardial tissue. Furthermore, these agents have been used in the treatment of endotoxic and hemorrhagic shock in an effort to minimize cardiac depression that frequently occurs in these types of circulatory shock.

The therapeutic value of cardiac glycosides in any type of circulatory shock in questionable, especially if the hemodynamic effect of the glycosides is examined independently of any other supportive regimen such as fluid therapy (113). Although cardiac glycosides exert a positive inotropic action on the myocardium, digitalization produces only slight increases in the cardiac output of patients in cardiogenic shock (114). Moreover, ouabain has been shown to increase infarct size in dogs following coronary artery embolization (92). Apparently, cardiac glycosides increase cardiac metabolism out of proportion to any increase in coronary artery flow. Thus, digitalization can actually aggravate the deleterious effects of myocardial ischemia. Furthermore, cardiac glycosides markedly increase peripheral vascular resistance especially in the splanchnic vascular bed (54,115), increasing the work of the normal and damaged myocardium.

The question of digitalization is particularly important in conditions of primary cardiovascular disease where a reduced cardiac output is often encountered. Thus, increased splanchnic vascular resistance in the digitalized patient, and particularly the overdigitalized patient, may be so extreme as to cause intestinal necrosis (116). Compounding the deleterious effect of increased splanchnic vascular resistance is the possible secondary decrease in cardiac output following induction of cardiac arrhythmias with administration of digitalis. A further complication of cardiac complication of cardiac glycoside therapy in states of circulatory shock is the alteration in myocardial excitability that may occur in cardiogenic, septic, or hemorrhagic shock. Allgood and Ebert (117) demonstrated an increased incidence of arrhythmias after acetyl-strophanthidin during endotoxin shock.

ANGIOTENSIN, VASOPRESSIN, AND THEIR ANALOGUES

The use of vasopressin, angiotensin, or analogues of these drugs has been advocated in various types of circulatory shock. Cort et al. (118) found increased blood pressure, cardiac output, and renal blood flow in hemorrhaged dogs given the vasopressin analogue. N-triglycy-1-8-lysine vasopressin. The authors attributed the improved survival of dogs treated with the vasopressin analogue to the improved cardiac output secondary to selective vasoconstriction and a generalized decrease in capacitance. Hershey et al. (119) also reported increased survival and decreased visceral congestion in hemorrhaged rats treated with the synthetic vasopressin analogue. The decreased visceral congestion may have been due to the specific ability of vasopressin to increase mesenteric vascular resistance and thus curtail splanchnic blood flow. This action is deleterious, as is the well-known coronary vasoconstrictor action of vasopressin. Caution is advised in the use of vasopressin analogues in the treatment of hemorrhagic shock, not only because of their vasoconstriction of splanchnic vessels, but because of bradycardia and other arrhythmias which may develop. Notwithstanding the possible deleterious effects of splanchnic vasoconstriction, selective, local vasopressin infusion has been used successfully to control gastrointestinal hemorrhage

(120). The infusion should be closely monitored and terminated when adequate hemostasis is achieved.

In addition to vasopressin, the most potent naturally occurring vasoconstrictor agent, angiotensin, has been administered to patients in various types of circulatory shock. Its usefulness in the treatment of cardiogenic shock is suspect because its inotropic effect is considerably less than its vasoconstrictor action. Administration of angiotensin would increase afterload out of proportion to any increase in contractility that may occur and in this way increase cardiac work. Moreover, its cardiac inotropic effect in increasing the metabolic demands of the heart would also tend to further injure ischemic myocardial tissue.

Although the ability of angiotensin to increase blood pressure has suggested its use in all forms of shock, the intense vasoconstriction which occurs within peripheral vascular beds is undesirable. Prolonged administration of angiotensin should be avoided in shock. Thus, the naturally occurring pressor peptides, vasopressin and angiotensin, are not particularly useful agents in the treatment of circulatory shock.

CORTICOSTEROIDS

Corticosteroids have received considerable attention as potential therapeutic agents in the treatment of a variety of types of circulatory shock. However, many clinicians and investigators are presently confused by much of the data that is available concerning the efficacy of corticosteroids in shock. A considerable degree of clarity can be achieved in this controversy if certain physiologic and pharmacologic principles are taken into consideration.

In reviewing the literature on the actions of corticosteroids in shock, one is initially overwhelmed by the diversity of shock models used, the multitude of different experimental conditions employed, and the variety of drug regimens attempted by the investigators in this field. Historically, corticosteroids were given for shock in the early 1940s with a notable lack of success. This occurred during the era when corticosteroids were not completely isolated or synthesized. In fact, the most prevalent preparation of tht time was adrenal cortical extract (ACE), which often contained considerable amounts of catecholamines and variable amounts of corticosteroids. Perhaps this early failure contributed to the skepticism of many scientists. Another deep-rooted criticism of the use of corticosteroids in shock is based on the well-documented findings that plasma corticosteroid concentrations become markedly elevated in response to stressful stimuli such as those which occur in shock (i.e., septicemia, hypotension, etc.). This is primarily due to an increased corticosteroid secretion rate.

Prolonged high corticosteroid secretion rate could theoretically result in functional exhaustion of the adrenal cortex. Because of this possibility, and since adrenal insufficiency results in a state of circulatory collapse similar to circulatory shock, adrenocortical failure has been suggested as an important mechanism in shock (121). Several investigators (122,123) have shown that hemorrhage results in a large increase in the rate of secretion of aldosterone and of cortisol.

Corticosteroid secretion is elevated in other forms of shock. Melby and coworkers (124) showed that the cortisol secretion rate increases markedly in endotoxin shock in dogs. Patients in bacteremic shock exhibit exhibit high plasma cortisol concentrations. Hokfelt and associates (125) showed that aldosterone secretion is also elevated in endotoxin shock.

In addition to the increase in corticosteroid secretion rates, shock results in impaired corticosteroid degradation mechanisms. These factors operate to elevate the circulating corticosteroid titers in shock. All available information indicates that adrenocortical insufficiency does not occur in shock. Rather, mobilization of corticosteroids appears to be the compensatory response to the stress. Therefore, the treatment of shock should not be corticosteroid replacement therapy as in adrenal insufficiency, but rather massive doses

of corticosteroids. One must look to a concept other than a normalizing role of corticosteroids to explain their protective effect in shock.

More recently, we have learned that five factors are important in considering the therapeutic actions of corticosteroids in shock. These are (a) type of steroid used, (b) dosage, (c) time of administration, (d) route of administration, and (e) rate of injection.

Certain corticosteroids have been found to be effective in all types of circulatory shock studied thus far. These corticosteroids prolong survival and exert beneficial actions in hemorrhagic shock (28,46,126–133), in endotoxin shock (134–145), in splanchnic ischemia shock (51,146), in cardiogenic shock (147–150), and in traumatic shock (151–153).

Corticosteroids are basically classified into two major groups of compounds, glucocorticoids and mineralocorticoids. Mineralocorticoids (e.g., aldosterone, desoxycorticosterone) primarily influence electrolyte metabolism, membrane transport of electrolytes and water, and exert certain cardiovascular effects at physiologic concentrations. At pharmacologic concentrations, they can exert imbalances in electrolyte metabolism as well as induce hypertension. In contrast, glucocorticoids (e.g., corticosterone, cortisol) primarily influence carbohydrate and lipid metabolism and exert very little or no acute cardiovascular action at physiologic concentrations. However, at extremely high concentrations, glucocorticoids, particularly the synthetic steroids, (e.g., methylprednisolone, dexamethasone) exert physical changes in biologic membranes so as to stabilize them from disruptive influences, without any significant circulatory action. High concentrations of glucocorticoids also exert other unusual effects (e.g., prevention of platelet aggregation, protection against the formation of toxic factors) which also may be of therapeutic value in circulatory shock.

In general, the glucocorticoids are effective in the treatment of circulatory shock states, whereas the mineralocorticoids are generally ineffective or aggravate the shock state. Thus, one must be specific in the use of the steroidal agent during shock.

A second major factor is the dose of steroid employed. Early investigators used very low doses (i.e., microgram quantities) of corticosteroids to treat shock. This may have been partially due to the erroneous assumption that "replacement doses" were required (i.e., that the steroids were being used to treat adrenal insufficiency during shock), and also to the unavailability of large quantities of these steroids. As the steroids became available in greater quantities, and as physicians overcame their fear of toxic effects of the steroids, they gradually increased the doses to 100 mg of steroids such as cortisol. We now know that these doses are only on the lower borderline of an effective dose. Considerable evidence (129,132,138–141,145,148) has been accumulated indicating that doses of 20 to 30 mg/kg of methylprednisolone or 4 to 8 mg/kg of dexamethasone are probably optimal in the treatment of shock.

Another vital consideration in evaluating the data on the effectiveness of steroids in circulatory shock is the time of administration of the steroid. Since many clinical investigators and physicians were skeptical of the efficacy of steroids in shock, they used other agents first and only when it was clear that the patient was deteriorating did they consider steroids as a last resort. Under these conditions, it is not surprising that several investigators were unable to find a salutary effect of corticosteroids in shock. Many of these clinicians chide the basic scientist by saying that they cannot pretreat their patients with steroids, as many investigators often do in animal models. However, pretreatment is not a prerequisite for efficacy of steroids in shock, but *early* treatment is essential. In general, the studies in which steroids were given relatively late in the course of the shock state resulted in little or no enhancement of survival and no significant beneficial effect developed. In contrast, there is a very high incidence of improvement of survival of other beneficial ef-

fects when the steroids were given early in the shock state. Clinical data indicate that this "effective period" for steroid administration is about to 4 to 6 hr after the onset of shock (113,147).

The route of administration is not a trivial consideration in the application of the steroid to the shock subject. Until recently, aqueous preparations of steroids were not readily available in quantities required to treat shock patients. This necessitated the administration of the steroid by less direct routes (i.e., intramuscular, intraperitoneal) which take considerably more time in which to accumulate sufficiently high circulating concentrations of the steroid to be effective in shock. The fact could also account for some of the failures to obtain a significant effect of steroids in shock. Now with the advent of methylprednisolone sodium succinate (Solu-Medrol®, Upjohn) and dexamethasone phosphate (Decadron®, Merck), one can administer the steroids intravenously and achieve a high blood concentration in a few minutes.

Fortunately, there are no deleterious side effects with acute intravenous infusion of massive doses of synthetic glucocorticoids such as methylprednisolone (154,155) and dexamethasone (156) when given slowly over about a 10-min period. Even in doses of about 2 g, these steroids do not exert any acute actions which would be a threat to the organism in shock. Of course, prolonged administration of these synthetic glucocorticoids can result in the well-known suppression of the immune mechanisms (157). However, these effects often require several days or weeks of chronic steroid administration to develop. Moreover, short-term administration (i.e., intravenously over 5 min) of up to 1 g of methylprednisolone did not impair phagocytosis or intracellular killing of ingested bacteria by leukocytes nor a change in total complement levels (155). These data speak eloquently for the relatively innocuous effects of these drugs. The major question that remains is why massive doses of steroids are required to protect in shock

TABLE 2. *Possible mechanisms of glucocorticoid action in shock*

Circulatory
  Direct positive inotropic effect
  Vasodilation
    Directly on vascular smooth muscle
    Indirectly via α-adrenergic blockage
Metabolic
  Makes more metabolic substrate available
  Alters electrolyte metabolism
  Antagonism of proteases
Cellular integrity
  Prevention of platelet aggregation
  Activation of phagocytosis (RE system)
  Preservation of capillary endothelium
  Protection against mast cell disruption
  Stabilization of lysosomal membranes
  Prevention of formation of toxic factors (e.g., MDF)

when amounts less than one-thousandth of that dose will sustain life in adrenal insufficiency.

The mechanism of the protective action of glucocorticoids (i.e., antiinflammatory steroids) in circulatory shock is by no means completely understood. Many potential theories have been proposed to explain the protective action of glucocorticoids in shock. These are summarized in Table 2.

Three basic types of hemodynamic effects have been proposed to explain the protective action of glucocorticoids in circulatory shock. These are (a) positive inotropic effect, (b) vasodilator action, and (c) potentiation of the circulatory effects of catecholamines. No convincing evidence exists for the occurrence of a significant positive inotropic effect of glucocorticoids. Thus, high doses of methylprednisolone and dexamethasone failed to augment the contractile state of isolated cardiac muscle under normal conditions, and were inactive under a variety of conditions which occur in shock (158). Moreover, these glucocorticoids were found to be inotropically inactive, even in depressed cardiac tissue taken from cats in a state of late shock. These data provide a strong argument against a direct inotropic effect of glucocorticoids as a significant protective mechanism in circulatory shock.

These results are in agreement with the ear-

lier findings of others who also failed to find an acute positive inotropic effect of glucocorticoids in isolated hearts as well as in intact cats. Only with chronic administration of glucocorticoids, particularly in animals after adrenalectomy, is a cardiotonic effect observed. Moreover, this cardiotonic action is capable of restoring cardiac performance to normal levels but not of exceeding those normal values. No published reports exist which show a significant, sustained, direct positive inotropic effect in response to the acute administration of pharmacologic concentrations of glucocorticoids that is independent of the steroid vehicle. Clearly, glucocorticoids, although they superficially resemble cardiac glycosides in stereochemical configuration, are not agents with high intrinsic activity.

Vasodilator properties also have been ascribed to pharmacologic concentrations of glucocorticoids by Lillehei and his co-workers (138,140) and an α-adrenergic blocking action has even been proposed by Dietzman and his collaborators (135,148). Several other investigators could not substantiate a vasodilator action of methylprednisolone or dexamethasone, either systemically or on the splanchnic vasculature (137,159). In this regard, these glucocorticoids neither dilated the splanchnic bed prior to hemorrhage (158) nor prevented the decrease in superior mesenteric arterial flow brought about by hemorrhage during the oligemic period.

Pharmacologic dosages of either methylprednisolone or dexamethasone do not induce a systemic vasodilation during hemorrhage, since the bleedout volumes of the steroid-treated dogs are not statistically different from those of the untreated dogs (51,129,158). If a significant vasodilation had occurred, as does with phenoxybenzamine (126), the bleedout volumes would have been significantly lower than for the nontreated dogs.

Kadowitz and Yard (137) also failed to demonstrate a vasodilator response to cortisol in hemodynamically isolated femoral, renal, and mesenteric beds perfused at constant flow.

This has been confirmed by Gorczynski et al. (159), who showed a lack of a vasodilator effect in the hemodynamically isolated *in situ* perfused pancreas. The apparent transient vasodilation that some investigtors allude to, often manifested by flushing of the patient, may be simply due to the benzyl alcohol in the vehicle. This lack of vasodilator effect also is consistent with the findings of Schmid and his colleagues (160) for dexamethasone, or Hakstian and his co-workers (126) for cortisone. No convincing data exist for a glucocorticoid-mediated vasodilator effect in normal dogs or in dogs in a state of shock, and no cogent evidence exists for an α-adrenergic blocking action of glucocorticoids at present, although Lillehei et al. (138) have suggested this as the primary mechanism of steroid action. Some of the alleged effects of glucocorticoids on improvement of vascular perfusion during shock can best be explained by their prevention of platelet aggregation or by prevention of the lysosomal enzyme-mediated vasoconstriction and capillary endothelial-damaging action induced by release of these acid hydrolases.

The third hemodynamic hypothesis, namely that glucocorticoids potentiate certain cardiovascular actions of catecholamines, is ambiguous. Presumably, the cardiac actions of catecholamines could be of value, if the net metabolic cost of such an inotropic effect is not too high and if arrhythmias do not occur, but, certainly, the predominant vasoconstriction brought about by increased α-adrenergic activity would reduce perfusion of many vascular beds and thus exaggerate the tissue hypoperfusion of the shock state. Spath et al. (158) were unable to observe a potentiation, or an inhibition, of the inotropic effects of norepinephrine or angiotensin in isolated cardiac tissue. This is consistent with the findings of Schmid and his co-workers (160) on the inotropic and pressor effects of dexamethasone in the intact animal. Kadowitz and Yard (137) found cortisol to be without effect on catecholamine responsivness in a variety of perfused vascular beds. These observations dispute the likelihood of a significant potentiation of naturally occurring pressor agents by glucocorticoids as a protective mechanism of shock.

Several other mechanisms purported to explain the beneficial effects of glucocorticoids in shock can be collectively termed membrane-stabilizing effects and involve the protection of membranes of cellular organelles, cells, or tissues, thereby preventing various deleterious actions in shock. These phenomena, which may be attenuated or inhibited by glucocorticoid action on membranes, include platelet aggregation, capillary endothelial leakage, lysosomal release of acid hydrolases, and formation of toxic factors (51,129).

No direct evidence to support or challenge the first two postulated mechanisms is available. These phenomena occur in varying degrees during shock, and these processes are curtailed by glucocorticoids. The direct bearing of these mechanisms on the major pathophysiologic pathways in shock must be established more firmly before a final evaluation can be made.

With regard to the latter two phenomena, considerble data indicate that both dexamethasone and methylprednisolone stabilize lysosomal membranes, thus preventing release of their endogenous hydrolases in shock, and as a consequence, prevent the plasma appearance of a myocardial depressant factor (66,158,161). There is considerable evidence to indicate that the splanchnic lysosomes exhibit an increased permeability or disrupt during shock, releasing several acid hydrolases which eventually appear in the circulating blood. Thus, pancreatic and hepatic lysosomal suspensions from animals in a state of shock have been shown to be more fragile than control preparations (51,162). Also, the total lysosomal enzyme content of liver and pancreas is reduced during shock (46), and the lost enzymes can be recovered in the lymph and, eventually, in peripheral blood (163). Moreover, electron microscopy has revealed that splanchnic lysosomes swell and many exhibit large autophagic vacuoles during shock. These data provide substantial evidence of lysosomal disruption during shock. All these phenomena can be prevented with prior massive dosages of glucocorticoid, consistent with a lysosomal membrane-stabilizing action of glucocorticoids.

The importance of lysosomal enzyme stabilization during shock can be readily appreciated, since lysosomal hydrolases, particularly the cathepsins, are intimately involved in the production of myocardial depressant factor (163,51). Moreover, lysosomal hydrolases curtail splanchnic blood flow, probably by damaging the endothelial lining of the small blood vessels (163), sensitize the heart to the depressant effect of myocardial depressant factor (67), and induce a general state of impaired circulatory performance not unlike shock itself (67). These manifold deleterious actions of lysosomal hydrolases are enhanced by the acidosis associated with shock, since these enzymes exhibit an optimal activity in an acid medium. Thus, many of the sequelae of circulatory shock appear to be related to the actions of lysosomal hydrolases.

One of the key mechanisms of the protective effect of glucocorticoids in shock appears to be the prevention of the accumulation of MDF in the plasma. All available data point to the stabilization of lysosomal membranes as the major step in this process. Figure 7 reviews the formation of MDF. This graph indicates that glucocorticoids do not prevent either the hypotension or the factors promoting pancreatic hypoperfusion with the possible exception of some action on platelet aggregation. Moreover, glucocorticoids do not reverse the effects of acidosis, hypoxia, or ischemia. However, they can circumvent the consequences of these events on the lysosomal membrane. They do not apparently have the capacity to prevent the activation of zymogenic proteases. Finally, glucocorticoids do not directly reverse the effects of MDF. Thus, these steroids cannot antagonize the negative inotropic or splachnic vasoconstrictor actions of MDF. They may modify the phagocytic properties of the reticuloendothelial system, but this ac-

tion has not yet shown to be an effective mechanism of enhancing survival in shock.

PROSTAGLANDINS

Prostaglandins are a family of ubiquitous acidic lipid compounds which are found in virtually all mammalian tissues and body fluids. Several of the prostglandins, notably PGE_1 and $PGF_{2\alpha}$ have received considerable attention since they exert prominent cardiovascular effects (164). PGE_1 has been found to vasodilate most peripheral vascular beds, whereas $PGF_{2\alpha}$ exerts a pressor effect, at least in dog in which many of the studies have been conducted. This pressor effect of $PGF_{2\alpha}$ appears to be exerted primarily on the venous segments. Both PGE_1 and $PGF_{2\alpha}$ exert a cardiotonic effect. However, this increase in cardiac output or cardiac work does not appear to result from a direct positive inotropic effect on cardiac muscle (165,166), but rather may result from positive chronotropic, venopressor, or vasodilator effects.

Despite several potentially beneficial cardiovascular effects, prostaglandins are considered by many to be mediators of inflammation (167). Moreover, prostaglandins are released during shock states such as hemorrhage (168) and endotoxemia (169). The finding that certain prostaglandins increase in the plasma during shock states is difficult to interpret at this time. Although part of the reason for the increased plasma concentrations is probably due to increased synthesis and release of prostaglandins in a variety of tissues (168,170), part of the increase may simply be due to a decreased rate of inactivation of prostaglandins (171) presumably due to a decrease in prostaglandin dehydrogenase activity. However, one must be extremely careful generalizing about prostaglandins, since closely related prostaglandins can exert very different effects. In this regard, PGE_1 is a potent antagonist of platelet aggregation, whereas $PGE_{2\alpha}$ appears to facilitate the aggregation of platelets into microthrombi. Moreover, prostaglandins can exert different effects at different concentrations, so that the same prostaglandin can exert opposite effects on the same organ system at different dose levels.

Evidence has been accumulating in recent years indicating that PGE_1 and $PGF_{2\alpha}$, administered exogenously, exert a beneficial effect in circulatory shock resulting in an increased survival time or rate. Thus, Glenn and co-workers (61,172) showed that PGE_1 and $PGF_{2\alpha}$ significantly prolonged survival in dogs from about 4 hr to 33 hr. Moreover, some permanent survivors were obtained with either PGE_1 and $PGF_{2\alpha}$ (172). Prostaglandin E_1 has also been shown to prevent almost completely the endotoxin-mediated increase in pulmonary vascular resistance (173). PGE_1 has been shown to significantly enhance survival in hemorrhagic shock (61,174,175). In one study PGE_1 increased survival rates from 25% to 75% (174).

These findings form a consensus that PGE_1 is a possible therapeutic agent in circulatory shock. However, the mechanism of the protective effect is not completely clear at this time. Cardiovascular effects of PGE_1 may play a supporting role in shock via a more sustained cardiac output over the course of the shock state (175). However, Hutton et al. (176) could find no significant hemodynamic action of PGE_1 in experimental myocardial infarction in cats.

A more likely mechanism of protection is the membrane-stabilizing effect of PGE_1 on lysosomal membranes. This effect prevents the release of deleterious acid hydrolases which usually are released in circulatory shock states (61,172–174). The effectiveness in preventing lysosomal hydrolase release appears to be related to prevention of (a) production of toxic factors such a MDF (61,172), (b) damage to pulmonary vessels and the development of pulmonary hypertension (173), and (c) ischemic damage to the microcirculation via endothelial damage or platelet aggregation (174). Thus, one can potentially explain many protective mechanisms by the lysosomal membrane-stabilizing action of PGE_1. Nevertheless, additional work is necessary to establish conclusively the effective dose range of PGE_1, the critical sites of action, and what combination of hemodynamic and cellular effects is important to their effectiveness in shock.

PROTEASE INHIBITORS

Proteolysis is a well-known consequence of circulatory shock and was recognized as an important phenomenon in the pathophysiology of shock states in 1945 by Sayers and co-workers (177). The most commonly measured indices of proteolysis are the plasma activity of a variety of acid protease (e.g., cathepsin D) and of free amino nitrogen groups in the circulating blood (i.e., ninhydrin-positive material). This increased activity is generally considered to be a result of ischemic damage to visceral organs, and is one key indication of enzymatically mediated protein and peptide breakdown. Indeed, proteolysis is a likely mechanism for the propagation of cellular damage in shock.

Proteolysis is involved in many events of shock which may contribute to the lethality of the shock state. Thus, proteolysis may be involved in platelet aggregation, microthrombus formation, endothelial damage to capillaries, release of kinins and other mediators of inflammation, depression of cardiac performance directly and via production of MDF, pulmonary hypertension and alveolar damage, metabolic acidosis, fibrinolysis, and edema (178). It is generally accepted that inhibition of proteolysis, or at least certain critical components of proteolysis, would represent a positive step in the therapeutics of the shock state.

Several types of protease inhibitors are known to the biochemist. However, most of these are either not in a form suitable for systemic administration to an intact animal or else exert severe side effects which negate their potentially valuable antiprotease action. Two protease inhibitors have been studied *in vivo* by several investigators. These are: (a) aprotinin (Trasylol®, Bayer) and (b) epsilon-aminocaproic acid (EACA). EACA has received relatively little attention in contrast to aprotinin.

Aprotinin inhibits many proteolytic enzymes including trypsin, papain, chymotrypsin, kallikrein, plasmin, pronase, trypsin-like proteases, and others (179). This wide-spectrum protease inhibitor is itself a protein having a molecular weight of 6,700 and is quite stable in an acidic environment.

Aprotinin, also known as the Kunitz inhibitor, has been found to be quite effective in limiting proteolysis, and thus is thought to be a potentially valuable agent in shock. Many of the early reports of the effectiveness of aprotinin in shock (i.e., particularly acute pancreatitis) have been mixed, some investigators reporting no effect whereas others have shown a beneficial effect. As with glucocorticoids, much of this controversy can be attributed to inadequate dosage and late administration of the drug. Thus, early administration of an adequate dose of aprotinin is essential in order to allow the protease inhibitor to exert its effects.

Aprotinin has been found to enhance survival rates or prolong survival in hemorrhagic (180,181) endotoxic (182,183), cardiogenic (184), splanchnic artery occlusion (162), tourniquet (185), burn (186), and traumatic shock (187). Some of the results were very impressive. For example, in traumatic shock, Back and co-workers (187) found aprotinin to increase survival rates from 0% (untreated) to 80% (treated). Similarly, Massion and Erdos (182) reported aprotinin to increase survival rates from 9% (untreated) to 63% (treated). These and other results suggest that inhibition of proteolysis may be an important mechanism in the pathophysiology of circulatory shock. However, at this point, the precise proteolytic mechanisms responsible for lethality are only partially understood and the exact locus of aprotinin action is not known.

In contrast to aprotinin, the results obtained with EACA are not very impressive. EACA, a substituted amino acid, blocks plasminogen activation and only slightly inhibits trypsin and other potent proteases (188). Under conditions in which aprotinin was very effective in traumatic and burn shock, EACA was not effective or only partially effective (186). Thus, EACA is not the protease inhibitor of choice in the treatment of circulatory shock.

Several possible mechanisms have been proposed to explain the protective actions of aprotinin in shock states. Some of these mechanisms are not mutually exclusive. The major mechanisms are (a) prevention of kinin release (182); (b) direct enzymatic action on the integrity of the capillary endothelium (185,189); (c) prevention of local edema (185); (d) inhibition of lysosomal enzyme release or of lysosomal protease action (190); (e) prevention of hemorrhagic lesions of the intestine (191,192); (f) inhibition of fibrinolysis (186); (g) preservation of lung integrity (71); and (h) prevention against the formation of toxic factors such as MDF (162,181,188).

Many of these proposed mechanisms are interrelated in very complex ways, and would be difficult to prove directly. However, the available evidence seems to be against kinin formation being the key step, since kinin formation is not an absolute requirement in shock (193) and because infusion of kinins (i.e., bradykinin) does not produce most of the conditions of the shock state (194). Similarly, local edema, although important in burn and tourniquet shock, is not a usual sequela in most other forms of shock. The action on the endothelium of the microcirculation and that of the lung may be very similar, but as yet cannot be associated with a definite enzyme action or biological process. Moreover, the problem of "shock lung" is a difficult question to evaluate at present, and some investigators are becoming skeptical of the pulmonary pathology as a major factor in the pathophysiology of circulatory shock (195,196). Regarding the inhibitory action of aprotinin on lysosomal enzyme release, the proteases do not seem to be affected. Thus, cathepsin B, C, and D are only very slightly inhibited or inhibited not at all by aprotinin (188). Moreover, Glenn et al. (67) clearly showed that aprotinin in doses that protect in shock was totally ineffective in stabilizing isolated lysosomal mechanisms. This was confirmed *in vivo* by Lefer and Barenholz (162) in the cat pancreas as well as in the blood of animals in shock. Moreover, fibrinolysis, although an important mechanism, is also inhibited by EACA, which is not a very effective antishock agent. Thus, fibrinolysis is probably not the key step by which aprotinin protects in shock. Finally, hemorrhagic necrosis of the intestine is a major problem only in the dog, it being markedly reduced or absent in cats, monkeys, and man. Since aprotinin is effective in all these species, the fact that it protects the intestinal mucosa from ischemic damage is probably of only incidental therapeutic value in shock.

The mechanism which appears to have the most substantiation is the prevention of toxic factors engendered by certain proteases. Among these factors, MDF (58,68) and another toxic factor (71), appear to be the major possibilities at present. It is conceivable that these two factors may even be identical. In any event, by preventing the lethal cardiac depression, splanchnic vasoconstriction, and reticuloendothelial depression of MDF, survival can be significantly enhanced. More work is needed, however, to determine the precise mechanism of aprotinin in limiting these other toxic factors in shock.

MISCELLANEOUS AGENTS

Many other pharmacologic agents have been used in the treatment of one or more types of circulatory shock. However, most of these agents or classes of compounds have not been adequately studied, so that a clear statement on whether they significantly protect in shock cannot be made at this time. Moreover, the mechanisms of potential protective effects are not necessarily the classical mechanisms associated with that drug. Nevertheless, some of these agents deserve mention because questions concerning them have been raised in literature.

Parasympatholytics

Atropine, the classical antagonist of muscarinic agents (i.e., it blocks the cardiovascular and exocrine gland actions of acetylcholine), has been rarely used in circulatory shock. Crowell (6) and Smith et al. (197) have reported that clinical doses of atropine can largely block the fluid loss from the denuded intestinal mucosa of the dog in hemorrhagic shock. However, if no other pharmacological protection is given, the animals die in shock. The lack of protection of atropine on survival was also confirmed by Priano et al. (198), who reported that atropine failed to modify significantly the cardiovascular response of the dog to endotoxin shock, whether given prior to or following injection of endotoxin. Thus, atropine alone does not appear to be a major protective therapeutic agent in shock, although it may have useful properties as an adjunct agent. Further work is necessary to clarify the role of atropine in shock.

Surfactants

An interesting new group of compounds called pluronics have been recently used in the treatment of circulatory shock. Pluronic F-108 and F-68 are nonionic surfactants having molecular weights of 8,000 to 16,000. These agents theoretically can improve tissue perfusion by lowering surface tension and reducing intravascular sludging. Pluronic F-68 was found to increase survival in dogs in hemorrhagic shock (199). The treated animals exhibited a reduction in surface tension of the blood as well as a decline in renal vascular resistance reflected by an enhanced degree of urine formation. However, Siemssen et al. (200) reported that pluronic F-108 did not restore blood pressure or enhance capillary flow above that of saline and did not improve circulatory performance as well as the combination of dextran and saline in rabbits during hemorrhagic shock. These data are far from complete, and the question of the usefulness of surfactants in shock therapy remains to be answered.

Xanthine Oxidase Inhibitors

Crowell and co-workers (201–203) reported that plasma uric acid concentrations significantly increased during hemorrhagic shock.

Jones et al. (204) extended these findings and postulated that the basis for the increased uric acid in the blood was a reduction in the high-energy phosphate compounds [i.e., adenosine triphosphate (ATP), creatine phosphate (CrP)] of critical tissues such as the heart and other muscle where these compounds are stored (202). This hypothesis received considerable attention when they reported that allopurinol, a potent xanthine oxidase inhibitor, increased the survival rate of dogs in hemorrhagic shock (203). Presumably, inhibition of xanthine oxidase would prevent the conversion of purine metabolites (i.e., inosine, hypoxanthine, etc.) to uric acid and, therefore, allow these compounds to be reconverted to AMP, ADP, and ultimately ATP under favorable conditions where they can once again provide energy for metabolic processes.

Several problems exist with this mechanism. Firstly, allopurinol has not been clearly shown to improve survival in the dog (205,206). In Crowell's experiment, atropine and glucose were given in addition to the allopurinol. Baker (205) did find some improvement in shock when allopurinol was combined with hypoxanthine, adenine, inosine, α-ketoglutarate, and oxaloacetate. However, there are other fundamental discrepancies with the "energy-depletion hypothesis." The basic problem is that the major sources of ATP and CrP (i.e., skeletal and cardiac muscle) do not undergo significant loss during circulatory shock (206–208). Moreover, even if the ATP and CrP levels were to decrease markedly as they do in complete ischemia, they are merely converted to another nucleotide purine base such as IMP or inosine (209), and are not lost from the tissue as such. These data suggest that the increased plasma levels of uric acid in shock may be more directly related to impaired renal function and uric acid degradation in shock than to loss of high-energy compounds in muscle. In any event, allopurinol is of questionable value in circulatory shock.

Nonsteroidal Antiinflammatory Agents

Since glucocorticoids are of considerable value in the treatment of shock, nonsteroidal antiinflammatory agents have also received some attention. Several investigators have shown that various antiinflammatory agents such as aspirin, phenylbutazone, or indomethacin can prevent much of the cardiovascular actions of *E. coli* endotoxin or of live *E. coli* cells (210–213). These studies are of interest since they may yield information on the nature of the humoral component of the early phase of endotoxin shock which is thought to be mediated perhaps by the formation of histamine, serotonin, bradykinin, or some other vasoactive agent. However, these findings do not deal with the major underlying bases of the shock state. Thus, even if the early hypotensive phase of endotoxin shock is eliminated, the animals still develop the signs of shock (i.e., the secondary circulatory collapse as shown in Fig. 2 still ocurs). Moreover, the massive doses of agents such as aspirin required to prevent the early effects of endotoxin are not without severe side effects, nor are the problems of an appropriate vehicle for the drug completely solved (212).

Thus, considerable work must be done in order to evaluate more carefully the prospective role of these agents in circulatory shock.

ANGIOTENSIN INHIBITORS AND ANTAGONISTS

Angiotensin II has become implicated in the pathogenesis of circulatory shock. Infusion of angiotensin II intravenously into anesthetized rabbits has resulted in cardiac damage characterized by multifocal microscopic necrotic lesions (214). Indeed, high infusion rates of angiotensin have been found to induce acute myocardial infarction (215) or severe ischemic or anoxic injury (216). This deleterious effect is prevented by concomitant infusion of the angiotensin receptor antagonist, saralasin. The mechanism of this effect appears to be related to the marked degree of endothelial disruption produced by angiotensin in the coronary microcirculation (217) and perhaps in other vascular beds as well.

These studies led to the concept that angiotensin II may contribute to the pathogenesis of circulatory shock. Two angiotensin converting enzyme (kininase II) inhibitors, bradykinin poteniating factor (SQ 20,881) and captopril (SQ 14,225), have been shown to be beneficial agents in hemorrhagic shock (218–220). These inhibitors of angiotensin II and angiotensin III biosynthesis did not appear to protect via a direct hemodynamic action (e.g., by altering blood pressure, or increasing blood flow). Rather, they protected by preventing the deleterious effects of angiotensin on the microcirculation and by preventing the release of lysosomal hydrolases and the subsequent formation of myocardial depressant factor (MDF). The possibility exists that captopril protects in shock by potentiating the formation of bradykinin or prolonging the duration of bradykinin, because these converting enzyme inhibitors also enhance the appearance of bradykinin in circulating blood. However, this was shown not to be the case by Trachte and Lefer (221), who found that simultaneous infusion of angiotensin II and captopril negated the protective effects of captopril alone in hemorrhagic shock. Furthermore, captopril failed to potentiate the vascular effects of bradykinin in hemorrhagic hypotension, even though it did potentiate the vasodepressor action of bradykinin at normotensive levels (221). These and other findings point to the inhibition of angiotensin formation rather than other effects as the primary beneficial action of converting enzyme inhibitors in shock. This was further reinforced by the findings that antagonism of angiotensin II receptors with [Sar^1-Ala^8]angiotensin II (i.e., saralasin) also protected in hemorrhagic shock (222), largely by the same mechanism as that by captopril (i.e., prevention of the disruptive effects of angiotensin II on the heart and coronary microcirculation).

Additional investigation is necessary to clarify the precise mechanisms of the shock-promoting actions of angiotensin, but this peptide apparently has a clear deleterious role in the pathogenesis of hemorrhagic shock, and probably other types of shock as well.

OPIATE ANTAGONISTS

Infusion of opioid peptides like β-endorphin has been reported to markedly decrease blood pressure (223,224). Recently, studies have also shown that the opiate antagonist naloxone exerts beneficial effects in hemorrhagic and endotoxic shock (225–227). The initial reports suggested that naloxone at doses of 2 to 10 mg/kg specifically antagonized the hypotensive action of pituitary endorphins or exerted a positive inotropic effect (225,227) and therefore reversed the hypotension of hypovolemic shock (227). However, more recent studies suggest that the beneficial actions of naloxone is shock are more complicated than this simple hemodynamic explanation.

Gurll et al. (228) reported that the cardiac autonomic nerves are not essential for the purported cardiotonic effect of naloxone in hemorrhagic shock. Furthermore, Hilton (229) showed that naloxone in doses of 5 to 100 mg/kg failed to retard the cardiovascular actions of burn shock, including reduced blood pressure and cardiac output. These findings suggest that the beneficial effect of naloxone or naltrexone (230) in shock may not be simply a reversal of blood pressure or cardiac function by action of these agents in the central nervous system or by direct cardiotonic or vasoconstrictor actions. Curtis and Lefer (231) provided data that may help explain this potential dilemma. They reported that naloxone not only acts as a potential β-endorphin antagonist but also stabilizes lysosomal membranes and prevents acid-hydrolase-mediated proteolysis and thus prevents the formation of a myocardial depressant factor in hemorrhagic shock (231). In this manner, naloxone prevents the cardiotoxic-factor-induced cardiodepression usually observed in shock.

Although additional work needs to be done to clarify the role of the endorphins and enkephalins in the pathogenesis of circulatory shock, opiate antagonists appear to be potentially useful agents in the treatment of hemorrhagic shock (225,227,228,231), endotoxic shock (227), burn shock (229), and splanchnic artery occlusion shock (232). Further efforts directed toward determining the mechanisms of actions of opiate antagonists in circulatory shock will be viewed with considerable interest by investigators in the shock field.

SUMMARY

Treatment of circulatory shock is a very difficult assignment, partly because of the severe nature of the disorder and partly because of the involvement of so many organs and systems. Nevertheless, modern biomedical science has made significant progress in elucidating the basic pathophysiologic processes occurring in shock and in defining the major priorities necessary for the treatment of circulatory shock.

At present, we are at a point where we know that much of what we use is ineffective or useless. We have a few agents which appear to be helpful. The major job now appears to seek new drugs or combinations of drugs which will solve the problem of shock both from a hemodynamic and a subcellular viewpoint.

REFERENCES

1. Wiggers, H. G., and Ingraham, R. C. (1946): Hemorrhagic shock: Definition and criteria for its diagnosis. *J. Clin. Invest.,* 25:30–36.
2. Forsyth, R. P., Hoffbrand, B. I., and Melmon, K. K. (1970): Redistribution of cardiac output during hemorrhage in the unanesthetized monkey. *Circ. Res.,* 27:311–320.
3. Rutherford, R. B., and Trow, R. S. (1973): The pathophysiology of irreversible hemorrhagic shock in monkeys. *J. Surg. Res.,* 14:538–550.
4. Gomez, O. A., and Hamilton, W. F. (1964): Functional cardiac deterioration during development of hemorrhagic circulatory deficiency. *Circ. Res.,* 14:327–336.
5. Crowell, J. W., and Guyton, A. C. (1962): Further evidence favoring a cardiac mechanism in irreversible hemorrhagic shock. *Am. J. Physiol.,* 208:248–252.
6. Crowell, J. W. (1970): Oxygen transport in the hypotensive state. *Fed. Proc.,* 29:1848–1853.
7. Hollenberg, N. K., and Nickerson, M. (1970): Changes in pre- and post-capillary resistance in pathogenesis of hemorrhagic shock. *Am. J. Physiol.,* 219:1483–1489.
8. Wyler, F., Forsyth, R. P., Nies, A. S., Neutze, J. M., and Melmon, K. L. (1969): Endotoxin induced regional circulatory changes in the unanesthetized monkey. *Circ. Res.,* 24:777–786.
9. Winslow, E. J., Loeb, H. S., Rahimtoola, S. H., Kamath, S., and Gunnar, R. M. (1973): Hemodynamic studies and results of therapy in 50 patients with bacteremic shock. *Am. J. Med.,* 54:421–432.
10. Solis, R. T., and Downing, S. E. (1966): Effects of *E. coli* endotoxemia on ventricular performance. *Am. J. Physiol.,* 211:307–313.
11. Wangensteen, S. L., Geissinger, W. T., Lovett, W. L., Glenn, T. M., and Lefer, A. M. (1971): Relationship between splanchnic blood flow and a myocardial depressant factor in endotoxin shock. *Surgery,* 69:410–418.
12. Hinshaw, L. B., Greenfield, L. J., Owen, S. W., Archer, L. T., and Guenter, C. A. (1972): Precipitation of cardiac failure in endotoxin shock. *Am. J. Physiol.,* 22:1047–1053.
13. Elkins, L. B., McCurdy, J. R., Brown, P. P., and Greenfield, L. J. (1973): Effects of coronary perfusion pressure on myocardial performance during endotoxin shock. *Surg. Gynecol. Obstet.,* 137:991–996.
14. Marchetti, G., Longo, T., Merlo, L., and Noseda, V. (1973): The effects of dopamine on cardiogenic and endotoxin experimental shock. *Eur. Surg. Res.,* 5:175–185.
15. Deets, D. K., and Glaviano, V. V. (1973): Plasma and cardiac lactic dehydrogenase activity in burn shock. *Proc. Soc. Exp. Biol. Med.,* 142:412–416.
16. Shoemaker, W. C., Vladeck, B. C., Bassin, R., Printen, K., Brown, R. S., Amato, J. J., Reinhard J. M., and Kard, A. E. (1973): Burn pathology in man. I. Sequential hemodynamic alterations. *J. Surg. Res.,* 14:64–73.
17. Leffler, J. N., Litvin, Y., Barenholz, Y., and Lefer, A. M. (1973): Proteolysis in formation of a myocardial depressant factor during shock. *Am. J. Physiol.,* 224:824–831.
18. Clowes, G. H. A., Jr., Farrington, G. H., Zuschneid, W., Cossette, G. R., and Saravis, C. (1970): Circulating factors in the etiology of pulmonary insufficiency and right heart failure accompanying severe sepsis (peritonitis). *Ann. Surg.,* 171:663–678.
19. Hashimoto, E., and Thal, A. P. (1971): The lung lesion produced by materials released from the superior mesenteric vein after superior mesenteric arterial occlusion. *Jap. Circ. J.,* 35:1071–1080.
20. DePalma, R. G., Holden, W. D., and Robinson, A. V. (1972): Fluid therapy in experimental hemorrhagic shock: Ultrastructural effects in liver and muscle. *Ann. Surg.,* 175:539–551.
21. Holden, W. D., DePalma, R. G., Drucker, W. R., and McKalen, A. (1965): Ultrastructural changes in hemorrhagic shock: Electron microscopic study of liver, kidney and striated muscle cells in rats. *Ann. Surg.,* 162:517–536.
22. White, R. R., Mela, L., Bacalzo, L. V., Jr., Olofsson, K., and Miller, L. (1973): Hepatic ultrastructure in endotoxemia, hemorrhage, and hypoxia: Emphasis on mitochondrial changes. *Surgery,* 73:525–534.

23. White, R. R., Mela, L., Miller, L. D., and Berwick, L. (1971): Effect of *E. coli* endotoxin on mitochondrial form and function: Inability to complete succinate-induced condensed-to-orthodox conformational change. *Ann. Surg.,* 174:983–990.

24. Blair, O. M., Stenger, R. J., Hopkins, R. W., and Simeone, F. A. (1968): Hepatocellular ultrastructure in dogs with hypovolemic shock. *Lab. Invest.,* 18:172–178.

25. Rangel, D. M., Byfield, J. E., Adomian, G. E., Stevens, G. H., and Fonkalsrud, E. W. (1970): Hepatic ultrastructural response to endotoxin shock. *Surgery,* 68:503–511.

26. Packer, L., Michaelis, M., and Martin, W. R. (1958): Effect of shock on rat heart and brain mitochondria. *Proc. Soc. Exp. Med.,* 98:164–167.

27. Reed, P. C., Erve, P. R., Das Gupta, T. K., and Schumer, W. (1970): Endotoxemia effect of *Escherichia coli* on cardiac and skeletal muscle mitochondria. *Surg. Forum,* 21:13–14.

28. Schumer, W., Das Gupta, T. K., Moss, G. S., and Nyhus, L. M. (1970): Effect of endotoxemia on liver cell mitochondria in man. *Ann. Surg.,* 71:875–882.

29. DePalma, R. G., Levey, S., and Holden, W. D. (1970): Ultrastructure and oxidative phosphorylation of liver mitochondria in experimental hemorrhagic shock. *J. Trauma,* 10:122–134.

30. Baue, A. E., Wurth, M. A., and Sayeed, M. (1972): Alterations in hepatic cell function during hemorrhagic shock. *Bull. Soc. Int. Chir.,* 5:387–392.

31. Mela, L., Miller, L. D., Bacalzo, L. V., Jr., Olofsson, K., and White, R. R. (1973): Role of intracellular variations of lysosomal enzyme activity and oxygen tension in mitochondrial impairment in endotoxemia and hemorrhage in the rat. *Ann. Surg.,* 178:727–735.

32. Nicholas, G. G., Mela, L. M., and Miller, L. D. (1974): Early alterations in mitochondrial membrane transport during endotoxemia. *J. Surg. Res.,* 16:375–383.

33. Mellors, A., Tappel, A. L., Sawant, P. L. and Desai, I. D. (1967): Mitochondrial swelling and uncoupling of oxidative phosphorylation by lysosomes. *Biochem. Biophys. Acta,* 143:299–309.

34. Nicholas, G. G., Mela, L. M., and Miller, L. D. (1972): Shock-induced alterations of mitochondrial membrane transport: Effects of endotoxin and lysosomal enzymes on calcium transport. *Ann. Surg.,* 176:579–584.

35. Wurth, M. A., Sayeed, M. M., and Baue, A. E. (1972): $(Na^+ + K^+)$-ATPase activity in the liver with hemorrhagic shock. *Proc. Soc. Exp. Biol. Med.,* 139:1238–1241.

36. Baue, A. E., Wurth A., Chaudry, I. H., and Sayeed, M. M. (1973): Impairment of cell membrane transport during shock and after treatment. *Ann. Surg.,* 178:412–422.

37. Campion, D. S., Lynch, L. J., Rector, F. C., Carter, N., and Shires, G. T. (1969): Effect of hemorrhagic shock on transmembrane potential. *Surgery,* 66:1051–1059.

38. Cunningham, J. N., Jr., Shires, G. T., and Wagner, Y. (1971): Cellular transport defects in hemorrhagic shock. *Surgery,* 70:215–221.

39. Shires, G. T., Cunningham, J. N., Baker, C. R. F., Reeder, S. F., Illner, H., Wagner, I. Y., and Maher, J. (1972): Alterations in cellular membrane function during hemorrhagic shock in primates. *Ann. Surg.,* 176:288–295.

40. Trunkey, D. D., Illner, H., Wagner, I. Y., and Shires, G. T. (1973): The effect of hemorrhagic shock on intracellular muscle action potentials in the primate. *Surgery,* 74:241–250.

41. Janoff, A., Weissmann, G., Zweifach, B. W., and Thomas, L. (1962): Pathogenesis of experimental shock: IV. Studies on lysosomes in normal and tolerant animals subjected to lethal trauma and endotoxemia. *J. Exp. Med.,* 116:451–466.

42. Weissmann, G., and Thomas, L. (1962): Studies of lysosomes. I. The effects of endotoxin, endotoxin tolerance, and cortisone on the release of enzymes from a granular fraction of rabbit liver. *J. Exp. Med.,* 116:433–450.

43. Bitensky, L., Chayen, J., and Cunningham, G. J. (1963): Behaviour of lysosomes in haemorrhagic shock. *Nature,* 199:493–494.

44. Clermont, H. G., and Williams, J. S. (1972): Lymph lysosomal enzyme acid phosphatase in hemorrhagic shock. *Ann. Surg.,* 176:90–96.

45. Fredlund, P. E., Ockerman, P. A., and Vang, J. O. (1972): Plasma activities of acid hydrolases in experimental olingemic shock in the pig. *Am. J. Surg.,* 124:300–306.

46. Glenn, T. M., and Lefer, A. M.(1971): Significance of splanchnic proteases in the production of a toxic factor in hemorrhagic shock. *Circ. Res.,* 29:338–349.

47. Janoff, A., and Kaley, G. (1964):Studies on lysosomes in tolerance, shock, and local injury induced by endotoxin. *J. Exp. Med.,* 116:451–466.

48. Glenn, T. M., and Lefer, A. M., Martin, J. B., Lovett, W. L., Morris, J. N., and Wangensteen, S. L. (1971): Production of a myocardial depressant factor in cardiogenic shock. *Am. Heart J.,* 82:78–85.

49. Okuda, M., and Yamada, T. (1974): Activity of a myocardial depressant factor and associated lysosomal abnormalities in experimental cardiogenic shock. *Circ. Shock.* 1:17–29.

50. Abe, H., Carballo, J., Appert, H. E., and Howard, J. M. (1972): The release and fate of the intestinal lysosomal enzymes after acute ischemic injury of the intestine. *Surg. Gynecol. Obstet.,* 135:581–585.

51. Glenn, T. M., and Lefer, A. M. (1970): Role of lysosomes in the pathogenesis of splanchnic ischemia shock in cats. *Circ. Res.,* 27:783–797.

52. Alho, A. (1970): Lysosomal enzymes in murine tourniquet shock. *Acta Chir. Scand.,* 136:555–560.

53. Karady, S., Horpacsy, G., and Ottlecz, A. (1968): Lysosomale veranderungen im tourniquet-schock-resistenz. *Enzym. Biol. Clin.,* 9:261–275.

54. Lefer, A. M., Glenn, T. M., Lopez-Rasi, A. M., Kiechel, S. F., Ferguson, W. W., and Wangensteen, S. L. (1971): Mechanism of the lack of a beneficial response to inotropic drugs in hemorrhagic shock. *Clin. Pharmacol. Ther.,* 12:506–516.

55. Clermont, H. G., Adams, J. T., and Williams, J. S. (1972): Source of a lysosomal enzyme acid phosphatase in hemorrhagic shock. *Ann. Surg.,* 175:19–25.

56. Brand, E. D., and Lefer, A. M. (1966): Myocardial depressant factor in plasma from cats in irreversible post-oligemic shock. *Proc. Soc. Exp. Biol. Med.,* 122:200–203.

57. Lefer, A. M., and Glenn. T. M. (1974): Corticosteroids and the lysosomal protease-MDF system. In: *Steroids and Shock,* edited by T. M. Glenn, pp. 233–248. University Park Press, Baltimore.

58. Lefer, A. M. (1974): Myocardial depressant factor and circulatory shock. *Klin. Wochenschr.,* 52:358–370.

59. Baxter, C. R., Cook, W. A., and Shires, G. T. (1966): Serum myocardial depressant factor of burn shock. *Surg. Forum,* 17:1–2.

60. Fisher, W. D., Heimbach, D. W., McArdle, C. S., Maddern, M., Hutcheson, M. M., and Ledingham, I. McA. (1973): A circulating depressant effect following canine haemorrhagic shock. *Br. J. Surg.,* 60:392–394.

61. Glenn, T. M. (1972): Studies on the mechanism of the protective action of prostaglandins in circulatory shock. *5th International Congress Pharmacol., July 23–28.*

62. Haglund, U., and Lundgren, O. (1973): Cardiovascular effects of blood borne material released from the cat small intestine during simulated shock conditions. *Acta Physiol. Scand.,* 89:558–570.

63. Okada, K., Kosugi, I., Yamaguchi, Y., Inami, H., Kawashima, Y., and Yamamura, H. (1974): The myocardial depressant factor in hemorrhagic or endotoxin shock in dogs. *Jap. J. Anesthesiol.,* 22:414–422.

64. Williams, L. F., Jr., Goldberg, A. H., Polansky, B. J., and Byrne, J. J. (1969): Myocardial effects of acute intestinal ischemia. *Surgery,* 66:138–144.

65. Lefer, A. M., and Glenn, T. M. (1972): Role of the pancreas in the pathogenesis of circulatory shock. In: *The Fundamental Mechanisms of Shock,* edited by L. B. Hinshaw and B. G. Cox, pp. 311–335. Plenum Press, New York.

66. Lefer, A. M., and Glenn, T. M. (1972): Interaction of lysosomal hydrolases and a myocardial depressant factor in the pathogenesis of circulatory shock. In: *Shock in Low- and High-Flow States,* edited by B. K. Forscher, R. C. Lillehei, and S. S. Stubbs, pp. 88–105. Excerpta Medica, Amsterdam.

67. Glenn, T. M., Lefer, A. M., Beardsley, A. C., Ferguson. W. W., Lopez-Rasi, A. M., Serate, T. S., Morris, J. R., and Wangensteen, S. L. (1972): Circulatory responses to splanchnic lysosomal hydrolases in the dog. *Ann. Surg.,* 176:120–127.

68. Lefer, A. M., (1973): Blood-borne humoral factors in the pathophysiology of circulatory shock. *Circ. Res.,* 32:129–139.

69. Fukuda, T. (1965): Endogenous shock-inducing factor in canine hemorrhagic shock. *Nature,* 205:392–395.

70. Kobold, E. E., and Thal, A. P. (1963): Quantitation and identification of vasoactive substances liberated during various types of experimental and clinical intestinal ischemia. *Surg. Gynecol. Obstet.,* 117:315–322.

71. Clowes, G. H. A., Jr., MacNichol, M., Voss, H., Altug, K., and Savaris, C. (1973): Inhibition by trasylol of the production of plasma factors (probably peptides) which cause pneumonitis and metabolic disorders in severe sepsis. In: *New Aspects of Trasylol Therapy: Protease Inhibition in Shock Therapy,* edited by W. Brendel and G. L. Haberland, pp. 209–222. F. K. Schattauer Verlag, Stuttgart, New York.

72. Rush, F. B., Jr. (1967): Treatment of experimental shock: Comparison of the effects of norepinephrine, dibenzyline, dextran, whole blood, and balanced saline solutions. *Surgery,* 61:938–944.

73. Rao, B. N. B., Upadhyaya, P., Nayak, N. C., and Kalhan, J. N. (1968): Effect of prolonged administration of noradrenaline, with and without heparinization in irreversible haemorrhagic shock in dogs. *Indian J. Med., Res.,* 56:163–170.

74. Nickerson, M. (1962): Drug therapy in shock. In: *Shock-Pathogenesis and Therapy,* edited by K. D. Bock, pp. 356–370. Academic Press, New York.

75. Grega, G. J., Kinnard, W. J., and Buckley, J. P. (1967): Effects of nylidrin, isoproterenol and phenoxybenzamine on dogs subjected to hemorrhagic shock. *Circ. Res.,* 20:253–261.

76. Myers, K. A., Paul, H. A., and Julian, O. C. (1968): Responses to isoproterenol and THAM during experimental hemorrhagic shock. *Surgery,* 64:653–660.

77. Rona, G., Chappel, C. I., and Kahn, D. S. (1963): The significance of factors modifying the development of isoproterenol-induced myocardial necrosis. *Am. Heart J.,* 66:389–395.

78. Goldberg, L. I. (1972): Cardiovascular and renal actions of dopamine: Potential clinical applications. *Pharmacol. Rev.,* 24:1–29.

79. Carvalho, M., Vyden, J. K., Bernstein, H., Gold, H., and Corday, E. (1969): Hemodynamic effects of 3-hydroxytryramine (dopamine) in experimentally induced shock. *Am. J. Cardiol.,* 23:217–223.

80. Gifford, R. M., MacCannell, K. L., McNay, J. L., and Haas, J. A. (1968): Changes in regional blood flows induced in dopamine and by isoproterenol during experimental hemorrhagic shock. *Can. J. Physiol. Pharmacol.,* 46:847–851.

81. Lansing, E. J., and Hinshaw, L. B. (1969): Hemodynamic effects of dopamine in endotoxin shock. *Proc. Soc. Exp. Biol. Med.,* 130:311–313.

82. Shanbour, L. L., and Parker, D. (1972): Effects of dopamine and other catecholamines on the splanchnic circulation. *Can. J. Physiol. Pharmacol.,* 50:594–602.

83. Cohn, J. N., and Luria, M. H. (1965): Studies in clinical shock and hypotension. II. Hemodynamic effects of norepinephrine and angiotensin. *J. Clin. Invest.,* 44:1949–1504.

84. Starzecki, B., and Spink, W. W. (1968): Hemodynamic effects of isoproterenol in canine endotoxin shock. *J. Clin. Invest.,* 47:2193–2205.

85. Tadepalli, A. S., and Buckley, J. P. (1972): Effects of nylidrin in endotoxin shock. *J. Pharm. Sci.,* 61:1844–1846.

86. Binder, M. J. (1965): Effect of vasopressor drugs on circulatory dynamics in shock following myocardial infarction. *Am. J. Cardiol.,* 16:834–840.

87. Gunnar, R. M., Peitras, R. J., Stavrakos, C., Loeb, H. S., and Tobin, J. R. (1967): The physiologic basis

for treatment of shock associated with myocardial infarction. *Med. Clin. North Am.,* 50:69–81.

88. Gunnar, R. M., Loeb, H. S., Pietras, R. J., and Tobin, J. R., Jr. (1967): Ineffectiveness of isoproterenol in shock due to acute myocardial infarction. *JAMA,* 202:1124–1128.

89. Gunnar, R. M., and Loeb, H. S. (1972): Use of drugs in cardiogenic shock due to acute myocardial infarction. *Circulation,* 45:1111–1124.

90. Puri, P. S. (1974): Modification of experimental myocardial infarct size by cardiac drugs. *Am. J. Cardiol.,* 33:521–528.

91. Lefer, A. M., and Spath, J. A. (1975): Comparison of surgical and humoral methods of induction of cardiogenic shock in cats. *J. Surg. Res.,* 18:43–50.

92. Maroko, P. R., Kjekshus, J. K., Sobel, B. E., Watanabe, T., Covell, J. W., Ross, J., Jr., and Braunwald, E. (1971): Factors influencing infarct size following experimental coronary artery occlusions. *Circulation,* 43:67–82.

93. Shell, W. E., and Sobel, B. E. (1973): Deleterious effects of increased heart rate on infarct size in the conscious dog. *Am. J. Cardiol.,* 31:474–479.

94. Gould, L., Ettinger, S., Carmichael, A., Lord, P., and Hofstra, P. (1970): The use of phentolamine in experimental hemorrhagic shock. *Angiology,* 21:330–335.

95. Bond, R. F., Manning, E. S., Gonzalez, N. M., Gonzales, R. R., Jr., and Becker, V. E. (1973): Myocardial and skeletal muscle responses to hemorrhage and shock during α-adrenergic blockade. *Am. J. Physiol.,* 225:247–257.

96. Spoerel, W. E. (1958): Adrenergic blocking agents in shock. *Can. Anaesth. Soc. J.,* 5:170–176.

97. Lotz, F., Beck, L., and Stevenson, J. A. F. (1955): The influence of adrenergic blocking agents on metabolic events in hemorrhagic shock in the dog. *Can. J. Biochem. Physiol.,* 33:741–752.

98. Schumer, W. (1966): The microcirculatory and metabolic effects of dibenzyline in oligemic shock. *Surg. Gynecol. Obstet.,* 123:787–791.

99. Wilson, R. F., Jablonski, D. V., and Thal, A. P. (1964): The usage of dibenzyline in clinical shock. *Surgery,* 56:172–183.

100. Zierott, G., Riedwyl, H., and Lundsgaard-Hansen, P. (1969): Optimum level of combined adrenergic blockade for the experimental study of hemorrhagic shock. *Experentia,* 25:823–824.

101. Bloch, J. H., Pierce, C. H., and Lillehei, R. C. (1966): Adrenergic blocking agents in the treatment of shock. *Ann. Rev. Med.,* 17:483–508.

102. Berk, J. L., Hagen, J. F., Beyer, W. H., Kochat, G. R., and LaPointe, R. (1967): The treatment of hemorrhagic shock by beta adrenergic receptor blockade. *Surg. Gynecol. Obstet.,* 125:311–318.

103. Halmagyi, D. F. J., Kennedy, M., Goodman, A. H., and Varga, D. (1971): Simple and combined adrenergic receptor blockade in canine endotoxinemia. *Eur. Surg. Res.,* 3:326–339.

104. Berk, J. L., Hagen, J. F., and Dunn, J. M. (1970): The role of beta adrenergic blockade in the treatment of septic shock. *Surg. Gynecol. Obstet.,* 130:1025–1034.

105. Hirsch, L. J., and Glick, G. (1973): Mesenteric cir-culation in cardiogenic shock with and without alpha-receptor blockade. *Am. J. Physiol.,* 225:356–359.

106. Libby, P., Maroko, P. R., Covell, J. W., Malloch, C. L., Ross, J., Jr., and Braunwald, E. (1973): Effect of practolol on the extent of myocardial ischaemic injury after experimental coronary occlusion and its effects on ventricular function in the normal and ischaemic heart. *Cardiovasc. Res.,* 7:167–173.

107. Bower, M. G., Okude, S., Jolley, W. B., and Smith, L. L. (1970): Hemodynamic effects of glucagon following hemorrhagic and endotoxic shock in the dog. *Arch. Surg.,* 101:411–415.

108. Alguire, P. A., Bowman, H. M., and Hook, J. B. (1972): Effect of glucagon on survival time of dogs in hemorrhagic shock. *Res. Commun. Chem. Pathol. Pharmacol.,* 4:235–245.

109. Bowman, H. M., Cowan, D., Kovach, G., Jr., and Hook, J. B. (1972): Renal effects of glucagon in rhesus monkeys during hypovolemia. *Surg. Gynecol. Obstet.,* 134:937–941.

110. Madden, J. J., Ludewig, R. M., and Wangesteen, S. L. (1971): Failure of glucagon in experimental hemorrhagic shock. *Am. J. Surg.,* 122:502–504.

111. Schumer, W., Miller, B., Nicholas, R. L., McDonald, G. O., and Nyhus, L. M. (1973): Metabolic and microcirculatory effects of glucagon in hypovolemic shock. *Arch. Surg.,* 107:176–180.

112. Tibblin, S., Kock, N. G., and Schenk, W. G., Jr. (1971): Central and peripheral circulatory responses to glucagon in hypovolemic dogs. *Acta Chir. Scand.,* 137:603–611.

113. Glasser, O., and Page, I. H. (1948): Experimental hemorrhagic shock: A study of its production and treatment. *Am. J. Physiol.,* 154:297–315.

114. Cohn, J. N., Tristani, F. E., and Khatri, I. M. (1969): Cardiac and peripheral vascular effects of digitalis in clinical cardiogenic shock. *Am. Heart J.,* 78:318–330.

115. Harrison, L. A., Blaschke, J., Phillips, R. S., Price, W. E., Cotton, M. DeV., and Jacobson, E. D. (1969): Effects of ouabain on the splanchnic circulation. *J. Pharmacol. Exp. Ther.,* 169:321–327.

116. Gazes, P. C., Holmes, C. R., Moseley, V., and Pratt-Thomas, H. R. (1961): Acute hemorrhage and necrosis of the intestines associated with digitalization. *Circulation,* 23:358–364.

117. Allgood, R. J., and Ebert, P. A. (1968): Digitalis tolerance during septic shock. *Arch. Surg.,* 96:91–94.

118. Cort, J. H., JeanJean, M. F., Thomson, A. E., and Nickerson, M. (1968): Effects of "hormonogen" forms of neurohypophysial peptides in hemorrhagic shock in dogs. *Am. J. Physiol.,* 214:455–462.

119. Hershey, S. G., Mazzia, W. D. B., Gyure, L., and Singer, K. (1974): Influence of a synthetic analogue of vasopressin on survival after hemorrhagic shock in rats. *Proc. Soc. Exp. Biol. Med.,* 115:325–328.

120. Covey, T. H., and Baue, A. E. (1974): Selective arterial infusion of vasopressin in the treatment of acute gastrointestinal hemorrhage. *Angiology,* 25:54–60.

121. Zweifach, B. W. (1961): Aspects of comparative physiology of laboratory animals relative to the

problem of experimental shock. *Fed. Proc.*, 20:18–27.

122. Hume, D. H., Nelson, D. H. (1954): Adrenal cortical function in surgical shock. *Surg. Forum*, 5:568–575.

123. Mulrow, P. J., and Ganong, W. F. (1962): Role of the kidney and the renin-angiotensin system in the response to aldosterone secretion to hemorrhage. *Circulation*, 25:213–220.

124. Melby, J. C., Egdahl, R. H., and Spink, W. W. (1960): Secretion and metabolism of cortisol after injection of endotoxin. *J. Lab. Clin. Med.*, 56:50–62.

125. Hokfelt, B., Bygdeman, S., and Sekkenes, J. (1962): The participation of the adrenal glands in endotoxin shock. In: *Shock*, edited by K. D. Bock, pp. 151–161. Academic Press, New York.

126. Hakstian, R. W., Hampson, L. G., and Gurd, F. N. (1961): Pharmacological agents in experimental hemorrhagic shock. *Arch. Surg.*, 83:335–347.

127. Halpern, B. N., Benacerraf, B., and Briot, M. (1952): The roles of cortisone, desoxycorticosterone, and adrenaline in protecting adrenalectomized animals against haemorrhagic, traumatic, and histaminic shock. *Br. J. Pharmacol.*, 7:287–297.

128. Horpacsy, G., Nagy, S., Barankay, T., Tarnoky, K., and Petri, G. (1970): Effect of a water-soluble corticosteroid derivative on plasma levels of various intracellular enzymes in haemorrhagic shock. *Enzym. Biol. Clin.*, 11:324–335.

129. Lefer, A. M., and Martin, J. (1969): Mechanism of the protective effect of corticosteroids in hemorrhagic shock. *Am. J. Physiol.*, 216:314–318.

130. Ogawa, R., Imai, T., and Fujita, R. (1973): The use of methylprednisolone in the treatment of shock. *Jap. J. Anesthesiol.*, 22:311–319.

131. Schumer, W. (1969): Dexamethasone in oligemic shock: Physiochemical effects in monkeys. *Arch. Surg.*, 98:259–261.

132. Weil, M. H., and Whigham, H. (1965): Corticosteroids for reversal of hemorrhagic shock in rats. *Am. J. Physiol.*, 209:815–818.

133. Williams, J. S. and Clermont, H. G. (1973): Thoracic duct lymph flow and acid phosphatase response to steroid in experimental shock. *Ann. Surg.*, 178:777–780.

134. Ashford, T., Palmerio, C., and Fine, J. (1966): Structural analogue in vascular muscle to the functional disorder in refractory traumatic shock and reversal by corticosteroid: electron microscopic evaluation. *Ann. Surg.*, 164:575–586.

135. Dietzman, R. H., and Lillehei, R. C. (1968): The treatment of cardiogenic shock. V. The use of corticosteroids in the treatment of cardiogenic shock. *Am. Heart J.*, 75:274–277.

136. Fukuda, R., Okada, M., and Kobayashi, T. (1964): On the mechanism of protection of endotoxin shock by glucocorticoids, *Jap. J. Physiol.*, 15:560–572.

137. Kadowitz, P. J., and Yard, A. C. (1970): Circulatory effects of hydorcortisone and protection against endotoxin shock in cats. *Eur. J. Pharmacol.*, 9:311–318.

138. Lillehei, R. C., Longerbeam, J. K., Bloch, J. H., and Manax, W. G. (1964): The modern treatment

of shock based on physiologic principles. *Clin. Pharmacol. Ther.*, 5:63–101.

139. Massion, W. H., Rosenbluth, B., and Kux, M. (1972): Protective effect of methylprednisolone against lung complications in endotoxin shock. *South. Med. J.*, 65:941–944.

140. Motsay, G. L., Alho, A., Jaeger, T., Dietzman, R. H., and Lillehei, R. C. (1970): Effects of corticosteroids on the circulation in shock: Experimental and clinical results. *Fed. Proc.*, 29:1861–1873.

141. Schumer, W., Erve, P. R., and Obernolte, R. P. (1972): Mechanisms of steroid protection in septic shock. *Surgery*, 72:119–124.

142. Spink, W. W., and Vick, J. (1961): Evaluation of plasma, metaraminol, and hydrocortisone in experimental endotoxin shock. *Circ. Res.*, 9:184–188.

143. Thomas, C. S., and Brockman, S. K. (1968): The role of adrenal corticosteroid therapy in *Escherichia coli* endotoxin shock. *Surg. Gynecol. Obstet.*, 126:1–9.

144. Weil, M. H. (1961): Adrenocortical steroid for therapy of acute hypotension. *Am. Prac. Dig. Treat.*, 12:162–168.

145. Wilson, J. W. (1972): Pulmonary factors produced by septic shock: Cause or consequence of shock lung? *J. Reprod. Med.*, 8:307–312.

146. Ogawa, R., Imai, T., Nakao, H., and Jujuita, T. (1973): Effect of corticosteroids on plasma lysosomal enzymes during splanchnic ischemic. *Jap. J. Anesthesiol.*, 22:11–15.

147. Crampton, R. S., Wangesteen, S. L., Lovett, W. L., Morris, J. N., Jr., Harris, R. H., Weitzmann, R., Glenn, T. M., and Lefer, A. M. (1972): Production of a myocardial depressant factor in shock following acute muocardial infarction: Preliminary evaluation of treatment with methylprednisolone. *Am. J. Cardiol.*, 29:257–258.

148. Dietzman, R. H., Lillehei, R. C., and Shatney, C. H. (1973): Therapeutic effects of corticosteroids in septic shock. *Acta Chir. Belg.* 72:308–330.

149. Moses, M. L., Camishion, R. C., Tokunaga, K., Pierucci, L., Jr., Davies, A. L., and Nealon, T. F., Jr. (1966): Effect of corticosteroid on the acidosis of prolonged cardiopulmonary bypass. *J. Surg. Res.*, 6:354–360.

150. Pierce, C. H., Briggs, B. T., and Gutelius, J. R. (1972): Methylprednisolone and phenoxybenzamine in experimental shock: cardiovascular dynamics and platelet function. In: *Shock in Low- and High-Flow States*, edited by B. K. Forscher, R. C. Lillehei, and S. S. Stubbs, pp. 183–195. Excerpta Medica, Amsterdam.

151. Novelli, G. P., Marsill, M., and Pieraccioli, E. (1973): Anti-shock action of steroids other than cortisone. *Eur. Surg. Res.*, 5:169–174.

152. Replogle, R. L., Gazzaniga, A. B., and Gross, R. E. (1966): Use of corticosteroids during cardiopulmonary bypass: possible lysosome stabilization. *Circulation*, Suppl. 1, 33, & 34:86–91.

153. Rokkanen, P., Alho, A., Avikainen, V., Karaharju, E., Kataja, J., Lahdensuu, M., Lepisto, P., and Tervo, T. (1974): The efficacy of corticosteroids in severe trauma. *Surg. Gynecol. Obstet.*, 138:69–73.

154. Novak, E., Stubbs, S. S., Seckman, C. E., and Hear-

ron, M. S. (1970): Effects of a single large intravenous dose of methylprednisolone sodium succinate. *Clin. Pharmacol. Ther.,* 11:711–717.

155. Webel, M. L., Ritts, R. E., Jr., Taswell, H. F., Donadio, J. V., Jr., and Woods, J. E. (1974): Cellular immunity after intravenous administration of methylprednisolone. *J. Lab. Clin. Med.,* 83:383–392.

156. Czerwinski, A. W., Czerwinski, A. B., Whitsett, T. L., and Clark, M. L. (1972): Effects of a single, large, intravenous injection of dexamethasone. *Clin. Pharmacol. Ther.,* 13:638–642.

157. Zurier, R. B., and Weissmann, G. (1973): Anti-immunologic and anti-inflammatory effects of steroid therapy. *Med. Clin. North Am.,* 57:1295–1307.

158. Spath, J. A., Jr., Gorczynski, R. J., and Lefer, A. M. (1973): Possible mechanisms of the beneficial action of glucocorticoids in circulatory shock. *Surg. Gynecol. Obstet.,* 137:597–607.

159. Gorczynski, R. J., Spath, J. A., Jr., and Lefer, A. M. (1974): Vascular responsiveness of the *in situ* perfused dog pancreas. *Eur. J. Pharmacol.,* 27:68–77.

160. Schmid, P. G., Eckstein, J. W., and Abboud, F. M. (1967): Comparison of effects of deoxycorticosterone and dexamethasone on cardiovascular responses to norepinephrine. *J. Clin. Invest.,* 46:590–598.

161. Glenn, T. M., and Lefer, A. M. (1970): Anti-toxic action of methylprednisolone in hemorrhagic shock. *Eur. J. Pharmacol.,* 13:230–238.

162. Lefer, A. M., and Barenholz, Y. (1972): Pancreatic hydrolases and the formation of a myocardial depressant factor in shock. *Am. J. Physiol.,* 223:1103–1109.

163. Ferguson, W. W., Glenn, T. M., and Lefer, A. M. (1972): Mechanisms of production of circulatory shock factors in isolated perfused pancreas. *Am. J. Physiol.,* 222:450–457.

164. Nakano, J. (1973): Cardiovascular actions. In: *The Prostaglandins,* edited by Peter W. Ramwell, pp. 239–316. Plenum Press, New York.

165. Ogletree, M. L., Beardsley, A. C., and Lefer, A. M. (1976): Myocardial actions of prostaglandins in isolated cat cardiac tissue. *Life Sci. (in press).*

166. Su, J. Y., Higgins, C. B., and Friedman, W. F. (1973): Chronotropic and inotropic effects of prostaglandins E_1, A_1 and F_2 on isolated mammalian cardiac tissue. *Proc. Soc. Exp. Biol. Med.,* 143:1227–1230.

167. Zurier, R. B. (1974): Prostaglandins, inflammation and asthma. *Arch. Intern. Med.,* 133: 101–110.

168. Flynn, J. T., and Reed, E. A. (1974): Arterial prostaglandin levels following hemorrhagic shock in the dog. *Fed. Proc.,* 33:317.

169. Anderson, F. L., Jubiz, W., Tsagaris, T. J., and Kuida, H. (1975): Endotoxin induced prostaglandin E and F release in dogs. *Am. J. Physiol.,* 228:410–414.

170. Parratt, J. R., and Sturgess, R. M. (1974): The effect of indomethacin on the cardiovascular and metabolic response to *E. coli* endotoxin in the cat. *Br. J. Pharmacol.,* 50:177–183.

171. Nakano, J., and Prancan, A. V. (1973): Metabolic degradation of prostaglandin E_1 in the lung and kid-

ney of rats in endotoxin shock. *Proc. Soc. Exp. Biol. Med.,* 144:506–508.

172. Raflo, G. T., Wangensteen, S. L., Glenn, T. M., and Lefer, A. M. (1973): Mechanism of the protective effects of prostaglandins E_1 and $F_{2\alpha}$ in canine endotoxin shock. *Eur. J. Pharmacol.,* 24:86–95.

173. Sorrells, K., Erdos, E. G., and Massion, W. H. (1972): Effect of prostaglandin E_1 on the pulmonary vascular response to endotoxin. *Proc. Soc. Exp. Biol. Med.,* 140:310–313.

174. Machiedo, G. W., Lavigne, J. E., and Rush, B. F., Jr. (1973): Prostaglandin E_1 as a therapeutic agent in hemorrhagic shock. *Surg. Forum,* 24:12–14.

175. Priano, L. L., Miller, T. H., and Traber, D. L. (1974): Use of prostaglandin E_1 in the treatment of experimental hypovolemic shock. *Circ. Shock,* 1:221–230.

176. Hutton, I., Paratt, J. R., and Lawrie, T. D. V. (1973): Cardiovascular effects of prostaglandin E_1 in experimental myocardial infarction. *Cardiovasc. Res.,* 7:149–155.

177. Sayers, G., Sayers, M. A., Liang, T. Y., and Long, C. N. H. (1945): The cholesterol and ascorbic acid content of the adrenal, liver, brain and plasma following hemorrhage. *Endocrinology,* 37:96–110.

178. Haberland, G. L., Koslowski, L., and Matis, P. (1972): Trasylol in der schock-therapie. *Med. Welt.,* 23:1049–1056.

179. Trautschold, I., Werle, E., and Zickgraf-Rudel, G. (1967): Trasylol. *Biochem. Pharmacol.,* 16:59–72.

180. Glenn, T. M., Herlihy, B. L., and Lefer, A. M. (1973): Protective action of a protease inhibitor in hemorrhagic shock. *Arch. Int. Pharmacol. Ther.,* 203:292–304.

181. Lefer, A. M., and Martin, J. (1970): Relationship of plasma peptides to the myocardial depressant factor in hemorrhagic shock in cats. *Circ. Res.,* 26:59–69.

182. Massion, W. H., and Erdos, E. G. (1966): The effects of ATP and a proteolytic enzyme inhibitor in irreversible shock. *J. Okla. State Med. Assoc.,* 59:467–471.

183. Meyer, A. (1966): Die Wirkung von Trasylol bei schockzuständen. In: *Neue Aspekte der Trasylol Therapie,* edited by R. Gross, pp. 142–146. F. K. Schattauer Verlag, Stuttgart, New York.

184. Massion, W. H., Blumel, G., Peschl, L., and Rettenbacher-Daubner, H. (1970): The role of the plasma kinin system in cardiogenic shock and related conditions. In: *Proteases and Antiproteases in Cardioangiology,* edtied by L. Donatelli, A. Marino, G. L. Haberland, and P. Matis, pp. 111–120. F. K. Schattauer Verlag, Stuttgart, New York.

185. Eigler, F. W., Stock, W., and Hofer, I. (1969): Wirkung eines proteinasen-inhibitors auf das tourniquet-syndrom der ratte. I. Beeinflussung des posteschamischen odems in abhangigkeit von dosis und zeitpunkt der trasylogabe. *Z. Ges. Exp. Med.,* 151: 55–63.

186. Back, N., Wilkens, H., and Steger, R. (1968): Proteinases and proteinase inhibitors in experimental shock states. *Ann. N.Y. Acad. Sci.,* 146:491–516.

187. Back, N., Wilkens, H., Munson, A. E., and Steger, R. (1966): Trasylol in experimental shock states.

In: *Neue Aspekte der Trasylol Therapie,* edited by R. Gross, pp. 170–175. F. K. Schättauer-Verlag, Stuttgart, New York.

188. Herlihy, B. L., and Lefer, A. M. (1974): Selective inhibition of pancreatic proteases and prevention of toxic factors in shock. *Circ. Shock,* 1:51–60.

189. Sherry, S., (1961): Hemostatic mechanisms and proteolysis in shock. *Fed. Proc.,* 20:209–218.

190. Horpacsy, G., Barankay, T., Nagy, S., Szabo, I., and Benlo, K. (1973): Beeinflussung des plasma-enzymniveaus im experimentallen hamorrhagischen schock durch Trasylol. *Med. Welt.,* 24:459–461.

191. Messmer, K., Kloverkorn, W. P., Sunder-Plassmann, L., and Brendel, W. (1972): Studies concerning the effect of trasylol in a standardized model of hemorrhagic shock in dogs. In: *New Aspects of Tyrasylol Therapy: Protease Inhibition in Shock Therapy,* edited by W. Brendel and G. L. Haberland, pp. 25–32. F. K. Schattauer Verlag, Stuttgart, New York.

192. Sutherland, N. G., Bounous, G., and Gurd, F. N. (1968): Role of intestinal mucosal lysosomal enzymes in the pathogenesis of shock. *J. Trauma,* 8:350–380.

193. Webster, M. E., and Clark, W. R. (1959): Significance of the callicrein:callidinogen-callidin system in shock. *Am. J. Physiol.,* 197:406–412.

194. Reichgott, M. J., and Melmon, K. L. (1972): Does bradykinin play a pathogenetic role in endotoxemia? In: *Shock in Low- and High-Flow States,* edited by B. K. Forscher, R. C. Lillehei, and S. S. Stubbs, pp. 59–64. Excerpta Medica, Amsterdam.

195. Fulton, R. L., and Fischer, R. P. (1974): Pulmonary changes due to hemorrhagic shock resuscitation with isotonic and hypertonic saline. *Surgery,* 75:881–890.

196. Tobey, R. E., Kopriva, C. J., Homer, L. D., Solis, R. T., Dickson, L. G., and Herman, C. M. (1974): Pulmonary gas exchange following hemorrhagic shock and massive blood transfusion in the baboon. *Ann. Surg.,* 179:316–321.

197. Smith, E. E., Crowell, J. W., Moran, C. J., and Smith, R. A. (1967): Intestinal fluid loss in dogs during irreversible hemorrhagic shock. *Surg. Gynecol. Obstet.,* 125:45–49.

198. Priano, L. L., Miller, T. H., Wilson, R. D., and Traber, D. L. (1972): Effects of atropine on the cardiorespiratory alterations of endotoxic shock in unanesthetized dogs. *Tex Rep. Biol. Med.,* 30:57–72.

199. Hymes, A. C., Safavian, M. H., and Gunther, T. (1971): The influence of an industrial surfactant pluronic F-68, in the treatment of hemorrhagic shock. *J. Surg. Res.,* 11:191–197.

200. Siemssen, S., Huland, H., and Nagel, G. P. (1973): Microcirculatory effects of pluronic F108 in hemorrhagic shock. In: *Bibliotheca Anatomica,* edited by J. Ditzel and D. H. Lewis, pp. 322–326. Karger, Basel.

201. Cowsert, M. K., Jr., Carrier, O., Jr., and Corwell, J. W. (1966): The effect of hemorrhagic shock on blood uric acid level. *Can. J. Physiol. Pharmacol.,* 44:861–864.

202. Crowell, J. W., Jones, C. E., and Smith, E. E. (1969):

Effect of allopurinol on hemorrhagic shock. *Physiologist,* 10:150.

203. Crowell, J. W., Jones, C. E., and Smith, E. E. (1969): Effect of allopurinol on hemorrhagic shock. *Am. J. Physiol.,* 216:744–748.

204. Jones, C. E., Crowell, J. W., and Smith, E. E. (1968): Significance of increased blood uric acid following extensive hemorrhage. *Am. J. Physiol.,* 214:1374–1377.

205. Baker, C. H. (1972): Protection against irreversible hemorrhagic shock by allopurinol. *Proc. Soc. Exp. Biol. Med.,* 141:694–698.

206. Lefer, A. M., Daw, C., and Berne, R. M. (1969): Cardiac and skeletal muscle metabolic energy stores in hemorrhagic shock. *Am. J. Physiol.,* 216:483–486.

207. Bollman, J. L., and Flock, E. V. (1944): Changes in phosphate of muscle during tourniquet shock. *Am. J. Physiol.,* 142:290–297.

208. LePage, G. A. (1946): The effects of hemorrhage on tissue metabolites. *Am. J. Physiol.,* 147:446–454.

209. Deuticke, B., Gerlach, E., and Dierkesmann, R. (1966): Nucleotid-abbau in verschiedenen organen bei O_2-mangel. *Pflugers Arch.,* 292:239–254.

210. Culp, J. R., Erdos, E. G., Hinshaw, L. B., and Holmes, D. D. (1971): Effects of anti-inflammatory drugs in shock caused by injection of living *E. coli* cells. *Proc. Soc. Exp. Biol. Med.,* 137:219–233.

211. Erdos, E. G., Hinshaw, L. B., and Gill, C. C. (1967): Effect of indomethacin in endotoxin shock in the dog. *Proc. Soc. Exp. Biol. Med.,* 125:916–919.

212. Hinshaw, L. B., Solomon, L. A., Erdos, E. G., Reins, D. A., and Gunter, B. J. (1967): Effects of acetylsalicylic acid on the canine response to endotoxin. *J. Pharmacol. Exp. Ther.,* 157:665–671.

213. Murthy, V. S., and Greenway, C. V. (1972): Aspirin and pulmonary lesions in endotoxin shock. *Am. Heart J.,* 84:581–582.

214. Gavras, H., Kremer, D., Brown, J. J., Gray, B., Lever, A. F., MacAdam, R. F., Medina, A., Mortin, J. J., and Robertson, J. I. S. (1975): Angiotensin and norepinephrine induced myocardial lesions; experimental and clinical studies in rabbits and man. *Am. Heart J.,* 89:321–332.

215. Gavras, H., Brown, J. J., Lever, A. F., MacAdam, R. F., and Robertson, J. I. S. (1971): Acute renal failure, tubular necrosis, and myocardial infarction induced in the rabbit by intravenous angiotensin II. *Lancet,* 2:19–22.

216. Giacomelli, F., Anversa, P., and Wiener, J. (1976): Effect of angiotensin-induced hypertension on rat coronary arteries and myocardium. *Am. J. Pathol.,* 84:111–128.

217. Trachte, G. J., and Lefer, A. M. (1980): Shock potentiating actions of angiotensin II infusion in cats. *Circ. Shock,* 7:343–351.

218. Morton, J. J., Semple, P. F., Ledingham, I. M., Stuart, B., Tehrani, M., Garcia A., and McGarrity, G. (1977): Effect of angiotensin-converting enzyme inhibitor (SQ 20,881) on plasma concentration of angiotensin I, angiotensin II, and arginine vasopressin in the dog during hemorrhagic shock. *Circ. Res.,* 41:301–308.

219. Errington, M. L., and Rocha e Silva, M. (1974): On the role of vasopressin and angiotensin in the

development of irreversible haemorrhagic shock. *J. Physiol. (Lond.)*, 242:119–141.

220. Trachte, G. J., and Lefer, A. M. (1978): Beneficial action of a new angiotensin-converting enzyme inhibitor (SQ 14,255) in hemorrhagic shock in cats. *Circ. Res.*, 43:577–582.

221. Trachte, G. J., and Lefer, A. M. (1979): Mechanism of the protective effect of angiotensin-converting enzyme inhibition in hemorrhagic shock. *Proc. Soc. Exp. Biol. Med.*, 162:54–57.

222. Trachte, G. J., and Lefer, A. M. (1979): Effect of angiotensin II receptor blockade by [Sar^1-Ala^8]angiotensin II (saralasin) in hemorrhagic shock. *Am. J. Physiol.*, 236:280–285.

223. Bolme, P., Fuxe, K., Agnati, L. F., Bradley, R., and Smythies. J. (1978): Cardiovascular effects of morphine and opioid peptides following intracisternal administration in chloralose-anesthetized rats. *Eur. J. Pharmacol.*, 48:319–324.

224. Lemaire, I., Tsend, R., and Lemaire, S. (1978): Systemic administration of β-endorphin: Potent hypotensive effect involving a serotonergic pathway. *Proc. Natl. Acad. Sci. U.S.A.*, 75:6240–6242.

225. Faden, A. I., and Holaday, J. W. (1979): Opiate antagonists: A role in the treatment of hypovolemic shock. *Science*, 205:317–318.

226. Holaday, J. W., And Faden, A. I. (1978): Naloxone reversal of endotoxin hypotension suggests a role of endorphins in shock. *Nature*, 275:450–451.

227. Holaday, J. W., and Faden, A. I. (1979): Hypophysectomy inhibits the therapeutic effects of naloxone in endotoxic and hypovolemic shock. *Physiologist*, 22:57.

228. Gurll, N., Lechner, R., Reynolds, D., and Jenkins, J. (1980): Autonomic innervation in the cardiovascular responses to naloxone in hypovolemic shock. *Fed. Proc.*, 39:975.

229. Hilton, J. G. (1980): Effects of naloxone upon thermal trauma induced cardiac changes. *Fed. Proc.*, 39:974.

230. Gurll, N., Lechner, R., Reynolds, D., and Vargish, T. (1979): Specific opiate receptor blockade improves cardiac performance and survival in canine hypovolemic shock. *Physiologist*, 22:49.

231. Curtis, M. T., and Lefer, A. M. (1980): Protective effect of naloxone in hemorrhagic shock. *Am. J. Physiol.* 239:H416–H421.

232. Curtis, M. T., and Lefer, A. M. (1981): Beneficial action of naloxone in splanchnic artery occlusion shock. *Experientia*, 37:403–404.

Subject Index